## Books by Corinne T. Netzer

The Corinne T. Netzer Annual Calorie Counter
The Complete Book of Food Counts
Corinne T. Netzer's Big Book of Miracle Cures
The Corinne T. Netzer Carbohydrate Dieter's Diary
The Complete Book of Vitamin and Mineral Counts
The Corinne T. Netzer Carbohydrate Counter
The Corinne T. Netzer Dieter's Diary
The Corinne T. Netzer Encyclopedia of Food Values
The Corinne T. Netzer Fat Gram Counter
The Corinne T. Netzer Low-Fat Diary
The Dieter's Calorie Counter
The Corinne T. Netzer Dieter's Activity Diary

D0311064

*Ninth Edition*

# THE
# COMPLETE
## BOOK
## OF
# FOOD COUNTS

## Corinne T. Netzer

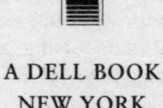

A DELL BOOK
NEW YORK

A Dell Mass Market Original

Copyright © 2012 by Corinne T. Netzer

Published in the United States by Dell, an imprint of The Random House Publishing Group, a division of Random House, Inc., New York.

DELL is a registered trademark of Random House, Inc., and the colophon is a trademark of Random House, Inc.

ISBN 978-0-440-24561-2
eBook ISBN 978-0-345-53247-3

Cover design: Gerald J. Pfeifer

Printed in the United States of America

www.bantamdell.com

9  8  7  6  5  4  3  2  1

Dell mass market edition: January 2012

To Joy

# THE
# COMPLETE
## BOOK
## OF
# FOOD COUNTS

*Ninth Edition*

# Introduction

The ninth edition of *The Complete Book of Food Counts* is the largest compilation of essential food data in this format. It contains data (calories, protein, carbohydrates, fat, cholesterol, sodium, and fiber) for basic generic foods, brand-name foods, and restaurant chains. Whether you are interested in dieting or nutrition—or both—you will find this book unique and invaluable as a reference.

Since this book is alphabetized, you should have no difficulty finding whatever you wish to look up. There are, however, times when you may have to look in more than one place. If you are searching for a particular food and cannot find it immediately, look for it under a category, such as cakes, puddings, cookies, soups. Wherever sensible, I have cross-referenced listings, but the pressure of space has made it impossible to do that for every item.

Compare only foods listed in similar measures. This rule particularly applies to the confusion between measures by capacity and measures by weight. Eight ounces is not necessarily equivalent to eight fluid ounces or one cup. Eight ounces is a measure of how much something weighs; one cup is a measure of how much space it occupies. For instance, a cup of lightweight food, such as puffed rice or popcorn, weighs about one ounce, and eight ounces of the same product would fill many cups. Naturally, you can convert a similar unit of measure into a smaller or larger amount. The following table may be useful in making such conversions.

**Equivalents by Capacity**
(all measures level)
1 quart = 4 cups
1 cup = 8 fluid ounces
= ½ pint
= 16 tablespoons
2 tablespoons = 1 fluid ounce
1 tablespoon = 3 teaspoons

**Equivalents by Weight**
1 pound = 16 ounces
3.57 ounces = 100 grams
1 ounce = 28.35 grams

All the material contained in *The Complete Book of Food Counts* is based on information from the U.S. government, from producers and processors of brand-name foods, and from food chains. The data contained herein is the most complete and accurate information available as this book goes to press. Please bear in mind that seasonal and regional differences can affect the nutritional value of foods. Also, the food industry often changes recipes and sizes and may discontinue products or add new ones. In the future I will revise and update this book to keep you completely informed.

Good luck and good dieting.

Corinne T. Netzer

# ABBREVIATIONS AND SYMBOLS

| | |
|---|---|
| cal. | calories |
| carbo. | carbohydrates |
| chol. | cholesterol |
| cont. | container |
| diam. | diameter |
| fl. | fluid |
| gms. | grams |
| " | inch |
| < | less than |
| > | more than |
| mgs. | milligrams |
| lb(s). | pound(s) |
| n.a. | not available |
| oz. | ounce(s) |
| pc(s). | piece(s) |
| pkg. | package |
| pkt. | packet |
| prot. | protein |
| sod. | sodium |
| sq. | square |
| tbsp. | tablespoon |
| tsp. | teaspoon |
| tr. | trace |
| w/ | with |
| * | prepared according to basic package directions, except as noted |

*Note:* Brand-name foods and restaurants listed in italics denote registered trademarks.

# A

| Food and Measure | cal. | prot. (gms) | carbo. (gms) | fat (gms) | chol. (mgs) | sod. (mgs) | fiber (gms) |
|---|---|---|---|---|---|---|---|
| **Abalone**, meat only, raw, 4 oz. . . . . . . . . . . | 119 | 19.4 | 6.8 | .9 | 96 | 341 | 0 |
| **Abalone, canned:** | | | | | | | |
| (*Roland* Abalone-like Limpets), ⅓ cup . . . . . | 45 | 9.0 | 1.0 | 0 | 117 | 350 | 0 |
| imitation (*Ocean Prince* Calamari), ¼ cup . . . . | 80 | 13.0 | 1.0 | 3.0 | 20 | 240 | <1.0 |
| **Abiyuch**, ½ cup, 4 oz. . . . | 79 | 1.7 | 20.1 | .1 | 0 | 23 | 6.0 |
| **Abruzzese sausage** (*Boar's Head*), 1 oz. . . . . . | 100 | 8.0 | <1.0 | 8.0 | 25 | 500 | 0 |
| **Acai drink blend,** 8 fl. oz.: | | | | | | | |
| berry, mixed (*V8 V-Fusion* Light) . . . . . . | 50 | 0 | 13.0 | 0 | 0 | 70 | 0 |
| blackberry (*Snapple*) . . . . | 110 | 0 | 27.0 | 0 | 0 | 5 | 0 |
| **Acai juice** (*Bossa Nova*), 8 fl. oz. . . . . . . | 95 | 0 | 23.0 | 0 | 0 | 15 | 0 |
| **Acai juice blend,** 8 fl. oz.: | | | | | | | |
| blueberry (*Bossa Nova*) . | 90 | 0 | 21.0 | 0 | 0 | 14 | 0 |
| berry, mixed: | | | | | | | |
| (*R.W. Knudsen* Organic) . . . . . . . . . | 100 | 1.0 | 24.0 | 0 | 0 | 15 | 0 |
| (*V8 V-Fusion*) . . . . . . . | 110 | 0 | 27.0 | 0 | 0 | 70 | 0 |
| mango (*Bossa Nova*) . . . | 90 | 1.0 | 23.0 | 0 | 0 | 14 | 0 |
| passion fruit or raspberry (*Bossa Nova*) | 90 | 0 | 23.0 | 0 | 0 | 14 | 0 |
| **Acerola**, fresh: | | | | | | | |
| 10 fruits . . . . . . . . . . . . | 15 | .2 | 3.7 | .1 | 0 | 3 | .5 |
| peeled, 1 cup . . . . . . . . . | 31 | .4 | 7.5 | .3 | 0 | 7 | 1.1 |
| **Acerola juice**, fresh, 8 fl. oz. . . . . . . . . . . | 56 | 1.0 | 11.6 | .7 | 0 | 7 | .7 |

| Food and Measure | cal. | prot. (gms) | carbo. (gms) | fat (gms) | chol. (mgs) | sod. (mgs) | fiber (gms) |
|---|---|---|---|---|---|---|---|
| **Acerola juice blend**, all fruits (*Bossa Nova*), 8 fl. oz. ...... | 85 | 0 | 22.0 | 0 | 0 | 0 | 0 |
| **Acorn squash**: | | | | | | | |
| raw: | | | | | | | |
| 4" squash, 15.2 oz. ... | 172 | 3.5 | 44.9 | .4 | 0 | 13 | 6.6 |
| cubed, 1 cup ........ | 56 | 1.1 | 14.6 | .1 | 0 | 4 | 2.1 |
| baked, cubed, ½ cup .... | 57 | 1.1 | 14.9 | .1 | 0 | 4 | 4.5 |
| boiled, mashed, ½ cup .. | 42 | .8 | 10.8 | .1 | 0 | 4 | 3.2 |
| cooked (*Frieda's*), 1 cup . | 115 | 2.0 | 30.0 | 0 | 0 | 8 | 9.0 |
| **Adobo sauce** (*Doña Maria*), 2 tbsp. ...... | 210 | 2.0 | 9.0 | 14.0 | 0 | 340 | 2.0 |
| **Adzuki beans**, dry: | | | | | | | |
| (*Arrowhead Mills* Organic), ¼ cup ..... | 130 | 8.0 | 26.0 | 0 | 0 | 0 | 5.0 |
| (*Bob's Red Mill*), ½ cup . | 323 | 19.0 | 61.0 | .5 | 0 | 3 | 5.0 |
| boiled, ½ cup ......... | 147 | 8.7 | 28.5 | .1 | 0 | 9 | 8.4 |
| **Adzuki beans**, canned (*Eden* Aduki Organic), ½ cup ............ | 110 | 7.0 | 19.0 | 0 | 0 | 10 | 5.0 |
| **Agave melon drink** (*Snapple* Antioxidant Water), 8 fl. oz. ...... | 60 | 0 | 13.0 | 0 | 0 | 0 | 0 |
| **Agave nectar** (*Madhava*), 1 tbsp. .... | 60 | 0 | 16.0 | 0 | 0 | 0 | 1.0 |
| **Agnolotti**, see "Ravioli" | | | | | | | |
| **Alfredo sauce**, in jars, ¼ cup: | | | | | | | |
| (*Bertolli*) ............. | 110 | 2.0 | 2.0 | 10.0 | 40 | 410 | 0 |
| (*Classico* Creamy) ...... | 100 | 2.0 | 3.0 | 9.0 | 50 | 410 | 0 |
| (*Newman's Own*) ....... | 90 | 1.0 | 3.0 | 8.0 | 40 | 460 | 0 |
| cheese, four: | | | | | | | |
| (*Bertolli*) ........... | 110 | 2.0 | 4.0 | 10.0 | 30 | 310 | 0 |
| (*Classico*) .......... | 80 | 2.0 | 4.0 | 6.0 | 40 | 390 | 0 |
| garlic (*Bertolli*) ........ | 100 | 2.0 | 2.0 | 10.0 | 30 | 320 | 0 |
| garlic, roasted: | | | | | | | |
| (*Classico*) .......... | 70 | 1.0 | 3.0 | 6.0 | 30 | 430 | 1.0 |
| (*Newman's Own*) .... | 90 | 1.0 | 4.0 | 8.0 | 40 | 450 | .0 |
| mushroom: | | | | | | | |
| (*Bertolli*) ........... | 80 | 2.0 | 2.0 | 7.0 | 30 | 380 | 0 |
| (*Classico*) .......... | 70 | 2.0 | 3.0 | 5.0 | 35 | 300 | 2.0 |
| red pepper, roasted (*Classico*) ..........:. | 60 | 1.0 | 3.0 | 5.0 | 35 | 310 | 0 |

| Food and Measure | cal. | prot. (gms) | carbo. (gms) | fat (gms) | chol. (mgs) | sod. (mgs) | fiber (gms) |
|---|---|---|---|---|---|---|---|
| sun-dried tomato | | | | | | | |
| (*Classico*) .......... | 90 | 2.0 | 4.0 | 7.0 | 35 | 430 | 0 |
| **Alfredo sauce, chilled:** | | | | | | | |
| (*Buitoni*), ¼ cup ....... | 130 | 4.0 | 4.0 | 11.0 | 35 | 390 | 0 |
| (*Buitoni* Light), ¼ cup ... | 90 | 4.0 | 5.0 | 6.0 | 15 | 350 | 0 |
| **Alfredo sauce mix,** | | | | | | | |
| creamy garlic | | | | | | | |
| (*McCormick*), 2 tbsp. . | 80 | 3.0 | 9.0 | 3.5 | 10 | 690 | 0 |
| **Allspice**, 1 tsp. ........ | 5 | .1 | 1.4 | .2 | 0 | 1 | .4 |
| **Almond**, shelled, 1 oz., | | | | | | | |
| except as noted: | | | | | | | |
| (*Beer Nuts*) ........... | 170 | 6.0 | 6.0 | 14.0 | 0 | 65 | 3.0 |
| (*Blue Diamond*) ........ | 160 | 6.0 | 6.0 | 14.0 | 0 | 0 | 3.0 |
| (*Blue Diamond* Lightly | | | | | | | |
| Salted) ............. | 170 | 6.0 | 5.0 | 16.0 | 0 | 40 | 3.0 |
| (*Diamond*), ¼ cup ...... | 170 | 6.0 | 6.0 | 15.0 | 0 | 0 | 4.0 |
| (*Planters* Go-Nuts) ..... | 170 | 6.0 | 6.0 | 15.0 | 0 | 40 | 3.0 |
| (*Planters* Harvest) ..... | 160 | 6.0 | 6.0 | 14.0 | 0 | 95 | 3.0 |
| (*Planters* NUT-rition) .... | 170 | 6.0 | 6.0 | 15.0 | 0 | 120 | 3.0 |
| (*Planters* NUT-rition 12 oz.) | 160 | 6.0 | 5.0 | 15.0 | 0 | 40 | 3.0 |
| (*Planters* NUT-rition | | | | | | | |
| Lightly Salted) ...... | 170 | 6.0 | 6.0 | 15.0 | 0 | 40 | 3.0 |
| barbecue (*Blue* | | | | | | | |
| *Diamond* Bold): | | | | | | | |
| Carolina ........... | 170 | 6.0 | 5.0 | 15.0 | 0 | 180 | 3.0 |
| Habanero .......... | 170 | 6.0 | 5.0 | 15.0 | 0 | 100 | 3.0 |
| dried ................ | 167 | 5.7 | 5.8 | 14.8 | 0 | 3 | 3.1 |
| dry-roasted, salted ..... | 167 | 4.6 | 6.9 | 14.7 | 0 | 221 | 3.9 |
| honey-roasted: | | | | | | | |
| (*Blue Diamond*) ..... | 160 | 5.0 | 9.0 | 13.0 | 0 | 60 | 2.0 |
| 1 oz. .............. | 168 | 5.2 | 7.9 | 14.2 | 0 | 37 | 3.9 |
| lime chili: | | | | | | | |
| (*Blue Diamond* Bold) . | 170 | 6.0 | 5.0 | 16.0 | 0 | 120 | 3.0 |
| (*Planters*) .......... | 170 | 6.0 | 6.0 | 15.0 | 0 | 160 | 3.0 |
| oil-roasted, salted ...... | 176 | 5.8 | 4.5 | 16.4 | 0 | 221 | 3.2 |
| pepper, cracked, w/garlic, | | | | | | | |
| onion (*Planters*) ..... | 170 | 6.0 | 6.0 | 15.0 | 0 | 135 | 3.0 |
| roasted: | | | | | | | |
| (*Blue Diamond*) ..... | 170 | 6.0 | 5.0 | 18.0 | 0 | 85 | 3.0 |
| (*Blue Diamond* | | | | | | | |
| Oven Unsalted) ... | 170 | 6.0 | 5.0 | 15.0 | 0 | 0 | 3.0 |
| (*Frito-Lay*) ......... | 190 | 6.0 | 5.0 | 16.0 | 0 | 170 | 3.0 |
| (*Nut Harvest*) ....... | 180 | 6.0 | 6.0 | 15.0 | 0 | 150 | 3.0 |
| honey (*Blue Diamond*) | 160 | 5.0 | 9.0 | 13.0 | 0 | 30 | 3.0 |

| Food and Measure | cal. | prot. (gms) | carbo. (gms) | fat (gms) | chol. (mgs) | sod. (mgs) | fiber (gms) |
|---|---|---|---|---|---|---|---|
| **Almond** *(cont.)* | | | | | | | |
| sea salt (*Blue Diamond*) ......... | 170 | 6.0 | 5.0 | 15.0 | 0 | 135 | 3.0 |
| salt and vinegar (*Blue Diamond* Bold) ...... | 170 | 6.0 | 5.0 | 15.0 | 0 | 140 | 3.0 |
| sea salt and olive oil (*Planters*) ........... | 170 | 6.0 | 5.0 | 15.0 | 0 | 190 | 3.0 |
| sliced (see also "Salad Toppers"): | | | | | | | |
| (*Blue Diamond*) ..... | 160 | 6.0 | 6.0 | 14.0 | 0 | 0 | 3.0 |
| (*Diamond*), 1.1 oz. ... | 180 | 6.0 | 6.0 | 15.0 | 0 | 0 | 3.0 |
| (*Planters*), 1.2 oz. .... | 190 | 7.0 | 7.0 | 17.0 | 0 | 0 | 4.0 |
| slivered: | | | | | | | |
| (*Blue Diamond*) ..... | 160 | 6.0 | 6.0 | 14.0 | 0 | 10 | 3.0 |
| (*Diamond*), ¼ cup, 1.1 oz. .......... | 170 | 7.0 | 6.0 | 15.0 | 0 | 0 | 4.0 |
| (*Planters*), 2 oz. ..... | 330 | 12.0 | 11.0 | 28.0 | 0 | 0 | 7.0 |
| smoked: | | | | | | | |
| (*Blue Diamond Smokehouse*) ..... | 170 | 6.0 | 5.0 | 16.0 | 0 | 150 | 3.0 |
| (*Frito-Lay*), 1 pkg. .... | 260 | 8.0 | 13.0 | 19.0 | 0 | 125 | 4.0 |
| (*Planters*), 1.5 oz. .... | 250 | 9.0 | 8.0 | 22.0 | 0 | 370 | 5.0 |
| jalapeño (*Blue Diamond Smokehouse*) ..... | 170 | 6.0 | 5.0 | 15.0 | 0 | 180 | 3.0 |
| tamari (*Eden* Organic) ... | 160 | 8.0 | 8.0 | 11.0 | 0 | 65 | 4.0 |
| toasted .............. | 167 | 5.8 | 6.5 | 14.4 | 0 | 3 | 3.2 |
| wasabi and soy sauce (*Blue Diamond* Bold) . | 170 | 6.0 | 6.0 | 15.0 | 0 | 115 | 3.0 |
| **Almond beverage**, 8 fl. oz.: | | | | | | | |
| (*Almond Dream*): | | | | | | | |
| original ............ | 50 | 1.0 | 6.0 | 2.5 | 0 | 100 | <1.0 |
| unsweetened ....... | 30 | 1.0 | 1.0 | 2.5 | 0 | 100 | <1.0 |
| (*Pacific* Organic): | | | | | | | |
| original ............ | 60 | 1.0 | 8.0 | 2.5 | 0 | 140 | 0 |
| unsweetened ....... | 35 | 1.0 | 2.0 | 2.5 | 0 | 180 | 0 |
| vanilla ............. | 70 | 1.0 | 11.0 | 2.5 | 0 | 140 | 0 |
| vanilla, unsweetened . | 40 | 1.0 | 3.0 | 2.5 | 0 | 180 | 0 |
| (*Silk PureAlmond*): | | | | | | | |
| original ............ | 60 | 1.0 | 8.0 | 2.5 | 0 | 150 | 1.0 |
| dark chocolate ...... | 120 | 1.0 | 23.0 | 3.0 | 0 | 190 | 1.0 |
| unsweetened ....... | 35 | 1.0 | 1.0 | 2.5 | 0 | 150 | 1.0 |
| vanilla ............. | 90 | 1.0 | 16.0 | 2.5 | 0 | 150 | 1.0 |

| Food and Measure | cal. | prot. (gms) | carbo. (gms) | fat (gms) | chol. (mgs) | sod. (mgs) | fiber (gms) |
|---|---|---|---|---|---|---|---|
| **Almond butter**, 2 tbsp.: | | | | | | | |
| creamy/crunchy: | | | | | | | |
| (*Arrowhead Mills*) .... | 200 | 7.0 | 6.0 | 17.0 | 0 | 0 | 4.0 |
| (*Blue Diamond* Homestyle) ....... | 190 | 7.0 | 6.0 | 17.0 | 0 | 75 | 4.0 |
| (*Blue Diamond* ReadySpread) .... | 190 | 7.0 | 7.0 | 17.0 | 0 | 75 | 3.0 |
| (*Kettle Roaster Fresh*) . | 180 | 5.0 | 6.0 | 17.0 | 0 | 55 | 2.0 |
| (*MaraNatha* Natural Hint of Sea Salt) ... | 180 | 7.0 | 6.0 | 16.0 | 0 | 60 | 4.0 |
| (*MaraNatha* Natural No Stir) ........ | 190 | 6.0 | 7.0 | 17.0 | 0 | 65 | 3.0 |
| raw (*MaraNatha* Natural/Organic) ... | 190 | 7.0 | 6.0 | 17.0 | 0 | 0 | 4.0 |
| roasted (*MaraNatha* Natural/Organic) ... | 190 | 7.0 | 6.0 | 16.0 | 0 | 0 | 4.0 |
| honey: | | | | | | | |
| (*Blue Diamond* Homestyle) ....... | 180 | 6.0 | 11.0 | 14.0 | 0 | 75 | 3.0 |
| (*Blue Diamond* ReadySpread) .... | 180 | 5.0 | 10.0 | 14.0 | 0 | 75 | 3.0 |
| (*MaraNatha*) ........ | 180 | 6.0 | 9.0 | 14.0 | 0 | 70 | 3.0 |
| **Almond flour/meal:** | | | | | | | |
| fine ground (*Bob's Red Mill*), ¼ cup ..... | 160 | 6.0 | 6.0 | 14.0 | 0 | 10 | 3.0 |
| meal, 1 oz. ........... | 116 | 11.2 | 8.2 | 5.2 | 0 | 2 | n.a. |
| **Almond paste** (*Roland*), 2 tbsp. ............ | 180 | 4.0 | 19.0 | 10.0 | 0 | 0 | 2.0 |
| **Amaranth**, whole grain, organic, ¼ cup: | | | | | | | |
| (*Arrowhead Mills*) ....... | 180 | 7.0 | 31.0 | 3.0 | 0 | 10 | 7.0 |
| (*Bob's Red Mill*) ....... | 190 | 8.0 | 34.0 | 3.5 | 0 | 10 | 7.0 |
| **Amaranth flakes**, see "Cereal" | | | | | | | |
| **Amaranth flour**, whole grain (*Bob's Red Mill* Organic), ¼ cup .. | 110 | 4.0 | 20.0 | 2.0 | 0 | 6 | 3.0 |
| **Amaranth leaves:** | | | | | | | |
| raw, trimmed, ½ cup .... | 4 | .3 | .6 | <.1 | 0 | 3 | n.a. |
| boiled, drained, ½ cup .. | 14 | 1.4 | 2.7 | .1 | 0 | 14 | n.a. |
| **Anasazi bean**, dry: | | | | | | | |
| (*Arrowhead Mills* organic), ¼ cup ..... | 140 | 7.0 | 26.0 | 1.0 | 0 | 10 | 6.0 |
| (*Bob's Red Mill*), ¼ cup . | 150 | 10.0 | 27.0 | .5 | 0 | 0 | 9.0 |

| Food and Measure | cal. | prot. (gms) | carbo. (gms) | fat (gms) | chol. (mgs) | sod. (mgs) | fiber (gms) |
|---|---|---|---|---|---|---|---|
| **Anchovy**, European, raw, meat only, 1 oz. . . . . | 37 | 5.8 | 0 | 1.4 | 17 | 29 | 0 |
| **Anchovy, can/jar**, in olive oil, drained: | | | | | | | |
| flat fillets: | | | | | | | |
| (*Crown Prince*), 6 pcs. | 40 | 4.0 | 0 | 2.5 | 15 | 1050 | 0 |
| (*Crown Prince Natural* jar), 9 pcs. . | 35 | 4.0 | 0 | 2.5 | 15 | 1050 | 0 |
| (*King Oscar*), 6 pcs. . . | 25 | 3.0 | 0 | 1.5 | 15 | 900 | 0 |
| (*Roland*), 6 pcs. . . . . . | 25 | 4.0 | 0 | 1.0 | 16 | 860 | 0 |
| (*Roland* jar), 4 pcs. . . . | 20 | 3.0 | 0 | 0 | 15 | 920 | 0 |
| (*Vigo*), 6 pcs. . . . . . . . | 25 | 3.0 | 0 | 1.5 | 15 | 700 | 0 |
| 5 medium, .7 oz. . . . . . | 42 | 5.8 | 0 | 1.9 | 3 | 734 | 0 |
| rolled, w/capers: | | | | | | | |
| (*Crown Prince*), 6 pcs. | 40 | 4.0 | 0 | 2.0 | 15 | 970 | 0 |
| (*Roland*), 6 pcs. . . . . . | 25 | 4.0 | 0 | 1.0 | 16 | 860 | 0 |
| (*Vigo*), 4 pcs. . . . . . . . | 25 | 3.0 | 0 | 1.5 | 12 | 880 | 0 |
| **Anchovy paste**, 1 tbsp.: | | | | | | | |
| (*Alessi*) . . . . . . . . . . . . . | 30 | 2.0 | 0 | 2.5 | 55 | 940 | 0 |
| (*Crown Prince*) . . . . . . . . | 40 | 2.0 | 0 | 3.5 | 5 | 660 | 0 |
| (*Roland*) . . . . . . . . . . . . | 30 | 2.0 | 0 | 2.0 | 24 | 1140 | 0 |
| **Angel-hair pasta**, see "Pasta" | | | | | | | |
| **Angel-hair pasta dish mix**, 1 cup*, except as noted: | | | | | | | |
| w/herbs (*Pasta Roni*) . . . | 310 | 9.0 | 41.0 | 13.0 | 5 | 750 | 2.0 |
| primavera (*Pasta Roni*) . . | 310 | 9.0 | 38.0 | 15.0 | 5 | 910 | 2.0 |
| tomato, spicy (*Near East*), 2 oz. mix . . . . . . | 190 | 7.0 | 38.0 | 2.0 | 0 | 530 | 3.0 |
| **Angel-hair pasta entree**, frozen, 1 pkg.: | | | | | | | |
| marinara (*Smart Ones*), 10 oz. . . . . . . . | 230 | 9.0 | 40.0 | 4.0 | 0 | 640 | 4.0 |
| meat sauce (*Michelina's Budget Gourmet*), 8 oz. | 290 | 11.0 | 48.0 | 5.0 | 10 | 410 | 4.0 |
| pomodoro (*Lean Cuisine*), 10 oz. . . . . . . | 250 | 8.0 | 42.0 | 5.0 | 5 | 620 | 4.0 |
| **Anise seed**, 1 tsp. . . . . . . | 7 | .4 | 1.1 | .3 | 0 | <1 | .3 |
| **Antelope**, meat only, roasted, 4 oz. . . . . . . . | 170 | 33.4 | 0 | 3.0 | 143 | 51 | 0 |
| **Apple, fresh**: | | | | | | | |
| (*Chiquita*), 6.4-oz. pc. . . . | 95 | 0 | 25.0 | 0 | 0 | 2 | 4.0 |
| (*Dole*), 5.4-oz. pc. . . . . . . | 80 | 0 | 21.0 | 0 | 0 | 0 | 4.0 |

| Food and Measure | cal. | prot. (gms) | carbo. (gms) | fat (gms) | chol. (mgs) | sod. (mgs) | fiber (gms) |
|---|---|---|---|---|---|---|---|
| (*Frieda's* Lady), 5 oz. .... | 80 | 0 | 21.0 | .5 | 0 | 0 | 3.0 |
| raw, w/peel: | | | | | | | |
|   2¾" apple .......... | 81 | .3 | 21.1 | .5 | 0 | 1 | 3.7 |
|   sliced, ½ cup ....... | 32 | .1 | 8.4 | .2 | 0 | 0 | 3.0 |
| raw, peeled: | | | | | | | |
|   2¾" apple .......... | 72 | .2 | 19.0 | .4 | 0 | <1 | 2.4 |
|   sliced, ½ cup ....... | 31 | .1 | 8.2 | .2 | 0 | 0 | 1.0 |
| cooked, peeled, sliced, | | | | | | | |
|   boiled, ½ cup ....... | 45 | .2 | 11.7 | .3 | 0 | 1 | 2.0 |
| **Apple, can/jar** (see | | | | | | | |
|   also "Applesauce"): | | | | | | | |
| baby, in light syrup | | | | | | | |
|   (*Roland*), ½ cup ..... | 50 | 0 | 12.0 | 0 | 0 | 20 | 2.0 |
| and crème (*Dole* | | | | | | | |
|   Parfait), 4.3-oz. cup .. | 120 | 1.0 | 23.0 | 2.0 | 0 | 10 | 1.0 |
| fried, ½ cup: | | | | | | | |
|   (*Lucky Leaf*) ........ | 170 | 0 | 43.0 | 0 | 0 | 20 | 2.0 |
|   cinnamon (*Glory*) .... | 80 | 0 | 21.0 | 0 | 0 | 170 | 1.0 |
| and oranges (*Del Monte* | | | | | | | |
|   Fruit Naturals), ½ cup . | 70 | 0 | 18.0 | 0 | 0 | 10 | <2.0 |
| sliced, in water (*Lucky* | | | | | | | |
|   Leaf/Musselman's*), | | | | | | | |
|   ½ cup ............. | 50 | 0 | 12.0 | 0 | 0 | 20 | 1.0 |
| spiced (*Lucky Leaf/* | | | | | | | |
|   Musselman's*), 1 ring . | 35 | 0 | 9.0 | 0 | 0 | 5 | 0 |
| **Apple, coated**, candy | | | | | | | |
|   or caramel, w/nuts | | | | | | | |
|   (*Tastee*), 3-oz. pc. .... | 160 | 3.0 | 26.0 | 5.0 | 0 | 20 | 4.0 |
| **Apple, dried**: | | | | | | | |
| (*Mariani*), ⅓ cup, 1.4 oz. . | 100 | 1.0 | 25.0 | 0 | 0 | 130 | 3.0 |
| (*Sun•Maid*), ¼ cup, | | | | | | | |
|   1.4 oz. ........... | 120 | 1.0 | 29.0 | 0 | 0 | 135 | 2.0 |
| dehydrated, ½ cup ..... | 104 | .4 | 28.1 | .2 | 0 | 74 | 7.4 |
| sulfured, 1 ring ........ | 16 | .1 | 4.2 | 0 | 0 | 6 | 4.2 |
| sulfured, ½ cup ........ | 104 | .4 | 28.3 | .1 | 0 | 75 | 7.5 |
| **Apple, fried**, see "Apple, | | | | | | | |
|   can/jar" | | | | | | | |
| **Apple, frozen/chilled**: | | | | | | | |
| (*Stouffer's* Harvest), | | | | | | | |
|   ½ of 12-oz. pkg. ..... | 190 | 0 | 40.0 | 3.0 | 0 | 5 | 2.0 |
| cinnamon (*Hormel* | | | | | | | |
|   Country Crock), ½ cup . | 130 | 0 | 26.0 | 2.5 | 0 | 150 | 1.0 |
| glazed (*Bob Evans*), | | | | | | | |
|   ½ cup ............. | 120 | 0 | 33.0 | 2.0 | 0 | 35 | 1.0 |

| Food and Measure | cal. | prot. (gms) | carbo. (gms) | fat (gms) | chol. (mgs) | sod. (mgs) | fiber (gms) |
|---|---|---|---|---|---|---|---|
| **Apple, frozen/chilled,** *(cont.)* | | | | | | | |
| unheated, ½ cup ....... | 42 | 0 | 10.7 | 0 | 0 | 3 | 1.6 |
| **Apple butter**, 1 tbsp.: | | | | | | | |
| (*Apple Time/Lucky* | | | | | | | |
| *Leaf/Musselman's*) ... | 30 | 0 | 8.0 | 0 | 0 | 0 | 0 |
| (*Eden* Organic) ........ | 20 | 0 | 4.0 | 0 | 0 | 0 | 1.0 |
| (*R.W. Knudsen* Organic) . | 35 | 0 | 9.0 | 0 | 0 | 0 | 0 |
| cherry (*Eden* Organic) ... | 25 | 0 | 6.0 | 0 | 0 | 0 | <1.0 |
| cider (*Smucker's*) ...... | 45 | 0 | 11.0 | 0 | 0 | 10 | 0 |
| **Apple cider**, see "Apple juice" | | | | | | | |
| **Apple cinnamon topping** | | | | | | | |
| (*Smucker's*), 2 tbsp. .. | 100 | 0 | 25.0 | 0 | 0 | 10 | 0 |
| **Apple crisp**, 4 oz.: | | | | | | | |
| cinnamon (*Dole*) ....... | 160 | 1.0 | 29.0 | 3.5 | 0 | 20 | 2.0 |
| pear (*Dole*) .......... | 150 | 2.0 | 29.0 | 3.5 | 0 | 25 | 2.0 |
| **Apple crisp mix** (*Betty* | | | | | | | |
| *Crocker*), ⅙ batch .... | 270 | 1.0 | 54.0 | 6.0 | 0 | 210 | 2.0 |
| **Apple crisp topping** | | | | | | | |
| (*Marzetti*), ⅛ pkg. ..... | 120 | 1.0 | 27.0 | 0 | 0 | 90 | 1.0 |
| **Apple dip**, see "Fruit dip" | | | | | | | |
| **Apple drink**: | | | | | | | |
| (*Snapple*), 8 fl. oz. ... | 110 | 0 | 27.0 | 0 | 0 | 5 | 0 |
| sparkling (*Kristian* | | | | | | | |
| *Regale*), 8 fl. oz. ... | 100 | 0 | 25.0 | 0 | 0 | 7 | 0 |
| **Apple drink blend**: | | | | | | | |
| cranberry (*Welch's*), | | | | | | | |
| 10 fl. oz. ......... | 180 | 0 | 45.0 | 0 | 0 | 25 | 0 |
| raspberry (*Odwalla Seri-* | | | | | | | |
| *ous Focus*), 8 fl. oz. | 170 | 0 | 40.0 | 0 | 0 | 15 | 0 |
| **Apple juice**, 8 fl. oz., except as noted: | | | | | | | |
| (*After the Fall* Organic) .. | 90 | 0 | 22.0 | 0 | 0 | 20 | 0 |
| (*Apple & Eve*), | | | | | | | |
| 6.75 fl. oz. ......... | 90 | 0 | 21.0 | 0 | 0 | 5 | 0 |
| (*Apple & Eve* Clear/ | | | | | | | |
| Natural/On-the-Go) ... | 110 | 1.0 | 26.0 | 0 | 0 | 5 | 0 |
| (*Apple Time/Lincoln/* | | | | | | | |
| *Lucky Leaf/Mussel-* | | | | | | | |
| *man's* Juice/Cider) . | 120 | 0 | 31.0 | 0 | 0 | 25 | 0 |
| (*Dole*) .............. | 110 | <1.0 | 27.0 | 0 | 0 | 10 | 0 |
| (*Eden* Organic) ........ | 90 | 0 | 24.0 | 0 | 0 | 0 | 0 |
| (*Florida's Natural*) ...... | 120 | 0 | 29.0 | 0 | 0 | 0 | 0 |

| Food and Measure | cal. | prot. (gms) | carbo. (gms) | fat (gms) | chol. (mgs) | sod. (mgs) | fiber (gms) |
|---|---|---|---|---|---|---|---|
| (*Fragile Planet* Organic) .......... | 120 | 0 | 28.0 | 0 | 0 | 15 | 0 |
| (*Langers* Cider/Juice) .... | 120 | 0 | 28.0 | 0 | 0 | 0 | 0 |
| (*Martinelli's* Juice/ Cider/Organic/ Unfiltered) ......... | 140 | 1.0 | 35.0 | 0 | 0 | 0 | 0 |
| (*Martinelli's* Juice), 10 fl. oz. ........... | 180 | 1.0 | 43.0 | 0 | 0 | 0 | 0 |
| (*Minute Maid*) ......... | 110 | 0 | 28.0 | 0 | 0 | 20 | 0 |
| (*Minute Maid*), 10 fl. oz. ........... | 140 | 0 | 35.0 | 0 | 0 | 25 | 0 |
| (*Mott's* Natural) ........ | 110 | 0 | 27.0 | 0 | 0 | 10 | 0 |
| (*Mott's* Original) ....... | 120 | 0 | 29.0 | 0 | 0 | 10 | 0 |
| (*Nantucket Nectars* Organic Cloudy) ..... | 120 | 0 | 29.0 | 0 | 0 | 30 | 0 |
| (*Nantucket Nectars* Pressed) ........... | 120 | 0 | 30.0 | 0 | 0 | 15 | 1.0 |
| (*R.W. Knudsen* Natural/Organic/Cider & Spice) ........... | 120 | <1.0 | 30.0 | 0 | 0 | 25 | 0 |
| (*R.W. Knudsen* Organic Filtered) .......... | 150 | <1.0 | 30.0 | 0 | 0 | 25 | 0 |
| (*Santa Cruz Organic*) .... | 120 | <1.0 | 30.0 | 0 | 0 | 25 | 0 |
| (*Simply Apple*) ........ | 120 | 0 | 30.0 | 0 | 0 | 5 | 0 |
| (*Snapple* Green Apple), 11.5 fl. oz. ......... | 160 | 0 | 41.0 | 0 | 0 | 20 | 0 |
| (*Tropicana*) ............ | 110 | <1.0 | 27.0 | 0 | 0 | 10 | 0 |
| (*Tropicana Pure Premium*), 12 fl. oz. .. | 170 | 0 | 43.0 | 0 | 0 | 20 | 0 |
| (*Veryfine*) ............. | 120 | 0 | 29.0 | 0 | 0 | 35 | 0 |
| (*Veryfine*), 10 fl. oz. .... | 140 | 0 | 36.0 | 0 | 0 | 40 | 0 |
| all varieties (*Litehouse* Cider) .... | 120 | 0 | 30.0 | 0 | 0 | 60 | 0 |
| frozen*: | | | | | | | |
| (*Cascadian Farm* Organic) ......... | 120 | 0 | 29.0 | 0 | 0 | 0 | 0 |
| (*Langers*) .......... | 120 | 0 | 28.0 | 0 | 0 | 15 | 0 |
| (*Minute Maid*) ....... | 110 | 0 | 28.0 | 0 | 0 | 0 | 0 |
| sparkling: | | | | | | | |
| (*Langers* Cider) ....... | 120 | 0 | 28.0 | 0 | 0 | 15 | 0 |
| (*Martinelli's* Cider/ Organic) ......... | 140 | 1.0 | 35.0 | 0 | 0 | 0 | 0 |
| (*Martinelli's* Juice), 10 fl. oz. ......... | 180 | 1.0 | 43.0 | 0 | 0 | 0 | 0 |

| Food and Measure | cal. | prot. (gms) | carbo. (gms) | fat (gms) | chol. (mgs) | sod. (mgs) | fiber (gms) |
|---|---|---|---|---|---|---|---|
| **Apple juice** *(cont.)* | | | | | | | |
| (*R.W. Knudsen* | | | | | | | |
| Crisp/Organic) ......... | 120 | <1.0 | 30.0 | 0 | 0 | 25 | 0 |
| **Apple juice blend**, | | | | | | | |
| 8 fl. oz., except | | | | | | | |
| as noted: | | | | | | | |
| berry cherry (*Ceres*) .... | 130 | 0 | 32.0 | 0 | 0 | 10 | 0 |
| caramel (*Litehouse* | | | | | | | |
| Cider) ............. | 120 | 0 | 30.0 | 0 | 0 | 60 | 0 |
| carrot (*Mott's* Medleys) .. | 110 | 0 | 25.0 | 0 | 0 | 80 | 0 |
| cranberry (*Veryfine* | | | | | | | |
| Cocktail), 10 fl. oz. ... | 190 | 0 | 48.0 | 0 | 0 | 25 | 0 |
| grape: | | | | | | | |
| (*Apple & Eve*), | | | | | | | |
| 6.75 fl. oz. ....... | 130 | 0 | 32.0 | 0 | 0 | 15 | 0 |
| (*Martinelli's*), | | | | | | | |
| 10 fl. oz. ......... | 150 | 0 | 39.0 | 0 | 0 | 18 | 0 |
| white (*Minute Maid*), | | | | | | | |
| 6.75 fl. oz. ........ | 100 | 0 | 25.0 | 0 | 0 | 15 | 0 |
| sparkling (*Martinelli's*): | | | | | | | |
| berry, wild .......... | 150 | 0 | 36.0 | 0 | 0 | 0 | 0 |
| black currant ........ | 120 | 0 | 28.0 | 0 | 0 | 10 | 0 |
| cherry ............. | 140 | 0 | 31.0 | 0 | 0 | 15 | 0 |
| cranberry .......... | 110 | 0 | 27.0 | 0 | 0 | 4 | 0 |
| grape ............. | 120 | 0 | 31.0 | 0 | 0 | 14 | 0 |
| mango ............. | 150 | 0 | 38.0 | 0 | 0 | 0 | 0 |
| marionberry ........ | 130 | 0 | 32.0 | 0 | 0 | 0 | <1.0 |
| peach ............. | 120 | 0 | 29.0 | 0 | 0 | 0 | 0 |
| pear .............. | 120 | 1.0 | 29.0 | 0 | 0 | 15 | 0 |
| pomegranate ....... | 150 | 0 | 38.0 | 0 | 0 | 10 | 0 |
| raspberry .......... | 120 | 0 | 30.0 | 0 | 0 | 4 | 0 |
| strawberry: | | | | | | | |
| (*Minute Maid*), | | | | | | | |
| 6.75 fl. oz. ....... | 100 | 0 | 25.0 | 0 | 0 | 15 | 0 |
| (*Veryfine*), 11.5 fl. oz. . | 190 | 0 | 48.0 | 0 | 0 | 40 | 0 |
| **Apple pastry**, see | | | | | | | |
| specific listings | | | | | | | |
| **Apple snack**, fresh: | | | | | | | |
| (*Chiquita Fruit Bites*), | | | | | | | |
| 2.5-oz. pkg.: | | | | | | | |
| red and green ...... | 30 | 0 | 8.0 | 0 | 0 | 0 | 2.0 |
| w/caramel .......... | 70 | 0 | 17.0 | 0 | 0 | 55 | 2.0 |
| w/cinnamon cream ... | 60 | 0 | 11.0 | 1.0 | 5 | 20 | 2.0 |
| and grapes ........ | 40 | 0 | 10.0 | 0 | 0 | 0 | 1.0 |

| Food and Measure | cal. | prot. (gms) | carbo. (gms) | fat (gms) | chol. (mgs) | sod. (mgs) | fiber (gms) |
|---|---|---|---|---|---|---|---|
| (*Ready Pac*), 1 cont.: | | | | | | | |
|   caramel, 6 oz. . . . . . . . | 200 | 2.0 | 52.0 | 0 | 0 | 200 | 2.0 |
|   peanut butter, 5.75 oz. | 340 | 12.0 | 28.0 | 24.0 | 0 | 230 | 6.0 |
| **Applesauce**, ½ cup, | | | | | | | |
|   except as noted: | | | | | | | |
| unsweetened//natural: | | | | | | | |
|   (*Eden* Organic) . . . . . . | 60 | 0 | 13.0 | 0 | 0 | 10 | 2.0 |
|   (*Langers*) . . . . . . . . . . | 50 | 0 | 13.0 | 0 | 0 | 5 | 2.0 |
|   (*Lucky Leaf*) . . . . . . . . | 50 | 0 | 13.0 | 0 | 0 | 20 | 2.0 |
|   (*Mott's* Natural) . . . . . | 50 | 0 | 14.0 | 0 | 0 | 0 | 1.0 |
|   (*Musselman's* Organic), | | | | | | | |
|     4-oz. cont. . . . . . . . | 50 | 0 | 12.0 | 0 | 0 | 10 | 2.0 |
|   (*Santa Cruz Organic*) . | 60 | 0 | 13.0 | 0 | 0 | 20 | 2.0 |
|   (*Santa Cruz Organic*), | | | | | | | |
|     4-oz. cont. . . . . . . . | 50 | 0 | 12.0 | 0 | 0 | 17 | 2.0 |
|   cinnamon (*Eden* | | | | | | | |
|     Organic) . . . . . . . . . | 60 | 0 | 14.0 | 0 | 0 | 10 | 2.0 |
|   cinnamon (*Santa Cruz* | | | | | | | |
|     *Organic*) . . . . . . . . . | 90 | 0 | 21.0 | 0 | 0 | 25 | 2.0 |
|   cinnamon (*Santa Cruz* | | | | | | | |
|     *Organic*), 4 oz. . . . . | 70 | 0 | 19.0 | 0 | 0 | 15 | 2.0 |
|   Granny Smith (*Mott's* | | | | | | | |
|     Healthy Harvest | | | | | | | |
|     Sauce), 4-oz. cont. . | 50 | 0 | 13.0 | 0 | 0 | 0 | 1.0 |
|   Granny Smith | | | | | | | |
|     (*Musselman's* Healthy | | | | | | | |
|     Picks), 4-oz. cont. . | 70 | 0 | 17.0 | 0 | 0 | 10 | 3.0 |
| sweetened: | | | | | | | |
|   (*Lucky Leaf/* | | | | | | | |
|     *Musselman's*) . . . . . | 90 | 0 | 22.0 | 0 | 0 | 10 | 2.0 |
|   (*Lucky Leaf/* | | | | | | | |
|     *Musselman's* Lite) . | 50 | 0 | 13.0 | 0 | 0 | 10 | 2.0 |
|   (*Lucky Leaf/* | | | | | | | |
|     *Musselman's*), | | | | | | | |
|     4-oz. cont. . . . . . . . | 80 | 0 | 20.0 | 0 | 0 | 10 | 2.0 |
|   (*Mott's* Classic) . . . . . . | 110 | 0 | 27.0 | 0 | 0 | 0 | 1.0 |
|   (*Mott's* Classic), 4 oz. . . | 100 | 0 | 24.0 | 0 | 0 | 0 | 1.0 |
|   (*Mott's* Chunky/ | | | | | | | |
|     Homestyle) . . . . . . . | 90 | 0 | 23.0 | 0 | 0 | 0 | 1.0 |
|   (*Musselman's* Organic), | | | | | | | |
|     4-oz. cont. . . . . . . . | 80 | 0 | 20.0 | 0 | 0 | 10 | 2.0 |
|   cinnamon (*Lucky Leaf/* | | | | | | | |
|     *Musselman's*) . . . . . | 100 | 0 | 25.0 | 0 | 0 | 10 | 2.0 |
|   cinnamon (*Mott's*) . . . | 120 | 0 | 29.0 | 0 | 0 | 0 | 1.0 |

| Food and Measure | cal. | prot. (gms) | carbo. (gms) | fat (gms) | chol. (mgs) | sod. (mgs) | fiber (gms) |
|---|---|---|---|---|---|---|---|
| **Applesauce, sweetened** *(cont.)* | | | | | | | |
| cinnamon (*Mott's*), | | | | | | | |
| 4 oz. . . . . . . . . . . | 100 | 0 | 24.0 | 0 | 0 | 0 | 1.0 |
| **Applesauce fruit blend**, | | | | | | | |
| 4-oz. cont., except | | | | | | | |
| as noted: | | | | | | | |
| all varieties (*Mott's* | | | | | | | |
| *Healthy Harvest Sauce*) | 50 | 0 | 13.0 | 0 | 0 | 0 | 1.0 |
| all varieties, except: | | | | | | | |
| blueberry (*Santa Cruz* | | | | | | | |
| *Organic*), ½ cup . . . | 60 | 0 | 15.0 | 0 | 0 | 20 | 2.0 |
| blueberry and | | | | | | | |
| raspberry (*Santa* | | | | | | | |
| *Cruz Organic*) . . . . . | 60 | 0 | 14.0 | 0 | 0 | 17 | 2.0 |
| mixed berry (*Mott's*) . . | 90 | 0 | 23.0 | 0 | 0 | 0 | 1.0 |
| berry, mixed: | | | | | | | |
| (*Mott's*) . . . . . . . . . . . | 100 | 0 | 25.0 | 0 | 0 | 0 | 1.0 |
| (*Musselman's Totally* | | | | | | | |
| *Fruit*) . . . . . . . . . . | 90 | 0 | 21.0 | 0 | 0 | 10 | 1.0 |
| blueberry: | | | | | | | |
| (*Santa Cruz Organic*), | | | | | | | |
| ½ cup . . . . . . . . . . | 70 | 0 | 16.0 | 0 | 0 | 20 | 2.0 |
| (*Santa Cruz Organic*) . | 60 | 0 | 14.0 | 0 | 0 | 20 | 2.0 |
| cherry (*Eden* Organic), | | | | | | | |
| ½ cup . . . . . . . . . . . | 70 | 0 | 17.0 | 0 | 0 | 10 | 3.0 |
| cranberry raspberry | | | | | | | |
| (*Mott's* Plus) . . . . . . . . | 50 | 0 | 13.0 | 0 | 0 | 0 | 3.0 |
| peach (*Musselman's* | | | | | | | |
| *Totally Fruit*) . . . . . . . . | 90 | 0 | 22.0 | 0 | 0 | 10 | 2.0 |
| pomegranate: | | | | | | | |
| (*Mott's* Plus) . . . . . . . . | 50 | 0 | 13.0 | 0 | 0 | 0 | 1.0 |
| (*Musselman's* Healthy | | | | | | | |
| Picks Blue Pom) . . . | 70 | 0 | 17.0 | 0 | 0 | 10 | 3.0 |
| raspberry: | | | | | | | |
| (*Santa Cruz Organic*) . | 60 | 0 | 13.0 | 0 | 0 | 20 | 2.0 |
| acai (*Musselman's* | | | | | | | |
| Healthy Picks) . . . . | 70 | 0 | 17.0 | 0 | 0 | 10 | 3.0 |
| strawberry: | | | | | | | |
| (*Eden* Organic), ½ cup | 60 | 0 | 13.0 | 0 | 0 | 10 | 2.0 |
| (*Musselman's Totally* | | | | | | | |
| *Fruit*) . . . . . . . . . . | 90 | 0 | 21.0 | 0 | 0 | 10 | 2.0 |
| **Apricot**, fresh: | | | | | | | |
| (*Dole*), 3 medium, 4 oz. . | 60 | 0 | 11.0 | 1.0 | 0 | 0 | 1.0 |
| 3 medium, 12 per lb. . . . . | 51 | 1.5 | 11.8 | .4 | 0 | 1 | 2.5 |

| Food and Measure | cal. | prot. (gms) | carbo. (gms) | fat (gms) | chol. (mgs) | sod. (mgs) | fiber (gms) |
|---|---|---|---|---|---|---|---|
| pitted, halves, ½ cup .... | 37 | 1.1 | 8.6 | .3 | 0 | 1 | 1.9 |
| pitted, sliced, ½ cup .... | 40 | 1.2 | 9.2 | .3 | 0 | 2 | 2.0 |
| **Apricot, can/jar**, ½ cup: | | | | | | | |
| in juice, w/liquid ....... | 59 | .8 | 15.1 | <.1 | 0 | 5 | 2.0 |
| in extra light syrup | | | | | | | |
| (*Del Monte* Lite) ..... | 60 | 0 | 16.0 | 0 | 0 | 10 | 1.0 |
| in light syrup: | | | | | | | |
| (*Del Monte Orchard* | | | | | | | |
| *Select*) .......... | 80 | <1.0 | 21.0 | 0 | 0 | 10 | 1.0 |
| chunks (*S&W* Sun) ... | 90 | 1.0 | 22.0 | 0 | 0 | 25 | 1.0 |
| almond flavor (*Del* | | | | | | | |
| *Monte*) .......... | 90 | 0 | 22.0 | 0 | 0 | 10 | 1.0 |
| in heavy syrup: | | | | | | | |
| (*Del Monte*) ........ | 100 | 0 | 26.0 | 0 | 0 | 10 | 1.0 |
| whole (*S&W*) ....... | 120 | <1.0 | 29.0 | 0 | 0 | 10 | 1.0 |
| **Apricot, dried**: | | | | | | | |
| (*Mariani* California), | | | | | | | |
| ¼ cup, 1.4 oz. ....... | 110 | 1.0 | 25.0 | 0 | 0 | 15 | 4.0 |
| (*Mariani* Mediterranean), | | | | | | | |
| ¼ cup, 1.4 oz. ....... | 110 | 1.0 | 25.0 | 0 | 0 | 0 | 2.0 |
| (*Mariani* Ultimate), | | | | | | | |
| ¼ cup, 1.4 oz. ....... | 110 | 1.0 | 24.0 | 0 | 0 | 100 | 6.0 |
| (*Sun•Maid* California), | | | | | | | |
| ¼ cup, 1.4 oz. ....... | 100 | 1.0 | 26.0 | 0 | 0 | 0 | 3.0 |
| (*Sun•Maid* Mediter- | | | | | | | |
| ranean), 1.4 oz. ...... | 100 | 1.0 | 23.0 | 0 | 0 | 15 | 3.0 |
| (*Sunsweet* Mediter- | | | | | | | |
| ranean), 1.4 oz. ...... | 100 | 1.0 | 23.0 | 0 | 0 | 25 | 3.0 |
| dehydrated, ½ cup ..... | 190 | 2.9 | 49.3 | .4 | 0 | 15 | n.a. |
| sulfured, ½ cup ........ | 155 | 2.4 | 40.1 | .3 | 0 | 7 | 5.9 |
| **Apricot, frozen**, | | | | | | | |
| sweetened, ½ cup ... | 119 | .9 | 30.4 | .1 | 0 | 5 | 2.1 |
| **Apricot glaze** (*Roland* | | | | | | | |
| Nappage), 2 tbsp. .... | 90 | 0 | 23.0 | 0 | 0 | 75 | 0 |
| **Apricot juice**, 8 fl. oz.: | | | | | | | |
| (*Ceres*) ............ | 130 | 0 | 32.0 | 0 | 0 | 15 | 0 |
| (*R.W. Knudsen* | | | | | | | |
| Nectar) ............ | 130 | <1.0 | 30.0 | 0 | 0 | 30 | 0 |
| (*Santa Cruz Organic* | | | | | | | |
| Nectar) ............ | 120 | 0 | 29.0 | 0 | 0 | 35 | <1.0 |
| **Apricot mango juice** | | | | | | | |
| (*Santa Cruz Organic*), | | | | | | | |
| 8 fl. oz. ............ | 120 | 0 | 29.0 | 0 | 0 | 10 | <1.0 |

| Food and Measure | cal. | prot. (gms) | carbo. (gms) | fat (gms) | chol. (mgs) | sod. (mgs) | fiber (gms) |
|---|---|---|---|---|---|---|---|
| **Arby's, dressing** 1 serving: | | | | | | | |
| breakfast biscuit: | | | | | | | |
| plain .............. | 250 | 6.0 | 32.0 | 11.0 | 0 | 780 | 1.0 |
| bacon/egg/cheese .... | 450 | 18.0 | 34.0 | 26.0 | 165 | 1610 | 1.0 |
| chicken ............ | 530 | 18.0 | 60.0 | 24.0 | 45 | 1310 | 1.0 |
| ham/egg/cheese ..... | 420 | 22.0 | 34.0 | 22.0 | 180 | 1720 | 1.0 |
| sausage ........... | 460 | 13.0 | 33.0 | 31.0 | 40 | 1230 | 1.0 |
| sausage gravy ....... | 590 | 14.0 | 48.0 | 38.0 | 40 | 1930 | 1.0 |
| sausage/egg/cheese .. | 590 | 20.0 | 35.0 | 42.0 | 195 | 1680 | 1.0 |
| breakfast croissant: | | | | | | | |
| bacon/egg/cheese .... | 390 | 16.0 | 24.0 | 24.0 | 190 | 1010 | 1.0 |
| ham/cheese ........ | 270 | 15.0 | 22.0 | 14.0 | 60 | 920 | 1.0 |
| ham/egg/cheese ..... | 360 | 19.0 | 24.0 | 20.0 | 205 | 1130 | 1.0 |
| sausage/egg/cheese .. | 530 | 18.0 | 24.0 | 40.0 | 220 | 1090 | 1.0 |
| breakfast platter: | | | | | | | |
| bacon/egg/biscuit .... | 570 | 23.0 | 43.0 | 30 | 280 | 1690 | 2.0 |
| bacon/egg/muffin .... | 600 | 21.0 | 44.0 | 33.0 | 335 | 1170 | 2.0 |
| ham/egg/biscuit ..... | 530 | 24.0 | 43.0 | 26.0 | 290 | 1730 | 2.0 |
| ham/egg/muffin ..... | 560 | 23.0 | 44.0 | 29.0 | 345 | 1200 | 2.0 |
| sausage/egg/biscuit .. | 700 | 23.0 | 43.0 | 44.0 | 305 | 1640 | 2.0 |
| sausage/egg/muffin .. | 720 | 22.0 | 44.0 | 48.0 | 360 | 1120 | 2.0 |
| breakfast sourdough: | | | | | | | |
| bacon/egg/cheese .... | 490 | 24.0 | 46.0 | 22.0 | 170 | 1450 | 2.0 |
| egg/cheese ......... | 392 | 17.0 | 40.0 | 12.0 | 166 | 1058 | 2.0 |
| ham/egg/cheese ..... | 440 | 26.0 | 45.0 | 17.0 | 180 | 1440 | 2.0 |
| sausage/egg/cheese .. | 610 | 25.0 | 46.0 | 37.0 | 195 | 1390 | 2.0 |
| sausage/omelet/cheese | 580 | 25.0 | 45.0 | 34.0 | 185 | 1280 | 2.0 |
| breakfast *Toastix*: | | | | | | | |
| w/bacon, platter ..... | 430 | 13.0 | 48.0 | 19.0 | 10 | 990 | 2.0 |
| w/ham, platter ...... | 380 | 14.0 | 48.0 | 15.0 | 20 | 1030 | 2.0 |
| w/sausage, platter ... | 550 | 13.0 | 48.0 | 33.0 | 35 | 940 | 2.0 |
| syrup .............. | 120 | 0 | 31.0 | 0 | 0 | 35 | 0 |
| breakfast wrap: | | | | | | | |
| bacon/egg/cheese .... | 560 | 21.0 | 45.0 | 29.0 | 170 | 1870 | 3.0 |
| ham/egg/cheese ..... | 520 | 22.0 | 45.0 | 24.0 | 180 | 1900 | 3.0 |
| sausage/egg/cheese .. | 690 | 21.0 | 45.0 | 43.0 | 195 | 1810 | 3.0 |
| sandwiches/melts: | | | | | | | |
| beef, roast: | | | | | | | |
| *Arby's* melt ....... | 370 | 23.0 | 40.0 | 13.0 | 50 | 1150 | 2.0 |
| beef, roast ....... | 340 | 23.0 | 38.0 | 11.0 | 45 | 970 | 2.0 |
| large ......... | 560 | 45.0 | 47.0 | 22.0 | 110 | 1870 | 3.0 |
| medium ....... | 430 | 33.0 | 39.0 | 16.0 | 80 | 1380 | 2.0 |
| super ......... | 420 | 23.0 | 45.0 | 17.0 | 45 | 1080 | 3.0 |
| beef 'n cheddar ... | 420 | 23.0 | 43.0 | 18.0 | 50 | 1260 | 2.0 |

| Food and Measure | cal. | prot. (gms) | carbo. (gms) | fat (gms) | chol. (mgs) | sod. (mgs) | fiber (gms) |
|---|---|---|---|---|---|---|---|
| large | 630 | 44.0 | 47.0 | 29.0 | 115 | 2270 | 2.0 |
| medium | 510 | 34.0 | 44.0 | 23.0 | 80 | 1670 | 2.0 |
| pepper bacon | 90 | 7.0 | 1.0 | 6.0 | 10 | 340 | 0 |
| *Roastburger*: | | | | | | | |
| All-American | 390 | 20.0 | 44.0 | 15.0 | 45 | 1730 | 2.0 |
| bacon cheddar | 420 | 26.0 | 42.0 | 16.0 | 60 | 1840 | 2.0 |
| double meat | 110 | 13.0 | 1.0 | 6.0 | 40 | 520 | 0 |
| chicken, crispy | 530 | 25.0 | 52.0 | 25.0 | 60 | 1310 | 4.0 |
| bacon/Swiss | 600 | 33.0 | 55.0 | 27.0 | 75 | 1750 | 4.0 |
| Cordon Bleu | 620 | 36.0 | 53.0 | 30.0 | 95 | 2040 | 3.0 |
| chicken, roast | 400 | 24.0 | 40.0 | 16.0 | 50 | 870 | 3.0 |
| bacon/Swiss | 470 | 32.0 | 43.0 | 19.0 | 65 | 1310 | 2.0 |
| club | 500 | 31.0 | 41.0 | 23.0 | 70 | 1320 | 2.0 |
| Cordon Bleu | 490 | 35.0 | 40.0 | 21.0 | 85 | 1600 | 2.0 |
| ham/Swiss melt | 300 | 18.0 | 37.0 | 8.0 | 35 | 1070 | 2.0 |
| *Market Fresh*: | | | | | | | |
| BLT ultimate | 820 | 32.0 | 78.0 | 44.0 | 45 | 1690 | 5.0 |
| pecan chicken salad | 750 | 29.0 | 85.0 | 34.0 | 55 | 1350 | 4.0 |
| Reuben | 700 | 38.0 | 64.0 | 32.0 | 65 | 1870 | 4.0 |
| roast beef/Swiss | 770 | 38.0 | 78.0 | 35.0 | 85 | 1680 | 5.0 |
| roast ham/Swiss | 710 | 36.0 | 78.0 | 30.0 | 75 | 2010 | 5.0 |
| turkey/ranch/bacon | 810 | 46.0 | 78.0 | 36.0 | 95 | 2270 | 5.0 |
| turkey/Swiss | 710 | 39.0 | 78.0 | 28.0 | 75 | 1780 | 5.0 |
| toasted subs: | | | | | | | |
| French dip/Swiss | 500 | 29.0 | 61.0 | 15.0 | 60 | 2220 | 2.0 |
| Italian, classic | 590 | 24.0 | 57.0 | 30.0 | 55 | 1870 | 3.0 |
| Philly beef | 560 | 28.0 | 56.0 | 25.0 | 65 | 1490 | 3.0 |
| turkey bacon club | 560 | 32.0 | 56.0 | 23.0 | 60 | 1710 | 3.0 |
| *Prime-Cut* chicken: | | | | | | | |
| tenders, regular | 360 | 21.0 | 31.0 | 17.0 | 50 | 1160 | 2.0 |
| tenders, large | 610 | 35.0 | 52.0 | 28.0 | 85 | 1940 | 3.0 |
| barbecue sauce | 45 | 0 | 11.0 | 0 | 0 | 350 | 0 |
| Buffalo sauce | 10 | 0 | 1.0 | 1.0 | 0 | 720 | 0 |
| honey Dijon sauce | 140 | 0 | 5.0 | 13.0 | 10 | 130 | 0 |
| ranch sauce | 160 | 1.0 | 2.0 | 16.0 | 30 | 280 | 0 |
| *Market Fresh* chopped | | | | | | | |
| Farmhouse salad: | | | | | | | |
| chicken, crispy | 430 | 27.0 | 30.0 | 24.0 | 65 | 1150 | 4.0 |
| chicken, roast | 250 | 23.0 | 11.0 | 13.0 | 60 | 680 | 3.0 |
| turkey and ham | 250 | 23.0 | 10.0 | 14.0 | 60 | 910 | 3.0 |
| side salad | 120 | 4.0 | 4.0 | 5.0 | 15 | 100 | 1.0 |
| dressings: | | | | | | | |
| balsamic vinaigrette | 130 | 0 | 5.0 | 12.0 | 0 | 470 | 0 |

| Food and Measure | cal. | prot. (gms) | carbo. (gms) | fat (gms) | chol. (mgs) | sod. (mgs) | fiber (gms) |
|---|---|---|---|---|---|---|---|
| **Arby's** *(cont.)* | | | | | | | |
| buttermilk ranch ... | 210 | 1.0 | 2.0 | 23.0 | 10 | 380 | 0 |
| honey mustard .... | 180 | 0 | 8.0 | 16.0 | 15 | 260 | 0 |
| sides/*Sidekickers*: | | | | | | | |
| fries, curly: | | | | | | | |
| large ............ | 710 | 7.0 | 87.0 | 37.0 | 30 | 1840 | 6.0 |
| medium ........ | 600 | 6.0 | 74.0 | 31.0 | 25 | 1550 | 5.0 |
| small ........... | 450 | 4.0 | 55.0 | 24.0 | 20 | 1160 | 4.0 |
| w/cheddar ....... | 50 | 1.0 | 4.0 | 3.5 | 0 | 360 | 0 |
| *Jalapeno Bites*, 5 .... | 300 | 5.0 | 31.0 | 17.0 | 25 | 740 | 2.0 |
| large, 8 ........ | 470 | 8.0 | 49.0 | 27.0 | 40 | 1180 | 4.0 |
| *Bronco Berry* sauce | 90 | 0 | 22.0 | 0 | 0 | 30 | 0 |
| *Loaded Potato Bites*, 5 | 350 | 9.0 | 32.0 | 21.0 | 40 | 810 | 3.0 |
| large, 8 .......... | 570 | 14.0 | 51.0 | 34.0 | 60 | 1300 | 5.0 |
| ranch sauce ...... | 160 | 1.0 | 2.0 | 16.0 | 30 | 280 | 0 |
| mozzarella sticks, 4 .. | 440 | 21.0 | 39.0 | 23.0 | 5 | 1190 | 2.0 |
| large, 6 .......... | 660 | 31.0 | 59.0 | 34.0 | 5 | 1780 | 3.0 |
| marinara sauce ... | 35 | 1.0 | 5.0 | 1.5 | 0 | 160 | 1.0 |
| onion rings, 5 ....... | 460 | 6.0 | 56.0 | 24.0 | 0 | 1400 | 3.0 |
| potato cakes, large ... | 510 | 4.0 | 57.0 | 30.0 | 0 | 790 | 4.0 |
| potato cakes, medium | 390 | 3.0 | 42.0 | 23.0 | 0 | 600 | 3.0 |
| potato cakes, small ... | 260 | 2.0 | 28.0 | 15.0 | 0 | 400 | 2.0 |
| shake, regular: | | | | | | | |
| chocolate .......... | 570 | 15.0 | 98.0 | 15.0 | 55 | 450 | 1.0 |
| Jamocha ........... | 570 | 14.0 | 97.0 | 15.0 | 55 | 440 | 1.0 |
| vanilla ............. | 480 | 14.0 | 74.0 | 15.0 | 55 | 390 | 0 |
| chocolate chunk cookies . | 420 | 4.0 | 54.0 | 21.0 | 30 | 320 | 2.0 |
| **Arctic char**, raw, meat | | | | | | | |
| only, 4 oz. .......... | 207 | 25.0 | 0 | 9.1 | 30 | 91 | 0 |
| **Arrowhead**: | | | | | | | |
| raw, 1 medium, 2⅝" .... | 12 | .6 | 2.4 | <.1 | 0 | 3 | .<1.0 |
| boiled, drained, | | | | | | | |
| 1 medium, .4 oz. ..... | 9 | .5 | 1.9 | <.1 | 0 | 2 | <1.0 |
| **Arrowroot**, raw, 1 cup: | | | | | | | |
| (*Frieda's*), sliced ....... | 80 | 5.0 | 16.0 | 0 | 0 | 31 | 2.0 |
| sliced ............... | 78 | 5.1 | 16.1 | .2 | 0 | 31 | 1.6 |
| **Arrowroot flour**, 1 cup .. | 457 | .4 | 112.8 | .1 | 0 | 2 | 4.4 |
| **Artichoke**, globe, fresh: | | | | | | | |
| raw: | | | | | | | |
| (*Dole*), ⅔ medium, | | | | | | | |
| 3 oz. ............ | 40 | 3.0 | 9.0 | 0 | 0 | 80 | 4.0 |
| (*Green Giant* Fresh), | | | | | | | |
| 5-oz. choke ...... | 70 | 5.0 | 15.0 | 0 | 0 | 135 | 8.0 |

| Food and Measure | cal. | prot. (gms) | carbo. (gms) | fat (gms) | chol. (mgs) | sod. (mgs) | fiber (gms) |
|---|---|---|---|---|---|---|---|
| 4.5-oz. choke ..... | 60 | 4.2 | 13.5 | .2 | 0 | 120 | 6.9 |
| 5.7-oz. choke ..... | 76 | 5.3 | 17.0 | .2 | 0 | 152 | 8.9 |
| boiled, drained, | | | | | | | |
| 1 medium, 4.2 oz. .... | 60 | 4.2 | 13.4 | .2 | 0 | 114 | 6.5 |
| hearts, boiled, drained, | | | | | | | |
| 2 cup ............ | 42 | 2.9 | 9.4 | .1 | 0 | 80 | 4.5 |
| **Artichoke, can/jar**, | | | | | | | |
| hearts, except as | | | | | | | |
| noted: | | | | | | | |
| in brine/water: | | | | | | | |
| (*Progresso*), 2 pcs., | | | | | | | |
| 4.6 oz. .......... | 30 | 1.0 | 7.0 | 0 | 0 | 400 | 2.0 |
| (*Vigo*), 2 whole or | | | | | | | |
| 8 quarters ....... | 30 | 2.0 | 6.0 | 0 | 0 | 240 | 1.0 |
| all varieties (*Roland*), | | | | | | | |
| ½ cup ........... | 35 | 2.0 | 6.0 | 0 | 0 | 420 | 4.0 |
| in brine, bottoms | | | | | | | |
| (*Roland*), large or | | | | | | | |
| medium, ⅔ cup ..... | 50 | 2.0 | 10.0 | 0 | 0 | 380 | 5.0 |
| marinated, in oil: | | | | | | | |
| (*Progresso*), 2 pcs. .... | 60 | 1.0 | 3.0 | 5.0 | 0 | 80 | 1.0 |
| (*Vigo* 6 oz.), 2 pcs. ... | 25 | 1.0 | 3.0 | 1.5 | 0 | 105 | 0 |
| (*Vigo* 12 oz.), 3 pcs. .. | 25 | 5.0 | 2.0 | 1.5 | 0 | 90 | 5.0 |
| grilled (*Roland*), 1.1 oz. | 45 | 0 | 2.0 | 4.0 | 0 | 250 | 2.0 |
| quartered, 2 pcs., 1 oz.: | | | | | | | |
| (*S&W*) .......... | 20 | 0 | 2.0 | 2.0 | 0 | 80 | 1.0 |
| or whole (*Roland*) . | 20 | 1.0 | 2.0 | 2.0 | 0 | 130 | 1.0 |
| Roman style (*Roland*): | | | | | | | |
| grilled, ½ cup ..... | 130 | 3.0 | 3.0 | 7.0 | 0 | 1040 | 4.0 |
| w/stem, ½ cup .... | 140 | 3.0 | 11.0 | 10.0 | 0 | 910 | 6.0 |
| w/stem, 1.4-oz. pc. | 60 | 1.0 | 2.0 | 5.0 | 0 | 330 | 2.0 |
| salad (*Roland*), 1 oz. ... | 20 | 1.0 | 2.0 | 2.0 | 0 | 130 | 1.0 |
| **Artichoke, frozen**: | | | | | | | |
| hearts: | | | | | | | |
| (*Birds Eye*), 12 pcs., | | | | | | | |
| 3 oz. ............ | 40 | 2.0 | 7.0 | .5 | 0 | 55 | 5.0 |
| (*C&W*), ½ cup ...... | 25 | 2.0 | 4.0 | 0 | 0 | 55 | 5.0 |
| 9-oz. pkg. .......... | 96 | 6.7 | 19.8 | 1.1 | 0 | 120 | 9.9 |
| grilled, butter sauce | | | | | | | |
| (*Contessa*), ¼ of | | | | | | | |
| 6-oz. pkg. .......... | 210 | 4.0 | 16.0 | 16.0 | 35 | 510 | 5.0 |
| **Artichoke, Jerusalem**, | | | | | | | |
| see "Jerusalem | | | | | | | |
| artichoke" | | | | | | | |

| Food and Measure | cal. | prot. (gms) | carbo. (gms) | fat (gms) | chol. (mgs) | sod. (mgs) | fiber (gms) |
|---|---|---|---|---|---|---|---|
| **Artichoke, marinated,** see "Artichoke, can/jar" | | | | | | | |
| **Artichoke appetizer:** | | | | | | | |
| canned: | | | | | | | |
| caponata (*Alessi*), | | | | | | | |
| ⅓ cup . . . . . . . . . . | 130 | 2.0 | 7.0 | 6.0 | 0 | 460 | 3.0 |
| pâté (*Alessi*), 2 tbsp. . . . | 120 | 1.0 | 1.0 | 12.0 | 0 | 310 | 3.0 |
| frozen, and spinach | | | | | | | |
| (*Pillsbury Savorings*), | | | | | | | |
| 4 pcs., 2.6 oz. . . . . . . | 190 | 7.0 | 21.0 | 9.0 | 20 | 450 | 1.0 |
| **Arugula, fresh:** | | | | | | | |
| 10 leaves . . . . . . . . . . . | 5 | .5 | .7 | .1 | 0 | 5 | .3 |
| ½ cup . . . . . . . . . . . . . . | 3 | .3 | .4 | <.1 | 0 | <1 | .2 |
| baby (*Ready Pac*), 3 oz. . | 20 | 2.0 | 3.0 | 0 | 0 | 25 | 1.0 |
| **Asparagus, fresh:** | | | | | | | |
| raw, spears, trimmed: | | | | | | | |
| (*Dole*), 5 pcs., 2.8 oz. . | 15 | 2.0 | 3.0 | 0 | 0 | 0 | 2.0 |
| (*Green Giant*), 3.3 oz. . | 20 | 2.0 | 4.0 | 0 | 0 | 0 | 2.0 |
| 4 small, 1.8 oz. . . . . . . | 14 | 1.3 | 2.6 | .1 | 0 | 1 | 1.2 |
| purple (*Frieda's*), 3 oz. | 20 | 4.0 | 4.0 | 0 | 0 | 0 | 1.0 |
| white (*Frieda's*), 3 oz. . | 20 | 2.0 | 4.0 | 0 | 0 | 0 | 2.0 |
| boiled, 4 spears, | | | | | | | |
| ½"-diam. base . . . . . . | 14 | 1.6 | 2.5 | .2 | 0 | 7 | 1.3 |
| boiled, drained, cuts, | | | | | | | |
| ½ cup . . . . . . . . . . . . . | 22 | 2.3 | 3.8 | .3 | 0 | 10 | 1.9 |
| **Asparagus, can/jar:** | | | | | | | |
| all styles (*Del Monte*), | | | | | | | |
| ½ cup . . . . . . . . . . . . | 20 | 2.0 | 3.0 | 0 | 0 | 365 | 1.0 |
| spears: | | | | | | | |
| (*Green Giant*), 4.5 oz., | | | | | | | |
| approx. 5 pcs. . . . . | 20 | 2.0 | 3.0 | 0 | 0 | 420 | 1.0 |
| (*Le Sueur* Extra | | | | | | | |
| Large), 4.3 oz., | | | | | | | |
| approx. 3 pcs. . . . . | 20 | 2.0 | 3.0 | 0 | 0 | 420 | 1.0 |
| (*Roland*), ⅔ cup . . . . . | 20 | 2.0 | 3.0 | 0 | 0 | 450 | 2.0 |
| (*S&W*), ½ cup . . . . . . | 20 | 2.0 | 3.0 | 0 | 0 | 365 | 1.0 |
| marinated (*Vigo*), | | | | | | | |
| 3 pcs. . . . . . . . . . . . | 10 | 1.0 | 1.0 | 0 | 0 | 75 | 0 |
| white: | | | | | | | |
| (*Roland*), ⅔ cup . . . | 20 | 2.0 | 3.0 | 0 | 0 | 510 | 2.0 |
| grilled (*Roland*), | | | | | | | |
| 3 pcs., 1.1 oz. . . | 15 | 1.0 | 1.0 | 0 | 0 | 310 | 1.0 |

| Food and Measure | cal. | prot. (gms) | carbo. (gms) | fat (gms) | chol. (mgs) | sod. (mgs) | fiber (gms) |
|---|---|---|---|---|---|---|---|
| cuts, ½ cup: | | | | | | | |
| (*Green Giant*) ....... | 20 | 2.0 | 3.0 | 0 | 0 | 420 | 1.0 |
| (*Green Giant* Low Sodium) ......... | 20 | 2.0 | 3.0 | 0 | 0 | 210 | 1.0 |
| (*Green Giant Simply Steam*) .......... | 20 | 2.0 | 3.0 | 0 | 0 | 90 | <1.0 |
| drained, ½ cup ....... | 23 | 2.6 | 3.0 | .8 | 0 | 350 | 2.0 |
| **Asparagus, frozen:** | | | | | | | |
| boiled, drained, 1 cup ... | 50 | 5.3 | 8.8 | .8 | 0 | 7 | 2.9 |
| spears: | | | | | | | |
| (*Birds Eye/C&W*), 7 pcs., 3 oz. ...... | 20 | 2.0 | 3.0 | 0 | 0 | 0 | <1.0 |
| 4 pcs. ............. | 14 | 1.9 | 2.4 | .1 | 0 | 5 | 1.1 |
| cuts, ⅔ cup: | | | | | | | |
| (*Cascadian Farm Organic*) ......... | 20 | 2.0 | 3.0 | 0 | 0 | 85 | <1.0 |
| (*Green Giant Simply Steam*) .......... | 20 | 2.0 | 3.0 | 0 | 0 | 90 | <1.0 |
| **Asparagus, pickled,** in jars, white (*Roland*), ⅔ cup ..... | 40 | 2.0 | 8.0 | 0 | 0 | 510 | 2.0 |
| **Asparagus bean**, see "Winged bean" | | | | | | | |
| **Asparagus combinations,** frozen: | | | | | | | |
| (*Birds Eye* Stir-fry), 1 cup cooked ....... | 90 | 4.0 | 16.0 | 0 | 0 | 30 | 2.0 |
| baby blend (*Freshlike*), ¾ cup ............. | 50 | 2.0 | 10.0 | 0 | 0 | 15 | 1.0 |
| corn, baby carrots (*Birds Eye Steamfresh*), ⅔ cup | 70 | 2.0 | 13.0 | .5 | 0 | 15 | 1.0 |
| **Atemoya**, fresh (*Frieda's*), 3-oz. pc. .... | 80 | 2.0 | 20.0 | 0 | 0 | 10 | 4.0 |
| **Au jus gravy,** ¼ cup: | | | | | | | |
| (*Campbell's*) .......... | 5 | 1.0 | 0 | 0 | 0 | 230 | 0 |
| (*Heinz* Bistro) ........ | 20 | 1.0 | 2.0 | .5 | 0 | 340 | 0 |
| **Au jus gravy mix:** | | | | | | | |
| (*Lawry's*), ¼ cup* ..... | 25 | <1.0 | 4.0 | 1.0 | 0 | 320 | 0 |
| (*McCormick*), ½ tsp. .... | 5 | 0 | 1.0 | 0 | 0 | 310 | 0 |
| **Aubergine**, see "Eggplant" | | | | | | | |
| **Australian blue squash** (*Frieda's*), cubes, cooked, 1 cup . | 50 | 2.0 | 12.0 | 0 | 0 | 2 | 3.0 |

| Food and Measure | cal. | prot. (gms) | carbo. (gms) | fat (gms) | chol. (mgs) | sod. (mgs) | fiber (gms) |
|---|---|---|---|---|---|---|---|
| **Avocado**, fresh: | | | | | | | |
| (*Chiquita*), 7-oz. pc. .... | 322 | 4.0 | 17.0 | 29.0 | 0 | 14 | 13.0 |
| (*Dole*), ⅕ medium, | | | | | | | |
|   1.1 oz. ............ | 50 | <1.0 | 3.0 | 5.0 | 0 | 0 | 2.0 |
| (*Green Giant*), 1.1 oz. ... | 50 | 1.0 | 3.0 | 4.5 | 0 | 0 | 2.0 |
| all varieties: | | | | | | | |
|   cubed, 1 cup ........ | 240 | 3.0 | 12.8 | 22.0 | 0 | 11 | 10.1 |
|   pureed, ½ cup ...... | 184 | 2.3 | 9.8 | 16.6 | 0 | 8 | 7.7 |
| California: | | | | | | | |
|   pulp from 1 medium, | | | | | | | |
|     6.1 oz. .......... | 289 | 3.4 | 14.9 | 26.7 | 0 | 14 | 11.8 |
|   pureed, ½ cup ...... | 192 | 2.3 | 9.9 | 17.7 | 0 | 9 | 7.8 |
| Florida, pureed, ½ cup .. | 138 | 2.6 | 9.0 | 11.6 | 0 | 2 | 6.4 |
| seedless (*Frieda's* | | | | | | | |
|   Cocktail), 1.4-oz. pc. .. | 60 | 1.0 | 3.0 | 6.0 | 0 | 0 | 2.0 |
| **Avocado, frozen**, pulp | | | | | | | |
|   (*Calavo*), 2 tbsp. ...... | 60 | 1.0 | 7.0 | 3.0 | 0 | 150 | 1.0 |
| **Avocado dip**, see | | | | | | | |
|   "Guacamole" | | | | | | | |
| **Avocado sauce**, frozen | | | | | | | |
|   (*Calavo*), 2 tbsp. ...... | 15 | <1.0 | 2.0 | .5 | 0 | 150 | 1.0 |

# B

| Food and Measure | cal. | prot. (gms) | carbo. (gms) | fat (gms) | chol. (mgs) | sod. (mgs) | fiber (gms) |
|---|---|---|---|---|---|---|---|
| **Baba ganoush**, see "Eggplant appetizer" | | | | | | | |
| **Bacon**, 2 slices cooked, except as noted: | | | | | | | |
| (*Applegate Farms*) . . . . . . | 60 | 4.0 | 0 | 5.0 | 10 | 290 | 0 |
| (*Black Label*) . . . . . . . . . . | 80 | 5.0 | 0 | 7.0 | 15 | 330 | 0 |
| (*Black Label* Center) . . . . | 70 | 5.0 | 0 | 5.0 | 15 | 300 | 0 |
| (*Boar's Head*) . . . . . . . . . | 70 | 4.0 | 0 | 6.0 | 10 | 190 | 0 |
| (*Hormel* Micro) . . . . . . . . | 80 | 5.0 | 0 | 7.0 | 20 | 300 | 0 |
| (*Jimmy Dean*), 1 slice . . . | 50 | 4.0 | 0 | 4.0 | 10 | 230 | 0 |
| (*Jimmy Dean* Lower Sodium), 1 slice . . . . . | 50 | 4.0 | 0 | 4.0 | 10 | 105 | 0 |
| (*Oscar Mayer*) . . . . . . . . . | 60 | 4.0 | 0 | 5.0 | 10 | 250 | 0 |
| (*Oscar Mayer* Center) . . . | 50 | 4.0 | 0 | 4.0 | 15 | 270 | 0 |
| (*Oscar Mayer* Hardwood) | 70 | 4.0 | 0 | 6.0 | 15 | 290 | 0 |
| (*Oscar Mayer* Lower Sodium) . . . . . . . . . . . | 70 | 4.0 | 0 | 6.0 | 10 | 170 | 0 |
| maple: | | | | | | | |
| (*Hormel*) . . . . . . . . . . . | 80 | 5.0 | 0 | 7.0 | 15 | 270 | 0 |
| (*Jimmy Dean*), 3 slices | 80 | 4.0 | 0 | 7.0 | 15 | 105 | 0 |
| mesquite (*Hormel*) . . . . . | 80 | 5.0 | 0 | 7.0 | 15 | 330 | 0 |
| precooked: | | | | | | | |
| (*Hormel*) . . . . . . . . . . . | 70 | 5.0 | 0 | 5.0 | 20 | 290 | 0 |
| (*Oscar Mayer*), .5 oz. . | 70 | 5.0 | 0 | 6.0 | 15 | 320 | 0 |
| hickory (*Jimmy Dean*), 3 slices . . . . . . . . . | 70 | 4.0 | 0 | 5.0 | 10 | 200 | 0 |
| hickory (*Tyson*) . . . . . | 90 | 5.0 | 0 | 7.0 | 15 | 240 | 0 |
| maple (*Jimmy Dean*), 3 slices . . . . . . . . . . | 80 | 4.0 | 1.0 | 7.0 | 15 | 280 | 0 |
| thick (*Oscar Mayer*), .5 oz. . . . . . . . . . . . | 70 | 5.0 | 0 | 5.0 | 15 | 300 | 0 |
| thick cut, 1 slice: | | | | | | | |
| (*Black Label*) . . . . . . . . | 110 | 7.0 | 0 | 9.0 | 20 | 460 | 0 |

| Food and Measure | cal. | prot. (gms) | carbo. (gms) | fat (gms) | chol. (mgs) | sod. (mgs) | fiber (gms) |
|---|---|---|---|---|---|---|---|
| **Bacon, thick cut** *(cont.)* | | | | | | | |
| (*Jimmy Dean*) . . . . . . . | 80 | 5.0 | 0 | 6.0 | 15 | 320 | 0 |
| (*Oscar Mayer* | | | | | | | |
| Smokehouse Center) | 70 | 7.0 | 0 | 5.0 | 20 | 320 | 0 |
| turkey: | | | | | | | |
| (*Applegate Farms*), | | | | | | | |
| 1-oz. slice . . . . . . . . | 35 | 6.0 | 0 | 1.5 | 25 | 200 | 0 |
| (*Jenny-O*), .5 oz. . . . . . | 35 | 3.0 | 1.0 | 3.0 | 15 | 150 | 0 |
| (*Jennie-O* Extra | | | | | | | |
| Lean), .5 oz. . . . . . . | 20 | 3.0 | 0 | .5 | 10 | 120 | 0 |
| (*Oscar Mayer*), .5 oz. . | 35 | 2.0 | 0 | 3.0 | 15 | 180 | 0 |
| uncured: | | | | | | | |
| (*Hormel Natural* | | | | | | | |
| *Choice*) . . . . . . . . . . | 80 | 5.0 | 0 | 7.0 | 20 | 360 | 0 |
| (*Oscar Mayer*) . . . . . . | 70 | 6.0 | 0 | 5.0 | 15 | 250 | 0 |
| **Bacon, Canadian**, 2 oz.: | | | | | | | |
| (*Applegate Farms*) . . . . . . | 90 | 12.0 | 1.0 | 4.0 | 35 | 500 | 0 |
| (*Boar's Head*) . . . . . . . . | 70 | 12.0 | 1.0 | 2.0 | 35 | 570 | 0 |
| (*Hormel*) . . . . . . . . . . . . | 70 | 11.0 | 1.0 | 2.0 | 30 | 680 | 0 |
| (*Hormel Pillow Pack*) . . . | 80 | 10.0 | 2.0 | 3.5 | 30 | 700 | 0 |
| unheated . . . . . . . . . . . . | 89 | 11.7 | 1.9 | 4.0 | 28 | 799 | 0 |
| **Bacon, Italian**, pancetta: | | | | | | | |
| (*Applegate Farms*), 1 oz. . | 100 | 6.0 | 0 | 8.0 | 20 | 550 | 0 |
| (*Beretta*), 2 oz. . . . . . . . . | 200 | 9.0 | 0 | 18.0 | 35 | 1280 | 0 |
| **"Bacon," vegetarian**, | | | | | | | |
| frozen, 2 slices, | | | | | | | |
| except as noted: | | | | | | | |
| (*MorningStar Farms* | | | | | | | |
| Veggie Strips) . . . . . . . | 60 | 2.0 | 2.0 | 4.5 | 0 | 230 | 1.0 |
| (*Worthington Stripples*) . | 60 | 2.0 | 2.0 | 4.5 | 0 | 220 | <1.0 |
| Canadian (*Yves*), 2 oz. . . | 80 | 17.0 | 2.0 | .5 | 0 | 400 | 0 |
| **Bacon bits**, 1 tbsp.: | | | | | | | |
| (*Oscar Mayer*) . . . . . . . . . | 25 | 2.0 | 0 | 1.5 | 5 | 170 | 0 |
| (*Hormel* Bits) . . . . . . . . . | 25 | 3.0 | 0 | 1.5 | 5 | 240 | 0 |
| crumbled (*Hormel*) . . . . . | 25 | 3.0 | 0 | 1.5 | 10 | 190 | 0 |
| pieces (*Hormel*) . . . . . . . | 25 | 3.0 | 0 | 1.5 | 10 | 180 | 0 |
| **"Bacon" bits**, imitation: | | | | | | | |
| (*Bac'n Pieces*), 1 tbsp. . . | 30 | 3.0 | 2.0 | 1.0 | 0 | 180 | 0 |
| (*Bac-Os* Bits), 1½ tbsp. . . | 30 | 3.0 | 2.0 | 1.5 | 0 | 120 | 0 |
| chips (*Bac-Os*), 1 tbsp. . . | 30 | 3.0 | 2.0 | 1.5 | 0 | 115 | 0 |
| **Bacon dip**, 2 tbsp.: | | | | | | | |
| cheddar (*Kraft*) . . . . . . . . | 60 | 1.0 | 3.0 | 5.0 | 5 | 170 | 0 |
| horseradish: | | | | | | | |
| (*Cabot*) . . . . . . . . . . . . | 50 | 1.0 | 1.0 | 5.0 | 15 | 190 | 0 |

| Food and Measure | cal. | prot. (gms) | carbo. (gms) | fat (gms) | chol. (mgs) | sod. (mgs) | fiber (gms) |
|---|---|---|---|---|---|---|---|
| (*Heluva Good!*) ...... | 60 | 1.0 | 2.0 | 5.0 | 20 | 200 | 0 |
| **Bagel**, 1 pc.: | | | | | | | |
| plain: | | | | | | | |
| (*Nature's Own*) ...... | 270 | 10.0 | 56.0 | 1.0 | 0 | 410 | 2.0 |
| (*Nature's Own* Thin) .. | 150 | 5.0 | 30.0 | 0 | 0 | 230 | 1.0 |
| (*Pepperidge Farm*) ... | 260 | 9.0 | 54.0 | 1.0 | 0 | 500 | 3.0 |
| (*Thomas'*) .......... | 260 | 9.0 | 51.0 | 2.0 | 0 | 500 | 2.0 |
| (*Thomas'* Whole Grain) | 260 | 10.0 | 52.0 | 2.0 | 0 | 480 | 3.0 |
| (*Thomas' Bagel Thins*) | 110 | 4.0 | 25.0 | 1.0 | 0 | 210 | 4.0 |
| plain, mini: | | | | | | | |
| (*Pepperidge Farm*) ... | 110 | 4.0 | 22.0 | .5 | 0 | 200 | 1.0 |
| (*Thomas'*) .......... | 120 | 4.0 | 24.0 | 1.0 | 0 | 240 | <1.0 |
| (*Thomas'* Whole Grain) | 120 | 4.0 | 23.0 | 1.0 | 0 | 220 | 2.0 |
| plain, onion, poppy, or sesame, 2 oz. ...... | 157 | 6.0 | 30.4 | .9 | 0 | 304 | 1.3 |
| blueberry: | | | | | | | |
| (*Nature's Own*) ...... | 260 | 9.0 | 55.0 | 1.0 | 0 | 350 | 3.0 |
| (*Thomas'*) .......... | 270 | 9.0 | 54.0 | 2.0 | 0 | 440 | 3.0 |
| mini (*Thomas'*) ...... | 120 | 4.0 | 25.0 | 1.0 | 0 | 200 | 1.0 |
| brown sugar cinnamon, mini: | | | | | | | |
| (*Pepperidge Farm*) ... | 120 | 4.0 | 24.0 | .5 | 0 | 150 | 2.0 |
| (*Thomas'*) .......... | 130 | 4.0 | 24.0 | 1.0 | 0 | 220 | 1.0 |
| chocolatey chip, mini (*Thomas'*) .......... | 120 | 4.0 | 24.0 | 1.0 | 0 | 260 | 2.0 |
| cinnamon raisin: | | | | | | | |
| (*Nature's Own*) ...... | 300 | 9.0 | 60.0 | 3.0 | 0 | 350 | 3.0 |
| (*Pepperidge Farm*) ... | 270 | 8.0 | 57.0 | 1.0 | 0 | 450 | 3.0 |
| (*Thomas' Bagel Thins*) | 110 | 4.0 | 25.0 | 1.0 | 0 | 160 | 5.0 |
| mini (*Pepperidge Farm*) .......... | 110 | 3.0 | 23.0 | .5 | 0 | 180 | 1.0 |
| mini (*Thomas'*) ...... | 120 | 4.0 | 24.0 | 1.0 | 0 | 210 | 1.0 |
| swirl (*Thomas'*) ..... | 250 | 8.0 | 50.0 | 1.5 | 0 | 410 | 4.0 |
| cinnamon swirl (*Thomas'*) | 270 | 9.0 | 52.0 | 2.5 | 0 | 450 | 3.0 |
| everything: | | | | | | | |
| (*Pepperidge Farm*) ... | 260 | 9.0 | 53.0 | 1.5 | 0 | 480 | 2.0 |
| (*Thomas'*) .......... | 270 | 10.0 | 50.0 | 4.0 | 0 | 470 | 3.0 |
| (*Thomas' Bagel Thins*) | 110 | 5.0 | 24.0 | 1.0 | 0 | 190 | 5.0 |
| fruit, harvest (*Thomas'*) . | 240 | 10.0 | 44.0 | 3.5 | 0 | 430 | 4.0 |
| honey wheat: | | | | | | | |
| (*Nature's Own*) ...... | 260 | 10.0 | 56.0 | 1.0 | 0 | 380 | 4.0 |
| (*Thomas'*) .......... | 250 | 10.0 | 51.0 | 1.5 | 0 | 460 | 4.0 |
| multigrain (*Thomas'* Fiber) | 250 | 10.0 | 51.0 | 3.0 | 0 | 480 | 8.0 |
| onion (*Thomas'*) ....... | 260 | 10.0 | 51.0 | 2.0 | 0 | 470 | 3.0 |

| Food and Measure | cal. | prot. (gms) | carbo. (gms) | fat (gms) | chol. (mgs) | sod. (mgs) | fiber (gms) |
|---|---|---|---|---|---|---|---|
| **Bagel** *(cont.)* | | | | | | | |
| whole wheat: | | | | | | | |
| (*Nature's Own*) ...... | 250 | 11.0 | 57.0 | 1.5 | 0 | 380 | 9.0 |
| (*Nature's Own* Thin) .. | 140 | 6.0 | 31.0 | 1.0 | 0 | 210 | 5.0 |
| (*Pepperidge Farm*) ... | 250 | 11.0 | 49.0 | 1.5 | 0 | 450 | 6.0 |
| (*Thomas'*) .......... | 240 | 10.0 | 49.0 | 2.0 | 0 | 400 | 7.0 |
| mini (*Pepperidge Farm*) | 100 | 4.0 | 20.0 | .5 | 0 | 180 | 3.0 |
| mini (*Thomas'*) ...... | 110 | 5.0 | 22.0 | 1.0 | 0 | 180 | 3.0 |
| **Bagel chips/crisps**, 1 oz.: | | | | | | | |
| plain: | | | | | | | |
| (*New York Style*) ..... | 130 | 3.0 | 18.0 | 5.0 | 0 | 70 | 1.0 |
| (*Stacy's Simply* | | | | | | | |
| *Naked*) .......... | 130 | 4.0 | 19.0 | 4.5 | 0 | 320 | 1.0 |
| cinnamon raisin (*New* | | | | | | | |
| *York Style*) ......... | 130 | 2.0 | 19.0 | 5.0 | 0 | 80 | 1.0 |
| everything: | | | | | | | |
| (*New York Style*) ..... | 130 | 3.0 | 16.0 | 6.0 | 0 | 340 | 1.0 |
| (*Stacy's*) ........... | 130 | 4.0 | 19.0 | 4.0 | 0 | 320 | 1.0 |
| garlic: | | | | | | | |
| roasted (*New York* | | | | | | | |
| *Style*) ........... | 130 | 3.0 | 17.0 | 5.0 | 0 | 320 | 1.0 |
| toasted (*Stacy's*) ..... | 130 | 3.0 | 19.0 | 4.5 | 0 | 300 | 1.0 |
| multigrain (*New York* | | | | | | | |
| *Style*) ............ | 130 | 3.0 | 17.0 | 5.0 | 0 | 340 | 1.0 |
| sea salt (*New York* | | | | | | | |
| *Style*) ............ | 130 | 3.0 | 17.0 | 5.0 | 0 | 350 | 1.0 |
| sesame (*New York* | | | | | | | |
| *Style*) ............ | 130 | 3.0 | 16.0 | 6.0 | 0 | 340 | 1.0 |
| **Bagel w/cream cheese** | | | | | | | |
| (*Philadelphia* To | | | | | | | |
| Go), ½ pkg., 3.2 oz.: | | | | | | | |
| plain cream cheese ..... | 240 | 6.0 | 34.0 | 9.0 | 30 | 420 | 2.0 |
| chive and onion ........ | 240 | 6.0 | 34.0 | 8.0 | 30 | 440 | 2.0 |
| strawberry ........... | 230 | 5.0 | 37.0 | 7.0 | 25 | 400 | 2.0 |
| **Baked beans**, ½ cup: | | | | | | | |
| (*Allens* Homestyle) ..... | 140 | 6.0 | 29.0 | 1.0 | 0 | 410 | 5.0 |
| (*Allens* Original) ....... | 150 | 6.0 | 29.0 | 1.0 | 0 | 350 | 8.0 |
| (*B&M* Country) ........ | 170 | 7.0 | 35.0 | 1.5 | <5 | 710 | 7.0 |
| (*B&M* Original 8 oz.) .... | 180 | 7.0 | 31.0 | 3.0 | <5 | 420 | 8.0 |
| (*B&M* Original 16 oz.) ... | 170 | 7.0 | 31.0 | 2.0 | <5 | 400 | 8.0 |
| (*Bush's* Bold & Spicy) ... | 110 | 6.0 | 24.0 | 1.0 | 0 | 560 | 5.0 |
| (*Bush's* Boston) ....... | 150 | 6.0 | 31.0 | 1.0 | 0 | 440 | 5.0 |
| (*Bush's* Country) ....... | 160 | 6.0 | 33.0 | 1.0 | 0 | 680 | 5.0 |
| (*Bush's* Homestyle) ..... | 140 | 6.0 | 29.0 | 1.0 | 0 | 550 | 5.0 |

| Food and Measure | cal. | prot. (gms) | carbo. (gms) | fat (gms) | chol. (mgs) | sod. (mgs) | fiber (gms) |
|---|---|---|---|---|---|---|---|
| (*Bush's* Original) ....... | 140 | 6.0 | 29.0 | 1.0 | 0 | 550 | 5.0 |
| (*Bush's Grillin' Beans* Smokehouse) ....... | 170 | 7.0 | 34.0 | 1.0 | 0 | 570 | 5.0 |
| (*Bush's Grillin' Beans* Steakhouse) ........ | 180 | 6.0 | 39.0 | .5 | 0 | 510 | 5.0 |
| (*S&W*) .............. | 160 | 8.0 | 32.0 | 1.0 | 0 | 510 | 8.0 |
| (*Van Camp's* Homestyle) . | 160 | 7.0 | 30.0 | 1.0 | 0 | 470 | 5.0 |
| (*Van Camp's* Original) ... | 160 | 7.0 | 30.0 | 1.0 | 0 | 510 | 5.0 |
| bacon, maple cured: | | | | | | | |
| (*Allens*) .......... | 140 | 6.0 | 27.0 | 1.0 | 0 | 450 | 4.0 |
| (*Bush's*) .......... | 140 | 6.0 | 28.0 | 1.0 | 0 | 620 | 5.0 |
| bacon onion w/brown sugar (*B&M*) ....... | 190 | 8.0 | 36.0 | 2.0 | <5 | 450 | 8.0 |
| barbecue: | | | | | | | |
| (*Allens*) ............ | 150 | 6.0 | 29.0 | 1.0 | 0 | 410 | 5.0 |
| (*B&M* 16 oz.) ....... | 190 | 8.0 | 39.0 | .5 | 0 | 570 | 9.0 |
| (*Bush's Grillin' Beans* Southern Pit) ..... | 170 | 6.0 | 35.0 | .5 | 0 | 550 | 6.0 |
| bourbon brown sugar (*Bush's Grillin' Beans*) | 170 | 7.0 | 35.0 | .5 | 0 | 480 | 6.0 |
| brown sugar bacon (*Campbell's*) ........ | 160 | 5.0 | 30.0 | 2.5 | <5 | 470 | 8.0 |
| hickory and bacon (*Van Camp's*) | 170 | 7.0 | 32.0 | 1.0 | 0 | 470 | 5.0 |
| honey (*Bush's*) ........ | 160 | 6.0 | 32.0 | 1.0 | 0 | 540 | 6.0 |
| maple (*B&M* 16 oz.) .... | 160 | 7.0 | 31.0 | 1.0 | 0 | 340 | 8.0 |
| maple sugar (*S&W*) .... | 140 | 6.0 | 28.0 | .5 | 0 | 440 | 4.0 |
| onion: | | | | | | | |
| (*Allens*) ............ | 140 | 5.0 | 25.0 | 1.5 | 0 | 410 | 4.0 |
| (*Bush's*) ........... | 140 | 6.0 | 29.0 | 1.0 | 0 | 550 | 5.0 |
| w/pork: | | | | | | | |
| (*Campbell's*) ........ | 140 | 6.0 | 25.0 | 1.5 | 5 | 440 | 7.0 |
| (*Van Camp's*) ....... | 110 | 6.0 | 23.0 | 1.0 | 0 | 390 | 6.0 |
| (*Van Camp's* Classic) . | 140 | 8.0 | 26.0 | 1.0 | 0 | 460 | 9.0 |
| (*Wagon Master*) ..... | 130 | 7.0 | 23.0 | 1.0 | 0 | 420 | 9.0 |
| (*Wagon Master* 1 lb.) . | 130 | 7.0 | 21.0 | 1.0 | 0 | 330 | 6.0 |
| maple brown sugar (*Van Camp's*) ..... | 160 | 7.0 | 30.0 | 1.0 | 0 | 440 | 8.0 |
| red kidney (*B&M*) ...... | 200 | 8.0 | 36.0 | 3.0 | <5 | 460 | 6.0 |
| w/sorghum and mustard (*Eden* Organic) | 150 | 8.0 | 27.0 | 0 | 0 | 130 | 7.0 |
| vegetarian: | | | | | | | |
| (*Allens*) ............ | 140 | 6.0 | 28.0 | 0 | 0 | 460 | 4.0 |
| (*Allens* Extra Fancy) .. | 130 | 6.0 | 24.0 | 0 | 0 | 360 | 7.0 |

| Food and Measure | cal. | prot. (gms) | carbo. (gms) | fat (gms) | chol. (mgs) | sod. (mgs) | fiber (gms) |
|---|---|---|---|---|---|---|---|
| **Baked beans, vegetarian** *(cont.)* | | | | | | | |
| (*Amy's* Organic) ..... | 140 | 7.0 | 28.0 | .5 | 0 | 480 | 6.0 |
| (*B&M* 8 oz.) ........ | 160 | 7.0 | 31.0 | 1.0 | 0 | 380 | 8.0 |
| (*B&M* 16 oz.) ....... | 160 | 7.0 | 28.0 | 1.0 | 0 | 380 | 8.0 |
| (*Bush's*) ........... | 130 | 6.0 | 29.0 | 0 | 0 | 550 | 5.0 |
| **Baking mix** (see also "Biscuit mix"), ⅓ cup, except as noted: | | | | | | | |
| (*Arrowhead Mills* Organic All Purpose) . | 130 | 5.0 | 28.0 | 1.0 | 0 | 390 | 2.0 |
| (*Bob's Red Mill* Low-Carb), ¼ cup ... | 100 | 14.0 | 11.0 | 2.0 | 0 | 115 | 5.0 |
| (*Bisquick* Original) ..... | 160 | 3.0 | 26.0 | 4.5 | 0 | 410 | 1.0 |
| (*Hodgson Mill* Multi Purpose) ........... | 100 | 3.0 | 22.0 | 1.0 | 0 | 0 | 3.0 |
| (*"Jiffy"*), ¼ cup ........ | 130 | 2.0 | 21.0 | 4.5 | 0 | 310 | <1.0 |
| gluten free (*Arrowhead Mills* Organic), ¼ cup . | 140 | 2.0 | 32.0 | .5 | 0 | 350 | <1.0 |
| whole wheat (*Hodgson Mill* Insta-Bake) ..... | 130 | 4.0 | 29.0 | 1.0 | 0 | 270 | 3.0 |
| **Baking powder**, ¼ tsp. .. | 0 | 0 | 0 | 0 | 0 | 100 | 0 |
| **Baking soda**, ½ tsp. .... | 0 | 0 | 0 | 0 | 0 | 630 | 0 |
| **Baklava**, frozen: | | | | | | | |
| (*Apollo*), 2 oz. ......... | 230 | 3.0 | 30.0 | 11.0 | 0 | 75 | 1.0 |
| (*Kontos*), 3.1-oz. pc. .... | 188 | 3.0 | 25.0 | 6.0 | 0 | 91 | <1.0 |
| walnut (*The Fillo Factory*), 2 oz. ....... | 220 | 3.0 | 34.0 | 9.0 | 5 | 90 | 1.0 |
| **Balsam pear**: | | | | | | | |
| (*Frieda's* Bittermelon), 1 cup, 3 oz. ......... | 15 | 1.0 | 3.0 | 0 | 0 | 5 | 2.0 |
| leafy-tips, ½ cup: | | | | | | | |
| raw .............. | 7 | 1.3 | .8 | .2 | 0 | 3 | .6 |
| boiled, drained ...... | 10 | 1.0 | 2.0 | .1 | 0 | 4 | .6 |
| pods, ½" pcs., ½ cup: | | | | | | | |
| raw .............. | 8 | .5 | 1.7 | .1 | 0 | 3 | 1.3 |
| boiled, drained ...... | 12 | .5 | 2.7 | .1 | 0 | 4 | 1.2 |
| **Balsamic glaze**, see "Vinegar" | | | | | | | |
| **Bamboo shoots**, fresh: | | | | | | | |
| raw, slices, ½ cup .... | 21 | 2.0 | 4.0 | .2 | 0 | 3 | .7 |
| boiled, drained, ½ cup .. | 8 | .9 | 1.2 | .1 | 0 | 3 | <1.0 |
| **Bamboo shoots, canned**, ½ cup: | | | | | | | |
| (*La Choy*) ............. | 10 | <1.0 | 2.0 | 0 | 0 | 10 | <1.0 |

| Food and Measure | cal. | prot. (gms) | carbo. (gms) | fat (gms) | chol. (mgs) | sod. (mgs) | fiber (gms) |
|---|---|---|---|---|---|---|---|
| slices/strips (*Roland*) ... | 25 | 1.0 | 3.0 | 0 | 0 | 15 | 2.0 |
| drained .............. | 13 | 1.1 | 2.1 | .3 | 0 | 5 | 2.0 |
| **Banana** (see also "Plantain"), fresh: | | | | | | | |
| (*Chiquita*), 4.1-oz. pc. ... | 105 | 1.0 | 27.0 | 0 | 0 | 1 | 3.0 |
| (*Dole*), 4.4-oz. pc. ...... | 110 | 1.0 | 29.0 | 0 | 0 | 0 | 3.0 |
| (*Frieda's* Baby Nino/ Burro), 3-oz. pc. ..... | 80 | 1.0 | 20.0 | 0 | 0 | 0 | 1.0 |
| 1 medium, 8¾" long .... | 105 | 1.2 | 26.7 | .6 | 0 | 1 | 2.7 |
| sliced, ½ cup .......... | 69 | .8 | 17.6 | .4 | 0 | 1 | 1.8 |
| mashed, ½ cup ........ | 104 | 1.2 | 26.4 | .5 | 0 | 1 | 2.7 |
| red (*Frieda's*), 5 oz. ..... | 130 | 1.0 | 33.0 | .5 | 0 | 0 | 2.0 |
| red, 7¼" long ......... | 118 | 1.6 | 30.7 | .3 | 0 | 1 | n.a. |
| **Banana, dried**: | | | | | | | |
| (*Frieda's*), 1.2-oz. pc. ... | 130 | 1.0 | 33.0 | .5 | 0 | 0 | 2.0 |
| chips (*Mariani*), 1.1 oz. ............. | 150 | 1.0 | 21.0 | 7.0 | 0 | 0 | 0 |
| dehydrated, ¼ cup ..... | 87 | 1.0 | 22.1 | .5 | 0 | 1 | 1.9 |
| **Banana drink blend**, 8 fl. oz.: | | | | | | | |
| (*Snapple* Go Bananas) .. | 110 | 0 | 28.0 | 0 | 0 | 5 | 0 |
| colada (*Chiquita*) ....... | 125 | 0 | 25.0 | 2.0 | 0 | 35 | 1.0 |
| **Banana juice blend**, 8 fl. oz.: | | | | | | | |
| (*After the Fall Banana Casablanca*) .. | 150 | 1.0 | 37.0 | 0 | 0 | 20 | 0 |
| mango carrot (*Nantucket Nectars*) .. | 120 | 0 | 30.0 | 0 | 0 | 30 | 0 |
| **Banana squash** (*Frieda's*), 3 oz. ...... | 30 | 1.0 | 7.0 | 0 | 0 | 0 | 1.0 |
| **Barbecue sauce** (see also "Grilling sauce"), 2 tbsp.: | | | | | | | |
| (*Annie's Naturals* Organic Original) .... | 50 | 0 | 9.0 | 1.0 | 0 | 260 | 0 |
| (*Buccaneer Blends* Sticky Rum) ........ | 50 | 0 | 13.0 | 0 | 0 | 340 | 0 |
| (*Bull's-Eye* Original) .... | 60 | 0 | 14.0 | 0 | 0 | 370 | 0 |
| (*Bull's-Eye* Guinness Draught Blend) ...... | 50 | 0 | 13.0 | 0 | 0 | 360 | 0 |
| (*Emeril's* Kicked Up) .... | 40 | 0 | 11.0 | 0 | 0 | 360 | 0 |
| (*Hunt's* Original) ....... | 60 | 0 | 15.0 | 0 | 0 | 280 | <1.0 |
| (*Hunt's* Original Bold) ... | 50 | 0 | 13.0 | 0 | 0 | 310 | <1.0 |

| Food and Measure | cal. | prot. (gms) | carbo. (gms) | fat (gms) | chol. (mgs) | sod. (mgs) | fiber (gms) |
|---|---|---|---|---|---|---|---|
| **Barbecue sauce** *(cont.)* | | | | | | | |
| (*KC Masterpiece* | | | | | | | |
| Original) . . . . . . . . . . . | 60 | 0 | 15.0 | 0 | 0 | 240 | 0 |
| (*Kraft* Char-Grill) . . . . . . . | 60 | 0 | 12.0 | 0 | 0 | 430 | 0 |
| (*Kraft* Original) . . . . . . . . | 60 | 0 | 15.0 | 0 | 0 | 450 | 0 |
| (*Kraft* Original Light) . . . . | 20 | 0 | 5.0 | 0 | 0 | 340 | 0 |
| (*Mrs. Renfro's*) . . . . . . . . | 35 | <1.0 | 8.0 | 0 | 0 | 220 | 0 |
| (*Sweet Baby Ray's* | | | | | | | |
| Original) . . . . . . . . . . . | 70 | 0 | 17.0 | 0 | 0 | 290 | 0 |
| (*Woody's* Cook-In) . . . . . | 50 | <1.0 | 4.0 | 4.0 | 0 | 490 | 1.0 |
| (*World Harbors* | | | | | | | |
| Australian) . . . . . . . . . | 70 | 0 | 16.0 | 0 | 0 | 540 | 0 |
| all varieties (*Maull's*) . . . . | 60 | 0 | 13.0 | 0 | 0 | 300 | 0 |
| apple maple (*Buccaneer* | | | | | | | |
| *Blends*) . . . . . . . . . . . | 60 | 0 | 14.0 | 0 | 0 | 200 | 0 |
| Asian: | | | | | | | |
| (*Roland* Char Siu) . . . . | 75 | 1.0 | 15.0 | 1.0 | 0 | 800 | 1.0 |
| (*San-J*) . . . . . . . . . . . | 50 | 1.0 | 12.0 | 0 | 0 | 420 | 0 |
| brown sugar (*Kraft* | | | | | | | |
| *Thick 'n Spicy*) . . . . . . | 60 | 0 | 16.0 | 0 | 0 | 450 | 0 |
| Carolina (*Bull's-Eye*) . . . . | 50 | 0 | 11.0 | 0 | 0 | 360 | 0 |
| Chinese style: | | | | | | | |
| (*Ah-So* Original) . . . . . | 70 | 0 | 24.0 | 0 | 0 | 480 | 0 |
| (*Sun Luck*), 1 tbsp. . . . | 30 | 0 | 5.0 | .5 | 0 | 250 | 0 |
| smoky (*Ah-So*) . . . . . . | 100 | 0 | 24.0 | 0 | 0 | 480 | 0 |
| chipotle, hot (*Annie's* | | | | | | | |
| *Naturals* Organic) . . . . | 50 | 0 | 10.0 | 1.0 | 0 | 260 | 0 |
| garlic, honey (*Roland*) . . . | 100 | 0 | 22.0 | 1.0 | 0 | 160 | 0 |
| hickory: | | | | | | | |
| (*Hunt's*) . . . . . . . . . . | 45 | 0 | 11.0 | 0 | 0 | 350 | <1.0 |
| brown sugar (*Hunt's*) . | 70 | 0 | 18.0 | 0 | 0 | 390 | <1.0 |
| brown sugar (*Sweet* | | | | | | | |
| *Baby Ray's*) . . . . . . | 70 | 0 | 18.0 | 0 | 0 | 240 | 0 |
| honey (*Hunt's*) . . . . . . | 50 | 0 | 13.0 | 0 | 0 | 420 | <1.0 |
| smoke (*Bull's-Eye*) . . . | 60 | 0 | 14.0 | 0 | 0 | 360 | 0 |
| smoke (*Kraft*) . . . . . . . | 60 | 0 | 13.0 | 0 | 0 | 430 | 0 |
| smoke, honey (*Kraft*) . | 70 | 0 | 16.0 | 0 | 0 | 460 | 0 |
| honey: | | | | | | | |
| (*Kraft* 16 oz.) . . . . . . . | 60 | 0 | 15.0 | 0 | 0 | 460 | 0 |
| (*Kraft* 18 oz.) . . . . . . . | 60 | 0 | 16.0 | 0 | 0 | 450 | 0 |
| (*Kraft* 28 oz.) . . . . . . . | 50 | 0 | 13.0 | 0 | 0 | 360 | 0 |
| (*Sweet Baby Ray's*) . . . | 70 | 0 | 17.0 | 0 | 0 | 300 | 0 |
| chipotle (*Sweet Baby* | | | | | | | |
| *Ray's*) . . . . . . . . . . . | 70 | 0 | 18.0 | 0 | 0 | 310 | 0 |

| Food and Measure | cal. | prot. (gms) | carbo. (gms) | fat (gms) | chol. (mgs) | sod. (mgs) | fiber (gms) |
|---|---|---|---|---|---|---|---|
| mango (*Buccaneer* *Blends*) .......... | 60 | 0 | 13.0 | 0 | 0 | 250 | 0 |
| mustard (*Hunt's*) .... | 50 | 0 | 13.0 | 0 | 0 | 330 | <1.0 |
| mustard (*Kraft*) ...... | 60 | 0 | 14.0 | 0 | 0 | 410 | 0 |
| roasted garlic (*Kraft*) . | 50 | 0 | 13.0 | 0 | 0 | 370 | 0 |
| spicy (*Kraft*) ........ | 60 | 0 | 15.0 | 0 | 0 | 440 | 0 |
| hot: | | | | | | | |
| (*Buccaneer Blends* Fra Diavlo) ....... | 45 | 1.0 | 11.0 | 0 | 0 | 260 | 0 |
| (*Kraft*) ............. | 50 | 0 | 12.0 | 0 | 0 | 460 | 0 |
| Kansas City (*Bull's-Eye*) . | 50 | 0 | 12.0 | 0 | 0 | 280 | 0 |
| Korean (*Annie Chun's*), 1 tbsp. ........... | 30 | 1.0 | 6.0 | 0 | 0 | 380 | 0 |
| maple, smoky (*Annie's Naturals Organic*) .... | 50 | 0 | 10.0 | 1.0 | 0 | 240 | 0 |
| Memphis (*Bull's-Eye*) ... | 50 | 0 | 12.0 | 0 | 0 | 290 | 0 |
| mesquite: | | | | | | | |
| (*Buccaneer Blends*) .. | 45 | 1.0 | 11.0 | 0 | 0 | 250 | 0 |
| smoke (*Kraft*) ....... | 50 | 0 | 12.0 | 0 | 0 | 450 | 0 |
| molasses (*Emeril's Sweet 'n Easy*) ...... | 50 | 0 | 15.0 | 0 | 0 | 400 | 0 |
| spare rib (*Mee Tu*) ...... | 80 | 0 | 19.0 | 0 | 0 | 260 | 1.0 |
| sweet (*Emeril's Original*) . | 45 | 0 | 12.0 | 0 | 0 | 390 | 0 |
| sweet/spicy: | | | | | | | |
| (*Annie's Naturals Organic*) ......... | 45 | 0 | 11.0 | 0 | 0 | 330 | 0 |
| (*Sweet Baby Ray's*) ... | 70 | 0 | 16.0 | 0 | 0 | 290 | 0 |
| sweet/tangy (*Bull's-Eye*) ......... | 60 | 0 | 13.0 | 0 | 0 | 310 | 0 |
| Texas (*Bull's-Eye*) ...... | 45 | 0 | 10.0 | 0 | 0 | 270 | 0 |
| **Barbecue seasoning** | | | | | | | |
| (*Grill Mates*), ¼ tsp. .. | 0 | 0 | 0 | 0 | 0 | 85 | 0 |
| **Barley** (see also "Cereal, cooking"): | | | | | | | |
| raw, ¼ cup: | | | | | | | |
| pearled (*Arrowhead Mills Organic*) .... | 160 | 5.0 | 32.0 | 1.0 | 0 | 5 | 8.0 |
| pearled (*Bob's Red Mill*) ............. | 180 | 5.0 | 39.0 | 1.0 | 0 | 4 | 8.0 |
| pearled ............. | 176 | 5.0 | 38.9 | .6 | 0 | 5 | 7.8 |
| whole (*Bob's Red Mill Hulled*) .......... | 170 | 6.0 | 34.0 | 1.0 | 0 | 5 | 8.0 |
| cooked, pearled, ½ cup .. | 97 | 1.8 | 22.2 | .4 | 0 | 3 | 3.0 |

| Food and Measure | cal. | prot. (gms) | carbo. (gms) | fat (gms) | chol. (mgs) | sod. (mgs) | fiber (gms) |
|---|---|---|---|---|---|---|---|
| **Barley flour:** | | | | | | | |
| (*Arrowhead Mills Organic*), ⅓ cup ..... | 95 | 3.0 | 19.0 | 1.0 | 0 | 0 | 4.0 |
| (*Bob's Red Mill* Whole Grain), ¼ cup ....... | 106 | 3.0 | 23.0 | 0 | 0 | 3 | 5.0 |
| malted (*Bob's Red Mill*), ¼ cup ........ | 105 | 4.0 | 20.0 | 1.0 | 0 | 3 | 3.0 |
| **Barley lentil dish** (*Tasty Bite*), ½ of 8-oz. pkg. . | 210 | 9.0 | 41.0 | 2.0 | 0 | 350 | 9.0 |
| **Barley malt syrup** (*Eden Organic*), 1 tbsp. ..... | 60 | 1.0 | 14.0 | 0 | 0 | 0 | 0 |
| **Basella**, see "Vine spinach" | | | | | | | |
| **Basil**, fresh: | | | | | | | |
| 1 oz. ............... | 8 | .7 | 1.2 | .2 | 0 | 0 | .3 |
| 5 medium leaves ....... | 1 | .1 | .1 | <.1 | 0 | 0 | .1 |
| chopped, 2 tbsp. ....... | 1 | .1 | .2 | <.1 | 0 | 0 | .2 |
| **Basil, dried**, ground, 1 tsp. ............. | 4 | .2 | .9 | .1 | 0 | <1 | .2 |
| ***Baskin-Robbins***, 4-oz. scoop, except as noted: | | | | | | | |
| ice cream: | | | | | | | |
| butter pecan ........ | 280 | 5.0 | 24.0 | 18.0 | 50 | 95 | 1.0 |
| cherries jubilee ...... | 240 | 4.0 | 30.0 | 12.0 | 45 | 80 | 1.0 |
| chocolate .......... | 260 | 5.0 | 33.0 | 14.0 | 50 | 130 | 0 |
| chocolate, *World Class* ........... | 280 | 5.0 | 31.0 | 16.0 | 45 | 95 | 0 |
| chocolate chip cookie dough .......... | 310 | 5.0 | 36.0 | 15.0 | 50 | 135 | 0 |
| coconut, nutty ...... | 300 | 6.0 | 28.0 | 20.0 | 45 | 90 | 1.0 |
| cookies 'n cream, *Oreo* ............ | 280 | 5.0 | 32.0 | 15.0 | 50 | 150 | 1.0 |
| *Gold Medal Ribbon* ... | 260 | 5.0 | 34.0 | 13.0 | 45 | 150 | 0 |
| *Jamoca* ............ | 240 | 5.0 | 26.0 | 13.0 | 55 | 90 | 0 |
| *Jamoca* almond fudge | 270 | 6.0 | 31.0 | 15.0 | 40 | 80 | 1.0 |
| mint chocolate chip .. | 270 | 5.0 | 28.0 | 16.0 | 55 | 95 | 1.0 |
| peanut butter 'n chocolate ........ | 320 | 7.0 | 31.0 | 20.0 | 45 | 180 | 1.0 |
| peanut butter cup, *Reese's* .......... | 300 | 6.0 | 31.0 | 18.0 | 50 | 130 | 0 |
| pistachio almond .... | 290 | 7.0 | 25.0 | 19.0 | 50 | 85 | 1.0 |
| pralines 'n cream .... | 280 | 5.0 | 35.0 | 14.0 | 45 | 170 | 1.0 |
| rocky road ........ | 290 | 5.0 | 36.0 | 15.0 | 45 | 120 | 1.0 |

| Food and Measure | cal. | prot. (gms) | carbo. (gms) | fat (gms) | chol. (mgs) | sod. (mgs) | fiber (gms) |
|---|---|---|---|---|---|---|---|
| strawberry, very ..... | 220 | 4.0 | 28.0 | 11.0 | 40 | 70 | 0 |
| vanilla ............. | 260 | 4.0 | 26.0 | 16.0 | 65 | 70 | 0 |
| ice cream, *BRight Choices,* light: | | | | | | | |
| brownie, Aloha ...... | 250 | 6.0 | 42.0 | 8.0 | 20 | 150 | 2.0 |
| cappuccino chip ..... | 220 | 6.0 | 32.0 | 8.0 | 25 | 110 | 1.0 |
| dulce de leche ....... | 230 | 5.0 | 37.0 | 7.0 | 25 | 140 | 1.0 |
| light mint *Oreo* ...... | 250 | 5.0 | 40.0 | 7.0 | 20 | 150 | 1.0 |
| peachy raspberry .... | 200 | 4.0 | 35.0 | 5.0 | 20 | 85 | 1.0 |
| raspberry chip ...... | 230 | 5.0 | 38.0 | 6.0 | 20 | 100 | 1.0 |
| ice cream, *BRight Choices,* No Sugar: | | | | | | | |
| berry banana ....... | 150 | 4.0 | 27.0 | 6.0 | 20 | 70 | 3.0 |
| butter almond crunch . | 220 | 7.0 | 31.0 | 11.0 | 25 | 140 | 4.0 |
| caramel turtle truffle .. | 200 | 5.0 | 38.0 | 8.0 | 25 | 115 | 3.0 |
| lemon cream pie ..... | 200 | 5.0 | 36.0 | 8.0 | 30 | 115 | 3.0 |
| mocha blackberry chip | 190 | 5.0 | 34.0 | 9.0 | 20 | 70 | 6.0 |
| pineapple coconut ... | 160 | 5.0 | 29.0 | 6.0 | 25 | 75 | 3.0 |
| ice cream, soft-serve, *31° Below,* 16 oz.: | | | | | | | |
| *Butterfinger* ........ | 860 | 20.0 | 132.0 | 31.0 | 85 | 550 | 1.0 |
| chocolate chip cookie dough ........... | 940 | 20.0 | 143.0 | 34.0 | 100 | 660 | 1.0 |
| chocolate *Oreo* ...... | 1290 | 22.0 | 187.0 | 55.0 | 85 | 1080 | 3.0 |
| fudge brownie ...... | 1390 | 26.0 | 199.0 | 58.0 | 175 | 990 | 2.0 |
| *Heath* ............. | 1160 | 21.0 | 151.0 | 54.0 | 115 | 860 | 1.0 |
| *Jamoca* almond fudge | 960 | 24.0 | 133.0 | 40.0 | 85 | 590 | 4.0 |
| *Jamoca Oreo* ....... | 860 | 19.0 | 128.0 | 33.0 | 85 | 710 | 2.0 |
| *Oreo* .............. | 1000 | 21.0 | 143.0 | 41.0 | 85 | 920 | 3.0 |
| peanut butter 'n chocolate ........ | 1190 | 27.0 | 149.0 | 58.0 | 85 | 810 | 4.0 |
| *Reese's* ........... | 1220 | 33.0 | 134.0 | 67.0 | 90 | 870 | 5.0 |
| strawberry banana ... | 710 | 19.0 | 112.0 | 23.0 | 85 | 440 | 3.0 |
| ice cream cone, unfilled: | | | | | | | |
| cake ............. | 25 | 0 | 5.0 | 0 | 0 | 15 | 0 |
| sugar ............. | 45 | 1.0 | 9.0 | .5 | 0 | 35 | 0 |
| waffle ............. | 160 | 2.0 | 28.0 | 4.0 | 10 | 5 | 0 |
| sherbet, rainbow: | | | | | | | |
| 4-oz. scoop ......... | 160 | 1.0 | 34.0 | 2.0 | 10 | 40 | 0 |
| prepacked, ½ cup .... | 120 | 1.0 | 26.0 | 1.5 | 5 | 30 | 0 |
| soft-serve cup, vanilla: | | | | | | | |
| plain, 9 oz. ........ | 430 | 13.0 | 58.0 | 17.0 | 65 | 320 | 0 |
| w/berry or watermelon sprinkles, 9 oz. ..... | 430 | 12.0 | 58.0 | 17.0 | 65 | 300 | 0 |

| Food and Measure | cal. | prot. (gms) | carbo. (gms) | fat (gms) | chol. (mgs) | sod. (mgs) | fiber (gms) |
|---|---|---|---|---|---|---|---|
| **Baskin-Robbins** *(cont.)* | | | | | | | |
| soft-serve pie, *31° Below*, 4 oz.: | | | | | | | |
|   *Heath* . . . . . . . . . . . . | 310 | 5.0 | 43.0 | 14.0 | 20 | 290 | 1.0 |
|   made from *Snickers* . . | 250 | 5.0 | 33.0 | 12.0 | 20 | 180 | 1.0 |
|   *Oreo* . . . . . . . . . . . . . | 290 | 5.0 | 40.0 | 13.0 | 20 | 180 | 1.0 |
|   *Reese's* . . . . . . . . . . . | 340 | 7.0 | 38.0 | 18.0 | 20 | 160 | 1.0 |
| sorbet, pink grapefruit . . . | 130 | 0 | 34.0 | 0 | 0 | 15 | 0 |
| yogurt, frozen: | | | | | | | |
|   lemon blueberry . . . . . | 200 | 4.0 | 33.0 | 6.0 | 25 | 75 | 0 |
|   vanilla, nonfat . . . . . . . | 150 | 6.0 | 32.0 | 0 | 5 | 105 | 0 |
|   vanilla pomegranate . . | 240 | 5.0 | 37.0 | 8.0 | 25 | 85 | 0 |
| *Cappuccino Blast*, 24 oz.: | | | | | | | |
|   caramel . . . . . . . . . . . | 670 | 10.0 | 111.0 | 23.0 | 85 | 370 | 0 |
|   mocha . . . . . . . . . . . | 610 | 9.0 | 104.0 | 19.0 | 75 | 150 | 0 |
|   mocha, whipped cream | 620 | 9.0 | 100.0 | 21.0 | 80 | 160 | 0 |
|   nonfat . . . . . . . . . . . . | 340 | 11.0 | 78.0 | 0 | 5 | 190 | 0 |
|   turtle . . . . . . . . . . . . | 780 | 10.0 | 137.0 | 22.0 | 75 | 470 | 1.0 |
|   w/soft-serve . . . . . . . . | 410 | 10.0 | 65.0 | 13.0 | 55 | 210 | 0 |
|   w/whipped cream . . . | 500 | 9.0 | 74.0 | 21.0 | 80 | 160 | 0 |
| float, root beer, vanilla ice cream, medium . . . | 680 | 8.0 | 99.0 | 30.0 · | 120 | 190 | 0 |
| freeze, orange sherbet, medium . . . . . . . . . . | 510 | 3.0 | 112.0 | 5.0 | 20 | 160 | 1.0 |
| fruit blast, 24 oz.: | | | | | | | |
|   peach passion fruit . . . | 370 | 2.0 | 94.0 | .5 | 0 | 10 | 3.0 |
|   strawberry citrus . . . . | 330 | 1.0 | 83.0 | 0 | 0 | 10 | 1.0 |
|   wild mango . . . . . . . . . | 470 | 1.0 | 116.0 | 1.5 | 0 | 15 | 2.0 |
| fruit blast smoothie, 24 oz.: | | | | | | | |
|   mango . . . . . . . . . . . | 620 | 7.0 | 148.0 | 2.0 | 5 | 120 | 3.0 |
|   peach passion banana | 540 | 8.0 | 131.0 | 1.0 | 5 | 110 | 5.0 |
|   strawberry banana . . . | 560 | 8.0 | 135.0 | 1.0 | 0 | 110 | 5.0 |
| fruit cream, soft-serve: | | | | | | | |
|   mango, 16 oz. . . . . . . . | 640 | 13.0 | 110.0 | 18.0 | 65 | 320 | 1.0 |
|   passion fruit, 16 oz. . . | 630 | 14.0 | 109.0 | 17.0 | 65 | 32 | 2.0 |
|   strawberry, 16 oz. . . . . | 630 | 15.0 | 102.0 | 19.0 | 70 | 360 | 1.0 |
| shakes, 24 oz.: | | | | | | | |
|   chocolate, chocolate ice cream . . . . . . . . | 990 | 20.0 | 149.0 | 40.0 | 135 | 440 | 1.0 |
|   chocolate, vanilla ice cream . . . . . . . . | 990 | 19.0 | 131.0 | 44.0 | 175 | 270 | 0 |
|   chocolate chip . . . . . . | 900 | 20.0 | 108.0 | 44.0 | 150 | 320 | 2.0 |

| Food and Measure | cal. | prot. (gms) | carbo. (gms) | fat (gms) | chol. (mgs) | sod. (mgs) | fiber (gms) |
|---|---|---|---|---|---|---|---|
| chocolate chip cookie | | | | | | | |
|   dough | 1030 | 19.0 | 137.0 | 42.0 | 140 | 430 | 1.0 |
| mint chocolate chip | 930 | 20.0 | 116.0 | 44.0 | 150 | 330 | 2.0 |
| mint *Oreo* | 860 | 20.0 | 151.0 | 22.0 | 70 | 480 | 2.0 |
| raspberry chip | 760 | 19.0 | 125.0 | 21.0 | 70 | 370 | 3.0 |
| strawberry | 770 | 17.0 | 105.0 | 31.0 | 125 | 290 | 1.0 |
| vanilla | 980 | 19.0 | 125.0 | 45.0 | 175 | 640 | 0 |
| soda, vanilla ice cream, | | | | | | | |
|   medium | 720 | 8.0 | 103.0 | 30.0 | 120 | 190 | 0 |
| sundae, soft-serve: | | | | | | | |
| caramel, 16 oz. | 850 | 20.0 | 132.0 | 29.0 | 100 | 700 | 1.0 |
| hot fudge, 16 oz. | 900 | 21.0 | 128.0 | 36.0 | 90 | 630 | 2.0 |
| strawberry, 16 oz. | 640 | 18.0 | 87.0 | 26.0 | 90 | 460 | 1.0 |
| sundae cup, 1 cont.: | | | | | | | |
| *Oreo* | 330 | 4.0 | 45.0 | 15.0 | 40 | 190 | 0 |
| pralines 'n cream | 330 | 4.0 | 44.0 | 16.0 | 40 | 170 | 1.0 |
| *Reese's* | 390 | 8.0 | 36.0 | 24.0 | 40 | 190 | 2.0 |
| desserts, 1 slice: | | | | | | | |
| apple pie à la mode | 280 | 3.0 | 34.0 | 14.0 | 25 | 120 | 1.0 |
| brownie à la mode | 260 | 3.0 | 36.0 | 13.0 | 20 | 130 | 2.0 |
| chocolate indulgence | 330 | 4.0 | 41.0 | 18.0 | 30 | 200 | 2.0 |
| chocolate temptation | 420 | 6.0 | 49.0 | 23.0 | 45 | 230 | 2.0 |
| raspberry fudge truffle | 280 | 3.0 | 36.0 | 15.0 | 20 | 115 | 2.0 |
| strawberry 'n cream | 220 | 2.0 | 25.0 | 13.0 | 20 | 40 | 0 |
| **Bass** (see also "Sea | | | | | | | |
| Bass"), meat only: | | | | | | | |
| freshwater, 4 oz.: | | | | | | | |
| raw | 129 | 21.4 | 0 | 4.2 | 77 | 79 | 0 |
| baked or broiled | 166 | 27.4 | 0 | 5.4 | 99 | 102 | 0 |
| striped, 4 oz.: | | | | | | | |
| raw | 110 | 20.1 | 0 | 2.7 | 91 | 78 | 0 |
| baked or broiled | 141 | 25.8 | 0 | 3.4 | 117 | 100 | 0 |
| **Batter/breading mix** | | | | | | | |
| (see also "Panko | | | | | | | |
| coating mix" and specific | | | | | | | |
| listings), ¼ cup: | | | | | | | |
| batter: | | | | | | | |
| (*Don's Chuck Wagon*) | 100 | 4.0 | 20.0 | 0 | 0 | 580 | 1.0 |
| (*Golden Dipt* Fry Easy | | | | | | | |
|   All-Purpose) | 100 | 2.0 | 20.0 | 0 | 0 | 770 | 0 |
| (*Old Bay* Better Batter) | 110 | 2.0 | 13.0 | .5 | 0 | 690 | 0 |
| batter, tempura: | | | | | | | |
| (*Kikkoman*) | 110 | 1.0 | 25.0 | 0 | 0 | 75 | 0 |
| (*Roland*) | 100 | 2.0 | 24.0 | 0 | 0 | 210 | 0 |

| Food and Measure | cal. | prot. (gms) | carbo. (gms) | fat (gms) | chol. (mgs) | sod. (mgs) | fiber (gms) |
|---|---|---|---|---|---|---|---|
| **Batter/breading mix** *(cont.)* | | | | | | | |
| breading: | | | | | | | |
| (*Golden Dipt* Fry Easy | | | | | | | |
| All Purpose) . . . . . . | 120 | 3.0 | 23.0 | 1.0 | 0 | 830 | 0 |
| (*Old Bay* Dip & Crisp) . | 100 | 3.0 | 19.0 | 1.5 | 0 | 500 | 1.0 |
| **Bay leaf**, dried, | | | | | | | |
| crumbled, 1 tsp. . . . . . | 5 | .1 | .3 | .1 | 0 | <1 | <1.0 |
| **Bean dip**, 2 tbsp.: | | | | | | | |
| (*Fritos* Original) . . . . . . . . | 35 | 2.0 | 5.0 | 1.0 | 0 | 190 | 2.0 |
| black bean: | | | | | | | |
| (*Emerald Valley* | | | | | | | |
| Organic) . . . . . . . . . | 45 | 2.0 | 6.0 | 1.5 | 0 | 120 | 1.0 |
| (*Guiltless Gourmet*) . . | 40 | 2.0 | 7.0 | 0 | 0 | 125 | 2.0 |
| cheese, see "Cheese dip" | | | | | | | |
| hot (*Fritos*) . . . . . . . . . . . | 35 | 2.0 | 5.0 | 1.0 | 0 | 230 | 2.0 |
| jalapeño (*Fritos* Hot) . . . . | 35 | 2.0 | 5.0 | 1.0 | 0 | 230 | 2.0 |
| spicy (*Mission*) . . . . . . . . | 35 | 2.0 | 4.0 | 1.0 | 0 | 125 | 1.0 |
| three-bean (*Emerald* | | | | | | | |
| *Valley* Organic) . . . . . . | 35 | 2.0 | 6.0 | 0 | 0 | 140 | 2.0 |
| **Bean entree,** see | | | | | | | |
| specific bean listings | | | | | | | |
| **Bean salad,** see | | | | | | | |
| "Beans, mixed" | | | | | | | |
| **Bean sauce**, Asian: | | | | | | | |
| black bean, 2 tbsp., | | | | | | | |
| except as noted: | | | | | | | |
| (*Ka•Me*) . . . . . . . . . . . | 25 | 1.0 | 6.0 | 0 | 0 | 690 | 0 |
| chili (*Heaven and* | | | | | | | |
| *Earth*), 1 tbsp. . . . . | 30 | 1.0 | 4.0 | 1.5 | 0 | 400 | 0 |
| garlic (*Kikkoman*) . . . . | 50 | 3.0 | 6.0 | 1.0 | 0 | 1120 | 2.0 |
| garlic (*Sun Luck*), | | | | | | | |
| 1 tbsp. . . . . . . . . . . | 25 | 1.0 | 2.0 | 1.5 | 0 | 820 | 0 |
| spicy (*Roland* 7 oz.) . . | 60 | 2.0 | 9.0 | 2.0 | 0 | 1090 | 2.0 |
| spicy (*Roland* 12 oz.) . | 60 | 2.0 | 9.0 | 2.0 | 0 | 920 | 2.0 |
| black bean, cooking | | | | | | | |
| (*Tiger Tiger* | | | | | | | |
| Cantonese), ½ cup . . . | 222 | 5.0 | 37.0 | 6.0 | 0 | 904 | <1.0 |
| brown bean, spicy | | | | | | | |
| (*House of Tsang*), | | | | | | | |
| 1 tsp. . . . . . . . . . . . . | 15 | 0 | 3.0 | 0 | 0 | 140 | 0 |
| **Bean sprouts**, fresh, | | | | | | | |
| see specific listings | | | | | | | |
| **Bean sprouts, canned:** | | | | | | | |
| (*La Choy*), ⅔ cup . . . . . . | 15 | <1.0 | 3.0 | 0 | 0 | 60 | 1.0 |

| Food and Measure | cal. | prot. (gms) | carbo. (gms) | fat (gms) | chol. (mgs) | sod. (mgs) | fiber (gms) |
|---|---|---|---|---|---|---|---|
| (*Roland*), ½ cup ........ | 25 | 3.0 | 4.0 | 0 | 0 | 270 | 2.0 |
| **Beans**, see specific listings | | | | | | | |
| **Beans, baked**, see "Baked beans" | | | | | | | |
| **Beans, mixed**, can/jar, ½ cup: | | | | | | | |
| (*Bush's*) .............. | 110 | 7.0 | 19.0 | 0 | 0 | 500 | 6.0 |
| (*S&W* San Antonio) .... | 120 | 7.0 | 20.0 | 1.0 | 0 | 610 | 6.0 |
| salad, three-bean (*Green Giant*) ........ | 80 | 3.0 | 18.0 | 0 | 0 | 470 | 3.0 |
| seasoned (*Glory* Crock Pot) .......... | 130 | 7.0 | 25.0 | 0 | 0 | 620 | 7.0 |
| **Beans, snap or string**, see "Green bean" | | | | | | | |
| **Beans and franks** (*Van Camp's Beenie Weenees*), 7.75-oz. can: | | | | | | | |
| baked .............. | 290 | 13.0 | 42.0 | 8.0 | 40 | 1160 | 6.0 |
| original .............. | 240 | 14.0 | 29.0 | 8.0 | 40 | 990 | 8.0 |
| smoked hickory ....... | 320 | 14.0 | 45.0 | 9.0 | 40 | 1140 | 8.0 |
| **Beans and rice**, see "Rice and beans" and "Rice dish/entree" | | | | | | | |
| **Bear**, meat only, simmered, 4 oz. ..... | 294 | 36.8 | 0 | 15.2 | 111 | 81 | 0 |
| **Béarnaise sauce**, in jars (*Reese*), 2 tbsp. .. | 80 | 1.0 | 1.0 | 8.0 | 70 | 360 | 0 |
| **Béarnaise sauce mix** (*McCormick*), 1 tsp. .. | 10 | 0 | 1.0 | 0 | 0 | 130 | 0 |
| **Beaver**, meat only, roasted, 4 oz. ....... | 240 | 39.5 | 0 | 7.9 | 133 | 67 | 0 |
| **Bee pollen** (*Shiloh Farms*), 1 tsp. ....... | 30 | 2.0 | 5.0 | 0 | 0 | 0 | 2.0 |
| **Beechnuts**, dried, shelled, 1 oz. ....... | 164 | 1.8 | 9.5 | 14.2 | 0 | 11 | n.a. |
| **Beef**, choice grade, trimmed to ¼" fat, except as noted, meat only, 4 oz.: | | | | | | | |
| brisket, whole: | | | | | | | |
| braised, lean w/fat ... | 437 | 26.6 | 0 | 35.8 | 107 | 69 | 0 |
| braised, lean only .... | 274 | 33.7 | 0 | 14.5 | 105 | 79 | 0 |

| Food and Measure | cal. | prot. (gms) | carbo. (gms) | fat (gms) | chol. (mgs) | sod. (mgs) | fiber (gms) |
|---|---|---|---|---|---|---|---|
| **Beef** *(cont.)* | | | | | | | |
| chuck, arm pot roast: | | | | | | | |
|   braised, lean w/fat ... | 395 | 30.6 | 0 | 29.2 | 112 | 67 | 0 |
|   braised, lean only .... | 255 | 37.4 | 0 | 10.5 | 115 | 75 | 0 |
| chuck, blade roast: | | | | | | | |
|   braised, lean w/fat ... | 412 | 29.7 | 0 | 31.5 | 117 | 73 | 0 |
|   braised, lean only .... | 298 | 35.2 | 0 | 16.3 | 120 | 81 | 0 |
| flank steak, trimmed to 0" fat: | | | | | | | |
|   braised, lean only .... | 269 | 31.8 | 0 | 14.7 | 81 | 82 | 0 |
|   broiled, lean only .... | 256 | 30.0 | 0 | 14.2 | 77 | 92 | 0 |
| ground, see "Beef, ground" | | | | | | | |
| porterhouse steak: | | | | | | | |
|   broiled, lean w/fat .... | 346 | 28.2 | 0 | 25.1 | 94 | 69 | 0 |
|   broiled, lean only .... | 247 | 31.9 | 0 | 12.2 | 91 | 75 | 0 |
| rib, whole: | | | | | | | |
|   roasted, lean w/fat ... | 426 | 25.1 | 0 | 35.4 | 96 | 71 | 0 |
|   roasted, lean only .... | 276 | 30.9 | 0 | 15.9 | 91 | 82 | 0 |
| rib, large end (ribs 6–9): | | | | | | | |
|   roasted, lean w/fat ... | 434 | 25.3 | 0 | 36.2 | 96 | 71 | 0 |
|   roasted, lean only .... | 284 | 31.2 | 0 | 16.7 | 92 | 83 | 0 |
| rib, small end (ribs 10–12): | | | | | | | |
|   broiled, lean w/fat .... | 376 | 26.7 | 0 | 31.3 | 95 | 70 | 0 |
|   broiled, lean only .... | 264 | 31.8 | 0 | 14.3 | 91 | 78 | 0 |
| round, bottom: | | | | | | | |
|   braised, lean w/fat ... | 322 | 32.5 | 0 | 20.3 | 109 | 57 | 0 |
|   braised, lean only .... | 249 | 35.8 | 0 | 10.7 | 109 | 58 | 0 |
| round, eye of: | | | | | | | |
|   roasted, lean w/fat ... | 273 | 30.2 | 0 | 16.0 | 82 | 67 | 0 |
|   roasted, lean only .... | 198 | 32.9 | 0 | 6.5 | 78 | 70 | 0 |
| round, full cut: | | | | | | | |
|   broiled, lean w/fat .... | 272 | 31.0 | 0 | 15.4 | 91 | 69 | 0 |
|   broiled, lean only .... | 217 | 33.1 | 0 | 8.3 | 88 | 73 | 0 |
| round, tip: | | | | | | | |
|   roasted, lean w/fat ... | 280 | 30.1 | 0 | 16.9 | 94 | 70 | 0 |
|   roasted, lean only .... | 213 | 32.6 | 0 | 8.3 | 92 | 74 | 0 |
| round, top: | | | | | | | |
|   broiled, lean w/fat .... | 254 | 34.2 | 0 | 12.0 | 96 | 68 | 0 |
|   broiled, lean only .... | 214 | 35.9 | 0 | 6.7 | 95 | 69 | 0 |
|   fried, lean w/fat ...... | 314 | 36.7 | 0 | 17.4 | 110 | 77 | 0 |
|   fried, lean only ...... | 257 | 39.8 | 0 | 9.7 | 110 | 81 | 0 |

| Food and Measure | cal. | prot. (gms) | carbo. (gms) | fat (gms) | chol. (mgs) | sod. (mgs) | fiber (gms) |
|---|---|---|---|---|---|---|---|
| shank, crosscuts: | | | | | | | |
| braised, lean w/fat ... | 298 | 34.8 | 0 | 16.6 | 91 | 69 | 0 |
| braised, lean only .... | 228 | 38.2 | 0 | 7.2 | 88 | 73 | 0 |
| shortribs: | | | | | | | |
| braised, lean w/fat ... | 534 | 24.5 | 0 | 47.6 | 107 | 57 | 0 |
| braised, lean only .... | 335 | 34.9 | 0 | 20.6 | 105 | 66 | 0 |
| sirloin, top: | | | | | | | |
| broiled, lean w/fat .... | 305 | 31.3 | 0 | 19.0 | 102 | 70 | 0 |
| broiled, lean only .... | 229 | 34.4 | 0 | 9.1 | 101 | 75 | 0 |
| fried, lean w/fat ...... | 370 | 31.9 | 0 | 25.9 | 111 | 79 | 0 |
| fried, lean only ...... | 270 | 36.8 | 0 | 12.4 | 112 | 87 | 0 |
| T-bone steak: | | | | | | | |
| broiled, lean w/fat .... | 338 | 28.3 | 0 | 24.0 | 94 | 69 | 0 |
| broiled, lean only .... | 243 | 31.9 | 0 | 11.8 | 91 | 75 | 0 |
| tenderloin: | | | | | | | |
| broiled, lean w/fat .... | 345 | 28.4 | 0 | 24.8 | 98 | 67 | 0 |
| broiled, lean only .... | 252 | 32.0 | 0 | 12.7 | 95 | 71 | 0 |
| top loin: | | | | | | | |
| broiled, lean w/fat .... | 338 | 28.8 | 0 | 23.8 | 90 | 71 | 0 |
| broiled, lean only .... | 243 | 32.5 | 0 | 11.5 | 86 | 77 | 0 |
| **Beef**, choice grade, trimmed to 1/8" fat, meat only, lean w/fat, 4 oz.: | | | | | | | |
| brisket, braised: | | | | | | | |
| whole ............. | 375 | 29.3 | 0 | 27.8 | 105 | 73 | 0 |
| flat half ............ | 338 | 32.5 | 0 | 22.1 | 91 | 52 | 0 |
| point half .......... | 396 | 27.7 | 0 | 30.8 | 104 | 78 | 0 |
| chuck, braised: | | | | | | | |
| arm ............... | 350 | 34.2 | 0 | 22.6 | 93 | 56 | 0 |
| blade .............. | 407 | 29.9 | 0 | 30.9 | 117 | 73 | 0 |
| ground, see "Beef, ground" | | | | | | | |
| rib, whole, broiled ...... | 399 | 25.2 | 0 | 32.3 | 81 | 71 | 0 |
| rib, whole, roasted ..... | 414 | 25.6 | 0 | 33.8 | 95 | 73 | 0 |
| rib, large end: | | | | | | | |
| broiled ............ | 420 | 23.7 | 0 | 35.4 | 82 | 71 | 0 |
| roasted ............ | 429 | 25.5 | 0 | 35.5 | 96 | 71 | 0 |
| rib, small end: | | | | | | | |
| broiled ............ | 345 | 27.8 | 0 | 25.1 | 132 | 56 | 0 |
| roasted ............ | 407 | 25.3 | 0 | 33.1 | 94 | 71 | 0 |
| round, full cut, broiled ... | 266 | 31.2 | 0 | 14.7 | 90 | 70 | 0 |
| round, bottom: | | | | | | | |
| braised ............ | 288 | 37.3 | 0 | 14.2 | 91 | 48 | 0 |

| Food and Measure | cal. | prot. (gms) | carbo. (gms) | fat (gms) | chol. (mgs) | sod. (mgs) | fiber (gms) |
|---|---|---|---|---|---|---|---|
| **Beef, round, bottom** *(cont.)* | | | | | | | |
| roasted ........... | 253 | 29.5 | 0 | 14.1 | 91 | 42 | 0 |
| round, eye, roasted ..... | 240 | 32.3 | 0 | 11.4 | 73 | 42 | 0 |
| round, tip, roasted ..... | 259 | 30.9 | 0 | 14.0 | 93 | 71 | 0 |
| round, top: | | | | | | | |
| braised ........... | 284 | 38.7 | 0 | 13.2 | 102 | 51 | 0 |
| broiled ........... | 254 | 34.8 | 0 | 11.6 | 75 | 45 | 0 |
| pan-fried .......... | 302 | 37.4 | 0 | 15.7 | 110 | 77 | 0 |
| sirloin, top: | | | | | | | |
| broiled ........... | 291 | 30.4 | 0 | 17.9 | 94 | 61 | 0 |
| pan-fried .......... | 355 | 32.6 | 0 | 23.9 | 111 | 81 | 0 |
| steak, broiled: | | | | | | | |
| porterhouse ........ | 339 | 26.4 | 0 | 25.1 | 84 | 73 | 0 |
| T-bone ............ | 324 | 27.3 | 0 | 20.0 | 74 | 75 | 0 |
| tenderloin: | | | | | | | |
| broiled ........... | 310 | 30.0 | 0 | 20.2 | 74 | 59 | 0 |
| roasted ........... | 375 | 27.1 | 0 | 28.8 | 96 | 74 | 0 |
| top loin, broiled ....... | 315 | 29.7 | 0 | 20.9 | 110 | 59 | 0 |
| **Beef, canned**, see specific listings | | | | | | | |
| **Beef, corned** (see also "Beef lunch meat"), brisket, cooked, 4 oz. . | 285 | 20.6 | .5 | 21.5 | 111 | 1286 | 0 |
| **Beef, corned, canned**: | | | | | | | |
| (*Hormel*), 2 oz. ........ | 120 | 15.0 | 0 | 6.0 | 20 | 490 | 0 |
| (*Libby's*), 2 oz. ........ | 120 | 14.0 | 0 | 7.0 | 40 | 490 | 0 |
| hash, see "Beef hash" | | | | | | | |
| **Beef, dried** (see also "Beef jerky/stick"): | | | | | | | |
| (*Hormel/Hormel Pillow Pack*), 1 oz. ......... | 50 | 8.0 | 1.0 | 1.5 | 25 | 1200 | 0 |
| cured, 1 oz. ........... | 47 | 8.3 | .4 | 1.1 | n.a. | 984 | 0 |
| **Beef, frozen/chilled, raw** (*Always Tender*), marinated sirloin fillet, 4 oz.: | | | | | | | |
| peppercorn ........... | 130 | 18.0 | 2.0 | 5.0 | 45 | 450 | 0 |
| tequila lime ........... | 130 | 18.0 | 2.0 | 5.0 | 45 | 480 | 0 |
| teriyaki ............. | 130 | 18.0 | 4.0 | 5.0 | 45 | 450 | 0 |
| **Beef, frozen/chilled, cooked** (see also "Beef entree, frozen"): | | | | | | | |
| brisket (*Tyson*), 5 oz.: | | | | | | | |
| braised, chili sauce ... | 150 | 19.0 | 7.0 | 5.0 | 55 | 770 | 0 |

| Food and Measure | cal. | prot. (gms) | carbo. (gms) | fat (gms) | chol. (mgs) | sod. (mgs) | fiber (gms) |
|---|---|---|---|---|---|---|---|
| fire-roasted onion sauce ......... | 150 | 19.0 | 7.0 | 5.0 | 55 | 770 | 0 |
| burger (*Applegate Farms Organic*), 3 oz. ...... | 195 | 21.0 | 0 | 12.0 | 70 | 85 | 0 |
| pot roast, in gravy: | | | | | | | |
| (*Bob Evans*), 5 oz. ... | 190 | 23.0 | 4.0 | 8.0 | 60 | 580 | 0 |
| (*Tyson*), 5 oz. ....... | 170 | 23.0 | 2.0 | 8.0 | 65 | 730 | 0 |
| ribs, barbecue sauce (*Lloyd's*), 2 ribs w/sauce, 7.5 oz. ..... | 620 | 32.0 | 25.0 | 43.0 | 140 | 1730 | 0 |
| roast, 5 oz.: | | | | | | | |
| (*Hormel*) ........... | 210 | 28.0 | 3.0 | 10.0 | 80 | 500 | 0 |
| Italian style, au jus (*Hormel*) ...... | 220 | 28.0 | 2.0 | 11.0 | 85 | 350 | 0 |
| sliced, and gravy (*Hormel*) ........ | 110 | 18.0 | 3.0 | 3.0 | 45 | 790 | 0 |
| Salisbury steak, gravy (*Hormel*), 5 oz. ...... | 170 | 15.0 | 6.0 | 10.0 | 60 | 890 | 0 |
| steak strips, seasoned (*Tyson*), 3 oz. ...... | 140 | 18.0 | 1.0 | 6.0 | 55 | 500 | 1.0 |
| steak tips, 5 oz.: | | | | | | | |
| bourbon sauce (*Tyson*) | 180 | 20.0 | 12.0 | 8.0 | 45 | 480 | 0 |
| Burgundy sauce (*Tyson*) .......... | 180 | 19.0 | 6.0 | 9.0 | 50 | 520 | 0 |
| w/gravy (*Hormel*) .... | 180 | 21.0 | 5.0 | 8.0 | 60 | 700 | 1.0 |
| in gravy (*Tyson*) ..... | 200 | 17.0 | 5.0 | 12.0 | 55 | 530 | 0 |
| stew, w/vegetables (*Bob Evans*), 1 cup ... | 190 | 15.0 | 16.0 | 7.0 | 35 | 900 | 2.0 |
| Stroganoff (*Hormel*), 5 oz. ............. | 220 | 22.0 | 4.0 | 13.0 | 75 | 520 | 0 |
| **Beef, ground**, 4 oz.: | | | | | | | |
| raw: | | | | | | | |
| 95% lean .......... | 155 | 24.3 | 0 | 6.0 | 70 | 75 | 0 |
| 90% lean .......... | 199 | 22.7 | 0 | 11.3 | 74 | 75 | 0 |
| 85% lean .......... | 244 | 21.1 | 0 | 17.0 | 77 | 75 | 0 |
| 80% lean .......... | 288 | 19.5 | 0 | 22.7 | 81 | 76 | 0 |
| 75% lean .......... | 332 | 17.9 | 0 | 28.4 | 85 | 76 | 0 |
| crumbles, pan-browned: | | | | | | | |
| 95% lean .......... | 219 | 33.1 | 0 | 8.6 | 101 | 96 | 0 |
| 90% lean .......... | 261 | 32.3 | 0 | 13.7 | 101 | 99 | 0 |
| 85% lean .......... | 290 | 31.4 | 0 | 17.4 | 102 | 101 | 0 |
| 80% lean .......... | 308 | 30.6 | 0 | 19.7 | 101 | 103 | 0 |
| 75% lean .......... | 314 | 30.4 | 0 | 20.7 | 101 | 105 | 0 |

| Food and Measure | cal. | prot. (gms) | carbo. (gms) | fat (gms) | chol. (mgs) | sod. (mgs) | fiber (gms) |
|---|---|---|---|---|---|---|---|
| **Beef, ground** *(cont.)* | | | | | | | |
| patty, broiled: | | | | | | | |
| 95% lean .......... | 202 | 29.8 | 0 | 8.0 | 86 | 74 | 0 |
| 90% lean .......... | 246 | 29.6 | 0 | 13.3 | 96 | 77 | 0 |
| 85% lean .......... | 284 | 29.4 | 0 | 17.6 | 102 | 82 | 0 |
| 80% lean .......... | 307 | 29.2 | 0 | 20.2 | 103 | 85 | 0 |
| 75% lean .......... | 315 | 29.0 | 0 | 21.3 | 101 | 88 | 0 |
| patty, pan-broiled: | | | | | | | |
| 95% lean .......... | 186 | 29.3 | 0 | 7.0 | 86 | 81 | 0 |
| 90% lean .......... | 231 | 28.6 | 0 | 12.1 | 93 | 85 | 0 |
| 85% lean .......... | 263 | 27.9 | 0 | 15.9 | 98 | 90 | 0 |
| 80% lean .......... | 274 | 27.3 | 0 | 18.1 | 98 | 94 | 0 |
| 75% lean .......... | 281 | 26.6 | 0 | 18.6 | 94 | 99 | 0 |
| **"Beef," vegetarian, canned** (see also "Burger, vegetarian"): | | | | | | | |
| (*Worthington* Prime Stakes), 3.2-oz. pc. .... | 120 | 9.0 | 7.0 | 6.0 | 0 | 440 | 1.0 |
| (*Worthington Vegetable Steaks* Low Fat), 2 slices, 2.5 oz. .. | 80 | 15.0 | 2.0 | 1.0 | 0 | 300 | 2.0 |
| **"Beef," vegetarian, frozen/chilled**: | | | | | | | |
| (*Loma Linda* Swiss Stake), 3.25-oz. pc. .. | 130 | 9.0 | 9.0 | 6.0 | 0 | 430 | 3.0 |
| (*Worthington Stakelets*), 2.5-oz. pc. . | 150 | 14.0 | 7.0 | 7.0 | 0 | 480 | 2.0 |
| burger, see "Burger patty, vegetarian" | | | | | | | |
| corned (*Worthington*), ⅜" slice, 2 oz. ....... | 140 | 10.0 | 5.0 | 8.0 | 0 | 450 | 0 |
| ground, ⅓ cup: | | | | | | | |
| (*Yves* Lettuce Wrap) .. | 60 | 7.0 | 8.0 | .5 | 0 | 350 | 2.0 |
| (*Yves* Original) ...... | 60 | 10.0 | 5.0 | .5 | 0 | 270 | 2.0 |
| (*Yves* Taco Stuffer) ... | 90 | 11.0 | 5.0 | 2.5 | 0 | 300 | 3.0 |
| "Philly steak" (*Tofurky*) 5 slices, 1.8 oz. ....... | 100 | 12.0 | 7.0 | 3.0 | 0 | 370 | 3.0 |
| strips (*Yves* Heart's Desire), 3 oz. ....... | 120 | 23.0 | 4.0 | 1.0 | 0 | 370 | 1.0 |
| **Beef appetizer**, frozen (*Original Rangoon*): | | | | | | | |
| beef Wellington, puff pastry, 4 pcs., 3.7 oz. . | 360 | 10.0 | 22.0 | 26.0 | 25 | 180 | <1.0 |

| Food and Measure | cal. | prot. (gms) | carbo. (gms) | fat (gms) | chol. (mgs) | sod. (mgs) | fiber (gms) |
|---|---|---|---|---|---|---|---|
| filet mignon, bacon wrapped, 4 pcs. ..... | 250 | 21.0 | 0 | 18.0 | 55 | 540 | 0 |
| steak/cheese wontons. 2-oz. pc. .......... | 225 | 11.0 | 40.0 | 12.0 | 40 | 470 | 0 |
| **Beef dinner**, see "Beef entree" | | | | | | | |
| **"Beef" dinner, vegetarian**, frozen, Salisbury steak (*Amy's* Whole Meal), 11 oz. .. | 380 | 12.0 | 50.0 | 16.0 | 30 | 680 | 7.0 |
| **Beef entree, canned**: | | | | | | | |
| chow mein (*La Choy*), 1 cup ........ | 80 | 7.0 | 11.0 | 1.0 | 10 | 920 | 3.0 |
| pepper, Oriental (*La Choy*), 1 cup ..... | 80 | 7.0 | 11.0 | 1.0 | 15 | 1240 | <1.0 |
| roast, w/gravy: | | | | | | | |
| (*Hormel*), ⅔ cup ..... | 130 | 18.0 | 8.0 | 3.0 | 40 | 740 | 0 |
| (*Libby's*), ⅔ cup ..... | 140 | 25.0 | 3.0 | 3.5 | 60 | 750 | 0 |
| stew, 1 cup: | | | | | | | |
| (*Dinty Moore*) ....... | 200 | 10.0 | 17.0 | 10.0 | 30 | 970 | 1.0 |
| (*Dinty Moore* Steakhouse) ...... | 190 | 14.0 | 16.0 | 8.0 | 35 | 900 | 2.0 |
| **Beef entree, frozen** (see also "Beef, frozen/chilled"), 1 pkg., except as noted: | | | | | | | |
| bourbon, Dijon (*Healthy Choice*), 11 oz. ...... | 280 | 17.0 | 38.0 | 6.0 | 40 | 600 | 6.0 |
| broccoli (*Contessa On the Stove*), 9.6 oz. ... | 370 | 14.0 | 52.0 | 11.0 | 30 | 500 | 3.0 |
| w/out sauce, 7.6 oz. .. | 300 | 12.0 | 38.0 | 11.0 | 30 | 140 | 3.0 |
| and broccoli: | | | | | | | |
| (*Lean Cuisine Cafe*), 9 oz. ............ | 260 | 14.0 | 39.0 | 5.0 | 20 | 580 | 2.0 |
| (*Marie Callender's*), 13 oz. ........... | 400 | 22.0 | 52.0 | 14.0 | 45 | 1200 | 3.0 |
| (*Stouffer's Easy Express* ½ of 25-oz. pkg. ... | 350 | 18.0 | 57.0 | 6.0 | 25 | 1660 | 2.0 |
| (*Wanchai Ferry*), ½ of 24-oz. pkg. ....... | 390 | 18.0 | 68.0 | 6.0 | 10 | 1320 | 3.0 |
| w/rice (*Zatarain's*), 12 oz. ........... | 400 | 18.0 | 63.0 | 5.0 | 15 | 1260 | 2.0 |

| Food and Measure | cal. | prot. (gms) | carbo. (gms) | fat (gms) | chol. (mgs) | sod. (mgs) | fiber (gms) |
|---|---|---|---|---|---|---|---|
| **Beef entree, frozen** *(cont.)* | | | | | | | |
| chipped, creamed (*Stouffer's*), ½ of 11-oz. pkg. ......... | 140 | 9.0 | 9.0 | 7.0 | 35 | 590 | 0 |
| chow fun (*Lean Cuisine Cafe*), 9 oz. .... | 320 | 15.0 | 54.0 | 5.0 | 20 | 520 | 3.0 |
| country fried (*Marie Callender's*), 15 oz. ... | 550 | 18.0 | 54.0 | 29.0 | 65 | 1330 | 7.0 |
| fajita steak (*Healthy Choice*), 12.3 oz. .... | 360 | 17.0 | 56.0 | 6.0 | 40 | 590 | 7.0 |
| fried steak (*Banquet*), 10 oz. ............. | 390 | 14.0 | 43.0 | 18.0 | 25 | 1030 | 5.0 |
| Hunan stir-fry w/ (*Lean Cuisine Spa Cuisine*), 8.5 oz. ..... | 260 | 17.0 | 37.0 | 5.0 | 20 | 490 | 5.0 |
| lo mein (*Birds Eye Voila!*), 1 cup* ...... | 230 | 12.0 | 37.0 | 3.0 | 25 | 1120 | 2.0 |
| Merlot (*Healthy Choice Café Steamers*), 10.6 oz. .. | 230 | 17.0 | 21.0 | 8.0 | 35 | 500 | 5.0 |
| Mongolian (*Contessa On the Stove*), ⅓ pkg.: | | | | | | | |
| w/sauce, 8 oz. ........ | 310 | 13.0 | 48.0 | 7.0 | 25 | 680 | 2.0 |
| w/out sauce ......... | 220 | 12.0 | 35.0 | 3.5 | 25 | 140 | 2.0 |
| orange (*Contessa On the Stove*), 9.6 oz. ... | 410 | 13.0 | 64.0 | 12.0 | 25 | 550 | 3.0 |
| w/out sauce, 8 oz. ... | 320 | 12.0 | 48.0 | 9.0 | 25 | 130 | 3.0 |
| patty: | | | | | | | |
| grilled (*Banquet Homestyle*), 8 oz. .. | 280 | 12.0 | 23.0 | 15.0 | 35 | 860 | 2.0 |
| smothered, cheesy (*Banquet*), 7.1 oz. . | 310 | 13.0 | 30.0 | 16.0 | 35 | 1160 | 3.0 |
| smothered, zesty (*Banquet*), 8.5 oz. . | 300 | 11.0 | 30.0 | 15.0 | 25 | 860 | 4.0 |
| pepper steak: | | | | | | | |
| green (*Stouffer's*), 10.5 oz. ......... | 240 | 18.0 | 32.0 | 4.0 | 30 | 910 | 3.0 |
| and rice (*Michelina's*), 8 oz. ............. | 260 | 9.0 | 46.0 | 4.0 | 15 | 690 | 2.0 |
| pineapple teriyaki (*Smart Ones Fruit Inspirations*), 9 oz. ... | 260 | 16.0 | 40.0 | 5.0 | 25 | 620 | 2.0 |
| portobello (*Lean Cuisine Cafe*), 9 oz. ... | 210 | 15.0 | 24.0 | 6.0 | 30 | 580 | 2.0 |

| Food and Measure | cal. | prot. (gms) | carbo. (gms) | fat (gms) | chol. (mgs) | sod. (mgs) | fiber (gms) |
|---|---|---|---|---|---|---|---|
| pot pie: | | | | | | | |
| (*Banquet*), 7 oz. ..... | 300 | 12.0 | 36.0 | 22.0 | 25 | 1010 | 3.0 |
| (*Marie Callender's*), | | | | | | | |
| 1 cup .......... | 510 | 14.0 | 48.0 | 29.0 | 25 | 780 | 3.0 |
| (*Pacific* Organic), 1 cup | 410 | 17.0 | 40.0 | 21.0 | 80 | 660 | 6.0 |
| pot roast: | | | | | | | |
| (*Banquet*), 9.6 oz. .... | 170 | 13.0 | 19.0 | 5.0 | 20 | 860 | 5.0 |
| (*Boston Market* | | | | | | | |
| Dinner), 16 oz. .... | 440 | 27.0 | 40.0 | 19.0 | 65 | 1520 | 5.0 |
| (*Healthy Choice*), | | | | | | | |
| 11 oz. .......... | 290 | 17.0 | 45.0 | 4.5 | 40 | 500 | 6.0 |
| (*Lean Cuisine*), 9 oz. .. | 210 | 14.0 | 26.0 | 6.0 | 25 | 550 | 3.0 |
| (*Marie Callender's*), | | | | | | | |
| 15 oz. .......... | 260 | 20.0 | 31.0 | 6.0 | 45 | 1130 | 7.0 |
| (*Smart Ones*), 9 oz. .. | 180 | 17.0 | 18.0 | 5.0 | 25 | 670 | 4.0 |
| (*Stouffer's*), 16 oz. ... | 320 | 20.0 | 41.0 | 8.0 | 30 | 1570 | 8.0 |
| Yankee (*Stouffer's* | | | | | | | |
| *Easy Express* Skillets), | | | | | | | |
| ½ of 24-oz. pkg. .... | 300 | 18.0 | 38.0 | 8.0 | 40 | 930 | 4.0 |
| roast, in gravy (*Smart* | | | | | | | |
| *Ones*), 9 oz. ........ | 230 | 16.0 | 18.0 | 11.0 | 40 | 530 | 2.0 |
| roasted, slow (*Marie* | | | | | | | |
| *Callender's*), 14.5 oz. . | 330 | 20.0 | 37.0 | 12.0 | 45 | 1320 | 7.0 |
| Salisbury steak: | | | | | | | |
| (*Banquet*), 9.5 oz. ..... | 290 | 1.0 | 25.0 | 16.0 | 30 | 1100 | 4.0 |
| (*Boston Market* | | | | | | | |
| Dinner), 16 oz. .... | 710 | 34.0 | 53.0 | 40.0 | 95 | 1760 | 5.0 |
| (*Healthy Choice* | | | | | | | |
| Complete Homestyle), | | | | | | | |
| 12.5 oz. .......... | 310 | 18.0 | 46.0 | 6.0 | 35 | 590 | 9.0 |
| (*Healthy Choice* | | | | | | | |
| Select), 8 oz. ...... | 190 | 14.0 | 18.0 | 6.0 | 30 | 520 | 5.0 |
| (*Lean Cuisine* | | | | | | | |
| Dinnertime Cuisine), | | | | | | | |
| 15.5 oz. .......... | 270 | 19.0 | 27.0 | 9.0 | 45 | 650 | 5.0 |
| (*Marie Callender's*), | | | | | | | |
| 14 oz. ........... | 370 | 24.0 | 35.0 | 15.0 | 60 | 1040 | 5.0 |
| (*Michelina's*), 8 oz. ... | 330 | 11.0 | 25.0 | 18.0 | 40 | 1010 | 2.0 |
| (*Michelina's Lean* | | | | | | | |
| *Gourmet*), 8 oz. ... | 190 | 11.0 | 23.0 | 6.0 | 35 | 760 | 2.0 |
| (*Smart Ones*), 9 oz. .. | 200 | 20.0 | 12.0 | 7.0 | 55 | 740 | 4.0 |
| (*Smart Ones*), 9.5 oz. . | 280 | 18.0 | 33.0 | 9.0 | 40 | 840 | 3.0 |
| (*Stouffer's*), 9.63 oz. .. | 360 | 25.0 | 22.0 | 19.0 | 50 | 1160 | 2.0 |
| (*Stouffer's*), 16 oz. ... | 630 | 39.0 | 41.0 | 34.0 | 100 | 1674 | 3.0 |

| Food and Measure | cal. | prot. (gms) | carbo. (gms) | fat (gms) | chol. (mgs) | sod. (mgs) | fiber (gms) |
|---|---|---|---|---|---|---|---|
| **Beef entree, frozen, Salisbury steak** *(cont.)* | | | | | | | |
| and gravy (*Banquet Family*), 1 pc. w/gravy | 180 | 9.0 | 9.0 | 13.0 | 25 | 710 | 2.0 |
| w/mac and cheese (*Lean Cuisine Comfort*), 9.5 oz. .. | 260 | 23.0 | 23.0 | 8.0 | 40 | 540 | 3.0 |
| shepherd's pie (*Blake's Organic*), 8 oz. ...... | 240 | 14.0 | 26.0 | 9.0 | 30 | 520 | 2.0 |
| sirloin, roasted (*Michelina's Lean Gourmet Supreme*), 8 oz. ..... | 230 | 13.0 | 34.0 | 5.0 | 15 | 950 | 2.0 |
| sliced (*Banquet*), 7.4 oz. . | 270 | 14.0 | 36.0 | 8.0 | 40 | 960 | 1.0 |
| steak: | | | | | | | |
| country fried (*Boston Market* Dinner), 13 oz. ........... | 540 | 24.0 | 51.0 | 27.0 | 60 | 910 | 5.0 |
| grilled whiskey (*Healthy Choice Café Steamers*), 9.5 oz. .......... | 250 | 18.0 | 34.0 | 4.0 | 30 | 580 | 6.0 |
| w/potatoes (*Boston Market*), 9.5 oz. ... | 290 | 17.0 | 29.0 | 12.0 | 40 | 1200 | 2.0 |
| and noodles (*Boston Market* Dinner), 14 oz. ........... | 460 | 29.0 | 58.0 | 12.0 | 70 | 960 | 4.0 |
| teriyaki (*Stouffer's Easy Express*), ½ of 23.5-oz. pkg. . | 310 | 17.0 | 49.0 | 5.0 | 25 | 1090 | 6.0 |
| steak tips: | | | | | | | |
| bourbon (*Stouffer's*), 14 oz. ........... | 490 | 22.0 | 61.0 | 17.0 | 40 | 1170 | 3.0 |
| Dijon (*Lean Cuisine Dinnertime Cuisine*), 12 oz. ........... | 280 | 18.0 | 35.0 | 7.0 | 30 | 600 | 5.0 |
| portobello (*Lean Cuisine Cafe*), 7.5 oz. | 160 | 15.0 | 10.0 | 7.0 | 40 | 450 | 3.0 |
| stew (*Contessa MicroSteam*), 1 cup* . | 190 | 11.0 | 19.0 | 8.0* | 25 | 660 | 3.0 |
| stir-fry (*Contessa On the Stove*), ⅓ pkg.: | | | | | | | |
| w/sauce, 8 oz. ....... | 180 | 15.0 | 23.0 | 3.0 | 35 | 700 | 4.0 |
| w/out sauce ........ | 120 | 13.0 | 11.0 | 3.0 | 35 | 260 | 4.0 |
| Stroganoff: | | | | | | | |
| (*Stouffer's*), 9.75 oz. ... | 380 | 22.0 | 34.0 | 17.0 | 70 | 990 | 2.0 |

| Food and Measure | cal. | prot. (gms) | carbo. (gms) | fat (gms) | chol. (mgs) | sod. (mgs) | fiber (gms) |
|---|---|---|---|---|---|---|---|
| (*Zatarain's*), 10 oz. . . . | 360 | 16.0 | 37.0 | 15.0 | 15 | 1530 | 2.0 |
| teriyaki, pineapple | | | | | | | |
| (*Smart Ones*), 9 oz. . . | 260 | 16.0 | 40.0 | 5.0 | 25 | 620 | 2.0 |
| tips: | | | | | | | |
| (*Marie Callender's*), | | | | | | | |
| 13.5 oz. . . . . . . . . | 310 | 16.0 | 44.0 | 36.0 | 35 | 880 | 3.0 |
| portobello (*Healthy* | | | | | | | |
| *Choice*), 11.25 oz. . | 270 | 18.0 | 34.0 | 7.0 | 45 | 600 | 5.0 |
| and vegetables: | | | | | | | |
| (*Stouffer's Easy* | | | | | | | |
| *Express* Skillets), | | | | | | | |
| ½ of 25-oz. pkg. . . . | 340 | 21.0 | 37.0 | 12.0 | 40 | 1180 | 6.0 |
| Asian (*Smart Ones*), | | | | | | | |
| 9 oz. . . . . . . . . . . . | 220 | 17.0 | 27.0 | 5.0 | 30 | 550 | 3.0 |
| **Beef entree, microwave**, | | | | | | | |
| 10-oz. cont., except | | | | | | | |
| as noted: | | | | | | | |
| (*Hormel Compleats* | | | | | | | |
| Homestyle) . . . . . . . . | 220 | 11.0 | 30.0 | 6.0 | 15 | 600 | 3.0 |
| pot roast, w/potato, | | | | | | | |
| carrots (*Hormel* | | | | | | | |
| *Compleats*) . . . . . . . . | 270 | 24.0 | 29.0 | 6.0 | 50 | 1470 | 3.0 |
| roast, w/gravy, potato | | | | | | | |
| (*Hormel Compleats*) . . | 220 | 22.0 | 27.0 | 3.0 | 50 | 830 | 3.0 |
| Salisbury steak | | | | | | | |
| (*Hormel Compleats*) . . | 280 | 16.0 | 30.0 | 11.0 | 50 | 980 | 2.0 |
| steak: | | | | | | | |
| and peppers (*Hormel* | | | | | | | |
| *Compleats*) . . . . . . . | 210 | 20.0 | 22.0 | 5.0 | 50 | 580 | 2.0 |
| portobello (*Healthy* | | | | | | | |
| *Choice Fresh* | | | | | | | |
| *Mixers*), 7.6 oz. . . . | 290 | 16.0 | 42.0 | 6.0 | 15 | 600 | 5.0 |
| tips (*Hormel Compleats*) | 270 | 17.0 | 29.0 | 9.0 | 45 | 800 | 2.0 |
| stew: | | | | | | | |
| (*Dinty Moore* Cup), | | | | | | | |
| 7.5 oz. . . . . . . . . . | 150 | 10.0 | 15.0 | 6.0 | 25 | 890 | 2.0 |
| (*Hormel* Microcup), | | | | | | | |
| 7.5 oz. . . . . . . . . . | 150 | 10.0 | 15.0 | 6.0 | 25 | 890 | 2.0 |
| (*Hormel Compleats*) . . | 250 | 15.0 | 22.0 | 11.0 | 45 | 1300 | 2.0 |
| Szechwan (*Healthy* | | | | | | | |
| *Choice Fresh* | | | | | | | |
| *Mixers*), 6.9 oz. . . . . . | 370 | 14.0 | 65.0 | 6.0 | 15 | 600 | 4.0 |
| **Beef entree mix**, see | | | | | | | |
| "Hamburger entree mix" | | | | | | | |

| Food and Measure | cal. | prot. (gms) | carbo. (gms) | fat (gms) | chol. (mgs) | sod. (mgs) | fiber (gms) |
|---|---|---|---|---|---|---|---|
| **Beef gravy**, ¼ cup: | | | | | | | |
| (*Campbell's*) .......... | 25 | 1.0 | 3.0 | 1.0 | 5 | 270 | 0 |
| (*Campbell's* Fat Free) ... | 20 | 1.0 | 3.0 | 0 | 0 | 300 | 0 |
| (*Franco-American* | | | | | | | |
| Slow Roast) ........ | 25 | 1.0 | 3.0 | .5 | 5 | 310 | 0 |
| (*Heinz* Home Style | | | | | | | |
| Savory) ............ | 30 | 1.0 | 4.0 | 1.0 | <5 | 380 | 0 |
| (*Imagine* Organic) ...... | 20 | 0 | 4.0 | 0 | 0 | 240 | 0 |
| **Beef hash**, canned: | | | | | | | |
| corned beef: | | | | | | | |
| (*Armour*), 1 cup ..... | 440 | 19.0 | 23.0 | 30.0 | 100 | 840 | 2.0 |
| (*Mary Kitchen*), 1 cup . | 390 | 21.0 | 22.0 | 24.0 | 80 | 1000 | 2.0 |
| (*Mary Kitchen*), 7.5 oz. | 350 | 18.0 | 20.0 | 22.0 | 70 | 900 | 2.0 |
| (*Mary Kitchen* Less | | | | | | | |
| Fat), 1 cup ....... | 290 | 21.0 | 24.0 | 12.0 | 60 | 1070 | 2.0 |
| (*Libby's*), 1 cup ...... | 420 | 19.0 | 33.0 | 24.0 | 55 | 1230 | 3.0 |
| roast beef (*Mary* | | | | | | | |
| *Kitchen*), 1 cup ...... | 390 | 21.0 | 22.0 | 24.0 | 70 | 790 | 2.0 |
| **Beef jerky/stick**, 1 oz.: | | | | | | | |
| (*Matador* Original | | | | | | | |
| Jerky) ............. | 80 | 1.0 | 6.0 | 1.5 | 30 | 610 | 0 |
| (*Matador* Original | | | | | | | |
| Snack Stick) ........ | 150 | 6.0 | 2.0 | 13.0 | 30 | 420 | 0 |
| (*Pemmican* Original) .... | 80 | 13.0 | 5.0 | .5 | 25 | 650 | 1.0 |
| hot/spicy (*Pemmican*) ... | 80 | 11.0 | 5.0 | 2.0 | 20 | 390 | 0 |
| mesquite (*Pemmican* | | | | | | | |
| Brisket) ............ | 90 | 12.0 | 6.0 | 1.5 | 35 | 530 | 0 |
| mild (*Matador* Snack | | | | | | | |
| Stick) ............. | 150 | 6.0 | 2.0 | 13.0 | 30 | 420 | 0 |
| peppered (*Pemmican*) ... | 80 | 12.0 | 5.0 | .5 | 25 | 560 | 1.0 |
| teriyaki: | | | | | | | |
| (*Matador* Jerky) ..... | 90 | 11.0 | 7.0 | 1.5 | 30 | 760 | 0 |
| (*Pemmican*) ........ | 80 | 13.0 | 5.0 | .5 | 25 | 790 | 1.0 |
| **Beef lunch meat** (see | | | | | | | |
| also "Bologna" and | | | | | | | |
| "Pastrami"), 2 oz., | | | | | | | |
| except as noted: | | | | | | | |
| corned: | | | | | | | |
| (*Black Bear*) ........ | 60 | 10.0 | 2.0 | 1.5 | 30 | 550 | 0 |
| (*Black Bear* Brisket) .. | 90 | 9.0 | 2.0 | 5.0 | 35 | 550 | 0 |
| (*Boar's Head* First | | | | | | | |
| Cut Brisket) ...... | 80 | 12.0 | 0 | 4.0 | 40 | 460 | 0 |
| (*Boar's Head* Top | | | | | | | |
| Round) .......... | 80 | 14.0 | 0 | 2.5 | 30 | 490 | 0 |

| Food and Measure | cal. | prot. (gms) | carbo. (gms) | fat (gms) | chol. (mgs) | sod. (mgs) | fiber (gms) |
|---|---|---|---|---|---|---|---|
| (*Di Lusso*) | 90 | 10.0 | 0 | 6.0 | 30 | 620 | 0 |
| (*Hebrew National*) | 80 | 13.0 | 1.0 | 3.5 | 35 | 520 | 0 |
| (*Thumann's* Cap/ Capless) | 70 | 14.0 | 0 | 1.5 | 30 | 560 | 0 |
| (*Thumann's* Bottom Round) | 80 | 14.0 | 0 | 3.0 | 30 | 520 | 0 |
| (*Thumann's* Brisket/ Top Round) | 70 | 14.0 | 0 | 2.0 | 32 | 500 | 0 |
| London broil: | | | | | | | |
| (*Black Bear*) | 60 | 12.0 | 0 | 1.5 | 30 | 390 | 0 |
| (*Thumann's*) | 100 | 13.0 | 0 | 3.0 | 32 | 400 | 0 |
| peppered eye round: | | | | | | | |
| (*Applegate Farms*) | 80 | 12.0 | 0 | 3.0 | 30 | 200 | 0 |
| (*Boar's Head*) | 90 | 14.0 | 0 | 3.0 | 40 | 190 | 0 |
| roast/roasted: | | | | | | | |
| (*Applegate Farms* Deli Counter) | 80 | 12.0 | 0 | 3.0 | 30 | 200 | 0 |
| (*Applegate Farms* Natural/Organic) | 80 | 12.0 | 0 | 3.0 | 35 | 320 | 0 |
| (*Black Bear*) | 60 | 12.0 | 0 | 1.5 | 30 | 290 | 0 |
| (*Black Bear* Choice) | 80 | 12.0 | 0 | 3.5 | 30 | 240 | 0 |
| (*Black Bear* Eye Round) | 70 | 12.0 | 0 | 2.0 | 30 | 390 | 0 |
| (*Boar's Head* All Natural) | 80 | 14.0 | 0 | 2.0 | 35 | 140 | 0 |
| (*Boar's Head* No Salt) | 90 | 14.0 | 0 | 3.5 | 30 | 40 | 0 |
| (*Boar's Head* Top Round Cap-Off) | 80 | 15.0 | <1.0 | 2.5 | 30 | 80 | 0 |
| (*Boar's Head* Londonport) | 80 | 14.0 | 2.0 | 2.0 | 40 | 350 | 0 |
| (*Hormel Natural Choice*) | 60 | 11.0 | 0 | 2.0 | 25 | 520 | 0 |
| (*Thumann's* Capless) | 70 | 14.0 | 0 | 1.5 | 20 | 160 | 0 |
| (*Thumann's* Ripple/ Top Round) | 80 | 14.0 | 0 | 3.0 | 30 | 150 | 0 |
| Cajun (*Boar's Head*) | 80 | 14.0 | 0 | 2.0 | 35 | 260 | 0 |
| Cajun (*Di Lusso*) | 80 | 11.0 | 0 | 4.0 | 30 | 370 | 0 |
| Cajun (*Thumann's*) | 100 | 12.0 | 0 | 2.5 | 32 | 250 | 0 |
| Italian (*Black Bear*) | 60 | 12.0 | 0 | 1.5 | 30 | 390 | 0 |
| Italian (*Boar's Head*) | 80 | 12.0 | 1.0 | 2.0 | 40 | 370 | 0 |
| Italian (*Di Lusso*) | 80 | 13.0 | 0 | 3.0 | 35 | 160 | 0 |
| Italian (*Thumann's*) | 100 | 13.0 | 0 | 4.0 | 38 | 400 | 0 |
| seasoned (*Di Lusso*) | 80 | 12.0 | 0 | 3.0 | 30 | 210 | 0 |

| Food and Measure | cal. | prot. (gms) | carbo. (gms) | fat (gms) | chol. (mgs) | sod. (mgs) | fiber (gms) |
|---|---|---|---|---|---|---|---|
| **Beef lunch meat, roast/roasted** *(cont.)* | | | | | | | |
| seasoned (*Di Lusso* Rare) . . . . . . . . . . | 80 | 12.0 | 0 | 4.0 | 35 | 250 | 0 |
| Slow-roasted (*Oscar Mayer*), 1.8 oz. . . . . | 60 | 10.0 | 0 | 2.0 | 30 | 530 | 0 |
| **"Beef" lunch meat, vegetarian** (*Yves*), 4 slices, 2.2 oz. . . . . . . | 110 | 15.0 | 4.0 | 2.0 | 0 | 360 | 1.0 |
| **Beef sandwich** (see also "Melts" and "Panini"), frozen, 1 pc., except as noted: | | | | | | | |
| w/cheddar (*Oscar Mayer Deli Creations*), 7.2 oz. . . . . . . . . . . . | 430 | 28.0 | 47.0 | 16.0 | 60 | 1560 | 5.0 |
| cheeseburgers, mini (*Smart Ones*), ½ of 12-oz. pkg. . . . . . . . . | 200 | 10.0 | 20.0 | 9.0 | 25 | 360 | 3.0 |
| pepper jack/focaccia (*Oscar Mayer Deli Creations*), 6 oz. . . . . . | 430 | 22.0 | 45.0 | 18.0 | 50 | 910 | 2.0 |
| Philly steak/cheese sub (*Stouffer's Corner Bistro*), 6 oz. . . | 370 | 20.0 | 39.0 | 16.0 | 40 | 550 | 3.0 |
| roast beef/cheddar sub (*Stouffer's Corner Bistro*), 6 oz. . . | 380 | 20.0 | 40.0 | 16.0 | 30 | 880 | 3.0 |
| **Beef sausage**, see "Sausage" and specific listings | | | | | | | |
| **Beef seasoning mix**: | | | | | | | |
| and broccoli, Asian (*Lawry's*), 1 tbsp. . . . | 25 | <1.0 | 5.0 | 0 | 0 | 360 | 0 |
| burger (*McCormick All-American*), 1 tsp. . . | 15 | 0 | 3.0 | 0 | 0 | 470 | 0 |
| pot roast: | | | | | | | |
| (*McCormick Slow Cookers*), 2 tsp. . . . | 10 | 0 | 2.0 | 0 | 0 | 460 | 0 |
| (*McCormick Bag 'n Season*), 1 tsp. . . | 10 | 0 | 1.0 | 0 | 0 | 400 | 0 |
| stew: | | | | | | | |
| (*Adolph's Meal Makers*), 1 tbsp. . . . | 20 | <1.0 | 4.0 | 0 | 0 | 710 | 0 |
| (*Lawry's*), 1 tsp. . . . . . | 10 | 0 | 2.0 | 0 | 0 | 500 | 0 |

| Food and Measure | cal. | prot. (gms) | carbo. (gms) | fat (gms) | chol. (mgs) | sod. (mgs) | fiber (gms) |
|---|---|---|---|---|---|---|---|
| (*McCormick*), 2 tsp. . . | 15 | 0 | 2.0 | 0 | 0 | 480 | 0 |
| (*McCormick* Slow Cookers), 2 tsp. . . . | 15 | <1.0 | 2.0 | 0 | 0 | 650 | 0 |
| (*McCormick Bag 'n Season*), 2 tsp. . . . . | 10 | <1.0 | 2.0 | 0 | 0 | 500 | 0 |
| Stroganoff: | | | | | | | |
| (*Lawry's*), 1 tbsp. . . . . | 20 | 0 | 5.0 | 0 | 0 | 520 | 0 |
| (*McCormick*), 1 tbsp. . | 20 | <1.0 | 4.0 | 0 | 0 | 500 | 0 |
| (*McCormick* Slow Cookers), 1 tsp. . . . | 10 | 0 | 2.0 | 0 | 0 | 460 | 0 |
| Swiss steak (*McCormick Bag 'n Season*), 1 tsp. | 15 | 0 | 3.0 | 0 | 0 | 500 | 0 |
| **Beef spread**, roast (*Underwood*), ¼ cup . | 130 | 8.0 | 2.0 | 10.0 | 30 | 370 | 0 |
| **Beef stew**, see "Beef entree" | | | | | | | |
| **Beefalo**, meat only, roasted, 4 oz. . . . . . . . | 213 | 34.8 | 0 | 7.2 | 66 | 93 | 0 |
| **Beer**, 12 fl. oz.: | | | | | | | |
| regular . . . . . . . . . . . . . | 146 | .9 | 13.2 | 0 | 0 | 19 | 0 |
| light . . . . . . . . . . . . . . . . | 100 | .7 | 4.8 | 0 | 0 | 10 | 0 |
| **Beerwurst**, pork and beef, 2 oz. . . . . . . . . . | 155 | 7.8 | 2.4 | 12.6 | 35 | 410 | .5 |
| **Beet**, fresh: | | | | | | | |
| raw: | | | | | | | |
| (*Frieda's*), ½ cup, 3 oz. . . . . . . . . . . | 35 | 1.0 | 8.0 | 0 | 0 | 65 | 2.0 |
| 2 medium, 2" diam. . . | 70 | 2.6 | 15.6 | .3 | 0 | 126 | 4.6 |
| trimmed, sliced, ½ cup . . . . . . . . . . | 29 | 1.1 | 6.5 | .1 | 0 | 53 | 1.9 |
| boiled, drained: | | | | | | | |
| 2 medium, 2" diam. . . | 44 | 1.7 | 10.0 | .2 | 0 | 77 | 1.7 |
| sliced, ½ cup . . . . . . . | 38 | 1.4 | 8.5 | .2 | 0 | 65 | 1.4 |
| **Beet, can/jar**, ½ cup, except as noted: | | | | | | | |
| whole (*Freshlike*), 3 small, 4.4 oz. . . . . . . | 40 | 1.0 | 9.0 | 0 | 0 | 240 | 2.0 |
| sliced: | | | | | | | |
| (*Del Monte*) . . . . . . . . | 35 | 1.0 | 8.0 | 0 | 0 | 290 | 2.0 |
| (*Freshlike* Small) . . . . . | 35 | 1.0 | 9.0 | 0 | 0 | 230 | 2.0 |
| (*Veg-All*) . . . . . . . . . . | 40 | <1.0 | 8.0 | 0 | 0 | 300 | 1.0 |
| or julienne (*S&W*) . . . . | 35 | 1.0 | 8.0 | 0 | 0 | 290 | 2.0 |
| Harvard (*Greenwood* Sweet & Tangy) . . . . . | 100 | 1.0 | 27.0 | 0 | 0 | 370 | 1.0 |

| Food and Measure | cal. | prot. (gms) | carbo. (gms) | fat (gms) | chol. (mgs) | sod. (mgs) | fiber (gms) |
|---|---|---|---|---|---|---|---|
| **Beet, can/jar** *(cont.)* | | | | | | | |
| pickled: | | | | | | | |
| whole (*Roland*) . . . . . . | 30 | 2.0 | 5.0 | 0 | 0 | 650 | 2.0 |
| whole or sliced | | | | | | | |
| (*Greenwood*), 1 oz. | 25 | 0 | 6.0 | 0 | 0 | 100 | 0 |
| sliced (*Del Monte*) . . . | 80 | 1.0 | 19.0 | 0 | 0 | 380 | 2.0 |
| sliced (*Freshlike*), | | | | | | | |
| 4 pcs., 1 oz. . . . . . . | 20 | 0 | 4.0 | 0 | 0 | 20 | 0 |
| sliced (*S&W*), 1 oz. . . . | 15 | 0 | 4.0 | 0 | 0 | 50 | 1.0 |
| **Beet greens**, ½ cup: | | | | | | | |
| raw, 1" pcs. . . . . . . . . . . | 4 | .4 | .8 | <.1 | 0 | 38 | .7 |
| boiled, drained, 1" pcs. . . | 20 | 1.9 | 3.9 | .1 | 0 | 173 | 2.1 |
| **Bellini drink mixer**, | | | | | | | |
| peach (*Stirrings*), | | | | | | | |
| 1 fl. oz. . . . . . . . . . . . . | 30 | 0 | 8.0 | 0 | 0 | 0 | 0 |
| **Berliner**, pork and | | | | | | | |
| beef, 1 oz. . . . . . . . . . | 65 | 4.3 | .7 | 4.9 | 13 | 368 | 0 |
| **Berries, mixed, dried**, | | | | | | | |
| 1.4 oz., ¼ cup, | | | | | | | |
| except as noted: | | | | | | | |
| (*Mariani* Berries 'N | | | | | | | |
| Apples), ⅓ cup . . . . . . | 130 | 0 | 32.0 | 0 | 0 | 30 | 2.0 |
| (*Mariani* Berries 'N | | | | | | | |
| Cherries), ⅓ cup . . . . . | 130 | 1.0 | 31.0 | 0 | 0 | 10 | 2.0 |
| (*Sunsweet* Blend) . . . . . . | 120 | 1.0 | 32.0 | 0 | 0 | 5 | 3.0 |
| (*Welch's* Medley) . . . . . . | 135 | 1.0 | 32.0 | 0 | 0 | 5 | 1.0 |
| w/green tea extract | | | | | | | |
| (*Mariani* Defense) . . . . | 130 | 1.0 | 31.0 | 0 | 0 | 0 | 3.0 |
| w/omega-3 (*Mariani* | | | | | | | |
| Thrive) . . . . . . . . . . . . | 140 | 1.0 | 32.0 | 0 | 0 | 0 | 2.0 |
| w/prunes (*Sunsweet* | | | | | | | |
| Antioxidant) . . . . . . . . | 130 | 1.0 | 31.0 | 0 | 0 | 5 | 1.0 |
| **Berries, mixed, frozen**, | | | | | | | |
| 1 cup, except as | | | | | | | |
| noted: | | | | | | | |
| (*Birds Eye/C&W* | | | | | | | |
| Medley), 1¼ cup . . . . | 70 | 1.0 | 16.0 | 0 | 0 | 20 | 6.0 |
| (*Cascadian Farm* | | | | | | | |
| Organic Harvest) . . . . | 60 | 1.0 | 17.0 | 0 | 0 | 0 | 4.0 |
| (*Dole Wildly Nutritious*) . | 70 | 0 | 17.0 | 0 | 0 | 0 | 5.0 |
| **Berry drink blend**, | | | | | | | |
| 8 fl. oz.: | | | | | | | |
| (*Bolthouse Farms* Berry | | | | | | | |
| Boost Smoothie) . . . . | 130 | 0 | 30.0 | 1.0 | 0 | 20 | 4.0 |

| Food and Measure | cal. | prot. (gms) | carbo. (gms) | fat (gms) | chol. (mgs) | sod. (mgs) | fiber (gms) |
|---|---|---|---|---|---|---|---|
| (*Bolthouse Farms Blue Goodness* Smoothie) . | 170 | 1.0 | 41.0 | 0 | 0 | 5 | 8.0 |
| (*Honest Tea* Organic Black Forest) ........ | 30 | 0 | 8.0 | 0 | 0 | 5 | 0 |
| (*SoBe Black & Blue Berry Brew*) ........ | 120 | 0 | 31.0 | 0 | 0 | 25 | 0 |
| (*Tropicana* Light) ....... | 10 | 0 | 2.0 | 0 | 0 | 25 | 0 |
| (*V8 Splash*) ............ | 70 | 0 | 18.0 | 0 | 0 | 50 | 0 |
| (*Welch's* Mountain) ..... | 140 | 0 | 34.0 | 0 | 0 | 20 | 0 |
| frozen* (*Chiquita* Smoothies) ......... | 120 | 0 | 28.0 | 0 | 0 | 40 | 0 |
| pineapple passion fruit (*Welch's*) .......... | 140 | 0 | 34.0 | 0 | 0 | 5 | 0 |
| punch: | | | | | | | |
| (*Minute Maid*) ....... | 120 | 0 | 32.0 | 0 | 0 | 15 | 0 |
| (*Tropicana*) ......... | 130 | 0 | 32.0 | 0 | 0 | 15 | 0 |
| frozen* (*Minute Maid*) ........... | 110 | 0 | 31.0 | 0 | 0 | 0 | 0 |
| **Berry juice blend**, 8 fl. oz., except as noted: | | | | | | | |
| (*After the Fall* Oregon) ... | 130 | 0 | 32.0 | 0 | 0 | 15 | 0 |
| (*Apple & Eve* Very), 6.75 fl. oz. ........ | 100 | 0 | 24.0 | 0 | 0 | 15 | 0 |
| (*Langers*) ............ | 120 | 0 | 30.0 | 0 | 0 | 15 | 0 |
| (*Minute Maid*), 10 fl. oz. . | 150 | 0 | 36.0 | 0 | 0 | 25 | 0 |
| (*Santa Cruz Organic* Nectar) ............ | 110 | <1.0 | 30.0 | 0 | 0 | 25 | 0 |
| **Berry topping**, triple (*Smucker's*), 2 tbsp. .. | 90 | 0 | 23.0 | 0 | 0 | 0 | 1.0 |
| **Bialy** (*Bell*), 2.5-oz. pc. .. | 180 | 7.0 | 38.0 | .5 | 0 | 240 | 3.0 |
| **Biryani paste**, see "Curry paste" | | | | | | | |
| **Biscuit**, plain or buttermilk, 2 oz. ..... | 206 | 3.5 | 27.5 | 9.4 | <1 | 596 | .7 |
| **Biscuit, frozen/chilled**, 1 pc., except as noted: | | | | | | | |
| (*Grands!* Extra Large Easy Split) ......... | 190 | 6.0 | 35.0 | 11.0 | 0 | 840 | <1.0 |
| (*Grands!* Flaky Layers Original Chilled) ..... | 180 | 3.0 | 25.0 | 8.0 | 0 | 540 | <1.0 |
| (*Grands!* Flaky Layers Original Frozen) ..... | 170 | 4.0 | 20.0 | 8.0 | 0 | 490 | 0 |

| Food and Measure | cal. | prot. (gms) | carbo. (gms) | fat (gms) | chol. (mgs) | sod. (mgs) | fiber (gms) |
|---|---|---|---|---|---|---|---|
| **Biscuit, frozen/chilled** *(cont.)* | | | | | | | |
| (*Grands!* Flaky Layers | | | | | | | |
| Reduced Fat) ....... | 160 | 4.0 | 26.0 | 6.0 | 0 | 570 | <1.0 |
| (*Grands!* Homestyle | | | | | | | |
| Original) ........... | 170 | 3.0 | 25.0 | 7.0 | 0 | 580 | <1.0 |
| (*Grands!* Homestyle | | | | | | | |
| Reduced Fat Wheat) .. | 170 | 3.0 | 29.0 | 5.0 | 0 | 580 | 2.0 |
| (*Grands! Butter Tastin'* | | | | | | | |
| Flaky Layers) ....... | 180 | 3.0 | 25.0 | 8.0 | 0 | 550 | <1.0 |
| (*Grands! Butter Tastin'* | | | | | | | |
| Frozen) ............ | 170 | 4.0 | 23.0 | 7.0 | 0 | 560 | <1.0 |
| (*Grands! Butter Tastin'* | | | | | | | |
| Homestyle) ......... | 180 | 3.0 | 25.0 | 8.0 | 0 | 580 | <1.0 |
| (*Grands!jr* Golden | | | | | | | |
| Layers Flaky) ....... | 100 | 2.0 | 14.0 | 4.0 | 0 | 360 | <1.0 |
| (*Grands!jr Butter Tastin'* | | | | | | | |
| Golden Homestyle) ... | 100 | 2.0 | 14.0 | 3.5 | 0 | 360 | 0 |
| (*Grands!jr Butter Tastin'* | | | | | | | |
| Golden Layers) ...... | 100 | 2.0 | 14.0 | 4.0 | 0 | 360 | <1.0 |
| (*Pillsbury* Country Value | | | | | | | |
| Pack), 3 pcs. ........ | 150 | 4.0 | 29.0 | 2.0 | 0 | 570 | 1.0 |
| (*Pillsbury* Flaky Layers | | | | | | | |
| Value Pack), 3 pcs. ... | 160 | 4.0 | 28.0 | 4.0 | 0 | 550 | 1.0 |
| buttermilk: | | | | | | | |
| (*Grands!* Flaky | | | | | | | |
| Layers Chilled) .... | 180 | 3.0 | 25.0 | 8.0 | 0 | 540 | <1.0 |
| (*Grands!* Flaky | | | | | | | |
| Layers Frozen) .... | 170 | 3.0 | 22.0 | 8.0 | 0 | 490 | <1.0 |
| (*Grands!* Homestyle) . | 180 | 3.0 | 25.0 | 7.0 | 0 | 580 | <1.0 |
| (*Grands!* Homestyle | | | | | | | |
| Reduced Fat) ..... | 160 | 3.0 | 25.0 | 5.0 | 0 | 590 | <1.0 |
| (*Grands!jr* Golden | | | | | | | |
| Homestyle) ....... | 100 | 2.0 | 14.0 | 3.5 | 0 | 360 | 0 |
| (*Grands!jr* Golden | | | | | | | |
| Layers) .......... | 100 | 2.0 | 14.0 | 4.0 | 0 | 360 | <1.0 |
| (*Pillsbury* Value Pack), | | | | | | | |
| 3 pcs. ............ | 150 | 4.0 | 29.0 | 2.0 | 0 | 570 | 1.0 |
| (*Sister Shubert's*), 2 pcs. | 210 | 3.0 | 24.0 | 11.0 | 5 | 500 | 1.0 |
| cheddar garlic (*Grands!*) . | 180 | 4.0 | 22.0 | 9.0 | <5 | 660 | <1.0 |
| honey butter: | | | | | | | |
| (*Grands!* Flaky Layers) | 180 | 3.0 | 26.0 | 7.0 | 0 | 450 | <1.0 |
| (*Grands!jr* Golden | | | | | | | |
| Layers) .......... | 110 | 2.0 | 15.0 | 4.0 | 0 | 290 | 0 |

| Food and Measure | cal. | prot. (gms) | carbo. (gms) | fat (gms) | chol. (mgs) | sod. (mgs) | fiber (gms) |
|---|---|---|---|---|---|---|---|
| Southern style: | | | | | | | |
| (*Grands!*) ......... | 170 | 4.0 | 23.0 | 7.0 | 0 | 550 | <1.0 |
| (*Grands!* Homestyle) . | 170 | 3.0 | 24.0 | 7.0 | 0 | 580 | <1.0 |
| **Biscuit mix** (see also | | | | | | | |
| "Baking mix" and | | | | | | | |
| "Roll mix"), 1/3 cup: | | | | | | | |
| buttermilk: | | | | | | | |
| (*Bob's Red Mill*) ..... | 130 | 5.0 | 28.0 | .5 | 0 | 450 | 3.0 |
| (*Bisquick* Complete) .. | 150 | 3.0 | 21.0 | 6.0 | 0 | 370 | <1.0 |
| (*"Jiffy"*) ............ | 160 | 3.0 | 27.0 | 5.0 | <5 | 420 | <1.0 |
| cheese, 3 (*Bisquick* | | | | | | | |
| Complete) .......... | 160 | 3.0 | 22.0 | 7.0 | 0 | 350 | <1.0 |
| cheese garlic: | | | | | | | |
| (*Bisquick* Complete) .. | 160 | 2.0 | 22.0 | 7.0 | 0 | 350 | <1.0 |
| (*Martha White* | | | | | | | |
| Quick & Easy) .... | 190 | 3.0 | 21.0 | 11.0 | 0 | 420 | 1.0 |
| honey butter (*Bisquick* | | | | | | | |
| Complete) .......... | 150 | 2.0 | 24.0 | 5.0 | 0 | 290 | <1.0 |
| **Bison**, meat only, 4 oz.: | | | | | | | |
| roasted ............. | 162 | 32.3 | 0 | 2.7 | 93 | 65 | 0 |
| ground, pan-broiled .... | 270 | 27.0 | 0 | 17.2 | 94 | 83 | 0 |
| **Bitter melon**, see | | | | | | | |
| "Balsam pear" | | | | | | | |
| **Bitters** (*Angostura*), | | | | | | | |
| 2 tbsp. ............ | 50 | 0 | 14.0 | 0 | 0 | 390 | 0 |
| **Black bean**, dried: | | | | | | | |
| (*Bob's Red Mill*), 1/4 cup . | 150 | 10.0 | 28.0 | 0 | 0 | 0 | 11.0 |
| boiled, 1/2 cup ......... | 113 | 7.6 | 20.4 | .5 | 0 | 1 | 7.5 |
| turtle: | | | | | | | |
| (*Eden* Organic), 1/4 cup . | 160 | 11.0 | 29.0 | .5 | 0 | 10 | 16.0 |
| boiled, 1/2 cup ....... | 120 | 7.5 | 22.4 | .3 | 0 | 3 | 4.9 |
| **Black bean, canned** | | | | | | | |
| (see also "Refried | | | | | | | |
| beans"), 1/2 cup: | | | | | | | |
| (*Allens*) ............. | 100 | 6.0 | 19.0 | .5 | 0 | 400 | 8.0 |
| (*Bush's*) ............ | 110 | 8.0 | 23.0 | .5 | 0 | 450 | 7.0 |
| (*Bush's* Reduced | | | | | | | |
| Sodium) .......... | 105 | 7.0 | 23.0 | .5 | 0 | 240 | 6.0 |
| (*Eden* Organic) ....... | 110 | 7.0 | 18.0 | 1.0 | 0 | 15 | 6.0 |
| (*Ortega*) ............ | 110 | 7.0 | 19.0 | 1.0 | 0 | 400 | 7.0 |
| (*Progresso*) .......... | 100 | 6.0 | 17.0 | .5 | 0 | 400 | 5.0 |
| (*Ranch Style*) ........ | 110 | 6.0 | 19.0 | .5 | 0 | 400 | 7.0 |
| (*Roland*) ............ | 120 | 8.0 | 21.0 | 0 | 0 | 430 | 6.0 |
| (*Rosarita*) ........... | 100 | 6.0 | 19.0 | .5 | 0 | 420 | 5.0 |

| Food and Measure | cal. | prot. (gms) | carbo. (gms) | fat (gms) | chol. (mgs) | sod. (mgs) | fiber (gms) |
|---|---|---|---|---|---|---|---|
| **Black bean, canned** *(cont.)* | | | | | | | |
| (*S&W*) . . . . . . . . . . . . . . | 100 | 6.0 | 17.0 | 1.0 | 0 | 380 | 6.0 |
| (*S&W* Less Salt) . . . . . . . | 120 | 8.0 | 22.0 | .5 | 0 | 180 | 5.0 |
| (*S&W* Organic) . . . . . . . . | 110 | 6.0 | 17.0 | 1.0 | 0 | 380 | 6.0 |
| Caribbean: | | | | | | | |
| (*Eden* Organic) . . . . . . | 90 | 7.0 | 20.0 | .5 | 0 | 135 | 7.0 |
| (*S&W*) . . . . . . . . . . | 110 | 6.0 | 18.0 | 1.0 | 0 | 550 | 7.0 |
| w/jalapeños (*Ortega*) . . . . | 110 | 6.0 | 18.0 | 1.5 | 0 | 450 | 4.0 |
| and rice (*Glory*) . . . . . . . . | 90 | 4.0 | 16.0 | 1.5 | 0 | 450 | 2.0 |
| seasoned: | | | | | | | |
| (*Allens*) . . . . . . . . . . . . | 200 | 12.0 | 37.0 | 1.0 | 0 | 380 | 15.0 |
| (*Bush's*) . . . . . . . . . . . | 110 | 8.0 | 23.0 | .5 | 0 | 450 | 7.0 |
| (*Glory* Sensibly) . . . . . | 100 | 6.0 | 18.0 | 0 | 0 | 220 | 4.0 |
| (*Trappey's*) . . . . . . . . . | 120 | 7.0 | 20.0 | 1.5 | 0 | 410 | 7.0 |
| **Black bean, microwave**, seasoned (*Old El Paso*), 1 cup . . . . . . | 130 | 6.0 | 26.0 | 3.0 | 0 | 430 | 8.0 |
| **Black bean flour** (*Bob's Red Mill* Stoneground), ¼ cup . . . . . . . . . . . . | 120 | 8.0 | 22.0 | 0 | 0 | 0 | 5.0 |
| **Black bean mix** (*Fantastic*), ¼ cup . . . | 130 | 7.0 | 22.0 | 1.5 | 0 | 230 | 10.0 |
| **Black bean pancake**, frozen (*Golden*), 1.3-oz. pc. . . . . . . . . . | 70 | 3.0 | 10.0 | 2.5 | 0 | 180 | 0 |
| **Black bean sauce**, see "Bean sauce" | | | | | | | |
| **Black currant drink**, 8 fl. oz. | | | | | | | |
| blend, yuzu (*SoBe Lifewater*) . . . . . . . . . | 40 | 0 | 17.0 | 0 | 0 | 20 | 0 |
| sparkling (*Kristian Regale*) . . . . . . . . . . . | 95 | 0 | 24.0 | 0 | 0 | 10 | 0 |
| **Black currant juice**, 8 fl. oz.: | | | | | | | |
| (*R.W. Knudsen* Organic Nectar) . . . . . | 110 | 0 | 27.0 | 0 | 0 | 15 | <1.0 |
| (*R.W. Knudsen* Just Black Currant) . . . . . . . | 100 | 1.0 | 15.0 | 0 | 0 | 5 | 0 |
| **Black pepper sauce**, see "Pepper sauce" | | | | | | | |
| **Blackberry**, fresh: | | | | | | | |
| (*Dole*), 1 cup . . . . . . . . . | 60 | 2.0 | 14.0 | 1.0 | 0 | 0 | 8.0 |
| ½ cup . . . . . . . . . . . . . . | 37 | .5 | 9.2 | .3 | 0 | tr. | 3.6 |

| Food and Measure | cal. | prot. (gms) | carbo. (gms) | fat (gms) | chol. (mgs) | sod. (mgs) | fiber (gms) |
|---|---|---|---|---|---|---|---|
| **Blackberry, dried** | | | | | | | |
| (*Frieda's* Marionberry), | | | | | | | |
| ⅓ cup, 1.4 oz. ....... | 98 | 0 | 32.0 | .5 | 0 | 0 | 2.0 |
| **Blackberry, frozen**: | | | | | | | |
| (*Cascadian Farm* | | | | | | | |
| Organic), 1 cup ...... | 80 | 1.0 | 22.0 | .5 | 0 | 0 | 7.0 |
| (*Dole*), 1 cup .......... | 90 | 2.0 | 22.0 | 0 | 0 | 0 | 7.0 |
| unsweetened, ½ cup .... | 49 | .9 | 11.8 | .3 | 0 | 1 | 3.8 |
| **Blackberry grape** | | | | | | | |
| **drink** (*SoBe* | | | | | | | |
| *Lifewater*), | | | | | | | |
| 8 fl. oz. ............ | 40 | 0 | 16.0 | 0 | 0 | 20 | 0 |
| **Black-eyed peas** (see | | | | | | | |
| also "Cowpeas"): | | | | | | | |
| dry (*Frieda's*), ¼ cup .... | 110 | 8.0 | 21.0 | 0 | 0 | 5 | 4.0 |
| mature, boiled, ½ cup ... | 100 | 6.7 | 17.9 | .5 | 0 | 3 | 5.6 |
| **Black-eyed peas,** | | | | | | | |
| **canned**, ½ cup: | | | | | | | |
| (*Allens Dry*) ........... | 110 | 7.0 | 18.0 | 1.0 | 0 | 275 | 4.0 |
| (*Allens/East Texas Fair*) .. | 120 | 7.0 | 21.0 | 1.0 | 0 | 350 | 6.0 |
| (*Bush's*) .............. | 100 | 5.0 | 15.0 | 0 | 0 | 480 | 3.0 |
| (*Eden* Organic) ........ | 90 | 6.0 | 16.0 | 1.0 | 0 | 25 | 4.0 |
| (*Glory*) .............. | 100 | 6.0 | 17.0 | .5 | 0 | 570 | 3.0 |
| w/bacon: | | | | | | | |
| (*Allens*) ............ | 120 | 7.0 | 20.0 | 1.5 | 0 | 390 | 5.0 |
| (*Bush's*) ........... | 95 | 6.0 | 17.0 | 1.5 | 0 | 370 | 3.0 |
| (*Ranch Style*) ....... | 100 | 6.0 | 20.0 | 0 | 0 | 520 | 3.0 |
| (*Trappey's*) ......... | 120 | 7.0 | 19.0 | 2.0 | 0 | 350 | 5.0 |
| jalapeño (*Bush's*) .... | 110 | 6.0 | 18.0 | 1.0 | 5 | 630 | 5.0 |
| jalapeño (*Trappey's*) .. | 110 | 6.0 | 19.0 | 2.0 | 0 | 470 | 5.0 |
| w/pork (*Sunshine*) ..... | 120 | 7.0 | 20.0 | 1.5 | 0 | 390 | 5.0 |
| and rice (*Glory*) ........ | 90 | 5.0 | 17.0 | .5 | 0 | 680 | 2.0 |
| seasoned: | | | | | | | |
| (*Allens*) ............ | 80 | 5.0 | 14.0 | .5 | 0 | 550 | 4.0 |
| (*Glory* Sensibly) ..... | 100 | 7.0 | 17.0 | 0 | 0 | 250 | 3.0 |
| w/snaps: | | | | | | | |
| (*Allens/East Texas* | | | | | | | |
| *Fair*) ............. | 120 | 8.0 | 20.0 | 1.0 | 0 | 420 | 5.0 |
| (*Bush's*) ........... | 70 | 5.0 | 15.0 | 0 | 0 | 470 | 3.0 |
| tomato/onion/jalapeños: | | | | | | | |
| (*Allens* Hoppin' John) . | 60 | 3.0 | 12.0 | 0 | 0 | 380 | 2.0 |
| Vidalia onion (*Allens* | | | | | | | |
| Hoppin' John) .... | 90 | 5.0 | 17.0 | .5 | 0 | 340 | 5.0 |

| Food and Measure | cal. | prot. (gms) | carbo. (gms) | fat (gms) | chol. (mgs) | sod. (mgs) | fiber (gms) |
|---|---|---|---|---|---|---|---|
| **Black-eyed peas,** | | | | | | | |
| **frozen**, ½ cup: | | | | | | | |
| (*McKenzie's*) . . . . . . . . . . | 120 | 8.0 | 22.0 | .5 | 0 | 20 | 5.0 |
| boiled, drained . . . . . . . . | 112 | 7.2 | 20.2 | .6 | 0 | 5 | 4.3 |
| **Blackened seasoning** | | | | | | | |
| (*Zatarain's*), ¼ tsp. . . . | 0 | 0 | 0 | 0 | 0 | 170 | 0 |
| **Blini**, mini (*Blinis &* | | | | | | | |
| *Crepes*), 3 pcs., .8 oz. . | 70 | 2.0 | 9.0 | 3.0 | 0 | 30 | 1.0 |
| **Blintzes**, frozen/chilled | | | | | | | |
| (*Golden*), 1 pc.: | | | | | | | |
| apple raisin . . . . . . . . . . . | 80 | 3.0 | 16.0 | 2.0 | 10 | 150 | 1.0 |
| blueberry . . . . . . . . . . . . . | 90 | 2.0 | 18.0 | 1.0 | 10 | 150 | 1.0 |
| cheese, chilled . . . . . . . . | 100 | 8.0 | 14.0 | 1.5 | 5 | 190 | <1.0 |
| cheese, frozen . . . . . . . . . | 80 | 6.0 | 13.0 | 2.0 | 15 | 135 | 2.0 |
| cherry . . . . . . . . . . . . . . . | 100 | 3.0 | 16.0 | 1.0 | 5 | 150 | 2.0 |
| potato . . . . . . . . . . . . . . . | 90 | 3.0 | 15.0 | 4.0 | 5 | 170 | 2.0 |
| spinach broccoli . . . . . . . | 120 | 3.0 | 16.0 | 5.0 | 15 | 200 | 1.0 |
| **Blood sausage**, 1 oz. . . . | 107 | 4.1 | .4 | 9.8 | 34 | n.a. | 0 |
| **Bloody Mary mixer:** | | | | | | | |
| (*Angostura*), 4 fl. oz. . . . . | 20 | 0 | 4.0 | 0 | 0 | 560 | 0 |
| (*Sacramento*), 8 fl. oz. . . | 60 | 2.0 | 13.0 | 0 | 0 | 930 | 3.0 |
| (*Stirrings*), 4 fl. oz. . . . . . | 40 | 0 | 10.0 | 0 | 0 | 750 | 1.0 |
| (*Tabasco*), 8 fl. oz. . . . . . . | 70 | 2.0 | 13.0 | 1.0 | 0 | 1480 | 2.0 |
| extra spicy (*Tabasco*), | | | | | | | |
| 8 fl. oz. . . . . . . . | 70 | 2.0 | 15.0 | 1.0 | 0 | 1930 | 2.0 |
| **Blue squash**, see | | | | | | | |
| "Australian blue squash" | | | | | | | |
| **Blueberry**, fresh, ½ cup . | 41 | .5 | 10.2 | .3 | 0 | 5 | 2.0 |
| **Blueberry, canned**, in | | | | | | | |
| heavy syrup, ½ cup . . | 113 | .8 | 28.2 | .4 | 0 | 4 | 1.9 |
| **Blueberry, dried,** | | | | | | | |
| ¼ cup, 1.4 oz.: | | | | | | | |
| (*Frieda's*) . . . . . . . . . . . . . | 140 | 1.0 | 33.0 | 0 | 0 | 0 | 4.0 |
| (*Sunsweet*) . . . . . . . . . . . | 140 | 1.0 | 33.0 | 0 | 0 | 0 | 3.0 |
| wild: | | | | | | | |
| (*Eden* Organic) . . . . . . | 150 | <1.0 | 35.0 | 0 | 0 | 15 | 5.0 |
| (*Hodgson Mill*) . . . . . . | 120 | 1.0 | 32.0 | 1.0 | 0 | 0 | 6.0 |
| (*Mariani*) . . . . . . . . . . . | 140 | 0 | 37.0 | 0 | 0 | 0 | 1.0 |
| **Blueberry, frozen:** | | | | | | | |
| (*Birds Eye/C&W*), | | | | | | | |
| 1¼ cup . . . . . . . . . . . . | 70 | 0 | 16.0 | 0 | 0 | 0 | 3.0 |
| (*Cascadian Farm* | | | | | | | |
| Organic), 1 cup . . . . . . | 70 | <1.0 | 17.0 | 1.0 | 0 | 0 | 4.0 |
| (*Dole*), 1 cup . . . . . . . . . | 70 | 0 | 17.0 | 1.0 | 0 | 0 | 4.0 |

| Food and Measure | cal. | prot. (gms) | carbo. (gms) | fat (gms) | chol. (mgs) | sod. (mgs) | fiber (gms) |
|---|---|---|---|---|---|---|---|
| (*Dole* Wild), 1 cup ...... | 70 | 0 | 16.0 | 0 | 0 | 15 | 6.0 |
| unsweetened, ½ cup .... | 40 | .3 | 9.4 | .5 | 0 | 1 | 2.1 |
| sweetened, ½ cup ...... | 94 | .5 | 25.2 | .2 | 0 | 2 | 2.4 |
| **Blueberry drink blend,** 8 fl. oz.: | | | | | | | |
| (*Ocean Spray* Cocktail) .. | 110 | 0 | 28.0 | 0 | 0 | 35 | 0 |
| cranberry (*Langers*) .... | 135 | 0 | 34.0 | 0 | 0 | 10 | 0 |
| pomegranate (*Ocean Spray*) ............ | 120 | 0 | 30.0 | 0 | 0 | 35 | 0 |
| **Blueberry glaze:** | | | | | | | |
| (*Marie's*), 2 tbsp. ....... | 40 | 0 | 10.0 | 0 | 0 | 35 | 0 |
| (*Marzetti*), 3 tbsp. ...... | 60 | 0 | 15.0 | 0 | 0 | 65 | 0 |
| **Blueberry juice,** 8 fl. oz.: | | | | | | | |
| (*After the Fall* Maine Coast) ............. | 120 | 0 | 31.0 | 0 | 0 | 15 | 0 |
| (*R.W. Knudsen* Nectar) .. | 110 | 0 | 28.0 | 0 | 0 | 15 | 0 |
| (*R.W. Knudsen Just Blueberry*) .......... | 100 | 0 | 24.0 | 0 | 0 | 10 | 0 |
| (*Simply Nutritious Vita Blueberry*) ...... | 120 | 0 | 30.0 | 0 | 0 | 10 | 0 |
| sparkling (*R.W. Knudsen*) ........... | 110 | 0 | 28.0 | 0 | 0 | 15 | 0 |
| **Blueberry juice blend,** 8 fl. oz.: | | | | | | | |
| acai: | | | | | | | |
| (*Northland*) ......... | 130 | 0 | 32.0 | 0 | 0 | 15 | 0 |
| (*Santa Cruz Organic*) . | 130 | 1.0 | 33.0 | 0 | 0 | 15 | 0 |
| blackberry (*Northland*) | 130 | 0 | 32.0 | 0 | 0 | 20 | 0 |
| banana (*Nantucket Nectars* Organic) ..... | 110 | 0 | 28.0 | 0 | 0 | 30 | 1.0 |
| pomegranate (*R.W. Knudsen* Organic) .... | 130 | 0 | 33.0 | 0 | 0 | 10 | 0 |
| **Blueberry juice concentrate** (*R.W. Knudsen*), 8 fl. oz.* .. | 100 | 0 | 24.0 | 0 | 0 | 10 | 0 |
| **Blueberry syrup** (*Maple Grove Farms*), ¼ cup . | 210 | 0 | 52.0 | 0 | 0 | 0 | 0 |
| **Bluefish,** meat only: | | | | | | | |
| raw, 4 oz. ............ | 141 | 22.7 | 0 | 4.8 | 67 | 68 | 0 |
| baked or broiled, 4 oz. .. | 180 | 29.1 | 0 | 6.2 | 86 | 87 | 0 |
| **Boar, wild,** meat only, roasted, 4 oz. ........ | 181 | 32.1 | 0 | 5.0 | 87 | 68 | 0 |
| **Bockwurst,** raw, 1 oz. ... | 87 | 3.8 | .1 | 7.8 | 17 | 313 | 0 |

| Food and Measure | cal. | prot. (gms) | carbo. (gms) | fat (gms) | chol. (mgs) | sod. (mgs) | fiber (gms) |
|---|---|---|---|---|---|---|---|
| **Bok choy**, see "Cabbage, Chinese" | | | | | | | |
| **Bologna** (see also "Ham lunch meat," etc.), 2 oz., except as noted: | | | | | | | |
| (*Black Bear* Ring), 3 oz. | 240 | 12.0 | 2.0 | 20.0 | 50 | 690 | 0 |
| (*Boar's Head*) | 150 | 7.0 | 1.0 | 13.0 | 35 | 530 | 0 |
| (*Boar's Head* Lower Sodium) | 150 | 8.0 | 0 | 13.0 | 30 | 410 | 0 |
| (*Oscar Mayer*), 1 oz. | 90 | 3.0 | 1.0 | 8.0 | 30 | 300 | 0 |
| (*Oscar Mayer* 98% Fat Free), 1 oz. | 25 | 3.0 | 3.0 | .5 | 10 | 240 | 0 |
| (*Oscar Mayer* Light 8 oz.), 1 oz. | 60 | 3.0 | 2.0 | 4.0 | 20 | 300 | 0 |
| (*Thumann's*) | 150 | 7.0 | 1.0 | 13.0 | 28 | 470 | 0 |
| (*Thumann's* Lower Sodium) | 150 | 7.0 | 1.0 | 13.0 | 28 | 370 | 0 |
| beef: | | | | | | | |
| (*Boar's Head*) | 150 | 7.0 | 0 | 13.0 | 35 | 520 | 0 |
| (*Di Lusso*) | 140 | 8.0 | 1.0 | 11.0 | 35 | 680 | 0 |
| (*Hebrew National*) | 170 | 6.0 | 0 | 16.0 | 15 | 400 | 0 |
| (*Hebrew National*), 1-oz. slice | 80 | 3.0 | 0 | 8.0 | 15 | 240 | 0 |
| (*Hebrew National* Lean) | 90 | 8.0 | 1.0 | 5.0 | 20 | 440 | 0 |
| (*Oscar Mayer*), 1 oz. | 90 | 3.0 | 1.0 | 8.0 | 20 | 310 | 0 |
| (*Oscar Mayer* Light), 1 oz. | 60 | 3.0 | 2.0 | 4.0 | 15 | 240 | 0 |
| (*Thumann's*) | 140 | 13.0 | 1.0 | 11.0 | 30 | 470 | 0 |
| garlic: | | | | | | | |
| (*Boar's Head*) | 150 | 7.0 | 1.0 | 13.0 | 35 | 530 | 0 |
| (*Thumann's*) | 150 | 7.0 | 1.0 | 13.0 | 28 | 470 | 0 |
| German: | | | | | | | |
| (*Obermeiser*) | 180 | 6.0 | 6.0 | 15.0 | 40 | 700 | 0 |
| (*Wunderbar*) | 190 | 6.0 | 5.0 | 16.0 | 20 | 600 | 0 |
| garlic (*Black Bear*) | 160 | 7.0 | 1.0 | 14.0 | 30 | 450 | 0 |
| Lebanon (*Boar's Head*) | 100 | 11.0 | 1.0 | 6.0 | 40 | 700 | 0 |
| **"Bologna," vegetarian**, frozen (*Yves*), 4 slices | 80 | 14.0 | 2.0 | 2.5 | 0 | 480 | 0 |
| **Boniato** (*Frieda's*), 3 oz. | 100 | 1.0 | 24.0 | 0 | 0 | 10 | 3.0 |
| **Bonito**, meat only, raw, 4 oz. | 146 | 29.3 | .5 | 2.3 | n.a. | 50 | 0 |
| **Bonito, dried** (*Eden* Flakes), 2 tbsp. | 5 | 1.0 | 0 | 0 | 1 | 4 | 0 |

| Food and Measure | cal. | prot. (gms) | carbo. (gms) | fat (gms) | chol. (mgs) | sod. (mgs) | fiber (gms) |
|---|---|---|---|---|---|---|---|
| **Borage:** | | | | | | | |
| raw, 1" pcs., ½ cup ..... | 9 | .8 | 1.4 | .3 | 0 | 35 | <1.0 |
| boiled, drained, 4 oz. .... | 28 | 2.4 | 4.0 | .9 | 0 | 98 | <2.0 |
| **Bouillon,** 1 cube, pkt., or tsp., except as noted: | | | | | | | |
| beef: | | | | | | | |
| (*Herb-Ox* Cube) ..... | 5 | 0 | 1.0 | 0 | 0 | 910 | 0 |
| (*Herb-Ox* Instant) .... | 5 | 0 | 1.0 | 0 | 0 | 900 | 0 |
| (*Herb-Ox* Instant Broth/Seasoning) .. | 5 | 0 | 1.0 | 0 | 0 | 1040 | 0 |
| (*Herb-Ox* Instant Broth/Seasoning Sodium Free) ..... | 10 | 0 | 2.0 | 0 | 0 | 0 | 0 |
| (*Maggi*), ½ cube ..... | 15 | 0 | 2.0 | .5 | 0 | 1260 | 0 |
| beef rib: | | | | | | | |
| (*Maggi*), ½ cube ..... | 15 | 0 | 1.0 | 1.0 | 0 | 1170 | 0 |
| (*Maggi* Instant) ...... | 10 | 0 | 1.0 | .5 | 0 | 780 | 0 |
| chicken: | | | | | | | |
| (*Herb-Ox* Cube) ..... | 5 | 0 | 1.0 | 0 | 0 | 1100 | 0 |
| (*Herb-Ox* Instant) .... | 5 | 0 | 1.0 | 0 | 0 | 870 | 0 |
| (*Herb-Ox* Instant Sodium Free) ..... | 10 | 1.0 | 2.0 | 0 | 0 | 0 | 0 |
| (*Herb-Ox* Instant Broth/Seasoning) .. | 5 | 0 | 1.0 | 0 | 0 | 1100 | 0 |
| (*Herb-Ox* Instant Broth/Seasoning Sodium Free) ..... | 10 | 1.0 | 2.0 | 0 | 0 | 0 | 0 |
| (*Maggi* Cube) ....... | 5 | 0 | <1.0 | 0 | 0 | 970 | 0 |
| (*Maggi* Instant) ...... | 10 | 0 | <1.0 | 0 | 0 | 840 | 0 |
| chicken and tomato: | | | | | | | |
| (*Maggi* Cube), ½ cube | 10 | 0 | 1.0 | 1.0 | 0 | 1240 | 0 |
| (*Maggi* Instant) ...... | 10 | 0 | <1.0 | 0 | 0 | 840 | 0 |
| garlic herb (*Herb-Ox*) ... | 5 | 0 | 1.0 | 0 | 0 | 860 | 0 |
| vegetable (*Herb-Ox*) .... | 5 | 0 | 1.0 | 0 | 0 | 960 | 0 |
| **Boysenberry,** fresh, see "Blackberry" | | | | | | | |
| **Boysenberry, frozen,** unsweetened, ½ cup . | 33 | .7 | 8.1 | .1 | 0 | 1 | 2.6 |
| **Boysenberry nectar** (*R.W. Knudsen*), 8 fl. oz. ............ | 130 | <1.0 | 31.0 | 0 | 0 | 20 | 0 |
| **Boysenberry syrup** (*Maple Grove Farms*), ¼ cup ............. | 210 | 0 | 53.0 | 0 | 0 | 0 | 0 |

| Food and Measure | cal. | prot. (gms) | carbo. (gms) | fat (gms) | chol. (mgs) | sod. (mgs) | fiber (gms) |
|---|---|---|---|---|---|---|---|
| **Brains**, 4 oz.: | | | | | | | |
| beef, fried ........... | 222 | 14.3 | 0 | 18.0 | 2262 | 179 | 0 |
| lamb, fried ......... | 310 | 19.2 | 0 | 25.2 | 2840 | 178 | 0 |
| pork, braised ......... | 156 | 13.8 | 0 | 10.8 | 2894 | 103 | 0 |
| veal, fried ........... | 242 | 16.4 | 0 | 19.0 | 2404 | 200 | 0 |
| **Bran**, see "Cereal" and specific grains | | | | | | | |
| **Bratwurst**, grilled, 1 link: | | | | | | | |
| (*Black Bear*), 3.2 oz. .... | 240 | 11.0 | 0 | 22.0 | 40 | 670 | 0 |
| (*Boar's Head*), 4 oz. .... | 300 | 19.0 | 0 | 25.0 | 75 | 650 | 0 |
| (*Hillshire Farm Miller High Life*), 2.7 oz. .... | 260 | 8.0 | 5.0 | 22.0 | 50 | 700 | 0 |
| (*Johnsonville* Beer Brats), 2.7 oz. ....... | 260 | 11.0 | 3.0 | 23.0 | 50 | 600 | 0 |
| (*Johnsonville* Original/ Beer 'n Bratwurst/ Irish O'Garlic), 3 oz. .. | 270 | 15.0 | 2.0 | 22.0 | 60 | 810 | 0 |
| (*Johnsonville* Stadium/ Smoked), 2.7 oz. .... | 220 | 10.0 | 3.0 | 19.0 | 45 | 700 | 0 |
| (*Thumann's*), 3.2 oz. .... | 290 | 19.0 | 0 | 25.0 | 65 | 750 | 0 |
| beef (*Johnsonville*), 2.3 oz. | 210 | 8.0 | 3.0 | 18.0 | 40 | 630 | 0 |
| cheddar (*Johnsonville*), 3 oz. ............... | 270 | 15.0 | 3.0 | 22.0 | 60 | 890 | 0 |
| hot and spicy (*Johnsonville*), 3 oz. .. | 280 | 16.0 | 3.0 | 22.0 | 55 | 840 | 0 |
| pork (*Applegate Farms* Organic), 3 oz. ...... | 170 | 12.0 | 2.0 | 12.0 | 45 | 660 | 0 |
| smoked (*Hillshire Farm*), 2.7 oz. ....... | 240 | 8.0 | 4.0 | 22.0 | 50 | 780 | 0 |
| turkey (*Jennie-O*), 3.8 oz. ............... | 170 | 17.0 | 2.0 | 10.0 | 70 | 670 | 0 |
| **"Bratwurst," vegetarian**, frozen: | | | | | | | |
| (*Tofurky* Beer Brats), 3.5 oz. ............ | 260 | 27.0 | 8.0 | 13.0 | 0 | 620 | 5.0 |
| (*Yves*), 3.4-oz. link ..... | 160 | 19.0 | 9.0 | 5.0 | 0 | 840 | 1.0 |
| (*Yves* Zesty Italian), 3.4-oz. link ....... | 150 | 19.0 | 9.0 | 5.0 | 0 | 650 | 2.0 |
| **Bratwurst patty**, grilled (*Johnsonville*), 3 oz. .. | 250 | 17.0 | 2.0 | 17.0 | 60 | 680 | 0 |
| **Braunschweiger** (see also "Liverwurst"), 2 oz.: | | | | | | | |
| (*Black Bear*) .......... | 180 | 9.0 | 2.0 | 15.0 | 55 | 500 | 0 |

| Food and Measure | cal. | prot. (gms) | carbo. (gms) | fat (gms) | chol. (mgs) | sod. (mgs) | fiber (gms) |
|---|---|---|---|---|---|---|---|
| (*Boar's Head* Lite) ...... | 120 | 9.0 | 1.0 | 8.0 | 50 | 450 | 0 |
| (*Thumann's*) .......... | 160 | 9.0 | 3.0 | 12.0 | 80 | 580 | 0 |
| **Brazil nuts**, shelled: | | | | | | | |
| (*Diamond*), 10 pcs., | | | | | | | |
| ¼ cup ............. | 200 | 4.0 | 4.0 | 20.0 | 0 | 0 | 2.0 |
| shelled, 8 medium or | | | | | | | |
| 6 large, 1 oz. ........ | 186 | 4.1 | 3.6 | 18.8 | 0 | <1 | 1.6 |
| **Bread**, fresh, 1 pc., | | | | | | | |
| except as noted: | | | | | | | |
| apple cinnamon | | | | | | | |
| swirl (*Thomas'* | | | | | | | |
| Toasting) .......... | 110 | 3.0 | 20.0 | 2.0 | 0 | 170 | <1.0 |
| berry, mixed (*Thomas'* | | | | | | | |
| Toasting) .......... | 110 | 4.0 | 20.0 | 1.5 | 0 | 170 | <1.0 |
| buttermilk: | | | | | | | |
| (*Wonder*) .......... | 70 | 2.0 | 13.0 | 1.0 | 0 | 150 | 0 |
| sweet (*Pepperidge* | | | | | | | |
| *Farm Farmhouse*) .. | 120 | 4.0 | 23.0 | 1.5 | 0 | 190 | 1.0 |
| chapatti, 1.2-oz. pc.: | | | | | | | |
| wheat (*Kontos*) ...... | 100 | 3.0 | 17.0 | 2.5 | 0 | 150 | 2.0 |
| white (*Kontos*) ...... | 100 | 2.0 | 18.0 | 2.5 | 0 | 150 | 1.0 |
| cinnamon raisin: | | | | | | | |
| (*Fiber One*), 2 pcs. ... | 150 | 5.0 | 35.0 | 2.0 | 0 | 170 | 7.0 |
| (*Glutino* Gluten Free) . | 110 | <1.0 | 22.0 | 1.5 | 0 | 170 | 1.0 |
| cinnamon raisin swirl: | | | | | | | |
| (*Pepperidge Farm*) ... | 80 | 2.0 | 15.0 | 1.5 | 0 | 100 | <1.0 |
| (*Pepperidge Farm* | | | | | | | |
| Whole Wheat) .... | 80 | 2.0 | 13.0 | 1.0 | 0 | 105 | 2.0 |
| (*Sun•Maid*) ........: | 100 | 3.0 | 18.0 | 1.5 | 5 | 130 | 1.0 |
| cinnamon swirl: | | | | | | | |
| (*Nature's Own*), 2 pcs. | 170 | 5.0 | 33.0 | 2.0 | 0 | 210 | 2.0 |
| (*Pepperidge Farm*) ... | 80 | 2.0 | 15.0 | 1.5 | 0 | 110 | <1.0 |
| brown sugar | | | | | | | |
| (*Pepperidge Farm*) . | 110 | 3.0 | 21.0 | 2.0 | 0 | 140 | <1.0 |
| corn: | | | | | | | |
| (*Glutino* Gluten Free) . | 90 | <1.0 | 16.0 | 2.0 | 0 | 200 | <1.0 |
| (*Thomas'* Toasting) ... | 110 | 4.0 | 19.0 | 2.0 | 0 | 210 | 1.0 |
| cranberry swirl (*Thomas'* | | | | | | | |
| Toasting) .......... | 160 | 5.0 | 30.0 | 2.0 | 0 | 240 | 1.0 |
| English muffin bread | | | | | | | |
| (*Thomas'* Toasting) ... | 90 | 4.0 | 18.0 | 1.0 | 0 | 200 | 1.0 |
| fiber (*Glutino* Gluten | | | | | | | |
| Free) ............. | 90 | <1.0 | 17.0 | 1.5 | 0 | 160 | 2.0 |

| Food and Measure | cal. | prot. (gms) | carbo. (gms) | fat (gms) | chol. (mgs) | sod. (mgs) | fiber (gms) |
|---|---|---|---|---|---|---|---|
| **Bread** *(cont.)* | | | | | | | |
| flatbread (see also specific bread): | | | | | | | |
| (*Kontos*), 2.8-oz. pc.: | | | | | | | |
| multigrain . . . . . . . . | 250 | 10.0 | 41.0 | 5.0 | 0 | 330 | 5.0 |
| olive . . . . . . . . . . . . | 233 | 7.0 | 22.0 | 6.0 | 0 | 586 | 4.0 |
| onion, Missy Roti . . | 250 | 9.0 | 36.0 | 8.0 | 0 | 370 | 3.0 |
| panini, grilled . . . . . | 250 | 9.0 | 46.0 | 3.0 | 0 | 570 | 2.0 |
| (*Kontos* Pan Plano), 3-oz. pc.: | | | | | | | |
| chipotle . . . . . . . . | 200 | 14.0 | 25.0 | 5.0 | 0 | 490 | 6.0 |
| jalapeño cilantro . . . | 220 | 13.0 | 27.0 | 7.0 | 0 | 480 | 7.0 |
| pico de gallo . . . . . . | 220 | 13.0 | 27.0 | 7.0 | 0 | 480 | 7.0 |
| sweet onion . . . . . . | 200 | 14.0 | 25.0 | 5.0 | 0 | 480 | 6.0 |
| flax: | | | | | | | |
| (*Glutino* Gluten Free) . | 90 | <1.0 | 17.0 | 2.5 | 0 | 210 | 1.0 |
| and fiber (*Arnold Grains & More*) . . . | 100 | 5.0 | 21.0 | 2.0 | 0 | 170 | 5.0 |
| French: | | | | | | | |
| (*Cobblestone Mill Sliced*), 2 pcs. . . . . | 130 | 5.0 | 26.0 | 1.0 | 0 | 290 | 1.0 |
| (*Pepperidge Farm* Twin Hearth), 4" pc. | 150 | 5.0 | 29.0 | 1.5 | 0 | 260 | 1.0 |
| Italian: | | | | | | | |
| (*Arnold* Premium) . . . | 90 | 2.0 | 16.0 | 1.5 | 0 | 180 | <1.0 |
| (*Pepperidge Farm*) . . . | 80 | 3.0 | 15.0 | 1.0 | 0 | 130 | 1.0 |
| (*Pepperidge Farm* Hearth), 2" pc. . . . . | 150 | 5.0 | 29.0 | 2.0 | 0 | 250 | 1.0 |
| sesame seeds (*Pepperidge Farm*) . | 90 | 3.0 | 15.0 | 1.0 | 0 | 130 | <1.0 |
| multigrain: | | | | | | | |
| (*Arnold* Whole Grains Healthy) . . . | 110 | 5.0 | 20.0 | 1.5 | 0 | 160 | 4.0 |
| (*Arnold Carb Counting*) | 60 | 5.0 | 9.0 | 1.5 | 0 | 120 | 3.0 |
| (*Arnold Grains & More* Ancient Grains) . . . . . . . . . | 110 | 5.0 | 21.0 | 1.5 | 0 | 170 | 3.0 |
| (*Arnold Health Nut*) . . | 120 | 5.0 | 21.0 | 2.0 | 0 | 170 | 2.0 |
| (*Fiber One*) . . . . . . . . | 110 | 4.0 | 25.0 | 1.5 | 0 | 135 | 6.0 |
| (*Nature's Own* Grains & Granola) . . . . . . . | 120 | 5.0 | 20.0 | 2.0 | 0 | 180 | 2.0 |
| (*Roman Meal*), 2 pcs. . | 130 | 6.0 | 25.0 | 1.5 | 0 | 240 | 3.0 |
| 7 (*Arnold*) . . . . . . . . . . | 110 | 4.0 | 21.0 | 1.5 | 0 | 170 | 3.0 |
| 7 (*Healthy Choice*) . . . | 80 | 4.0 | 18.0 | 1.0 | 0 | 170 | 3.0 |

| Food and Measure | cal. | prot. (gms) | carbo. (gms) | fat (gms) | chol. (mgs) | sod. (mgs) | fiber (gms) |
|---|---|---|---|---|---|---|---|
| 7 (*Pepperidge Farm Light*), 3 pcs. ..... | 130 | 7.0 | 26.0 | 1.0 | 0 | 270 | 4.0 |
| 7 (*Pepperidge Farm Farmhouse*) ...... | 110 | 4.0 | 21.0 | 1.5 | 0 | 170 | 2.0 |
| 7, honey (*Nature's Own* 20 oz.) ...... | 70 | 3.0 | 14.0 | 1.0 | 0 | 105 | 1.0 |
| 7, honey (*Nature's Own* 24 oz.) ...... | 90 | 4.0 | 16.0 | 1.5 | 0 | 125 | 2.0 |
| 9 (*Pepperidge Farm* 100% Natural) .... | 100 | 4.0 | 17.0 | 1.5 | 0 | 110 | 3.0 |
| 12 (*Arnold*) ......... | 110 | 5.0 | 21.0 | 1.5 | 0 | 170 | 3.0 |
| 12 (*Nature's Own* Specialty) ........ | 110 | 5.0 | 20.0 | 2.5 | 0 | 180 | 3.0 |
| 12 (*Pepperidge Farm Farmhouse*) ...... | 120 | 4.0 | 21.0 | 2.0 | 0 | 180 | 3.0 |
| 12 (*Roman Meal*) .... | 110 | 4.0 | 19.0 | 2.0 | 0 | 190 | 2.0 |
| 15 (*Pepperidge Farm*) . | 100 | 5.0 | 20.0 | 2.0 | 0 | 115 | 4.0 |
| 15 (*Pepperidge Farm Small*) .......... | 70 | 3.0 | 13.0 | 1.5 | 0 | 75 | 3.0 |
| dark (*Nature's Own* Specialty) ........ | 130 | 5.0 | 21.0 | 3.0 | 0 | 180 | 3.0 |
| nan (*Kontos*), 2.8-oz. pc.: |  |  |  |  |  |  |  |
| kulcha ............. | 250 | 9.0 | 40.0 | 3.0 | 0 | 570 | 2.0 |
| massala ........... | 242 | 7.0 | 39.0 | 6.0 | 0 | 353 | 2.0 |
| onion, oval ........ | 240 | 14.0 | 30.0 | 7.0 | 0 | 320 | 2.0 |
| tandoori or roghani ... | 255 | 9.0 | 40.0 | 6.0 | 0 | 510 | 2.0 |
| oat (*Arnold Oatnut*) ..... | 120 | 4.0 | 22.0 | 2.5 | 0 | 170 | 2.0 |
| oat, honey (*Pepperidge Farm Soft*) ......... | 100 | 5.0 | 19.0 | 2.0 | 0 | 115 | 4.0 |
| oat bran: |  |  |  |  |  |  |  |
| (*Arnold Country*) .... | 110 | 4.0 | 21.0 | 1.5 | 0 | 180 | 1.0 |
| honey (*Roman Meal*) . | 110 | 4.0 | 20.0 | 1.5 | 0 | 200 | 2.0 |
| oatmeal: |  |  |  |  |  |  |  |
| (*Fiber One Soft*) ..... | 110 | 4.0 | 25.0 | 1.5 | 0 | 210 | 6.0 |
| (*Pepperidge Farm*) ... | 70 | 2.0 | 12.0 | 1.0 | 0 | 85 | 1.0 |
| (*Pepperidge Farm Light*), 3 pcs. ...... | 140 | 7.0 | 27.0 | 1.0 | 0 | 260 | 2.0 |
| (*Pepperidge Farm Whole Grain*) ..... | 100 | 4.0 | 20.0 | 1.5 | 0 | 110 | 4.0 |
| (*Pepperidge Farm Farmhouse Soft*) .. | 120 | 4.0 | 21.0 | 1.5 | 0 | 200 | 1.0 |
| pita, 1 pc.: |  |  |  |  |  |  |  |
| (*Garden of Eatin' Organic Bible Bread*) | 145 | 5.0 | 30.0 | .5 | 0 | 115 | 1.0 |

| Food and Measure | cal. | prot. (gms) | carbo. (gms) | fat (gms) | chol. (mgs) | sod. (mgs) | fiber (gms) |
|---|---|---|---|---|---|---|---|
| **Bread, pita** *(cont.)* | | | | | | | |
| (*Kontos*), 2 oz. . . . . . . | 160 | 7.0 | 33.0 | 0 | 0 | 160 | 1.0 |
| (*Kontos Pocket-Less* | | | | | | | |
| Pita), 2.8 oz. . . . . . . | 200 | 7.0 | 42.0 | 2.0 | 0 | 516 | 2.0 |
| (*Thomas' Sahara*), 2 oz. | 170 | 5.0 | 32.0 | 1.5 | 0 | 350 | 2.0 |
| (*Kontos Carbsmart*), | | | | | | | |
| 2.5 oz. . . . . . . . . . | 170 | 14.0 | 20.0 | 3.5 | 0 | 410 | 7.0 |
| multigrain (*Thomas'* | | | | | | | |
| Sahara), 2 oz. . . . . . | 140 | 6.0 | 27.0 | 2.0 | 0 | 320 | 4.0 |
| whole wheat (*Kontos*), | | | | | | | |
| 2 oz. . . . . . . . . . . . . | 140 | 6.0 | 31.0 | 0 | 0 | 130 | 3.0 |
| whole wheat (*Kontos* | | | | | | | |
| Pocket-Less Pita), | | | | | | | |
| 2.8 oz. . . . . . . . . . | 210 | 10.0 | 38.0 | 2.0 | 0 | 510 | 4.0 |
| whole wheat (*Thomas'* | | | | | | | |
| Sahara), 2 oz. . . . . . | 140 | 6.0 | 28.0 | 1.5 | 0 | 320 | 4.0 |
| potato: | | | | | | | |
| (*Arnold Dutch Country*) | 100 | 3.0 | 18.0 | 1.5 | 0 | 170 | <1.0 |
| (*Cobblestone Mill*) . . . | 80 | 3.0 | 15.0 | 1.0 | 0 | 130 | <1.0 |
| (*Wonder*) . . . . . . . . . | 70 | 2.0 | 14.0 | 1.0 | 0 | 150 | 0 |
| pumpernickel: | | | | | | | |
| (*Pepperidge Farm*) . . . | 80 | 3.0 | 15.0 | 1.0 | 0 | 190 | 1.0 |
| (*Pepperidge Farm* | | | | | | | |
| Party), 5 pcs. . . . . . | 130 | 5.0 | 23.0 | 1.5 | 0 | 320 | 3.0 |
| rice, brown (*Glutino*) . . . . | 110 | 1.0 | 21.0 | 2.5 | 0 | 85 | 3.0 |
| rye: | | | | | | | |
| (*Arnold* Real Jewish | | | | | | | |
| Everything) . . . . . . | 90 | 3.0 | 16.0 | 2.0 | 0 | 210 | <1.0 |
| (*Cobblestone Mill* | | | | | | | |
| Jewish) . . . . . . . . . | 80 | 3.0 | 15.0 | 1.0 | 0 | 240 | 1.0 |
| (*Pepperidge Farm* | | | | | | | |
| Party), 5 pcs. . . . . . | 130 | 4.0 | 25.0 | 2.0 | 0 | 460 | 2.0 |
| (*Rubschlager* Cocktail), | | | | | | | |
| 3 pcs. . . . . . . . . . . | 70 | 2.0 | 14.0 | 1.0 | 0 | 180 | 2.0 |
| seeded (*Arnold* Real | | | | | | | |
| Jewish) . . . . . . . . . | 80 | 3.0 | 14.0 | 1.0 | 0 | 220 | <1.0 |
| seeded (*Pepperidge* | | | | | | | |
| Farm) . . . . . . . . . . . | 80 | 3.0 | 15.0 | 1.0 | 0 | 170 | 2.0 |
| seeded (*Pepperidge* | | | | | | | |
| Farm Whole Grain) . | 70 | 3.0 | 14.0 | 1.0 | 0 | 190 | 2.0 |
| seedless (*Arnold* Real | | | | | | | |
| Jewish), 2 pcs. . . . . | 110 | 3.0 | 20.0 | 1.5 | 0 | 290 | <1.0 |
| seedless (*Pepperidge* | | | | | | | |
| Farm) . . . . . . . . . . . | 80 | 3.0 | 14.0 | 1.0 | 0 | 170 | 1.0 |

| Food and Measure | cal. | prot. (gms) | carbo. (gms) | fat (gms) | chol. (mgs) | sod. (mgs) | fiber (gms) |
|---|---|---|---|---|---|---|---|
| thin (*Arnold* Real Jewish Melba), 2 pcs. | 110 | 3.0 | 20.0 | 1.5 | 0 | 290 | <1.0 |
| rye/pumpernickel: | | | | | | | |
| (*Arnold* Real Jewish Dark Rye) ........ | 80 | 2.0 | 15.0 | 1.0 | 0 | 220 | <1.0 |
| (*Pepperidge Farm* Deli Swirl) ....... | 80 | 3.0 | 14.0 | 1.0 | 0 | 180 | 1.0 |
| marble (*Arnold* Real Jewish) ......... | 80 | 2.0 | 14.0 | 1.0 | 0 | 210 | <1.0 |
| sourdough: | | | | | | | |
| (*Cobblestone Mill* San Francisco) .... | 80 | 3.0 | 16.0 | .5 | 0 | 180 | <1.0 |
| (*Pepperidge Farm* Farmhouse Soft) .. | 120 | 4.0 | 22.0 | 1.5 | 0 | 220 | 1.0 |
| wheat: | | | | | | | |
| (*Arnold* Country) .... | 120 | 4.0 | 22.0 | 1.5 | 0 | 170 | 2.0 |
| (*Country Kitchen* Split Top) ........ | 80 | 2.0 | 16.0 | 1.0 | 0 | 170 | 1.0 |
| (*Nature's Own* Double Fiber) ........... | 50 | 3.0 | 13.0 | .5 | 0 | 135 | 5.0 |
| (*Nature's Own* Double Fiber Specialty) ... | 100 | 5.0 | 22.0 | 1.5 | 0 | 190 | 6.0 |
| (*Pepperidge Farm* Light Extra Fiber), 3 pcs. ........... | 120 | 6.0 | 26.0 | 1.0 | 0 | 250 | 6.0 |
| (*Pepperidge Farm* Light Soft), 3 pcs. . | 130 | 8.0 | 25.0 | 1.0 | 0 | 270 | 4.0 |
| (*Wonder* Light) ...... | 40 | 3.0 | 9.0 | 0 | 0 | 120 | 3.0 |
| dark (*Arnold* German) . | 110 | 5.0 | 20.0 | 2.0 | 0 | 170 | 3.0 |
| dark (*Pepperidge Farm* Natural German) .. | 100 | 3.0 | 17.0 | 1.5 | 0 | 130 | 3.0 |
| honey (*Arnold* Soft), 2 pcs. ........... | 140 | 5.0 | 25.0 | 2.0 | 0 | 240 | 2.0 |
| honey (*Nature's Own*) . | 70 | 2.0 | 14.0 | .5 | 0 | 120 | <1.0 |
| honey (*Nature's Own* Specialty) ........ | 100 | 4.0 | 22.0 | 1.0 | 0 | 190 | 3.0 |
| wheat, whole: | | | | | | | |
| (*Arnold* Light), 2 pcs. . | 80 | 5.0 | 18.0 | .5 | 0 | 170 | 5.0 |
| (*Arnold* Soft), 2 pcs. ... | 130 | 6.0 | 23.0 | 2.5 | 0 | 240 | 3.0 |
| (*Arnold* Stoneground), 2 pcs. ........... | 130 | 6.0 | 22.0 | 2.0 | 0 | 260 | 3.0 |
| (*Arnold* Whole Grain) . | 110 | 5.0 | 20.0 | 1.0 | 0 | 170 | 3.0 |
| (*Arnold* Dutch Country) | 100 | 4.0 | 18.0 | 1.5 | 0 | 200 | 3.0 |

| Food and Measure | cal. | prot. (gms) | carbo. (gms) | fat (gms) | chol. (mgs) | sod. (mgs) | fiber (gms) |
|---|---|---|---|---|---|---|---|
| **Bread, wheat, whole** *(cont.)* | | | | | | | |
| (*Arnold Grains & More Active Health*) | 110 | 5.0 | 22.0 | 1.5 | 0 | 180 | 5.0 |
| (*Arnold Grains & More Grain Lovers*) | 120 | 5.0 | 21.0 | 2.5 | 0 | 170 | 3.0 |
| (*Fiber One*) ......... | 100 | 5.0 | 23.0 | 1.5 | 0 | 170 | 7.0 |
| (*Healthy Choice*) ..... | 80 | 3.0 | 18.0 | 1.0 | 0 | 170 | 3.0 |
| (*Nature's Own* 20 oz.) . | 50 | 4.0 | 10.0 | 1.0 | 0 | 115 | 2.0 |
| (*Nature's Own* 24 oz.) . | 70 | 4.0 | 13.0 | 1.5 | 0 | 150 | 2.0 |
| (*Nature's Own* Specialty) ........ | 110 | 5.0 | 20.0 | 1.5 | 0 | 190 | 3.0 |
| (*Nature's Own* Whole Grain) .......... | 70 | 4.0 | 12.0 | 1.5 | 0 | 115 | 2.0 |
| (*Nature's Own* Whole Grain Sugar Free) .. | 50 | 3.0 | 11.0 | 1.0 | 0 | 110 | 2.0 |
| (*Pepperidge Farm* 100% Soft) ...... | 100 | 4.0 | 18.0 | 1.5 | 0 | 130 | 3.0 |
| (*Pepperidge Farm* 100% Whole Grain) | 100 | 5.0 | 20.0 | 1.5 | 0 | 105 | 4.0 |
| (*Pepperidge Farm* 100% Whole Grain Double Fiber) ..:.. | 100 | 4.0 | 21.0 | 1.0 | 0 | 115 | 6.0 |
| (*Pepperidge Farm* 100% Whole Grain Small) .......... | 70 | 3.0 | 13.0 | 1.0 | 0 | 70 | 3.0 |
| (*Pepperidge Farm* 100% Very Thin), 3 slices .......... | 110 | 4.0 | 20.0 | 2.0 | 0 | 230 | 3.0 |
| (*Pepperidge Farm* Whole Grain) ..... | 100 | 4.0 | 20.0 | 1.5 | 0 | 150 | 3.0 |
| (*Pepperidge Farm* Farmhouse 100%) . | 110 | 5.0 | 19.0 | 2.0 | 0 | 150 | 3.0 |
| (*Roman Meal* 100%) . | 100 | 5.0 | 10.0 | 1.5 | 0 | 200 | 3.0 |
| (*Roman Meal* Whole Grain), 2 pcs. ..... | 130 | 5.0 | 24.0 | 2.0 | 0 | 250 | 2.0 |
| (*Wonder* Soft 100%), 2 pcs. ........... | 110 | 5.0 | 20.0 | 1.5 | 0 | 220 | 3.0 |
| (*Wonder* Stoneground 100%), 2 pcs. .... | 180 | 7.0 | 32.0 | 2.5 | 0 | 400 | 4.0 |
| (*Wonder* Whole Grain), 2 pcs. ..... | 130 | 6.0 | 26.0 | 1.5 | 0 | 320 | 4.0 |
| fiber, double (*Arnold Grains & More*) ... | 100 | 4.0 | 21.0 | 1.5 | 0 | 170 | 6.0 |

| Food and Measure | cal. | prot. (gms) | carbo. (gms) | fat (gms) | chol. (mgs) | sod. (mgs) | fiber (gms) |
|---|---|---|---|---|---|---|---|
| fiber, extra (*Arnold Dutch Country*) ... | 90 | 4.0 | 18.0 | 1.5 | 0 | 190 | 4.0 |
| honey (*Arnold* Whole Grains) .......... | 110 | 5.0 | 20.0 | 1.0 | 0 | 170 | 3.0 |
| honey (*Nature's Own*), 2 pcs. ........... | 110 | 6.0 | 20.0 | 1.5 | 0 | 150 | 3.0 |
| honey (*Pepperidge Farm* Soft) ....... | 110 | 4.0 | 21.0 | 1.5 | 0 | 115 | 4.0 |
| protein, double (*Arnold Grains & More*) .......... | 110 | 7.0 | 18.0 | 1.5 | 0 | 170 | 3.0 |
| and rye (*Roman Meal*) | 100 | 5.0 | 19.0 | 1.0 | 0 | 200 | 2.0 |
| stoneground (*Pepperidge Farm* 100%) ...... | 70 | 2.0 | 12.0 | 1.0 | 0 | 65 | 2.0 |
| wheat berry, honey (*Roman Meal*) ....... | 100 | 5.0 | 19.0 | 1.5 | 0 | 180 | 2.0 |
| white: | | | | | | | |
| (*Arnold* Country) .... | 120 | 3.0 | 22.0 | 1.5 | 0 | 180 | 1.0 |
| (*Arnold* Country Whole Grain) ..... | 110 | 4.0 | 21.0 | 1.5 | 0 | 170 | 2.0 |
| (*Arnold* Soft), 2 pcs. ... | 140 | 5.0 | 26.0 | 1.5 | 0 | 270 | 1.0 |
| (*Arnold* Soft Whole Grain), 2 pcs. ...... | 140 | 5.0 | 25.0 | 2.0 | 0 | 260 | 2.0 |
| (*Arnold Brick Oven*) .. | 90 | 3.0 | 17.0 | 1.5 | 0 | 190 | <1.0 |
| (*Arnold Dutch Country Butter Split Top*) ... | 90 | 3.0 | 18.0 | 1.0 | 0 | 180 | <1.0 |
| (*Arnold Dutch Country* Premium) . | 90 | 3.0 | 17.0 | 1.5 | 0 | 200 | <1.0 |
| (*Fiber One* Country) .. | 100 | 4.0 | 24.0 | 1.0 | 0 | 200 | 6.0 |
| (*Nature's Own* Butterbread 20 oz.) | 60 | 3.0 | 12.0 | .5 | 0 | 140 | 1.0 |
| (*Nature's Own* Butterbread 24 oz.) | 70 | 4.0 | 14.0 | .5 | 0 | 160 | <1.0 |
| (*Nature's Own* Whole Grain), 2 pcs. ...... | 130 | 5.0 | 26.0 | 1.5 | 0 | 230 | 2.0 |
| (*Nature's Own Whitewheat*), 2 pcs. | 130 | 6.0 | 27.0 | 1.5 | 0 | 270 | 5.0 |
| (*Pepperidge Farm* Original) ......... | 70 | 2.0 | 13.0 | 1.0 | 0 | 75 | 1.0 |
| (*Pepperidge Farm* Sandwich), 2 pcs. . | 130 | 4.0 | 23.0 | 2.5 | 0 | 250 | <1.0 |
| (*Pepperidge Farm* Very Thin), 3 pcs. ... | 120 | 4.0 | 24.0 | 1.0 | 0 | 250 | 1.0 |

| Food and Measure | cal. | prot. (gms) | carbo. (gms) | fat (gms) | chol. (mgs) | sod. (mgs) | fiber (gms) |
|---|---|---|---|---|---|---|---|
| **Bread, white** *(cont.)* | | | | | | | |
| (*Pepperidge Farm Whole Grain*), 2 pcs. . . . . . . . . . . | 110 | 4.0 | 22.0 | 2.0 | 0 | 200 | 3.0 |
| (*Pepperidge Farm Farmhouse* Hearty) | 120 | 4.0 | 22.0 | 1.5 | 0 | 210 | 1.0 |
| (*Pepperidge Farm Farmhouse* Whole Grain Soft) . . . . . . . | 110 | 4.0 | 21.0 | 2.0 | 0 | 180 | 3.0 |
| (*Wonder* Classic) . . . . | 70 | 2.0 | 14.0 | 1.0 | 0 | 150 | 0 |
| (*Wonder* Light), 2 pcs. . . . . . . . . . . | 80 | 4.0 | 18.0 | .5 | 0 | 260 | 5.0 |
| (*Wonder* Sandwich) . . | 60 | 2.0 | 13.0 | .5 | 0 | 135 | 0 |
| (*Wonder* Smartwhite), 2 pcs. . . . . . . . . . . | 100 | 5.0 | 23.0 | 1.0 | 0 | 200 | 5.0 |
| (*Wonder* Texas Toast) . | 100 | 3.0 | 19.0 | 1.0 | 0 | 200 | <1.0 |
| (*Wonder* Whole Grain), 2 pcs. . . . . . | 140 | 6.0 | 25.0 | 2.0 | 0 | 200 | 3.0 |
| **Bread, brown** (*B&M*): | | | | | | | |
| plain, ½" slice, 2 oz. . . . . | 130 | 3.0 | 29.0 | .5 | 0 | 400 | 2.0 |
| raisin, ½" slice, 2 oz. . . . . | 130 | 3.0 | 29.0 | .5 | 0 | 380 | 2.0 |
| **Bread, frozen/chilled:** | | | | | | | |
| French, crusty (*Pillsbury*), ⅛ loaf . . . . | 120 | 4.0 | 24.0 | 1.5 | 0 | 300 | <1.0 |
| garlic bread, 2 pcs., except as noted: | | | | | | | |
| (*Mamma Bella*) . . . . . . | 150 | 3.0 | 17.0 | 9.0 | 5 | 230 | 1.0 |
| (*Mamma Bella* Cholesterol Free) . . | 150 | 3.0 | 16.0 | 8.0 | 0 | 220 | 1.0 |
| (*New York*), 1" pcs. . . . | 180 | 5.0 | 25.0 | 7.0 | 0 | 400 | 1.0 |
| (*New York* Presliced) . | 150 | 3.0 | 17.0 | 9.0 | <5 | 230 | 1.0 |
| (*Pepperidge Farm*), 2½" pc. . . . . . . . . . | 180 | 4.0 | 21.0 | 8.0 | 0 | 270 | 1.0 |
| baguette, buttery (*Alexia* Artisan) . . . | 130 | 3.0 | 18.0 | 5.0 | 15 | 260 | <1.0 |
| cheese (*Mamma Bella*) | 150 | 3.0 | 17.0 | 8.0 | 5 | 230 | 1.0 |
| cheese, 5 (*Pepperidge Farm*), 2¼" pc. . . . . | 210 | 6.0 | 21.0 | 11.0 | 5 | 320 | 1.0 |
| ciabatta (*New York*), 1" pcs. . . . . . . . . . . | 160 | 4.0 | 22.0 | 6.0 | 0 | 330 | 1.0 |
| mozzarella (*Pepperidge Farm*), 2¼" pc. . . . . | 160 | 5.0 | 22.0 | 6.0 | 0 | 250 | 2.0 |
| Parmesan (*Pepperidge Farm*), 2½" pc. . . . . | 160 | 5.0 | 23.0 | 6.0 | 0 | 270 | 2.0 |

| Food and Measure | cal. | prot. (gms) | carbo. (gms) | fat (gms) | chol. (mgs) | sod. (mgs) | fiber (gms) |
|---|---|---|---|---|---|---|---|
| roasted (*Pepperidge Farm* Premium), 2½" pc. | 170 | 4.0 | 21.0 | 8.0 | 0 | 320 | 2.0 |
| Italian, (*Pillsbury Country*), ⅛ loaf | 110 | 4.0 | 22.0 | 1.5 | 0 | 270 | <1.0 |
| sourdough, 2" pc.: | | | | | | | |
| (*Pepperidge Farm* Rome Inspired) | 170 | 5.0 | 21.0 | 8.0 | 0 | 330 | 1.0 |
| (*Pepperidge Farm* Tuscan Inspired) | 170 | 4.0 | 22.0 | 7.0 | 0 | 310 | 1.0 |
| toast, 1 pc.: | | | | | | | |
| 5 cheese (*Mamma Bella*) | 180 | 5.0 | 20.0 | 9.0 | 5 | 350 | 1.0 |
| cheese garlic (*Mamma Bella*) | 150 | 2.0 | 13.0 | 10.0 | 0 | 260 | 0 |
| garlic (*Mamma Bella* Traditional) | 160 | 2.0 | 12.0 | 11.0 | 0 | 250 | 0 |
| garlic, roasted (*Pepperidge Farm*) | 150 | 4.0 | 18.0 | 7.0 | 0 | 260 | 1.0 |
| toast, Texas, 1 pc.: | | | | | | | |
| cheese (*New York*) | 170 | 5.0 | 16.0 | 10.0 | 5 | 360 | 1.0 |
| 5 cheese (*New York*) | 180 | 5.0 | 20.0 | 9.0 | 5 | 350 | 1.0 |
| 5 cheese (*Pepperidge Farm*) | 150 | 5.0 | 17.0 | 7.0 | 5 | 200 | 2.0 |
| garlic (*New York*) | 150 | 3.0 | 15.0 | 9.0 | 0 | 260 | 1.0 |
| garlic (*New York* Lite) | 130 | 3.0 | 18.0 | 4.5 | 0 | 270 | 1.0 |
| garlic (*Pepperidge Farm*) | 150 | 3.0 | 18.0 | 7.0 | 0 | 190 | 2.0 |
| mozzarella Monterey Jack (*Pepperidge Farm*) | 140 | 5.0 | 17.0 | 6.0 | 5 | 250 | 2.0 |
| Parmesan (*New York*) | 180 | 6.0 | 18.0 | 10.0 | 5 | 370 | 1.0 |
| Parmesan (*Pepperidge Farm*) | 140 | 3.0 | 15.0 | 7.0 | 0 | 210 | <1.0 |
| **Bread mix** (see also "Bread mix, sweet"), dry mix, ¼ cup, except as noted: | | | | | | | |
| (*Bob's Red Mill* Wonderful Bread Gluten Free), 1 pc.* | 150 | 4.0 | 23.0 | 4.5 | 15 | 210 | 3.0 |
| barley (*Hodgson Mill*) | 120 | 5.0 | 23.0 | 1.0 | 0 | 215 | 2.0 |

| Food and Measure | cal. | prot. (gms) | carbo. (gms) | fat (gms) | chol. (mgs) | sod. (mgs) | fiber (gms) |
|---|---|---|---|---|---|---|---|
| **Bread mix** *(cont.)* | | | | | | | |
| cheese and herb | | | | | | | |
| (*Hodgson Mill*) ...... | 110 | 5.0 | 22.0 | 0 | 0 | 225 | 1.0 |
| gluten free (*Hodgson* | | | | | | | |
| *Mill*) ............. | 120 | 2.0 | 26.0 | 1.0 | 0 | 135 | 2.0 |
| multigrain: | | | | | | | |
| (*Arrowhead Mills* | | | | | | | |
| Organic) ......... | 140 | 6.0 | 28.0 | .5 | 0 | 115 | 3.0 |
| 9 (*Hodgson Mill*) .... | 120 | 6.0 | 22.0 | 0 | 0 | 180 | 2.0 |
| 10 (*Bob's Red Mill*), | | | | | | | |
| ½" pc.* .......... | 180 | 7.0 | 29.0 | 4.0 | 0 | 250 | 2.0 |
| potato: | | | | | | | |
| (*Bob's Red Mill*), | | | | | | | |
| ½" pc.* .......... | 140 | 5.0 | 23.0 | 2.5 | 0 | 230 | 1.0 |
| (*Hodgson Mill*) ...... | 120 | 5.0 | 24.0 | 0 | 0 | 170 | 1.0 |
| rye: | | | | | | | |
| (*Bob's Red Mill*), | | | | | | | |
| ½" pc.* .......... | 150 | 6.0 | 25.0 | 3.0 | 0 | 210 | 1.0 |
| caraway (*Hodgson* | | | | | | | |
| *Mill*) ............ | 110 | 5.0 | 22.0 | 1.0 | 0 | 190 | 3.0 |
| soda, Irish (*Bob's Red* | | | | | | | |
| *Mill*), ½" pc.* ....... | 190 | 5.0 | 30.0 | 6.0 | 15 | 330 | 1.0 |
| white (*Hodgson Mill*) ... | 120 | 5.0 | 22.0 | .5 | 0 | 170 | 1.0 |
| whole wheat: | | | | | | | |
| (*Arrowhead Mills* | | | | | | | |
| Organic) ......... | 140 | 6.0 | 27.0 | 1.0 | 0 | 140 | 4.0 |
| (*Bob's Red Mill*), | | | | | | | |
| ½" pc.* .......... | 170 | 7.0 | 27.0 | 4.0 | 0 | 230 | 2.0 |
| honey (*Hodgson Mill*) . | 120 | 5.0 | 22.0 | .5 | 0 | 160 | 2.0 |
| **Bread mix, sweet**, ¹⁄₁₄ pkg. | | | | | | | |
| mix, except as noted: | | | | | | | |
| apple cinnamon | | | | | | | |
| (*Pillsbury* Quick) ..... | 130 | 1.0 | 26.0 | 2.0 | 0 | 115 | <1.0 |
| banana: | | | | | | | |
| (*Betty Crocker* Quick), | | | | | | | |
| ¹⁄₁₂ loaf* ......... | 170 | 3.0 | 25.0 | 7.0 | 35 | 210 | 0 |
| (*Pillsbury* Quick) ..... | 110 | 2.0 | 22.0 | 1.0 | 0 | 160 | <1.0 |
| blueberry (*Pillsbury* | | | | | | | |
| Quick) ............. | 120 | 1.0 | 24.0 | 1.5 | 0 | 100 | <1.0 |
| chocolate chip swirl | | | | | | | |
| (*Pillsbury* Quick) ..... | 150 | 1.0 | 26.0 | 4.5 | 0 | 140 | <1.0 |
| cinnamon raisin (*Bob's* | | | | | | | |
| *Red Mill* Gluten | | | | | | | |
| Free), ¹⁄₁₆ pkg. ....... | 130 | 2.0 | 29.0 | 1.5 | 0 | 230 | 2.0 |

| Food and Measure | cal. | prot. (gms) | carbo. (gms) | fat (gms) | chol. (mgs) | sod. (mgs) | fiber (gms) |
|---|---|---|---|---|---|---|---|
| cinnamon streusel (*Betty Crocker* Quick), ¹⁄₁₄ loaf* | 180 | 2.0 | 28.0 | 7.0 | 30 | 160 | 0 |
| cinnamon swirl (*Pillsbury* Quick) | 150 | 1.0 | 27.0 | 4.0 | 0 | 140 | 0 |
| corn, see "Cornbread" | | | | | | | |
| cranberry: | | | | | | | |
| (*Pillsbury* Quick) | 120 | 2.0 | 26.0 | 1.5 | 0 | 135 | <1.0 |
| orange (*Betty Crocker* Quick), ¹⁄₁₂ loaf* | 180 | 3.0 | 29.0 | 6.0 | 35 | 180 | <1.0 |
| date (*Pillsbury* Quick) | 130 | 2.0 | 28.0 | 1.5 | 0 | 115 | 1.0 |
| gingerbread, whole wheat (*Hodgson Mill*), ¼ cup | 110 | 2.0 | 24.0 | 0 | 0 | 260 | 2.0 |
| lemon poppy seed (*Pillsbury* Quick) | 130 | 2.0 | 25.0 | 2.5 | 0 | 120 | <1.0 |
| nut (*Pillsbury* Quick) | 120 | 2.0 | 23.0 | 3.0 | 0 | 135 | <1.0 |
| pecan swirl (*Pillsbury* Quick) | 150 | 1.0 | 25.0 | 5.0 | 0 | 140 | <1.0 |
| pumpkin (*Pillsbury* Quick), ¹⁄₁₂ pkg. | 130 | 2.0 | 27.0 | 1.5 | 0 | 190 | 1.0 |
| **Bread crumbs**, ¼ cup, except as noted: | | | | | | | |
| plain: | | | | | | | |
| (*Contadina*) | 110 | 4.0 | 19.0 | 1.5 | 0 | 200 | 1.0 |
| (*Old London*) | 110 | 4.0 | 19.0 | 1.5 | 0 | 200 | 1.0 |
| (*Progresso*) | 110 | 4.0 | 20.0 | 1.5 | 0 | 220 | 1.0 |
| (*Vigo*) | 110 | 4.0 | 19.0 | 1.5 | 0 | 200 | 1.0 |
| cheese, 3 (*Contadina*) | 110 | 4.0 | 19.0 | 1.5 | 0 | 510 | 1.0 |
| corn (*Glutino*), ⅓ cup | 110 | 3.0 | 25.0 | 0 | 0 | 135 | 0 |
| w/garlic, roasted, spices *Contadina* | 110 | 4.0 | 19.0 | 1.5 | 0 | 530 | 1.0 |
| garlic herb (*Progresso*) | 110 | 4.0 | 20.0 | 1.5 | 0 | 540 | 1.0 |
| Italian: | | | | | | | |
| (*Contadina*) | 100 | 4.0 | 19.0 | 1.5 | 0 | 720 | 1.0 |
| (*Progresso*) | 110 | 4.0 | 20.0 | 1.5 | 0 | 470 | 1.0 |
| (*Vigo*) | 110 | 4.0 | 21.0 | 1.5 | 0 | 520 | 1.0 |
| panko crumbs: | | | | | | | |
| (*Kikkoman*), ½ cup | 110 | 3.0 | 24.0 | .5 | 0 | 40 | <1.0 |
| (*Roland*), ⅓ cup | 70 | 3.0 | 15.0 | 0 | 0 | 45 | 0 |
| plain (*Progresso*) | 110 | 2.0 | 19.0 | 2.5 | 0 | 50 | 0 |
| Italian (*Progresso*) | 120 | 2.0 | 18.0 | 4.5 | 0 | 430 | 0 |
| lemon pepper (*Progresso*) | 120 | 2.0 | 17.0 | 4.5 | 0 | 430 | <1.0 |

| Food and Measure | cal. | prot. (gms) | carbo. (gms) | fat (gms) | chol. (mgs) | sod. (mgs) | fiber (gms) |
|---|---|---|---|---|---|---|---|
| **Bread crumbs** *(cont.)* | | | | | | | |
| Parmesan (*Progresso*) .. | 110 | 4.0 | 19.0 | 1.5 | 0 | 870 | 1.0 |
| seasoned (*Old London*) .. | 110 | 4.0 | 19.0 | 1.5 | 0 | 560 | 1.0 |
| **Bread pudding** (*Kozy Shack*), 4-oz. cont.: | | | | | | | |
| apple cinnamon ........ | 150 | 5.0 | 27.0 | 3.5 | 40 | 105 | 0 |
| cinnamon raisin ....... | 160 | 5.0 | 29.0 | 3.5 | 45 | 105 | 1.0 |
| peach ............... | 150 | 5.0 | 25.0 | 3.5 | 40 | 100 | 0 |
| **Bread stick**: | | | | | | | |
| (*Alessi*), 1 oz.: | | | | | | | |
| plain, thin, 9 pcs. .... | 110 | 3.0 | 22.0 | 1.5 | 0 | 280 | 1.0 |
| garlic, 5 pcs. ........ | 120 | 4.0 | 24.0 | 1.5 | 0 | 210 | 2.0 |
| rosemary, 9 pcs. ..... | 110 | 3.0 | 22.0 | 1.5 | 0 | 280 | 1.0 |
| sea salt dippers, 3 pcs. | 80 | 2.0 | 12.0 | 3.0 | 0 | 150 | 0 |
| sesame, 4 pcs. ...... | 110 | 4.0 | 22.0 | 2.0 | 0 | 210 | 2.0 |
| (*Glutino* Gluten Free): | | | | | | | |
| pizza, 9 pcs., .5 oz. ... | 60 | 0 | 13.0 | 1.0 | 0 | 105 | 0 |
| sesame, .5 oz. ........ | 60 | 0 | 13.0 | 1.5 | 0 | 100 | 0 |
| **Bread stick, frozen/ chilled**: | | | | | | | |
| (*Pillsbury* Original), 2 pcs. ............. | 130 | 4.0 | 26.0 | 2.0 | 0 | 380 | <1.0 |
| dipping, 2 pcs.: | | | | | | | |
| (*New York* Pizzeria Dip'n Sticks), w/2 tbsp. sauce ... | 140 | 4.0 | 21.0 | 4.5 | 0 | 460 | 1.0 |
| cheese (*New York* Pizzeria Dip'n Sticks), w/1⅓ tbsp. sauce .. | 160 | 7.0 | 21.0 | 6.0 | 5 | 420 | 1.0 |
| garlic: | | | | | | | |
| (*Mamma Bella/ New York*), 1 pc. .. | 170 | 5.0 | 24.0 | 6.0 | 0 | 300 | 1.0 |
| (*Pillsbury*), 2 pcs. .... | 180 | 4.0 | 23.0 | 9.0 | 0 | 560 | <1.0 |
| **Breadfruit**, raw, ½ cup .. | 113 | 1.2 | 29.8 | .3 | 0 | 2 | 5.4 |
| **Breadfruit seeds**: | | | | | | | |
| raw, 1 oz. ............ | 54 | 2.1 | 8.3 | 1.6 | 0 | 7 | 1.5 |
| boiled, shelled, 1 oz. .... | 48 | 1.5 | 9.1 | .7 | 0 | 7 | 1.4 |
| roasted, shelled, 1 oz. ... | 59 | 1.8 | 11.4 | .8 | 0 | 8 | 1.7 |
| **Breading**, see "Batter/ breading mix," "Panko coating mix" and specific listings | | | | | | | |
| **Breadnut tree seeds**, dried, 1 oz. ......... | 104 | 2.4 | 22.5 | .5 | 0 | 15 | 4.2 |

| Food and Measure | cal. | prot. (gms) | carbo. (gms) | fat (gms) | chol. (mgs) | sod. (mgs) | fiber (gms) |
|---|---|---|---|---|---|---|---|
| **Breakfast bar**, see "Granola/cereal bar" | | | | | | | |
| **Breakfast dish** (see also "Egg breakfast" and specific listings) (*Jimmy Dean* Skillets), ¼ of 18-oz. pkg.: | | | | | | | |
| bacon . . . . . . . . . . . . . . | 230 | 10.0 | 14.0 | 13.0 | 20 | 710 | 2.0 |
| ham . . . . . . . . . . . . . . . | 130 | 8.0 | 16.0 | 4.0 | 20 | 670 | 2.0 |
| sausage . . . . . . . . . . . | 220 | 6.0 | 16.0 | 15.0 | 25 | 590 | 2.0 |
| **Breakfast sandwich** (see also "Burrito, breakfast," "Panini," "Quesadilla," etc.), frozen, 1 pc., except as noted: | | | | | | | |
| (*Smart Ones* Stuffed) . . . | 240 | 15.0 | 30.0 | 7.0 | 30 | 570 | 3.0 |
| bagel, turkey sausage/ egg/cheese (*Jimmy Dean* D-lights) . . . . . . | 260 | 18.0 | 31.0 | 8.0 | 40 | 860 | 4.0 |
| biscuit: | | | | | | | |
| gravy/sausage (*Michelina's* Snackers) . . . | 150 | 3.0 | 15.0 | 9.0 | 15 | 370 | 1.0 |
| sausage (*Jimmy Dean*) | 360 | 8.0 | 26.0 | 24.0 | 30 | 600 | 1.0 |
| biscuit, egg/cheese: | | | | | | | |
| bacon (*Jimmy Dean*) . | 320 | 12.0 | 27.0 | 18.0 | 100 | 800 | 1.0 |
| bacon (*MorningStar Farms*) . . . . . . . . . . | 270 | 9.0 | 40.0 | 8.0 | 25 | 630 | 1.0 |
| sausage (*Aunt Jemima*) | 340 | 12.0 | 27.0 | 21.0 | 110 | 830 | <1.0 |
| sausage (*Jimmy Dean*) | 440 | 13.0 | 27.0 | 31.0 | 120 | 850 | 1.0 |
| sausage (*MorningStar Farms*) . . . . . . . . . . | 270 | 9.0 | 40.0 | 8.0 | 25 | 630 | 1.0 |
| cheese sauce/egg, and (*Toaster Scrambles*): | | | | | | | |
| bacon . . . . . . . . . . . . | 180 | 4.0 | 16.0 | 12.0 | 20 | 310 | 0 |
| bacon, reduced fat . . . | 170 | 4.0 | 17.0 | 9.0 | 20 | 340 | <1.0 |
| ham . . . . . . . . . . . . . | 170 | 3.0 | 16.0 | 11.0 | 20 | 310 | 0 |
| sausage . . . . . . . . . . | 180 | 3.0 | 16.0 | 11.0 | 20 | 300 | 0 |
| croissant, ham/cheese (*Jimmy Dean*) . . . . . . . | 280 | 12.0 | 29.0 | 13.0 | 25 | 760 | 1.0 |
| croissant, sausage/ egg/cheese: | | | | | | | |
| (*Aunt Jemima*) . . . . . . | 350 | 13.0 | 23.0 | 23.0 | 145 | 680 | <1.0 |
| (*Jimmy Dean*) . . . . . . . | 430 | 13.0 | 30.0 | 29.0 | 115 | 740 | 1.0 |

| Food and Measure | cal. | prot. (gms) | carbo. (gms) | fat (gms) | chol. (mgs) | sod. (mgs) | fiber (gms) |
|---|---|---|---|---|---|---|---|
| **Breakfast sandwich** *(cont.)* | | | | | | | |
| (*Jimmy Dean* | | | | | | | |
| D-lights) . . . . . . . . | 290 | 17.0 | 30.0 | 12.0 | 30 | 830 | 4.0 |
| croissant entree, w/hash | | | | | | | |
| browns, apples | | | | | | | |
| (*Jimmy Dean* Entrees), | | | | | | | |
| 7.5-oz. pkg.: | | | | | | | |
| ham/cheese . . . . . . . . | 440 | 13.0 | 62.0 | 16.0 | 25 | 1130 | 4.0 |
| sausage/egg/cheese . . | 560 | 11.0 | 62.0 | 30.0 | 35 | 1050 | 4.0 |
| French toast: | | | | | | | |
| (*Jimmy D's* | | | | | | | |
| Griddlers) . . . . . . . . | 210 | 8.0 | 27.0 | 8.0 | 60 | 390 | 0 |
| sausage/egg/cheese | | | | | | | |
| (*Aunt Jemima*) . . . . | 310 | 15.0 | 23.0 | 18.0 | 205 | 690 | <1.0 |
| griddlecake: | | | | | | | |
| ham/egg/cheese | | | | | | | |
| (*Aunt Jemima*) . . . . | 240 | 9.0 | 33.0 | 8.0 | 110 | 870 | <1.0 |
| maple cakes, sausage | | | | | | | |
| (*Jimmy Dean*) . . . . | 370 | 8.0 | 32.0 | 23.0 | 40 | 640 | 1.0 |
| sausage/egg/cheese | | | | | | | |
| (*Aunt Jemima*) . . . . | 350 | 13.0 | 30.0 | 20.0 | 150 | 900 | <1.0 |
| muffin, egg/cheese: | | | | | | | |
| (*Smart Ones*) . . . . . . . | 210 | 13.0 | 27.0 | 5.0 | 15 | 610 | 2.0 |
| Canadian bacon | | | | | | | |
| (*Jimmy Dean* | | | | | | | |
| D-lights) . . . . . . . . | 230 | 15.0 | 30.0 | 4.5 | 15 | 760 | 2.0 |
| Canadian bacon | | | | | | | |
| (*Michelina's Lean* | | | | | | | |
| Gourmet) . . . . . . . . | 170 | 7.0 | 23.0 | 5.0 | 40 | 360 | 1.0 |
| Canadian bacon | | | | | | | |
| (*Smart Ones*) . . . . . | 210 | 14.0 | 27.0 | 6.0 | 25 | 700 | 2.0 |
| sausage (*Jimmy Dean*) | 350 | 13.0 | 28.0 | 21.0 | 110 | 720 | 1.0 |
| sausage (*Michelina's* | | | | | | | |
| Lean Gourmet) . . . . | 170 | 7.0 | 23.0 | 5.0 | 40 | 360 | 1.0 |
| turkey sausage (*Jimmy* | | | | | | | |
| Dean D-lights) . . . . | 260 | 18.0 | 29.0 | 8.0 | 35 | 760 | 2.0 |
| tofu scramble (*Amy's* | | | | | | | |
| Pocket) . . . . . . . . . . . | 180 | 11.0 | 23.0 | 6.0 | 0 | 520 | <1.0 |
| **Breakfast syrup**, see | | | | | | | |
| "Pancake syrup" | | | | | | | |
| **Broad bean**, fresh: | | | | | | | |
| raw, ½ cup . . . . . . . . . . . | 40 | 3.1 | 6.4 | .4 | 0 | 28 | 2.3 |
| boiled, drained, 4 oz. . . . . | 64 | 5.4 | 11.5 | .6 | 0 | 47 | <3.0 |

| Food and Measure | cal. | prot. (gms) | carbo. (gms) | fat (gms) | chol. (mgs) | sod. (mgs) | fiber (gms) |
|---|---|---|---|---|---|---|---|
| **Broad bean, mature**: | | | | | | | |
| dry: | | | | | | | |
| (*Bob's Red Mill* | | | | | | | |
| Fava), ¼ cup ..... | 140 | 10.0 | 23.0 | .5 | 0 | 5 | 10.0 |
| (*Frieda's* Habas), | | | | | | | |
| ½ cup, 3 oz. ...... | 100 | 6.0 | 17.0 | 0 | 0 | 5 | 4.0 |
| boiled, ½ cup ......... | 93 | 6.5 | 16.7 | .3 | 0 | 4 | 4.6 |
| **Broad bean, mature,** | | | | | | | |
| **canned**, ½ cup: | | | | | | | |
| (*Progresso* Fava) ....... | 100 | 6.0 | 17.0 | .5 | 0 | 250 | 5.0 |
| w/liquid ............. | 91 | 7.0 | 15.9 | .3 | 0 | 580 | 4.7 |
| **Broccoli**, fresh: | | | | | | | |
| raw: | | | | | | | |
| (*Dole*), 5.2-oz. stalk .. | 50 | 4.0 | 10.0 | 1.0 | 0 | 50 | 4.0 |
| untrimmed, 8.7-oz. stalk | 42 | 4.5 | 7.9 | .5 | 0 | 40 | 4.5 |
| chopped, ½ cup ..... | 12 | 1.3 | 2.3 | .2 | 0 | 12 | 1.3 |
| raw, baby (*Green Giant Sweet Baby Broccoli*), | | | | | | | |
| 8 stalks, 3 oz. ....... | 35 | 3.0 | 6.0 | 0 | 0 | 25 | 1.0 |
| boiled, drained: | | | | | | | |
| 1 stalk, 6.3 oz. ...... | 51 | 5.4 | 9.1 | .6 | 0 | 46 | 5.2 |
| chopped, ½ cup ..... | 22 | 2.3 | 3.9 | .2 | 0 | 20 | 2.3 |
| **Broccoli, Chinese**, see "Kale, Chinese" | | | | | | | |
| **Broccoli, frozen**: | | | | | | | |
| spears: | | | | | | | |
| (*Birds Eye*), 2 spears, | | | | | | | |
| 3.1 oz. .......... | 30 | 2.0 | 4.0 | 0 | 0 | 25 | 2.0 |
| (*Green Giant*), 3.5 oz., | | | | | | | |
| approx. 3 spears .. | 25 | 2.0 | 4.0 | 0 | 0 | 120 | 2.0 |
| 10-oz. pkg. ........ | 84 | 8.7 | 15.2 | 1.0 | 0 | 49 | 8.5 |
| or chopped, boiled, | | | | | | | |
| drained, 1 cup .... | 52 | 5.7 | 9.8 | .2 | 0 | 44 | 5.5 |
| florets: | | | | | | | |
| (*Allens* SteamSupreme), | | | | | | | |
| 1 cup ........... | 30 | 2.0 | 4.0 | 0 | 0 | 5 | 2.0 |
| (*Birds Eye/Birds Eye Steamfresh/C&W*), | | | | | | | |
| 1 cup ........... | 30 | 1.0 | 4.0 | 0 | 0 | 20 | 2.0 |
| (*Cascadian Farm* Organic Bag), ⅔ cup, 3 oz. . | 25 | 2.0 | 4.0 | 0 | 0 | 20 | 2.0 |
| (*Cascadian Farm* Organic Box), | | | | | | | |
| 1⅓ cups, 3 oz. .... | 20 | 1.0 | 3.0 | 0 | 0 | 120 | 2.0 |

| Food and Measure | cal. | prot. (gms) | carbo. (gms) | fat (gms) | chol. (mgs) | sod. (mgs) | fiber (gms) |
|---|---|---|---|---|---|---|---|
| **Broccoli, frozen, florets** (cont.) | | | | | | | |
| (Green Giant Valley Fresh Steamers), | | | | | | | |
| ¾ cup cooked .... | 20 | 2.0 | 4.0 | 0 | 0 | 20 | 2.0 |
| cuts: | | | | | | | |
| (Birds Eye Steamfresh/ Freshlike), 1 cup .. | 30 | 2.0 | 4.0 | 0 | 0 | 20 | 2.0 |
| (Cascadian Farm Organic), ⅔ cup ... | 20 | 2.0 | 4.0 | 0 | 0 | 20 | 2.0 |
| (Green Giant Simply Steam), ⅔ cup .... | 20 | 1.0 | 4.0 | 0 | 0 | 105 | 2.0 |
| chopped: | | | | | | | |
| (Birds Eye), ¾ cup ... | 30 | 1.0 | 4.0 | 0 | 0 | 20 | 2.0 |
| (Green Giant Valley Fresh Steamers), | | | | | | | |
| ⅔ cup cooked .... | 20 | 2.0 | 4.0 | 0 | 0 | 20 | 2.0 |
| 10-oz. pkg. ......... | 75 | 8.0 | 13.6 | .8 | 0 | 68 | 8.5 |
| in butter sauce, | | | | | | | |
| spears (Green Giant), | | | | | | | |
| 4 oz., approx. 3 pcs. ... | 40 | 2.0 | 6.0 | 1.5 | <5 | 330 | 2.0 |
| in cheese sauce: | | | | | | | |
| (Allens Steam- Supreme), | | | | | | | |
| ⅔ cup ........... | 70 | 4.0 | 6.0 | 3.0 | 10 | 330 | 2.0 |
| (Birds Eye), ½ cup ... | 90 | 3.0 | 8.0 | 5.0 | 5 | 490 | 1.0 |
| (Birds Eye Steamfresh Lightly Sauced), 1 cup .... | 60 | 2.0 | 7.0 | 2.0 | 5 | 370 | 2.0 |
| (Green Giant), ⅔ cup . | 60 | 2.0 | 7.0 | 2.5 | 0 | 460 | 2.0 |
| (Green Giant Zesty), | | | | | | | |
| ¾ cup ........... | 60 | 2.0 | 8.0 | 2.0 | 0 | 470 | 1.0 |
| (Green Giant Just for One), 1 tray .... | 40 | 2.0 | 7.0 | 1.0 | <5 | 410 | 3.0 |
| (Green Giant Valley Fresh Steamers), | | | | | | | |
| ½ cup cooked .... | 45 | 2.0 | 7.0 | 1.5 | 0 | 380 | 2.0 |
| 3 (Green Giant), | | | | | | | |
| ½ cup cooked .... | 45 | 3.0 | 7.0 | 1.5 | 0 | 420 | 2.0 |
| cheddar, white (Green Giant), ¾ cup ..... | 60 | 2.0 | 9.0 | 2.0 | 0 | 470 | 1.0 |
| **Broccoli combinations, fresh** (Green Giant Fresh): | | | | | | | |
| carrots, 3 oz. .......... | 30 | 2.0 | 6.0 | 0 | 0 | 35 | 2.0 |

| Food and Measure | cal. | prot. (gms) | carbo. (gms) | fat (gms) | chol. (mgs) | sod. (mgs) | fiber (gms) |
|---|---|---|---|---|---|---|---|
| carrots, baby, 1 cup: | | | | | | | |
|   w/cheese sauce ..... | 90 | 3.0 | 7.0 | 7.0 | 15 | 200 | 3.0 |
|   w/garlic butter ...... | 110 | 3.0 | 7.0 | 9.0 | 20 | 220 | 3.0 |
| carrots, cauliflower, 3 oz. | 25 | 2.0 | 5.0 | 0 | 0 | 30 | 2.0 |
| cauliflower, 3 oz. ....... | 25 | 2.0 | 4.0 | 0 | 0 | 25 | 2.0 |
| **Broccoli combinations, frozen**, 1 cup, except as noted: | | | | | | | |
| baby blend (*Birds Eye Steamfresh*) ........ | 60 | 4.0 | 8.0 | 1.5 | 0 | 30 | 3.0 |
| carrots: | | | | | | | |
|   (*Cascadian Farm Purely Steam*), Organic), ¾ cup* | 60 | 2.0 | 8.0 | 3.0 | 0 | 250 | 3.0 |
|   (*Green Giant Simply Steam*), ¾ cup* ... | 60 | 2.0 | 8.0 | 3.0 | 0 | 260 | 3.0 |
|   w/garlic, herbs (*Green Giant*), ½ cup cooked .... | 40 | 2.0 | 7.0 | .5 | 0 | 200 | 2.0 |
|   w/Italian seasoning (*Green Giant Just for One*), 1 tray .... | 40 | 1.0 | 7.0 | 1.5 | 0 | 200 | 3.0 |
| carrots, cauliflower, cheese sauce: | | | | | | | |
|   (*Green Giant*), ½ cup cooked ......... | 45 | 2.0 | 7.0 | 1.0 | 0 | 380 | 2.0 |
|   (*Green Giant Valley Fresh Steamers*), ½ cup cooked .... | 45 | 2.0 | 8.0 | 1.0 | 0 | 290 | 2.0 |
|   (*Veg-All Steam-Supreme*), ⅔ cup .......... | 70 | 4.0 | 6.0 | 3.0 | 10 | 330 | 2.0 |
| carrots, water chestnuts: | | | | | | | |
|   (*Birds Eye*) ........ | 35 | 1.0 | 6.0 | 0 | 0 | 35 | 2.0 |
|   sugar snaps (*Birds Eye Steamfresh*), ¾ cup .......... | 35 | 1.0 | 6.0 | 0 | 0 | 25 | 2.0 |
| cauliflower: | | | | | | | |
|   (*Birds Eye*) ........ | 25 | 1.0 | 4.0 | 0 | 0 | 25 | 2.0 |
|   (*Birds Eye Steamfresh*) | 30 | 1.0 | 4.0 | 0 | 0 | 25 | 2.0 |
| cauliflower, carrots: | | | | | | | |
|   (*Birds Eye*) ........ | 30 | 1.0 | 5.0 | 0 | 0 | 35 | 2.0 |
|   (*Birds Eye Steamfresh*), ¾ cup | 30 | 1.0 | 5.0 | 0 | 0 | 30 | 2.0 |

| Food and Measure | cal. | prot. (gms) | carbo. (gms) | fat (gms) | chol. (mgs) | sod. (mgs) | fiber (gms) |
|---|---|---|---|---|---|---|---|
| **Broccoli combinations, frozen, cauliflower, carrots** *(cont.)* | | | | | | | |
| (*Veg-All SteamSupreme*), | | | | | | | |
| ⅔ cup ........... | 30 | 2.0 | 5.0 | 0 | 0 | 15 | 2.0 |
| in cheese sauce (*Birds Eye Steamfresh Lightly Sauced*), | | | | | | | |
| ¾ cup ........... | 50 | 1.0 | 7.0 | 1.5 | 5 | 330 | 1.0 |
| corn and peppers | | | | | | | |
| (*Birds Eye*), ¾ cup ... | 50 | 2.0 | 10.0 | 0 | 0 | 10 | 1.0 |
| stir-fry: | | | | | | | |
| (*Birds Eye*) ......... | 35 | 1.0 | 6.0 | 0 | 0 | 30 | 2.0 |
| (*Freshlike*) ......... | 30 | 1.0 | 5.0 | 0 | 0 | 35 | 2.0 |
| **Broccoli dish**, frozen/ chilled: | | | | | | | |
| bites, breaded: | | | | | | | |
| (*Dr. Praeger's*), | | | | | | | |
| 2 pcs., 2 oz. ...... | 110 | 3.0 | 17.0 | 3.5 | 0 | 220 | 2.0 |
| w/chedder (*Veggie Patch/Bistro au Naturel*), 3 pcs., | | | | | | | |
| 2.6 oz. .......... | 150 | 5.0 | 17.0 | 8.0 | 10 | 380 | 4.0 |
| and cheese (*Bob Evans*), | | | | | | | |
| ½ cup ............. | 120 | 6.0 | 8.0 | 7.0 | 15 | 570 | 1.0 |
| pancake, 1 pc.: | | | | | | | |
| (*Dr. Praeger's*) ...... | 80 | 2.0 | 9.0 | 3.5 | 0 | 170 | 2.0 |
| (*Golden*) ........... | 70 | 2.0 | 10.0 | 3.0 | <5 | 210 | <1.0 |
| **Broccoli pot pie**, | | | | | | | |
| frozen (*Amy's*), 7.5 oz. | 430 | 11.0 | 46.0 | 22.0 | 45 | 630 | 4.0 |
| **Broccoli rabe**, fresh: | | | | | | | |
| (*Frieda's Rapini*), 3 oz. .. | 25 | 3.0 | 4.0 | 0 | 0 | 25 | 0 |
| (*Ready Pac Microwave*), | | | | | | | |
| ½ cup cooked ....... | 30 | 3.0 | 3.0 | 0 | 0 | 50 | 2.0 |
| **Broccoli-cheese pocket**, frozen, 1 pc.: | | | | | | | |
| (*Amy's*), 4.5 oz. ........ | 270 | 8.0 | 37.0 | 10.0 | 15 | 560 | 3.0 |
| cheddar (*Aunt Trudy's*), | | | | | | | |
| 5 oz. .............. | 320 | 12.0 | 34.0 | 15.0 | 30 | 480 | 3.0 |
| **Broccolini**, fresh: | | | | | | | |
| (*Frieda's Asparation*), | | | | | | | |
| 8 stalks, 2.9 oz. ..... | 35 | 3.0 | 6.0 | 0 | 0 | 25 | 1.0 |
| (*Mann's*), 8 stalks, 2.9 oz. | 35 | 3.0 | 6.0 | 0 | 0 | 25 | 1.0 |
| **Brown gravy**, w/onion, canned (*Campbell's*), | | | | | | | |
| ¼ cup .............. | 25 | 0 | 4.0 | 1.0 | 0 | 330 | 0 |

| Food and Measure | cal. | prot. (gms) | carbo. (gms) | fat (gms) | chol. (mgs) | sod. (mgs) | fiber (gms) |
|---|---|---|---|---|---|---|---|
| **Brown gravy mix**, ¼ cup*: | | | | | | | |
| (*Lawry's*) | 20 | 0 | 4.0 | 0 | 0 | 340 | 0 |
| (*McCormick*) | 20 | <1.0 | 3.0 | .5 | 0 | 340 | 0 |
| (*McCormick* Less Sodium) | 25 | <1.0 | 3.0 | .5 | 0 | 230 | 0 |
| Cajun (*Zatarain's*) | 20 | <1.0 | 3.0 | 1.0 | 0 | 280 | 0 |
| **Brownie, frozen/chilled:** | | | | | | | |
| chocolate chip (*Duncan Hines* Oven Ready!), ¹⁄₁₂ pkg. | 170 | 2.0 | 24.0 | 8.0 | 15 | 85 | <1.0 |
| chocolate fudge: | | | | | | | |
| bite size (*Sweet Moments*), 3 pcs. | 180 | 2.0 | 25.0 | 9.0 | 15 | 85 | <1.0 |
| or milk chocolate (*Duncan Hines* Oven Ready!), ¹⁄₁₂ pkg. | 170 | 2.0 | 23.0 | 8.0 | 20 | 85 | <1.0 |
| **Brownie, microwave:** | | | | | | | |
| (*Sweet Moments* Molten Lava), 3 oz.: | | | | | | | |
| chocolate caramel | 360 | 4.0 | 48.0 | 17.0 | 40 | 200 | 1.0 |
| chocolate fudge | 370 | 4.0 | 47.0 | 19.0 | 45 | 180 | 1.0 |
| chocolate, hot (*Guiltless Gourmet*), 2 oz. | 200 | 4.0 | 42.0 | 3.0 | 20 | 190 | 3.0 |
| fudge (*Betty Crocker Warm Delights*): | | | | | | | |
| hot, 3.1 oz. | 370 | 5.0 | 61.0 | 12.0 | 0 | 270 | 3.0 |
| peanut butter, 3.3 oz. | 400 | 7.0 | 63.0 | 14.0 | 0 | 290 | 2.0 |
| **Brownie mix:** | | | | | | | |
| (*Arrowhead Mills* Organic), ¹⁄₂₀ pkg. | 90 | 1.0 | 21.0 | 1.5 | 0 | 65 | <1.0 |
| (*Arrowhead Mills* Organic Bake with Me), ¹⁄₁₅ pkg. | 90 | 1.0 | 21.0 | 1.5 | 0 | 45 | 1.0 |
| (*Arrowhead Mills* Organic Gluten Free), ¹⁄₂₀ pkg. | 110 | 1.0 | 21.0 | 2.0 | 0 | 40 | <1.0 |
| (*Betty Crocker* Gluten Free), ¹⁄₁₆ pkg.* | 150 | 2.0 | 24.0 | 5.0 | 35 | 85 | 1.0 |
| (*Betty Crocker* Supreme Original), ¹⁄₂₀ pkg.* | 160 | 2.0 | 27.0 | 5.0 | 15 | 105 | <1.0 |
| (*Hodgson Mill* Gluten Free), ¹⁄₁₅ pkg. | 100 | 1.0 | 24.0 | .5 | 0 | 106 | 1.7 |

| Food and Measure | cal. | prot. (gms) | carbo. (gms) | fat (gms) | chol. (mgs) | sod. (mgs) | fiber (gms) |
|---|---|---|---|---|---|---|---|
| **Brownie mix, cauliflower, carrots** *(cont.)* | | | | | | | |
| caramel filled (*Pillsbury Minis*), ⅓ tray ....... | 140 | 1.0 | 25.0 | 4.0 | 0 | 85 | 1.0 |
| caramel swirl (*Pillsbury Premium*), 1/12 pkg. .... | 130 | 1.0 | 26.0 | 2.5 | 0 | 95 | <1.0 |
| cheesecake swirl (*Pillsbury* Premium), 1/18 pkg. ............. | 100 | 1.0 | 19.0 | 2.5 | 0 | 70 | <1.0 |
| chocolate: | | | | | | | |
| (*Pillsbury* Premium Extreme), 1/16 pkg. . | 120 | 1.0 | 22.0 | 3.0 | 0 | 65 | 1.0 |
| dark (*Betty Crocker*), 1/20 pkg.* ........ | 160 | 1.0 | 25.0 | 6.0 | 15 | 105 | <1.0 |
| dark (*Duncan Hines*), 1/18 pkg.* ........ | 190 | 2.0 | 25.0 | 9.0 | 25 | 135 | <1.0 |
| double (*Pillsbury* Premium), 1/16 pkg. . | 110 | 1.0 | 23.0 | 2.0 | 0 | 85 | <1.0 |
| marble swirl (*Duncan Hines*), 1/18 pkg.* .. | 170 | 2.0 | 23.0 | 9.0 | 25 | 115 | <1.0 |
| milk (*Duncan Hines*), 1/20 pkg* ......... | 170 | 2.0 | 22.0 | 9.0 | 25 | 75 | <1.0 |
| milk (*Pillsbury* Classics), 1/20 pkg. ......... | 110 | 1.0 | 23.0 | 2.5 | 0 | 80 | <1.0 |
| mint (*Pillsbury* Premium), 1/15 pkg. . | 110 | 1.0 | 22.0 | 2.5 | 0 | 75 | <1.0 |
| triple (*Duncan Hines*), 1/16 pkg.* .. | 180 | 2.0 | 25.0 | 8.0 | 15 | 115 | 1.0 |
| chocolate chunk: | | | | | | | |
| (*Betty Crocker*), 1/16 pkg.* | 170 | 2.0 | 27.0 | 7.0 | 15 | 100 | 1.0 |
| (*Pillsbury* Premium), 1/16 pkg. ........ | 120 | 1.0 | 21.0 | 3.5 | 0 | 70 | <1.0 |
| milk (*Duncan Hines*), 1/16 pkg.* ........ | 170 | 2.0 | 24.0 | 7.0 | 15 | 75 | <1.0 |
| milk (*Pillsbury* Reduced Sugar), 1/12 pkg. ... | 100 | 1.0 | 23.0 | 2.0 | 0 | 90 | 1.0 |
| milk (*Pillsbury* Sugar Free), 1/12 pkg. .... | 90 | 1.0 | 23.0 | 2.5 | 0 | 85 | 3.0 |
| milk (*Pillsbury Minis*), ⅓ tray .......... | 150 | 2.0 | 25.0 | 5.0 | 0 | 95 | 1.0 |
| triple (*Betty Crocker*), 1/16 pkg.* ........ | 170 | 2.0 | 28.0 | 6.0 | 15 | 105 | 1.0 |
| chocolate walnut: | | | | | | | |
| (*Betty Crocker*), 1/20 pkg.* ........ | 160 | 2.0 | 25.0 | 7.0 | 15 | 90 | 1.0 |

| Food and Measure | cal. | prot. (gms) | carbo. (gms) | fat (gms) | chol. (mgs) | sod. (mgs) | fiber (gms) |
|---|---|---|---|---|---|---|---|
| (*Pillsbury* Premium), 1/12 pkg. | 140 | 2.0 | 24.0 | 4.5 | 0 | 85 | 1.0 |
| cookie bar (*Betty Crocker*), 1/16 pkg.* | 200 | 2.0 | 28.0 | 9.0 | 30 | 170 | 0 |
| fudge, all varieties (*No Pudge!*), 1/12 pkg. | 110 | 2.0 | 28.0 | 0 | 0 | 100 | 1.0 |
| fudge/chocolate fudge: | | | | | | | |
| (*Betty Crocker* Family Size), 1/20 pkg.* | 170 | 2.0 | 23.0 | 9.0 | 20 | 95 | <1.0 |
| (*Betty Crocker* Pouch), 1/9 pkg.* | 200 | 2.0 | 27.0 | 10.0 | 25 | 120 | 1.0 |
| (*Betty Crocker* Ultimate), 1/16 pkg.* | 160 | 2.0 | 26.0 | 6.0 | 15 | 110 | <1.0 |
| (*Dr. Oetker* Organics), 1/9 pkg. | 160 | 1.0 | 36.0 | 1.0 | 0 | 90 | 0 |
| (*Duncan Hines* Chewy Snack Size), 1/12 pkg.* | 140 | 2.0 | 20.0 | 7.0 | 20 | 90 | 0 |
| (*"Jiffy"*), 1/8 pkg. | 120 | 1.0 | 22.0 | 3.5 | 0 | 120 | <1.0 |
| (*Pillsbury* Classics Family), 1/20 pkg. | 110 | 1.0 | 23.0 | 2.5 | 0 | 80 | <1.0 |
| (*Pillsbury* Reduced Sugar), 1/12 pkg. | 100 | 1.0 | 24.0 | 2.5 | 0 | 90 | 1.0 |
| (*Pillsbury* Sugar Free), 1/12 pkg. | 90 | 1.0 | 23.0 | 2.5 | 0 | 85 | 3.0 |
| (*Pillsbury Funfetti* Premium), 1/20 pkg. | 110 | 1.0 | 23.0 | 2.5 | 0 | 80 | 1.0 |
| (*Pillsbury Minis*), 1/3 tray | 150 | 1.0 | 25.0 | 4.5 | 0 | 80 | 1.0 |
| chewy (*Duncan Heinz*), 1/20 pkg.* | 170 | 2.0 | 24.0 | 8.0 | 20 | 105 | <1.0 |
| dark, chunk (*Duncan Hines*), 1/16 pkg.* | 160 | 2.0 | 24.0 | 7.0 | 15 | 120 | <1.0 |
| double (*Duncan Hines*), 1/16 pkg.* | 170 | 2.0 | 25.0 | 8.0 | 15 | 105 | <1.0 |
| frosted (*Dr. Oetker* Organics), 1/9 pkg. | 210 | 2.0 | 45.0 | .5 | 0 | 120 | 1.0 |
| peanut butter, 1/16 pkg.*: | | | | | | | |
| (*Betty Crocker*) | 160 | 2.0 | 25.0 | 6.0 | 15 | 110 | <1.0 |
| chocolate (*Duncan Hines*) | 160 | 2.0 | 23.0 | 8.0 | 15 | 100 | <1.0 |
| raspberry filled (*Pillsbury Minis*), 1/3 tray | 130 | 1.0 | 24.0 | 3.5 | 0 | 75 | 1.0 |
| turtle, 1/16 pkg.*: | | | | | | | |
| (*Betty Crocker*) | 160 | 2.0 | 25.0 | 6.0 | 15 | 110 | <1.0 |

| Food and Measure | cal. | prot. (gms) | carbo. (gms) | fat (gms) | chol. (mgs) | sod. (mgs) | fiber (gms) |
|---|---|---|---|---|---|---|---|
| **Brownie mix, turtle** *(cont.)* | | | | | | | |
| caramel (*Duncan Hines*) ......... | 150 | 2.0 | 23.0 | 7.0 | 15 | 100 | <1.0 |
| walnut (*Duncan Hines*), 1/16 pkg.* ........... | 160 | 2.0 | 23.0 | 8.0 | 15 | 100 | 1.0 |
| w/whole wheat flour, flax seed (*Hodgson Mill*), 3 tbsp. ........ | 120 | 3.0 | 28.0 | .5 | 0 | 80 | 2.0 |
| **Browning sauce** (*Gravy Master*), 1/4 tsp. | 0 | 0 | <1.0 | 0 | 0 | 30 | 0 |
| **Bruschetta**, frozen, pesto, mozzarella, tomato (*Cedarlane*), 1.25-oz. pc. ........ | 100 | 3.0 | 10.0 | 5.0 | 5 | 190 | .5 |
| **Bruschetta spread**: | | | | | | | |
| (*Progressso*), 2 tbsp. ... | 10 | 0 | 1.0 | 1.0 | 0 | 100 | 0 |
| basil tomato or garlic (*Classico*), 1 tbsp. ... | 15 | 0 | 1.0 | 1.0 | 0 | 55 | 0 |
| tomato, eggplant, peppers (*Roland*), 2 tbsp. ............. | 60 | 0 | 7.0 | 1.0 | 0 | 0 | 0 |
| **Brussels sprouts**: | | | | | | | |
| (*Dole*), 4 pcs., 3 oz. ..... | 30 | 2.0 | 6.0 | 0 | 0 | 20 | 2.0 |
| raw, 1/2 cup ........... | 19 | 1.5 | 3.9 | .1 | 0 | 11 | 1.8 |
| boiled, .7-oz. pc. ....... | 8 | .5 | 1.8 | .1 | 0 | 4 | .9 |
| boiled, drained, 1/2 cup .. | 30 | 2.0 | 6.8 | .4 | 0 | 17 | 3.4 |
| **Brussels sprouts, frozen**: | | | | | | | |
| (*Birds Eye/Birds Eye Steamfresh* Baby/ *C&W*), 10 pcs., 3 oz. . | 45 | 3.0 | 8.0 | 0 | 0 | 15 | 3.0 |
| (*Birds Eye Steamfresh* Baby Singles), 3.25-oz. bag ........ | 50 | 3.0 | 9.0 | 0 | 0 | 20 | 3.0 |
| butter sauce, baby: | | | | | | | |
| (*Green Giant* Bag), 1/2 cup cooked .... | 70 | 4.0 | 10.0 | 1.0 | <5 | 320 | 3.0 |
| (*Green Giant* Box), 2/3 cup ........... | 60 | 3.0 | 9.0 | 1.0 | <5 | 320 | 3.0 |
| **Brussels sprouts combination**, frozen, cauliflower, carrots (*Birds Eye*), 1 cup .... | 40 | 2.0 | 7.0 | 0 | 0 | 35 | 2.0 |

| Food and Measure | cal. | prot. (gms) | carbo. (gms) | fat (gms) | chol. (mgs) | sod. (mgs) | fiber (gms) |
|---|---|---|---|---|---|---|---|
| **Buckwheat**, grain: | | | | | | | |
| (*Eden* Organic), ¼ cup .. | 160 | 5.0 | 31.0 | 1.0 | 0 | 0 | 5.0 |
| 1 oz. ............... | 97 | 3.8 | 20.3 | 1.0 | 0 | <1 | 2.8 |
| 1 cup ............... | 584 | 22.5 | 121.6 | 5.8 | 0 | 1 | 17.0 |
| **Buckwheat flour:** | | | | | | | |
| (*Arrowhead Mills* | | | | | | | |
| Organic), ⅓ cup ..... | 115 | 5.0 | 20.0 | 1.5 | 0 | 0 | 6.0 |
| (*Bob's Red* Mill | | | | | | | |
| Organic), ¼ cup ..... | 100 | 4.0 | 21.0 | 1.0 | 0 | 0 | 4.0 |
| (*Hodgson Mill*), <¼ cup . | 100 | 2.0 | 22.0 | 1.0 | 0 | 0 | 3.0 |
| 1 cup ............. | 402 | 15.1 | 84.7 | 3.7 | 0 | 13 | 12.0 |
| **Buckwheat groats:** | | | | | | | |
| (*Arrowhead Mills* | | | | | | | |
| Organic), ¼ cup ..... | 150 | 5.0 | 31.0 | 1.0 | 0 | 0 | 4.0 |
| (*Bob's Red Mill* | | | | | | | |
| Organic), ¼ cup ..... | 150 | 6.0 | 32.0 | 1.5 | 0 | 0 | 5.0 |
| (*Wolff's* Kasha), ¼ cup .. | 170 | 6.0 | 35.0 | 1.0 | 0 | 10 | 2.0 |
| roasted, cooked, 1 cup .. | 182 | 6.7 | 39.5 | 1.2 | 0 | 8 | 4.5 |
| **Buffalo wing sauce,** | | | | | | | |
| see "Wing sauce" | | | | | | | |
| **Bulgur:** | | | | | | | |
| dry (*Roland*), ¼ cup .... | 150 | 5.0 | 34.0 | 1.0 | 0 | 0 | 3.0 |
| dry, ¼ cup ............ | 120 | 4.3 | 26.6 | .5 | 0 | 6 | 6.4 |
| cooked, 1 cup ......... | 152 | 5.6 | 33.8 | .4 | 0 | 9 | 8.2 |
| **Bulgur salad**, see | | | | | | | |
| "Tabouli" | | | | | | | |
| **Bun**, see "Roll" | | | | | | | |
| **Bun, sweet**, fresh | | | | | | | |
| (*Entenmann's*), 1 pc., | | | | | | | |
| except as noted: | | | | | | | |
| cheese topped ........ | 320 | 6.0 | 40.0 | 15.0 | 55 | 320 | 1.0 |
| cinnamon, ½ bun: | | | | | | | |
| super, 3 oz. ......... | 330 | 5.0 | 49.0 | 13.0 | 35 | 260 | 1.0 |
| ultimate, 2.25 oz. .... | 250 | 4.0 | 36.0 | 11.0 | 30 | 190 | 1.0 |
| cinnamon raisin swirl ... | 320 | 5.0 | 44.0 | 14.0 | 45 | 280 | 2.0 |
| honey, ½ bun, 2.5 oz.: | | | | | | | |
| glazed ............. | 310 | 4.0 | 34.0 | 18.0 | 0 | 180 | <1.0 |
| iced .............. | 330 | 4.0 | 36.0 | 19.0 | 0 | 180 | 1.0 |
| **Bun, sweet, frozen/** | | | | | | | |
| **chilled**, 1 pc., | | | | | | | |
| except as noted: | | | | | | | |
| blueberry (*Sister* | | | | | | | |
| *Schubert's*), 2 pcs. .... | 190 | 3.0 | 33.0 | 6.0 | 15 | 210 | 1.0 |
| caramel (*Pillsbury*) ..... | 170 | 2.0 | 25.0 | 7.0 | 0 | 330 | <1.0 |

| Food and Measure | cal. | prot. (gms) | carbo. (gms) | fat (gms) | chol. (mgs) | sod. (mgs) | fiber (gms) |
|---|---|---|---|---|---|---|---|
| **Bun, sweet, frozen/chilled** *(cont.)* | | | | | | | |
| cinnamon, w/icing: | | | | | | | |
| (*Grands!* Frozen) .... | 290 | 4.0 | 45.0 | 11.0 | 0 | 460 | 1.0 |
| (*Grands! Cinnabon*) .. | 310 | 4.0 | 54.0 | 9.0 | 0 | 650 | 1.0 |
| (*Grands! Cinnabon* | | | | | | | |
| Extra Flaky) ...... | 370 | 4.0 | 46.0 | 19.0 | 0 | 650 | 1.0 |
| (*Pillsbury*) .......... | 140 | 2.0 | 23.0 | 5.0 | 0 | 340 | <1.0 |
| (*Pillsbury* Reduced | | | | | | | |
| Fat) .......... | 130 | 2.0 | 24.0 | 3.5 | 0 | 330 | <1.0 |
| (*Sister Schubert's*), | | | | | | | |
| 2 pcs. ........... | 220 | 3.0 | 37.0 | 7.0 | 20 | 200 | 1.0 |
| buttercream or cream | | | | | | | |
| cheese iced (*Grands!* | | | | | | | |
| *Cinnabon*) ....... | 310 | 4.0 | 54.0 | 9.0 | 0 | 650 | 1.0 |
| cream cheese icing | | | | | | | |
| (*Pillsbury*) ....... | 140 | 2.0 | 23.0 | 5.0 | 0 | 340 | <1.0 |
| mini (*Grands!* Frozen) | 110 | 2.0 | 18.0 | 4.0 | 0 | 170 | 0 |
| mini (*Pillsbury*), | | | | | | | |
| 3 pcs. ........... | 160 | 2.0 | 26.0 | 6.0 | 0 | 370 | <1.0 |
| cinnamon twists, flaky: | | | | | | | |
| iced (*Pillsbury*) ...... | 180 | 2.0 | 22.0 | 9.0 | 0 | 330 | <1.0 |
| chocolate iced | | | | | | | |
| (*Pillsbury*) ....... | 180 | 2.0 | 22.0 | 9.0 | 0 | 310 | <1.0 |
| orange, w/icing: | | | | | | | |
| (*Pillsbury*) .......... | 160 | 2.0 | 26.0 | 6.0 | 0 | 350 | <1.0 |
| (*Sister Schubert's*), | | | | | | | |
| 2 pcs. ........... | 190 | 2.0 | 31.0 | 6.0 | 15 | 200 | 0 |
| **Bun, sweet, mix**, see | | | | | | | |
| "Roll mix" | | | | | | | |
| **Burbot**, meat only: | | | | | | | |
| raw, 4 oz. ............ | 102 | 21.9 | 0 | .9 | 68 | 110 | 0 |
| baked or broiled, 4 oz. .. | 130 | 28.1 | 0 | 1.2 | 87 | 141 | 0 |
| **Burdock root**: | | | | | | | |
| raw: | | | | | | | |
| (*Frieda's* Gobo Root), | | | | | | | |
| chopped, 1 cup ... | 85 | 2.0 | 20.0 | 0 | 0 | 6 | 4.0 |
| 7.3-oz. pc. ......... | 112 | 1.3 | 13.6 | .1 | 0 | 4 | 5.1 |
| pieces, ½ cup ....... | 43 | .9 | 10.3 | .1 | 0 | 3 | 1.9 |
| boiled, 1" pcs., ½ cup ... | 55 | 1.3 | 13.2 | .1 | 0 | 3 | 1.1 |
| **Burger, vegetarian** (see | | | | | | | |
| also "Burger patty, | | | | | | | |
| vegetarian" and | | | | | | | |
| "'Beef,' vegetarian"): | | | | | | | |

| Food and Measure | cal. | prot. (gms) | carbo. (gms) | fat (gms) | chol. (mgs) | sod. (mgs) | fiber (gms) |
|---|---|---|---|---|---|---|---|
| canned: | | | | | | | |
| (*Loma Linda* Redi-Burger), | | | | | | | |
| ⅝" slice, 3 oz. . . . . . | 120 | 18.0 | 7.0 | 2.5 | 0 | 450 | 4.0 |
| (*Loma Linda* | | | | | | | |
| *VegeBurger*), ¼ cup | 60 | 12.0 | 2.0 | .5 | 0 | 130 | 2.0 |
| (*Worthington Vegetarian* | | | | | | | |
| *Burger*), ¼ cup . . . . | 70 | 10.0 | 3.0 | 1.5 | 0 | 250 | 1.0 |
| frozen/chilled: | | | | | | | |
| ground (*Boca*), 2 oz. . . | 60 | 13.0 | 6.0 | .5 | 0 | 270 | 3.0 |
| ground (*MorningStar* | | | | | | | |
| *Farms Meal Starters* | | | | | | | |
| *Grillers Recipe* | | | | | | | |
| *Crumbles*), ⅔ cup . | 80 | 10.0 | 5.0 | 2.5 | 0 | 230 | 3.0 |
| mix (*Fantastic* Nature's | | | | | | | |
| Burger), ¼ cup . . . . . . | 170 | 8.0 | 30.0 | 3.0 | 0 | 450 | 5.0 |
| **Burger patty, vege-** | | | | | | | |
| **tarian**, frozen, | | | | | | | |
| 1 pc., 2.5 oz., | | | | | | | |
| except as noted: | | | | | | | |
| (*Amy's* Bistro) . . . . . . . . . | 110 | 5.0 | 16.0 | 2.5 | 0 | 370 | 2.0 |
| (*Amy's* ¼ Pound), 4 oz. . | 200 | 21.0 | 23.0 | 3.5 | 0 | 600 | 6.0 |
| (*Boca* Organic Vegan) . . . | 100 | 13.0 | 9.0 | 2.5 | 0 | 470 | 4.0 |
| (*Boca* Original), 3.5 oz. . . | 100 | 19.0 | 8.0 | 1.0 | 0 | 520 | 6.0 |
| (*Boca* Original Vegan) . . . | 70 | 13.0 | 6.0 | .5 | 0 | 260 | 4.0 |
| (*Gardenburger* Garden | | | | | | | |
| Vegan) . . . . . . . . . . . . | 80 | 9.0 | 12.0 | 1.0 | 0 | 270 | 4.0 |
| (*Gardenburger* The | | | | | | | |
| Original) . . . . . . . . . . . | 100 | 5.0 | 18.0 | 3.0 | 0 | 400 | 5.0 |
| (*MorningStar Farms* | | | | | | | |
| *Garden Veggie* | | | | | | | |
| *Patties*), 2.36 oz. . . . . | 110 | 10.0 | 9.0 | 3.5 | 0 | 350 | 3.0 |
| (*MorningStar Farms* | | | | | | | |
| *Grillers* Original), | | | | | | | |
| 2.25 oz. . . . . . . . . . . | 130 | 15.0 | 5.0 | 6.0 | 0 | 260 | 2.0 |
| (*MorningStar Farms* | | | | | | | |
| *Grillers* Quarter | | | | | | | |
| Pounder), 4 oz. . . . . . . | 250 | 26.0 | 10.0 | 12.0 | 0 | 490 | 3.0 |
| (*MorningStar Farms* | | | | | | | |
| *Grillers* Vegan) . . . . . . | 100 | 12.0 | 7.0 | 2.5 | 0 | 280 | 4.0 |
| (*MorningStar Farms* | | | | | | | |
| *Grillers Prime*) . . . . . . | 170 | 17.0 | 4.0 | 9.0 | 0 | 360 | 2.0 |
| (*Worthington FriPats*), | | | | | | | |
| 2.25 oz. . . . . . . . . . . . | 130 | 15.0 | 5.0 | 6.0 | 0 | 320 | 3.0 |
| (*Worthington Stakelets*) . | 150 | 14.0 | 7.0 | 7.0 | 0 | 480 | 2.0 |

| Food and Measure | cal. | prot. (gms) | carbo. (gms) | fat (gms) | chol. (mgs) | sod. (mgs) | fiber (gms) |
|---|---|---|---|---|---|---|---|
| **Burger patty, vegetarian** *(cont.)* | | | | | | | |
| (*Yves*), 2.6 oz. . . . . . . . . | 110 | 14.0 | 8.0 | 4.0 | 0 | 440 | 2.0 |
| all American: | | | | | | | |
| (*Amy's*) . . . . . . . . . . . . | 130 | 12.0 | 12.0 | 3.5 | 0 | 390 | 4.0 |
| (*Boca* Organic) . . . . . . | 140 | 15.0 | 9.0 | 5.0 | 5 | 500 | 4.0 |
| (*Dr. Praeger's*) . . . . . . | 130 | 15.0 | 9.0 | 4.0 | 0 | 350 | 3.0 |
| flame grilled (*Boca*) . . | 120 | 14.0 | 6.0 | 5.0 | 5 | 380 | 5.0 |
| Asian (*MorningStar* | | | | | | | |
| *Farms*), 2.36 oz. . . . . . | 100 | 7.0 | 10.0 | 4.0 | 0 | 490 | 2.0 |
| black bean: | | | | | | | |
| chipotle | | | | | | | |
| (*Gardenburger*) . . . | 100 | 5.0 | 16.0 | 3.0 | 0 | 390 | 5.0 |
| chipotle (*MorningStar* | | | | | | | |
| *Farms*), 4.2 oz. . . . . | 210 | 17.0 | 24.0 | 7.0 | 0 | 700 | 7.0 |
| spicy (*MorningStar* | | | | | | | |
| *Farms*), 2.36 oz. . . . | 120 | 11.0 | 13.0 | 4.0 | 0 | 350 | 4.0 |
| Bombay (*Dr. Praeger's* | | | | | | | |
| *Veggie*), 2.8 oz. . . . . . . | 110 | 6.0 | 13.0 | 4.5 | 0 | 250 | 5.0 |
| bruschetta (*Boca*) . . . . . . | 90 | 13.0 | 9.0 | 1.5 | 5 | 440 | 5.0 |
| California: | | | | | | | |
| (*Amy's*) . . . . . . . . . . . . | 150 | 6.0 | 21.0 | 5.0 | 0 | 500 | 4.0 |
| (*Amy's* Light Sodium) . | 110 | 5.0 | 16.0 | 4.0 | 0 | 250 | 3.0 |
| (*Dr. Praeger's Veggie*), | | | | | | | |
| 2.75 oz. . . . . . . . . | 110 | 6.0 | 13.0 | 4.5 | 0 | 250 | 5.0 |
| (*Dr. Praeger's Veggie* | | | | | | | |
| Gluten Free), | | | | | | | |
| 2.75 oz. . . . . . . . . | 120 | 5.0 | 13.0 | 6.0 | 0 | 180 | 4.0 |
| (*Gardenburger*) . . . . . . | 110 | 3.0 | 15.0 | 3.5 | 0 | 400 | 3.0 |
| (*MorningStar Farms* | | | | | | | |
| *Grillers* Turk'y), | | | | | | | |
| 2.25 oz. . . . . . . . . | 90 | 9.0 | 7.0 | 5.0 | 0 | 390 | 5.0 |
| cheddar (*Amy's*) . . . . . . . | 150 | 8.0 | 16.0 | 5.0 | 5 | 440 | 3.0 |
| cheeseburger: | | | | | | | |
| (*Boca*) . . . . . . . . . . . . . | 100 | 13.0 | 6.0 | 4.5 | 10 | 320 | 4.0 |
| (*Boca* Organic) . . . . . . | 120 | 15.0 | 7.0 | 4.5 | 5 | 650 | 3.0 |
| "chicken," see " 'Chicken,' | | | | | | | |
| vegetarian" | | | | | | | |
| garlic, roasted: | | | | | | | |
| (*Boca*) . . . . . . . . . . . . . | 70 | 12.0 | 6.0 | 1.5 | 0 | 370 | 4.0 |
| (*Boca* Organic) . . . . . . | 130 | 16.0 | 9.0 | 3.0 | 0 | 470 | 4.0 |
| garlic portobello: | | | | | | | |
| (*Veggie Patch*) . . . . . . | 120 | 11.0 | 8.0 | 6.0 | 0 | 320 | 4.0 |
| (*Veggie Patch* | | | | | | | |
| Family), 3.2 oz. . . . | 140 | 15.0 | 7.0 | 6.0 | 0 | 390 | 5.0 |

| Food and Measure | cal. | prot. (gms) | carbo. (gms) | fat (gms) | chol. (mgs) | sod. (mgs) | fiber (gms) |
|---|---|---|---|---|---|---|---|
| Italian (*Dr. Praeger's Veggie*), 2.75 oz. ..... | 110 | 6.0 | 13.0 | 5.0 | 0 | 250 | 5.0 |
| mushroom: | | | | | | | |
| (*MorningStar Farms Mushroom Lovers*), 2.25 oz. ......... | 110 | 7.0 | 8.0 | 6.0 | 0 | 220 | <1.0 |
| mozzarella (*Boca Savory*) ......... | 110 | 13.0 | 8.0 | 2.5 | 0 | 320 | 4.0 |
| onion, roasted: | | | | | | | |
| (*Boca*) ............. | 70 | 11.0 | 7.0 | 1.0 | 0 | 300 | 4.0 |
| (*Boca* Organic) ...... | 130 | 15.0 | 10.0 | 3.0 | 0 | 420 | 4.0 |
| portobello (*Gardenburger*) ...... | 100 | 4.0 | 17.0 | 2.5 | <5 | 490 | 5.0 |
| Sonoma (*Amy's*) ....... | 140 | 5.0 | 18.0 | 5.0 | 0 | 500 | 3.0 |
| Southwest (*Dr. Praeger's*) | 120 | 12.0 | 11.0 | 3.5 | 0 | 260 | 3.0 |
| sun-dried tomato basil (*Gardenburger*) ...... | 100 | 4.0 | 17.0 | 2.5 | <5 | 270 | 4.0 |
| Texas (*Amy's*) ......... | 130 | 12.0 | 14.0 | 2.5 | 0 | 350 | 3.0 |
| Tex-Mex (*Dr. Praeger's Veggie*), 2.75 oz. ..... | 110 | 6.0 | 13.0 | 4.5 | 0 | 250 | 5.0 |
| vegetable, soy (*Boca*): | | | | | | | |
| garden, organic ..... | 130 | 15.0 | 9.0 | 3.0 | 0 | 400 | 4.0 |
| grilled ............. | 80 | 12.0 | 7.0 | 1.0 | 0 | 300 | 4.0 |
| veggie medley: | | | | | | | |
| (*Gardenburger*) ...... | 100 | 3.0 | 17.0 | 2.5 | 0 | 380 | 5.0 |
| (*Golden* Baja), 1.3 oz. . | 100 | 2.0 | 14.0 | 4.0 | 10 | 200 | 1.0 |
| ***Burger King:*** | | | | | | | |
| breakfast: | | | | | | | |
| *BK* breakfast bowl .... | 540 | 24.0 | 17.0 | 42.0 | 375 | 1020 | 2.0 |
| *BK* ciabatta club ..... | 480 | 24.0 | 41.0 | 23.0 | 210 | 1270 | 2.0 |
| *BK* muffin sandwich .. | 410 | 17.0 | 24.0 | 26.0 | 125 | 680 | 1.0 |
| *BK* platter .......... | 810 | 25.0 | 57.0 | 54.0 | 360 | 1790 | 4.0 |
| *BK* platter, ultimate ...1310 | 1310 | 32.0 | 134.0 | 72.0 | 455 | 2490 | 5.0 |
| *BK Wrapper* cheesy bacon ............ | 380 | 13.0 | 28.0 | 24.0 | 185 | 1020 | 2.0 |
| biscuit: | | | | | | | |
| bacon/egg/cheese . | 420 | 16.0 | 34.0 | 25.0 | 185 | 1360 | 1.0 |
| ham/egg/cheese ... | 420 | 16.0 | 33.0 | 22.0 | 185 | 1410 | 1.0 |
| sausage ......... | 420 | 13.0 | 32.0 | 27.0 | 35 | 1090 | 1.0 |
| sausage/egg/cheese | 570 | 20.0 | 34.0 | 37.0 | 210 | 1510 | 1.0 |
| *Croissan'wich:* | | | | | | | |
| egg/cheese ....... | 320 | 11.0 | 26.0 | 16.0 | 180 | 680 | 0 |
| bacon/egg/cheese . | 360 | 14.0 | 26.0 | 19.0 | 190 | 830 | 0 |

| Food and Measure | cal. | prot. (gms) | carbo. (gms) | fat (gms) | chol. (mgs) | sod. (mgs) | fiber (gms) |
|---|---|---|---|---|---|---|---|
| **Burger King,** Croissan'wich *(cont.)* | | | | | | | |
| ham/egg/cheese ... | 350 | 18.0 | 27.0 | 17.0 | 200 | 1110 | 0 |
| sausage/cheese ... | 380 | 14.0 | 26.0 | 24.0 | 50 | 780 | 0 |
| sausage/egg/cheese | 490 | 18.0 | 27.0 | 31.0 | 215 | 990 | 0 |
| *Double Croissan'wich,* | | | | | | | |
| egg/cheese, and: | | | | | | | |
| bacon ........... | 440 | 20.0 | 27.0 | 25.0 | 210 | 1190 | 0 |
| ham ............ | 440 | 26.0 | 28.0 | 22.0 | 230 | 1740 | 0 |
| ham/bacon ....... | 440 | 23.0 | 28.0 | 24.0 | 220 | 1470 | 0 |
| ham/sausage ..... | 320 | 28.0 | 28.0 | 35.0 | 240 | 1630 | 0 |
| sausage ......... | 700 | 29.0 | 29.0 | 49.0 | 255 | 1510 | 0 |
| sausage/bacon .... | 570 | 24.0 | 28.0 | 37.0 | 235 | 1350 | 0 |
| omelet sandwich, | | | | | | | |
| enormous ........ | 760 | 35.0 | 44.0 | 44.0 | 405 | 1840 | 2.0 |
| French toast sticks, 3 . | 230 | 3.0 | 29.0 | 11.0 | 0 | 260 | 1.0 |
| pancakes w/syrup, 3 .. | 500 | 7.0 | 77.0 | 19.0 | 95 | 700 | 1.0 |
| platter w/sausage .. | 670 | 14.0 | 78.0 | 34.0 | 125 | 1010 | 1.0 |
| potatoes, Southwest .. | 90 | 2.0 | 12.0 | 3.5 | 0 | 220 | 2.0 |
| hash browns, large ... | 670 | 5.0 | 65.0 | 44.0 | 0 | 1080 | 9.0 |
| medium ......... | 500 | 4.0 | 48.0 | 33.0 | 0 | 810 | 7.0 |
| small ........... | 250 | 2.0 | 24.0 | 16.0 | 0 | 410 | 3.0 |
| cini-minis, 4 ........ | 400 | 7.0 | 52.0 | 18.0 | 20 | 380 | 2.0 |
| vanilla icing ...... | 90 | 0 | 22.0 | 0 | 0 | 25 | 0 |
| burgers: | | | | | | | |
| *BK* double stacker .... | 560 | 30.0 | 29.0 | 36.0 | 110 | 1040 | 1.0 |
| triple stacker ..... | 740 | 43.0 | 30.0 | 50.0 | 165 | 1390 | 1.0 |
| quad stacker ..... | 920 | 58.0 | 31.0 | 63.0 | 220 | 1730 | 1.0 |
| buck double ........ | 410 | 24.0 | 28.0 | 22.0 | 85 | 740 | 1.0 |
| cheeseburger ....... | 300 | 16.0 | 28.0 | 14.0 | 45 | 710 | 1.0 |
| bacon ........... | 330 | 18.0 | 28.0 | 16.0 | 55 | 810 | 1.0 |
| double .......... | 450 | 26.0 | 29.0 | 26.0 | 95 | 960 | 1.0 |
| double bacon ..... | 510 | 31.0 | 29.0 | 30.0 | 105 | 1150 | 1.0 |
| rodeo ........... | 350 | 16.0 | 37.0 | 17.0 | 45 | 600 | 2.0 |
| hamburger ......... | 260 | 13.0 | 28.0 | 10.0 | 35 | 490 | 1.0 |
| double .......... | 360 | 22.0 | 28.0 | 18.0 | 70 | 520 | 1.0 |
| *Steakhouse XT* ...... | 770 | 36.0 | 52.0 | 46.0 | 115 | 1330 | 3.0 |
| *A.1* .............. | 970 | 42.0 | 54.0 | 61.0 | 135 | 1920 | 4.0 |
| *Whopper* ........... | 670 | 29.0 | 51.0 | 40.0 | 75 | 980 | 3.0 |
| no mayo ......... | 510 | 28.0 | 51.0 | 23.0 | 65 | 840 | 3.0 |
| w/cheese ........ | 760 | 33.0 | 53.0 | 47.0 | 100 | 1410 | 3.0 |
| *Whopper, Jr.* ........ | 340 | 14.0 | 28.0 | 19.0 | 40 | 510 | 2.0 |
| no mayo ......... | 260 | 13.0 | 28.0 | 10.0 | 35 | 440 | 2.0 |
| w/cheese. ........ | 380 | 16.0 | 29.0 | 23.0 | 55 | 730 | 2.0 |

| Food and Measure | cal. | prot. (gms) | carbo. (gms) | fat (gms) | chol. (mgs) | sod. (mgs) | fiber (gms) |
|---|---|---|---|---|---|---|---|
| *Double Whopper* ..... | 900 | 47.0 | 51.0 | 57.0 | 140 | 1050 | 3.0 |
| no mayo ......... | 740 | 47.0 | 51.0 | 39.0 | 130 | 910 | 3.0 |
| w/cheese ........ | 990 | 52.0 | 53.0 | 65.0 | 160 | 1480 | 3.0 |
| *Triple Whopper* ...... | 1140 | 67.0 | 51.0 | 75.0 | 205 | 1110 | 3.0 |
| no mayo ......... | 980 | 66.0 | 51.0 | 57.0 | 190 | 970 | 3.0 |
| w/cheese ........ | 1230 | 71.0 | 53.0 | 82.0 | 225 | 1550 | 3.0 |
| mustard *Whopper* .... | 530 | 29.0 | 52.0 | 23.0 | 65 | 1080 | 3.0 |
| Texas *Whopper* ...... | 800 | 37.0 | 50.0 | 51.0 | 110 | 1700 | 3.0 |
| double .......... | 1040 | 56.0 | 50.0 | 69.0 | 175 | 1770 | 3.0 |
| triple .......... | 1270 | 76.0 | 50.0 | 86.0 | 240 | 1840 | 3.0 |
| sandwiches/wrap: | | | | | | | |
| *BK Big Fish* ........ | 640 | 23.0 | 67.0 | 31.0 | 45 | 1560 | 3.0 |
| no tarter sauce .... | 460 | 23.0 | 64.0 | 13.0 | 30 | 1320 | 3.0 |
| *BK Veggie* burger .... | 410 | 22.0 | 44.0 | 16.0 | 5 | 1030 | 7.0 |
| no mayo ......... | 320 | 22.0 | 43.0 | 7.0 | 0 | 960 | 7.0 |
| w/cheese ........ | 450 | 24.0 | 44.0 | 20.0 | 20 | 1250 | 7.0 |
| chicken, original ..... | 630 | 24.0 | 46.0 | 39.0 | 65 | 1390 | 3.0 |
| no mayo ......... | 420 | 24.0 | 46.0 | 16.0 | 45 | 1210 | 3.0 |
| American ........ | 730 | 29.0 | 49.0 | 47.0 | 85 | 1830 | 3.0 |
| Italian .......... | 520 | 32.0 | 50.0 | 22.0 | 65 | 1670 | 3.0 |
| chicken *BK Wrapper* .. | 360 | 14.0 | 32.0 | 19.0 | 30 | 1010 | 2.0 |
| *Chicken Tenders* ..... | 440 | 12.0 | 35.0 | 28.0 | 35 | 610 | 1.0 |
| *Chick'n Crisp*, spicy .. | 460 | 13.0 | 34.0 | 30.0 | 30 | 810 | 2.0 |
| no mayo ......... | 300 | 12.0 | 35.0 | 12.0 | 20 | 670 | 2.0 |
| pork, country ....... | 810 | 29.0 | 78.0 | 42.0 | 75 | 1910 | 4.0 |
| tacos, 2 ............ | 330 | 14.0 | 18.0 | 23.0 | 30 | 750 | 5.0 |
| *Tendercrisp* chicken .. | 800 | 32.0 | 68.0 | 46.0 | 70 | 1640 | 3.0 |
| no mayo ......... | 590 | 31.0 | 68.0 | 22.0 | 55 | 1450 | 3.0 |
| *Tendergrill* chicken ... | 470 | 37.0 | 40.0 | 18.0 | 85 | 1100 | 2.0 |
| no mayo ......... | 360 | 37.0 | 40.0 | 7.0 | 75 | 1010 | 2.0 |
| *BK* chicken fries, 6 pcs. ... | 250 | 14.0 | 16.0 | 15.0 | 30 | 820 | 1.0 |
| 9 pcs. ............. | 380 | 21.0 | 24.0 | 22.0 | 40 | 1220 | 2.0 |
| 12 pcs. ............ | 500 | 28.0 | 32.0 | 29.0 | 55 | 1630 | 3.0 |
| *Chicken Tenders*, 4 pcs. . | 180 | 9.0 | 13.0 | 11.0 | 30 | 310 | 0 |
| 5 pcs. ............. | 230 | 11.0 | 16.0 | 13.0 | 35 | 380 | 0 |
| 6 pcs. ............. | 270 | 14.0 | 19.0 | 16.0 | 45 | 460 | 0 |
| 8 pcs. ............. | 360 | 18.0 | 25.0 | 21.0 | 60 | 610 | 0 |
| dipping sauce, 1 oz.: | | | | | | | |
| barbecue .......... | 40 | 0 | 11.0 | 0 | 0 | 310 | 0 |
| Buffalo ........... | 80 | 0 | 2.0 | 8.0 | 5 | 360 | 0 |
| honey mustard ...... | 90 | 0 | 8.0 | 6.0 | 10 | 180 | 0 |
| ranch ............ | 140 | 1.0 | 1.0 | 15.0 | 5 | 230 | 0 |
| sweet and sour ...... | 45 | 0 | 11.0 | 0 | 0 | 55 | 0 |

| Food and Measure | cal. | prot. (gms) | carbo. (gms) | fat (gms) | chol. (mgs) | sod. (mgs) | fiber (gms) |
|---|---|---|---|---|---|---|---|
| **Burger King** (cont.) | | | | | | | |
| sides: | | | | | | | |
|   *BK* apple fries ....... | 25 | 0 | 6.0 | 0 | 0 | 0 | 1.0 |
|     caramel sauce .... | 45 | 0 | 10.0 | .5 | 0 | 35 | 0 |
|   fries, salted, large .... | 540 | 6.0 | 69.0 | 27.0 | 0 | 830 | 6.0 |
|     medium ......... | 440 | 5.0 | 56.0 | 22.0 | 0 | 670 | 5.0 |
|     small .......... | 340 | 4.0 | 44.0 | 17.0 | 0 | 530 | 4.0 |
|     value .......... | 220 | 2.0 | 28.0 | 11.0 | 0 | 340 | 2.0 |
|   ketchup pkt. ........ | 10 | 0 | 3.0 | 0 | 0 | 125 | 0 |
|   mayo pkt. .......... | 80 | 0 | 1.0 | 9.0 | 10 | 75 | 0 |
|   mozzarella | | | | | | | |
|     sticks, 4 ......... | 280 | 11.0 | 24.0 | 15.0 | 35 | 650 | 2.0 |
|     marinara sauce ... | 15 | 1.0 | 4.0 | 0 | 0 | 170 | 1.0 |
|   onion rings, large .... | 490 | 7.0 | 57.0 | 26.0 | 0 | 770 | 5.0 |
|     medium ......... | 400 | 6.0 | 47.0 | 21.0 | 0 | 630 | 4.0 |
|     small .......... | 310 | 4.0 | 36.0 | 17.0 | 0 | 490 | 3.0 |
|     value .......... | 150 | 2.0 | 17.0 | 8.0 | 0 | 230 | 1.0 |
|   onion ring sauce ..... | 150 | 0 | 3.0 | 15.0 | 15 | 210 | 1.0 |
|   picante/taco sauce ... | 10 | 0 | 2.0 | 0 | 0 | 115 | 0 |
| salad, garden, no | | | | | | | |
|   dressing/extras: | | | | | | | |
|   *Tendercrisp* chicken .. | 410 | 27.0 | 27.0 | 23.0 | 65 | 1060 | 4.0 |
|   *Tendergrill* chicken ... | 230 | 34.0 | 9.0 | 8.0 | 85 | 930 | 3.0 |
|   w/out chicken ....... | 70 | 4.0 | 7.0 | 4.0 | 10 | 100 | 3.0 |
|   side salad .......... | 40 | 3.0 | 2.0 | 2.0 | 5 | 45 | 1.0 |
| croutons ............. | 60 | 1.0 | 9.0 | 2.0 | 0 | 120 | 0 |
| dressing (*Ken's*), 2 oz.: | | | | | | | |
|   Caesar, creamy ...... | 210 | 3.0 | 4.0 | 21.0 | 25 | 610 | 0 |
|   honey mustard ...... | 270 | 1.0 | 15.0 | 23.0 | 20 | 510 | 0 |
|   Italian, light ........ | 120 | 0 | 5.0 | 11.0 | 0 | 440 | 0 |
|   ranch ............. | 190 | 1.0 | 2.0 | 20.0 | 20 | 550 | 0 |
|   ranch, fat free ....... | 60 | 0 | 15.0 | 0 | 0 | 740 | 2.0 |
| shakes, 16 fl. oz.: | | | | | | | |
|   chocolate .......... | 570 | 12.0 | 99.0 | 15.0 | 50 | 470 | 1.0 |
|   strawberry ......... | 560 | 11.0 | 98.0 | 15.0 | 50 | 400 | 0 |
|   vanilla ............. | 480 | 11.0 | 78.0 | 15.0 | 50 | 390 | 0 |
| desserts: | | | | | | | |
|   Dutch apple pie ...... | 320 | 2.0 | 46.0 | 14.0 | 0 | 300 | 1.0 |
|   *Hershey's* sundae pie . | 300 | 3.0 | 31.0 | 18.0 | 10 | 210 | 1.0 |
|   funnel cake sticks, | | | | | | | |
|     w/icing .......... | 300 | 2.0 | 49.0 | 11.0 | 10 | 210 | 1.0 |
| **Burger seasoning** | | | | | | | |
|   (*Grill Mates*), ¼ tsp. .. | 0 | 0 | 0 | 0 | 0 | 115 | 0 |

| Food and Measure | cal. | prot. (gms) | carbo. (gms) | fat (gms) | chol. (mgs) | sod. (mgs) | fiber (gms) |
|---|---|---|---|---|---|---|---|
| **Burrito** (see also "Burrito, breakfast"), frozen, 1 pc.: | | | | | | | |
| (*Amy's* Especial), 6 oz. . . | 300 | 9.0 | 50.0 | 7.0 | 5 | 620 | 4.0 |
| (*Amy's* Gluten Free Nondairy), 5.5 oz. . . . . | 240 | 7.0 | 38.0 | 6.0 | 0 | 430 | 5.0 |
| bean/cheese: | | | | | | | |
| (*Amy's*), 6 oz. . . . . . . . | 310 | 11.0 | 46.0 | 9.0 | 10 | 580 | 7.0 |
| (*Amy's* Gluten Free), 6 oz. . . . . . . . . . . . | 260 | 9.0 | 37.0 | 8.0 | 5 | 430 | 5.0 |
| (*Amy's* Light Sodium) . | 330 | 12.0 | 51.0 | 9.0 | 10 | 290 | 7.0 |
| (*El Monterey*), 5 oz. . . | 280 | 10.0 | 43.0 | 8.0 | 5 | 560 | 5.0 |
| (*El Monterey* Family Pack), 4 oz. . . . . . . | 240 | 8.0 | 35.0 | 7.0 | 5 | 270 | 2.0 |
| (*El Monterey* 2 Pack), 4 oz. . . . . . . . . . . . | 240 | 8.0 | 35.0 | 7.0 | 5 | 380 | 2.0 |
| (*El Monterey* XX Large!), 10 oz. . . . . | 600 | 21.0 | 89.0 | 17.0 | 10 | 740 | 5.0 |
| bean/rice, 6 oz.: | | | | | | | |
| (*Amy's*) . . . . . . . . . . . | 300 | 10.0 | 48.0 | 8.0 | 0 | 580 | 6.0 |
| (*Amy's* Gluten Free) . . | 240 | 7.0 | 38.0 | 6.0 | 0 | 430 | 5.0 |
| (*Amy's* Light Sodium) . | 320 | 10.0 | 52.0 | 8.0 | 0 | 290 | 8.0 |
| cheese (*Cedarlane*) . . . | 260 | 13.0 | 48.0 | 1.0 | 0 | 490 | 7.0 |
| beef/bean: | | | | | | | |
| (*El Monterey*), 5 oz. . . | 370 | 10.0 | 42.0 | 17.0 | 20 | 610 | 4.0 |
| (*El Monterey*), 8 oz. . . | 590 | 17.0 | 68.0 | 27.0 | 30 | 980 | 7.0 |
| (*El Monterey* Family Pack), 4 oz. . . . . . . | 300 | 9.0 | 33.0 | 14.0 | 15 | 300 | 2.0 |
| (*El Monterey* Gigante), ½ of 14-oz. pkg. . . . | 520 | 16.0 | 58.0 | 25.0 | 30 | 830 | 3.0 |
| (*El Monterey* 2 Pack), 4 oz. . . . . . . . . . . . | 300 | 9.0 | 34.0 | 14.0 | 15 | 410 | 2.0 |
| (*El Monterey* XX Large!), 10 oz. . . . . | 760 | 24.0 | 84.0 | 35.0 | 40 | 810 | 4.0 |
| spicy (*El Monterey* Red Hot), 5 oz. . . . . | 380 | 11.0 | 42.0 | 18.0 | 20 | 700 | 4.0 |
| spicy (*El Monterey* Red Hot), 8 oz. . . . . | 600 | 17.0 | 68.0 | 29.0 | 35 | 1120 | 7.0 |
| spicy (*El Monterey* Red Hot Gigante), ½ of 14-oz. pkg. . . . | 520 | 16.0 | 58.0 | 25.0 | 25 | 800 | 3.0 |
| spicy (*El Monterey* Red Hot XX Large!), 10 oz. . . . . | 760 | 24.0 | 85.0 | 35.0 | 40 | 770 | 5.0 |

| Food and Measure | cal. | prot. (gms) | carbo. (gms) | fat (gms) | chol. (mgs) | sod. (mgs) | fiber (gms) |
|---|---|---|---|---|---|---|---|
| **Burrito** *(cont.)* | | | | | | | |
| beef/bean, green chili: | | | | | | | |
| (*El Monterey*), 5 oz. .. | 360 | 10.0 | 41.0 | 17.0 | 20 | 610 | 4.0 |
| (*El Monterey* Family | | | | | | | |
| Pack), 4 oz. ...... | 290 | 9.0 | 32.0 | 14.0 | 15 | 300 | 2.0 |
| (*El Monterey* Gigante), | | | | | | | |
| ½ of 14-oz. pkg. ... | 520 | 16.0 | 58.0 | 24.0 | 25 | 700 | 4.0 |
| (*El Monterey* XX | | | | | | | |
| Large!), 10 oz. .... | 740 | 23.0 | 84.0 | 34.0 | 40 | 790 | 5.0 |
| beef/bean, red chili | | | | | | | |
| (*El Monterey* Family/ | | | | | | | |
| 2 Pack), 4 oz. ....... | 300 | 9.0 | 34.0 | 14.0 | 15 | 270 | 2.0 |
| black bean/vegetable | | | | | | | |
| (*Amy's*), 6 oz. ....... | 290 | 7.0 | 45.0 | 8.0 | 0 | 680 | 5.0 |
| cheddar (*Amy's* Gluten | | | | | | | |
| Free), 5.5 oz. ........ | 260 | 9.0 | 37.0 | 8.0 | 5 | 430 | 5.0 |
| chicken: | | | | | | | |
| (*Cedarlane* Low Fat), | | | | | | | |
| 6 oz. ........... | 270 | 15.0 | 47.0 | 3.0 | 15 | 500 | 6.0 |
| (*José Olé* Monterey), | | | | | | | |
| 5 oz. ........... | 270 | 11.0 | 41.0 | 6.0 | 20 | 600 | 2.0 |
| w/chili verde sauce | | | | | | | |
| (*Cedarlane* Grande), | | | | | | | |
| 10 oz. .......... | 460 | 26.0 | 62.0 | 14.0 | 45 | 980 | 11.0 |
| fajita (*Cedarlane*), 6 oz. | 310 | 15.0 | 47.0 | 8.0 | 25 | 710 | 4.0 |
| tequila lime flavor | | | | | | | |
| (*Cedarlane*), 6 oz. .. | 330 | 16.0 | 49.0 | 8.0 | 25 | 830 | 5.0 |
| chicken/cheese (*El* | | | | | | | |
| *Monterey* Butcher | | | | | | | |
| Wrap), 8 oz. ........ | 460 | 22.0 | 60.0 | 15.0 | 35 | 1090 | 3.0 |
| chicken/rice/beans | | | | | | | |
| (*El Monterey* Family/ | | | | | | | |
| 2-Pack), 4 oz. ....... | 240 | 10.0 | 33.0 | 7.0 | 10 | 460 | 1.0 |
| w/chili verde sauce | | | | | | | |
| (*Cedarlane* Grande), | | | | | | | |
| ½ of 10-oz. pkg. ..... | 230 | 9.0 | 27.0 | 10.0 | 20 | 540 | 2.0 |
| jalapeño/beef/cheese | | | | | | | |
| (*El Monterey* XX | | | | | | | |
| Large!), 10 oz. ...... | 720 | 23.0 | 82.0 | 35.0 | 40 | 840 | 4.0 |
| w/salsa roja (*Cedarlane* | | | | | | | |
| Grande), ½ of | | | | | | | |
| 10-oz. pkg. ......... | 220 | 9.0 | 27.0 | 9.0 | 20 | 610 | 2.0 |
| Southwestern (*Amy's*), | | | | | | | |
| 5.5 oz. ............. | 290 | 12.0 | 38.0 | 10.0 | 15 | 680 | 6.0 |

| Food and Measure | cal. | prot. (gms) | carbo. (gms) | fat (gms) | chol. (mgs) | sod. (mgs) | fiber (gms) |
|---|---|---|---|---|---|---|---|
| steak, shredded/cheese: | | | | | | | |
| (*José Olé*), 5 oz. ..... | 300 | 12.0 | 40.0 | 10.0 | 25 | 570 | 2.0 |
| (*El Monterey* Butcher Wrap), 8 oz. ...... | 450 | 21.0 | 58.0 | 14.0 | 50 | 920 | 2.0 |
| (*El Monterey* Supreme), 5 oz. ... | 290 | 12.0 | 41.0 | 9.0 | 20 | 590 | 1.0 |
| steak/jalapeño (*José Olé*), 5 oz. .......... | 290 | 11.0 | 43.0 | 9.0 | 15 | 700 | 3.0 |
| taco picante, spicy (*El Monterey* Family Pack), 4 oz. ......... | 290 | 9.0 | 31.0 | 14.0 | 15 | 340 | 1.0 |
| vegetable, roasted, and cheese (*Cedarlane* Organic), 6 oz. ...... | 330 | 14.0 | 48.0 | 8.0 | 15 | 590 | 3.0 |
| **Burrito, breakfast**, frozen, 1 pc.: | | | | | | | |
| (*Amy's*), 6 oz. ......... | 270 | 11.0 | 38.0 | 8.0 | 0 | 540 | 5.0 |
| egg/bacon (*José Olé*), 4 oz. ............... | 260 | 11.0 | 33.0 | 9.0 | 90 | 630 | 1.0 |
| egg/bacon/cheese/ salsa (*El Monterey* Butcher Wrap), 8 oz. ... | 480 | 19.0 | 58.0 | 19.0 | 60 | 590 | 0 |
| egg/cheese/salsa/ bacon (*El Monterey* Supreme), 4.5 oz. .... | 290 | 13.0 | 36.0 | 11.0 | 120 | 740 | 1.0 |
| egg/ham (*José Olé*), 4 oz. ............... | 250 | 10.0 | 34.0 | 8.0 | 80 | 640 | 2.0 |
| egg/sausage (*José Olé*), 4 oz. .......... | 270 | 9.0 | 34.0 | 10.0 | 85 | 630 | 2.0 |
| egg/sausage/cheese: | | | | | | | |
| (*El Monterey* Supreme), 4.5 oz. . | 300 | 10.0 | 34.0 | 13.0 | 75 | 630 | 1.0 |
| potato (*El Monterey* Butcher Wrap), 8 oz. ............ | 510 | 17.0 | 60.0 | 22.0 | 145 | 1150 | 2.0 |
| egg white/vegetable/ cheese (*Cedarlane*), 6 oz. .............. | 290 | 15.0 | 39.0 | 9.0 | 15 | 650 | <1.0 |
| turkey bacon/egg white/ vegetable/cheese (*Cedarlane*), 6 oz. .... | 300 | 16.0 | 37.0 | 9.0 | 25 | 690 | <1.0 |
| **Burrito bites**, frozen (*Dr. Praeger's*), 2 oz. .. | 130 | 5.0 | 20.0 | 3.0 | 0 | 210 | 4.0 |

| Food and Measure | cal. | prot. (gms) | carbo. (gms) | fat (gms) | chol. (mgs) | sod. (mgs) | fiber (gms) |
|---|---|---|---|---|---|---|---|
| **Burrito entree kit** (*Old El Paso*), ⅛ pkg.* .... | 260 | 14.0 | 31.0 | 10.0 | 35 | 880 | 2.0 |
| **Burrito seasoning**: | | | | | | | |
| (*Lawry's*), 2 tsp. ....... | 20 | <1.0 | 4.0 | 0 | 0 | 390 | <1.0 |
| (*McCormick*), 1 tbsp. ... | 25 | <1.0 | 5.0 | .5 | 0 | 470 | 0 |
| (*Old El Paso*), 2 tsp. .... | 20 | 0 | 4.0 | 0 | 0 | 780 | 0 |
| (*Ortega*), 1½ tsp. ....... | 20 | 0 | 3.0 | 0 | 0 | 230 | <1.0 |
| **Butter**: | | | | | | | |
| regular, unsalted: | | | | | | | |
| 1 stick or 4 oz. ...... | 813 | 1.0 | 0 | 92.0 | 248 | 12 | 0 |
| 1 tbsp. ........... | 100 | .1 | 0 | 11.4 | 31 | 1 | 0 |
| 1 tsp. ............ | 34 | <.1 | 0 | 3.8 | 10 | <1 | 0 |
| regular, salted: | | | | | | | |
| 1 stick or 4 oz. ...... | 813 | 1.0 | 0 | 92.0 | 248 | 937 | 0 |
| 1 tbsp. ........... | 100 | .1 | 0 | 11.4 | 31 | 115 | 0 |
| 1 tsp. ............ | 34 | <.1 | 0 | 3.8 | 10 | 39 | 0 |
| whipped, unsalted: | | | | | | | |
| ½ cup or 1 stick ..... | 542 | .6 | <.1 | 61.3 | 165 | 8 | 0 |
| 1 tbsp. ........... | 67 | .1 | tr. | 7.6 | 20 | 1 | 0 |
| 1 tsp. ............ | 23 | tr. | tr. | 2.6 | 7 | <1 | 0 |
| whipped, salted: | | | | | | | |
| ½ cup or 1 stick ..... | 542 | .6 | <.1 | 61.3 | 165 | 625 | 0 |
| 1 tbsp. ........... | 67 | .1 | tr. | 7.6 | 20 | 78 | 0 |
| 1 tsp. ............ | 23 | tr. | tr. | 2.6 | 7 | 26 | 0 |
| **Butter, blend**, 1 tbsp.: | | | | | | | |
| w/canola oil: | | | | | | | |
| (*Land O Lakes*) ...... | 100 | 0 | 0 | 11.0 | 15 | 85 | 0 |
| (*Land O Lakes* Light) ........... | 50 | 0 | 0 | 5.0 | 5 | 90 | 0 |
| (*Shedd's Country Crock* Spreadable) . | 80 | 0 | 0 | 9.0 | 15 | 65 | 0 |
| w/olive oil (*Land O Lakes*) ........... | 90 | 0 | 0 | 10.0 | 15 | 90 | 0 |
| **Butter, flavored**, 1 tbsp.: | | | | | | | |
| garlic (*Land O Lakes*) ... | 90 | 0 | 0 | 10.0 | 20 | 110 | 0 |
| honey: | | | | | | | |
| (*Downey's*) ......... | 60 | 0 | 11.0 | 1.0 | 5 | 10 | 0 |
| (*Land O Lakes*) ...... | 90 | 0 | 4.0 | 8.0 | 15 | 40 | 0 |
| **Butter beans** (see also "Lima beans"), canned, ½ cup: | | | | | | | |
| (*Bush's* Speckled) ...... | 110 | 6.0 | 19.0 | .5 | 0 | 420 | 5.0 |
| (*Eden* Organic) ........ | 100 | 5.0 | 17.0 | 1.0 | 0 | 35 | 4.0 |

| Food and Measure | cal. | prot. (gms) | carbo. (gms) | fat (gms) | chol. (mgs) | sod. (mgs) | fiber (gms) |
|---|---|---|---|---|---|---|---|
| (*Glory*) ............. | 100 | 6.0 | 18.0 | 0 | 0 | 570 | 5.0 |
| (*S&W*) .............. | 110 | 6.0 | 19.0 | .5 | 0 | 480 | 5.0 |
| baby: | | | | | | | |
| (*Allens*) ........... | 120 | 7.0 | 22.0 | .5 | 0 | 460 | 6.0 |
| (*Bush's*) .......... | 120 | 7.0 | 19.0 | .5 | 0 | 510 | 5.0 |
| green (*Sunshine*) ...... | 120 | 7.0 | 22.0 | .5 | 0 | 460 | 6.0 |
| large: | | | | | | | |
| (*Allens*) ........... | 120 | 7.0 | 20.0 | 1.0 | 0 | 290 | 7.0 |
| (*Bush's*) .......... | 100 | 6.0 | 18.0 | .5 | 0 | 450 | 5.0 |
| white, w/sausage | | | | | | | |
| (*Trappey's*) ....... | 110 | 6.0 | 21.0 | 1.0 | 0 | 300 | 6.0 |
| seasoned: | | | | | | | |
| (*Allens*) ........... | 100 | 5.0 | 18.0 | 0 | 0 | 610 | 3.0 |
| w/Vidalia onion | | | | | | | |
| (*Allens*) ......... | 100 | 5.0 | 19.0 | 0 | 0 | 470 | 4.0 |
| **Butter beans, frozen,** ½ cup: | | | | | | | |
| (*McKenzie's*) .......... | 100 | 5.0 | 18.0 | 0 | 0 | 220 | 4.0 |
| speckled (*McKenzie's*) ... | 100 | 6.0 | 19.0 | 0 | 0 | 130 | 6.0 |
| **Butter seasoning** (*Molly McButter*), 1 tsp. .... | 5 | 0 | 1.0 | 0 | 0 | 180 | 0 |
| **Butterbur**, fresh: | | | | | | | |
| raw, .2-oz. stalk ........ | 1 | <.1 | .2 | <.1 | 0 | <1 | <1.0 |
| boiled, drained, 4 oz. .... | 9 | .3 | 2.4 | <.1 | 0 | 5 | n.a. |
| **Butterbur, canned,** | | | | | | | |
| chopped, ½ cup ..... | 2 | .1 | .2 | .1 | 0 | 3 | n.a. |
| **Buttercup squash** (*Frieda's*), 3 oz. ...... | 30 | 1.0 | 7.0 | 0 | 0 | 0 | 1.0 |
| **Butterfish**, meat only: | | | | | | | |
| raw, 4 oz. ............. | 166 | 19.6 | 0 | 9.1 | 74 | 100 | 0 |
| baked or broiled, 4 oz. .. | 212 | 25.1 | 0 | 11.7 | 94 | 129 | 0 |
| **Buttermilk**, see "Milk" | | | | | | | |
| **Butternut**, dried: | | | | | | | |
| in shell, 1 lb. .......... | 750 | 30.5 | 14.8 | 69.8 | 0 | 1 | 5.8 |
| shelled, 1 oz. .......... | 174 | 7.1 | 3.4 | 16.2 | 0 | <1 | 1.3 |
| **Butternut squash**, raw, except as noted: | | | | | | | |
| (*Frieda's*), 3 oz. ........ | 30 | 1.0 | 7.0 | 0 | 0 | 0 | 1.0 |
| w/cinnamon sauce (*Green Giant*), ⅔ cup . | 90 | 1.0 | 14.0 | 4.5 | 10 | 350 | 2.0 |
| cubed, ½ cup ......... | 32 | .7 | 8.1 | .1 | 0 | 3 | 1.1 |
| cubed, baked, ½ cup .... | 41 | .9 | 10.7 | .1 | 0 | 4 | 2.9 |
| **Butternut squash, frozen**: | | | | | | | |
| diced (*C&W*), ⅔ cup .... | 40 | 1.0 | 7.0 | 0 | 0 | 0 | 1.0 |

| Food and Measure | cal. | prot. (gms) | carbo. (gms) | fat (gms) | chol. (mgs) | sod. (mgs) | fiber (gms) |
|---|---|---|---|---|---|---|---|
| **Butternut squash, frozen** *(cont.)* | | | | | | | |
| cooked, seasoned | | | | | | | |
| (*McKenzie's* Southland), | | | | | | | |
| ½ cup . . . . . . . . . . . . | 70 | 1.0 | 10.0 | 3.0 | 0 | 270 | 1.0 |
| boiled, drained, | | | | | | | |
| mashed, ½ cup . . . . . . | 47 | 1.5 | 12.1 | .1 | 0 | 2 | n.a. |
| **Butterscotch baking** | | | | | | | |
| **chips**, .5 oz.: | | | | | | | |
| (*Hershey's*) . . . . . . . . . . | 80 | 1.0 | 9.0 | 4.0 | 0 | 35 | 0 |
| (*Nestlé Toll House*) . . . . . | 70 | 0 | 9.0 | 4.0 | 0 | 15 | 0 |
| **Butterscotch syrup** | | | | | | | |
| (*Smucker's Sundae* | | | | | | | |
| *Syrup*), 2 tbsp. . . . . . . . . | 100 | 1.0 | 25.0 | 0 | 0 | 110 | 0 |
| **Butterscotch topping**, | | | | | | | |
| 2 tbsp.: | | | | | | | |
| (*Smucker's*) . . . . . . . . . . | 120 | 0 | 30.0 | 0 | 0 | 105 | 0 |
| caramel (*Smucker's* | | | | | | | |
| Special Recipe) . . . . . . | 140 | 1.0 | 31.0 | 1.0 | <5 | 70 | 0 |

# C

| Food and Measure | cal. | prot. (gms) | carbo. (gms) | fat (gms) | chol. (mgs) | sod. (mgs) | fiber (gms) |
|---|---|---|---|---|---|---|---|
| **Cabbage**, fresh: | | | | | | | |
| raw: | | | | | | | |
| (*Glory*), 1 cup, 3 oz. . . | 20 | 1.0 | 5.0 | 0 | 0 | 15 | 2.0 |
| 5¾" head, 2½ lbs. . . . . | 228 | 13.1 | 49.3 | 2.4 | 0 | 164 | 20.9 |
| shredded, ½ cup . . . . | 9 | .5 | 1.9 | .1 | 0 | 6 | .8 |
| boiled, drained, | | | | | | | |
| shredded, ½ cup . . . . | 17 | .8 | 3.4 | .3 | 0 | 6 | 2.1 |
| **Cabbage**, can/jar: | | | | | | | |
| red, sweet/sour | | | | | | | |
| (*Greenwood*), ½ cup . | 100 | 1.0 | 24.0 | 0 | 0 | 380 | 0 |
| seasoned, ½ cup: | | | | | | | |
| (*Allens*) . . . . . . . . . . . | 30 | 1.0 | 7.0 | 0 | 0 | 350 | 2.0 |
| (*Glory* Country) . . . . . | 30 | 1.0 | 6.0 | 0 | 0 | 350 | 1.0 |
| **Cabbage, Chinese**, fresh: | | | | | | | |
| bok-choy: | | | | | | | |
| raw (*Frieda's* Baby/ | | | | | | | |
| Bok Choy/Choy | | | | | | | |
| Sum), sliced, 1 cup | 9 | 1.0 | 2.0 | 0 | 0 | 46 | 1.0 |
| raw, shredded, ½ cup . | 5 | .5 | .8 | .1 | 0 | 23 | .4 |
| boiled, drained, | | | | | | | |
| shredded, ½ cup . . | 10 | 1.3 | 1.5 | .1 | 0 | 29 | 1.4 |
| napa, cooked (*Frieda's*), | | | | | | | |
| 1 cup . . . . . . . . . . . . | 10 | 1.0 | 2.0 | 0 | 0 | 12 | 4.0 |
| pe-tsai, shredded, | | | | | | | |
| boiled, drained, ½ cup | 8 | .9 | 1.4 | .1 | 0 | 6 | 1.0 |
| **Cabbage, marinated**, | | | | | | | |
| see "Kim chee" | | | | | | | |
| **Cabbage, mustard**, | | | | | | | |
| raw (*Frieda's* Gai | | | | | | | |
| Choy), chopped, 1 cup | 15 | 2.0 | 3.0 | 0 | 0 | 14 | 2.0 |
| **Cabbage, napa**, see | | | | | | | |
| "Cabbage, Chinese" | | | | | | | |

| Food and Measure | cal. | prot. (gms) | carbo. (gms) | fat (gms) | chol. (mgs) | sod. (mgs) | fiber (gms) |
|---|---|---|---|---|---|---|---|
| **Cabbage, red**, fresh: | | | | | | | |
| raw, whole, 1 lb. ....... | 100 | 5.0 | 22.2 | .9 | 0 | 38 | 7.3 |
| raw, shredded, ½ cup ... | 10 | .5 | 2.1 | .1 | 0 | 4 | .7 |
| boiled, drained, | | | | | | | |
|   shredded, ½ cup .... | 16 | .8 | 3.5 | .2 | 0 | 6 | 1.5 |
| **Cabbage,** *Salad Savoy* | | | | | | | |
|   (*Frieda's*), 3 oz. ...... | 25 | 2.0 | 5.0 | 0 | 0 | 25 | 3.0 |
| **Cabbage, savoy**, fresh: | | | | | | | |
| raw, whole, 1 lb. ....... | 100 | 7.3 | 22.1 | .4 | 0 | 102 | 11.2 |
| raw, shredded, ½ cup ... | 10 | .7 | 2.1 | <.1 | 0 | 10 | 1.1 |
| boiled, drained, | | | | | | | |
|   shredded, ½ cup .... | 18 | 1.3 | 4.0 | .1 | 0 | 17 | n.a. |
| **Cabbage, stuffed,** | | | | | | | |
|   **entree**, frozen (*Lean* | | | | | | | |
|   *Cuisine*), 9.5-oz. pkg. . | 210 | 10.0 | 28.0 | 6.0 | 15 | 670 | 3.0 |
| **Cabbage, Tuscan** | | | | | | | |
|   (*Frieda's*), 3 oz. ...... | 20 | 1.0 | 5.0 | 0 | 0 | 15 | 2.0 |
| **Cactus pads**, fresh: | | | | | | | |
| raw, sliced: | | | | | | | |
|   (*Frieda's*), 3 oz. ...... | 14 | 1.0 | 3.0 | 0 | 0 | 18 | 2.0 |
|   1 cup ............. | 14 | 1.1 | 2.9 | .1 | 0 | 19 | 2.0 |
| cooked: | | | | | | | |
|   1 pad ............. | 4 | .4 | 1.0 | <.1 | 0 | 6 | .6 |
|   1 cup ............. | 22 | 2.0 | 4.9 | .1 | 0 | 30 | 3.0 |
| **Cactus pads, can/jar** | | | | | | | |
|   (nopalitos), 2 tbsp., | | | | | | | |
|   except as noted: | | | | | | | |
| chopped (*Doña Maria*) .. | 5 | 0 | 1.0 | 0 | 0 | 500 | 0 |
| pickled (*Sabores* | | | | | | | |
|   *Aztecas*), 2.1 oz. ..... | 40 | 2.0 | 6.0 | 0 | 0 | 240 | 5.0 |
| sliced (*Embasa*) ....... | 5 | 0 | 1.0 | 0 | 0 | 830 | 2.0 |
| **Cactus pear**, see | | | | | | | |
|   "Prickly pear" | | | | | | | |
| **Cajun seasoning** | | | | | | | |
|   (*McCormick*), ¼ tsp. . | 0 | 0 | 0 | 0 | 0 | 130 | 0 |
| **Cake**, fresh (*Entenmann's*), | | | | | | | |
|   ⅛ cake, except | | | | | | | |
|   as noted: | | | | | | | |
| apple strudel, ¼ cake ... | 350 | 3.0 | 52.0 | 15.0 | 0 | 260 | 2.0 |
| banana crunch ........ | 230 | 2.0 | 33.0 | 10.0 | 30 | 270 | <1.0 |
| black and white ........ | 300 | 2.0 | 41.0 | 15.0 | 30 | 210 | <1.0 |
| butter loaf, ⅙ cake ..... | 220 | 3.0 | 30.0 | 9.0 | 70 | 270 | 0 |
| carrot, iced, ⅛ cake ..... | 310 | 3.0 | 39.0 | 16.0 | 30 | 250 | <1.0 |

| Food and Measure | cal. | prot. (gms) | carbo. (gms) | fat (gms) | chol. (mgs) | sod. (mgs) | fiber (gms) |
|---|---|---|---|---|---|---|---|
| chocolate chip, Swiss, | | | | | | | |
| ⅛ cake | 320 | 3.0 | 44.0 | 15.0 | 40 | 240 | 1.0 |
| chocolate chip crumb: | | | | | | | |
| filled, ⅑ cake | 380 | 3.0 | 48.0 | 21.0 | 35 | 230 | 1.0 |
| loaf | 240 | 3.0 | 33.0 | 11.0 | 35 | 220 | <1.0 |
| chocolate fudge | 270 | 3.0 | 40.0 | 11.0 | 25 | 230 | 2.0 |
| chocolate truffle, | | | | | | | |
| ⅙ cake | 400 | 3.0 | 55.0 | 19.0 | 40 | 290 | 2.0 |
| coffee cake, crumb, | | | | | | | |
| ⅒ cake | 260 | 3.0 | 34.0 | 13.0 | 15 | 210 | 1.0 |
| crumb cake: | | | | | | | |
| all butter, French | 210 | 2.0 | 29.0 | 10.0 | 50 | 230 | <1.0 |
| ultimate, ⅒ cake | 250 | 2.0 | 33.0 | 13.0 | 25 | 270 | <1.0 |
| Danish cake: | | | | | | | |
| cheese twist | 230 | 3.0 | 29.0 | 12.0 | 25 | 210 | <1.0 |
| cherry cheese, ⅑ cake | 200 | 3.0 | 25.0 | 9.0 | 25 | 170 | <1.0 |
| cinnamon hazelnut | | | | | | | |
| ring, ⅙ cake | 270 | 4.0 | 28.0 | 16.0 | 25 | 190 | 1.0 |
| pecan ring | 240 | 3.0 | 24.0 | 15.0 | 20 | 150 | 1.0 |
| raspberry twist | 220 | 3.0 | 29.0 | 11.0 | 15 | 170 | <1.0 |
| walnut ring | 240 | 4.0 | 24.0 | 14.0 | 20 | 150 | 2.0 |
| devil's food, | | | | | | | |
| marshmallow iced | 280 | 2.0 | 40.0 | 13.0 | 25 | 250 | <1.0 |
| golden, fudge iced | 290 | 3.0 | 41.0 | 13.0 | 35 | 210 | 1.0 |
| lemon coconut | 320 | 2.0 | 38.0 | 18.0 | 35 | 240 | <1.0 |
| lemon or Louisiana | | | | | | | |
| crunch, ⅑ cake | 330 | 3.0 | 49.0 | 14.0 | 45 | 300 | <1.0 |
| marble loaf | 180 | 2.0 | 26.0 | 8.0 | 35 | 240 | <1.0 |
| raisin loaf | 210 | 2.0 | 33.0 | 8.0 | 35 | 220 | 1.0 |
| sour cream oval | 220 | 2.0 | 26.0 | 13.0 | 45 | 160 | 0 |
| **Cake, frozen,** ⅛ cake, | | | | | | | |
| except as noted: | | | | | | | |
| cheese, see "Cheesecake" | | | | | | | |
| chocolate, ⅙ cake: | | | | | | | |
| (*Amy's* Organic) | 170 | 2.0 | 27.0 | 6.0 | 0 | 130 | 1.0 |
| (*Amy's* Organic | | | | | | | |
| Gluten Free) | 180 | 3.0 | 27.0 | 7.0 | 0 | 200 | 2.0 |
| chocolate, 3 layer | | | | | | | |
| (*Pepperidge Farm*): | | | | | | | |
| fudge | 230 | 2.0 | 33.0 | 10.0 | 20 | 130 | 1.0 |
| German | 240 | 2.0 | 34.0 | 10.0 | 15 | 200 | 1.0 |
| stripe | 240 | 2.0 | 34.0 | 10.0 | 20 | 150 | 2.0 |
| coconut, 3 layer | | | | | | | |
| (*Pepperidge Farm* | 240 | 1.0 | 35.0 | 10.0 | 20 | 120 | <1.0 |

| Food and Measure | cal. | prot. (gms) | carbo. (gms) | fat (gms) | chol. (mgs) | sod. (mgs) | fiber (gms) |
|---|---|---|---|---|---|---|---|
| **Cake, frozen** *(cont.)* | | | | | | | |
| devil's food, 3 layer | | | | | | | |
|   (*Pepperidge Farm*) ... | 220 | 2.0 | 34.0 | 9.0 | 20 | 170 | <1.0 |
| fudge, double (*Smart* | | | | | | | |
|   *Ones*), 2.2 oz. ....... | 170 | 3.0 | 31.0 | 4.0 | 30 | 260 | 3.0 |
| golden, 3 layer | | | | | | | |
|   (*Pepperidge Farm*) ... | 230 | 2.0 | 34.0 | 9.0 | 15 | 130 | 1.0 |
| lemon, 3 layer | | | | | | | |
|   (*Pepperidge Farm*) ... | 240 | 2.0 | 34.0 | 11.0 | 25 | 130 | <1.0 |
| lemon poppy seed | | | | | | | |
|   (*Amy's* Organic), | | | | | | | |
|   ⅙ cake ............ | 200 | 2.0 | 31.0 | 7.0 | 0 | 240 | 1.0 |
| orange (*Amy's* Organic), | | | | | | | |
|   ⅙ cake ............ | 180 | 2.0 | 28.0 | 6.0 | 0 | 130 | 0 |
| pound (*Sara Lee*), ¼ cake: | | | | | | | |
|   all butter ........... | 300 | 4.0 | 35.0 | 16.0 | 110 | 220 | <1.0 |
|   chocolate swirl ...... | 310 | 4.0 | 42.0 | 15.0 | 70 | 280 | <1.0 |
| strawberry shortcake | | | | | | | |
|   (*Smart Ones*), 3.3 oz. . | 170 | 4.0 | 26.0 | 6.0 | 35 | 280 | 1.0 |
| vanilla bean, 3 layer | | | | | | | |
|   (*Pepperidge Farm*) ... | 230 | 1.0 | 35.0 | 9.0 | 15 | 120 | <1.0 |
| **Cake, microwave**, 1 pkg., | | | | | | | |
|   except as noted: | | | | | | | |
| (*Betty Crocker Warm* | | | | | | | |
|   *Delights*): | | | | | | | |
|   caramel, molten ..... | 360 | 5.0 | 64.0 | 10.0 | 5 | 490 | 3.0 |
|   chocolate: | | | | | | | |
|     dark, mini, ½ pkg. . | 150 | 2.0 | 25.0 | 4.0 | 0 | 170 | 2.0 |
|     milk ............ | 340 | 5.0 | 59.0 | 10.0 | 0 | 450 | 3.0 |
|     molten ......... | 370 | 6.0 | 61.0 | 12.0 | 5 | 490 | 3.0 |
|   cinnamon swirl ...... | 390 | 4.0 | 72.0 | 10.0 | 0 | 500 | 1.0 |
|   lemon swirl ......... | 380 | 4.0 | 72.0 | 9.0 | 5 | 410 | 1.0 |
|   raspberry, mini, ½ pkg. | 150 | 2.0 | 26.0 | 3.5 | 0 | 160 | 1.0 |
| (*Guiltless Gourmet* | | | | | | | |
|   Dessert Bowls): | | | | | | | |
|   bananas Foster ...... | 200 | 3.0 | 42.0 | 2.0 | 15 | 250 | <1.0 |
|   black velvet ........ | 200 | 4.0 | 42.0 | 2.5 | 20 | 190 | 3.0 |
| **Cake, mix**, ¹⁄₁₂ cake*, | | | | | | | |
|   except as noted: | | | | | | | |
| (*Duncan Hines Moist* | | | | | | | |
|   *Deluxe* Tres Leches) .. | 210 | 6.0 | 30.0 | 7.0 | 80 | 230 | 0 |
| (*Pillsberry Funfetti*), | | | | | | | |
|   ¹⁄₁₂ pkg. ............ | 180 | 1.0 | 36.0 | 3.5 | 0 | 300 | <1.0 |

| Food and Measure | cal. | prot. (gms) | carbo. (gms) | fat (gms) | chol. (mgs) | sod. (mgs) | fiber (gms) |
|---|---|---|---|---|---|---|---|
| angel food: | | | | | | | |
| (*Betty Crocker*) ...... | 140 | 3.0 | 32.0 | 0 | 0 | 310 | 0 |
| (*Pillsbury*) .......... | 140 | 3.0 | 31.0 | 0 | 0 | 360 | 0 |
| (*Duncan Hines*) ...... | 140 | 3.0 | 31.0 | 0 | 0 | 280 | 0 |
| confetti (*Betty Crocker*) ......... | 150 | 2.0 | 34.0 | 0 | 0 | 320 | 0 |
| banana supreme (*Duncan Hines Moist Deluxe*) ....... | 270 | 3.0 | 36.0 | 12.0 | 55 | 310 | 0 |
| Black Forest (*Dr. Oetker*), 1/16 pkg. ..... | 110 | 1.0 | 25.0 | 1.0 | 0 | 70 | 0 |
| butter pecan (*SuperMoist*) ....... | 230 | 3.0 | 35.0 | 9.0 | 55 | 290 | 0 |
| caramel: | | | | | | | |
| (*Dr. Oetker* Lava), 1/4 pkg. ......... | 240 | 2.0 | 58.0 | 1.5 | 0 | 50 | 0 |
| (*Duncan Hines Moist Deluxe*) .......... | 270 | 3.0 | 34.0 | 12.0 | 55 | 310 | 0 |
| carrot: | | | | | | | |
| (*Duncan Hines Moist Deluxe*) .......... | 260 | 4.0 | 37.0 | 11.0 | 55 | 260 | 1.0 |
| (*SuperMoist*) ....... | 260 | 3.0 | 35.0 | 12.0 | 55 | 280 | 0 |
| cherry chip (*SuperMoist*) | 230 | 3.0 | 35.0 | 9.0 | 55 | 310 | <1.0 |
| chocolate: | | | | | | | |
| (*Arrowhead Mills* Organic), 1/12 pkg. .. | 160 | 3.0 | 37.0 | 1.0 | 0 | 190 | 1.0 |
| (*Bob's Red Mill* Gluten Free), 1/16 pkg. | 110 | 2.0 | 24.0 | .5 | 0 | 85 | 2.0 |
| (*Dr. Oetker* Lava), 1/4 pkg. .......... | 250 | 2.0 | 55.0 | 1.5 | 0 | 60 | 2.0 |
| (*Dr. Oetker* Organics), 1/12 pkg. ......... | 150 | 2.0 | 32.0 | .5 | 0 | 280 | 2.0 |
| (*Dr. Oetker* Organics Lava), 1/4 pkg. ..... | 240 | 3.0 | 56.0 | 1.0 | 0 | 150 | 2.0 |
| (*Glutino* Gluten Free), 1/10 pkg. ......... | 130 | 2.0 | 36.0 | 1.0 | 0 | 100 | 0 |
| (*Hodgson Mill* Gluten Free), 1/10 pkg. .... | 153 | 3.0 | 35.0 | 1.0 | 0 | 197 | 2.5 |
| (*Moist Supreme*), 1/12 pkg. ......... | 170 | 2.0 | 35.0 | 2.5 | 0 | 330 | 1.0 |
| butter recipe (*SuperMoist*) ...... | 250 | 4.0 | 35.0 | 11.0 | 75 | 440 | 1.0 |
| dark (*Moist Supreme*), 1/12 pkg. ......... | 170 | 2.0 | 33.0 | 4.0 | 0 | 360 | 1.0 |

| Food and Measure | cal. | prot. (gms) | carbo. (gms) | fat (gms) | chol. (mgs) | sod. (mgs) | fiber (gms) |
|---|---|---|---|---|---|---|---|
| **Cake, mix, chocolate** *(cont.)* | | | | | | | |
| dark (*SuperMoist*) ... | 270 | 4.0 | 37.0 | 12.0 | 55 | 420 | 1.0 |
| German (*Duncan Hines* | | | | | | | |
| *Moist Deluxe*) ..... | 270 | 4.0 | 35.0 | 12.0 | 55 | 410 | <1.0 |
| German (*Moist* | | | | | | | |
| *Supreme*), 1/12 pkg. . | 170 | 1.0 | 34.0 | 3.5 | 0 | 280 | <1.0 |
| German (*SuperMoist*) . | 260 | 3.0 | 35.0 | 12.0 | 55 | 360 | <1.0 |
| milk (*SuperMoist*) .... | 230 | 3.0 | 35.0 | 9.0 | 55 | 300 | <1.0 |
| Swiss (*Duncan Hines* | | | | | | | |
| *Moist Deluxe*) ..... | 290 | 4.0 | 35.0 | 15.0 | 55 | 380 | 1.0 |
| chocolate fudge: | | | | | | | |
| (*SuperMoist*) ...... | 260 | 3.0 | 35.0 | 12.0 | 55 | 380 | 1.0 |
| dark (*Duncan Hines* | | | | | | | |
| *Moist Deluxe*) ..... | 290 | 4.0 | 35.0 | 15.0 | 55 | 380 | 1.0 |
| triple (*SuperMoist*) ... | 270 | 4.0 | 34.0 | 13.0 | 55 | 380 | 1.0 |
| chocolate molten lava | | | | | | | |
| (*Decadent Supreme*), | | | | | | | |
| 1/8 pkg. ........... | 200 | 2.0 | 38.0 | 4.5 | 0 | 15 | 2.0 |
| chocolate mousse | | | | | | | |
| (*Decadent Supreme*) .. | 290 | 5.0 | 39.0 | 13.0 | 70 | 250 | 3.0 |
| chocolate raspberry | | | | | | | |
| (*Dr. Oetker* Lava), | | | | | | | |
| 1/4 pkg. ........... | 260 | 2.0 | 55.0 | 1.5 | 0 | 50 | 2.0 |
| cinnamon swirl | | | | | | | |
| (*Decadent Supreme*) .. | 240 | 3.0 | 37.0 | 9.0 | 65 | 310 | <1.0 |
| coconut supreme (*Duncan* | | | | | | | |
| *Hines Moist Deluxe*) .. | 250 | 3.0 | 34.0 | 11.0 | 55 | 300 | 0 |
| coffee cake: | | | | | | | |
| (*Aunt Jemima* Easy | | | | | | | |
| Mix), 1/8 pkg. ...... | 140 | 2.0 | 27.0 | 5.0 | 0 | 240 | 1.0 |
| blueberry streusel | | | | | | | |
| (*Martha White*), | | | | | | | |
| 1/12 pkg. ......... | 180 | 2.0 | 35.0 | 4.0 | 0 | 160 | <1.0 |
| cinnamon streusel | | | | | | | |
| (*Martha White*), | | | | | | | |
| 1/12 pkg. ......... | 220 | 2.0 | 38.0 | 6.0 | 0 | 190 | <1.0 |
| corn, see "Corn cake mix" | | | | | | | |
| devil's food: | | | | | | | |
| (*Betty Crocker* Gluten | | | | | | | |
| Free), 1/10 cake* ... | 240 | 4.0 | 36.0 | 8.0 | 60 | 140 | 0 |
| (*Duncan Hines Moist* | | | | | | | |
| *Deluxe*) .......... | 290 | 4.0 | 35.0 | 15.0 | 55 | 380 | 1.0 |
| (*"Jiffy"*), 1/5 pkg. ..... | 210 | 3.0 | 39.0 | 5.0 | 0 | 450 | 1.0 |

| Food and Measure | cal. | prot. (gms) | carbo. (gms) | fat (gms) | chol. (mgs) | sod. (mgs) | fiber (gms) |
|---|---|---|---|---|---|---|---|
| (*Moist Supreme*), 1/12 pkg. ......... | 160 | 2.0 | 34.0 | 2.5 | 0 | 330 | 1.0 |
| (*Moist Supreme* No Sugar), 1/12 pkg. ... | 120 | 2.0 | 29.0 | 3.5 | 0 | 250 | 1.0 |
| (*Moist Supreme* Reduced Sugar), 1/12 pkg. ......... | 150 | 2.0 | 35.0 | 2.0 | 0 | 340 | 1.0 |
| (*SuperMoist*) ....... | 260 | 4.0 | 35.0 | 12.0 | 55 | 390 | 1.0 |
| fudge: | | | | | | | |
| butter recipe (*Duncan Hines Moist Deluxe*) | 250 | 3.0 | 34.0 | 14.0 | 75 | 310 | 1.0 |
| hot (*Betty Crocker Complete Desserts*), 1/6 cake* | 440 | 5.0 | 78.0 | 13.0 | 5 | 550 | 3.0 |
| marble (*Duncan Hines Moist Deluxe*) ..... | 240 | 3.0 | 34.0 | 11.0 | 55 | 280 | 0 |
| funnel (*Golden Dipt Batter Mix*), 1/4 cup ... | 120 | 0 | 23.0 | 1.0 | 20 | 200 | 0 |
| gingerbread (*Betty Crocker Cake & Cookie*), 1/8 cake* .... | 210 | 3.0 | 39.0 | 6.0 | 25 | 360 | 0 |
| golden, butter recipe: | | | | | | | |
| (*Duncan Hines Moist Deluxe*) .......... | 270 | 3.0 | 35.0 | 14.0 | 75 | 240 | 0 |
| (*Moist Supreme*), 1/12 pkg. ......... | 170 | 1.0 | 35.0 | 3.5 | 0 | 290 | <1.0 |
| lemon: | | | | | | | |
| (*Dr. Oetker* Organics), 1/12 pkg. ......... | 140 | 1.0 | 32.0 | 0 | 0 | 200 | 0 |
| (*Moist Supreme*), 1/12 pkg. ......... | 170 | 1.0 | 35.0 | 3.5 | 0 | 300 | <1.0 |
| (*SuperMoist*) ....... | 240 | 3.0 | 35.0 | 9.0 | 55 | 300 | 0 |
| lemon or orange supreme (*Duncan Hines Moist Deluxe*) ....... | 270 | 3.0 | 36.0 | 12.0 | 55 | 310 | 0 |
| marble: | | | | | | | |
| (*Dr. Oetker*), 1/8 pkg. .. | 180 | 2.0 | 41.0 | 1.5 | 0 | 220 | 0 |
| (*Dr. Oetker* Organics), 1/12 pkg. ......... | 140 | 1.0 | 33.0 | 0 | 0 | 290 | 0 |
| pineapple: | | | | | | | |
| (*Moist Supreme*), 1/12 pkg. ......... | 170 | 1.0 | 35.0 | 3.5 | 0 | 290 | <1.0 |
| supreme (*Duncan Hines Moist Deluxe*) ..... | 270 | 3.0 | 36.0 | 12.0 | 55 | 310 | 0 |

| Food and Measure | cal. | prot. (gms) | carbo. (gms) | fat (gms) | chol. (mgs) | sod. (mgs) | fiber (gms) |
|---|---|---|---|---|---|---|---|
| **Cake, mix, pineapple** *(cont.)* | | | | | | | |
| upside-down (*Betty Crocker*), ⅙ cake* | 390 | 3.0 | 65.0 | 14.0 | 35 | 330 | >1.0 |
| pound (*Betty Crocker*), ⅛ cake* | 290 | 4.0 | 48.0 | 10.0 | 70 | 250 | <1.0 |
| rainbow chip (*SuperMoist* Party) | 230 | 3.0 | 35.0 | 9.0 | 55 | 320 | 0 |
| red velvet (*Duncan Hines Moist Deluxe*) | 270 | 4.0 | 35.0 | 13.0 | 55 | 280 | 1.0 |
| spice: | | | | | | | |
| (*Duncan Hines Moist Deluxe*) | 270 | 3.0 | 36.0 | 12.0 | 55 | 310 | 0 |
| (*SuperMoist*) | 270 | 4.0 | 34.0 | 13.0 | 55 | 380 | 1.0 |
| strawberry: | | | | | | | |
| (*Moist Supreme*), 1/12 pkg. | 170 | 1.0 | 35.0 | 3.5 | 0 | 290 | <1.0 |
| (*SuperMoist*) | 240 | 3.0 | 34.0 | 10.0 | 55 | 290 | 0 |
| supreme (*Duncan Hines Moist Deluxe*) | 270 | 3.0 | 36.0 | 12.0 | 55 | 310 | 0 |
| streusel, German (*Dr. Oetker*), ⅑ pkg. | 170 | 3.0 | 38.0 | 0 | 0 | 240 | 1.0 |
| tiramisu (*Dr. Oetker*), ⅕ pkg. | 150 | 2.0 | 24.0 | 4.5 | 5 | 80 | 0 |
| vanilla: | | | | | | | |
| (*Arrowhead Mills Gluten Free*), 1/12 pkg. | 180 | 2.0 | 41.0 | 0 | 0 | 170 | 0 |
| (*Arrowhead Mills Organic*), 1/12 pkg. | 160 | 2.0 | 37.0 | 0 | 0 | 140 | <1.0 |
| (*Bob's Red Mill Gluten Free*), 1/16 pkg. | 120 | 0 | 29.0 | 0 | 0 | 180 | 0 |
| (*Dr. Oetker Organics*), 1/12 pkg. | 140 | 1.0 | 32.0 | 0 | 0 | 280 | 0 |
| (*SuperMoist*) | 230 | 3.0 | 35.0 | 9.0 | 55 | 310 | 0 |
| French (*Duncan Hines Moist Deluxe*) | 270 | 3.0 | 34.0 | 12.0 | 55 | 310 | 0 |
| French or golden (*SuperMoist*) | 230 | 3.0 | 35.0 | 9.0 | 55 | 300 | 0 |
| white: | | | | | | | |
| (*Duncan Hines Moist Deluxe Classic*) | 200 | 2.0 | 34.0 | 6.0 | 0 | 290 | 0 |
| (*Moist Supreme Classic*), 1/12 pkg. | 170 | 1.0 | 34.0 | 3.5 | 0 | 290 | <1.0 |
| (*SuperMoist*) | 230 | 3.0 | 35.0 | 8.0 | 0 | 310 | 0 |

| Food and Measure | cal. | prot. (gms) | carbo. (gms) | fat (gms) | chol. (mgs) | sod. (mgs) | fiber (gms) |
|---|---|---|---|---|---|---|---|
| white or golden yellow | | | | | | | |
| ("Jiffy"), ⅕ pkg. . . . . . | 210 | 2.0 | 40.0 | 4.5 | 0 | 340 | 0 |
| yellow: | | | | | | | |
| (Betty Crocker Gluten | | | | | | | |
| Free), ¹⁄₁₁ cake* . . . | 250 | 3.0 | 34.0 | 6.0 | 25 | 360 | 0 |
| (Duncan Hines Moist | | | | | | | |
| Deluxe Classic) . . . | 270 | 3.0 | 36.0 | 12.0 | 55 | 310 | 0 |
| (Hodgson Mill Gluten | | | | | | | |
| Free), ¹⁄₁₀ pkg. . . . . | 160 | 2.0 | 38.0 | 0 | 0 | 185 | 1.0 |
| (Moist Supreme), | | | | | | | |
| ¹⁄₁₂ pkg. . . . . . . . . | 170 | 1.0 | 34.0 | 3.5 | 0 | 290 | <1.0 |
| (Moist Supreme No | | | | | | | |
| Sugar), ¹⁄₁₂ pkg. . . . | 120 | 1.0 | 29.0 | 3.5 | 0 | 280 | <1.0 |
| (Moist Supreme | | | | | | | |
| Reduced Sugar), | | | | | | | |
| ¹⁄₁₂ pkg. . . . . . . . . | 160 | 1.0 | 34.0 | 3.0 | 0 | 300 | 1.0 |
| (SuperMoist) . . . . . . . | 230 | 3.0 | 35.0 | 9.0 | 55 | 300 | 0 |
| butter recipe | | | | | | | |
| (SuperMoist) . . . . . | 250 | 3.0 | 35.0 | 10.0 | 75 | 350 | 0 |
| **Cake, snack** , 2 pcs., | | | | | | | |
| except as noted: | | | | | | | |
| apple puffs | | | | | | | |
| (Entenmann's), 1 pc. . | 290 | 3.0 | 39.0 | 14.0 | 0 | 260 | 1.0 |
| carrot (Enten-Mini's) . . . . | 330 | 3.0 | 46.0 | 15.0 | 40 | 320 | 1.0 |
| chocolate, w/crème: | | | | | | | |
| (Ding Dongs) . . . . . . . | 360 | 3.0 | 44.0 | 19.0 | 15 | 240 | 2.0 |
| (Hostess Ho-Hos) . . . . | 250 | 2.0 | 34.0 | 12.0 | 20 | 150 | 1.0 |
| (Oreo Cakesters) . . . . . | 250 | 2.0 | 36.0 | 12.0 | 5 | 250 | 1.0 |
| (Oreo Cakesters | | | | | | | |
| Double Stuf) . . . . . . | 350 | 2.0 | 48.0 | 18.0 | 5 | 260 | 1.0 |
| (Ring Dings) . . . . . . . . | 330 | 2.0 | 44.0 | 17.0 | 0 | 230 | 2.0 |
| (Sno Balls) . . . . . . . . . | 360 | 3.0 | 61.0 | 11.0 | 5 | 440 | 2.0 |
| (Yodels) . . . . . . . . . . . | 270 | 2.0 | 37.0 | 14.0 | 10 | 140 | 1.0 |
| chocolate chip (Entenmann's | | | | | | | |
| Mini), 1 pc. . . . . . . . . | 190 | 2.0 | 24.0 | 9.0 | 20 | 120 | <1.0 |
| coffee cake (Drake's) . . . . | 260 | 3.0 | 42.0 | 10.0 | 10 | 170 | 1.0 |
| crumb (Entenmann's | | | | | | | |
| Mini Cake), 1 pc. . . . . . | 260 | 2.0 | 34.0 | 13.0 | 25 | 230 | <1.0 |
| cupcake, w/crème.: | | | | | | | |
| chocolate | | | | | | | |
| (Enten-Mini's) . . . . | 310 | 2.0 | 50.0 | 11.0 | 50 | 350 | 2.0 |
| chocolate (Hostess) . . | 360 | 3.0 | 59.0 | 14.0 | 10 | 480 | 2.0 |
| chocolate (Yankee | | | | | | | |
| Doodles), 1 pc. . . . . | 190 | 2.0 | 37.0 | 4.5 | 0 | 200 | 1.0 |

| Food and Measure | cal. | prot. (gms) | carbo. (gms) | fat (gms) | chol. (mgs) | sod. (mgs) | fiber (gms) |
|---|---|---|---|---|---|---|---|
| **Cake, snack, cupcake** *(cont.)* | | | | | | | |
| golden (*Sunny* | | | | | | | |
| *Doodles*), 1 pc. . . . . | 210 | 2.0 | 32.0 | 8.0 | 10 | 230 | 0 |
| orange (*Hostess*) . . . . | 410 | 2.0 | 68.0 | 14.0 | 25 | 410 | 0 |
| Danish (*Entenmann's* | | | | | | | |
| Single Serve), 1 pc.: | | | | | | | |
| cheese . . . . . . . . . . . | 400 | 6.0 | 52.0 | 19.0 | 10 | 390 | 1.0 |
| cherry cheese . . . . . . . | 450 | 6.0 | 52.0 | 24.0 | 10 | 540 | 1.0 |
| cinnamon . . . . . . . . . . | 460 | 6.0 | 61.0 | 22.0 | 10 | 470 | 2.0 |
| pineapple cheese . . . . | 460 | 6.0 | 53.0 | 24.0 | 10 | 530 | 1.0 |
| raspberry twist . . . . . . | 480 | 6.0 | 61.0 | 24.0 | 10 | 470 | 2.0 |
| golden, w/crème: | | | | | | | |
| (*Oreo Cakesters*) . . . . . | 220 | 2.0 | 32.0 | 10.0 | 5 | 135 | 0 |
| (*Twinkies*), 1 pc. . . . . . | 150 | 1.0 | 27.0 | 4.5 | 20 | 220 | 0 |
| guava cheese puffs | | | | | | | |
| (*Entenmann's*), 1 pc. . | 300 | 4.0 | 34.0 | 17.0 | 10 | 270 | 1.0 |
| peanut butter (*Oreo* | | | | | | | |
| *Cakesters*) . . . . . . . . . | 220 | 3.0 | 30.0 | 10.0 | 5 | 280 | 1.0 |
| pound (*Entenmann's* | | | | | | | |
| Mini Cake), 1 pc. . . . . . | 170 | 2.0 | 20.0 | 9.0 | 35 | 160 | 0 |
| **Calabaza** (*Frieda's*), | | | | | | | |
| ½ cup, 3 oz. . . . . . . . . | 10 | 1.0 | 2.0 | 0 | 0 | 0 | 1.0 |
| **Calamari**, fresh, | | | | | | | |
| see "Squid" | | | | | | | |
| **Calamari, canned**, | | | | | | | |
| see "Cuttlefish" | | | | | | | |
| **Calamari rings**, frozen, | | | | | | | |
| breaded, fried: | | | | | | | |
| (*Margaritaville* Captain's), | | | | | | | |
| 3 pcs., 3 oz. . . . . . . . . | 220 | 9.0 | 22.0 | 11.0 | 90 | 570 | 1.0 |
| sauce, 2 tbsp. . . . . . . . | 100 | 0 | 3.0 | 10.0 | 10 | 240 | 0 |
| (*Tiger Thai*), 3 oz. . . . . . . | 220 | 7.0 | 16.0 | 14.0 | 95 | 300 | 2.0 |
| marinara sauce, 1 oz. . | 120 | <1.0 | 17.0 | <1.0 | 0 | 10 | <1.0 |
| w/sauce (*Contessa*), | | | | | | | |
| ¼ of 12-oz. pkg. . . . . . | 160 | 5.0 | 21.0 | 6.0 | 55 | 370 | 3.0 |
| tempura (*Tiger Thai*), | | | | | | | |
| 3 oz. . . . . . . . . . . . . . . | 220 | 7.0 | 16.0 | 14.0 | 95 | 300 | 2.0 |
| chili sauce, 1.1 oz. . . . | 100 | 0 | 32.0 | 0 | 0 | 410 | 2.0 |
| **Calzone**, frozen | | | | | | | |
| (*Smart Ones* Italiano), | | | | | | | |
| 5-oz. pc. . . . . . . . . . . . | 290 | 14.0 | 47.0 | 6.0 | 25 | 620 | 6.0 |
| *Camouflage* **melon**, | | | | | | | |
| see "Christmas melon" | | | | | | | |

| Food and Measure | cal. | prot. (gms) | carbo. (gms) | fat (gms) | chol. (mgs) | sod. (mgs) | fiber (gms) |
|---|---|---|---|---|---|---|---|
| **Candy**: | | | | | | | |
| almond, 1 oz.: | | | | | | | |
|   butter toffee (*Blue* | | | | | | | |
|     *Diamond*) ........ | 160 | 5.0 | 9.0 | 12.0 | 0 | 35 | 3.0 |
|   cinnamon brown sugar | | | | | | | |
|     (*Blue Diamond*) ... | 160 | 6.0 | 7.0 | 14.0 | 0 | 30 | 3.0 |
| almond, chocolate | | | | | | | |
|   coated: | | | | | | | |
|   dark (*Dove*), 13 pcs. .. | 210 | 3.0 | 19.0 | 15.0 | 5 | 10 | 3.0 |
|   dark/mint dark (*Blue* | | | | | | | |
|     *Diamond*), 1 oz. .... | 160 | 5.0 | 9.0 | 13.0 | 0 | 35 | 3.0 |
|   milk (*Dove*), 13 pcs. ... | 220 | 4.0 | 19.0 | 15.0 | 5 | 20 | 2.0 |
| almond, chocolate/ | | | | | | | |
|   candy coated | | | | | | | |
|   (*M&M's*), 1.5 oz. ..... | 220 | 3.0 | 25.0 | 12.0 | 5 | 20 | 2.0 |
| butter rum (*Life Savers*), | | | | | | | |
|   .5 oz. .............. | 60 | 0 | 15.0 | 0 | 0 | 105 | 0 |
| candy corn (*Brach's*), | | | | | | | |
|   22 pcs., 1.4 oz. ...... | 140 | 0 | 36.0 | 0 | 0 | 115 | 0 |
| caramel, 1.4 oz.: | | | | | | | |
|   (*Sugar Babies* | | | | | | | |
|     Caramel Apple) ... | 160 | 0 | 37.0 | 1.0 | 0 | 30 | 0 |
|   (*Sugar Babies* | | | | | | | |
|     Original) .......... | 160 | 0 | 37.0 | 1.5 | 0 | 40 | 0 |
|   (*Sugar Daddy* Pop) ... | 170 | 1.0 | 36.0 | 2.0 | 0 | 55 | 0 |
|   assortment (*Pot of* | | | | | | | |
|     *Gold*), 4 pcs. ..... | 190 | 2.0 | 25.0 | 10.0 | 5 | 75 | 1.0 |
| caramel, chocolate | | | | | | | |
|   coated: | | | | | | | |
|   (*Junior*), 1.4 oz. ..... | 190 | 1.0 | 33.0 | 6.0 | 5 | 45 | 1.0 |
|   (*Milk Duds*), 1.8 oz. .. | 230 | 2.0 | 38.0 | 8.0 | 0 | 135 | 0 |
|   (*Milky Way*), .3-oz. pc. | 40 | 0 | 6.0 | 1.5 | 0 | 20 | 0 |
|   (*Milky Way* Simply | | | | | | | |
|     Caramel), 1.9 oz. .. | 250 | 2.0 | 37.0 | 11.0 | 5 | 60 | 0 |
|   (*Rolo*), 1.7-oz. pkg. ... | 220 | 2.0 | 33.0 | 10.0 | 5 | 80 | 0 |
|   (*Sugar Babies*), 1.4 oz. | 180 | 1.0 | 33.0 | 4.5 | 5 | 35 | 0 |
| cookie bar (*Twix*), | | | | | | | |
|   .9-oz. bar ......... | 130 | 1.0 | 17.0 | 6.0 | 0 | 50 | 0 |
| cookie bar (*Twix*), | | | | | | | |
|   2 bars, 1.8 oz. ..... | 250 | 2.0 | 33.0 | 12.0 | 5 | 115 | 1.0 |
| cookie bar, dark | | | | | | | |
|   (*Twix*), .4-oz. pc. .. | 50 | 0 | 6.0 | 2.5 | 0 | 20 | 0 |
| peanut, nougat, chocolate | | | | | | | |
|   (*Zero*), 1.8 oz. .... | 230 | 3.0 | 37.0 | 8.0 | 0 | 115 | 0 |

| Food and Measure | cal. | prot. (gms) | carbo. (gms) | fat (gms) | chol. (mgs) | sod. (mgs) | fiber (gms) |
|---|---|---|---|---|---|---|---|
| **Candy** *(cont.)* | | | | | | | |
| caramel corn, see "Popcorn, popped" | | | | | | | |
| cashew, chocolate coated: | | | | | | | |
| (*Planters* Chocolate Lovers), 1.5 oz. . . . | 230 | 5.0 | 20.0 | 16.0 | 5 | 25 | 1.0 |
| dark (*Planters* Forest Blend), 1.2 oz. . . . . | 170 | 4.0 | 17.0 | 11.0 | 0 | 40 | 3.0 |
| cherry, chocolate coated, 3 pcs., 1.5 oz.: | | | | | | | |
| dark (*Cella's*) . . . . . . . . | 160 | 1.0 | 27.0 | 7.0 | 0 | 0 | 2.0 |
| milk (*Cella's*) . . . . . . . . | 160 | 1.0 | 27.0 | 6.0 | 0 | 15 | 1.0 |
| cherry flavor: | | | | | | | |
| (*Twizzlers* Bites), 17 pcs., 1.4 oz. . . . | 140 | 1.0 | 32.0 | .5 | 0 | 95 | 0 |
| (*Twizzlers* Nibs), 29 pcs., 1.4 oz. . . . | 140 | 1.0 | 32.0 | 1.0 | 0 | 65 | 0 |
| (*Twizzlers Pull 'n' Peel*), 1.2-oz. pc. . . | 110 | 1.0 | 26.0 | .5 | 0 | 70 | 0 |
| twists (*Twizzlers*), 4 pcs., 1.6 oz. . . . . | 160 | 1.0 | 36.0 | 1.0 | 0 | 105 | 0 |
| chocolate, dark: | | | | | | | |
| (*Cadbury* Royal), 7 blocks, 1.4 oz. . . . | 170 | 2.0 | 23.0 | 12.0 | 5 | 0 | 3.0 |
| (*Dagoba Eclipse Organic*), 2-oz. bar . | 290 | 7.0 | 19.0 | 27.0 | 0 | 0 | 8.0 |
| (*Dagoba New Moon Organic*), 1.4 oz. . . | 200 | 4.0 | 17.0 | 17.0 | 0 | 0 | 5.0 |
| (*Dove*), 1 bar, ⅓ pkg. . | 170 | 2.0 | 20.0 | 11.0 | 5 | 0 | 3.0 |
| (*Dove*), large bar . . . . . | 190 | 2.0 | 22.0 | 12.0 | 5 | 0 | 3.0 |
| (*Dove* 63%), large bar | 180 | 2.0 | 17.0 | 13.0 | 0 | 0 | 3.0 |
| (*Dove* 71%), large bar | 200 | 2.0 | 14.0 | 16.0 | 0 | 0 | 3.0 |
| (*Dove Promises*), 5 pcs., 1.4 oz. . . . . | 210 | 3.0 | 21.0 | 14.0 | 5 | 10 | 2.0 |
| (*Hershey's* Extra Dark Bar), 3 blocks, 1.3 oz. | 170 | 3.0 | 19.0 | 13.0 | 5 | 0 | 4.0 |
| (*Hershey's* Extra Dark Pouch), 4 pcs., 1.4 oz. | 180 | 3.0 | 21.0 | 14.0 | 5 | 0 | 4.0 |
| (*Hershey's Bliss*), 6 pcs., 1.5 oz. . . . . | 210 | 3.0 | 25.0 | 14.0 | 5 | 10 | 3.0 |
| (*Hershey's Kisses Special Dark*), 9 pcs., 1.4 oz. . . . . | 210 | 2.0 | 25.0 | 12.0 | 5 | 15 | 3.0 |

| Food and Measure | cal. | prot. (gms) | carbo. (gms) | fat (gms) | chol. (mgs) | sod. (mgs) | fiber (gms) |
|---|---|---|---|---|---|---|---|
| (*Hershey's Special Dark*), 1.4-oz. bar .. | 180 | 2.0 | 25.0 | 12.0 | 5 | 15 | 3.0 |
| (*Hershey's Special Dark* Miniatures), 5 pcs., 1.4 oz. .... | 200 | 3.0 | 24.0 | 13.0 | 5 | 25 | 3.0 |
| (*Seeds of Change* Organic), 1 oz. .... | 140 | 2.0 | 14.0 | 11.0 | 0 | 0 | 2.0 |
| almond (*Dove Promises*), 5 pcs. ...... | 200 | 2.0 | 14.0 | 16.0 | 0 | 0 | 3.0 |
| almond (*Hershey's Nuggets Special Dark*), 4 pcs. ..... | 200 | 4.0 | 20.0 | 13.0 | 10 | 25 | 2.0 |
| almond, roasted (*Dove*), 1 bar, ⅓ pkg. ..... | 180 | 3.0 | 18.0 | 12.0 | 5 | 10 | 1.0 |
| candy coated (*Hershey's Special Dark Pieces*), 1.4 oz. ... | 180 | 1.0 | 29.0 | 8.0 | 10 | 10 | 2.0 |
| candy coated (*M&M's*), 1.5 oz. .. | 210 | 2.0 | 29.0 | 10.0 | 5 | 10 | 2.0 |
| w/cherries, vanilla (*Seeds of Change* Organic), 1 oz. .... | 140 | 2.0 | 15.0 | 10.0 | 0 | 0 | 2.0 |
| w/coconut (*Seeds of Change* Organic), 1 oz. ............ | 140 | 2.0 | 14.0 | 11.0 | 0 | 0 | 3.0 |
| cranberry, blueberry, almonds (*Hershey's* Extra Dark), 1.3 oz. | 170 | 3.0 | 19.0 | 13.0 | 5 | 0 | 4.0 |
| cranberry almond (*Dove*), 1 bar ..... | 170 | 2.0 | 20.0 | 10.0 | 5 | 10 | 2.0 |
| crèmes, all flavors (*Dove* Sugar Free), 5 pcs. ........... | 190 | 2.0 | 22.0 | 15.0 | 5 | 0 | 3.0 |
| honey almond nougat (*Toblerone* Bittersweet), 1.2 oz. | 170 | 1.0 | 20.0 | 9.0 | 5 | 5 | 2.0 |
| w/mango and cashews (*Seeds of Change* Organic), 1 oz. .... | 140 | 2.0 | 14.0 | 10.0 | 0 | 0 | 2.0 |
| orange (*Terry's*), 1.5 oz. .......... | 240 | 1.0 | 28.0 | 13.0 | 5 | 5 | 3.0 |
| tiramisu (*Dove Promises*), 5 pcs. .. | 200 | 2.0 | 24.0 | 11.0 | 5 | 30 | 2.0 |

| Food and Measure | cal. | prot. (gms) | carbo. (gms) | fat (gms) | chol. (mgs) | sod. (mgs) | fiber (gms) |
|---|---|---|---|---|---|---|---|
| **Candy** *(cont.)* | | | | | | | |
| chocolate, milk: | | | | | | | |
| (*Cadbury Dairy Milk*), | | | | | | | |
| 7 blocks, 1.4 oz. ... | 200 | 3.0 | 23.0 | 11.0 | 10 | 40 | 1.0 |
| (*Dove*), 1.3-oz. | | | | | | | |
| bar ............. | 200 | 2.0 | 22.0 | 12.0 | 5 | 0 | 1.0 |
| (*Dove*), 1 bar, ⅓ pkg. . | 180 | 2.0 | 20.0 | 11.0 | 5 | 20 | 1.0 |
| (*Dove* Extra Creamy), | | | | | | | |
| 1 bar, ⅓ pkg. ..... | 170 | 2.0 | 20.0 | 10.0 | 5 | 10 | 2.0 |
| (*Dove Promises*), | | | | | | | |
| 5 pcs., 1.4 oz. .... | 220 | 2.0 | 24.0 | 13.0 | 5 | 25 | 1.0 |
| (*Hershey's*), 1.5 oz. ... | 210 | 3.0 | 26.0 | 13.0 | 10 | 35 | 1.0 |
| (*Hershey's* Drops), | | | | | | | |
| 15 pcs., 1.4 oz. ... | 200 | 3.0 | 25.0 | 12.0 | 10 | 35 | 1.0 |
| (*Hershey's Bliss*),. | | | | | | | |
| 6 pcs., 1.5 oz. .... | 210 | 3.0 | 24.0 | 14.0 | 5 | 40 | 1.0 |
| (*Hershey's Bliss* Melt- | | | | | | | |
| away), 6 pcs., 1.5 oz. | 220 | 3.0 | 24.0 | 15.0 | 5 | 65 | 1.0 |
| (*Hershey's Hugs*), | | | | | | | |
| 9 pcs., 1.4 oz. .... | 210 | 3.0 | 24.0 | 12.0 | 10 | 45 | 0 |
| (*Hershey's Kisses*), | | | | | | | |
| 9 pcs., 1.4 oz. .... | 200 | 3.0 | 25.0 | 12.0 | 10 | 35 | 1.0 |
| (*Hershey's Nuggets*), | | | | | | | |
| 4 pcs., 1.4 oz. .... | 200 | 3.0 | 25.0 | 12.0 | 10 | 35 | 1.0 |
| (*Symphony*), 5 blocks, | | | | | | | |
| 1.3 oz. .......... | 200 | 3.0 | 22.0 | 12.0 | 10 | 40 | 1.0 |
| (*Terry's*), 1.5 oz. ..... | 230 | 3.0 | 27.0 | 12.0 | 10 | 35 | 1.0 |
| almond (*Cadbury* | | | | | | | |
| Roast Almond), | | | | | | | |
| 7 blocks, 1.4 oz. ... | 210 | 4.0 | 21.0 | 13.0 | 10 | 35 | 1.0 |
| almond (*Dove Promises*), | | | | | | | |
| 5 pcs. ........... | 210 | 3.0 | 21.0 | 13.0 | 5 | 20 | 2.0 |
| almond (*Hershey's*), | | | | | | | |
| 1.4-oz. bar ....... | 210 | 4.0 | 21.0 | 14.0 | 10 | 25 | 2.0 |
| almond (*Hershey's Kis-* | | | | | | | |
| *ses*), 9 pcs., 1.4 oz. | 200 | 4.0 | 21.0 | 14.0 | 10 | 30 | 1.0 |
| almond (*Hershey's Nug-* | | | | | | | |
| *gets*), 4 pcs., 1.3 oz. | 180 | 3.0 | 20.0 | 13.0 | 5 | 10 | 3.0 |
| almond, roasted (*Dove*), | | | | | | | |
| 1 bar, ⅓ pkg. ..... | 180 | 3.0 | 18.0 | 12.0 | 5 | 20 | 1.0 |
| almond/toffee chips | | | | | | | |
| (*Symphony*), 5 blocks, | | | | | | | |
| 1.3 oz. .......... | 200 | 3.0 | 21.0 | 13.0 | 10 | 60 | 1.0 |

| Food and Measure | cal. | prot. (gms) | carbo. (gms) | fat (gms) | chol. (mgs) | sod. (mgs) | fiber (gms) |
|---|---|---|---|---|---|---|---|
| bananas Foster (*Dove Promises*), 5 pcs., 1.4 oz. .... | 200 | 2.0 | 24.0 | 11.0 | 5 | 45 | 1.0 |
| blueberry almond (*Dove*), ⅓ pkg. .... | 180 | 2.0 | 20.0 | 10.0 | 5 | 20 | 1.0 |
| candy coated (*M&M's*), ¼ cup, 1.5 oz. .... | 210 | 2.0 | 30.0 | 9.0 | 5 | 25 | 1.0 |
| candy coated, mini (*M&M's*), 1.1 oz. .. | 150 | 1.0 | 21.0 | 7.0 | 5 | 20 | 1.0 |
| caramel (*Caramello*), 1.6-oz. bar ....... | 220 | 3.0 | 29.0 | 10.0 | 10 | 45 | 1.0 |
| caramel (*Dove Promises*), 5 pcs., 1.4 oz. .... | 200 | 2.0 | 24.0 | 11.0 | 5 | 45 | 1.0 |
| caramel filled (*Hershey's Kisses*), 9 pcs., 1.5 oz. .......... | 190 | 3.0 | 27.0 | 9.0 | 15 | 75 | .0 |
| cherry cordial (*Hershey's Kisses*), 9 pcs., 1.5 oz. | 180 | 2.0 | 30.0 | 7.0 | 5 | 25 | 0 |
| crisps (*Crunch*), 1.55-oz. bar ...... | 220 | 2.0 | 30.0 | 11.0 | 5 | 60 | 1.0 |
| crisps (*Crunch* Fun Size), 3 pcs., 1.3 oz. | 180 | 2.0 | 26.0 | 9.0 | <5 | 55 | <1.0 |
| crisps, wafers (*Crunch Crisp*), 1 pkg. ...... | 190 | 2.0 | 24.0 | 11.0 | 5 | 60 | 1.0 |
| egg, caramel (*Cadbury*), 1.2 oz. .......... | 170 | 2.0 | 22.0 | 8.0 | 5 | 45 | 0 |
| egg, créme (*Cadbury*), 1.2 oz. .......... | 150 | 2.0 | 24.0 | 6.0 | 5 | 15 | <1.0 |
| egg, mini (*Cadbury*), 12 pcs, 1.4 oz. .... | 190 | 2.0 | 28.0 | 8.0 | 5 | 30 | 1.0 |
| fruit and nut (*Cadbury*), 7 blocks, 1.4 oz. ... | 190 | 3.0 | 23.0 | 10.0 | 5 | 30 | 1.0 |
| hazelnut, roasted (*Dove*), 1 bar, ⅓ pkg. ...... | 190 | 2.0 | 18.0 | 12.0 | 5 | 20 | 1.0 |
| honey almond nougat (*Toblerone*), 1.2 oz. | 170 | 2.0 | 21.0 | 9.0 | 10 | 15 | 1.0 |
| honey almond nougat (*Toblerone*), ⅕ of 7.05-oz. bar ...... | 210 | 2.0 | 26.0 | 11.0 | 20 | 20 | 1.0 |
| honey almond nougat (*Toblerone*), 1.76 oz. | 260 | 3.0 | 32.0 | 13.0 | 10 | 25 | 1.0 |
| mint, crispy, candy coated (*M&M's*), ⅓ cup, 1.5 oz. .... | 210 | 2.0 | 29.0 | 10.0 | 5 | 40 | 2.0 |

| Food and Measure | cal. | prot. (gms) | carbo. (gms) | fat (gms) | chol. (mgs) | sod. (mgs) | fiber (gms) |
|---|---|---|---|---|---|---|---|
| **Candy, chocolate, milk** *(cont.)* | | | | | | | |
| orange (*Terry's*), | | | | | | | |
| 1.5 oz. . . . . . . . . . | 230 | 3.0 | 27.0 | 12.0 | 10 | 30 | 1.0 |
| peanut (*Mr. Goodbar*), | | | | | | | |
| 1.7-oz. bar . . . . . . . | 250 | 5.0 | 26.0 | 17.0 | 5 | 65 | 2.0 |
| peanut butter (*Dove* | | | | | | | |
| *Promises*), 5 pcs. . . | 220 | 4.0 | 20.0 | 14.0 | 5 | 85 | 1.0 |
| peanut toffee crunch | | | | | | | |
| (*Dove*), 1 bar, ⅓ pkg. | 180 | 2.0 | 19.0 | 11.0 | 5 | 35 | 1.0 |
| puffed grains (*Seeds of* | | | | | | | |
| *Change* Organic), 1 oz. | 150 | 2.0 | 15.0 | 10.0 | 5 | 20 | 1.0 |
| toffee/almonds | | | | | | | |
| (*Hershey's Nuggets*), | | | | | | | |
| 4 pcs., 1.4 oz. . . . . | 200 | 3.0 | 25.0 | 12.0 | 10 | 35 | 1.0 |
| truffle (*Milka* Alpine | | | | | | | |
| Milk), ⅓ of | | | | | | | |
| 3.52-oz. bar . . . . . . | 180 | 2.0 | 19.0 | 11.0 | 5 | 25 | 1.0 |
| chocolate, white: | | | | | | | |
| honey almond nougat | | | | | | | |
| (*Toblerone*), 1.2 oz. | 180 | 2.0 | 20.0 | 10.0 | 5 | 30 | 0 |
| (*Hershey's Bliss*), | | | | | | | |
| 6 pcs., 1.5 oz. . . . . | 230 | 3.0 | 24.0 | 14.0 | 10 | 70 | 0 |
| chocolate chews | | | | | | | |
| (*Tootsie Roll*), 1.4 oz. . | 140 | 1.0 | 28.0 | 3.0 | 0 | 15 | 0 |
| chocolate thins | | | | | | | |
| (*Andes*), 8 pcs., 1.3 oz.: | | | | | | | |
| cherry jubilee . . . . . . . | 190 | 2.0 | 22.0 | 12.0 | 0 | 20 | 1.0 |
| crème de menthe . . . . | 200 | 2.0 | 22.0 | 13.0 | 0 | 20 | 1.0 |
| mint parfait . . . . . . . . | 210 | 2.0 | 22.0 | 13.0 | 0 | 20 | 0 |
| toffee crunch . . . . . . . | 200 | 2.0 | 24.0 | 11.0 | 0 | 45 | 0 |
| chocolate truffle, crème/ | | | | | | | |
| cookies (*Milka*), ⅓ of | | | | | | | |
| 3.52-oz. bar . . . . . . . . | 180 | 2.0 | 19.0 | 11.0 | 5 | 25 | 1.0 |
| chocolate twists (*Twizzlers*), | | | | | | | |
| 4 pcs., 1.6 oz. . . . . . . . | 160 | 2.0 | 35.0 | 2.0 | 0 | 85 | 1.0 |
| circus peanuts | | | | | | | |
| (*Brach's*), 1.5 oz. . . . . | 160 | <1.0 | 39.0 | 0 | 0 | 0 | 0 |
| coconut, w/chocolate: | | | | | | | |
| (*Mounds*), 1.7 oz. . . . . | 230 | 2.0 | 29.0 | 13.0 | 0 | 55 | 3.0 |
| (*Mounds/Almond Joy* | | | | | | | |
| Snack Size), .6 oz. . | 80 | 1.0 | 10.0 | 4.5 | 0 | 20 | 1.0 |
| almond (*Almond* | | | | | | | |
| *Joy*), 1.6 oz. . . . . . . | 220 | 2.0 | 26.0 | 13.0 | 0 | 50 | 2.0 |

| Food and Measure | cal. | prot. (gms) | carbo. (gms) | fat (gms) | chol. (mgs) | sod. (mgs) | fiber (gms) |
|---|---|---|---|---|---|---|---|
| almond, candy coated (*Almond Joy Pieces*), 1.4 oz. | 200 | 2.0 | 27.0 | 10.0 | 5 | 10 | 1.0 |
| candy coated (*M&M's*), 1.5 oz. | 210 | 2.0 | 30.0 | 9.0 | 5 | 30 | 1.0 |
| cookies and cream: | | | | | | | |
| (*Hershey's*), 1.5 oz. | 220 | 3.0 | 27.0 | 11.0 | 5 | 110 | 0 |
| (*Hershey's* Drops), 14 pcs., 1.4 oz. | 210 | 3.0 | 26.0 | 11.0 | 5 | 75 | 0 |
| (*Hershey's* Miniatures), 5 pcs., 1.4 oz. | 200 | 3.0 | 24.0 | 11.0 | 10 | 60 | 1.0 |
| cotton candy (*Tear Jerkers/Fluffy Stuff*), 1.4 oz. | 150 | 0 | 40.0 | 0 | 0 | 0 | 0 |
| cranberries, chocolate coated (*Raisinets*), ¼ cup, 1.58 oz. | 200 | 1.0 | 33.0 | 8.0 | 5 | 10 | 1.0 |
| fruit flavor, assorted: | | | | | | | |
| (*Skittles* Crazy Cores), 2-oz. pkg. | 230 | 0 | 52.0 | 2.5 | 0 | 10 | 0 |
| (*Skittles* Fizzl'd Fruit), 1.8-oz. pkg. | 200 | 0 | 46.0 | 2.0 | 0 | 10 | 0 |
| (*Skittles* Fun Size), .5-oz. pkg. | 60 | 0 | 14.0 | .5 | 0 | 0 | 0 |
| (*Skittles* Original/ Wild Berry/ Tropical), 2.2 oz. | 250 | 0 | 56.0 | 2.5 | 0 | 10 | 0 |
| (*Swedish Fish*), 1.5 oz. | 140 | 0 | 36.0 | 0 | 0 | 30 | 0 |
| sour (*Skittles*), 1.8-oz. pkg. | 200 | 0 | 44.0 | 2.0 | 0 | 5 | 0 |
| fruit flavor, chews: | | | | | | | |
| (*Frooties*), 1.4 oz. | 160 | 0 | 32.0 | 0 | 0 | 20 | 0 |
| (*Mike & Ike*), 1.4 oz. | 140 | 0 | 36.0 | 0 | 0 | 25 | 0 |
| (*Jolly Rancher* Soft & Chewy), 2 oz. | 200 | 0 | 43.0 | 0 | 0 | 25 | 0 |
| (*Starburst*), 1.4 oz. | 160 | 0 | 34.0 | 3.0 | 0 | 0 | 0 |
| (*Tootsie Roll*), 1.4 oz. | 140 | 0 | 28.0 | 3.0 | 0 | 15 | 0 |
| sour (*Starburst*), 8 pcs., 1.4 oz. | 160 | 0 | 34.0 | 3.0 | 0 | 20 | 0 |
| tropical (*Starburst*), 8 pcs., 1.4 oz. | 160 | 0 | 33.0 | 3.5 | 0 | 0 | 0 |
| fruit flavor, gummy, 1.4 oz.: | | | | | | | |
| (*Dots*) | 130 | 0 | 33.0 | 0 | 0 | 15 | 0 |

| Food and Measure | cal. | prot. (gms) | carbo. (gms) | fat (gms) | chol. (mgs) | sod. (mgs) | fiber (gms) |
|---|---|---|---|---|---|---|---|
| **Candy, fruit flavor, gummy** *(cont.)* | | | | | | | |
| (*Jolly Rancher*) . . . . . . | 120 | 2.0 | 28.0 | 0 | 0 | 35 | 0 |
| (*Jujubes*), 52 pcs. . . . . . | 110 | 0 | 28.0 | 0 | 0 | 0 | 0 |
| (*RealFruit* Medley) . . . | 120 | 2.0 | 28.0 | 0 | 0 | 5 | 0 |
| (*Starburst Gummibursts*), | | | | | | | |
|   9 pcs. . . . . . . . . . . | 130 | 2.0 | 31.0 | 0 | 0 | 40 | 0 |
| orchard or tropical | | | | | | | |
|   fruit (*RealFruit*) . . . | 120 | 2.0 | 28.0 | 0 | 0 | 10 | 0 |
| fruit flavor, gummy | | | | | | | |
|   sour (*Starburst* | | | | | | | |
|   *Gummibursts*), | | | | | | | |
|   1.5 oz. . . . . . . . . . | 140 | 2.0 | 32.0 | 0 | 0 | 25 | 0 |
| fruit flavor, hard: | | | | | | | |
|   (*Jolly Rancher*), | | | | | | | |
|     3 pcs., .6 oz. . . . . . | 70 | 0 | 17.0 | 0 | 0 | 10 | 0 |
|   (*Jolly Rancher* Sugar | | | | | | | |
|     Free), .6 oz. . . . . . . | 40 | 0 | 16.0 | 0 | 0 | 0 | 0 |
|   (*Life Savers*), 4 pcs., | | | | | | | |
|     .5 oz. . . . . . . . . . . | 45 | 0 | 11.0 | 0 | 0 | 0 | 0 |
| fudge, maple walnut | | | | | | | |
|   (*Maple Grove Farms*), | | | | | | | |
|   1 oz. . . . . . . . . . . . . . | 110 | 0 | 19.0 | 4.5 | 5 | 25 | 0 |
| ginger: | | | | | | | |
|   (*Gin-gins* Boost), | | | | | | | |
|     6 pcs., .5 oz. . . . . . | 60 | 0 | 15.0 | 0 | 0 | 15 | 0 |
|   chews (*Ginger People*), | | | | | | | |
|     2 pcs., .4 oz. . . . . . | 40 | 0 | 10.0 | 0 | 0 | 0 | 0 |
| gum, chewing, 1 pc.: | | | | | | | |
|   (*Big Red/Juicy Fruit/* | | | | | | | |
|     *Wrigley's Spearmint/* | | | | | | | |
|     *Doublemint/* | | | | | | | |
|     *Winterfresh*) . . . . . . | 10 | 0 | 2.0 | 0 | 0 | 0 | 0 |
|   (*Bubble Yum*) . . . . . . . | 25 | 0 | 6.0 | 0 | 0 | 0 | 0 |
|   (*Charms* Bubble Gum) | 15 | 0 | 4.0 | 0 | 0 | 5 | 0 |
|   (*Double Bubble* Ball) . . | 20 | 0 | 5.0 | 0 | 0 | 0 | 0 |
|   (*Double Bubble* Twist) | 50 | 0 | 13.0 | 0 | 0 | 0 | 0 |
|   (*Ice Breakers*) . . . . . . . | 5 | 0 | 2.0 | 0 | 0 | 0 | 0 |
|   (*Razzles*) . . . . . . . . . . . | 15 | 0 | 3.0 | 0 | 0 | 0 | 0 |
| jelly beans: | | | | | | | |
|   (*Jelly Belly*), 35 pcs., | | | | | | | |
|     1.4 oz. . . . . . . . . . | 140 | 0 | 37.0 | 0 | 0 | 10 | 0 |
|   (*Jolly Rancher*), | | | | | | | |
|     30 pcs., 1.4 oz. . . . | 140 | 0 | 36.0 | 0 | 0 | 65 | 0 |

| Food and Measure | cal. | prot. (gms) | carbo. (gms) | fat (gms) | chol. (mgs) | sod. (mgs) | fiber (gms) |
|---|---|---|---|---|---|---|---|
| (*Starburst* Original/ Red/Tropical), ¼ cup, 1.5 oz. . . . . | 150 | 0 | 37.0 | 0 | 0 | 20 | 0 |
| sour (*Starburst*), ¼ cup, 1.5 oz. . . . . | 150 | 0 | 39.0 | 0 | 0 | 20 | 0 |
| licorice, black: | | | | | | | |
| (*Crows*), 1.4 oz. . . . . . | 130 | 0 | 33.0 | 0 | 0 | 15 | 0 |
| (*Darrell Lea* Original), 3 pcs., 1.5 oz. . . . . | 130 | 1.0 | 28.0 | 1.0 | 0 | 40 | 0 |
| (*Twizzlers*), 4 pcs., 1.6 oz. . . . . . . . . . | 150 | 1.0 | 35.0 | .5 | 0 | 210 | 0 |
| (*Twizzlers* Bites), 17 pcs., 1.4 oz. . . . | 130 | 1.0 | 31.0 | .5 | 0 | 180 | 0 |
| (*Twizzlers* Nibs), 29 pcs., 1.4 oz. . . . | 140 | 1.0 | 30.0 | 1.0 | 0 | 180 | 0 |
| (*Young & Smylie*), 11 pcs., 1.5 oz. . . . | 150 | 1.0 | 32.0 | 1.5 | 0 | 190 | 0 |
| candy coated (*Good & Plenty*), 33 pcs., 1.4 oz. . . . | 140 | 1.0 | 35.0 | 0 | 0 | 120 | 0 |
| candy coated (*Good & Fruity*), 1.8 oz. . . | 180 | 1.0 | 45.0 | 0 | 0 | 160 | 1.0 |
| soft (*Lucky Country*), 4 pcs., 1.4 oz. . . . . | 130 | 1.0 | 30.0 | 1.0 | 0 | 30 | 0 |
| lollipop, .6-oz. pop, except as noted: | | | | | | | |
| (*Caramel Apple Pops*) . | 60 | 0 | 15.0 | .5 | 0 | 15 | 0 |
| (*Charms Blow Pop*) . . | 60 | 0 | 17.0 | 0 | 0 | 0 | 0 |
| (*Dum Dum Pops*), 2 pcs., .5 oz. . . . . . | 70 | 0 | 13.0 | 0 | 0 | 0 | 0 |
| (*Jolly Rancher*) . . . . . . | 60 | 0 | 15.0 | 0 | 0 | 15 | 0 |
| (*Tootsie Bunch Pops*), .45-oz. pop . . . . . . . | 45 | 0 | 12.0 | 0 | 0 | 0 | 0 |
| (*Tootsie Pops*) . . . . . . | 60 | 0 | 15.0 | 0 | 0 | 0 | 0 |
| (*Tootsie Pops* Mini), 3 pcs., .5 oz. . . . . . | 50 | 0 | 13.0 | 0 | 0 | 0 | 0 |
| macadamias, coated (*Mauna Loa*): | | | | | | | |
| butter candy, ¼ cup . . | 180 | 1.0 | 11.0 | 16.0 | 5 | 90 | 1.0 |
| chocolate, dark, ¼ cup | 200 | 2.0 | 21.0 | 15.0 | 5 | 5 | 2.0 |
| chocolate, dark, sugar free, 6 pcs., 1.4 oz. | 170 | 3.0 | 20.0 | 16.0 | 5 | 5 | 4.0 |
| chocolate, milk, ¼ cup | 210 | 3.0 | 19.0 | 15.0 | 10 | 30 | 1.0 |

| Food and Measure | cal. | prot. (gms) | carbo. (gms) | fat (gms) | chol. (mgs) | sod. (mgs) | fiber (gms) |
|---|---|---|---|---|---|---|---|
| **Candy, macadamias, coated** *(cont.)* | | | | | | | |
| chocolate, milk, sugar | | | | | | | |
| free, 6 pcs., 1.4 oz. | 180 | 2.0 | 21.0 | 16.0 | 5 | 10 | 3.0 |
| chocolate, milk, toffee, | | | | | | | |
| ¼ cup . . . . . . . . . . . | 210 | 3.0 | 19.0 | 15.0 | 10 | 45 | 1.0 |
| malt balls, chocolate | | | | | | | |
| coated (*Whoppers*), | | | | | | | |
| 18 pcs., 1.4 oz. . . . . . . | 190 | 1.0 | 31.0 | 7.0 | 0 | 115 | 1.0 |
| maple flavor drops | | | | | | | |
| (*Maple Grove Farms*), | | | | | | | |
| 2 pcs., .4 oz. . . . . . . . . | 50 | 0 | 12.0 | 0 | 0 | 1 | 0 |
| marshmallow, 1.1 oz., | | | | | | | |
| except as noted: | | | | | | | |
| (*FunMallows*) . . . . . . . | 100 | 1.0 | 24.0 | 0 | 0 | 20 | 0 |
| (*Jet-Puffed*) . . . . . . . . | 100 | 1.0 | 24.0 | 0 | 0 | 25 | 0 |
| caramel/vanilla swirl | | | | | | | |
| (*Jet-Puffed*) . . . . . . | 100 | 1.0 | 24.0 | 0 | 0 | 15 | 0 |
| chocolate (*Jet-Puffed* | | | | | | | |
| *ChocoMallows*) . . . | 100 | 1.0 | 25.0 | 0 | 0 | 30 | 0 |
| coconut, toasted | | | | | | | |
| (*Jet-Puffed*), 1.6 oz. | 170 | 1.0 | 32.0 | 4.5 | 0 | 55 | 0 |
| mini (*Jet-Puffed*) . . | 100 | 1.0 | 25.0 | 0 | 0 | 25 | 0 |
| mini, chocolate or | | | | | | | |
| strawberry | | | | | | | |
| (*Jet-Puffed*), 1 oz. . | 90 | 1.0 | 23.0 | 0 | 0 | 25 | 0 |
| strawberry (*Jet-Puffed*) | 100 | 1.0 | 24.0 | 0 | 0 | 25 | 0 |
| vanilla (*Jet-Puffed* | | | | | | | |
| *StarMallows*) . . . . . | 100 | 1.0 | 24.0 | 0 | 0 | 25 | 0 |
| marzipan (*Biermann*), | | | | | | | |
| .42-oz. pc. . . . . . . . . . | 50 | 1.0 | 10.0 | 1.0 | 0 | 5 | 1.0 |
| mint: | | | | | | | |
| (*Altoids*), 3 pcs. . . . . . | 10 | 0 | 2.0 | 0 | 0 | 0 | 0 |
| (*BreathSavers*), 1 pc. . | 5 | 0 | 2.0 | 0 | 0 | 5 | 0 |
| mint, chocolate coated: | | | | | | | |
| (*Junior* Mints), | | | | | | | |
| 16 pcs., 1.4 oz. . . . | 170 | 1.0 | 35.0 | 3.0 | 0 | 30 | 1.0 |
| (*York* Peppermint | | | | | | | |
| Pattie), 1.4-oz. pc. . | 140 | 1.0 | 31.0 | 2.5 | 0 | 10 | 1.0 |
| (*York* Miniatures), | | | | | | | |
| 3 pcs., 1.45 oz. . . . | 150 | 1.0 | 33.0 | 3.0 | 0 | 15 | 1.0 |
| (*York* Snack / | | | | | | | |
| Snowflake), 1.2 oz. | 120 | 1.0 | 27.0 | 2.5 | 0 | 10 | 1.0 |
| candy coated (*York* | | | | | | | |
| Pieces), 1.4 oz. . . . | 170 | 2.0 | 28.0 | 8.0 | 5 | 0 | 3.0 |

| Food and Measure | cal. | prot. (gms) | carbo. (gms) | fat (gms) | chol. (mgs) | sod. (mgs) | fiber (gms) |
|---|---|---|---|---|---|---|---|
| nonpareils (*Sno-Caps*), | | | | | | | |
| ¼ cup, 1.4 oz. ....... | 180 | 1.0 | 30.0 | 8.0 | <5 | 0 | 2.0 |
| nougat, w/chocolate: | | | | | | | |
| (*Milky Way* Classic), | | | | | | | |
| 2-oz. bar ......... | 260 | 2.0 | 41.0 | 10.0 | 5 | 95 | 1.0 |
| (*Milky Way* Fun Size), | | | | | | | |
| 2 bars, 1.2 oz. .... | 150 | 1.0 | 24.0 | 6.0 | 5 | 55 | 0 |
| (*Milky Way Midnight*), | | | | | | | |
| 1.76-oz. bar ...... | 220 | 2.0 | 36.0 | 8.0 | 5 | 90 | 1.0 |
| (*Milky Way 2 To Go*), | | | | | | | |
| 1.9-oz. bar ....... | 230 | 2.0 | 36.0 | 9.0 | 5 | 85 | 1.0 |
| (*3 Musketeers*), | | | | | | | |
| 2.13-oz. bar ...... | 260 | 2.0 | 46.0 | 8.0 | 5 | 110 | 1.0 |
| chocolate (*Charleston* | | | | | | | |
| *Chew*), 1.4 oz. .... | 170 | 1.0 | 32.0 | 5.0 | 0 | 25 | 1.0 |
| minis (*Charleston* | | | | | | | |
| *Chew*), 1.5 oz. .... | 190 | 1.0 | 34.0 | 6.0 | 0 | 30 | 0 |
| minis (*Milky Way*), | | | | | | | |
| 5 pcs., 1.5 oz. .... | 190 | 2.0 | 30.0 | 7.0 | 5 | 70 | 0 |
| minis (*Milky Way Midnight*), | | | | | | | |
| 5 pcs., 1.4 oz. .... | 180 | 1.0 | 29.0 | 7.0 | 5 | 70 | 1.0 |
| minis (*3 Musketeers*), | | | | | | | |
| 7 pcs., 1.4 oz. .... | 170 | 1.0 | 32.0 | 5.0 | 5 | 80 | 1.0 |
| strawberry (*Charleston* | | | | | | | |
| *Chew*), 1.4 oz. .... | 170 | 1.0 | 33.0 | 4.5 | 0 | 25 | 0 |
| vanilla (*Charleston* | | | | | | | |
| *Chew*), 1.4 oz. .... | 160 | 1.0 | 30.0 | 4.5 | 0 | 25 | 0 |
| peanut, chocolate | | | | | | | |
| coated: | | | | | | | |
| (*Goober's*), 1.4 oz. ... | 200 | 4.0 | 21.0 | 13.0 | 5 | 14 | 4.0 |
| (*Planters*), 1.4 oz. .... | 210 | 5.0 | 18.0 | 15.0 | 5 | 80 | 2.0 |
| dark, and candy | | | | | | | |
| (*M&M's*), 1.5 oz. .. | 220 | 4.0 | 25.0 | 12.0 | 0 | 10 | 2.0 |
| milk, and candy | | | | | | | |
| (*M&M's*), 1.74 oz. . | 250 | 5.0 | 30.0 | 13.0 | 5 | 25 | 2.0 |
| peanut bar: | | | | | | | |
| (*Munch*), 1.4-oz. bar .. | 220 | 6.0 | 18.0 | 15.0 | 10 | 140 | 2.0 |
| (*Planters*), 1.6 oz. .... | 230 | 7.0 | 22.0 | 14.0 | 0 | 100 | 2.0 |
| caramel chocolate | | | | | | | |
| (*Planters* Carb | | | | | | | |
| Well), 1.35 oz. .... | 180 | 6.0 | 17.0 | 13.0 | 0 | 140 | 2.0 |
| peanut brittle, 1 oz. ...... | 130 | 2.0 | 20.0 | 5.0 | 5 | 130 | 1.0 |
| peanut butter, w/chocolate: | | | | | | | |
| (*Butterfinger*), 2.1 oz. . | 270 | 4.0 | 43.0 | 11.0 | 0 | 135 | 1.0 |

| Food and Measure | cal. | prot. (gms) | carbo. (gms) | fat (gms) | chol. (mgs) | sod. (mgs) | fiber (gms) |
|---|---|---|---|---|---|---|---|
| **Candy, peanut butter, w/chocolate** *(cont.)* | | | | | | | |
| (*Butterfinger* Fun Size), .75-oz. bar .. | 100 | 1.0 | 15.0 | 4.0 | 0 | 50 | 0 |
| (*Butterfinger Crisp*), 2.1-oz. bar ....... | 270 | 4.0 | 43.0 | 11.0 | 0 | 135 | 1.0 |
| (*Butterfinger Snackerz*), 1.3-oz. pouch ..... | 170 | 2.0 | 23.0 | 8.0 | 0 | 80 | 2.0 |
| (*5th Avenue*), 2 oz. ... | 260 | 4.0 | 38.0 | 12.0 | 0 | 120 | 1.0 |
| (*Reese's Fast Break*), 2-oz. bar ......... | 260 | 5.0 | 35.0 | 12.0 | 0 | 190 | 2.0 |
| (*Reese's NutRageous*), 2-oz. bar ......... | 260 | 6.0 | 28.0 | 16.0 | 0 | 100 | 2.0 |
| (*Reese's Peanut Butter Cups*), 1.5 oz. ..... | 210 | 5.0 | 24.0 | 13.0 | 5 | 150 | 1.0 |
| (*Reese's Peanut Butter Cups Big Cup*), 1.4 oz. .......... | 200 | 5.0 | 22.0 | 12.0 | 5 | 150 | 1.0 |
| (*Reese's Pieces*), 1.4 oz. .......... | 190 | 4.0 | 25.0 | 9.0 | 0 | 75 | 1.0 |
| (*Reese's Whipps*), 1.9-oz. bar ....... | 230 | 3.0 | 37.0 | 9.0 | 0 | 110 | 1.0 |
| candy coated (*M&M's*), 1.63 oz. .......... | 240 | 5.0 | 26.0 | 14.0 | 5 | 100 | 2.0 |
| clusters (*Reese's*), 3 pcs., 1.5 oz. .... | 220 | 4.0 | 24.0 | 12.0 | 5 | 80 | 1.0 |
| coconut (*Zagnut*), 1.7-oz. bar ....... | 220 | 3.0 | 35.0 | 9.0 | 0 | 100 | 1.0 |
| cookie bar (*Twix*), .8-oz. bar ........ | 120 | 2.0 | 13.0 | 7.0 | 0 | 70 | 1.0 |
| cookie bar (*Twix*), 2 bars, 1.7 oz. .... | 250 | 5.0 | 26.0 | 15.0 | 0 | 135 | 2.0 |
| crèmes (*Reese's*), 3 pcs., 1.25 oz. ... | 190 | 3.0 | 18.0 | 13.0 | 5 | 95 | 1.0 |
| crispy crunch bar (*Reese's*), 1.7 oz. .. | 260 | 7.0 | 22.0 | 18.0 | 5 | 140 | 3.0 |
| dark (*Reese's*), 1.5 oz. | 210 | 4.0 | 23.0 | 14.0 | 5 | 130 | 2.0 |
| wafer bar (*Reese's Sticks*), 1.5 oz. .... | 220 | 4.0 | 23.0 | 13.0 | 0 | 130 | 1.0 |
| white (*Reese's*), 1.5 oz. | 220 | 5.0 | 22.0 | 13.0 | 5 | 170 | 1.0 |
| peanut butter crunch: | | | | | | | |
| (*Old Dominion*), 1 oz. . | 135 | 4.0 | 14.0 | 7.2 | 0 | 45 | 2.0 |
| bar (*Planters* Carb Well), 1.35 oz. ...... | 160 | 6.0 | 16.0 | 12.0 | 0 | 140 | 2.0 |

| Food and Measure | cal. | prot. (gms) | carbo. (gms) | fat (gms) | chol. (mgs) | sod. (mgs) | fiber (gms) |
|---|---|---|---|---|---|---|---|
| peanut caramel bar: | | | | | | | |
| (*Baby Ruth*), 2.1-oz. .. | 280 | 4.0 | 39.0 | 14.0 | 0 | 130 | 1.0 |
| (*Baby Ruth* Fun | | | | | | | |
| Size), 2 pc., 1.3 oz. | 170 | 2.0 | 24.0 | 8.0 | 0 | 85 | <1.0 |
| (*PayDay*), 1.8 oz. .... | 240 | 7.0 | 27.0 | 13.0 | 0 | 120 | 2.0 |
| (*Snickers*), 2.oz. ..... | 280 | 4.0 | 35.0 | 14.0 | 5 | 140 | 1.0 |
| (*Snickers* Dark), | | | | | | | |
| 1.8 oz. ......... | 240 | 5.0 | 31.0 | 12.0 | 0 | 125 | 2.0 |
| (*Snickers* Fun Size), | | | | | | | |
| 2 bars, 1.2 oz. .... | 160 | 3.0 | 21.0 | 8.0 | 5 | 85 | 1.0 |
| (*Snickers* Marathon), | | | | | | | |
| 2 oz. ........... | 220 | 10.0 | 31.0 | 7.0 | 5 | 180 | 3.0 |
| (*Snickers* Miniatures), | | | | | | | |
| 4 pcs., 1.2 oz. .... | 170 | 3.0 | 22.0 | 8.0 | 5 | 80 | 1.0 |
| (*Snickers* Xtreme), | | | | | | | |
| 2 oz. ........... | 290 | 5.0 | 33.0 | 16.0 | 10 | 110 | 2.0 |
| (*Whatchamacallit*), | | | | | | | |
| 1.6-oz. bar ....... | 230 | 3.0 | 28.0 | 12.0 | 5 | 140 | 1.0 |
| almond (*Snickers*), | | | | | | | |
| 1.76-oz. bar ...... | 230 | 3.0 | 32.0 | 11.0 | 5 | 115 | 1.0 |
| fudge (*Snickers*), | | | | | | | |
| 1.76-oz. bar ...... | 250 | 4.0 | 31.0 | 13.0 | 10 | 90 | 1.0 |
| pecan caramel (*Pot of* | | | | | | | |
| *Gold*), 4 pcs., 1.4 oz. . | 200 | 2.0 | 23.0 | 12.0 | 5 | 60 | 1.0 |
| plum bites, chocolate | | | | | | | |
| coated (*Sunsweet* | | | | | | | |
| *PlumSweets*), 1.1 oz. . | 120 | 1.0 | 19.0 | 6.0 | 0 | 5 | 2.0 |
| pretzel, caramel, | | | | | | | |
| peanut, chocolate | | | | | | | |
| (*Take 5*), 1.5-oz. bar .. | 210 | 4.0 | 25.0 | 11.0 | <5 | 180 | 1.0 |
| pretzel, chocolate/candy | | | | | | | |
| coated (*M&M's*), | | | | | | | |
| 1.14 oz. .......... | 150 | 2.0 | 24.0 | 5.0 | 0 | 150 | 1.0 |
| pretzel, coated (*Glutino* | | | | | | | |
| Gluten Free), 1.1 oz.: | | | | | | | |
| chocolate ......... | 160 | 1.0 | 19.0 | 8.0 | 5 | 200 | 0 |
| yogurt ............ | 150 | 1.0 | 19.0 | 9.0 | 5 | 160 | 0 |
| pretzel, coated | | | | | | | |
| (*Snyder's Hershey's* | | | | | | | |
| Dips), 1 oz.: | | | | | | | |
| dark chocolate ...... | 140 | 2.0 | 22.0 | 4.5 | <5 | 130 | 2.0 |
| milk chocolate ...... | 140 | 2.0 | 19.0 | 6.0 | <5 | 100 | <1.0 |
| milk chocolate peanut | | | | | | | |
| butter ........... | 150 | 3.0 | 18.0 | 7.0 | <5 | 100 | 0 |

| Food and Measure | cal. | prot. (gms) | carbo. (gms) | fat (gms) | chol. (mgs) | sod. (mgs) | fiber (gms) |
|---|---|---|---|---|---|---|---|
| **Candy, pretzel, coated** *(cont.)* | | | | | | | |
| milk chocolate | | | | | | | |
|   sandwich . . . . . . . . | 150 | 3.0 | 18.0 | 7.0 | <5 | 100 | 0 |
|   white chocolate . . . . . . | 140 | 3.0 | 19.0 | 6.0 | <5 | 110 | 0 |
|   white crème peanut | | | | | | | |
|     butter . . . . . . . . . . . | 150 | 3.0 | 18.0 | 7.0 | <5 | 85 | <1.0 |
| pretzel, fudge dipped | | | | | | | |
| (*Fudge Shoppe Right* | | | | | | | |
| *Bites*), .75-oz. pkg. . . . | 100 | 2.0 | 15.0 | 3.5 | 0 | 125 | <1.0 |
| rainbow (*Twizzlers*), | | | | | | | |
| 3 pcs., 1.2 oz. . . . . . . | 120 | 1.0 | 27.0 | .5 | 0 | 75 | 0 |
| raisins, chocolate | | | | | | | |
| coated: | | | | | | | |
| (*Raisinets*), 1.58 oz. . . | 190 | 2.0 | 32.0 | 8.0 | 5 | 15 | 1.0 |
| (*Sun•Maid*), 1.1 oz. . . | 170 | 2.0 | 26.0 | 6.0 | 5 | 20 | 1.0 |
| dark (*Raisinets*), | | | | | | | |
| ¼ cup, 1.58 oz. . . . | 180 | 2.0 | 32.0 | 8.0 | 5 | 5 | 2.0 |
| raisins, yogurt coated, | | | | | | | |
| ¼ cup, 1.1 oz.: | | | | | | | |
| chocolate (*Sun•Maid*) . | 120 | 1.0 | 22.0 | 4.0 | 0 | 20 | 1.0 |
| vanilla (*Mariani*) . . . . . | 150 | 2.0 | 19.0 | 7.0 | 0 | 25 | <1.0 |
| vanilla (*Sun•Maid*) . . . | 130 | 1.0 | 21.0 | 5.0 | 0 | 20 | 1.0 |
| soy nuts, w/chocolate: | | | | | | | |
| (*Genisoy*), 1 oz. . . . . . | 140 | 5.0 | 15.0 | 8.0 | 0 | 20 | 1.0 |
| dark (*South Beach* | | | | | | | |
| *Living*), .67 oz. . . . . | 100 | 3.0 | 9.0 | 6.0 | 0 | 0 | 2.0 |
| spearmint (*Brach's* | | | | | | | |
| Leaves), 5 pcs., 1.4 oz. | 130 | 0 | 34.0 | 0 | 0 | 15 | 0 |
| spice drops (*Brach's*), | | | | | | | |
| 12 pcs., 1.4 oz. . . . . . . | 130 | 0 | 33.0 | 0 | 0 | 15 | 0 |
| strawberry flavor: | | | | | | | |
| (*Young & Smylie*), | | | | | | | |
| 11 pcs., 1.5 oz. . . . | 150 | 1.0 | 33.0 | 1.5 | 0 | 30 | 0 |
| twists (*Twizzlers*), | | | | | | | |
| 4 pcs., 1.6 oz. . . . . | 160 | 1.0 | 36.0 | .5 | 0 | 95 | 0 |
| taffy (*Brach's* Salt | | | | | | | |
| Water), 5 pcs. . . . . . . . | 170 | 0 | 36.0 | 2.5 | 00 | 35 | 0 |
| toffee bar, chocolate: | | | | | | | |
| (*Heath*), 1.4 oz. . . . . . . | 210 | 1.0 | 24.0 | 13.0 | 10 | 135 | 1.0 |
| (*Skor*), 1.4 oz. . . . . . . | 200 | 1.0 | 25.0 | 12.0 | 20 | 130 | 1.0 |
| truffle, w/chocolate: | | | | | | | |
| (*Toblerone* Truffle | | | | | | | |
| Peaks), 1.4 oz. . . . . | 240 | 2.0 | 23.0 | 15.0 | 10 | 20 | 1.0 |

| Food and Measure | cal. | prot. (gms) | carbo. (gms) | fat (gms) | chol. (mgs) | sod. (mgs) | fiber (gms) |
|---|---|---|---|---|---|---|---|
| assortment (*Pot of Gold*), 4 pcs., 1.4 oz. | 200 | 3.0 | 23.0 | 13.0 | 5 | 40 | 1.0 |
| wafer, w/chocolate: | | | | | | | |
| (*KitKat*), 1.5-oz. bar .. | 210 | 3.0 | 28.0 | 11.0 | 5 | 30 | 1.0 |
| extra crispy | | | | | | | |
| (*KitKat*), 1.6-oz. bar | 220 | 3.0 | 29.0 | 12.0 | 5 | 30 | 1.0 |
| white (*KitKat*), 1.5 oz.. | 220 | 3.0 | 26.0 | 12.0 | 5 | 45 | 0 |
| watermelon flavor (*Twizzlers Pull 'n' Peel*), 1.2-oz. pc. .... | 110 | 1.0 | 26.0 | .5 | 0 | 70 | 0 |
| **Cane syrup**: | | | | | | | |
| (*Mrs. Renfro's*), ¼ cup .. | 250 | 0 | 63.0 | 0 | 0 | 15 | 0 |
| 1 tbsp. ............... | 52 | 0 | 13.4 | 0 | 0 | <1 | 0 |
| **Cannellini beans**, see "Kidney beans" | | | | | | | |
| **Cannelloni entree**, frozen: | | | | | | | |
| cheese: | | | | | | | |
| 5 (*Buitoni*), ½ of 26-oz. pkg. ....... | 560 | 27.0 | 52.0 | 27.0 | 115 | 1560 | 5.0 |
| 4 (*Lean Cuisine*), 9.125-oz. pkg. .... | 240 | 17.0 | 30.0 | 6.0 | 20 | 690 | 3.0 |
| chicken, grilled, and spinach (*Buitoni*), ½ of 22-oz. pkg. ..... | 560 | 35.0 | 46.0 | 26.0 | 145 | 1070 | 3.0 |
| **Cannoli shells**: | | | | | | | |
| (*Alessi*), 1 pc. ......... | 90 | 2.0 | 16.0 | 1.5 | 10 | 100 | 2.0 |
| mini (*Alessi*), 1 pc. ..... | 50 | 1.0 | 9.0 | 1.0 | 5 | 60 | 0 |
| **Cantaloupe**: | | | | | | | |
| (*Dole*), ¼ medium ...... | 45 | 1.0 | 11.0 | 0 | 0 | 20 | 1.0 |
| (*Earthbound Farm Organic*), ¼ medium, 4.75 oz. ........... | 50 | 1.0 | 12.0 | 0 | 0 | 25 | 1.0 |
| (*Frieda's French Kiss*), 10 balls, 4.8 oz. ..... | 80 | 1.0 | 17.0 | 0 | 0 | 35 | 1.0 |
| (*Green Giant*), 4.75 oz. .. | 45 | 1.0 | 11.0 | 0 | 0 | 20 | 2.0 |
| ½ of 5" melon ......... | 94 | 2.3 | 22.3 | .7 | 0 | 23 | 2.1 |
| cubed, 1 cup ......... | 56 | 1.4 | 13.4 | .5 | 0 | 14 | 1.3 |
| **Caper berries**: | | | | | | | |
| (*Roland*), 2 tbsp. ....... | 0 | 0 | 1.0 | 0 | 0 | 410 | 0 |
| in balsamic vinegar (*Alessi*), .5 oz. ....... | 0 | 0 | 0 | 0 | 0 | 120 | 0 |
| **Capers**, 1 tsp.: | | | | | | | |
| (*Crosse & Blackwell*) .... | 5 | 0 | 1.0 | 0 | 0 | 350 | 0 |

| Food and Measure | cal. | prot. (gms) | carbo. (gms) | fat (gms) | chol. (mgs) | sod. (mgs) | fiber (gms) |
|---|---|---|---|---|---|---|---|
| **Capers** *(cont.)* | | | | | | | |
| (*Roland* Capote/ | | | | | | | |
| Nonpareille/Surfines) . | 0 | 0 | 0 | 0 | 0 | 85 | 0 |
| (*Vigo*) . . . . . . . . . . . . . . . | 0 | 0 | 0 | 0 | 0 | 140 | 0 |
| in salt (*Roland*) . . . . . . . . | 5 | 0 | 0 | 0 | 0 | 70 | 0 |
| in sherry wine | | | | | | | |
| vinegar (*Roland*) . . . . . | 5 | 0 | 1.0 | 0 | 0 | 85 | 0 |
| **Capocola/Coppa**, 1 oz.: | | | | | | | |
| (*Applegate Farms* | | | | | | | |
| Dry Cure Coppa) . . . . . | 100 | 8.0 | 0 | 7.0 | 20 | 510 | 0 |
| hot/sweet (*Boar's* | | | | | | | |
| *Head* Capocollo) . . . . . | 80 | 7.0 | 0 | 7.0 | 25 | 590 | 0 |
| **Capon**, see "Chicken" | | | | | | | |
| **Caponata**, see "Artichoke | | | | | | | |
| appetizer" and | | | | | | | |
| "Eggplant appetizer" | | | | | | | |
| **Cappuccino**, see | | | | | | | |
| "Coffee, iced/mix" | | | | | | | |
| **Carambola**, fresh: | | | | | | | |
| (*Frieda's* Starfruit), | | | | | | | |
| sliced, 1 cup . . . . . . . . | 30 | 1.0 | 7.0 | 0 | 0 | 2 | 3.0 |
| 1 medium, 4.7 oz. . . . . . . | 42 | .7 | 9.9 | .4 | 0 | 2 | 3.4 |
| sliced, ½ cup . . . . . . . . . | 18 | .3 | 1.0 | .2 | 0 | 1 | 1.5 |
| **Carambola**, dried | | | | | | | |
| (*Frieda's* Starfruit), | | | | | | | |
| ⅓ cup, 1.4 oz. . . . . . . . | 120 | 2.0 | 29.0 | 0 | 0 | 5 | 1.0 |
| **Caramel dip**, see | | | | | | | |
| "Fruit dip" | | | | | | | |
| **Caramel spread** | | | | | | | |
| (*Roland* Dulce de Leche), | | | | | | | |
| 1 tbsp.: | | | | | | | |
| banana flavor . . . . . . . . | 90 | 1.0 | 16.0 | 2.0 | 5 | 35 | 0 |
| coffee flavor . . . . . . . . . | 90 | 2.0 | 18.0 | 2.0 | 5 | 35 | 0 |
| for pastry . . . . . . . . . . . | 90 | 2.0 | 16.0 | 2.0 | 5 | 30 | 0 |
| **Caramel syrup**, 2 tbsp.: | | | | | | | |
| (*Hershey's*) . . . . . . . . . . . | 110 | 1.0 | 27.0 | 0 | 0 | 125 | 0 |
| (*Hershey's* Classic | | | | | | | |
| *Caramel* Sundae) . . . . | 100 | 0 | 25.0 | 0 | 0 | 100 | 0 |
| (*Smucker's* Sundae) . . . . | 100 | 1.0 | 25.0 | 0 | 0 | 110 | 0 |
| **Caramel topping** (see | | | | | | | |
| also "Butterscotch | | | | | | | |
| topping"), 2 tbsp.: | | | | | | | |
| (*Hershey's*) . . . . . . . . . . | 110 | 1.0 | 27.0 | 0 | 0 | 140 | 0 |
| (*Smucker's*) . . . . . . . . . . | 120 | 0 | 29.0 | 0 | 0 | 110 | 0 |

| Food and Measure | cal. | prot. (gms) | carbo. (gms) | fat (gms) | chol. (mgs) | sod. (mgs) | fiber (gms) |
|---|---|---|---|---|---|---|---|
| (*Smucker's* No Sugar) ... | 90 | 0 | 24.0 | 0 | 0 | 65 | 0 |
| (*Smucker's Magic Shell*) ............. | 220 | 1.0 | 14.0 | 18.0 | 5 | 45 | 0 |
| hot (*Smucker's*) ........ | 140 | 1.0 | 27.0 | 3.5 | 0 | 60 | 0 |
| **Caraway seeds:** | | | | | | | |
| whole (*Bobs Red Mill*), 1 tsp. ............. | 5 | 0 | 1.0 | 0 | 0 | 0 | 0 |
| 1 tsp. ................. | 7 | .4 | 1.1 | .3 | 0 | <1 | <1.0 |
| **Cardamom**, ground, 1 tsp. | 6 | .2 | 1.4 | .1 | 0 | <1 | .5 |
| **Cardoon:** | | | | | | | |
| raw, shredded: | | | | | | | |
| (*Frieda's*), 1 cup ..... | 30 | 1.0 | 7.0 | 0 | 0 | 303 | 3.0 |
| ½ cup .............. | 18 | .6 | 4.4 | .1 | 0 | 151 | 1.4 |
| boiled, drained, 4 oz. .... | 25 | .9 | 6.0 | .1 | 0 | 200 | n.a. |
| **Caribou**, meat only, roasted, 4 oz. ........ | 189 | 33.8 | 0 | 5.0 | 123 | 68 | 0 |
| **Carissa**, sliced, ½ cup .. | 46 | .4 | 10.2 | 1.0 | 0 | 2 | n.a. |
| **Carnival squash** (*Frieda's*), 3 oz. ....... | 30 | 1.0 | 7.0 | 0 | 0 | 0 | 1.0 |
| **Carob drink mix**, powder, 3 tsp. ....... | 45 | .2 | 11.2 | tr. | 0 | 12 | <1.0 |
| **Carob flour**, ¼ cup ..... | 99 | 1.2 | 22.9 | .2 | 0 | 9 | 10.2 |
| **Carob powder** (*Shiloh Farms*), 1 tbsp. ....... | 55 | 1.0 | 13.0 | 0 | 0 | 5 | 1.0 |
| **Carp**, meat only: | | | | | | | |
| raw, 4 oz. ............. | 144 | 20.2 | 0 | 6.4 | 75 | 58 | 0 |
| baked or broiled, 4 oz. .. | 184 | 25.9 | 0 | 8.1 | 95 | 71 | 0 |
| **Carrot**, fresh: | | | | | | | |
| raw: | | | | | | | |
| (*Bolthouse Farms*), 7" x 1¼" diam. .... | 30 | 1.0 | 7.0 | 0 | 0 | 60 | 2.0 |
| (*Bolthouse Farms* Baby/ Chips/Matchsticks/ *Sweet Petites*), 3 oz. | 35 | 1.0 | 8.0 | 0 | 0 | 65 | 2.0 |
| (*Dole*), 2.5-oz. pc. .... | 30 | <1.0 | 7.0 | 0 | 0 | 50 | 2.0 |
| (*Frieda's* Gold), 3 oz. ... | 35 | 1.0 | 9.0 | 0 | 0 | 30 | 3.0 |
| whole, 7½", 2.8 oz. .... | 31 | .7 | 7.3 | .1 | 0 | 25 | 2.2 |
| shredded (*Dole*), 3 oz. .. | 40 | 1.0 | 9.0 | 0 | 0 | 45 | 2.0 |
| shredded, ½ cup .... | 24 | .6 | 5.6 | .1 | 0 | 19 | 1.7 |
| raw, baby: | | | | | | | |
| (*Dole* Mini Cut), 8 pcs. | 30 | <1.0 | 7.0 | 0 | 0 | 65 | 2.0 |
| medium, 2¾" long ... | 4 | .1 | .8 | .1 | 0 | 3 | .2 |

| Food and Measure | cal. | prot. (gms) | carbo. (gms) | fat (gms) | chol. (mgs) | sod. (mgs) | fiber (gms) |
|---|---|---|---|---|---|---|---|
| **Carrot** *(cont.)* | | | | | | | |
| raw, w/ranch dip: | | | | | | | |
| (*Chiquita Fruit Bites*), | | | | | | | |
| 2.5-oz. pkt. . . . . . . . | 50 | 1.0 | 7.0 | 2.5 | 5 | 150 | 2.0 |
| (*Ready Pac Cool* | | | | | | | |
| *Cuts*), 2.25-oz. pkt. | 70 | 1.0 | 5.0 | 5.0 | 5 | 210 | 1.0 |
| boiled, drained, | | | | | | | |
| sliced, ½ cup . . . . . . | 35 | .9 | 8.2 | .1 | 0 | 52 | 2.6 |
| **Carrot, can/jar**, ½ cup: | | | | | | | |
| baby, whole: | | | | | | | |
| (*Le Sueur*) . . . . . . . . . | 35 | <1.0 | 8.0 | 0 | 0 | 410 | 2.0 |
| (*Roland*) . . . . . . . . . . . | 35 | 1.0 | 7.0 | 0 | 0 | 400 | 3.0 |
| (*S&W*) . . . . . . . . . . . . | 35 | 0 | 8.0 | 0 | 0 | 300 | 3.0 |
| crinkle (*Freshlike*) . . . . . . | 45 | 1.0 | 11.0 | 0 | 0 | 180 | 3.0 |
| julienne strips: | | | | | | | |
| (*Roland*) . . . . . . . . . . . | 45 | 1.0 | 9.0 | 0 | 0 | 310 | 3.0 |
| (*S&W*) . . . . . . . . . . . . | 35 | 0 | 8.0 | 0 | 0 | 300 | 3.0 |
| sliced: | | | | | | | |
| (*Allens* Tiny) . . . . . . . . | 35 | 0 | 8.0 | 0 | 0 | 40 | 3.0 |
| (*Del Monte*) . . . . . . . . | 35 | 0 | 8.0 | 0 | 0 | 300 | 3.0 |
| (*Veg-All*) . . . . . . . . . . . | 30 | 0 | 5.0 | 0 | 0 | 320 | 2.0 |
| w/liquid . . . . . . . . . . . . | 28 | .8 | 6.2 | .2 | 0 | 297 | 1.1 |
| drained . . . . . . . . . . . . | 17 | .5 | 4.0 | .1 | 0 | 176 | 1.1 |
| honey (*Glory*) . . . . . . . . . | 50 | 0 | 12.0 | 0 | 0 | 220 | 2.0 |
| honey glaze (*Del Monte* | | | | | | | |
| *Savory Sides*) . . . . . . . | 70 | 1.0 | 18.0 | 0 | 0 | 440 | 1.0 |
| **Carrot, frozen**: | | | | | | | |
| sliced: | | | | | | | |
| (*Freshlike*), ⅔ cup . . . | 35 | <1.0 | 7.0 | 0 | 0 | 55 | 2.0 |
| boiled, drained, ½ cup | 26 | .9 | 6.0 | .1 | 0 | 43 | 2.6 |
| honey glazed (*Green* | | | | | | | |
| *Giant*), 1 cup . . . . . . . . | 90 | 1.0 | 15.0 | 3.0 | 0 | 180 | 3.0 |
| **Carrot drink blend,** | | | | | | | |
| orange mango | | | | | | | |
| (*Nantucket Nectars*), | | | | | | | |
| 8 fl. oz. . . . . . . . . . . | 120 | 0 | 28.0 | 0 | 0 | 30 | 0 |
| **Carrot juice**, 8 fl. oz.: | | | | | | | |
| (*Bolthouse Farms*) . . . . . | 70 | 2.0 | 14.0 | 0 | 0 | 150 | <1.0 |
| (*Earthbound Farm* | | | | | | | |
| Organic) . . . . . . . . . . . | 70 | 2.0 | 14.0 | 0 | 0 | 150 | <1.0 |
| (*Odwalla*) . . . . . . . . . . . . | 70 | 2.0 | 15.0 | 0 | 0 | 160 | 1.0 |
| **Carrot juice blend** | | | | | | | |
| (see also specific | | | | | | | |
| listings), 8 fl. oz.: | | | | | | | |

| Food and Measure | cal. | prot. (gms) | carbo. (gms) | fat (gms) | chol. (mgs) | sod. (mgs) | fiber (gms) |
|---|---|---|---|---|---|---|---|
| orange (*After the Fall* 24 Karrot) .......... | 120 | 1.0 | 28.0 | 0 | 0 | 55 | 0 |
| tropical fruit (*Mott's* Medleys) ........... | 140 | 0 | 32.0 | 0 | 0 | 90 | 0 |
| **Casaba melon:** | | | | | | | |
| 1/10 of 7¾" melon ....... | 43 | 1.5 | 10.2 | .2 | 0 | 20 | 1.3 |
| cubed, 1 cup .......... | 44 | 1.5 | 10.5 | .2 | 0 | 10 | 1.4 |
| **Cashew**, 1 oz., except as noted: | | | | | | | |
| (*Beer Nuts*) ........... | 170 | 5.0 | 8.0 | 13.0 | 0 | 80 | 1.0 |
| (*Frito-Lay*), 1 pkg. ...... | 240 | 6.0 | 12.0 | 20.0 | 0 | 180 | 2.0 |
| (*Frito-Lay* Whole), 3 tbsp. ............ | 180 | 4.0 | 8.0 | 15.0 | 0 | 120 | 1.0 |
| (*Planters* Deluxe Whole Sea Salt) ..... | 160 | 5.0 | 8.0 | 13.0 | 0 | 115 | 1.0 |
| (*Planters* Jumbo Deluxe Sea Salt) ..... | 170 | 5.0 | 8.0 | 13.0 | 0 | 115 | 1.0 |
| (*Planters* Jumbo Natural Harvest) ..... | 160 | 5.0 | 9.0 | 13.0 | 0 | 100 | 1.0 |
| (*Planters* Salted) ....... | 170 | 5.0 | 8.0 | 14.0 | 0 | 115 | 1.0 |
| (*Planters* Salted), 1.5-oz. pkg. ........ | 250 | 8.0 | 11.0 | 20.0 | 0 | 170 | 1.0 |
| (*Planters* Salted), 2-oz. pkg. ........... | 330 | 10.0 | 16.0 | 28.0 | 0 | 320 | 3.0 |
| (*Planters* Whole) ....... | 160 | 5.0 | 8.0 | 13.0 | 0 | 115 | 1.0 |
| (*Planters* Whole Lightly Salted) ....... | 160 | 5.0 | 8.0 | 13.0 | 0 | 55 | 1.0 |
| dry-roasted: | | | | | | | |
| (*Planters*), .7 oz. ..... | 160 | 5.0 | 9.0 | 12.0 | 0 | 140 | 1.0 |
| 18 medium, 1 oz. .... | 163 | 4.4 | 9.3 | 13.2 | 0 | 4 | .9 |
| whole or halves, 1 cup ........... | 787 | 21.0 | 44.8 | 63.5 | 0 | 21 | 4.1 |
| halves and pieces: | | | | | | | |
| (*Planters*) .......... | 160 | 5.0 | 9.0 | 13.0 | 0 | 150 | 1.0 |
| (*Planters* 3 oz.) ...... | 160 | 5.0 | 9.0 | 13.0 | 0 | 115 | 1.0 |
| (*Planters* Lightly Salted) .......... | 160 | 5.0 | 9.0 | 13.0 | 0 | 60 | 1.0 |
| honey-roasted: | | | | | | | |
| (*Planters*) .......... | 150 | 4.0 | 11.0 | 11.0 | 0 | 120 | 1.0 |
| (*Planters*), 1.5 oz. .......... | 230 | 7.0 | 14.0 | 18.0 | 0 | 135 | 1.0 |
| (*Planters*), 2 oz. ............ | 310 | 9.0 | 23.0 | 24.0 | 0 | 170 | 3.0 |

| Food and Measure | cal. | prot. (gms) | carbo. (gms) | fat (gms) | chol. (mgs) | sod. (mgs) | fiber (gms) |
|---|---|---|---|---|---|---|---|
| **Cashew,** *(cont.)* | | | | | | | |
| oil-roasted: | | | | | | | |
| 18 medium, 1 oz. . . . . | 163 | 4.6 | 8.1 | 13.7 | 0 | 5 | 1.1 |
| whole/halves, 1 cup . . | 748 | 21.0 | 37.1 | 62.7 | 0 | 22 | 4.9 |
| **Cashew butter,** 2 tbsp.: | | | | | | | |
| (*Arrowhead Mills*) . . . . . . . | 160 | 4.0 | 9.0 | 13.0 | 0 | 0 | <1.0 |
| (*Kettle Roaster Fresh*) . . . | 160 | 5.0 | 8.0 | 14.0 | 0 | 0 | 1.0 |
| (*MaraNatha*) . . . . . . . . . . | 190 | 5.0 | 10.0 | 15.0 | 0 | 0 | 2.0 |
| **Cassava** (see also | | | | | | | |
| "Yuca root"), raw: | | | | | | | |
| 14.4-oz. root . . . . . . . . | 653 | 5.6 | 155.2 | 1.1 | 0 | 57 | 7.3 |
| 1 cup . . . . . . . . . . . . | 330 | 2.8 | 78.4 | .6 | 0 | 29 | 3.7 |
| **Catfish,** channel, | | | | | | | |
| meat only: | | | | | | | |
| farmed, 4 oz.: | | | | | | | |
| raw . . . . . . . . . . . . . | 153 | 17.7 | 0 | 8.6 | 15 | 60 | 0 |
| baked or broiled . . . . . | 172 | 21.2 | 0 | 9.1 | 73 | 91 | 0 |
| wild, 4 oz.: | | | | | | | |
| raw . . . . . . . . . . . . . | 108 | 18.6 | 0 | 3.2 | 66 | 49 | 0 |
| baked or broiled . . . . . | 119 | 20.9 | 0 | 3.2 | 82 | 57 | 0 |
| **Catjang,** boiled, ½ cup . . | 100 | 7.0 | 17.5 | .6 | 0 | 16 | 3.1 |
| **Cauliflower,** fresh: | | | | | | | |
| raw: | | | | | | | |
| (*Dole*), ⅙ medium | | | | | | | |
| head, 3.5 oz. . . . . . | 25 | 2.0 | 5.0 | 0 | 0 | 30 | 2.0 |
| florets (*Green Giant*), | | | | | | | |
| 3.5 oz. . . . . . . . . . | 25 | 2.0 | 5.0 | 0 | 0 | 30 | 2.0 |
| florets, 3 pcs. . . . . . . | 14 | 1.1 | 2.9 | .1 | 0 | 17 | 1.4 |
| 1" pcs., ½ cup . . . . . . | 13 | 1.0 | 2.6 | .1 | 0 | 15 | 1.3 |
| raw, cheese sauce | | | | | | | |
| (*Green Giant*), 1 cup . . | 90 | 3.0 | 6.0 | 7.0 | 15 | 190 | 2.0 |
| boiled, drained, | | | | | | | |
| 1" pcs., ½ cup . . . . . . | 14 | 1.1 | 2.6 | .3 | 0 | 9 | 1.7 |
| green: | | | | | | | |
| raw, ⅕ head . . . . . . . | 28 | 2.7 | 5.7 | .3 | 0 | 22 | 3.0 |
| raw, 1" pcs., ½ cup . . . | 16 | 1.5 | 3.0 | .2 | 0 | 12 | 1.6 |
| boiled, drained, | | | | | | | |
| 1" pcs., ½ cup . . . . | 20 | 1.9 | 3.9 | .2 | 0 | 14 | 2.0 |
| **Cauliflower,** frozen: | | | | | | | |
| florets (*Birds Eye/* | | | | | | | |
| *Freshlike*), 4 pcs., | | | | | | | |
| 3 oz. . . . . . . . . . . . . | 25 | 1.0 | 4.0 | 0 | 0 | 25 | 1.0 |
| boiled, drained, | | | | | | | |
| 1" pcs., ½ cup . . . . . . . | 17 | 1.5 | 3.4 | .2 | 0 | 16 | 2.0 |

| Food and Measure | cal. | prot. (gms) | carbo. (gms) | fat (gms) | chol. (mgs) | sod. (mgs) | fiber (gms) |
|---|---|---|---|---|---|---|---|
| cheese sauce: | | | | | | | |
| (*Allens SteamSupreme*), | | | | | | | |
| ½ cup . . . . . . . . . . . | 50 | 3.0 | 5.0 | 2.5 | 5 | 230 | 1.0 |
| (*Green Giant*), ½ cup . | 50 | 2.0 | 6.0 | 2.5 | 0 | 410 | 1.0 |
| (*Green Giant Just* | | | | | | | |
| *for One*), 1 tray . . . . | 40 | 2.0 | 8.0 | 1.0 | <5 | 410 | 3.0 |
| 3 (*Green Giant* Bag), | | | | | | | |
| ½ cup cooked . . . . | 45 | 2.0 | 7.0 | 1.5 | 0 | 390 | 1.0 |
| garlic (*Birds Eye* | | | | | | | |
| *Steamfresh*), 1 cup . . . | 40 | 1.0 | 5.0 | 1.5 | 0 | 330 | 1.0 |
| **Cauliflower combination**, | | | | | | | |
| frozen, w/carrots, | | | | | | | |
| snow peas (*Birds Eye*), | | | | | | | |
| 1 cup . . . . . . . . . . . | 30 | 1.0 | 6.0 | 0 | 0 | 35 | 2.0 |
| **Cavatappi entree**, frozen, | | | | | | | |
| Genovese (*Marie* | | | | | | | |
| *Callender's*), 11 oz. . . . | 410 | 24.0 | 44.0 | 15.0 | 50 | 980 | 5.0 |
| **Cavatelli pasta entree**, | | | | | | | |
| frozen, 1 cup: | | | | | | | |
| (*Celentano*) . . . . . . . . . . | 240 | 9.0 | 46.0 | 1.5 | 10 | 15 | 3.0 |
| (*Italian Village*) . . . . . . . | 200 | 8.0 | 39.0 | 1.0 | 15 | 10 | 3.0 |
| **Caviar** (see also | | | | | | | |
| "Roe"), 1 tbsp.: | | | | | | | |
| lumpfish: | | | | | | | |
| black (*Roland*) . . . . . . | 15 | 2.0 | 0 | .5 | 46 | 380 | 0 |
| black/red (*Romanoff*) . | 15 | 1.0 | 0 | 1.0 | 50 | 380 | 0 |
| red (*Roland*) . . . . . . . . | 15 | 2.0 | 0 | 1.0 | 44 | 410 | 0 |
| salmon (*Romanoff*) . . . . . | 35 | 3.0 | 0 | 1.5 | 55 | 310 | 0 |
| whitefish, black | | | | | | | |
| (*Romanoff*) . . . . . . . . . | 25 | 1.0 | 1.0 | 1.5 | 45 | 300 | 0 |
| **Cayenne**, see "Pepper" | | | | | | | |
| **Ceci bean**, see "Garbanzo | | | | | | | |
| bean" | | | | | | | |
| **Celeriac**, see "Celery | | | | | | | |
| root" | | | | | | | |
| **Celery**, fresh: | | | | | | | |
| raw: | | | | | | | |
| (*Dole* Hearts), 2 stalks, | | | | | | | |
| 3.9 oz. . . . . . . . . . | 15 | <1.0 | 3.0 | 0 | 0 | 90 | 2.0 |
| 7½" stalk, 1.6 oz. . . . . | 6 | .3 | 1.5 | .1 | 0 | 35 | .7 |
| diced, ½ cup . . . . . . . . | 10 | .5 | 2.2 | .1 | 0 | 52 | 1.0 |
| raw, w/dip (*Ready Pac* | | | | | | | |
| *Cool Cuts*), 2.25 oz.: | | | | | | | |
| peanut butter . . . . . . . | 160 | 5.0 | 9.0 | 13.0 | 0 | 170 | 2.0 |

| Food and Measure | cal. | prot. (gms) | carbo. (gms) | fat (gms) | chol. (mgs) | sod. (mgs) | fiber (gms) |
|---|---|---|---|---|---|---|---|
| **Celery, raw, w/dip** *(cont.)* | | | | | | | |
| ranch | 60 | 1.0 | 3.0 | 5.0 | 5 | 210 | 1.0 |
| boiled, drained, diced, | | | | | | | |
| ½ cup | 13 | .6 | 3.0 | .1 | 0 | 68 | 1.2 |
| **Celery, canned**, hearts | | | | | | | |
| (*Roland*), ½ cup | 15 | 1.0 | 2.0 | 0 | 0 | 360 | 1.0 |
| **Celery, dried**, flake/ | | | | | | | |
| seed (*Tone's*), 1 tsp. | 9 | .4 | .9 | .5 | 0 | 4 | .3 |
| **Celery root**, raw: | | | | | | | |
| (*Frieda's*), sliced, 1 cup | 65 | 2.0 | 14.0 | 0 | 0 | 156 | 3.0 |
| trimmed, 4 oz. | 44 | 1.7 | 10.4 | .3 | 0 | 113 | 2.0 |
| trimmed, ½ cup | 31 | 1.2 | 7.2 | .2 | 0 | 78 | 1.4 |
| **Celery root, canned**, | | | | | | | |
| strips (*Roland* Celery | | | | | | | |
| Knob), ½ cup | 45 | 1.0 | 10.0 | 0 | 0 | 550 | 3.0 |
| **Celery salt** | | | | | | | |
| (*McCormick*), ¼ tsp. | 0 | 0 | 0 | 0 | 0 | 290 | 0 |
| **Celtus**, raw, trimmed: | | | | | | | |
| 1 oz. | 6 | .2 | 1.0 | .1 | 0 | 3 | .3 |
| .3-oz. leaf | 1 | <.1 | .3 | 0 | 0 | 1 | .1 |
| **Cereal, ready-to-eat** | | | | | | | |
| (see also specific | | | | | | | |
| grains), 1 cup, | | | | | | | |
| except as noted: | | | | | | | |
| amaranth flakes: | | | | | | | |
| (*Arrowhead Mills* | | | | | | | |
| Organic) | 140 | 4.0 | 26.0 | 2.0 | 0 | 0 | 3.0 |
| (*Health Valley* | | | | | | | |
| Organic), 1¼ cup | 210 | 6.0 | 43.0 | 2.0 | 0 | 190 | 5.0 |
| bran: | | | | | | | |
| (*All-Bran*), ½ cup | 80 | 4.0 | 23.0 | 1.0 | 0 | 80 | 10.0 |
| (*All-Bran Bran Buds*), | | | | | | | |
| ⅓ cup | 70 | 2.0 | 24.0 | 1.0 | 0 | 200 | 13.0 |
| (*Fiber One*), ½ cup | 60 | 2.0 | 25.0 | 1.0 | 0 | 105 | 14.0 |
| flakes (*All-Bran* | | | | | | | |
| Complete), ¾ cup | 90 | 3.0 | 23.0 | .5 | 0 | 210 | 5.0 |
| flakes (*Post*), ¾ cup | 100 | 3.0 | 24.0 | .5 | 0 | 220 | 5.0 |
| strawberry medley | | | | | | | |
| (*All-Bran*) | 170 | 5.0 | 44.0 | 1.5 | 0 | 230 | 10.0 |
| bran, raisin: | | | | | | | |
| (*Cascadian Farm* | | | | | | | |
| Organic) | 180 | 5.0 | 43.0 | 1.0 | 0 | 340 | 6.0 |
| (*Erewhon* Organic) | 170 | 5.0 | 40.0 | 1.0 | 0 | 100 | 6.0 |
| (*Fiber One* Clusters) | 170 | 3.0 | 47.0 | 1.0 | 0 | 210 | 11.0 |

| Food and Measure | cal. | prot. (gms) | carbo. (gms) | fat (gms) | chol. (mgs) | sod. (mgs) | fiber (gms) |
|---|---|---|---|---|---|---|---|
| (*Kellogg's Raisin Bran*) .......... | 190 | 5.0 | 46.0 | 1.0 | 0 | 250 | 7.0 |
| (*Kellogg's Raisin Bran* Extra!) ...... | 170 | 4.0 | 38.0 | 2.5 | 0 | 310 | 6.0 |
| (*Kellogg's Raisin Bran Crunch*) ..... | 190 | 3.0 | 45.0 | 1.0 | 0 | 210 | 4.0 |
| (*Malt-O-Meal*) ....... | 220 | 5.0 | 49.0 | 1.5 | 0 | 340 | 6.0 |
| (*Post*) ............. | 190 | 4.0 | 46.0 | 1.0 | 0 | 250 | 8.0 |
| (*Skinner's*) ......... | 170 | 6.0 | 41.0 | 1.0 | 0 | 85 | 7.0 |
| (*Total*) ............. | 160 | 3.0 | 40.0 | 1.0 | 0 | 230 | 5.0 |
| nut (*General Mills*), ¾ cup ........... | 180 | 3.0 | 39.0 | 3.0 | 0 | 230 | 5.0 |
| buckwheat flakes, maple (*Arrowhead Mills* Organic) ....... | 170 | 4.0 | 35.0 | 1.0 | 0 | 190 | 1.0 |
| corn: | | | | | | | |
| (*Barbara's Puffins* Original), ¾ cup ... | 90 | 2.0 | 23.0 | 1.0 | 0 | 190 | 5.0 |
| (*Chex* Corn) ........ | 120 | 2.0 | 26.0 | .5 | 0 | 240 | 2.0 |
| (*Cocoa Puffs*), ¾ cup . | 100 | 1.0 | 23.0 | 1.5 | 0 | 150 | 2.0 |
| (*Cocoa Puffs* Combos), ¾ cup ........... | 110 | 1.0 | 23.0 | 1.5 | 0 | 160 | 1.0 |
| (*Colossal Crunch*), ¾ cup ........... | 120 | 1.0 | 26.0 | 1.5 | 0 | 230 | 0 |
| (*Corn Bursts*) ....... | 120 | 1.0 | 28.0 | 0 | 0 | 270 | 0 |
| (*Corn Pops*) ........ | 120 | 1.0 | 29.0 | 0 | 0 | 125 | 3.0 |
| (*Health Valley* Crunch-Ems!) .... | 110 | 2.0 | 27.0 | 0 | 0 | 160 | 2.0 |
| (*Kix*), 1¼ cups ...... | 110 | 2.0 | 25.0 | 1.0 | 0 | 190 | 3.0 |
| (*Trix*) .............. | 120 | 1.0 | 28.0 | 1.5 | 0 | 190 | 1.0 |
| apple cinnamon (*Glutino*), ½ cup ... | 120 | 1.0 | 26.0 | 1.0 | 0 | 120 | 1.0 |
| berry (*Colossal Crunch*), ¾ cup ... | 120 | 1.0 | 26.0 | 1.5 | 0 | 220 | <1.0 |
| berry berry (*Kix*), ¾ cup ........... | 100 | 1.0 | 22.0 | 1.0 | 0 | 180 | 1.0 |
| bran, crunchy (*Quaker*), ¾ cup ........... | 90 | 2.0 | 23.0 | 1.0 | 0 | 240 | 5.0 |
| cinnamon (*Barbara's Puffins*), ¾ cup ... | 90 | 2.0 | 26.0 | 1.0 | 0 | 150 | <6.0 |
| cocoa (*Barbara's Puffins*), ¾ cup ... | 120 | 2.0 | 24.0 | 1.0 | 0 | 80 | <3.0 |
| cocoa (*Mother's Bumpers*) ........ | 130 | 1.0 | 30.0 | .5 | 0 | 160 | 1.0 |

| Food and Measure | cal. | prot. (gms) | carbo. (gms) | fat (gms) | chol. (mgs) | sod. (mgs) | fiber (gms) |
|---|---|---|---|---|---|---|---|
| **Cereal, ready-to-eat, corn** *(cont.)* | | | | | | | |
| fruit medley (*Barbara's Puffins*), ¾ cup | 120 | 2.0 | 26.0 | 1.0 | 0 | 80 | <1.0 |
| graham (*Mother's Bumpers*), ¾ cup | 110 | 1.0 | 25.0 | .5 | 0 | 230 | 1.0 |
| honey (*Kix*), 1¼ cup | 120 | 2.0 | 28.0 | 1.0 | 0 | 190 | 3.0 |
| honey nut (*Chex*), ¾ cup | 120 | 2.0 | 28.0 | 1.0 | 0 | 200 | 1.0 |
| honey nut (*Glutino*), ½ cup | 120 | 1.0 | 26.0 | 1.5 | 0 | 120 | 1.0 |
| peanut butter (*Barbara's Puffins*), ¾ cup | 110 | 3.0 | 23.0 | 2.0 | 0 | 230 | 2.0 |
| peanut butter (*Mother's Bumpers*) | 130 | 3.0 | 26.0 | 2.5 | 0 | 260 | 1.0 |
| puffed (*Arrowhead Mills*) | 60 | 2.0 | 12.0 | 1.0 | 0 | 5 | 2.0 |
| puffed (*Nature's Path Organic*) | 60 | 2.0 | 12.0 | 0 | 0 | 0 | 1.0 |
| corn flakes: | | | | | | | |
| (*Arrowhead Mills Organic*) | 120 | 2.0 | 27.0 | 0 | 0 | 70 | 2.0 |
| (*Barbara's Organic*) | 110 | 2.0 | 25.0 | 1.0 | 0 | 80 | <1.0 |
| (*Erewhon Organic*) | 130 | 3.0 | 30.0 | 0 | 0 | 60 | 1.0 |
| (*Kellogg's Corn Flakes*) | 100 | 2.0 | 24.0 | 0 | 0 | 200 | 1.0 |
| (*Kellogg's Frosted Flakes*), ¾ cup | 110 | 1.0 | 27.0 | 0 | 0 | 140 | 1.0 |
| (*Kellogg's Frosted Flakes Less Sugar*) | 120 | 2.0 | 28.0 | 0 | 0 | 180 | <1.0 |
| cinnamon (*Kellogg's Corn Flakes*) | 120 | 2.0 | 27.0 | 0 | 0 | 210 | <1.0 |
| frosted (*Malt-O-Meal*), ¾ cup | 120 | 2.0 | 28.0 | 0 | 0 | 180 | 1.0 |
| frosted, chocolate (*Malt-O-Meal*), ¾ cup | 120 | 2.0 | 29.0 | 1.0 | 0 | 180 | 1.0 |
| corn and oat, ¾ cup: | | | | | | | |
| (*Cap'n Crunch*) | 110 | 1.0 | 23.0 | 1.5 | 0 | 200 | 1.0 |
| (*Health Valley Organic Cranberry Crunch*) | 190 | 4.0 | 38.0 | 4.0 | 0 | 100 | 3.0 |
| berries (*Cap'n Crunch*) | 110 | 1.0 | 22.0 | 1.5 | 0 | 190 | 1.0 |

| Food and Measure | cal. | prot. (gms) | carbo. (gms) | fat (gms) | chol. (mgs) | sod. (mgs) | fiber (gms) |
|---|---|---|---|---|---|---|---|
| cinna-graham (*Post Honeycomb*) ..... | 130 | 2.0 | 27.0 | 1.5 | 0 | 190 | 2.0 |
| corn and rice: | | | | | | | |
| (*Crispix*) ........... | 110 | 2.0 | 25.0 | 0 | 0 | 220 | <1.0 |
| flakes (*Glutino*) ...... | 120 | 2.0 | 27.0 | 0 | 0 | 130 | 1.0 |
| flakes, frosted (*Glutino*) ......... | 120 | 2.0 | 28.0 | 0 | 0 | 120 | 2.0 |
| strawberry crisp (*Erewhon* Organic), ¾ cup .......... | 120 | 2.0 | 28.0 | .5 | 0 | 125 | 1.0 |
| corn and wheat, ¾ cup: | | | | | | | |
| (*Malt-O-Meal Coco-Roos*) ...... | 120 | 1.0 | 26.0 | 1.5 | 0 | 135 | <1.0 |
| (*Malt-O-Meal Honey Graham Squares*) .. | 130 | 1.0 | 25.0 | 3.0 | 0 | 270 | 1.0 |
| granola, ½ cup, except as noted: | | | | | | | |
| (*Agave Plus* Organic), ¾ cup ........... | 250 | 6.0 | 37.0 | 9.0 | 0 | 95 | 4.0 |
| (*Bob's Red Mill* Organic) ......... | 180 | 5.0 | 35.0 | 2.5 | 0 | 10 | 4.0 |
| (*Breadshop* Crunchy Oat Bran) ....... | 210 | 5.0 | 33.0 | 8.0 | 0 | 0 | 4.0 |
| (*Breadshop* Honey Gone Nuts) ....... | 240 | 6.0 | 33.0 | 10.0 | 0 | 0 | 4.0 |
| (*Hemp Plus* Organic), ¾ cup ........... | 260 | 6.0 | 36.0 | 10.0 | 0 | 45 | 5.0 |
| (*Kashi* Mountain Medley) ......... | 220 | 6.0 | 38.0 | 7.0 | 0 | 120 | 7.0 |
| (*Kashi Cocoa Beach*) . | 230 | 6.0 | 36.0 | 9.0 | 0 | 140 | 7.0 |
| (*Nature's Path Love Crunch* Organic), ¾ cup ........... | 260 | 5.0 | 38.0 | 9.0 | 0 | 25 | 4.0 |
| (*Quaker* 100% Natural Low Fat), ⅔ cup ... | 210 | 4.0 | 45.0 | 3.0 | 0 | 135 | 3.0 |
| (*Special K* Low Fat) ... | 190 | 6.0 | 39.0 | 3.0 | 0 | 120 | 5.0 |
| almond (*Health Valley* Organic), ⅔ cup ... | 190 | 5.0 | 42.0 | 2.0 | 0 | 90 | 5.0 |
| almond raisins (*Breadshop* Crunchy Oat Bran) ........ | 210 | 5.0 | 33.0 | 8.0 | 0 | 0 | 4.0 |
| almond raisins (*Breadshop* SuperNatural) ..... | 220 | 5.0 | 34.0 | 8.0 | 0 | 5 | 3.0 |

| Food and Measure | cal. | prot. (gms) | carbo. (gms) | fat (gms) | chol. (mgs) | sod. (mgs) | fiber (gms) |
|---|---|---|---|---|---|---|---|
| **Cereal, ready-to-eat, granola** *(cont.)* | | | | | | | |
| ancient grains, almond *(Nature's Path Organic)*, ¾ cup ... | 250 | 5.0 | 39.0 | 9.0 | 0 | 135 | 6.0 |
| apple, all varieties *(Bob's Red Mill)* ... | 180 | 5.0 | 35.0 | 2.5 | 0 | 10 | 4.0 |
| berry, summer *(Kashi)* | 220 | 6.0 | 39.0 | 6.0 | 0 | 150 | 7.0 |
| berry crunch, triple *(Breadshop)* ...... | 210 | 5.0 | 34.0 | 8.0 | 0 | 65 | 4.0 |
| blueberry and cream *(Breadshop)* ...... | 210 | 6.0 | 36.0 | 6.0 | 0 | 0 | 4.0 |
| w/cherries *(Pomegran Plus* Organic), ¾ cup ......... | 250 | 5.0 | 38.0 | 9.0 | 0 | 60 | 4.0 |
| chocolate, dark, almond *(Cascadian Farm* Organic), ¾ cup ........... | 210 | 5.0 | 39.0 | 4.5 | 0 | 150 | 4.0 |
| cinnamon raisin *(Breadshop* Organic) | 220 | 4.0 | 39.0 | 7.0 | 0 | 65 | 4.0 |
| cinnamon raisin *(Cascadian Farm* Organic), ⅔ cup ... | 210 | 5.0 | 42.0 | 3.0 | 0 | 200 | 3.0 |
| coconut *(Bob's Red Mill)*, ¼ cup ...... | 130 | 4.0 | 18.0 | 5.0 | 0 | 0 | 3.0 |
| cranberry vanilla *(Post Trail Mix Crunch)* .. | 190 | 4.0 | 36.0 | 4.0 | 0 | 135 | 4.0 |
| flax and *(Barbara's Ultima)* .......... | 200 | 5.0 | 43.0 | 3.0 | 0 | 240 | <5.0 |
| fruit and nut *(Cascadian Farm* Organic), ¾ cup ... | 210 | 5.0 | 38.0 | 5.0 | 0 | 80 | 3.0 |
| honey almond *(Bob's Red Mill)* ........ | 230 | 7.0 | 38.0 | 7.0 | 0 | 0 | 4.0 |
| maple *(Breadshop* Organic Vermont) .. | 220 | 5.0 | 34.0 | 7.0 | 0 | 85 | 4.0 |
| maple brown sugar *(Cascadian Farm* Organic), ⅔ cup ... | 220 | 5.0 | 42.0 | 5.0 | 0 | 160 | 3.0 |
| mocha almond crunch *(Breadshop)* ...... | 210 | 5.0 | 33.0 | 8.0 | 0 | 40 | 4.0 |
| oats/honey *(Cascadian Farm* Organic), ⅔ cup ........... | 230 | 5.0 | 42.0 | 6.0 | 0 | 120 | 3.0 |

| Food and Measure | cal. | prot. (gms) | carbo. (gms) | fat (gms) | chol. (mgs) | sod. (mgs) | fiber (gms) |
|---|---|---|---|---|---|---|---|
| oats/honey (*Quaker*) .. | 210 | 5.0 | 35.0 | 6.0 | 0 | 25 | 3.0 |
| pralines and cream (*Breadshop*) ...... | 210 | 5.0 | 32.0 | 8.0 | 0 | 45 | 4.0 |
| pumpkin (*Flax Plus Organic*), ¾ cup ... | 260 | 6.0 | 37.0 | 10.0 | 0 | 45 | 5.0 |
| raisin almond (*Post Trail Mix Crunch*) .. | 180 | 4.0 | 37.0 | 2.5 | 0 | 210 | 5.0 |
| raisin cinnamon (*Health Valley Organic*), ⅔ cup ... | 190 | 5.0 | 42.0 | 2.0 | 0 | 90 | 5.0 |
| w/raisins (*Kellogg's Low Fat*), ⅔ cup ... | 230 | 5.0 | 48.0 | 3.0 | 0 | 140 | 4.0 |
| w/out raisins (*Kellogg's Low Fat*) ......... | 190 | 4.0 | 40.0 | 2.5 | 0 | 110 | 3.0 |
| raspberry and cream (*Breadshop*) ...... | 220 | 5.0 | 34.0 | 8.0 | 0 | 0 | 4.0 |
| spelt, apple cinnamon raisin (*VitaSpelt Organic*) ......... | 220 | 5.0 | 33.0 | 8.0 | 0 | 15 | 3.0 |
| spelt, cranberry vanilla walnut (*VitaSpelt Organic*) ......... | 220 | 5.0 | 33.0 | 9.0 | 0 | 0 | 3.0 |
| spelt, maple almond (*VitaSpelt* Organic) . | 220 | 5.0 | 34.0 | 8.0 | 0 | 0 | 3.0 |
| strawberry and cream (*Breadshop*) ...... | 220 | 5.0 | 34.0 | 8.0 | 0 | 0 | 4.0 |
| kamut, puffed, organic: | | | | | | | |
| (*Arrowhead Mills*) .... | 50 | 3.0 | 11.0 | 0 | 0 | 0 | 2.0 |
| (*Nature's Path*) ...... | 50 | 2.0 | 11.0 | 0 | 0 | 0 | 2.0 |
| kamut flakes: | | | | | | | |
| (*Arrowhead Mills Organic*) ......... | 120 | 4.0 | 25.0 | 1.0 | 0 | 70 | 2.0 |
| (*Shiloh Farms*), ½ cup | 140 | 6.0 | 28.0 | .5 | 0 | 0 | 4.0 |
| cranberries (*Arrowhead Mills* Organic) .... | 170 | 5.0 | 36.0 | 1.0 | 0 | 90 | 3.0 |
| millet, puffed: | | | | | | | |
| (*Arrowhead Mills*) .... | 60 | 2.0 | 11.0 | .5 | 0 | 0 | 1.0 |
| (*Nature's Path* Organic) | 50 | 2.0 | 14.0 | 0 | 0 | 0 | 1.0 |
| multigrain (see also "granola," above): | | | | | | | |
| (*Annie's Bunny O's Organic*), ¾ cup ... | 120 | 2.0 | 24.0 | 1.5 | 0 | 110 | 1.0 |
| (*Apple Jacks*) ....... | 100 | 1.0 | 25.0 | .5 | 0 | 130 | 3.0 |

| Food and Measure | cal. | prot. (gms) | carbo. (gms) | fat (gms) | chol. (mgs) | sod. (mgs) | fiber (gms) |
|---|---|---|---|---|---|---|---|
| **Cereal, ready-to-eat, multigrain** *(cont.)* | | | | | | | |
| (*Barbara's Puffins*), ¾ cup ........... | 110 | 2.0 | 25.0 | 0 | 0 | 80 | <3.0 |
| (*Barbara's Ultima* Original), ¾ cup ... | 180 | 5.0 | 42.0 | 1.5 | 0 | 140 | 10.0 |
| (*Basic 4*) ........... | 200 | 4.0 | 43.0 | 2.0 | 0 | 320 | 3.0 |
| (*Cascadian Farm* Organic Squares), ¾ cup ........... | 110 | 3.0 | 25.0 | 1.0 | 0 | 115 | 2.0 |
| (*Cascadian Farm Hearty Morning* Organic), ¾ cup ... | 200 | 5.0 | 43.0 | 3.0 | 0 | 360 | 8.0 |
| (*Cheerios*) .......... | 110 | 2.0 | 23.0 | 1.0 | 0 | 160 | 3.0 |
| (*Chex* Multi-Bran), ¾ cup ........... | 160 | 4.0 | 39.0 | 1.5 | 0 | 270 | 6.0 |
| (*Fiber One* Honey Clusters) ........ | 160 | 3.0 | 44.0 | 1.5 | 0 | 230 | 13.0 |
| (*Flax Plus* Organic Omega-3), ¾ cup .. | 110 | 4.0 | 23.0 | 1.5 | 0 | 135 | 5.0 |
| (*Froot Loops*) ....... | 110 | 1.0 | 25.0 | 1.0 | 0 | 135 | 3.0 |
| (*GoLean* Original) .... | 140 | 13.0 | 30.0 | 1.0 | 0 | 85 | 10.0 |
| (*GoLean Crunch!*) .... | 190 | 9.0 | 37.0 | 3.0 | 0 | 100 | 8.0 |
| (*Good Friends*) ...... | 160 | 5.0 | 42.0 | 1.5 | 0 | 110 | 12.0 |
| (*Grape-Nuts*), ½ cup . | 200 | 6.0 | 48.0 | 1.0 | 0 | 290 | 7.0 |
| (*Health Valley* Organic Fiber 7) ......... | 160 | 6.0 | 37.0 | 1.0 | 0 | 100 | 7.0 |
| (*Health Valley* Heart Wise) ........... | 200 | 11.0 | 37.0 | 3.0 | 0 | 140 | 5.0 |
| (*Health Valley* Organic Golden Flax) | 190 | 6.0 | 37.0 | 3.5 | 0 | 65 | 6.0 |
| (*Kashi Honey Sunshine*), ¾ cup .. | 100 | 2.0 | 25.0 | 1.0 | 0 | 135 | 5.0 |
| (*Kellogg's Müselix*), ⅔ cup ........... | 200 | 5.0 | 40.0 | 3.0 | 0 | 170 | 4.0 |
| (*Malt-O-Meal Apple Zings*) .......... | 120 | 1.0 | 30.0 | 1.0 | 0 | 150 | 1.0 |
| (*Malt-O-Meal Honey Buzzers*), 1⅓ cups . | 110 | 1.0 | 26.0 | .5 | 0 | 220 | 1.0 |
| (*Malt-O-Meal Honey & Oat Blenders*), ¾ cup ........... | 120 | 2.0 | 25.0 | 1.5 | 0 | 150 | 1.0 |
| (*Malt-O-Meal Tootie Fruities*) ........ | 130 | 2.0 | 28.0 | 1.0 | 0 | 150 | 1.0 |
| (*Product 19*) ........ | 100 | 2.0 | 25.0 | 0 | 0 | 210 | 1.0 |

| Food and Measure | cal. | prot. (gms) | carbo. (gms) | fat (gms) | chol. (mgs) | sod. (mgs) | fiber (gms) |
|---|---|---|---|---|---|---|---|
| (*Vive*), 1¼ cups ..... | 170 | 4.0 | 43.0 | 2.5 | 0 | 100 | 12.0 |
| (*Waffle Crisp*) ....... | 120 | 2.0 | 25.0 | 2.5 | 0 | 115 | <1.0 |
| acai apple (*Nature's Path* Organic), ¾ cup | 240 | 5.0 | 39.0 | 8.0 | 0 | 70 | 4.0 |
| all varieties (*Health Valley* Organic Square-Ems), 1¼ cups .......... | 210 | 5.0 | 44.0 | 3.0 | 0 | 125 | 8.0 |
| almond (*Honey Bunches of Oats*), ¾ cup ... | 130 | 2.0 | 25.0 | 2.5 | 0 | 140 | 2.0 |
| apple caramel pecan (*Post* Selects) .... | 210 | 4.0 | 41.0 | 3.5 | 0 | 220 | 5.0 |
| banana nut (*Post* Selects) ......... | 240 | 5.0 | 44.0 | 6.0 | 0 | 230 | 4.0 |
| berry crumble (*GoLean Crisp!*) ... | 180 | 9.0 | 35.0 | 3.5 | 0 | 125 | 8.0 |
| black currants, walnuts (*Kashi U*) ........ | 200 | 5.0 | 42.0 | 3.5 | 0 | 125 | 7.0 |
| blueberry (*Post* Selects Morning), 1¼ cups | 220 | 3.0 | 45.0 | 3.0 | 0 | 260 | 2.0 |
| chocolate (*Honey Bunches of Oats*), ¾ cup ........... | 120 | 2.0 | 25.0 | 1.5 | 0 | 140 | 2.0 |
| cinnamon (*Cinnabon*) . | 120 | 2.0 | 25.0 | 2.0 | 0 | 115 | 1.0 |
| cinnamon (*Honey Bunches of Oats*), ¾ cup ........... | 120 | 2.0 | 25.0 | 1.5 | 0 | 150 | 2.0 |
| cinnamon roll or fruity (*Annie's Bunny O's*), ¾ cup . | 120 | 2.0 | 25.0 | 1.0 | 0 | 85 | 1.0 |
| cinna-raisin crunch (*Good Friends*) .... | 170 | 4.0 | 41.0 | 1.5 | 0 | 105 | 8.0 |
| cocoa/vanilla (*Annie's Bunny O's*), ¾ cup . | 110 | 2.0 | 25.0 | 1.0 | 0 | 85 | 1.0 |
| cranberry (*Barbara's Ultima*) .......... | 190 | 5.0 | 42.0 | 1.5 | 0 | 140 | 10.0 |
| cranberry almond crunch (*Post* Selects), ¾ cup ........... | 200 | 4.0 | 40.0 | 3.0 | 0 | 115 | 3.0 |
| honey (*Annie's Bunny O's*), ¾ cup ...... | 110 | 2.0 | 25.0 | .5 | 0 | 90 | 1.0 |
| honey almond flax (*GoLean Crunch!*) . | 200 | 9.0 | 36.0 | 4.5 | 0 | 140 | 8.0 |
| honey nut (*Clusters*) .. | 210 | 4.0 | 49.0 | 1.0 | 0 | 290 | 3.0 |

| Food and Measure | cal. | prot. (gms) | carbo. (gms) | fat (gms) | chol. (mgs) | sod. (mgs) | fiber (gms) |
|---|---|---|---|---|---|---|---|
| **Cereal, ready-to-eat, multigrain** *(cont.)* | | | | | | | |
| honey-roasted (*Honey Bunches of Oats*), ¾ cup ..... | 120 | 2.0 | 25.0 | 1.5 | 0 | 150 | 2.0 |
| maple pecan crunch (*Flax Plus* Organic), ¾ cup .......... | 220 | 6.0 | 38.0 | 7.0 | 0 | 190 | 5.0 |
| maple pecan crunch (*Post* Selects), ¾ cup | 220 | 4.0 | 40.0 | 5.0 | 0 | 150 | 3.0 |
| maple or vanilla (*Nature's Path Sunrise* Organic), ⅔ cup ... | 110 | 2.0 | 25.0 | 1.0 | 0 | 130 | 3.0 |
| marshmallow (*Froot Loops*) .......... | 110 | 1.0 | 25.0 | 1.0 | 0 | 110 | 2.0 |
| nuggets (*Kashi*), ½ cup | 210 | 7.0 | 47.0 | 1.5 | 0 | 260 | 7.0 |
| oats and honey (*Special K*), ⅔ cup ........ | 100 | 2.0 | 25.0 | .5 | 0 | 140 | 3.0 |
| peach (*Honey Bunches of Oats*), ¾ cup ... | 120 | 2.0 | 26.0 | 1.5 | 0 | 130 | 2.0 |
| peanut butter (*Nature's Path* Organic), ¾ cup ... | 260 | 7.0 | 35.0 | 11.0 | 0 | 75 | 4.0 |
| pecans (*Honey Bunches of Oats*), ¾ cup ... | 110 | 2.0 | 24.0 | 1.5 | 0 | 140 | 2.0 |
| pecans, crunchy (*Post* Selects Great Grains), ¾ cup .... | 210 | 5.0 | 37.0 | 6.0 | 0 | 160 | 5.0 |
| puffed (*Kashi* Puffs) .. | 70 | 2.0 | 15.0 | .5 | 0 | 0 | 1.0 |
| puffed, honey (*Kashi* Puffs) .......... | 120 | 3.0 | 25.0 | 1.0 | 0 | 0 | 2.0 |
| pumpkin raisin crunch (*Flax Plus* Organic), ¾ cup .......... | 210 | 6.0 | 40.0 | 4.5 | 0 | 150 | 7.0 |
| raisins/dates/pecans (*Post* Selects Great Grains), ¾ cup .... | 200 | 4.0 | 40.0 | 4.0 | 0 | 160 | 5.0 |
| raspberry pomegranate (*Cascadian Farm Flax Right* Organic) | 210 | 5.0 | 45.0 | 1.5 | 0 | 190 | 4.0 |
| shredded (*Barbara's Spoonfuls*), ¾ cup . | 120 | 4.0 | 24.0 | 1.5 | 0 | 200 | 4.0 |
| strawberries (*Honey Bunches of Oats*), ¾ cup .......... | 120 | 2.0 | 26.0 | 1.5 | 0 | 135 | 2.0 |

| Food and Measure | cal. | prot. (gms) | carbo. (gms) | fat (gms) | chol. (mgs) | sod. (mgs) | fiber (gms) |
|---|---|---|---|---|---|---|---|
| vanilla (*Honey Bunches of Oats*) ......... | 220 | 4.0 | 45.0 | 3.0 | 0 | 180 | 4.0 |
| vanilla almond (*Newman's Own Sweet Enough*), ¾ cup ... | 110 | 2.0 | 24.0 | 1.0 | 0 | 125 | 2.0 |
| vanilla almond (*Flax Plus* Organic), ¾ cup | 250 | 6.0 | 36.0 | 9.0 | 0 | 80 | 5.0 |
| vanilla almond crunch (*Cascadian Farm* Organic), ¾ cup ... | 200 | 4.0 | 41.0 | 3.0 | 0 | 190 | 3.0 |
| multigrain flakes: | | | | | | | |
| (*Arrowhead Mills* Organic) ......... | 170 | 5.0 | 33.0 | 2.0 | 0 | 180 | 3.0 |
| (*Grape-Nuts*), ¾ cup . | 110 | 3.0 | 24.0 | 1.0 | 0 | 125 | 3.0 |
| (*Kashi*) ............ | 180 | 6.0 | 41.0 | 1.0 | 0 | 150 | 6.0 |
| (*Smart Start*) ....... | 190 | 3.0 | 43.0 | .5 | 0 | 280 | 3.0 |
| honey flax (*Newman's Own Sweet Enough*), ¾ cup ........... | 100 | 3.0 | 24.0 | 1.0 | 0 | 80 | 4.0 |
| strawberries (*Newman's Own Sweet Enough*), ¾ cup ... | 110 | 2.0 | 25.0 | 0 | 0 | 130 | 2.0 |
| oat/oats: | | | | | | | |
| (*Alpha-Bits*) ........ | 110 | 3.0 | 23.0 | 1.0 | 0 | 160 | 2.0 |
| (*Cascadian Farm Purely O's* Organic) ...... | 110 | 3.0 | 24.0 | 1.0 | 0 | 200 | 3.0 |
| (*Cheerios*) .......... | 100 | 3.0 | 20.0 | 2.0 | 0 | 160 | 3.0 |
| (*King Vitamin*), 1½ cups ......... | 120 | 2.0 | 26.0 | 1.0 | 0 | 260 | 1.0 |
| (*Life*), ¾ cup ........ | 120 | 3.0 | 25.0 | 1.5 | 0 | 160 | 2.0 |
| (*Lucky Charms*), ¾ cup ........... | 110 | 2.0 | 22.0 | 1.0 | 0 | 190 | 1.0 |
| (*Mother's* Crunch) ... | 230 | 6.0 | 48.0 | 3.0 | 0 | 250 | 5.0 |
| (*Oatios* Organic) ..... | 110 | 5.0 | 22.0 | 2.0 | 0 | 125 | 3.0 |
| almond, crunchy (*Oatmeal Crisp*) ... | 240 | 6.0 | 47.0 | 4.0 | 0 | 125 | 5.0 |
| apple cinnamon (*Cheerios*), ¾ cup . | 120 | 2.0 | 24.0 | 1.5 | 0 | 135 | 2.0 |
| banana nut (*Cheerios*), ¾ cup ........... | 100 | 1.0 | 23.0 | 1.0 | 0 | 160 | 1.0 |
| brown sugar (*Quaker Oatmeal Squares*) . | 210 | 6.0 | 44.0 | 2.5 | 0 | 250 | 5.0 |
| chocolate (*Cheerios*), ¾ cup ........... | 100 | 1.0 | 22.0 | 1.5 | 0 | 170 | 2.0 |

| Food and Measure | cal. | prot. (gms) | carbo. (gms) | fat (gms) | chol. (mgs) | sod. (mgs) | fiber (gms) |
|---|---|---|---|---|---|---|---|
| **Cereal, ready-to-eat, oat/oats** *(cont.)* | | | | | | | |
| cinnamon (*Heart to Heart*), ¾ cup ..... | 120 | 4.0 | 25.0 | 1.5 | 0 | 80 | 5.0 |
| cinnamon (*Life*), ¾ cup | 120 | 3.0 | 25.0 | 1.5 | 0 | 150 | 2.0 |
| cinnamon (*Quaker Oatmeal Squares*) . | 230 | 6.0 | 47.0 | 2.5 | 0 | 240 | 4.0 |
| cinnamon crunch (*FiberPlus*), ¾ cup . | 110 | 3.0 | 26.0 | 1.5 | 0 | 140 | 9.0 |
| flakes, blueberry cluster (*Heart to Heart*) ... | 200 | 6.0 | 44.0 | 2.0 | 0 | 135 | 4.0 |
| frosted (*Cheerios*), ¾ cup ........... | 110 | 2.0 | 23.0 | 1.0 | 0 | 170 | 2.0 |
| fruit juice (*Barbara's Hole 'n Oats*) ..... | 120 | 4.0 | 22.0 | 2.0 | 0 | 80 | 3.0 |
| fruit juice (Fruity *Cheerios*), ¾ cup .. | 100 | 1.0 | 23.0 | 1.5 | 0 | 135 | 2.0 |
| honey graham (*Quaker Oh!s*), ¾ cup ..... | 110 | 1.0 | 23.0 | 2.0 | 0 | 170 | 1.0 |
| honey nut (*Barbara's Hole 'n Oats*) ..... | 120 | 3.0 | 24.0 | 2.0 | 0 | 80 | <2.0 |
| honey nut (*Cascadian Farm* Organic O's) . | 110 | 2.0 | 25.0 | 1.0 | 0 | 180 | 3.0 |
| honey nut (*Cheerios*), ¾ cup ........... | 110 | 2.0 | 22.0 | 1.5 | 0 | 190 | 2.0 |
| honey nut (*Malt-O-Meal Scooters*) .... | 110 | 2.0 | 24.0 | 1.5 | 0 | 210 | 2.0 |
| honey toasted (*Heart to Heart*), ¾ cup ... | 120 | 4.0 | 25.0 | 1.5 | 0 | 85 | 5.0 |
| maple (*Quaker Oatmeal Squares*) . | 210 | 6.0 | 44.0 | 3.0 | 0 | 240 | 4.0 |
| maple brown sugar (*Life*), ¾ cup ..... | 120 | 3.0 | 25.0 | 1.5 | 0 | 150 | 2.0 |
| marshmallow (*Malt-O-Meal Mateys*) ..... | 120 | 2.0 | 25.0 | 1.0 | 0 | 200 | 1.0 |
| marshmallow, chocolate (*Malt-O-Meal Mateys*) ..... | 120 | 1.0 | 25.0 | 1.5 | 0 | 135 | 1.0 |
| raisin (*Oatmeal Crisp*) : | 240 | 5.0 | 51.0 | 2.5 | 0 | 120 | 5.0 |
| shredded (*Barbara's*): | | | | | | | |
| original, 1¼ cups .. | 220 | 6.0 | 46.0 | 2.5 | 0 | 260 | 5.0 |
| blueberry burst ... | 220 | 6.0 | 43.0 | 3.0 | 0 | 140 | 4.0 |
| cinnamon crunch .. | 230 | 6.0 | 43.0 | 3.0 | 0 | 220 | <4.0 |
| vanilla almond .... | 220 | 7.0 | 42.0 | 3.0 | 0 | 210 | <4.0 |

| Food and Measure | cal. | prot. (gms) | carbo. (gms) | fat (gms) | chol. (mgs) | sod. (mgs) | fiber (gms) |
|---|---|---|---|---|---|---|---|
| strawberry, yogurt (*Cheerios Yogurt Burst*), ¾ cup . . . . . | 120 | 2.0 | 24.0 | 1.5 | 0 | 180 | 2.0 |
| oat bran: | | | | | | | |
| (*Cracklin' Oat Bran*), ¾ cup . . . . . . . . . . | 200 | 4.0 | 35.0 | 7.0 | 0 | 150 | 6.0 |
| (*Quaker*), 1¼ cups . . . | 210 | 7.0 | 43.0 | 3.0 | 0 | 210 | 6.0 |
| almond crunch (*Health Valley* Organic), ½ cup . . . | 200 | 6.0 | 34.0 | 3.0 | 0 | 90 | 5.0 |
| crunch, toasted (*Mother's*), ¾ cup . | 120 | 4.0 | 24.0 | 1.5 | 0 | 200 | 3.0 |
| oat bran flakes: | | | | | | | |
| (*Arrowhead Mills* Organic) . . . . . . . . . | 140 | 5.0 | 24.0 | 2.5 | 0 | 80 | 4.0 |
| (*Health Valley* Organic) . . . . . . . . . | 190 | 5.0 | 39.0 | 1.5 | 0 | 190 | 4.0 |
| (*Smart Start* Toasted), 1¼ cups . . . . . . . . | 220 | 6.0 | 48.0 | 2.5 | 0 | 140 | 5.0 |
| maple brown sugar (*Smart Start*), 1¼ cups . . . . . . . . | 220 | 6.0 | 47.0 | 2.5 | 0 | 140 | 5.0 |
| raisins (*Health Valley* Organic) . . . . . . . . | 200 | 5.0 | 43.0 | 1.5 | 0 | 160 | 4.0 |
| oats and wheat, honey almond flax (*Total* Plus Omega-3) . . . . . . | 200 | 5.0 | 39.0 | 3.5 | 0 | 90 | 4.0 |
| rice: | | | | | | | |
| (*Chex* Rice) . . . . . . . . | 100 | 2.0 | 23.0 | 0 | 0 | 240 | 1.0 |
| (*Cocoa Krispies*), ¾ cup . . . . . . . . . | 120 | 1.0 | 27.0 | 1.0 | 0 | 130 | <1.0 |
| (*Cocoa/Fruity Pebbles*), ¾ cup . . . . . . . . . | 120 | 1.0 | 26.0 | 0 | 0 | 190 | 0 |
| (*Frosted Krispies*), ¾ cup . . . . . . . . . | 110 | 1.0 | 27.0 | 0 | 0 | 110 | 0 |
| (*Health Valley* Rice Crunch-Ems!) . . . . | 110 | 2.0 | 26.0 | 0 | 0 | 150 | 2.0 |
| (*Rice Krispies*), 1¼ cups . . . . . . . . | 130 | 2.0 | 29.0 | 0 | 0 | 190 | <1.0 |
| (*Rice Krispies Treats*), ¾ cup . . . . . . . . . | 120 | 1.0 | 26.0 | 1.5 | 0 | 170 | 0 |
| chocolate (*Chex*), ¾ cup . . . . . . . . . | 130 | 2.0 | 26.0 | 2.5 | 0 | 240 | <1.0 |

| Food and Measure | cal. | prot. (gms) | carbo. (gms) | fat (gms) | chol. (mgs) | sod. (mgs) | fiber (gms) |
|---|---|---|---|---|---|---|---|
| **Cereal, ready-to-eat, rice** *(cont.)* | | | | | | | |
| cinnamon (*Chex*), ¾ cup .......... | 120 | 1.0 | 25.0 | 2.0 | 0 | 180 | <1.0 |
| crispy (*Malt-O-Meal*), 1¼ cups ......... | 130 | 2.0 | 29.0 | 0 | 0 | 300 | 0 |
| flakes (*Arrowhead Mills* Organic Sweetened) ...... | 180 | 3.0 | 40.0 | 1.0 | 0 | 190 | 1.0 |
| honey (*Barbara's Puffins*), ¾ cup ... | 120 | 2.0 | 25.0 | 1.0 | 0 | 80 | 3.0 |
| puffed (*Arrowhead Mills*) ........... | 60 | 1.0 | 14.0 | 0 | 0 | 0 | <1.0 |
| puffed (*Quaker*) ..... | 40 | 1.0 | 9.0 | 0 | 0 | 0 | 0 |
| rice, brown, organic: | | | | | | | |
| (*Barbara's* Crisps) .... | 120 | 2.0 | 25.0 | 1.0 | 0 | 95 | <1.0 |
| (*Erewhon* Crispy): | | | | | | | |
| plain ............ | 110 | 2.0 | 25.0 | 0 | 0 | 180 | 1.0 |
| gluten free ....... | 110 | 2.0 | 25.0 | 0 | 0 | 160 | 0 |
| w/berries ........ | 120 | 2.0 | 27.0 | .5 | 0 | 100 | 1.0 |
| cocoa, gluten free . | 200 | 3.0 | 44.0 | 1.5 | 0 | 190 | 1.0 |
| crispy/puffs (*Erewhon Rice Twice* Gluten Free), ¾ cup ...... | 120 | 2.0 | 26.0 | 0 | 0 | 60 | 0 |
| puffed (*Nature's Path*) | 50 | 1.0 | 14.0 | 0 | 0 | 0 | 1.0 |
| rice and wheat flakes: | | | | | | | |
| (*Kashi Strawberry Fields* Organic) .... | 120 | 2.0 | 27.0 | 0 | 0 | 170 | 1.0 |
| (*Special K*) ......... | 120 | 6.0 | 23.0 | .5 | 0 | 220 | <1.0 |
| (*Special K* Protein Plus), ¾ cup ..... | 120 | 6.0 | 23.0 | .5 | 0 | 220 | <1.0 |
| blueberry (*Special K*), ¾ cup .......... | 110 | 2.0 | 26.0 | 0 | 0 | 140 | 3.0 |
| chocolate (*Special K*), ¾ cup .......... | 120 | 2.0 | 25.0 | 2.0 | 0 | 180 | 3.0 |
| cinnamon pecan (*Special K*), ¾ cup . | 120 | 2.0 | 24.0 | 2.0 | 0 | 180 | 3.0 |
| fruit and yogurt (*Special K*), ¾ cup . | 120 | 2.0 | 27.0 | 1.0 | 0 | 135 | 3.0 |
| red berry (*Special K*) . | 110 | 2.0 | 27.0 | 0 | 0 | 190 | 3.0 |
| strawberry blueberry (*Fruit Harvest*), ¾ cup .......... | 110 | 2.0 | 25.0 | 0 | 0 | 140 | 1.0 |
| vanilla almond (*Special K*), ¾ cup ........ | 110 | 2.0 | 25.0 | 1.5 | 0 | 160 | 3.0 |

| Food and Measure | cal. | prot. (gms) | carbo. (gms) | fat (gms) | chol. (mgs) | sod. (mgs) | fiber (gms) |
|---|---|---|---|---|---|---|---|
| spelt flakes: | | | | | | | |
| (*Arrowhead Mills* Organic) ......... | 120 | 4.0 | 24.0 | 1.0 | 0 | 100 | 3.0 |
| (*Eden* Organic), ½ cup | 180 | 6.0 | 35.0 | 1.5 | 0 | 0 | 4.0 |
| (*VitaSpelt*), ¼ cup ... | 93 | 3.5 | 20.0 | .5 | 0 | 1 | 3.0 |
| and cranberries (*Arrowhead Mills* Organic) ......... | 170 | 5.0 | 35.0 | 1.0 | 0 | 120 | 4.0 |
| wheat: | | | | | | | |
| (*Chex* Wheat), ¾ cup . | 160 | 5.0 | 39.0 | 1.0 | 0 | 300 | 5.0 |
| (*Golden Grahams*), ¾ cup ........... | 120 | 2.0 | 26.0 | 1.0 | 0 | 270 | 1.0 |
| (*Malt-O-Meal Blueberry Muffin Tops/ Cinnamon Toasters*), ¾ cup ........... | 130 | 1.0 | 24.0 | 3.5 | 0 | 140 | 1.0 |
| (*Malt-O-Meal Golden Puffs*), ¾ cup ..... | 110 | 2.0 | 24.0 | 0 | 0 | 65 | 0 |
| (*Total*), ¾ cup ....... | 100 | 2.0 | 23.0 | .5 | 0 | 190 | 3.0 |
| (*Wheaties*), ¾ cup ... | 100 | 3.0 | 22.0 | .5 | 0 | 190 | 3.0 |
| (*Wheaties Fuel*), ¾ cup | 210 | 3.0 | 46.0 | 3.0 | 0 | 150 | 5.0 |
| blueberry pomegranate (*Total*) ........... | 170 | 5.0 | 38.0 | 2.0 | 0 | 95 | 4.0 |
| cinnamon crunch (*Cascadian Farm* Organic) ......... | 110 | 2.0 | 22.0 | 2.5 | 0 | 105 | 3.0 |
| cinnamon fiber (*Newman's Own Sweet Enough*), ¾ cup ... | 90 | 2.0 | 25.0 | 5.0 | 0 | 0 | 8.0 |
| cranberry crunch (*Total*), 1¼ cups ... | 190 | 4.0 | 45.0 | 1.0 | 0 | 190 | 4.0 |
| whole, caramel (*Fiber One* Delight) ......: | 180 | 3.0 | 41.0 | 3.0 | 0 | 230 | 9.0 |
| whole, maple syrup (*Eggo*) .......... | 110 | 2.0 | 25.0 | 1.5 | 0 | 150 | 2.0 |
| wheat, puffed: | | | | | | | |
| (*Arrowhead Mills*) .... | 60 | 3.0 | 12.0 | 0 | 0 | 0 | 2.0 |
| (*Honey Smacks*), ¾ cup | 100 | 2.0 | 24.0 | .5 | 0 | 50 | 1.0 |
| (*Post* Golden Crisp), ¾ cup ........... | 110 | 2.0 | 24.0 | 0 | 0 | 25 | <1.0 |
| (*Quaker*) ........... | 50 | 2.0 | 11.0 | 0 | 0 | 0 | 1.0 |
| wheat, shredded: | | | | | | | |
| (*Arrowhead Mills* Organic) ......... | 190 | 6.0 | 38.0 | 1.0 | 0 | 5 | 6.0 |

| Food and Measure | cal. | prot. (gms) | carbo. (gms) | fat (gms) | chol. (mgs) | sod. (mgs) | fiber (gms) |
|---|---|---|---|---|---|---|---|
| **Cereal, ready-to-eat, wheat, shredded** *(cont.)* | | | | | | | |
| (*Arrowhead Mills* Organic Sweetened) | 200 | 5.0 | 42.0 | 1.0 | 0 | 5 | 5.0 |
| (*Barbara's*), 2 pcs. . . . | 140 | 4.0 | 31.0 | 1.0 | 0 | 0 | 5.0 |
| (*Kashi Autumn Wheat* Organic), 29 pcs. . . | 180 | 6.0 | 43.0 | 1.0 | 0 | 0 | 6.0 |
| (*Kashi Cinnamon Harvest* Organic), 28 pcs. . . . . . . . . . | 180 | 6.0 | 43.0 | 1.0 | 0 | 0 | 5.0 |
| (*Kashi Island Vanilla* Organic), 29 pcs. . . | 190 | 6.0 | 44.0 | 1.0 | 0 | 5 | 6.0 |
| (*Kellogg's Mini-Wheats*), 30 pcs. . . | 200 | 6.0 | 46.0 | 1.5 | 0 | 10 | 6.0 |
| (*Post* Original), 2 pcs. . | 160 | 5.0 | 37.0 | 1.0 | 0 | 0 | 6.0 |
| (*Post* Spoon Size) . . . . | 170 | 6.0 | 40.0 | 1.0 | 0 | 0 | 6.0 |
| (*Post* Wheat 'n Bran Spoon Size), 1¼ cups . . . . . . . . . | 200 | 6.0 | 49.0 | 1.0 | 0 | 0 | 8.0 |
| honey nut (*Post* Spoon Size) . . . . . . . . . . . . | 190 | 4.0 | 44.0 | 1.5 | 0 | 70 | 5.0 |
| strawberry cream (*Malt-O-Meal Mini Spooners*) . . . | 190 | 5.0 | 45.0 | 1.0 | 0 | 10 | 6.0 |
| vanilla almond (*Post* Spoon Size) . . . . . . | 190 | 4.0 | 43.0 | 1.5 | 0 | 45 | 5.0 |
| wheat, shredded, frosted: | | | | | | | |
| (*Fiber One*) . . . . . . . . . | 200 | 5.0 | 50.0 | 1.0 | 0 | 0 | 9.0 |
| (*Kellogg's Mini-Wheats* Big Bite), 5 pcs. . . . | 180 | 5.0 | 41.0 | 1.0 | 0 | 5 | 6.0 |
| (*Kellogg's Mini-Wheats* Bite Size), 24 pcs. . | 200 | 6.0 | 48.0 | 1.0 | 0 | 5 | 6.0 |
| (*Kellogg's Mini-Wheats* Little Bites), 51 pcs. | 190 | 5.0 | 46.0 | 1.0 | 0 | 0 | 6.0 |
| (*Malt-O-Meal Frosted Mini Spooners*) . . . | 190 | 5.0 | 45.0 | 1.0 | 0 | 10 | 6.0 |
| (*Post* Spoon Size) . . . . | 180 | 4.0 | 44.0 | 1.0 | 0 | 0 | 5.0 |
| blueberry muffin (*Kellogg's Mini-Wheats*), 24 pcs. . . | 180 | 4.0 | 43.0 | 1.0 | 0 | 0 | 5.0 |
| chocolate (*Kellogg's Mini-Wheats* Little Bites), 52 pcs. | 200 | 5.0 | 45.0 | 2.0 | 0 | 200 | 6.0 |
| chocolate (*Malt-O-Meal*), ¾ cup . . . . . | 120 | 1.0 | 29.0 | 1.0 | 0 | 180 | 1.0 |

| Food and Measure | cal. | prot. (gms) | carbo. (gms) | fat (gms) | chol. (mgs) | sod. (mgs) | fiber (gms) |
|---|---|---|---|---|---|---|---|
| cinnamon streusel (*Kellogg's Mini-Wheats*), 24 pcs. .. | 180 | 4.0 | 44.0 | 1.0 | 0 | 0 | 5.0 |
| maple brown sugar (*Kellogg's Mini-Wheats*), 24 pcs. .. | 190 | 4.0 | 44.0 | 1.0 | 0 | 0 | 5.0 |
| wheat and rice: | | | | | | | |
| (*Cinnamon Toast Crunch*), ¾ cup ... | 130 | 1.0 | 25.0 | 3.0 | 0 | 220 | 1.0 |
| berry yogurt crunch (*FiberPlus*) ....... | 170 | 3.0 | 45.0 | 1.0 | 0 | 200 | 10.0 |
| cinnamon crunch (*Total*) .......... | 190 | 4.0 | 40.0 | 2.5 | 0 | 200 | 4.0 |
| and soy, flakes (*Kellogg's Special K* Low Carb), ¾ cup ..... | 100 | 10.0 | 14.0 | 3.0 | 0 | 110 | 5.0 |
| **Cereal, cooking/hot** (see also specific grains), uncooked: | | | | | | | |
| barley: | | | | | | | |
| (*Erewhon Barley Plus Organic*), ¼ cup ... | 170 | 5.0 | 37.0 | 1.0 | 0 | 0 | 4.0 |
| (*Mother's* Quick), ⅓ cup ........... | 160 | 5.0 | 37.0 | .5 | 0 | 0 | 5.0 |
| flakes, rolled (*Bob's Red Mill*), ¼ cup .. | 80 | 3.0 | 18.0 | .5 | 0 | 5 | 3.0 |
| grits (*Bob's Red Mill*), ¼ cup .......... | 80 | 3.0 | 18.0 | .5 | 0 | 5 | 3.0 |
| buckwheat, ¼ cup: | | | | | | | |
| (*Hodgson Mill* Gluten Free) ............ | 150 | 2.0 | 33.0 | 1.0 | 0 | 0 | 1.0 |
| creamy (*Bob's Red Mill* Organic) ..... | 140 | 5.0 | 30.0 | 1.0 | 0 | 0 | 2.0 |
| bulgur, ¼ cup: | | | | | | | |
| (*Arrowhead Mills* Organic) ......... | 150 | 5.0 | 34.0 | .5 | 0 | 0 | 4.0 |
| w/soy (*Hodgson Mill*) . | 115 | 10.0 | 22.0 | 1.0 | 0 | 0 | 3.0 |
| grits, see "Corn grits" | | | | | | | |
| kamut (*Bob's Red Mill*), ¼ cup ............. | 120 | 5.0 | 26.0 | 1.0 | 0 | 0 | 4.0 |
| millet grits (*Bob's Red Mill*), ¼ cup ........ | 170 | 5.0 | 34.0 | 1.5 | 0 | 0 | 3.0 |

| Food and Measure | cal. | prot. (gms) | carbo. (gms) | fat (gms) | chol. (mgs) | sod. (mgs) | fiber (gms) |
|---|---|---|---|---|---|---|---|
| **Cereal, cooking/hot** *(cont.)* | | | | | | | |
| multigrain, ¼ cup, | | | | | | | |
| except as noted: | | | | | | | |
| (*Bob's Red Mill* | | | | | | | |
| Gluten Free Mighty | | | | | | | |
| Tasty) . . . . . . . . . . . | 150 | 8.0 | 27.0 | 5.0 | 0 | 0 | 10.0 |
| (*Bob's Red Mill* | | | | | | | |
| Organic High Fiber), | | | | | | | |
| ⅓ cup . . . . . . . . . . | 150 | 8.0 | 27.0 | 5.0 | 0 | 0 | 10.0 |
| (*Bob's Red Mill* Spice | | | | | | | |
| N' Nice) . . . . . . . . | 190 | 5.0 | 28.0 | 2.0 | 0 | 5 | 4.0 |
| (*Bob's Red Mill* | | | | | | | |
| Peppy Kernels) . . . . | 100 | 4.0 | 18.0 | 2.5 | 0 | 0 | 4.0 |
| (*Country Choice* | | | | | | | |
| Organic), ½ cup . . . | 130 | 5.0 | 29.0 | 1.0 | 0 | 0 | 5.0 |
| 4 (*Arrowhead Mills* | | | | | | | |
| Plus Flax) . . . . . . . . | 140 | 5.0 | 28.0 | 1.5 | 0 | 0 | 9.0 |
| 5 (*Bob's Red Mill* | | | | | | | |
| Rolled), ⅓ cup . . . . | 120 | 5.0 | 24.0 | 1.5 | 0 | 0 | 5.0 |
| 6 (*Bob's Red Mill* | | | | | | | |
| Organic Right Stuff) | 140 | 6.0 | 27.0 | 2.0 | 0 | 0 | 5.0 |
| 7 (*Arrowhead Mills* | | | | | | | |
| Organic), ⅓ cup . . . | 140 | 8.0 | 28.0 | 1.0 | 0 | 0 | 6.0 |
| 7 (*Bob's Red Mill*) . . . . | 140 | 6.0 | 28.0 | 1.5 | 0 | 0 | 6.0 |
| 8 (*Bob's Red Mill*) . . . . | 150 | 5.0 | 27.0 | 2.5 | 0 | 0 | 6.0 |
| 10 (*Bob's Red Mill*) . . . | 140 | 6.0 | 28.0 | 1.0 | 0 | 5 | 5.0 |
| apple cinnamon grains | | | | | | | |
| (*Bob's Red Mill*) . . . | 110 | 3.0 | 16.0 | 1.0 | 0 | 5 | 3.0 |
| w/flax, soy (*Hodgson* | | | | | | | |
| *Mill*), ⅓ cup . . . . . . | 160 | 7.0 | 25.0 | 3.0 | 0 | 0 | 6.0 |
| muesli (*Bob's Red Mill* | | | | | | | |
| Old Country) . . . . . | 110 | 4.0 | 21.0 | 3.0 | 0 | 02 | 4.0 |
| muesli, apples & more | | | | | | | |
| (*Hodgson Mill*) . . . . | 160 | 7.0 | 25.0 | 3.0 | 0 | 0 | 6.0 |
| nuts, grains and (*Bob's* | | | | | | | |
| *Red Mill*) . . . . . . . . | 110 | 4.0 | 19.0 | 2.0 | 0 | 2 | 2.0 |
| multigrain, instant, | | | | | | | |
| 1 pkt.: | | | | | | | |
| apple cinnamon (*Quaker* | | | | | | | |
| *Simple Harvest*) . . . | 150 | 4.0 | 33.0 | 1.5 | 0 | 90 | 4.0 |
| apple cranberry almond | | | | | | | |
| (*Quaker Hearty* | | | | | | | |
| *Medley*) . . . . . . . . . | 130 | 3.0 | 27.0 | 2.5 | 0 | 135 | 3.0 |

| Food and Measure | cal. | prot. (gms) | carbo. (gms) | fat (gms) | chol. (mgs) | sod. (mgs) | fiber (gms) |
|---|---|---|---|---|---|---|---|
| banana walnut (*Quaker Hearty Medley*) .... | 140 | 3.0 | 27.0 | 2.5 | 0 | 130 | 3.0 |
| cranberry honey (*Ocean Spray*) .......... | 160 | 4.0 | 32.0 | 2.0 | 0 | 170 | n.a. |
| honey cinnamon (*GoLean*) ........ | 150 | 8.0 | 26.0 | 2.0 | 0 | 100 | 5.0 |
| maple brown sugar pecan (*Quaker Simple Harvest*) ... | 160 | 4.0 | 30.0 | 3.5 | 0 | 75 | 4.0 |
| raisin spice (*Nature's Path* Organic) ..... | 180 | 4.0 | 39.0 | 1.0 | 0 | 100 | 4.0 |
| vanilla (*GoLean Truly Vanilla*) ..... | 150 | 9.0 | 25.0 | 2.0 | 0 | 100 | 7.0 |
| vanilla almond honey (*Quaker Simple Harvest*) ......... | 160 | 4.0 | 31.0 | 3.0 | 0 | 75 | 4.0 |
| oat/oats: | | | | | | | |
| (*Bob's Red Mill* Quick Gluten Free), ½ cup | 180 | 7.0 | 29.0 | 3.0 | 0 | 0 | 5.0 |
| (*Quaker* Quick/Old Fashioned), ½ cup . | 150 | 5.0 | 27.0 | 3.0 | 0 | 0 | 4.0 |
| flakes (*Arrowhead Mills* Organic), ⅓ cup .......... | 130 | 5.0 | 23.0 | 2.0 | 0 | 0 | 4.0 |
| groats (*Bob's Red Mill*), ¼ cup .......... | 110 | 7.0 | 27.0 | 2.5 | 0 | 0 | 4.0 |
| groats (*Bob's Red Mill* Organic), ¼ cup ... | 180 | 7.0 | 30.0 | 3.0 | 0 | 0 | 5.0 |
| oats, rolled: | | | | | | | |
| (*Bob's Red Mill* Gluten Free), ¼ cup | 190 | 7.0 | 32.0 | 3.5 | 0 | 0 | 5.0 |
| (*Bob's Red Mill* Instant), ⅓ cup ... | 120 | 5.0 | 21.0 | 2.0 | 0 | 0 | 3.0 |
| (*Bob's Red Mill* Old Fashioned/Extra Thick Regular/ Organic), ½ cup ... | 190 | 7.0 | 32.0 | 3.5 | 0 | 0 | 5.0 |
| (*Bob's Red Mill* Quick Regular/ Organic), ½ cup ... | 180 | 7.0 | 29.0 | 3.0 | 0 | 0 | 5.0 |
| (*Country Choice* Organic Old Fashioned/ Quick), ½ cup .... | 150 | 5.0 | 27.0 | 3.0 | 0 | 0 | 4.0 |
| (*Mother's*), ½ cup .... | 150 | 5.0 | 27.0 | 3.0 | 0 | 0 | 4.0 |

| Food and Measure | cal. | prot. (gms) | carbo. (gms) | fat (gms) | chol. (mgs) | sod. (mgs) | fiber (gms) |
|---|---|---|---|---|---|---|---|
| **Cereal, cooking/hot** *(cont.)* | | | | | | | |
| oats, steel cut, ¼ cup: | | | | | | | |
| (*Arrowhead Mills* Organic) . . . . . . . . | 160 | 6.0 | 27.0 | 3.0 | 0 | 0 | 8.0 |
| (*Bob's Red Mill* Regular/Gluten Free/Organic) . . . . . | 170 | 7.0 | 29.0 | 3.0 | 0 | 0 | 5.0 |
| (*Country Choice* Organic) . . . . . . . . . | 150 | 5.0 | 27.0 | 3.0 | 0 | 0 | 4.0 |
| (*Hodgson Mill*) . . . . . . | 150 | 5.0 | 27.0 | 2.5 | 0 | 0 | 4.0 |
| (*Quaker*) . . . . . . . . . . . | 150 | 5.0 | 27.0 | 2.5 | 0 | 0 | 4.0 |
| oat bran: | | | | | | | |
| (*Arrowhead Mills* Organic), ⅓ cup . . . | 130 | 6.0 | 21.0 | 2.5 | 0 | 0 | 4.0 |
| (*Bob's Red Mill*), ⅓ cup . . . . . . . . . . . | 120 | 5.0 | 21.0 | 2.0 | 0 | 0 | 6.0 |
| (*Bob's Red Mill* Organic), ⅓ cup . . . | 150 | 7.0 | 26.0 | 2.5 | 0 | 0 | 6.0 |
| (*Hodgson Mill*), ¼ cup | 120 | 6.0 | 23.0 | 3.0 | 0 | 3 | 6.0 |
| (*Mother's*), ½ cup . . . . | 150 | 7.0 | 25.0 | 3.0 | 0 | 0 | 6.0 |
| oatmeal: | | | | | | | |
| (*Arrowhead Mills* Organic Old Fashioned), ⅓ cup . | 130 | 5.0 | 23.0 | 2.0 | 0 | 0 | 4.0 |
| (*Bob's Red Mill* Scottish Regular/ Organic), ¼ cup . . . | 140 | 6.0 | 23.0 | 2.5 | 0 | 0 | 4.0 |
| (*Mother's*), ½ cup . . . . | 150 | 5.0 | 27.0 | 3.0 | 0 | 0 | 2.0 |
| oatmeal, instant, 1 pkt.: | | | | | | | |
| (*Arrowhead Mills* Organic Original) . . | 110 | 4.0 | 19.0 | 2.0 | 0 | 0 | 2.0 |
| (*Country Choice* Organic Original) . . | 110 | 4.0 | 19.0 | 2.0 | 0 | 0 | 3.0 |
| (*Nature's Path* Original Organic) . . . . . . . . . | 210 | 7.0 | 37.0 | 3.5 | 0 | 160 | 6.0 |
| (*Nature's Path* Hemp *Plus* Organic) . . . . . | 180 | 5.0 | 30.0 | 2.5 | 0 | 105 | 4.0 |
| (*Quaker* Organic) . . . . | 100 | 4.0 | 19.0 | 2.0 | 0 | 0 | 3.0 |
| (*Quaker* Original) . . . . | 100 | 4.0 | 19.0 | 2.0 | 0 | 75 | 3.0 |
| w/added oat bran (*Erewhon* Organic) . | 130 | 6.0 | 25.0 | 2.5 | 0 | 0 | 4.0 |
| apple, baked (*Quaker* Oatmeal Express*) . | 200 | 5.0 | 41.0 | 2.5 | 0 | 250 | 4.0 |

| Food and Measure | cal. | prot. (gms) | carbo. (gms) | fat (gms) | chol. (mgs) | sod. (mgs) | fiber (gms) |
|---|---|---|---|---|---|---|---|
| apple cinnamon (*Country Choice Organic*) ... | 140 | 4.0 | 22.0 | 1.5 | 0 | 60 | 3.0 |
| apple cinnamon (*Erewhon* Organic) . | 130 | 5.0 | 24.0 | 2.0 | 0 | 100 | 3.0 |
| apple cinnamon (*Heart to Heart*) ... | 160 | 4.0 | 33.0 | 2.0 | 0 | 110 | 5.0 |
| apple cinnamon (*Nature's Path* Organic) ......... | 210 | 5.0 | 40.0 | 2.5 | 0 | 100 | 4.0 |
| apple cinnamon (*Quaker*) ......... | 130 | 3.0 | 27.0 | 1.5 | 0 | 160 | 3.0 |
| blueberry muffin (*Quaker True Delights*) ..... | 150 | 5.0 | 29.0 | 2.0 | 0 | 200 | 4.0 |
| brown sugar, golden (*Quaker Oatmeal Express*) ......... | 200 | 5.0 | 42.0 | 2.5 | 0 | 290 | 3.0 |
| cinnamon (*Quaker Weight Control*) ... | 160 | 7.0 | 29.0 | 3.0 | 0 | 270 | 6.0 |
| cinnamon blueberry flax (*Nature's Path Optimum Organic*) . | 150 | 5.0 | 29.0 | 2.5 | 0 | 115 | 3.0 |
| cinnamon raisin flax (*Erewhon* Organic) . | 130 | 4.0 | 24.0 | 2.5 | 0 | 100 | 4.0 |
| cinnamon roll (*Quaker*) | 160 | 4.0 | 32.0 | 2.5 | 0 | 220 | 3.0 |
| cinnamon spice (*Quaker*) ......... | 160 | 4.0 | 32.0 | 2.5 | 0 | 210 | 3.0 |
| cinnamon swirl (*Quaker* High Fiber) | 160 | 4.0 | 34.0 | 2.0 | 0 | 210 | 10.0 |
| cranberry or cranberry pomegranate (*Ocean Spray*) .......... | 160 | 4.0 | 33.0 | 2.0 | 0 | 170 | n.a. |
| cranberry ginger (*Nature's Path Optimum Organic*) . | 150 | 5.0 | 30.0 | 2.0 | 0 | 160 | 3.0 |
| cranberry orange muffin (*Ocean Spray*) | 160 | 4.0 | 33.0 | 2.0 | 0 | 240 | n.a. |
| w/flax (*Arrowhead Mills* Organic) .... | 140 | 5.0 | 24.0 | 3.0 | 0 | 70 | 4.0 |
| w/flax (*Nature's Path* Flax Plus Organic) . | 210 | 6.0 | 38.0 | 3.0 | 0 | 140 | 5.0 |
| maple (*Country Choice* Organic) ......... | 170 | 4.0 | 32.0 | 2.0 | 0 | 60 | 3.0 |
| maple, golden brown (*Heart to Heart*) ... | 160 | 4.0 | 33.0 | 2.0 | 0 | 100 | 5.0 |

| Food and Measure | cal. | prot. (gms) | carbo. (gms) | fat (gms) | chol. (mgs) | sod. (mgs) | fiber (gms) |
|---|---|---|---|---|---|---|---|
| **Cereal, cooking/hot, oatmeal, instant** *(cont.)* | | | | | | | |
| maple apple spice (*Arrowhead Mills* Organic) ......... | 140 | 4.0 | 26.0 | 2.0 | 0 | 45 | 3.0 |
| maple brown sugar (*Quaker*) ......... | 160 | 4.0 | 32.0 | 2.5 | 0 | 260 | 3.0 |
| maple brown sugar (*Quaker* Fiber) .... | 160 | 4.0 | 34.0 | 2.0 | 0 | 260 | 10.0 |
| maple brown sugar (*Quaker* Lower Sugar) .......... | 120 | 4.0 | 24.0 | 2.0 | 0 | 290 | 3.0 |
| maple brown sugar (*Quaker* Organic) .. | 150 | 4.0 | 31.0 | 2.0 | 0 | 95 | 3.0 |
| maple brown sugar (*Quaker* Weight Control) ......... | 160 | 7.0 | 29.0 | 3.0 | 0 | 290 | 6.0 |
| maple nut (*Nature's Path* Organic) ..... | 210 | 5.0 | 38.0 | 4.0 | 0 | 100 | 4.0 |
| maple spice (*Erewhon* Organic) ......... | 130 | 5.0 | 25.0 | 2.0 | 0 | 100 | 3.0 |
| peaches and cream (*Quaker*) ......... | 130 | 3.0 | 27.0 | 2.0 | 0 | 180 | 2.0 |
| raisin, date, walnuts (*Quaker*) ......... | 140 | 3.0 | 27.0 | 2.5 | 0 | 190 | 3.0 |
| raisin spice (*Quaker*) . | 150 | 4.0 | 32.0 | 2.0 | 0 | 210 | 3.0 |
| strawberries and cream (*Quaker*) ... | 130 | 4.0 | 27.0 | 2.0 | 0 | 180 | 2.0 |
| rice, brown, organic, ¼ cup: | | | | | | | |
| (*Arrowhead Mills* Rice & Shine) ..... | 150 | 3.0 | 32.0 | 1.0 | 0 | 0 | 2.0 |
| (*Lundberg* Purely) ... | 160 | 3.0 | 36.0 | .5 | 0 | 0 | 2.0 |
| cream (*Erewhon*) .... | 170 | 5.0 | 36.0 | 1.0 | 0 | 30 | 1.0 |
| creamy (*Bob's Red Mill* Farina) ....... | 150 | 3.0 | 32.0 | 1.0 | 0 | 5 | 2.0 |
| rye: | | | | | | | |
| cracked (*Bob's Red Mill* Organic), ¼ cup ... | 110 | 4.0 | 21.0 | 1.0 | 0 | 0 | 7.0 |
| creamy flakes (*Bob's Red Mill*), ¼ cup .. | 100 | 4.0 | 21.0 | 0 | 0 | 0 | 4.0 |
| soy grits (*Bob's Red Mill* Defatted), ¼ cup . | 130 | 19.0 | 14.0 | 1.0 | 0 | 0 | 7.0 |
| spelt, rolled (*Bob's Red Mill*), ½ cup ........ | 130 | 5.0 | 28.0 | 1.5 | 0 | 0 | 3.0 |

| Food and Measure | cal. | prot. (gms) | carbo. (gms) | fat (gms) | chol. (mgs) | sod. (mgs) | fiber (gms) |
|---|---|---|---|---|---|---|---|
| triticale, rolled (*Bob's Red Mill*), ¼ cup ..... | 100 | 4.0 | 22.0 | .5 | 0 | 0 | 4.0 |
| wheat, ¼ cup, except as noted: | | | | | | | |
| (*Arrowhead Mills* Bear Mush) ...... | 150 | 5.0 | 32.0 | 1.0 | 0 | 0 | 2.0 |
| (*Bob's Red Mill* Rolled) .......... | 70 | 3.0 | 14.0 | 0 | 0 | 0 | 2.5 |
| (*Malt-O-Meal*), 3 tbsp. | 130 | 5.0 | 27.0 | .5 | 0 | 0 | 1.0 |
| chocolate or creamy hot (*Malt-O-Meal*), 3 tbsp. ..... | 130 | 4.0 | 27.0 | 0 | 0 | 0 | 1.0 |
| cracked (*Bob's Red Mill* Organic) ..... | 140 | 5.0 | 29.0 | .5 | 0 | 0 | 5.0 |
| cracked (*Hodgson Mill*) ............. | 110 | 5.0 | 25.0 | 1.0 | 0 | 0 | 5.0 |
| creamy (*Bob's Red Mill* Regular/ Organic) ......... | 160 | 5.0 | 33.0 | .5 | 0 | 0 | 1.0 |
| maple brown sugar (*Malt-O-Meal*) .... | 170 | 4.0 | 37.0 | 0 | 0 | 0 | 1.0 |
| whole wheat (*Bob's Red Mill* Farina Regular/Organic) .. | 160 | 5.0 | 33.0 | 1.0 | 0 | 1 | 4.0 |
| wheat, whole (*Mother's*), ½ cup . | 130 | 5.0 | 30.0 | 1.0 | 0 | 0 | 4.0 |
| wheat, instant, 1 pkt.: | | | | | | | |
| (*Cream of Wheat*) .... | 100 | 3.0 | 19.0 | 0 | 0 | 160 | 1.0 |
| (*Cream of Wheat Healthy Grain*) .... | 150 | 7.0 | 30.0 | 1.0 | 0 | 170 | 6.0 |
| cinnamon (*Cream of Wheat Cinnabon*) .. | 130 | 3.0 | 29.0 | 0 | 0 | 170 | 1.0 |
| cinnamon swirl (*Cream of Wheat*) ........ | 130 | 2.0 | 29.0 | 0 | 0 | 170 | 1.0 |
| maple brown sugar (*Cream of Wheat*) .. | 130 | 2.0 | 28.0 | 0 | 0 | 140 | 1.0 |
| maple brown sugar (*Cream of Wheat Healthy Grain*) .... | 130 | 2.0 | 28.0 | 0 | 0 | 140 | 1.0 |
| **Cereal, frozen/chilled:** | | | | | | | |
| (*Amy's* Organic), 9 oz.: | | | | | | | |
| cream of rice ....... | 170 | 2.0 | 39.0 | 1.0 | 0 | 220 | 2.0 |
| multigrain .......... | 190 | 4.0 | 40.0 | 1.5 | 0 | 300 | 5.0 |
| rolled oats .......... | 220 | 6.0 | 42.0 | 3.5 | 0 | 220 | 5.0 |

| Food and Measure | cal. | prot. (gms) | carbo. (gms) | fat (gms) | chol. (mgs) | sod. (mgs) | fiber (gms) |
|---|---|---|---|---|---|---|---|
| **Cereal, frozen/chilled** *(cont.)* | | | | | | | |
| steel cut oats ....... | 220 | 6.0 | 42.0 | 3.5 | 0 | 190 | 5.0 |
| multigrain (*Kozy Shack Ready Grains*), 7 oz.: | | | | | | | |
| apple cinnamon ..... | 210 | 8.0 | 38.0 | 2.0 | 20 | 190 | 7.0 |
| maple brown sugar ... | 190 | 7.0 | 32.0 | 2.0 | 20 | 170 | 7.0 |
| original ............ | 180 | 8.0 | 29.0 | 2.5 | 20 | 190 | 7.0 |
| strawberry ......... | 210 | 8.0 | 37.0 | 2.0 | 20 | 180 | 7.0 |
| **Cereal bar**, see "Granola/cereal bar" | | | | | | | |
| **Cervelat**, see "Summer sausage" | | | | | | | |
| **Channa masala**, see "Garbanzo dish" | | | | | | | |
| **Chapati**, see "Bread" | | | | | | | |
| **Chayote**: | | | | | | | |
| raw: | | | | | | | |
| 1 medium, 7.2 oz. .... | 49 | 1.8 | 11.0 | .6 | 0 | 8 | 6.1 |
| 1" pcs., ½ cup ....... | 16 | .6 | 3.6 | .2 | 0 | 3 | 2.0 |
| boiled, drained: | | | | | | | |
| (*Dole*), ½ cup ....... | 17 | 1.0 | 4.0 | 0 | 0 | 3 | 2.0 |
| 1" pcs., ½ cup ....... | 19 | .5 | 4.1 | .4 | 0 | 1 | 2.3 |
| **Cheddarwurst**, see "Sausage" | | | | | | | |
| **Cheese** (see also "Cheese food" and "Cheese spread"), 1 oz., except as noted: | | | | | | | |
| American: | | | | | | | |
| (*Alpine Lace*) ....... | 90 | 6.0 | 1.0 | 6.0 | 20 | 380 | 0 |
| (*Applegate Farms*) ... | 80 | 5.0 | 1.0 | 7.0 | 25 | 270 | 0 |
| (*Black Bear*) ........ | 100 | 6.0 | 1.0 | 9.0 | 30 | 410 | 0 |
| (*Boar's Head*) ....... | 100 | 6.0 | 1.0 | 9.0 | 25 | 380 | 0 |
| (*Boar's Head* Lower Sodium/Fat) ...... | 90 | 6.0 | 1.0 | 6.0 | 20 | 300 | 0 |
| (*Cabot*), ¾-oz. slice .. | 80 | 4.0 | 1.0 | 7.0 | 20 | 270 | 0 |
| (*Kraft* Singles), ⅔ oz. . | 60 | 3.0 | 1.0 | 4.5 | 15 | 250 | 0 |
| (*Kraft* Singles), ¾ oz. . | 70 | 4.0 | 2.0 | 5.0 | 20 | 270 | 0 |
| (*Kraft* Singles 2%), ⅔ oz. ............ | 45 | 4.0 | 2.0 | 2.5 | 10 | 280 | 0 |
| (*Kraft Deli Deluxe*) ... | 100 | 5.0 | 1.0 | 9.0 | 30 | 460 | 0 |
| (*Kraft Deli Deluxe*), ⅔ oz. ............ | 70 | 4.0 | 0 | 6.0 | 20 | 310 | 0 |

| Food and Measure | cal. | prot. (gms) | carbo. (gms) | fat (gms) | chol. (mgs) | sod. (mgs) | fiber (gms) |
|---|---|---|---|---|---|---|---|
| (*Kraft Deli Deluxe* 2%), ⅔ oz. | 60 | 4.0 | 0 | 4.0 | 15 | 340 | 0 |
| (*Land O Lakes*) | 110 | 5.0 | 2.0 | 9.0 | 25 | 400 | 0 |
| (*Land O Lakes* 2%) | 90 | 6.0 | 1.0 | 6.0 | 20 | 370 | 0 |
| (*Land O Lakes* Light) | 70 | 7.0 | 1.0 | 4.5 | 15 | 390 | 0 |
| (*Land O Lakes* Less Sodium) | 110 | 6.0 | 1.0 | 9.0 | 30 | 260 | 0 |
| (*Land O Lakes* Singles) | 110 | 6.0 | 1.0 | 9.0 | 30 | 390 | 0 |
| (*Thumann's*) | 100 | 6.0 | 1.0 | 9.0 | 25 | 430 | 0 |
| sharp (*Land O Lakes*) | 110 | 6.0 | 1.0 | 9.0 | 25 | 380 | 0 |
| sharp, extra (*Land O Lakes*) | 110 | 6.0 | 1.0 | 9.0 | 25 | 350 | 0 |
| white (*Kraft* Singles), ⅔ oz. | 60 | 4.0 | 2.0 | 4.0 | 15 | 240 | 0 |
| white (*Kraft* Singles 2%), ⅔ oz. | 45 | 4.0 | 2.0 | 2.5 | 10 | 260 | 0 |
| white (*Kraft Deli Deluxe*), ¾ oz. | 80 | 4.0 | 0 | 7.0 | 20 | 340 | 0 |
| asiago (*Boar's Head*) | 100 | 6.0 | 1.0 | 9.0 | 25 | 220 | 0 |
| blue (*Boar's Head*) | 90 | 6.0 | 0 | 8.0 | 30 | 280 | 0 |
| blue, crumbled: (*Athenos/Kraft Crumbles*), 3 tbsp. | 110 | 7.0 | 2.0 | 9.0 | 30 | 430 | 1.0 |
| (*Organic Valley*) | 100 | 6.0 | 1.0 | 8.0 | 25 | 380 | 0 |
| (*Sargento*), ¼ cup | 100 | 6.0 | 1.0 | 8.0 | 25 | 380 | 0 |
| brick (*Land O Lakes*) | 110 | 7.0 | 1.0 | 8.0 | 25 | 170 | 0 |
| Brie | 95 | 5.9 | .1 | 7.9 | 20 | 229 | 0 |
| Brie, goat (*Woolwich Dairy*) | 90 | 6.0 | 1.0 | 7.0 | 30 | 180 | 0 |
| butterKäse (*Boar's Head*) | 100 | 6.0 | 0 | 9.0 | 30 | 180 | 0 |
| Camembert | 85 | 5.6 | .1 | 6.9 | 20 | 239 | 0 |
| caraway | 107 | 7.1 | .9 | 8.3 | 2.6 | 196 | 0 |
| *Chedarella* (*Land O Lakes*) | 110 | 7.0 | 0 | 9.0 | 25 | 190 | 0 |
| cheddar: (*Alpine Lace*) | 90 | 7.0 | 0 | 7.0 | 20 | 170 | 0 |
| (*Applegate Farms*) | 110 | 7.0 | 0 | 9.0 | 30 | 180 | 0 |
| (*Boar's Head* Vermont) | 110 | 7.0 | 0 | 10.0 | 30 | 180 | 0 |
| (*Cabot* 50% Less Fat) | 70 | 8.0 | <1.0 | 4.5 | 15 | 170 | 0 |
| (*Cracker Barrel* Stick) | 120 | 6.0 | 0 | 10.0 | 30 | 180 | 0 |
| (*Cracker Barrel* Stick Reduced Fat) | 90 | 7.0 | 1.0 | 6.0 | 20 | 240 | 0 |
| (*Kraft* Organic) | 120 | 7.0 | 0 | 10.0 | 30 | 190 | 0 |

| Food and Measure | cal. | prot. (gms) | carbo. (gms) | fat (gms) | chol. (mgs) | sod. (mgs) | fiber (gms) |
|---|---|---|---|---|---|---|---|
| **Cheese, cheddar** *(cont.)* | | | | | | | |
| (*Kraft* Stick 2%) ..... | 90 | 7.0 | 1.0 | 3.5 | 20 | 240 | 0 |
| (*Land O Lakes*) ...... | 110 | 7.0 | 0 | 9.0 | 30 | 190 | 0 |
| (*Sargento*), ¾ oz. .... | 90 | 5.0 | 0 | 7.0 | 20 | 140 | 0 |
| all styles, except Longhorn (*Kraft* Natural Block) .... | 120 | 6.0 | 0 | 10.0 | 30 | 180 | 0 |
| all styles, except reduced fat (*Cabot*) | 110 | 7.0 | <1.0 | 9.0 | 30 | 180 | 0 |
| medium (*Applegate Farms*), ⅔ oz. ..... | 70 | 5.0 | 0 | 6.0 | 20 | 120 | 0 |
| medium (*Sargento* Reduced Fat), ⅔ oz. | 60 | 6.0 | 0 | 4.0 | 15 | 135 | 0 |
| mild (*Applegate Farms* Organic), ¾ oz. ... | 85 | 5.0 | 0 | 6.0 | 20 | 130 | 0 |
| mild (*Kraft* Longhorn) . | 110 | 7.0 | 0 | 9.0 | 30 | 180 | 0 |
| mild (*Kraft* Longhorn 2%) ............ | 90 | 7.0 | 1.0 | 6.0 | 20 | 240 | 0 |
| mild (*Kraft Deli Fresh*), .8 oz. ..... | 90 | 5.0 | 0 | 8.0 | 25 | 160 | 0 |
| mild (*Sargento* Bar), ¾-oz. pc. ........ | 90 | 5.0 | 1.0 | 7.0 | 20 | 140 | 0 |
| mild (*Sargento* Cube), 7 pcs., 1.1 oz. .... | 120 | 7.0 | 1.0 | 10.0 | 30 | 190 | 0 |
| mild or extra sharp (*Kraft* Stick) ...... | 120 | 6.0 | 0 | 10.0 | 30 | 180 | 0 |
| raw (*Organic Valley*) .. | 110 | 7.0 | 0 | 9.0 | 30 | 170 | 0 |
| sharp (*Boar's Head*) .. | 110 | 7.0 | <1.0 | 9.0 | 30 | 190 | 0 |
| sharp (*Cracker Barrel*) | 120 | 6.0 | 0 | 10.0 | 30 | 180 | 0 |
| sharp (*Cracker Barrel/ Kraft* Sticks Reduced Fat) ..... | 90 | 7.0 | 1.0 | 6.0 | 20 | 240 | 0 |
| sharp (*Kraft* Singles), ⅔ oz. ........... | 60 | 4.0 | 2.0 | 4.5 | 15 | 270 | 0 |
| sharp (*Kraft* Singles 2%), ⅔ oz. ....... | 45 | 4.0 | 1.0 | 3.0 | 10 | 250 | 0 |
| sharp (*Kraft Deli Deluxe*) .......... | 110 | 6.0 | 1.0 | 9.0 | 30 | 440 | 0 |
| sharp (*Kraft Deli Fresh*), .8 oz. ..... | 90 | 5.0 | 0 | 8.0 | 25 | 150 | 0 |
| sharp (*Thumann's*) ... | 110 | 7.0 | 0 | 9.0 | 25 | 180 | 0 |
| sharp, extra (*Applegate Farms*) . | 110 | 7.0 | 1.0 | 9.0 | 30 | 180 | 0 |

| Food and Measure | cal. | prot. (gms) | carbo. (gms) | fat (gms) | chol. (mgs) | sod. (mgs) | fiber (gms) |
|---|---|---|---|---|---|---|---|
| sharp, extra (*Cracker Barrel/Kraft*) ...... | 120 | 6.0 | 0 | 10.0 | 30 | 180 | 0 |
| sharp, extra (*Cracker Barrel* Reduced Fat) ............. | 90 | 7.0 | 1.0 | 6.0 | 20 | 240 | 0 |
| sharp, extra (*Land O Lakes* Deli) ..... | 110 | 6.0 | 1.0 | 9.0 | 25 | 350 | 0 |
| sharp, white (*Cracker Barrel* Vermont) ... | 110 | 7.0 | 1.0 | 9.0 | 30 | 180 | 0 |
| sharp, white (*Sargento* Vermont), .7 oz. ... | 80 | 5.0 | 0 | 7.0 | 20 | 125 | 0 |
| cheddar, crumbled (*Kraft Crumbles*) ..... | 110 | 6.0 | 1.0 | 10.0 | 25 | 190 | 0 |
| cheddar, flavored: | | | | | | | |
| all varieties, except horseradish and jalapeño (*Cabot*) ... | 110 | 7.0 | <1.0 | 9.0 | 30 | 180 | 0 |
| bacon (*Kraft*) ....... | 90 | 5.0 | 2.0 | 7.0 | 20 | 480 | 0 |
| chipotle (*Sargento*), ¾ oz. ............ | 80 | 5.0 | 1.0 | 6.0 | 10 | 150 | 0 |
| garlic, roasted (*Kraft*) . | 80 | 5.0 | 1.0 | 2.0 | 25 | 380 | 0 |
| horseradish (*Boar's Head*) ........... | 110 | 6.0 | 2.0 | 9.0 | 30 | 190 | 0 |
| horseradish (*Cabot*) .. | 110 | 6.0 | 1.0 | 9.0 | 30 | 270 | 0 |
| jalapeño (*Cabot* Reduced Fat) ..... | 70 | 8.0 | <1.0 | 4.5 | 15 | 170 | 0 |
| cheddar, goat cheese (*Woolrich Dairy*) ..... | 100 | 8.0 | 2.0 | 7.0 | 20 | 210 | 0 |
| cheddar, shredded, ¼ cup or 1 oz.: | | | | | | | |
| (*Cabot* Fancy) ....... | 100 | 7.0 | 1.0 | 7.0 | 20 | 180 | 0 |
| (*Kraft* Organic) ...... | 120 | 6.0 | 1.0 | 10.0 | 30 | 180 | 0 |
| double (*Sargento Artisan Blends*) ... | 110 | 7.0 | 1.0 | 9.0 | 30 | 190 | 0 |
| mild (*Kraft*) .......... | 110 | 6.0 | 1.0 | 10.0 | 30 | 180 | 0 |
| mild (*Kraft* Longhorn) . | 90 | 7.0 | 1.0 | 6.0 | 20 | 240 | 0 |
| mild (*Sargento* Reduced Fat) ..... | 80 | 7.0 | <1.0 | 6.0 | 20 | 180 | 0 |
| mild (*Sargento* Reduced Sodium) .. | 110 | 7.0 | 1.0 | 9.0 | 30 | 140 | 0 |
| mild or sharp (*Sargento* ChefStyle/ Classic) ......... | 110 | 7.0 | 1.0 | 9.0 | 30 | 190 | 0 |

| Food and Measure | cal. | prot. (gms) | carbo. (gms) | fat (gms) | chol. (mgs) | sod. (mgs) | fiber (gms) |
|---|---|---|---|---|---|---|---|
| **Cheese, cheddar, shredded** *(cont.)* | | | | | | | |
| mild or sharp, fine | | | | | | | |
| (*Kraft*) . . . . . . . . . | 110 | 6.0 | 1.0 | 9.0 | 25 | 180 | 0 |
| sharp (*Sargento* | | | | | | | |
| Reduced Fat) . . . . . | 90 | 8.0 | 1.0 | 6.0 | 20 | 200 | 0 |
| sharp (*Sargento* | | | | | | | |
| Artisan Blends) . . . | 110 | 7.0 | 2.0 | 9.0 | 25 | 180 | 0 |
| sharp or extra sharp | | | | | | | |
| (*Cracker Barrel*) . . . | 110 | 6.0 | 1.0 | 9.0 | 25 | 180 | 0 |
| cheddar blend, shredded | | | | | | | |
| ¼ cup: | | | | | | | |
| American (*Kraft* | | | | | | | |
| Classic Melts) . . . . | 120 | 7.0 | 1.0 | 10.0 | 30 | 310 | 0 |
| w/bacon, sharp | | | | | | | |
| (*Sargento Bistro*) . . | 110 | 7.0 | 1.0 | 9.0 | 25 | 220 | 0 |
| chipotle (*Sargento* | | | | | | | |
| Bistro) . . . . . . . . . | 100 | 6.0 | 1.0 | 8.0 | 15 | 190 | 0 |
| Jack (*Kraft* Mexican) . . | 100 | 6.0 | 1.0 | 9.0 | 25 | 170 | 0 |
| Jack (*Sargento*) . . . . . | 110 | 7.0 | 1.0 | 9.0 | 30 | 180 | 0 |
| Jack, w/jalapeño | | | | | | | |
| (*Kraft* Mexican) . . . | 110 | 6.0 | 1.0 | 9.0 | 25 | 190 | 0 |
| Monterey Jack | | | | | | | |
| (*Kraft*) . . . . . . . . . | 110 | 6.0 | 1.0 | 9.0 | 25 | 180 | 0 |
| Cheshire . . . . . . . . . . . . | 110 | 6.6 | 1.4 | 8.7 | 29 | 198 | 0 |
| Colby: | | | | | | | |
| (*Boar's Head*) . . . . . . . | 110 | 7.0 | <1.0 | 9.0 | 30 | 170 | 0 |
| (*Cracker Barrel* | | | | | | | |
| Slices), ¾ oz. . . . . . | 80 | 5.0 | 0 | 7.0 | 20 | 135 | 0 |
| (*Kraft*) . . . . . . . . . . . . | 110 | 7.0 | 1.0 | 9.0 | 30 | 180 | 0 |
| (*Land O Lakes*) . . . . . . | 110 | 7.0 | 1.0 | 9.0 | 25 | 190 | 0 |
| (*Sargento*), ¾ oz. . . . . | 80 | 5.0 | <1.0 | 7.0 | 20 | 140 | 0 |
| Colby Jack: | | | | | | | |
| (*Alpine Lace Co-Jack*), | | | | | | | |
| .8-oz. slice . . . . . . . | 70 | 5.0 | 0 | 5.0 | 15 | 150 | 0 |
| (*Boar's Head*) . . . . . . . | 110 | 6.0 | 0 | 9.0 | 25 | 180 | 0 |
| (*Cabot*) . . . . . . . . . . . . | 110 | 7.0 | 1.0 | 9.0 | 30 | 180 | 0 |
| (*Kraft*) . . . . . . . . . . . . | 100 | 6.0 | 0 | 9.0 | 25 | 220 | 0 |
| (*Kraft Deli Fresh*), .8 oz. | 90 | 5.0 | 0 | 7.0 | 25 | 150 | 0 |
| (*Land O Lakes* | | | | | | | |
| Co-Jack) . . . . . . . . . | 110 | 7.0 | 0 | 9.0 | 25 | 190 | 0 |
| (*Sargento*), ⅔ oz. . . . . | 70 | 4.0 | 0 | 6.0 | 15 | 125 | 0 |
| (*Sargento* Reduced | | | | | | | |
| Fat), ⅔ oz. . . . . . . . | 50 | 5.0 | 0 | 4.0 | 10 | 120 | 0 |

| Food and Measure | cal. | prot. (gms) | carbo. (gms) | fat (gms) | chol. (mgs) | sod. (mgs) | fiber (gms) |
|---|---|---|---|---|---|---|---|
| (*Sargento* Reduced | | | | | | | |
| Sodium), ⅔ oz. ... | 70 | 4.0 | 0 | 6.0 | 15 | 90 | 0 |
| stick (*Sargento*), ¾ oz. | 80 | 5.0 | <1.0 | 7.0 | 20 | 105 | 0 |
| Colby Jack, crumbled | | | | | | | |
| (*Kraft Crumbles*) ..... | 80 | 7.0 | 1.0 | 6.0 | 15 | 240 | 0 |
| Colby Jack, shredded, | | | | | | | |
| ¼ cup or 1 oz.: | | | | | | | |
| (*Kraft*) ............. | 110 | 6.0 | 1.0 | 8.0 | 25 | 190 | 0 |
| (*Sargento* Classic) ... | 110 | 6.0 | 1.0 | 9.0 | 25 | 190 | 0 |
| (*Sargento* Reduced | | | | | | | |
| Fat) ............. | 80 | 7.0 | 1.0 | 6.0 | 15 | 180 | 0 |
| Colby Monterey Jack, | | | | | | | |
| see "Colby Jack" | | | | | | | |
| cottage (*Breakstone/* | | | | | | | |
| *Knudsen Live Active*), | | | | | | | |
| 4 oz. ............. | 90 | 10.0 | 8.0 | 2.0 | 15 | 380 | 3.0 |
| cottage, 4%, ½ cup: | | | | | | | |
| (*Breakstone's*) ...... | 120 | 12.0 | 6.0 | 5.0 | 25 | 430 | 0 |
| (*Friendship*) ........ | 110 | 15.0 | 3.0 | 5.0 | 20 | 380 | 0 |
| (*Knudsen*) .......... | 120 | 13.0 | 5.0 | 5.0 | 25 | 430 | 0 |
| cottage, 2%, ½ cup: | | | | | | | |
| (*Breakstone's* Large | | | | | | | |
| Curd) ............ | 90 | 11.0 | 6.0 | 2.5 | 15 | 410 | 0 |
| (*Breakstone's* Small | | | | | | | |
| Curd) ............ | 90 | 12.0 | 6.0 | 2.5 | 15 | 400 | 0 |
| (*Cabot*) ............. | 100 | 13.0 | 4.0 | 4.5 | 15 | 400 | 0 |
| (*Fiber One*) ........ | 80 | 10.0 | 8.0 | 2.0 | 10 | 430 | 5.0 |
| (*Friendship*) ........ | 90 | 15.0 | 3.0 | 2.5 | 10 | 400 | 0 |
| (*Friendship* Digestive | | | | | | | |
| Health) .......... | 90 | 14.0 | 5.0 | 2.5 | 10 | 360 | 3.0 |
| cottage, 1%, ½ cup: | | | | | | | |
| (*Friendship*) ........ | 90 | 16.0 | 3.0 | 1.0 | 5 | 360 | 0 |
| (*Friendship* No Salt) .. | 90 | 16.0 | 4.0 | 1.0 | 5 | 50 | 0 |
| cottage, nonfat, ½ cup: | | | | | | | |
| (*Breakstone's*) ...... | 80 | 12.0 | 8.0 | 0 | 10 | 450 | 0 |
| (*Cabot*) ............. | 70 | 13.0 | 5.0 | 0 | 5 | 410 | 0 |
| (*Friendship*) ........ | 80 | 15.0 | 4.0 | 0 | <5 | 380 | 0 |
| (*Knudsen*) .......... | 80 | 13.0 | 7.0 | 0 | 5 | 430 | 0 |
| (*Light n' Lively*) ..... | 80 | 12.0 | 8.0 | 0 | 10 | 460 | 0 |
| cottage, low fat, 4 oz.: | | | | | | | |
| (*Light n' Lively*) ..... | 80 | 11.0 | 5.0 | 1.0 | 10 | 360 | 0 |
| mixed berry | | | | | | | |
| (*Breakstone/Knudsen* | | | | | | | |
| *LiveAction*) ....... | 120 | 8.0 | 18.0 | 1.5 | 10 | 310 | 3.0 |

| Food and Measure | cal. | prot. (gms) | carbo. (gms) | fat (gms) | chol. (mgs) | sod. (mgs) | fiber (gms) |
|---|---|---|---|---|---|---|---|
| **Cheese, cottage, low fat** *(cont.)* | | | | | | | |
| pineapple (*Breakstone's*) .... | 100 | 8.0 | 12.0 | 2.0 | 10 | 310 | 0 |
| pineapple (*Breakstone's/ Knudsen LiveAction*) ....... | 110 | 8.0 | 17.0 | 1.5 | 10 | 310 | 3.0 |
| pineapple (*Knudsen*) .. | 120 | 10.0 | 14.0 | 2.0 | 10 | 350 | 0 |
| cottage, low fat, w/ topping, 5.5-oz. cont.: | | | | | | | |
| apple cinnamon (*Breakstone's Cottage Doubles*) .. | 140 | 11.0 | 18.0 | 2.5 | 15 | 390 | 0 |
| apple cinnamon (*Knudsen Cottage Doubles*) ........ | 140 | 11.0 | 18.0 | 2.0 | 15 | 400 | 0 |
| blueberry (*Break-stone's/Knudsen Cottage Doubles*) .. | 140 | 11.0 | 18.0 | 2.5 | 15 | 400 | 1.0 |
| peach (*Knudsen Cottage Doubles*) .. | 140 | 11.0 | 17.0 | 2.5 | 15 | 390 | 1.0 |
| peach or pineapple (*Breakstone's Cottage Doubles*) .. | 130 | 11.0 | 16.0 | 2.0 | 15 | 400 | 0 |
| pineapple (*Knudsen Cottage Doubles*) .. | 130 | 11.0 | 17.0 | 2.5 | 15 | 390 | 0 |
| raspberry (*Breakstone's Cottage Doubles*) .. | 140 | 11.0 | 17.0 | 2.5 | 15 | 400 | 1.0 |
| raspberry (*Knudsen Cottage Doubles*) .. | 150 | 11.0 | 20.0 | 2.5 | 15 | 400 | 1.0 |
| strawberry (*Breakstone's Cottage Doubles*) .. | 130 | 11.0 | 17.0 | 2.0 | 15 | 400 | 0 |
| strawberry (*Knudsen Cottage Doubles*) .. | 140 | 11.0 | 17.0 | 2.5 | 15 | 390 | 0 |
| cream cheese, 2 tbsp.: | | | | | | | |
| (*Boar's Head*) ....... | 100 | 2.0 | 2.0 | 10.0 | 30 | 100 | 0 |
| (*Philadelphia*): | | | | | | | |
| bar ............. | 100 | 2.0 | 1.0 | 9.0 | 35 | 105 | 0 |
| bar, fat free ....... | 30 | 4.0 | 2.0 | 0 | 5 | 200 | 0 |
| light ............ | 70 | 2.0 | 2.0 | 5.0 | 20 | 140 | 0 |
| tub .............. | 90 | 2.0 | 2.0 | 9.0 | 35 | 125 | 0 |
| tub, fat free ....... | 30 | 4.0 | 2.0 | 0 | 5 | 210 | 0 |

| Food and Measure | cal. | prot. (gms) | carbo. (gms) | fat (gms) | chol. (mgs) | sod. (mgs) | fiber (gms) |
|---|---|---|---|---|---|---|---|
| (*Thumann's*) ........ | 100 | 2.0 | 2.0 | 9.0 | 30 | 100 | 0 |
| cream cheese, flavored | | | | | | | |
| (*Philadelphia*), 2 tbsp.: | | | | | | | |
| blueberry .......... | 90 | 1.0 | 5.0 | 7.0 | 30 | 110 | 0 |
| cheesecake ........ | 100 | 1.0 | 5.0 | 8.0 | 30 | 115 | 0 |
| chive/onion ........ | 90 | 2.0 | 2.0 | 9.0 | 35 | 150 | 0 |
| chive/onion, light .... | 60 | 2.0 | 2.0 | 5.0 | 20 | 170 | 0 |
| garlic, roasted, light .. | 60 | 3.0 | 3.0 | 4.5 | 15 | 180 | 0 |
| honey nut .......... | 90 | 1.0 | 4.0 | 8.0 | 30 | 110 | 0 |
| peaches and cream, | | | | | | | |
| *Cream Swirls* ..... | 90 | 1.0 | 5.0 | 7.0 | 30 | 110 | 0 |
| pineapple .......... | 90 | 1.0 | 4.0 | 7.0 | 30 | 110 | 0 |
| raspberry .......... | 90 | 1.0 | 5.0 | 8.0 | 30 | 110 | 0 |
| salmon ............ | 90 | 2.0 | 2.0 | 8.0 | 30 | 210 | 0 |
| strawberry ......... | 90 | 1.0 | 5.0 | 7.0 | 30 | 110 | 0 |
| strawberry, fat free ... | 40 | 4.0 | 6.0 | 0 | 5 | 180 | 0 |
| strawberry, light ..... | 70 | 2.0 | 6.0 | 4.5 | 20 | 120 | 0 |
| vegetable, garden .... | 90 | 2.0 | 2.0 | 8.0 | 35 | 160 | 0 |
| vegetable, garden, | | | | | | | |
| light ............. | 60 | 2.0 | 2.0 | 5.0 | 20 | 190 | 0 |
| cream cheese, whipped, | | | | | | | |
| 2 tbsp.: | | | | | | | |
| (*Philadelphia*) ....... | 60 | 1.0 | 1.0 | 6.0 | 20 | 90 | 0 |
| (*Temp Tee*) ......... | 80 | 1.0 | 1.0 | 8.0 | 25 | 65 | 0 |
| berry, mixed | | | | | | | |
| (*Philadelphia*) ..... | 70 | 1.0 | 3.0 | 5.0 | 15 | 55 | 0 |
| chive (*Philadelphia*) .. | 60 | 1.0 | 1.0 | 6.0 | 15 | 130 | 0 |
| cinnamon brown sugar | | | | | | | |
| (*Philadelphia*) ..... | 70 | 1.0 | 3.0 | 6.0 | 20 | 55 | 0 |
| garlic and herb | | | | | | | |
| (*Philadelphia*) ..... | 60 | 1.0 | 1.0 | 6.0 | 20 | 100 | 0 |
| ranch (*Philadelphia*) .. | 60 | 1.0 | 1.0 | 6.0 | 15 | 150 | 0 |
| Edam (*Boar's Head*) .... | 90 | 7.0 | 0 | 7.0 | 20 | 280 | 0 |
| farmer: | | | | | | | |
| (*Friendship*) ........ | 50 | 5.0 | 0 | 2.5 | 10 | 120 | 0 |
| (*Friendship* | | | | | | | |
| No Salt) ......... | 50 | 5.0 | 0 | 2.5 | 10 | 10 | 0 |
| feta: | | | | | | | |
| (*Athenos* | | | | | | | |
| Traditional in Brine) | 80 | 6.0 | 1.0 | 6.0 | 20 | 330 | 0 |
| (*Boar's Head*) ....... | 60 | 5.0 | 1.0 | 4.0 | 10 | 370 | 0 |
| (*Vigo*) ............. | 77 | 4.0 | 1.0 | 6.0 | 20 | 580 | 0 |
| feta, crumbled, ¼ cup: | | | | | | | |
| (*Athenos* Mild) ...... | 90 | 6.0 | 1.0 | 7.0 | 20 | 220 | <1.0 |

| Food and Measure | cal. | prot. (gms) | carbo. (gms) | fat (gms) | chol. (mgs) | sod. (mgs) | fiber (gms) |
|---|---|---|---|---|---|---|---|
| **Cheese, feta, crumbled** *(cont.)* | | | | | | | |
| (*Athenos* Reduced | | | | | | | |
| Fat) . . . . . . . . . . . . | 70 | 7.0 | 1.0 | 4.5 | 10 | 470 | 1.0 |
| (*Athenos* Traditional) . | 90 | 7.0 | 2.0 | 7.0 | 20 | 390 | 1.0 |
| (*Kraft Crumbles*) . . . . . | 90 | 7.0 | 2.0 | 7.0 | 25 | 390 | 1.0 |
| basil tomato | | | | | | | |
| (*Athenos*) . . . . . . . . | 90 | 7.0 | 2.0 | 7.0 | 25 | 380 | 1.0 |
| basil tomato (*Athenos* | | | | | | | |
| Reduced Fat) . . . . . | 70 | 7.0 | 1.0 | 4.5 | 10 | 460 | 1.0 |
| garlic herb (*Athenos*) . | 90 | 7.0 | 2.0 | 7.0 | 25 | 390 | 1.0 |
| feta, goat cheese | | | | | | | |
| (*Woolrich Dairy*) . . . . . | 90 | 6.0 | 1.0 | 7.0 | 25 | 280 | 0 |
| (*Finlandia Lappi*) . . . . . . . | 100 | 7.0 | <1.0 | 8.0 | 25 | 160 | 0 |
| fontina: | | | | | | | |
| (*Cracker Barrel* | | | | | | | |
| Slices), ¾ oz. . . . . . | 80 | 6.0 | 1.0 | 7.0 | 15 | 230 | 0 |
| (*Krönenost*) . . . . . . . . | 110 | 6.0 | 1.0 | 9.0 | 25 | 150 | 0 |
| garlic, roasted (*Black* | | | | | | | |
| *Bear* New York) . . . . . . | 110 | 6.0 | 1.0 | 9.0 | 25 | 270 | 0 |
| gjetost (*Ski Queen*) . . . . . | 130 | 3.0 | 11.0 | 9.0 | 30 | 90 | 0 |
| Gloucester, double: | | | | | | | |
| (*Boar's Head*) . . . . . . . | 110 | 7.0 | 0 | 10.0 | 35 | 200 | 0 |
| (*Finlandia*), .8 oz. . . . . | 83 | 5.0 | 1.0 | 7.0 | 23 | 115 | 0 |
| goat: | | | | | | | |
| (*Snofrisk*) . . . . . . . . . . | 70 | 2.0 | 2.0 | 8.0 | 15 | 170 | 0 |
| (*Woolwich Dairy* | | | | | | | |
| Castile*) . . . . . . . . . . | 90 | 5.0 | 1.0 | 7.0 | 30 | 30 | 0 |
| (*Woolwich Dairy* | | | | | | | |
| Crottin*) . . . . . . . . . . | 70 | 5.0 | 1.0 | 6.0 | 25 | 100 | 0 |
| ash log (*Woolwich* | | | | | | | |
| *Dairy Tre* | | | | | | | |
| *Fratello*) . . . . . . . . . | 80 | 5.0 | 1.0 | 6.0 | 25 | 135 | 0 |
| log, crumbles, or | | | | | | | |
| rounds | | | | | | | |
| (*Woolwich Dairy*) . . | 70 | 5.0 | 1.0 | 6.0 | 25 | 100 | 0 |
| hard type . . . . . . . . | 128 | 8.7 | .6 | 10.1 | 30 | 98 | 0 |
| semi-soft type . . . . . . . | 103 | 6.1 | .7 | 8.5 | 22 | 146 | 0 |
| soft type . . . . . . . . . . | 76 | 5.3 | .3 | 6.0 | 13 | 104 | 0 |
| goat, flavored (*Woolrich* | | | | | | | |
| *Dairy*): | | | | | | | |
| bruschetta . . . . . . . . . | 80 | 4.0 | 3.0 | 5.0 | 20 | 90 | 0 |
| cranberry cinnamon . . | 80 | 4.0 | 3.0 | 5.0 | 20 | 100 | 0 |
| cranberry port . . . . . . | 60 | 3.0 | 6.0 | 3.0 | 10 | 60 | 0 |
| fig . . . . . . . . . . . . . . . | 80 | 3.0 | 7.0 | 6.0 | 15 | 75 | 0 |

| Food and Measure | cal. | prot. (gms) | carbo. (gms) | fat (gms) | chol. (mgs) | sod. (mgs) | fiber (gms) |
|---|---|---|---|---|---|---|---|
| fine herb | 70 | 4.0 | 1.0 | 6.0 | 30 | 135 | 0 |
| garlic, roasted | 80 | 5.0 | 1.0 | 6.0 | 25 | 150 | 1.0 |
| herb garlic | 70 | 4.0 | 1.0 | 5.0 | 25 | 120 | 0 |
| red pepper, roasted | 50 | 3.0 | 2.0 | 3.0 | 10 | 150 | 0 |
| gorgonzola: | | | | | | | |
| (*Stella*) | 100 | 6.0 | <1.0 | 9.0 | 25 | 390 | 0 |
| crumbled (*Athenos*), 3 tbsp. | 110 | 7.0 | 2.0 | 9.0 | 30 | 400 | 1.0 |
| Gouda: | | | | | | | |
| (*Boar's Head*) | 110 | 6.0 | 0 | 9.0 | 30 | 280 | 0 |
| (*Finlandia* Slices), .8 oz. | 79 | 6.0 | 0 | 6.0 | 15 | 132 | 0 |
| (*Finlandia* Stick) | 100 | 7.0 | 0 | 8.0 | 19 | 168 | 0 |
| (*Sargento*), .7 oz. | 70 | 5.0 | 0 | 6.0 | 20 | 170 | 0 |
| Grana Padano | 108 | 9.0 | 0 | 8.0 | 24 | 170 | 0 |
| Gruyère | 117 | 8.5 | .1 | 9.2 | 31 | 95 | 0 |
| havarti: | | | | | | | |
| (*Applegate Farms*), 1.5-oz. slice | 180 | 7.0 | 0 | 15.0 | 37 | 225 | 0 |
| (*Cracker Barrel* Slices), ¾ oz. | 60 | 5.0 | 0 | 7.0 | 20 | 140 | 0 |
| (*Finlandia* Stick) | 109 | 7.0 | <1.0 | 9.0 | 23 | 168 | 0 |
| (*Land O Lakes*) | 110 | 6.0 | 0 | 9.0 | 25 | 180 | 0 |
| (*Sargento*), .7 oz. | 80 | 4.0 | 0 | 6.0 | 15 | 120 | 0 |
| cream, all varieties (*Boar's Head*) | 110 | 6.0 | 0 | 10.0 | 35 | 210 | 0 |
| Italian, crumbled (*Kraft Crumbles*) | 90 | 7.0 | 1.0 | 6.0 | 20 | 240 | 0 |
| Italian, shredded, ¼ cup: | | | | | | | |
| 4 cheese (*Sargento* Reduced Fat*) | 80 | 8.0 | 1.0 | 4.5 | 15 | 220 | 0 |
| 5 cheese (*Kraft*) | 90 | 7.0 | 1.0 | 6.0 | 20 | 240 | 0 |
| 6 cheese (*Sargento*) | 90 | 7.0 | 1.0 | 7.0 | 20 | 200 | 0 |
| pasta (*Sargento* Bistro) | 90 | 7.0 | 2.0 | 6.0 | 15 | 320 | 0 |
| Jack style, raw milk (*Organic Valley*) | 100 | 7.0 | 0 | 8.0 | 25 | 170 | 0 |
| jalapeño Jack (*Land O Lakes*) | 90 | 5.0 | 1.0 | 8.0 | 20 | 420 | 0 |
| (*Jarlsberg*): | | | | | | | |
| loaf | 100 | 7.0 | 0 | 8.0 | 25 | 130 | 0 |
| loaf, lite | 70 | 9.0 | 0 | 3.5 | 10 | 130 | 0 |
| thin sliced, ¾ oz. | 70 | 5.0 | 0 | 6.0 | 15 | 100 | 0 |

| Food and Measure | cal. | prot. (gms) | carbo. (gms) | fat (gms) | chol. (mgs) | sod. (mgs) | fiber (gms) |
|---|---|---|---|---|---|---|---|
| **Cheese, Jarlsberg** *(cont.)* | | | | | | | |
| thin sliced, lite, ¾ oz. . | 50 | 7.0 | 0 | 2.5 | 10 | 100 | 0 |
| wheel . . . . . . . . . . . . | 100 | 7.0 | 0 | 8.0 | 20 | 180 | 0 |
| Limburger . . . . . . . . . . . | 93 | 5.7 | .1 | 7.7 | 26 | 227 | 0 |
| mascarpone (*Vermont* | | | | | | | |
| *Butter & Cheese*) . . . . | 140 | <1.0 | 2.0 | 14.0 | 35 | 20 | 0 |
| Mediterranean style | | | | | | | |
| (*Kraft Crumbles*) . . . . . | 90 | 7.0 | 1.0 | 7.0 | 20 | 280 | 0 |
| Mexican (*Kraft* | | | | | | | |
| *Crumbles* Reduced Fat) | 80 | 7.0 | 1.0 | 5.0 | 15 | 250 | 0 |
| Mexican, shredded, | | | | | | | |
| ¼ cup: | | | | | | | |
| (*Sargento Artisan* | | | | | | | |
| *Blends* Authentic) . . | 110 | 7.0 | 1.0 | 9.0 | 25 | 190 | 0 |
| 4 cheese (*Kraft*) . . . . . | 100 | 8.0 | 1.0 | 8.0 | 25 | 180 | 0 |
| 4 cheese (*Sargento*) . . | 110 | 6.0 | 1.0 | 9.0 | 25 | 200 | 0 |
| 4 cheese (*Sargento* | | | | | | | |
| Reduced Fat) . . . . . | 80 | 8.0 | <1.0 | 6.0 | 20 | 200 | 0 |
| Monterey Jack: | | | | | | | |
| (*Applegate Farms* | | | | | | | |
| Organic), ¾ oz. . . . | 80 | 5.0 | 0 | 6.0 | 20 | 130 | 0 |
| (*Black Bear*) . . . . . . . . | 110 | 7.0 | 1.0 | 9.0 | 25 | 180 | 0 |
| (*Boar's Head*) . . . . . . . | 100 | 6.0 | 0 | 9.0 | 25 | 180 | 0 |
| (*Cabot*) . . . . . . . . . . . | 110 | 7.0 | <1.0 | 9.0 | 30 | 170 | 0 |
| (*Kraft*) . . . . . . . . . . . . | 100 | 6.0 | 0 | 9.0 | 30 | 190 | 0 |
| (*Land O Lakes*) . . . . . . | 110 | 7.0 | 0 | 9.0 | 25 | 190 | 0 |
| (*Sargento*), ¾ oz. . . . . | 80 | 5.0 | 0 | 6.0 | 20 | 135 | 0 |
| hot pepper (*Land* | | | | | | | |
| *O Lakes*) . . . . . . . . . | 110 | 6.0 | 1.0 | 9.0 | 25 | 190 | 0 |
| jalapeño (*Applegate* | | | | | | | |
| *Farms*), ⅔ oz. . . . . . | 70 | 5.0 | 0 | 5.0 | 20 | 110 | 0 |
| jalapeño (*Boar's* | | | | | | | |
| *Head*) . . . . . . . . . . . | 100 | 6.0 | 0 | 9.0 | 25 | 170 | 0 |
| Monterey Jack, crumbled, | | | | | | | |
| w/Colby, cheddar | | | | | | | |
| (*Kraft Crumbles*) . . . . . | 110 | 6.0 | 1.0 | 9.0 | 25 | 190 | 0 |
| Monterey Jack, shredded, | | | | | | | |
| ¼ cup: | | | | | | | |
| (*Kraft*) . . . . . . . . . . . . | 100 | 6.0 | 1.0 | 8.0 | 25 | 190 | 0 |
| (*Sargento* Classic) . . . | 110 | 7.0 | 1.0 | 9.0 | 30 | 190 | 0 |
| Morbier (*Montboisse*) . . . | 99 | 6.5 | .7 | 7.0 | 23 | 220 | 0 |
| mozzarella: | | | | | | | |
| (*Alpine Lace*), | | | | | | | |
| .8-oz. slice . . . . . . . | 60 | 5.0 | 1.0 | 4.0 | 15 | 160 | 0 |

| Food and Measure | cal. | prot. (gms) | carbo. (gms) | fat (gms) | chol. (mgs) | sod. (mgs) | fiber (gms) |
|---|---|---|---|---|---|---|---|
| (*Boar's Head*) ....... | 90 | 6.0 | 1.0 | 7.0 | 20 | 150 | 0 |
| (*Kraft Deli Fresh*), | | | | | | | |
| ¾ oz. .......... | 60 | 6.0 | 0 | 4.0 | 10 | 150 | 0 |
| (*Kraft String-ums*) ... | 80 | 7.0 | 1.0 | 6.0 | 20 | 220 | 1.0 |
| (*Land O Lakes*) ...... | 90 | 7.0 | 1.0 | 6.0 | 15 | 190 | 0 |
| (*Sargento*), ¾ oz. .... | 60 | 5.0 | 1.0 | 4.0 | 10 | 140 | 0 |
| (*Thumann's*) ........ | 90 | 6.0 | 1.0 | 7.0 | 25 | 290 | 0 |
| whole (*Polly-O*) ...... | 80 | 6.0 | 1.0 | 6.0 | 20 | 200 | 0 |
| part skim (*Kraft*) ..... | 90 | 7.0 | 1.0 | 6.0 | 20 | 170 | 0 |
| part skim (*Polly-O*) ... | 70 | 6.0 | 1.0 | 5.0 | 15 | 200 | 0 |
| nonfat (*Polly-O*) ..... | 35 | 7.0 | 1.0 | 0 | 5 | 220 | 0 |
| mozzarella, crumbled | | | | | | | |
| (*Kraft Crumbles*) ..... | 80 | 7.0 | 1.0 | 6.0 | 20 | 200 | 0 |
| mozzarella, fresh: | | | | | | | |
| (*BelGioioso*) ........ | 70 | 5.0 | <1.0 | 5.0 | 20 | 85 | 0 |
| (*Polly-O* Balls) ...... | 80 | 5.0 | 0 | 7.0 | 20 | 15 | 0 |
| (*Polly-O* Bite Size), | | | | | | | |
| 1.5 oz. .......... | 120 | 7.0 | 0 | 10.0 | 35 | 25 | 0 |
| mozzarella, shredded, | | | | | | | |
| ¼ cup: | | | | | | | |
| (*Cabot*) ............ | 80 | 8.0 | 1.0 | 6.0 | 15 | 170 | 0 |
| (*Kraft*) ............. | 80 | 6.0 | 1.0 | 5.0 | 20 | 220 | 0 |
| (*Kraft* 16 oz.) ....... | 80 | 7.0 | 1.0 | 6.0 | 20 | 200 | 0 |
| (*Kraft* Organic) ...... | 80 | 7.0 | 1.0 | 5.0 | 15 | 200 | 0 |
| (*Polly-O* Lite) ....... | 60 | 7.0 | 1.0 | 2.5 | 10 | 230 | 0 |
| (*Sargento* ChefStyle/ | | | | | | | |
| Classic) ........ | 80 | 7.0 | 1.0 | 6.0 | 15 | 190 | 0 |
| (*Sargento* Reduced | | | | | | | |
| Fat) ............. | 80 | 8.0 | <1.0 | 4.5 | 10 | 200 | 0 |
| (*Sargento* Reduced | | | | | | | |
| Sodium) ......... | 80 | 7.0 | 1.0 | 6.0 | 15 | 140 | 0 |
| whole (*Polly-O*) ...... | 90 | 6.0 | 1.0 | 7.0 | 20 | 190 | 0 |
| whole (*Sargento* | | | | | | | |
| Artisan Blends) ... | 90 | 7.0 | 1.0 | 7.0 | 25 | 190 | 0 |
| part skim (*Polly-O*) ... | 80 | 7.0 | 1.0 | 5.0 | 15 | 200 | 0 |
| nonfat (*Polly-O*) ..... | 40 | 8.0 | 1.0 | 0 | 5 | 240 | 0 |
| mozzarella blend, | | | | | | | |
| shredded, ¼ cup: | | | | | | | |
| asiago, roasted garlic | | | | | | | |
| (*Sargento Bistro*) .. | 80 | 7.0 | 2.0 | 5.0 | 15 | 270 | 0 |
| Parmesan (*Kraft*) .... | 90 | 6.0 | 1.0 | 6.0 | 20 | 210 | 0 |
| Parmesan, fine | | | | | | | |
| (*Polly-O*) ........ | 90 | 6.0 | 1.0 | 7.0 | 20 | 210 | 0 |
| pizza (*Polly-O*) ...... | 90 | 7.0 | 1.0 | 7.0 | 20 | 230 | 0 |

| Food and Measure | cal. | prot. (gms) | carbo. (gms) | fat (gms) | chol. (mgs) | sod. (mgs) | fiber (gms) |
|---|---|---|---|---|---|---|---|
| **Cheese, mozzarella blend** *(cont.)* | | | | | | | |
| provolone (*Sargento Artisan Blends*) ... | 90 | 6.0 | 0 | 7.0 | 20 | 170 | 0 |
| sun-dried tomato (*Sargento Bistro*) .. | 90 | 7.0 | 1.0 | 6.0 | 20 | 220 | 0 |
| Muenster: | | | | | | | |
| (*Alpine Lace*) ....... | 100 | 7.0 | 0 | 9.0 | 20 | 135 | 0 |
| (*Applegate Farms*), ¾-oz. slice ....... | 70 | 5.0 | 0 | 6.0 | 20 | 140 | 0 |
| (*Applegate Farms Organic*), ¾ oz. ... | 85 | 5.0 | 0 | 6.0 | 20 | 130 | 0 |
| (*Black Bear*) ........ | 110 | 7.0 | 1.0 | 9.0 | 25 | 180 | 0 |
| (*Boar's Head*) ....... | 100 | 6.0 | 0 | 8.0 | 25 | 180 | 0 |
| (*Cabot*) ........... | 110 | 7.0 | <1.0 | 9.0 | 30 | 180 | 0 |
| (*Finlandia*) ........ | 110 | 6.0 | <1.0 | 10.0 | 25 | 150 | 0 |
| (*Land O Lakes*) ...... | 100 | 7.0 | 0 | 8.0 | 25 | 180 | 0 |
| (*Sargento*), ¾ oz. .... | 80 | 5.0 | 0 | 6.0 | 20 | 135 | 0 |
| (*Thumann's*) ........ | 110 | 7.0 | 0 | 9.0 | 30 | 180 | 0 |
| baby (*Finlandia Oltermanni*) ...... | 100 | 7.0 | 0 | 8.0 | 20 | 160 | 0 |
| nacho and taco, shredded (*Sargento Bistro*), ¼ cup ............. | 110 | 7.0 | 1.0 | 9.0 | 30 | 200 | 0 |
| Neufchâtel, 2 tbsp.: | | | | | | | |
| (*Organic Valley* Bar) .. | 80 | 2.0 | 1.0 | 6.0 | 20 | 115 | 0 |
| (*Organic Valley* Tub) .. | 70 | 2.0 | 2.0 | 6.0 | 20 | 160 | 0 |
| (*Philadelphia*) ....... | 70 | 2.0 | 1.0 | 6.0 | 20 | 120 | 0 |
| Parmesan (*Sargento*) ... | 100 | 9.0 | <1.0 | 7.0 | 20 | 390 | 0 |
| Parmesan, grated, 2 tsp.: | | | | | | | |
| (*Kraft*) ............. | 20 | 2.0 | 0 | 1.5 | 5 | 85 | 0 |
| (*Kraft* Reduced Fat) .. | 20 | 1.0 | 2.0 | 1.0 | 5 | 80 | 0 |
| (*Polly-O*) ........... | 20 | 2.0 | 0 | 1.5 | 5 | 85 | 0 |
| (*Sargento*) ......... | 25 | 2.0 | 0 | 1.5 | 5 | 80 | 0 |
| Romano (*Kraft*) ..... | 20 | 2.0 | 0 | 1.5 | 5 | 85 | 0 |
| Romano (*Polly-O*) .... | 20 | 2.0 | 0 | 1.5 | 5 | 85 | 0 |
| Romano (*Sargento*) .. | 25 | 2.0 | 0 | 1.5 | 5 | 80 | 0 |
| Parmesan, shredded: | | | | | | | |
| (*Kraft*), ¼ cup ........ | 110 | 9.0 | 1.0 | 8.0 | 25 | 400 | 0 |
| (*Organic Valley*), ¼ cup ............ | 110 | 10.0 | 0 | 7.0 | 20 | 350 | 0 |
| (*Sargento Artisan Blends*), 2 tsp. .... | 20 | 2.0 | 0 | 1.5 | <5 | 55 | 0 |
| Romano (*Sargento Artisan Blends*), 2 tsp. | 20 | 2.0 | 0 | 1.5 | <5 | 60 | 0 |

| Food and Measure | cal. | prot. (gms) | carbo. (gms) | fat (gms) | chol. (mgs) | sod. (mgs) | fiber (gms) |
|---|---|---|---|---|---|---|---|
| Romano and asiago (*Kraft*), ¼ cup .... | 110 | 9.0 | 1.0 | 8.0 | 25 | 370 | 0 |
| pecorino, fresh: | | | | | | | |
| all varieties, except tri-color (*Gabriella*) | 120 | 8.0 | 0 | 10.0 | 25 | 220 | 0 |
| tri-color (*Gabriella*) ... | 130 | 8.0 | 1.0 | 10.0 | 25 | 220 | 0 |
| pecorino, grated, 1 tbsp.: | | | | | | | |
| (*Gabriella* Canestrato) . | 25 | 2.0 | 0 | 1.5 | 5 | 55 | 0 |
| (*Gabriella* Siciliano) .. | 20 | 1.0 | 0 | 1.5 | 5 | 220 | 0 |
| pepato (*Gabriella* Canestrato) ......... | 140 | 10.0 | 0 | 10.0 | 25 | 220 | 0 |
| pepper, hot (*Black Bear*) .............. | 110 | 6.0 | 1.0 | 9.0 | 27 | 270 | 0 |
| pepper Jack: | | | | | | | |
| (*Cabot*) ............. | 110 | 7.0 | <1.0 | 9.0 | 30 | 170 | 0 |
| (*Cabot* 50% Less Fat) . | 70 | 8.0 | <1.0 | 4.5 | 15 | 170 | 0 |
| (*Kraft*) ............. | 110 | 6.0 | 1.0 | 9.0 | 30 | 170 | 0 |
| (*Kraft* Singles 2%), ⅔ oz. ....... | 45 | 4.0 | 2.0 | 2.5 | 10 | 330 | 0 |
| (*Kraft Deli Fresh*), .8 oz. ........... | 90 | 5.0 | 0 | 7.0 | 25 | 150 | 0 |
| (*Land O Lakes*) ...... | 110 | 6.0 | 1.0 | 9.0 | 25 | 190 | 0 |
| (*Sargento*), ¾ oz. .... | 80 | 4.0 | 0 | 6.0 | 20 | 140 | 0 |
| (*Sargento* Reduced Fat), ⅔ oz. ....... | 50 | 6.0 | 0 | 4.0 | 10 | 125 | 0 |
| (*Thumann's*) ........ | 100 | 5.0 | 1.0 | 8.0 | 25 | 470 | 0 |
| pepperoni (*Black Bear*) .. | 90 | 5.0 | 2.0 | 7.0 | 20 | 480 | 0 |
| pizza, shredded, ¼ cup: | | | | | | | |
| (*Sargento Double Cheese*) ......... | 90 | 7.0 | 1.0 | 6.0 | 20 | 190 | 0 |
| 4 cheese (*Kraft*) ..... | 90 | 6.0 | 1.0 | 7.0 | 20 | 210 | 0 |
| mozzarella/cheddar (*Kraft*) .......... | 90 | 6.0 | 1.0 | 7.0 | 20 | 190 | 0 |
| Port du Salut ......... | 100 | 6.7 | .2 | 8.0 | 35 | 151 | 0 |
| provolone: | | | | | | | |
| (*Alpine Lace*) ....... | 80 | 7.0 | 1.0 | 6.0 | 15 | 160 | 0 |
| (*Applegate Farms*), ⅔-oz. slice ....... | 70 | 5.0 | 0 | 5.0 | 15 | 160 | 0 |
| (*Auricchio*) ......... | 110 | 7.0 | <1.0 | 9.0 | 25 | 280 | 0 |
| (*Black Bear*) ....... | 90 | 7.0 | 1.0 | 7.0 | 20 | 290 | 0 |
| (*Boar's Head* Lower Sodium) ... | 100 | 7.0 | 1.0 | 7.0 | 20 | 140 | 0 |

| Food and Measure | cal. | prot. (gms) | carbo. (gms) | fat (gms) | chol. (mgs) | sod. (mgs) | fiber (gms) |
|---|---|---|---|---|---|---|---|
| **Cheese, provolone** (cont.) | | | | | | | |
| (*Boar's Head* Picante) ......... | 100 | 7.0 | 1.0 | 8.0 | 25 | 250 | 0 |
| (*Kraft Deli Fresh*) .... | 100 | 7.0 | 0 | 8.0 | 25 | 230 | 0 |
| (*Sargento*), ⅔ oz. .... | 70 | 5.0 | 0 | 5.0 | 15 | 125 | 0 |
| (*Sargento* Reduced Fat), ⅔ oz. ....... | 50 | 5.0 | 0 | 3.5 | 10 | 140 | 0 |
| (*Sargento* Reduced Sodium), ⅔ oz. ... | 70 | 5.0 | 0 | 5.0 | 15 | 100 | 0 |
| (*Thumann's*) ......... | 100 | 7.0 | 1.0 | 8.0 | 25 | 250 | 0 |
| sharp (*Sargento*), .7 oz. | 80 | 5.0 | 0 | 7.0 | 20 | 125 | 0 |
| smoke flavor (*Land O Lakes*) ......... | 100 | 7.0 | 1.0 | 8.0 | 20 | 250 | 0 |
| quark (*Vermont Butter & Cheese*) .......... | 35 | 2.0 | 2.0 | 2.0 | 10 | 40 | 0 |
| ricotta, ¼ cup: | | | | | | | |
| (*Organic Valley*) ..... | 100 | 6.0 | 3.0 | 7.0 | 20 | 100 | 0 |
| (*Polly-O Lite*) ....... | 70 | 8.0 | 3.0 | 3.0 | 10 | 80 | 0 |
| (*Polly-O* Original) .... | 110 | 7.0 | 2.0 | 8.0 | 25 | 65 | 0 |
| (*Sargento* Light) ..... | 60 | 5.0 | 3.0 | 2.5 | 15 | 55 | 0 |
| whole (*Sargento*) .... | 90 | 7.0 | 3.0 | 6.0 | 25 | 75 | 0 |
| part skim (*Polly-O*) ... | 90 | 8.0 | 2.0 | 6.0 | 20 | 65 | 0 |
| part skim (*Sargento*) . | 70 | 6.0 | 3.0 | 4.5 | 25 | 85 | 0 |
| nonfat (*Polly-O*) ..... | 45 | 8.0 | 3.0 | 0 | 5 | 80 | 0 |
| nonfat (*Sargento*) .... | 50 | 5.0 | 5.0 | 0 | 10 | 65 | 0 |
| (*Ridder*) ............. | 120 | 5.0 | 4.0 | 10.0 | 30 | 210 | 0 |
| Romano: | | | | | | | |
| (*Gabriella* Pecorino) .. | 109 | 9.0 | 0 | 7.0 | 29 | 340 | 0 |
| grated (*Kraft*), 2 tsp. .. | 20 | 2.0 | 0 | 1.5 | 5 | 85 | 0 |
| Roquefort ............. | 105 | 6.1 | .6 | 8.7 | 26 | 513 | 0 |
| string cheese: | | | | | | | |
| (*Sargento*) ......... | 80 | 8.0 | 1.0 | 6.0 | 15 | 210 | 0 |
| (*Sargento*), .8-oz. pc. . | 70 | 6.0 | 1.0 | 4.5 | 15 | 170 | 0 |
| (*Sargento* Light), ¾-oz. pc. ........ | 50 | 6.0 | 1.0 | 2.5 | 10 | 160 | 0 |
| (*Sargento* Reduced Sodium), ¾-oz. pc. | 60 | 6.0 | <1.0 | 4.0 | 10 | 110 | 0 |
| Swiss: | | | | | | | |
| (*Alpine Lace*) ....... | 90 | 8.0 | 1.0 | 6.0 | 20 | 115 | 0 |
| (*Applegate Farms*), ⅔-oz. slice ....... | 80 | 5.0 | 0 | 6.0 | 15 | 35 | 0 |
| (*Boar's Head* Gold Label Import) ..... | 110 | 8.0 | <1.0 | 8.0 | 20 | 70 | 0 |
| (*Boar's Head* Lacey) .. | 90 | 9.0 | 0 | 6.0 | 15 | 35 | 0 |

| Food and Measure | cal. | prot. (gms) | carbo. (gms) | fat (gms) | chol. (mgs) | sod. (mgs) | fiber (gms) |
|---|---|---|---|---|---|---|---|
| (*Boar's Head* Natural No Salt) ........ | 110 | 8.0 | 1.0 | 8.0 | 25 | 10 | 0 |
| (*Cabot* Slices) ....... | 110 | 8.0 | 1.0 | 8.0 | 25 | 60 | 0 |
| (*Cracker Barrel* Emmentaler Slices), ¾ oz. ........... | 80 | 6.0 | 0 | 7.0 | 20 | 35 | 0 |
| (*Finlandia*) ......... | 110 | 8.0 | 0 | 8.0 | 20 | 80 | 0 |
| (*Finlandia* Light) ..... | 70 | 9.0 | 0 | 4.0 | 10 | 130 | 0 |
| (*Finlandia* Slices), .8 oz. ........... | 86 | 6.0 | 0 | 7.0 | 16 | 62 | 0 |
| (*Finlandia* Slices Light), .8 oz. ...... | 57 | 7.0 | 0 | 3.0 | 8 | 110 | 0 |
| (*Finlandia* Thin Slices), .5 oz. ...... | 55 | 4.0 | 0 | 4.0 | 10 | 39 | 0 |
| (*Kraft* Singles) ...... | 110 | 8.0 | 0 | 9.0 | 30 | 50 | 0 |
| (*Kraft* Singles 2% Milk), ⅔ oz. ...... | 45 | 4.0 | 2.0 | 2.5 | 10 | 270 | 0 |
| (*Kraft* Singles Fat Free), ⅔ oz. ...... | 25 | 4.0 | 2.0 | 0 | 5 | 250 | 0 |
| (*Kraft Deli Deluxe*), .8 oz. ........... | 90 | 6.0 | 0 | 7.0 | 25 | 40 | 0 |
| (*Kraft Deli Fresh*) .... | 110 | 8.0 | 0 | 9.0 | 30 | 50 | 0 |
| (*Kraft Deli Fresh* Natural), ¾ oz. .... | 80 | 6.0 | 0 | 7.0 | 20 | 35 | 0 |
| (*Kraft Deli Fresh* 2%), ¾ oz. ....... | 70 | 6.0 | 0 | 4.5 | 15 | 50 | 0 |
| (*Land O Lakes*) ...... | 110 | 8.0 | 1.0 | 8.0 | 25 | 115 | 0 |
| (*Sargento* Regular/ Aged), ⅔-oz. slice . | 70 | 5.0 | 0 | 5.0 | 20 | 40 | 0 |
| (*Sargento* Reduced Fat), ¾-oz. slice ... | 60 | 7.0 | 1.0 | 4.0 | 10 | 30 | 0 |
| (*Thumann's*) ........ | 100 | 8.0 | 1.0 | 8.0 | 25 | 60 | 0 |
| Swiss, baby: | | | | | | | |
| (*Black Bear*) ........ | 110 | 7.0 | 0 | 8.0 | 28 | 30 | 0 |
| (*Boar's Head*) ....... | 110 | 7.0 | <1.0 | 9.0 | 25 | 135 | 0 |
| (*Cracker Barrel*) ..... | 110 | 7.0 | 0 | 9.0 | 25 | 110 | 0 |
| (*Kraft Cracker Cuts*) .. | 110 | 7.0 | 0 | 9.0 | 25 | 110 | 0 |
| (*Land O Lakes*) ...... | 110 | 8.0 | 1.0 | 8.0 | 25 | 115 | 0 |
| (*Sargento*), ⅔ oz. .... | 70 | 5.0 | 0 | 5.0 | 15 | 40 | 0 |
| (*Thumann's*) ........ | 100 | 7.0 | 0 | 8.0 | 25 | 110 | 0 |
| Swiss, shredded: | | | | | | | |
| (*Kraft*), ¼ cup ....... | 110 | 7.0 | 1.0 | 8.0 | 25 | 45 | 0 |
| (*Sargento Artisan Blends*), ¼ cup .... | 110 | 8.0 | <1.0 | 8.0 | 25 | 60 | 0 |

| Food and Measure | cal. | prot. (gms) | carbo. (gms) | fat (gms) | chol. (mgs) | sod. (mgs) | fiber (gms) |
|---|---|---|---|---|---|---|---|
| **Cheese** *(cont.)* | | | | | | | |
| Swiss American | | | | | | | |
|   (*Land O Lakes*) . . . . . . | 100 | 6.0 | 1.0 | 8.0 | 25 | 400 | 0 |
| Swiss cheddar, smoky | | | | | | | |
|   (*Kraft*) . . . . . . . . . . . . . | 100 | 5.0 | 1.0 | 8.0 | 25 | 380 | 0 |
| taco, shredded, ¼ cup: | | | | | | | |
|   (*Kraft* Mexican) . . . . . . | 100 | 6.0 | 1.0 | 8.0 | 25 | 210 | 0 |
|   (*Sargento Bistro*) . . . . | 110 | 7.0 | 1.0 | 9.0 | 30 | 200 | 0 |
| yogurt (*Applegate* | | | | | | | |
|   Farms*), ¾-oz. slice . . . | 80 | 5.0 | <1.0 | 6.0 | 15 | 105 | 0 |
| **Cheese appetizer/** | | | | | | | |
| **snack**, frozen: | | | | | | | |
| in fillo: | | | | | | | |
|   Brie/raspberry (*The* | | | | | | | |
|     *Fillo Factory*), 3 oz. . | 270 | 10.0 | 27.0 | 14.0 | 40 | 320 | 1.0 |
|   feta/ricotta (*Kontos*), | | | | | | | |
|     1-oz. pc. . . . . . . . . . | 60 | 4.0 | 5.0 | 2.0 | 15 | 180 | 0 |
|   feta/sun-dried tomato | | | | | | | |
|     (*The Fillo Factory*), | | | | | | | |
|     3 oz. . . . . . . . . . . . . | 200 | 8.0 | 24.0 | 8.0 | 15 | 350 | 1.0 |
|   3 cheese (*Athens/* | | | | | | | |
|     *Apollo* Tyropita), | | | | | | | |
|     2 pcs., 2 oz. . . . . . . | 180 | 6.0 | 14.0 | 11.0 | 25 | 310 | 0 |
| mozzarella, breaded: | | | | | | | |
|   nuggets (*Banquet*), | | | | | | | |
|     7 pcs., 3.2 oz. . . . . | 290 | 10.0 | 22.0 | 18.0 | 15 | 330 | 3.0 |
|   sticks (*Alexia* Stix), | | | | | | | |
|     2 pcs., 1.3 oz. . . . . | 120 | 5.0 | 13.0 | 7.0 | 15 | 220 | <1.0 |
| pastry puffs (*Pillsbury* | | | | | | | |
|   *Savorings*), 4 pcs.: | | | | | | | |
|   cream cheese/jalapeño | 200 | 6.0 | 21.0 | 11.0 | 25 | 380 | 1.0 |
|   mozzarella/pepperoni . | 260 | 6.0 | 22.0 | 16.0 | 15 | 460 | 1.0 |
|   and spinach . . . . . . . . | 260 | 6.0 | 21.0 | 17.0 | 20 | 430 | 1.0 |
| **Cheese dip**, 2 tbsp.: | | | | | | | |
| (*Cheez Whiz* Light) . . . . . | 80 | 6.0 | 6.0 | 3.5 | 20 | 500 | 0 |
| (*Cheez Whiz* Original) . . . | 90 | 3.0 | 4.0 | 7.0 | 5 | 440 | 0 |
| (*Margaritaville* Con | | | | | | | |
|   Queso in Paradise) . . . | 45 | 2.0 | 2.0 | 3.0 | 10 | 210 | 0 |
| bean con queso: | | | | | | | |
|   (*Taco Bell*) . . . . . . . . . | 35 | 1.0 | 2.0 | 2.0 | 0 | 300 | 1.0 |
|   (*Tostitos*) . . . . . . . . . . | 45 | 2.0 | 5.0 | 2.0 | 0 | 230 | 2.0 |
| blue (*Marzetti's*) . . . . . . . | 140 | 1.0 | 1.0 | 15.0 | 15 | 250 | 0 |
| cheddar: | | | | | | | |
|   (*Mission*) . . . . . . . . . . | 45 | 1.0 | 4.0 | 3.0 | 0 | 280 | 0 |

| Food and Measure | cal. | prot. (gms) | carbo. (gms) | fat (gms) | chol. (mgs) | sod. (mgs) | fiber (gms) |
|---|---|---|---|---|---|---|---|
| jalapeño (*Fritos*) . . . . . | 50 | 1.0 | 3.0 | 3.5 | <5 | 320 | 0 |
| jalapeño (*Heluva Good!*) . . . . . . . . . . | 60 | 1.0 | 2.0 | 5.0 | 20 | 210 | 0 |
| mild (*Fritos*) . . . . . . . . | 50 | 1.0 | 4.0 | 3.5 | <5 | 340 | 0 |
| white, and bacon (*Heluva Good!*) . . . | 60 | 1.0 | 2.0 | 5.0 | 20 | 160 | 0 |
| chili (*Fritos*) . . . . . . . . . . | 45 | 1.0 | 3.0 | 3.0 | <5 | 290 | <1.0 |
| chili con queso (*Taco Bell* Home Originals) . . . . . . . . . . | 40 | 2.0 | 3.0 | 2.0 | 5 | 470 | 0 |
| cream, see "Fruit dip" | | | | | | | |
| Monterey Jack (*Tostitos* Queso) . . . . . . . . . . . . | 40 | 1.0 | 4.0 | 2.5 | <5 | 210 | 0 |
| nacho (*Mrs. Renfro's*) . . . | 30 | 1.0 | 4.0 | 1.5 | 0 | 150 | 0 |
| salsa con queso: | | | | | | | |
| (*Cheez Whiz*) . . . . . . . | 90 | 3.0 | 4.0 | 7.0 | 30 | 500 | 0 |
| (*Chi-Chi's*) . . . . . . . . . | 45 | 1.0 | 4.0 | 3.0 | 0 | 280 | 0 |
| (*Mission*) . . . . . . . . . . | 45 | 1.0 | 4.0 | 3.0 | 0 | 280 | 0 |
| (*Newman's Own*) . . . . | 40 | 0 | 3.0 | 3.0 | 5 | 200 | 0 |
| (*Old El Paso* Cheese n' Salsa) . . . . . . . . . | 35 | 0 | 3.0 | 3.0 | 0 | 280 | 0 |
| (*Ortega*) . . . . . . . . . . . | 45 | 1.0 | 4.0 | 3.0 | <5 | 280 | 0 |
| (*Taco Bell*) . . . . . . . . . | 25 | 1.0 | 1.0 | 2.0 | 0 | 220 | 0 |
| (*Tostitos*) . . . . . . . . . . | 40 | <1.0 | 5.0 | 2.5 | <5 | 280 | <1.0 |
| (*Wise*) . . . . . . . . . . . . | 45 | 1.0 | 3.0 | 3.0 | 5 | 280 | 0 |
| 4 cheese (*Pace*) . . . . . | 90 | 1.0 | 5.0 | 7.0 | 5 | 430 | 0 |
| **Cheese dip kit**, 1 pkg.: | | | | | | | |
| w/breadsticks (*Premium Handi-Snacks*) . . . . . . | 110 | 3.0 | 14.0 | 4.5 | 5 | 350 | 0 |
| w/crackers: | | | | | | | |
| (*Ritz Handi-Snacks*) . . | 100 | 2.0 | 11.0 | 6.0 | 5 | 330 | 0 |
| (*Sargento Mootown*) . | 100 | 2.0 | 12.0 | 5.0 | 5 | 350 | 0 |
| Colby Jack (*Kraft To Go!*) . . . . . . . . . | 170 | 8.0 | 10.0 | 11.0 | 30 | 280 | 1.0 |
| cheddar (*Kraft To Go!*) | 190 | 7.0 | 10.0 | 13.0 | 30 | 310 | 0 |
| w/pretzels (*Sargento Mootown*) . . . . . . . . . | 80 | 2.0 | 13.0 | 2.5 | 5 | 350 | <1.0 |
| w/sticks (*Sargento Mootown*) . . . . . . . . . | 100 | 2.0 | 14.0 | 4.0 | 10 | 340 | 0 |
| **Cheese entree, frozen** (see also "Spinach entree") (*Ethnic Gourmet* Shahi Paneer), 11-oz. pkg. . . . . . . . . | 560 | 22.0 | 49.0 | 30.0 | 60 | 400 | 7.0 |

| Food and Measure | cal. | prot. (gms) | carbo. (gms) | fat (gms) | chol. (mgs) | sod. (mgs) | fiber (gms) |
|---|---|---|---|---|---|---|---|
| **Cheese entree, microwave** (*Tasty Bite* Paneer Makhani), ½ of 10-oz. pkg. . . . . . | 120 | 6.0 | 10.0 | 8.0 | 10 | 440 | 2.0 |
| **Cheese food** (see also "Cheese spread") (*Velveeta*), 1 oz., except as noted: | | | | | | | |
| loaf, regular . . . . . . . . . . | 80 | 5.0 | 3.0 | 6.0 | 20 | 410 | 0 |
| loaf, 2% . . . . . . . . . . . . | 60 | 5.0 | 4.0 | 3.0 | 10 | 410 | 0 |
| Mexican, hot . . . . . . . . . | 90 | 5.0 | 3.0 | 6.0 | 25 | 430 | 0 |
| Mexican, mild . . . . . . . . | 80 | 5.0 | 3.0 | 6.0 | 25 | 400 | 0 |
| pepper jack . . . . . . . . . . | 80 | 5.0 | 3.0 | 6.0 | 25 | 430 | 0 |
| shredded, ¼ cup . . . . . . . | 130 | 8.0 | 3.0 | 9.0 | 30 | 500 | 0 |
| slices, ¾ oz. . . . . . . . . . | 60 | 4.0 | 2.0 | 4.0 | 15 | 270 | 0 |
| **Cheese powder** (*Cabot Cheddar Shake!*), 2 tsp. . . . . . | 25 | 1.0 | 1.0 | 1.5 | 5 | 220 | 0 |
| **Cheese sauce**, nacho (*Mrs. Renfro's*), ¼ cup | 60 | 1.0 | 7.0 | 3.5 | 0 | 310 | 0 |
| **Cheese seasoning** (*Molly McButter*), 1 tsp. | 5 | 0 | 1.0 | 0 | 0 | 125 | 0 |
| **Cheese spread** (see also "Cheese"), 2 tbsp.: (*Boursin*): | | | | | | | |
| apple, cranberry, cinnamon . . . . . . . . | 120 | 1.0 | 3.0 | 12.0 | 30 | 85 | <1.0 |
| garlic herb . . . . . . . . . | 120 | 2.0 | 1.0 | 12.0 | 30 | 180 | 0 |
| garlic herb, light . . . . . | 70 | 3.0 | 1.0 | 6.0 | 20 | 170 | 0 |
| pepper . . . . . . . . . . . | 120 | 2.0 | 1.0 | 12.0 | 30 | 210 | 0 |
| roasted red pepper and garlic . . . . . . . . | 120 | 2.0 | 2.0 | 12.0 | 30 | 115 | 0 |
| shallot and chive . . . . . | 120 | 2.0 | 1.0 | 12.0 | 30 | 190 | 0 |
| (*Finlandia Viola*) . . . . . . . | 87 | 3.0 | 1.0 | 8.0 | 19 | 280 | 0 |
| American (*Kraft Easy Cheese*) . . . . . . . . . . | 90 | 5.0 | 2.0 | 6.0 | 20 | 410 | 0 |
| bacon (*Kraft*) . . . . . . . . . | 90 | 5.0 | 1.0 | 8.0 | 25 | 570 | 0 |
| blue (*Kraft Roka*) . . . . . . | 80 | 3.0 | 2.0 | 7.0 | 20 | 340 | 0 |
| cheddar: | | | | | | | |
| (*Kraft Easy Cheese*) . . | 90 | 5.0 | 2.0 | 6.0 | 20 | 410 | 0 |
| all varieties (*Heluva Good!*) . . . . . . . . . . | 90 | 5.0 | 3.0 | 7.0 | 20 | 210 | 0 |
| sharp (*Kraft Easy Cheese*) . . . . . . . . | 80 | 4.0 | 2.0 | 6.0 | 10 | 450 | 0 |

| Food and Measure | cal. | prot. (gms) | carbo. (gms) | fat (gms) | chol. (mgs) | sod. (mgs) | fiber (gms) |
|---|---|---|---|---|---|---|---|
| cheddar and bacon | | | | | | | |
| (*Kraft Easy Cheese*) | 90 | 5.0 | 2.0 | 7.0 | 25 | 400 | 0 |
| olive pimento (*Kraft*) | 70 | 2.0 | 3.0 | 6.0 | 20 | 220 | 0 |
| pimento (*Kraft*) | 80 | 2.0 | 3.0 | 6.0 | 20 | 170 | 0 |
| pineapple (*Kraft*) | 70 | 2.0 | 4.0 | 5.0 | 15 | 120 | 0 |
| sharp (*Kraft Old* | | | | | | | |
| *English*) | 90 | 5.0 | 1.0 | 8.0 | 25 | 520 | 0 |
| **Cheesecake**, fresh | | | | | | | |
| (*Entenmann's*), ⅙ cake: | | | | | | | |
| French style | 390 | 6.0 | 39.0 | 24.0 | 40 | 400 | <1.0 |
| pineapple | 330 | 5.0 | 37.0 | 18.0 | 90 | 240 | <1.0 |
| **Cheesecake, frozen**: | | | | | | | |
| (*Sara Lee* New York): | | | | | | | |
| plain, ⅙ cake | 480 | 7.0 | 47.0 | 30.0 | 130 | 490 | <1.0 |
| pumpkin, ⅙ cake | 460 | 7.0 | 43.0 | 29.0 | 130 | 480 | 2.0 |
| (*Sara Lee* Original): | | | | | | | |
| plain, ¼ cake | 320 | 7.0 | 36.0 | 17.0 | 70 | 250 | <1.0 |
| cherry, ¼ cake | 320 | 6.0 | 50.0 | 11.0 | 50 | 240 | <1.0 |
| strawberry (*Sara Lee* | | | | | | | |
| French), ⅙ cake | 320 | 4.0 | 37.0 | 18.0 | 15 | 220 | <1.0 |
| **Cheesecake, mix**, dry: | | | | | | | |
| (*Dr. Oetker*), ⅑ pkg. | 170 | 3.0 | 38.0 | 0 | 0 | 240 | 1.0 |
| (*Jell-O* No Bake | | | | | | | |
| Homestyle), ⅙ pkg. | 230 | 2.0 | 44.0 | 4.5 | 0 | 380 | 1.0 |
| (*Jell-O* No Bake | | | | | | | |
| Real), ⅛ pkg. | 290 | 4.0 | 39.0 | 15.0 | 0 | 330 | 2.0 |
| cherry: | | | | | | | |
| (*Eagle Brand Cherry* | | | | | | | |
| *Cheesecake* | | | | | | | |
| *Treasures*), ⅙ pkg. | 380 | 6.0 | 72.0 | 8.0 | 15 | 400 | 1.0 |
| (*Jell-O* No Bake), | | | | | | | |
| ⅑ pkg. | 210 | 2.0 | 42.0 | 3.5 | 0 | 270 | 1.0 |
| strawberry (*Jell-O* | | | | | | | |
| No Bake), ⅑ pkg. | 200 | 2.0 | 42.0 | 3.5 | 0 | 270 | 1.0 |
| **Cheesecake snack**, 1 pc.: | | | | | | | |
| bars (*Philadelphia*): | | | | | | | |
| classic | 190 | 2.0 | 20.0 | 11.0 | 15 | 85 | 0 |
| marble brownie | 170 | 3.0 | 20.0 | 9.0 | 25 | 110 | 1.0 |
| strawberry | 180 | 2.0 | 22.0 | 9.0 | 10 | 80 | 0 |
| bites (*Philadelphia*): | | | | | | | |
| strawberry, chocolate | | | | | | | |
| coated | 130 | 1.0 | 15.0 | 7.0 | 10 | 55 | 0 |
| turtle | 130 | 2.0 | 14.0 | 7.0 | 10 | 70 | 0 |

| Food and Measure | cal. | prot. (gms) | carbo. (gms) | fat (gms) | chol. (mgs) | sod. (mgs) | fiber (gms) |
|---|---|---|---|---|---|---|---|
| **Cheesecake snack** *(cont.)* | | | | | | | |
| bites, battered (*El Monterey*): | | | | | | | |
|   dulce de leche ....... | 180 | 3.0 | 21.0 | 9.0 | 20 | 160 | 0 |
|   raspberry .......... | 160 | 2.0 | 23.0 | 7.0 | 15 | 160 | 0 |
| **Cherimoya** (see also "Custard apple"): | | | | | | | |
| (*Frieda's*), diced, 1 cup ............. | 115 | 3.0 | 28.0 | 1.0 | 0 | 6 | 4.0 |
| 1 medium, 1.9 lb. ...... | 515 | 7.1 | 131.3 | 2.2 | 0 | n.a. | 13.1 |
| **Cherry**, fresh: | | | | | | | |
| (*Chiquita*), 1 cup ....... | 87 | 1.0 | 22.0 | 0 | 0 | 0 | 3.0 |
| (*Dole*), 1 cup .......... | 90 | 1.0 | 22.0 | 0 | 0 | 0 | 3.0 |
| sour, red, ½ cup: | | | | | | | |
|   w/pits ............. | 26 | .5 | 6.3 | .2 | 0 | 2 | .6 |
|   red, pitted .......... | 39 | .8 | 9.4 | .2 | 0 | 3 | .9 |
| sweet, w/pits, ½ cup .... | 52 | .9 | 12.0 | .7 | 0 | 1 | 1.7 |
| sweet, 10 medium ...... | 49 | .8 | 11.3 | .7 | 0 | <1 | 1.6 |
| **Cherry, can/jar**, pitted, ½ cup, except as noted: | | | | | | | |
| dark, sweet: | | | | | | | |
|   in heavy syrup (*Del Monte*) .......... | 100 | <1.0 | 24.0 | 0 | 0 | 10 | <1.0 |
|   in extra heavy syrup (*S&W*) .......... | 140 | 1.0 | 34.0 | 0 | 0 | 10 | 1.0 |
| flavored, all varieties (*Roland*), .2-oz. pc. ... | 10 | 0 | 2.0 | 0 | 0 | 0 | 0 |
| jubilee dessert topping (*Lucky Leaf/ Musselman's*), ¼ cup | 80 | 0 | 20.0 | 0 | 0 | 10 | 1.0 |
| red, tart, in water (*Lucky Leaf/ Musselman's*) ..... | 50 | 0 | 12.0 | 0 | 0 | 10 | 1.0 |
| sour, w/liquid: | | | | | | | |
|   in light syrup ....... | 95 | .9 | 24.3 | .1 | 0 | 9 | 1.0 |
|   in heavy syrup ...... | 116 | .9 | 29.8 | .1 | 0 | 9 | 1.0 |
| sweet, w/liquid: | | | | | | | |
|   in juice ............. | 68 | 1.1 | 17.3 | <.1 | 0 | 4 | 1.9 |
|   in light syrup ....... | 84 | .8 | 21.8 | .2 | 0 | 4 | 1.9 |
| **Cherry, dried**: | | | | | | | |
| (*Mariani*), ¼ cup, 1.4 oz. . | 130 | 1.0 | 31.0 | 0 | 0 | 5 | 2.0 |
| (*Roland*), ⅓ cup ....... | 140 | 1.0 | 34.0 | 0 | 0 | 10 | 2.0 |
| (*Sunsweet*), ¼ cup, 1.4 oz. | 100 | 1.0 | 30.0 | 0 | 0 | 5 | 2.0 |

| Food and Measure | cal. | prot. (gms) | carbo. (gms) | fat (gms) | chol. (mgs) | sod. (mgs) | fiber (gms) |
|---|---|---|---|---|---|---|---|
| bing (*Frieda's*), ⅓ cup, 1.4 oz. . . . . . . . . . . . | 140 | 2.0 | 32.0 | 0 | 0 | 5 | 3.0 |
| sour/tart: | | | | | | | |
| (*Eden* Montmorency), ¼ cup, 1.6 oz. . . . . | 140 | 1.0 | 36.0 | 0 | 0 | 15 | 3.0 |
| (*Frieda's*), ⅓ cup, 1.4 oz. . . . . . . . . . | 140 | 3.0 | 31.0 | 0 | 0 | 0 | 4.0 |
| (*Roland* Amarena), 2 pcs., .2 oz. . . . . . | 15 | 0 | 4.0 | 0 | 0 | 0 | 0 |
| **Cherry, frozen:** | | | | | | | |
| dark sweet (*Dole*), 1 cup . . . . . . . . . . . | 90 | 2.0 | 22.0 | 0 | 0 | 0 | 3.0 |
| sweet (*Cascadian Farm* Organic), 1 cup . . . . . . | 90 | 1.0 | 22.0 | 0 | 0 | 0 | 3.0 |
| unsweetened, ½ cup . . . . | 36 | 7.1 | 8.5 | .3 | 0 | 1 | 1.2 |
| sweetened, ½ cup . . . . . . | 116 | 1.5 | 29.0 | .2 | 0 | 1 | 2.7 |
| **Cherry, West Indian**, see "Acerola" | | | | | | | |
| **Cherry butter**, tart (*Eden* Organic Montmorency), 1 tbsp. . | 35 | 0 | 9.0 | 0 | 0 | 0 | 1.0 |
| **Cherry drink blend:** | | | | | | | |
| (*Minute Maid* Clear Coolers), 6.75 fl. oz. . . . | 100 | 0 | 28.0 | 0 | 0 | 15 | 0 |
| (*Welch's* Burst), 8 fl. oz. . | 130 | 0 | 32.0 | 0 | 0 | 5 | 0 |
| (*Welch's* Tropical), 8 fl. oz. . . . . . . . . . . . | 140 | 0 | 36.0 | 0 | 0 | 5 | 0 |
| berry (*Tropicana Twister* Blast), 8 fl. oz. | 110 | 0 | 27.0 | 0 | 0 | 25 | 0 |
| **Cherry juice**, 8 fl. oz., except as noted: | | | | | | | |
| (*Veryfine* Twisted), 11.5 fl. oz. . . . . . . . . | 190 | 0 | 46.0 | 0 | 0 | 45 | 0 |
| all varieties (*Cherrish*), 11.5 fl. oz. . . . . . . . . | 130 | 2.0 | 32.0 | 0 | 0 | 35 | 0 |
| black (*R.W. Knudsen Just Black Cherry*) . . . | 160 | 2.0 | 36.0 | 0 | 0 | 10 | 0 |
| cider (*R.W. Knudsen*) . . . | 130 | <1.0 | 33.0 | 0 | 0 | 40 | 0 |
| sparkling (*R.W. Knudsen*) . . . . . . . . . . | 120 | <1.0 | 31.0 | 0 | 0 | 20 | 0 |
| tart: | | | | | | | |
| (*Eden* Organic Montmorency) . . . . | 140 | 1.0 | 33.0 | 1.0 | 0 | 30 | 0 |

| Food and Measure | cal. | prot. (gms) | carbo. (gms) | fat (gms) | chol. (mgs) | sod. (mgs) | fiber (gms) |
|---|---|---|---|---|---|---|---|
| **Cherry juice, tart** *(cont.)* | | | | | | | |
| (*R.W. Knudsen Just Tart Cherry*) | 130 | 1.0 | 32.0 | 0 | 0 | 20 | 0 |
| red (*Santa Cruz Organic*) | 120 | 0 | 30.0 | 0 | 0 | 25 | 0 |
| **Cherry juice blend,** black, goji (*Northland*), 8 fl. oz. | 130 | 0 | 32.0 | 0 | 0 | 10 | 0 |
| **Cherry juice concentrate:** | | | | | | | |
| (*Eden* Organic), 2 tbsp. | 110 | 1.0 | 26.0 | 0 | 0 | 20 | 0 |
| black (*R.W. Knudsen*), 8 fl. oz.* | 200 | 2.0 | 47.0 | 0 | 0 | 10 | 0 |
| **Cherry topping,** 2 tbsp.: | | | | | | | |
| (*Smucker's Magic Shell*) | 220 | 2.0 | 16.0 | 16.0 | 5 | 65 | 0 |
| black (*Smucker's*) | 90 | 0 | 23.0 | 0 | 0 | 0 | 0 |
| **Chervil,** dried, 1 tsp. | 1 | .1 | .3 | <.1 | 0 | <1 | .1 |
| **Chestnut, Chinese,** shelled, 1 oz.: | | | | | | | |
| dried | 103 | 1.9 | 22.7 | .5 | 0 | 2 | <1.0 |
| boiled or steamed | 44 | .8 | 9.6 | .2 | 0 | 1 | <1.0 |
| roasted | 68 | 1.3 | 14.9 | .3 | 0 | 1 | <1.0 |
| **Chestnut, European:** | | | | | | | |
| raw, in shell, 1 lb. | 714 | 8.1 | 152.8 | 7.6 | 0 | 9 | 27.2 |
| raw, shelled, w/peel, 1 cup, 13 pcs. | 308 | 3.5 | 66.0 | 3.3 | 0 | 4 | 11.7 |
| dried, peeled, 1 oz. | 105 | 1.4 | 23.3 | 1.1 | 0 | 11 | <2.0 |
| boiled, 1 oz. | 37 | .8 | 7.9 | .4 | 0 | 8 | <1.0 |
| roasted, peeled: | | | | | | | |
| 1 oz. | 70 | .9 | 15.0 | .6 | 0 | 1 | 3.3 |
| 1 cup, 17 kernels | 350 | 4.3 | 75.7 | 3.2 | 0 | 3 | 16.7 |
| **Chestnuts, European,** can/jar: | | | | | | | |
| plain, 4 pcs., 1.1 oz.: | | | | | | | |
| (*Minerve*) | 40 | <1.0 | 9.0 | 0 | 0 | 0 | 2.0 |
| (*Roland*) | 50 | 0 | 11.0 | 0 | 0 | 0 | 2.0 |
| in water (*Roland*) | 30 | 0 | 7.0 | 0 | 0 | 180 | 1.0 |
| cream (*Roland* Crème de Marrons), 2 tbsp. | 80 | 0 | 18.0 | 0 | 0 | 0 | 2.0 |
| puree (*Roland*), 2 tbsp. | 25 | 0 | 6.0 | 0 | 0 | 60 | 2.0 |
| **Chia bran** (*Shiloh Farms*), 2 tsp. | 83 | 5.0 | 0 | 8.0 | 0 | 0 | 10.0 |
| **Chia seeds,** dry: | | | | | | | |
| (*Bob's Red Mill*), 1 tbsp. | 70 | 3.0 | 6.0 | 5.0 | 0 | 0 | 5.0 |
| 1 oz. | 139 | 4.4 | 12.4 | 10.8 | 8 | 5 | 10.7 |

| Food and Measure | cal. | prot. (gms) | carbo. (gms) | fat (gms) | chol. (mgs) | sod. (mgs) | fiber (gms) |
|---|---|---|---|---|---|---|---|
| **Chicken**, fresh, 4 oz., except as noted: | | | | | | | |
| broiler-fryer, roasted: | | | | | | | |
|   w/skin, ½ chicken, 10.5 oz. (15.8 oz. w/bone) | 715 | 81.6 | 0 | 40.7 | 263 | 244 | 0 |
|   w/skin | 271 | 31.0 | 0 | 15.4 | 100 | 93 | 0 |
|   meat only | 215 | 32.8 | 0 | 8.4 | 101 | 98 | 0 |
|   meat only, chopped or diced, 1 cup | 266 | 40.5 | 0 | 10.4 | 125 | 120 | 0 |
|   skin only, 1 oz. | 129 | 5.8 | 0 | 11.5 | 24 | 18 | 0 |
|   dark meat only | 232 | 31.0 | 0 | 11.0 | 105 | 105 | 0 |
|   light meat only | 196 | 35.1 | 0 | 5.1 | 96 | 87 | 0 |
|   breast, w/skin, ½ breast, 3½ oz. (8½ oz. w/bone) | 193 | 29.2 | 0 | 7.6 | 83 | 69 | 0 |
|   drumstick, w/skin, 1.8 oz. (2.9 oz. w/bone) | 112 | 14.1 | 0 | 5.8 | 48 | 47 | 0 |
|   leg, w/skin (5.7 oz. w/bone) | 265 | 29.6 | 0 | 15.4 | 105 | 99 | 0 |
|   thigh, w/skin, 2.2 oz. (2.9 oz. w/bone) | 153 | 15.5 | 0 | 9.6 | 58 | 52 | 0 |
|   wing, w/skin, 1.2 oz. (2.3 oz. w/bone) | 99 | 9.1 | 0 | 6.6 | 29 | 28 | 0 |
| capon, roasted, w/skin: | | | | | | | |
|   ½ capon, 1.4 lbs. (2 lbs. w/bone) | 1457 | 184.5 | 0 | 74.2 | 549 | 313 | 0 |
|   w/skin | 260 | 32.8 | 0 | 13.2 | 98 | 56 | 0 |
| ground, see "Chicken, ground" | | | | | | | |
| roaster, roasted: | | | | | | | |
|   w/skin, ½ chicken, 1 lb. (1½ lbs. w/bone) | 1071 | 115.0 | 0 | 64.3 | 365 | 349 | 0 |
|   meat w/skin | 253 | 27.2 | 0 | 15.2 | 86 | 83 | 0 |
| stewing, stewed: | | | | | | | |
|   w/skin, ½ chicken, 9.2 oz. (13½ oz. w/bone) | 744 | 70.2 | 0 | 49.2 | 205 | 190 | 0 |
|   meat w/skin | 323 | 30.5 | 0 | 21.4 | 90 | 83 | 0 |
|   meat only | 269 | 34.5 | 0 | 13.5 | 94 | 88 | 0 |
|   meat only, chopped or diced, 1 cup | 332 | 42.6 | 0 | 16.6 | 117 | 109 | 0 |

| Food and Measure | cal. | prot. (gms) | carbo. (gms) | fat (gms) | chol. (mgs) | sod. (mgs) | fiber (gms) |
|---|---|---|---|---|---|---|---|
| **Chicken, can/pouch,** | | | | | | | |
| chunk, 2 oz.: | | | | | | | |
| (*Hormel*) . . . . . . . . . . . . | 70 | 10.0 | 0 | 3.0 | 45 | 250 | 0 |
| (*Tyson*) . . . . . . . . . . . . . | 60 | 10.0 | 0 | 2.5 | 30 | 200 | 0 |
| breast: | | | | | | | |
| (*Bumble Bee*) . . . . . . . | 70 | 13.0 | 1.0 | 1.0 | 35 | 140 | 0 |
| (*Hormel*) . . . . . . . . . . | 60 | 12.0 | 0 | 1.5 | 40 | 250 | 0 |
| (*Hormel* No Salt) . . . . | 50 | 11.0 | 0 | 1.0 | 40 | 70 | 0 |
| (*Swanson*) . . . . . . . . . | 50 | 9.0 | 1.0 | 1.0 | 25 | 260 | 0 |
| (*Tyson*) . . . . . . . . . . . . | 60 | 13.0 | 0 | 1.0 | 30 | 200 | 0 |
| (*Tyson* Pouch) . . . . . . | 70 | 14.0 | 0 | 1.5 | 45 | 210 | 0 |
| breast, seasoned (*Bumble Bee Prime Fillet*), 4-oz. pouch: | | | | | | | |
| barbecue sauce . . . . . . | 170 | 29.0 | 10.0 | 1.5 | 80 | 740 | 0 |
| garlic and herbs . . . . . | 110 | 24.0 | 1.0 | 1.5 | 75 | 490 | 0 |
| Southwest . . . . . . . . . | 120 | 25.0 | 3.0 | 1.5 | 60 | 670 | 0 |
| white (*Valley Fresh*) . . . . . | 70 | 12.0 | 0 | 2.0 | 40 | 240 | 0 |
| white and dark: | | | | | | | |
| (*Swanson*) . . . . . . . . . | 60 | 10.0 | 0 | 2.0 | 30 | 250 | 0 |
| (*Valley Fresh*) . . . . . . | 80 | 12.0 | 0 | 3.5 | 50 | 180 | 0 |
| **Chicken, frozen/chilled, raw**, 4 oz., except as noted: | | | | | | | |
| whole, seasoned: | | | | | | | |
| (*Perdue* Oven Ready Roaster) . . . . . . . . | 210 | 17.0 | 1.0 | 15.0 | 70 | 430 | 0 |
| garlic herb (*Empire Kosher*) . . . . . . . . . . | 230 | 23.0 | 2.0 | 10.0 | 70 | 470 | 0 |
| marinated (*Pilgrim's*) . | 200 | 18.0 | 0 | 14.0 | 70 | 210 | 0 |
| breast, bone-in, seasoned (*Perdue* Oven Ready) . . . . . . . . | 140 | 20.0 | 1.0 | 7.0 | 75 | 410 | 0 |
| breast, bone/skinless (*Perdue Perfect Portions*), 4.8-oz. pc.: | | | | | | | |
| regular . . . . . . . . . . . | 130 | 29.0 | 0 | 1.5 | 80 | 350 | 0 |
| all natural . . . . . . . . . | 140 | 32.0 | 0 | 1.5 | 90 | 60 | 0 |
| garlic, roasted, w/wine | 110 | 29.0 | 1.0 | 1.5 | 80 | 520 | 0 |
| herb and pepper . . . . . | 140 | 29.0 | 0 | 1.5 | 80 | 330 | 0 |
| Italian style . . . . . . . . | 130 | 27.0 | 2.0 | 1.5 | 105 | 480 | 0 |
| breast, breaded (*Bell & Evans*), 5.25-oz. pc.: | | | | | | | |
| plain . . . . . . . . . . . . . | 260 | 25.0 | 21.0 | 8.0 | 45 | 560 | 2.0 |

| Food and Measure | cal. | prot. (gms) | carbo. (gms) | fat (gms) | chol. (mgs) | sod. (mgs) | fiber (gms) |
|---|---|---|---|---|---|---|---|
| gluten free ......... | 270 | 27.0 | 19.0 | 9.0 | 55 | 530 | 3.0 |
| garlic Parmesan ..... | 270 | 25.0 | 16.0 | 12.0 | 60 | 640 | 2.0 |
| garlic Parmesan, gluten free ....... | 280 | 28.0 | 15.0 | 12.0 | 70 | 600 | 2.0 |
| breast chunks, breaded (*Pilgrim's* Blazin') .... | 170 | 19.0 | 15.0 | 3.5 | 40 | 970 | 1.0 |
| breast tenders, breaded: | | | | | | | |
| (*Bell & Evans*) ....... | 210 | 20.0 | 12.0 | 10.0 | 40 | 490 | 2.0 |
| (*Bell & Evans* Gluten Free) ............ | 180 | 19.0 | 12.0 | 6.0 | 45 | 440 | 1.0 |
| coconut (*Bell & Evans*) .......... | 210 | 19.0 | 22.0 | 5.0 | 45 | 360 | 2.0 |
| fingers, breaded, 1 pc.: | | | | | | | |
| (*Barber*), 3.2 oz. ..... | 170 | 13.0 | 14.0 | 7.0 | 25 | 620 | <1.0 |
| Italian (*Barber*), 3.1 oz. .......... | 170 | 13.0 | 13.0 | 8.0 | 25 | 640 | <1.0 |
| nuggets: | | | | | | | |
| (*Barber*), 5 pcs. ..... | 310 | 15.0 | 16.0 | 21.0 | 45 | 450 | <1.0 |
| (*Bell & Evans*) ....... | 220 | 21.0 | 13.0 | 9.0 | 45 | 360 | 1.0 |
| (*Bell & Evans* Gluten Free) ...... | 180 | 19.0 | 12.0 | 6.0 | 45 | 440 | 1.0 |
| (*Empire Kosher*), 3 oz. | 140 | 16.0 | 7.0 | 5.0 | 40 | 340 | 0 |
| patties, breaded: | | | | | | | |
| (*Bell & Evans*) ...... | 240 | 19.0 | 13.0 | 12.0 | 55 | 390 | 2.0 |
| (*Bell & Evans* Gluten Free) ...... | 230 | 19.0 | 13.0 | 12.0 | 55 | 390 | 2.0 |
| Italian (*Bell & Evans* Gluten Free) ...... | 270 | 18.0 | 15.0 | 16.0 | 55 | 610 | 2.0 |
| w/mozzarella (*Bell & Evans*) ...... | 270 | 18.0 | 14.0 | 16.0 | 55 | 540 | 1.0 |
| strips, breast, breaded: | | | | | | | |
| (*Barber*), 3.4-oz. pc. .. | 170 | 14.0 | 14.0 | 7.0 | 30 | 630 | <1.0 |
| (*Pilgrim's*), 4.4-oz. pc. | 220 | 19.0 | 16.0 | 9.0 | 45 | 650 | .5 |
| (*Pilgrim's* Blazin'), 2 pcs., 3.3 oz. .... | 170 | 15.0 | 13.0 | 7.0 | 35 | 810 | 0 |
| Southern (*Pilgrim's*) .. | 170 | 15.0 | 13.0 | 7.0 | 35 | 810 | 0 |
| stuffed (*Barber*), 5-oz. pc.: | | | | | | | |
| asparagus/cheese .... | 250 | 21.0 | 14.0 | 13.0 | 55 | 320 | 1.0 |
| broccoli/cheese ..... | 230 | 19.0 | 14.0 | 11.0 | 45 | 400 | 1.0 |
| broccoli/cheese, Seasoned Selects .. | 180 | 24.0 | 4.0 | 9.0 | 65 | 460 | <1.0 |
| Cordon Bleu ........ | 250 | 24.0 | 11.0 | 12.0 | 65 | 490 | <1.0 |
| Cordon Bleu, Seasoned Selects .. | 220 | 29.0 | 3.0 | 11.0 | 80 | 570 | 0 |

| Food and Measure | cal. | prot. (gms) | carbo. (gms) | fat (gms) | chol. (mgs) | sod. (mgs) | fiber (gms) |
|---|---|---|---|---|---|---|---|
| **Chicken, frozen/chilled, raw, stuffed** *(cont.)* | | | | | | | |
| crème brie/apple ..... | 290 | 20.0 | 21.0 | 14.0 | 55 | 590 | <1.0 |
| homestyle .......... | 240 | 19.0 | 15.0 | 12.0 | 45 | 480 | <1.0 |
| Kiev .............. | 370 | 20.0 | 13.0 | 27.0 | 95 | 480 | <1.0 |
| Parmesan .......... | 250 | 19.0 | 17.0 | 12.0 | 45 | 440 | <1.0 |
| w/scallops/lobster ... | 270 | 21.0 | 17.0 | 13.0 | 55 | 450 | <1.0 |
| spinach Florentine, Seasoned Selects .. | 210 | 24.0 | 7.0 | 10.0 | 60 | 570 | <1.0 |
| stuffed (*Barber* Fit & Flavorful), 4-oz. pc.: | | | | | | | |
| broccoli/cheese ..... | 190 | 17.0 | 9.0 | 9.0 | 35 | 270 | <1.0 |
| Cordon Bleu ........ | 210 | 20.0 | 9.0 | 11.0 | 50 | 340 | <1.0 |
| stuffed (*Barber* Premium), 6-oz. pc.: | | | | | | | |
| broccoli/cheese ..... | 300 | 24.0 | 16.0 | 16.0 | 60 | 400 | 1.0 |
| Cordon Bleu ........ | 320 | 29.0 | 16.0 | 16.0 | 75 | 500 | <1.0 |
| Kiev .............. | 450 | 24.0 | 18.0 | 32.0 | 95 | 460 | <1.0 |
| homestyle .......... | 360 | 22.0 | 26.0 | 19.0 | 50 | 470 | 1.0 |
| long grain/wild rice ... | 300 | 22.0 | 20.0 | 15.0 | 50 | 390 | <1.0 |
| Parmesan .......... | 290 | 25.0 | 17.0 | 15.0 | 60 | 400 | <1.0 |
| tenderloin or tenders, see "breast" above | | | | | | | |
| wings, breaded (*Pilgrim's Blazin'*), 3 pcs. ...... | 270 | 13.0 | 13.0 | 18.0 | 45 | 1070 | 0 |
| **Chicken, frozen/chilled, cooked** (see also "Chicken entree"), 3 oz., except as noted: | | | | | | | |
| whole, barbecue (*Empire Kosher*), 5 oz. | 230 | 22.0 | 8.0 | 12.0 | 85 | 780 | 0 |
| bites, breaded (*Foster Farms*): | | | | | | | |
| bourbon ........... | 190 | 16.0 | 17.0 | 7.0 | 30 | 810 | 0 |
| orange ............ | 190 | 15.0 | 12.0 | 9.0 | 35 | 430 | 0 |
| bites, breast, breaded (*Perdue*), 12 pcs. .... | 190 | 10.0 | 14.0 | 12.0 | 30 | 580 | 0 |
| bites, in pastry, Buffalo (*Pillsbury* Savorings), 4 pcs., 2.8 oz. ....... | 230 | 6.0 | 21.0 | 13.0 | 15 | 590 | 0 |
| breast, diced, roasted (*Tyson Grilled & Ready*) | 110 | 19.0 | 2.0 | 2.5 | 60 | 370 | 1.0 |
| breast, grilled: | | | | | | | |
| (*Bell & Evans*), 2.75 oz. ......... | 90 | 21.0 | 1.0 | .5 | 50 | 320 | 0 |

| Food and Measure | cal. | prot. (gms) | carbo. (gms) | fat (gms) | chol. (mgs) | sod. (mgs) | fiber (gms) |
|---|---|---|---|---|---|---|---|
| Buffalo (*Bell & Evans*) .......... | 110 | 24.0 | 0 | 1.0 | 65 | 340 | 0 |
| honey barbecue (*Bell & Evans*), 3.25 oz. . | 120 | 22.0 | 6.0 | 1.0 | 55 | 170 | 0 |
| breast, shredded, chipotle (*Hormel*), 5 oz. | 160 | 20.0 | 5.0 | 7.0 | 90 | 750 | 0 |
| breast chunks, glazed (*Perdue*): | | | | | | | |
| barbecue ........... | 190 | 11.0 | 17.0 | 8.0 | 25 | 630 | 0 |
| bourbon ........... | 180 | 11.0 | 20.0 | 6.0 | 25 | 490 | 0 |
| General Tso's ....... | 170 | 12.0 | 17.0 | 6.0 | 25 | 760 | 0 |
| honey barbecue ..... | 160 | 12.0 | 15.0 | 7.0 | 30 | 570 | 0 |
| honey Dijon ........ | 220 | 13.0 | 15.0 | 13.0 | 35 | 510 | 0 |
| honey mustard ...... | 140 | 11.0 | 19.0 | 3.0 | 25 | 630 | 0 |
| sweet and spicy Asian style, 3.2 oz. ...... | 190 | 11.0 | 23.0 | 6.0 | 30 | 530 | 0 |
| breast chunks, w/sauce (*Tyson Any'tizers*), chicken, 3 pcs. ...... | 170 | 11.0 | 19.0 | 6.0 | 25 | 580 | 0 |
| sauce, 2 tbsp.: | | | | | | | |
| General Tso's ..... | 70 | 1.0 | 16.0 | .5 | 0 | 180 | 0 |
| spicy sweet ...... | 90 | 0 | 23.0 | 0 | 0 | 30 | 0 |
| breast cutlet, breaded (*Perdue*): | | | | | | | |
| original ........... | 200 | 10.0 | 13.0 | 13.0 | 45 | 450 | 0 |
| baked, homestyle .... | 160 | 12.0 | 12.0 | 7.0 | 50 | 470 | 0 |
| baked, Italian ....... | 160 | 13.0 | 10.0 | 8.0 | 35 | 520 | 0 |
| breast fillet: | | | | | | | |
| (*Tyson Grilled & Ready*), 3.5-oz. pc. . | 110 | 24.0 | 1.0 | 1.5 | 60 | 230 | 0 |
| Alfredo sauce (*Hormel*), 5.7-oz. pc. | 200 | 20.0 | 3.0 | 12.0 | 90 | 1090 | 0 |
| breaded (*Tyson*), 4.6-oz. pc. ....... | 240 | 19.0 | 20.0 | 9.0 | 45 | 680 | 0 |
| w/gravy (*Hormel*), 5.7-oz. pc. ....... | 120 | 20.0 | 4.0 | 3.0 | 55 | 1070 | 0 |
| chunks w/sauce (*Simply Simmered*), 5 oz.: | | | | | | | |
| garlic ............. | 140 | 16.0 | 10.0 | 4.0 | 15 | 750 | 3.0 |
| General Tso's ....... | 157 | 18.0 | 23.0 | 3.0 | 20 | 750 | 1.0 |
| sesame ............ | 140 | 18.0 | 10.0 | 3.0 | 25 | 610 | 1.0 |
| sweet and sour ...... | 180 | 15.0 | 26.0 | 2.5 | 10 | 750 | 5.0 |
| Szechuan .......... | 180 | 19.0 | 16.0 | 4.5 | 10 | 810 | 5.0 |
| teriyaki ............ | 190 | 16.0 | 23.0 | 3.5 | 20 | 950 | 1.0 |

| Food and Measure | cal. | prot. (gms) | carbo. (gms) | fat (gms) | chol. (mgs) | sod. (mgs) | fiber (gms) |
|---|---|---|---|---|---|---|---|
| **Chicken, frozen/chilled, cooked** *(cont.)* | | | | | | | |
| cutlet or tenderloin, breaded (*Foster Farms*) ............ | 180 | 13.0 | 14.0 | 8.0 | 35 | 490 | 0 |
| cuts (*Oscar Mayer*): | | | | | | | |
| honey-roasted ...... | 130 | 22.0 | 3.0 | 2.5 | 60 | 780 | 0 |
| oven-roasted ....... | 130 | 22.0 | 1.0 | 2.5 | 60 | 790 | 0 |
| drumstick, breaded (*Banquet*) .......... | 200 | 16.0 | 8.0 | 12.0 | 65 | 700 | <1.0 |
| fried (*Banquet*), 4.25-oz. pc.: | | | | | | | |
| country ............ | 350 | 24.0 | 11.0 | 24.0 | 70 | 1180 | 1.0 |
| hot and spicy ....... | 340 | 25.0 | 12.0 | 22.0 | 70 | 1380 | 1.0 |
| original ............ | 330 | 24.0 | 12.0 | 21.0 | 75 | 890 | <1.0 |
| skinless ........... | 360 | 25.0 | 13.0 | 23.0 | 65 | 720 | 1.0 |
| Southern ........... | 360 | 22.0 | 14.0 | 24.0 | 65 | 1050 | 2.0 |
| nuggets, breast: | | | | | | | |
| (*Applegate Farms*), 7 pcs., 3.1 oz. .... | 180 | 12.0 | 12.0 | 9.0 | 35 | 210 | 0 |
| (*Applegate Farms* Gluten Free), 7 pcs., 3.1 oz. .... | 170 | 12.0 | 11.0 | 9.0 | 35 | 350 | 0 |
| (*Banquet*), 6 pcs. .... | 270 | 12.0 | 12.0 | 16.0 | 20 | 540 | 1.0 |
| (*Foster Farms*), 4 pcs., 2.8 oz. .......... | 160 | 13.0 | 9.0 | 9.0 | 25 | 360 | 1.0 |
| (*Foster Farms* Whole Grain), 4 pcs. ...... | 170 | 13.0 | 12.0 | 9.0 | 30 | 440 | 4.0 |
| (*Health is Wealth* Whole Wheat), 4 pcs. ............. | 170 | 13.0 | 12.0 | 9.0 | 30 | 440 | 4.0 |
| (*Perdue* Fresh), 5 pcs. | 200 | 10.0 | 13.0 | 13.0 | 45 | 450 | 0 |
| (*Perdue* Frozen Whole Grain), 5 pcs., 3.1 oz. | 210 | 12.0 | 13.0 | 13.0 | 35 | 480 | 0 |
| (*Pilgrim's*), 5 pcs., 3.3 oz. .......... | 170 | 15.0 | 10.0 | 8.0 | 35 | 480 | 0 |
| (*Tyson*), 5 pcs., 3.2 oz. | 270 | 14.0 | 15.0 | 17.0 | 40 | 470 | 0 |
| baked (*Perdue* Whole Grain), 4 pcs., 2.6 oz. | 170 | 11.0 | 14.0 | 7.0 | 30 | 420 | 0 |
| w/broccoli, cheddar (*Alexia*), 6 pcs. .... | 200 | 11.0 | 13.0 | 12.0 | 30 | 420 | >1.0 |
| w/cheese (*Perdue*), 5 pcs. ............. | 210 | 10.0 | 12.0 | 14.0 | 50 | 460 | 0 |
| Southern (*Tyson*), 6 pcs. ............ | 270 | 10.0 | 11.0 | 21.0 | 45 | 570 | 1.0 |

| Food and Measure | cal. | prot. (gms) | carbo. (gms) | fat (gms) | chol. (mgs) | sod. (mgs) | fiber (gms) |
|---|---|---|---|---|---|---|---|
| patties, breaded, 1 pc.: | | | | | | | |
| (*Applegate Farms*) ... | 180 | 12.0 | 12.0 | 9.0 | 35 | 210 | 0 |
| (*Banquet*), 2.4 oz. .... | 200 | 9.0 | 11.0 | 13.0 | 15 | 340 | 1.0 |
| (*Foster Farms*), 4 oz. . | 240 | 16.0 | 18.0 | 12.0 | 40 | 490 | 0 |
| (*Health is Wealth* Whole Wheat) .... | 170 | 13.0 | 11.0 | 9.0 | 30 | 440 | 4.0 |
| (*Perdue*), 2.9 oz. ...... | 230 | 18.0 | 14.0 | 12.0 | 75 | 750 | 0 |
| (*Tyson*), 2.6 oz. ...... | 180 | 10.0 | 12.0 | 11.0 | 25 | 390 | 1.0 |
| popcorn, breaded: | | | | | | | |
| (*Foster Farms*) ...... | 190 | 14.0 | 13.0 | 9.0 | 35 | 400 | 0 |
| (*Perdue* Chunks) ..... | 180 | 12.0 | 13.0 | 9.0 | 35 | 370 | 0 |
| (*Tyson Any'tizers Popcorn Chicken Bites*), 7 pcs. ..... | 180 | 13.0 | 11.0 | 9.0 | 30 | 560 | 0 |
| Buffalo (*Tyson Any'tizers Popcorn Chicken Bites*), 8 pcs. ..... | 190 | 15.0 | 12.0 | 9.0 | 40 | 960 | 1.0 |
| rolls, Buffalo, in crust (*Michelina's Lean Gourmet*), 11 pcs. ... | 190 | 10.0 | 23.0 | 7.0 | 10 | 480 | 1.0 |
| shredded, barbecue (*Lloyd's*), ¼ cup: | | | | | | | |
| honey hickory ....... | 80 | 6.0 | 10.0 | 2.0 | 20 | 450 | 0 |
| original sauce ....... | 80 | 6.0 | 9.0 | 2.0 | 15 | 360 | 0 |
| strips: | | | | | | | |
| (*Tyson Grilled & & Ready*) ........ | 110 | 17.0 | 1.0 | 4.0 | 55 | 540 | 0 |
| fajita (*Tyson Grilled & Ready*) ........ | 100 | 19.0 | 2.0 | 2.0 | 60 | 460 | 0 |
| strips, breast: | | | | | | | |
| grilled (*Foster Farms*) . | 100 | 19.0 | 2.0 | 1.5 | 25 | 550 | 0 |
| grilled (*Foster Farms* Chilled) .......... | 110 | 19.0 | 2.0 | 2.5 | 45 | 550 | 0 |
| grilled (*Oscar Mayer*) . | 110 | 19.0 | 1.0 | 2.5 | 55 | 770 | 0 |
| grilled (*Oscar Mayer Deli Fresh*) ....... | 100 | 22.0 | 0 | 1.5 | 55 | 690 | 0 |
| grilled (*Perdue*) ...... | 100 | 18.0 | 1.0 | 2.0 | 45 | 470 | 0 |
| grilled (*Tyson Grilled & Ready*) ........ | 100 | 21.0 | 1.0 | 2.0 | 50 | 470 | 0 |
| honey-roasted (*Foster Farms*) .......... | 130 | 22.0 | 6.0 | 1.5 | 50 | 500 | 0 |
| honey-roasted (*Oscar Mayer*) .......... | 110 | 21.0 | 1.0 | 1.0 | 60 | 660 | 0 |

| Food and Measure | cal. | prot. (gms) | carbo. (gms) | fat (gms) | chol. (mgs) | sod. (mgs) | fiber (gms) |
|---|---|---|---|---|---|---|---|
| **Chicken, frozen/chilled, cooked, strips, breast** *(cont.)* | | | | | | | |
| oven-roasted (*Oscar Mayer*) . . . . . . . . . | 100 | 23.0 | 0 | 1.5 | 60 | 670 | 0 |
| Southwest (*Foster Farms*) . . . . . . . . . . | 110 | 22.0 | 1.0 | 1.5 | 50 | 500 | 0 |
| Southwest (*Oscar Mayer*) . . . . . . . . . | 110 | 19.0 | 1.0 | 3.5 | 55 | 770 | 0 |
| Southwest (*Oscar Mayer Deli Fresh*) . . | 110 | 22.0 | 0 | 1.5 | 55 | 690 | 0 |
| Southwest (*Tyson Grilled & Ready*) . . . | 120 | 19.0 | 3.0 | 3.0 | 60 | 310 | 0 |
| strips, breast, breaded: | | | | | | | |
| (*Applegate Farms* Organic) . . . . . . . . | 160 | 12.0 | 11.0 | 7.0 | 35 | 180 | 0 |
| (*Banquet* Breast) . . . . . | 190 | 12.0 | 14.0 | 10.0 | 15 | 500 | 2.0 |
| (*Perdue* Homestyle), 2 pcs., 3.2 oz. . . . . | 170 | 18.0 | 13.0 | 9.0 | 35 | 550 | 0 |
| (*Perdue* Whole Grain) . | 160 | 15.0 | 13.0 | 6.0 | 35 | 470 | 0 |
| Buffalo (*Foster Farms*) | 190 | 14.0 | 15.0 | 8.0 | 30 | 1100 | 0 |
| Buffalo (*Perdue*) . . . . . | 140 | 11.0 | 12.0 | 6.0 | 25 | 860 | 0 |
| crispy (*Foster Farms*) . | 200 | 18.0 | 14.0 | 8.0 | 35 | 790 | 0 |
| crispy (*Tyson*) . . . . . . . | 190 | 15.0 | 12.0 | 9.0 | 30 | 480 | 1.0 |
| strips, breast, breaded, 2.6 oz.: | | | | | | | |
| (*Perdue*), 2 pcs. . . . . . . | 160 | 9.0 | 12.0 | 10.0 | 25 | 500 | 0 |
| (*Perdue* Whole Grain), 4 pcs. . . . . . | 170 | 11.0 | 14.0 | 7.0 | 30 | 420 | 0 |
| strips, carved breast (*Perdue Short Cuts*), ½ cup, 2.5 oz.: | | | | | | | |
| grilled, 9-oz. pkg. . . . . | 100 | 16.0 | 1.0 | 2.0 | 60 | 380 | 0 |
| grilled, 24-oz. pkg. . . . | 90 | 16.0 | 1.0 | 2.0 | 40 | 510 | 0 |
| grilled, 27-oz. pkg. . . . | 90 | 16.0 | 1.0 | 2.0 | 60 | 460 | 0 |
| Italian, grilled . . . . . . . | 100 | 17.0 | 2.0 | 2.0 | 75 | 480 | 0 |
| garlic, roasted . . . . . . . | 110 | 19.0 | 3.0 | 2.5 | 45 | 450 | 0 |
| honey-roasted . . . . . . | 90 | 17.0 | 2.0 | 2.0 | 55 | 440 | 0 |
| roasted, 9-oz. pkg. . . . | 90 | 16.0 | 1.0 | 2.0 | 60 | 460 | 0 |
| roasted, 24-oz. pkg. . . | 90 | 16.0 | 1.0 | 2.0 | 60 | 380 | 0 |
| Southwest . . . . . . . . . | 90 | 17.0 | 2.0 | 2.0 | 55 | 460 | 0 |
| stuffed (*Barber*), 5-oz. pc.: | | | | | | | |
| asparagus/cheese . . . . | 290 | 23.0 | 15.0 | 16.0 | 55 | 320 | 1.0 |
| broccoli/cheese . . . . . | 260 | 20.0 | 16.0 | 13.0 | 85 | 450 | 1.0 |
| broccoli/cheese/ham . | 280 | 22.0 | 15.0 | 15.0 | 55 | 540 | 1.0 |

| Food and Measure | cal. | prot. (gms) | carbo. (gms) | fat (gms) | chol. (mgs) | sod. (mgs) | fiber (gms) |
|---|---|---|---|---|---|---|---|
| Cordon Bleu ........ | 280 | 24.0 | 14.0 | 14.0 | 65 | 550 | <1.0 |
| Kiev .............. | 360 | 22.0 | 14.0 | 25.0 | 90 | 550 | <1.0 |
| Parmesan .......... | 290 | 22.0 | 19.0 | 14.0 | 55 | 530 | 1.0 |
| stuffed, mini (*Tyson Any'tizers*), 3 pcs.: | | | | | | | |
| Cordon Bleu ........ | 180 | 13.0 | 9.0 | 10.0 | 35 | 490 | 0 |
| pepperoni .......... | 200 | 15.0 | 10.0 | 11.0 | 40 | 420 | 0 |
| tenderloin, breaded, baked (*Perdue*) ...... | 160 | 13.0 | 14.0 | 6.0 | 35 | 490 | 0 |
| tenders, breast, breaded: | | | | | | | |
| (*Health is Wealth Whole Wheat*) .... | 170 | 13.0 | 11.0 | 9.0 | 30 | 440 | 4.0 |
| (*Perdue* Frozen), 3 pcs., 3.5 oz. .... | 240 | 13.0 | 15.0 | 15.0 | 45 | 480 | 0 |
| (*Perdue* Whole Grain), 3 pcs., 3.2 oz. .... | 220 | 12.0 | 15.0 | 12.0 | 35 | 480 | 0 |
| Buffalo (*Banquet*), 5 pcs. ........... | 220 | 12.0 | 15.0 | 13.0 | 15 | 330 | 2.0 |
| Southern (*Banquet*), 5 pcs. ........... | 220 | 12.0 | 15.0 | 12.0 | 15 | 360 | 0 |
| wings: | | | | | | | |
| Buffalo (*Bell & Evans*), 3 pcs. .... | 170 | 19.0 | 0 | 10.0 | 110 | 350 | 0 |
| Buffalo (*Perdue*) ..... | 180 | 15.0 | 1.0 | 12.0 | 60 | 550 | 0 |
| chipotle (*Foster Farms*), 4 pcs. .... | 190 | 15.0 | 1.0 | 14.0 | 80 | 430 | 0 |
| honey barbecue (*Bell & Evans*), 3 pcs. ... | 160 | 17.0 | 6.0 | 8.0 | 80 | 240 | 0 |
| honey barbecue (*Foster Farms*), 4 pcs. | 170 | 13.0 | 5.0 | 10.0 | 50 | 390 | 0 |
| honey barbecue (*Perdue*) ......... | 180 | 17.0 | 3.0 | 11.0 | 60 | 420 | 0 |
| hot and spicy (*Foster Farms*), 4 pcs. .... | 170 | 14.0 | 1.0 | 13.0 | 55 | 460 | 1.0 |
| hot and spicy (*Tyson Any'tizers*), 3 pcs. . | 220 | 20.0 | 1.0 | 15.0 | 110 | 560 | 0 |
| wings, breaded: | | | | | | | |
| (*Pilgrim's Pride Wing Dings*), 4 pcs. ..... | 210 | 13.0 | 9.0 | 13.0 | 50 | 520 | 0 |
| (*Pilgrim's Pride Wing Zings*), 4 pcs. ..... | 200 | 12.0 | 8.0 | 12.0 | 45 | 550 | 0 |
| Buffalo (*Pilgrim's Pride*), 5 pcs. ........... | 220 | 19.0 | 4.0 | 15.0 | 70 | 820 | 0 |

| Food and Measure | cal. | prot. (gms) | carbo. (gms) | fat (gms) | chol. (mgs) | sod. (mgs) | fiber (gms) |
|---|---|---|---|---|---|---|---|
| **Chicken, frozen/chilled, cooked** *(cont.)* | | | | | | | |
| Buffalo, boneless (*Tyson Any'tizers*), 3 pcs. . . . . . . . . . . . | 150 | 12.0 | 8.0 | 7.0 | 30 | 680 | 0 |
| honey barbecue (*Banquet*) . . . . . . . . | 270 | 16.0 | 11.0 | 18.0 | 50 | 540 | 1.0 |
| honey barbecue, boneless (*Tyson Any'tizers*), 3 pcs. . | 200 | 11.0 | 20.0 | 8.0 | 25 | 450 | 0 |
| honey barbecue, boneless (*Tyson Wyngs*), 3 pcs. . . . . | 210 | 11.0 | 13.0 | 12.0 | 25 | 400 | 0 |
| hot/spicy (*Banquet*) . . | 270 | 15.0 | 11.0 | 18.0 | 55 | 470 | 1.0 |
| orange peel (*Margaritaville*) . . . . | 170 | 11.0 | 3.0 | 11.0 | 75 | 510 | 0 |
| sauce, 2 tbsp. . . . . . . | 50 | 0 | 12.0 | 0 | 0 | 105 | 0 |
| **Chicken, ground,** raw, 4 oz.: | | | | | | | |
| (*Empire Kosher*) . . . . . . . | 220 | 19.0 | 0 | 16.0 | 85 | 200 | 0 |
| breast (*Barber*) . . . . . . . . | 140 | 23.0 | 2.0 | 5.0 | 65 | 430 | <1.0 |
| breast (*Perdue Fit & Easy*) . . . . . . . . . . . . | 100 | 24.0 | 0 | .5 | 65 | 75 | 0 |
| burgers (*Bell & Evans*) . . | 160 | 21.0 | 3.0 | 6.0 | 95 | 140 | 0 |
| white (*Empire Kosher*) . . | 160 | 23.0 | 0 | 8.0 | 65 | 125 | 0 |
| **"Chicken," vegetarian, canned**: | | | | | | | |
| (*Worthington FriChik*), 2 pcs., 3.2 oz. . . . . . . . | 140 | 12.0 | 3.0 | 8.0 | 0 | 430 | 1.0 |
| (*Worthington FriChik Low Fat*), 2 pcs., 3 oz. | 80 | 12.0 | 4.0 | 2.5 | 0 | 400 | 0 |
| diced, drained (*Worthington Chik*), ¼ cup . . . . . . . . . | 50 | 9.0 | 2.0 | 0 | 0 | 220 | 1.0 |
| **"Chicken," vegetarian, frozen/chilled** (see also "'Chicken' entree, vegetarian"): | | | | | | | |
| (*Worthington Chicketts*), 2 slices, 2 oz. . . . . . . . | 110 | 14.0 | 3.0 | 5.0 | 0 | 390 | 2.0 |
| burger (*Yves*) 2.6 oz. . . . | 100 | 15.0 | 5.0 | 3.0 | 0 | 420 | 2.0 |
| cutlet (*Veggie Patch Chick'n*), 2.5 oz. . . . . . | 140 | 10.0 | 15.0 | 6.0 | 0 | 380 | 3.0 |
| fried, w/gravy (*Loma Linda*), 2 pcs., 2.9 oz. . | 150 | 12.0 | 5.0 | 10.0 | 0 | 430 | 2.0 |

| Food and Measure | cal. | prot. (gms) | carbo. (gms) | fat (gms) | chol. (mgs) | sod. (mgs) | fiber (gms) |
|---|---|---|---|---|---|---|---|
| nuggets: | | | | | | | |
| (*Boca* Chik'n), 3 oz. ... | 180 | 14.0 | 17.0 | 7.0 | 0 | 500 | 3.0 |
| (*Dr. Praeger's*), 4 pcs., 2.5 oz. ......... | 170 | 11.0 | 14.0 | 7.0 | 0 | 230 | 3.0 |
| (*Health is Wealth*), 3 oz. ............ | 120 | 14.0 | 14.0 | 2.0 | 0 | 450 | 2.0 |
| (*MorningStar Farms* Chik'n), 4 pcs., 3 oz. | 190 | 12.0 | 19.0 | 9.0 | 0 | 320 | 4.0 |
| (*Veggie Patch* Chick'n), 4 pcs., 3 oz. ...... | 190 | 10.0 | 22.0 | 8.0 | 0 | 480 | 3.0 |
| Buffalo (*Dr. Praeger's*), 4 pcs., 2.5 oz. ......... | 160 | 11.0 | 13.0 | 7.0 | 0 | 460 | 3.0 |
| patties, 1 pc., 2.5 oz., except as noted: | | | | | | | |
| (*Boca* Chik'n) ....... | 160 | 11.0 | 15.0 | 6.0 | 0 | 430 | 2.0 |
| (*Dr. Praeger's*) .... | 160 | 13.0 | 13.0 | 7.0 | 0 | 250 | 3.0 |
| (*Health is Wealth*) .... | 110 | 12.0 | 12.0 | 1.5 | 0 | 400 | 2.0 |
| (*MorningStar Farms Chik Patties*) ...... | 140 | 8.0 | 16.0 | 5.0 | 0 | 590 | 2.0 |
| (*MorningStar Farms Grillers* Chik'n), 2.36 oz. ......... | 80 | 9.0 | 7.0 | 3.0 | 0 | 350 | 5.0 |
| Buffalo (*Dr. Praeger's*) ........ | 160 | 15.0 | 10.0 | 7.0 | 0 | 430 | 3.0 |
| Italian herb (*MorningStar Farms Chik Patties*) ...... | 170 | 10.0 | 22.0 | 5.0 | 0 | 480 | 2.0 |
| spicy (*Boca* Original Chick'n) ......... | 160 | 11.0 | 15.0 | 6.0 | 0 | 560 | 2.0 |
| roll (*Worthington*), ⅜" slice, 2 oz. ....... | 90 | 9.0 | 2.0 | 4.5 | 0 | 240 | 1.0 |
| skewers, lemon herb (*Yves*), 2.8-oz. pc. ... | 100 | 15.0 | 7.0 | 1.0 | 0 | 450 | 4.0 |
| slices, smoked (*Yves*), 4 pcs. ............. | 100 | 16.0 | 5.0 | 1.5 | 0 | 480 | 0 |
| strips, 3 oz.: | | | | | | | |
| (*MorningStar Farms Meal Starters*) .... | 140 | 23.0 | 6.0 | 3.5 | 0 | 510 | 1.0 |
| (*Yves* Heart's Desire) . | 110 | 22.0 | 3.0 | 1.0 | 0 | 440 | 1.0 |
| tenders (*MorningStar Farms* Chik'n), 2 pcs., 2.9 oz. ....... | 190 | 12.0 | 20.0 | 7.0 | 0 | 580 | 3.0 |

| Food and Measure | cal. | prot. (gms) | carbo. (gms) | fat (gms) | chol. (mgs) | sod. (mgs) | fiber (gms) |
|---|---|---|---|---|---|---|---|
| **"Chicken," vegetarian, frozen/chilled** *(cont.)* | | | | | | | |
| wings, Buffalo, 3 oz.: | | | | | | | |
| (*Boca* Chik'n Hot & Spicy) .......... | 160 | 14.0 | 14.0 | 7.0 | 0 | 700 | 3.0 |
| (*Health is Wealth*) .... | 130 | 13.0 | 18.0 | 2.5 | 0 | 690 | 4.0 |
| (*MorningStar Farms*) . | 200 | 12.0 | 20.0 | 8.0 | 0 | 640 | 3.0 |
| (*Veggie Patch*) ....... | 200 | 11.0 | 23.0 | 8.0 | 0 | 540 | 3.0 |
| **Chicken bologna** | | | | | | | |
| (*Empire Kosher*), 2 oz. | 50 | 11.0 | 1.0 | 0 | 30 | 300 | 0 |
| **Chicken coating mix** | | | | | | | |
| (see also "Chicken seasoning" and "Batter/breading mix"): | | | | | | | |
| (*Don's Chuck Wagon* Bake & Fry), ¼ cup ... | 95 | 3.0 | 21.0 | 0 | 0 | 665 | 1.0 |
| (*Golden Dipt* Extra Crispy), 1½ tbsp. .... | 60 | <1.0 | 9.0 | 0 | 0 | 310 | 0 |
| (*Golden Dipt* Fry Easy Homestyle), 2 tbsp. ... | 50 | 0 | 9.0 | 0 | 0 | 660 | 0 |
| (*McCormick* Season 'n Fry), 1 tbsp. ....... | 35 | <1.0 | 7.0 | 0 | 0 | 610 | 0 |
| (*Oven Fry* Extra Crispy), ⅛ pkg. ...... | 60 | 2.0 | 10.0 | 1.0 | 0 | 420 | 0 |
| (*Oven Fry* Homestyle Flour), ⅛ pkg. ........ | 40 | 1.0 | 7.0 | 1.0 | 0 | 470 | 0 |
| (*Shake 'n Bake* Extra Crispy), 1 tbsp. ...... | 35 | 1.0 | 7.0 | .5 | 0 | 280 | 0 |
| (*Shake 'n Bake* Original), 1 tbsp. ..... | 40 | 1.0 | 7.0 | 1.0 | 0 | 220 | 0 |
| (*Zatarain's* Bake & Crisp), 2 tbsp. ........ | 60 | 1.0 | 9.0 | 1.5 | 0 | 510 | 0 |
| (*Zatarain's Chick-Fri*), 3 tbsp. ............. | 50 | <1.0 | 12.0 | 0 | 0 | 350 | <1.0 |
| barbecue glaze (*Shake 'n Bake* Chicken/ Pork), 1 tbsp. ....... | 45 | 0 | 9.0 | 1.0 | 0 | 410 | 0 |
| garlic herb (*Shake 'n Bake*), 1 tbsp. ..... | 35 | 1.0 | 7.0 | 0 | 0 | 190 | 0 |
| herbs & spices (*Golden Dipt*), 2 tbsp. ....... | 70 | <1.0 | 13.0 | 0 | 0 | 490 | 0 |
| hot and spicy: | | | | | | | |
| (*Golden Dipt*), 2 tbsp. . | 50 | 0 | 9.0 | 0 | 0 | 430 | 0 |
| (*Shake 'n Bake*), 1 tbsp. ........... | 40 | 1.0 | 7.0 | 1.0 | 0 | 180 | 0 |

| Food and Measure | cal. | prot. (gms) | carbo. (gms) | fat (gms) | chol. (mgs) | sod. (mgs) | fiber (gms) |
|---|---|---|---|---|---|---|---|
| Italian (*Shake 'n Bake*), 1 tbsp. . . . . . . . . . . . | 35 | 1.0 | 7.0 | .5 | 0 | 280 | 0 |
| Parmesan crust (*Shake 'n Bake*), 1 tbsp. . . . . . | 35 | 1.0 | 7.0 | .5 | 0 | 290 | 0 |
| ranch herb crust (*Shake 'n Bake* Chicken/Pork), 1 tbsp. | 35 | 1.0 | 7.0 | 0 | 0 | 350 | 0 |
| Southern (*Zatarain's* Frying Mix), 4 tbsp. . . | 80 | 2.0 | 16.0 | 0 | 0 | 930 | <1.0 |
| **Chicken dinner**, see "Chicken entree" | | | | | | | |
| **Chicken entree, canned**, 1 cup, except as noted: | | | | | | | |
| chow mein (*La Choy*) . . . | 100 | 5.0 | 11.0 | 4.0 | 15 | 1520 | 3.0 |
| and dumplings (*Dinty Moore*) . . . . . . . . . . . | 230 | 12.0 | 28.0 | 8.0 | 35 | 900 | 1.0 |
| ravioli (*Dinty Moore American Classics*) . . . | 230 | 9.0 | 36.0 | 6.0 | 15 | 860 | 1.0 |
| stew (*Dinty Moore*) . . . . . | 220 | 12.0 | 17.0 | 11.0 | 35 | 1020 | 2.0 |
| sweet and sour (*La Choy* Family Meal), 1 cup* . . . . . . . | 340 | 28.0 | 51.0 | 2.0 | 45 | 500 | 2.0 |
| teriyaki: | | | | | | | |
| (*La Choy*) . . . . . . . . . . | 120 | 5.0 | 18.0 | 3.5 | 15 | 1510 | 3.0 |
| (*La Choy* Family Meal), 1 cup* . . . . . | 320 | 29.0 | 42.0 | 4.0 | 45 | 570 | 1.0 |
| vegetables, mixed (*La Choy*), ½ cup . . . . . . . | 100 | 5.0 | 11.0 | 4.0 | 15 | 1520 | 3.0 |
| **Chicken entree, frozen** (see also "Chicken, frozen/chilled, cooked"), 1 pkg., except as noted: | | | | | | | |
| à la king (*Stouffer's*), 11.5 oz. . . . . . . . . . . | 360 | 18.0 | 44.0 | 12.0 | 35 | 800 | 0 |
| Alfredo: | | | | | | | |
| (*Birds Eye Voila!*), 1 cup* . . . . . . . . . . | 280 | 14.0 | 27.0 | 12.0 | 55 | 600 | 2.0 |
| (*Contessa* MicroSteam), 1 cup* | 260 | 12.0 | 24.0 | 13.0 | 55 | 450 | 3.0 |
| (*Glutino* Gluten Free), 9.2 oz. . . . . . . . . . . | 340 | 15.0 | 48.0 | 8.0 | 50 | 830 | 3.0 |
| (*Lean Cuisine* Market Creations), 10.5 oz. | 280 | 20.0 | 33.0 | 7.0 | 35 | 680 | 4.0 |

| Food and Measure | cal. | prot. (gms) | carbo. (gms) | fat (gms) | chol. (mgs) | sod. (mgs) | fiber (gms) |
|---|---|---|---|---|---|---|---|
| **Chicken entree, frozen, Alfredo** *(cont.)* | | | | | | | |
| (*Stouffer's Easy Express* Skillets), ½ of 25-oz. pkg. . . . . . . . | 410 | 31.0 | 48.0 | 10.0 | 50 | 980 | 6.0 |
| blackened (*Zatarain's*), 10.5 oz. . . . . . . . . | 510 | 19.0 | 50.0 | 24.0 | 70 | 1200 | 2.0 |
| blackened w/roasted vegetables (*Zatarain's*), 10.5 oz. | 440 | 19.0 | 44.0 | 21.0 | 95 | 1080 | 2.0 |
| Florentine (*Healthy Choice*), 8.5 oz. . . . | 230 | 17.0 | 31.0 | 3.5 | 25 | 470 | 4.0 |
| Florentine (*Michelina's Lean Gourmet*), 8 oz. . . . . . . . . . . . | 250 | 12.0 | 34.0 | 7.0 | 40 | 690 | 2.0 |
| pesto (*Healthy Choice Complete*), 11.5 oz. | 300 | 20.0 | 39.0 | 7.0 | 45 | 580 | 7.0 |
| red pepper (*Healthy Choice Café Steamers*), 10.3 oz. | 250 | 20.0 | 30.0 | 5.0 | 35 | 520 | 4.0 |
| w/almonds (*Lean Cuisine Cafe*), 8.5 oz. . | 250 | 16.0 | 38.0 | 4.0 | 30 | 490 | 4.0 |
| apple cranberry (*Lean Cuisine Spa Cuisine*), 1 pkg. . . . . . . . . . . . . . | 300 | 14.0 | 54.0 | 4.0 | 20 | 500 | 6.0 |
| bacon, cheddar (*Healthy Choice*), 8.6 oz. . . . . . | 260 | 18.0 | 32.0 | 6.0 | 45 | 560 | 3.0 |
| baked: | | | | | | | |
| (*Lean Cuisine Comfort*), 8.5 oz. . . | 250 | 15.0 | 29.0 | 8.0 | 35 | 600 | 2.0 |
| breast (*Stouffer's*), 8.88 oz. . . . . . . . . | 250 | 20.0 | 20.0 | 10.0 | 60 | 730 | 1.0 |
| balsamic glazed (*Lean Cuisine Dinnertime Cuisine*), 12 oz. . . . . . . | 330 | 25.0 | 41.0 | 7.0 | 40 | 660 | 4.0 |
| balsamico (*Healthy Choice Complete*), 12 oz. . . . . . . . . . . . . | 350 | 16.0 | 56.0 | 6.0 | 40 | 520 | 6.0 |
| barbecue: | | | | | | | |
| (*Banquet*), 8 oz. . . . . . | 250 | 13.0 | 31.0 | 6.0 | 25 | 890 | 5.0 |
| (*Stouffer's*), 10 oz. . . . | 430 | 23.0 | 42.0 | 19.0 | 70 | 1120 | 3.0 |
| honey mango (*Smart Ones Fruit Inspirations*), 9 oz. . | 240 | 18.0 | 32.0 | 4.0 | 35 | 520 | 3.0 |

| Food and Measure | cal. | prot. (gms) | carbo. (gms) | fat (gms) | chol. (mgs) | sod. (mgs) | fiber (gms) |
|---|---|---|---|---|---|---|---|
| sweet/tangy (*Healthy Choice* Complete), 10.5 oz. | 310 | 16.0 | 54.0 | 3.5 | 30 | 470 | 6.0 |
| basil cream sauce (*Lean Cuisine* Cafe), 8.5 oz. . . . . . . . . . . | 250 | 19.0 | 31.0 | 6.0 | 30 | 420 | 2.0 |
| biryani (*Ethnic Gourmet*), 10 oz. . . . . | 390 | 16.0 | 54.0 | 12.0 | 20 | 1080 | 4.0 |
| blackened, w/: | | | | | | | |
| black beans, rice (*Zatarain's*), 10 oz. . | 410 | 16.0 | 59.0 | 11.0 | 25 | 1290 | 2.0 |
| yellow rice (*Zatarain's*), 10.5 oz. | 470 | 16.0 | 71.0 | 13.0 | 25 | 1310 | 3.0 |
| breaded, country (*Healthy Choice* Complete), 10.6 oz. | 340 | 14.0 | 50.0 | 9.0 | 30 | 560 | 6.0 |
| and broccoli (*Stouffer's Easy Express* 25.8 oz.), 7.38 oz. . . . . | 330 | 18.0 | 30.0 | 15.0 | 35 | 800 | 3.0 |
| broccoli and cheese casserole (*Boston Market*), 9.7 oz. . . . . . | 330 | 31.0 | 38.0 | 6.0 | 80 | 1010 | 1.0 |
| Cajun, and shrimp (*Healthy Choice Café Steamers*), 10.4 oz. . . | 260 | 15.0 | 40.0 | 4.0 | 50 | 570 | 3.0 |
| carbonara: | | | | | | | |
| (*Banquet*), 8 oz. . . . . . | 290 | 11.0 | 33.0 | 12.0 | 25 | 740 | 4.0 |
| (*Lean Cuisine*), 9 oz. . . | 270 | 21.0 | 33.0 | 6.0 | 30 | 600 | 3.0 |
| (*Smart Ones*), 9.25 oz. | 260 | 21.0 | 32.0 | 5.0 | 40 | 700 | 2.0 |
| Caribbean, spicy (*Healthy Choice*), 8.5 oz. . . . . . . . . . . | 310 | 15.0 | 56.0 | 2.0 | 20 | 290 | 6.0 |
| cheddar, potato (*Birds Eye Voila!*), 1 cup* . . . | 230 | 13.0 | 31.0 | 7.0 | 25 | 1170 | 4.0 |
| cheese, three: | | | | | | | |
| (*Birds Eye Voila!*), 1 cup* . . . . . . . . . | 210 | 13.0 | 21.0 | 8.0 | 30 | 940 | 2.0 |
| (*Lean Cuisine* Cafe), 8 oz. . . . . . . . . . . | 210 | 21.0 | 10.0 | 9.0 | 40 | 500 | 3.0 |
| (*Michelina's Lean Gourmet*), 8 oz. . . . | 300 | 14.0 | 41.0 | 8.0 | 40 | 750 | 1.0 |
| (*Stouffer's Easy Express* Skillets), ½ of 24-oz. pkg. . . . | 420 | 26.0 | 44.0 | 15.0 | 50 | 980 | 4.0 |

| Food and Measure | cal. | prot. (gms) | carbo. (gms) | fat (gms) | chol. (mgs) | sod. (mgs) | fiber (gms) |
|---|---|---|---|---|---|---|---|
| **Chicken entree, frozen** *(cont.)* | | | | | | | |
| cheesy, 1 cup*: | | | | | | | |
|   (*Birds Eye Voila!*) .... | 250 | 14.0 | 35.0 | 6.0 | 5 | 830 | 3.0 |
|   ranch (*Birds Eye* | | | | | | | |
|     *Voila!*) .......... | 210 | 12.0 | 30.0 | 4.5 | 25 | 760 | 2.0 |
| chow mein: | | | | | | | |
|   (*Contessa On the* | | | | | | | |
|     *Stove*), ⅓ pkg.: | | | | | | | |
|     w/sauce, 8.5 oz. ... | 260 | 14.0 | 44.0 | 2.5 | 30 | 670 | 3.0 |
|     w/out sauce ...... | 200 | 13.0 | 30.0 | 2.5 | 30 | 220 | 3.0 |
|   w/rice (*Lean Cuisine*), | | | | | | | |
|     9 oz. ............ | 240 | 13.0 | 39.0 | 4.0 | 25 | 550 | 3.0 |
| citron (*Organic Bistro*), | | | | | | | |
|   10.5 oz. ........... | 450 | 35.0 | 38.0 | 18.0 | 45 | 430 | 8.0 |
| country fried: | | | | | | | |
|   (*Boston Market* | | | | | | | |
|     Dinner), 14 oz. .... | 470 | 21.0 | 44.0 | 24.0 | 50 | 1430 | 6.0 |
|   (*Marie Callender's*), | | | | | | | |
|     16 oz. ........... | 570 | 24.0 | 60.0 | 27.0 | 70 | 1340 | 7.0 |
| curry: | | | | | | | |
|   Malay (*Ethnic* | | | | | | | |
|     *Gourmet*), 10 oz. .. | 410 | 18.0 | 59.0 | 11.0 | 35 | 530 | 3.0 |
|   red (*Kashi*), 9.5 oz. ... | 300 | 18.0 | 40.0 | 9.0 | 25 | 470 | 5.0 |
| and dumplings: | | | | | | | |
|   (*Stouffer's Easy* | | | | | | | |
|     *Express* Skillets), | | | | | | | |
|     ½ of 24-oz. pkg. ... | 370 | 22.0 | 40.0 | 13.0 | 70 | 1060 | 3.0 |
|   chunky (*Marie* | | | | | | | |
|     *Callender's*), 13 oz. . | 450 | 28.0 | 40.0 | 20.0 | 85 | 1230 | 3.0 |
| escalloped, w/noodles: | | | | | | | |
|   (*Stouffer's*), 12 oz. ... | 450 | 19.0 | 43.0 | 22.0 | 65 | 940 | 5.0 |
|   (*Stouffer's* Family), | | | | | | | |
|     ⅕ of 45-oz. pkg. ... | 280 | 15.0 | 28.0 | 12.0 | 30 | 770 | 2.0 |
| fettuccine: | | | | | | | |
|   (*Lean Cuisine*), | | | | | | | |
|     9.25 oz. ......... | 270 | 22.0 | 32.0 | 6.0 | 40 | 690 | 0 |
|   (*Lean Cuisine* | | | | | | | |
|     *Dinnertime Cuisine*), | | | | | | | |
|     12 oz. ............ | 330 | 26.0 | 42.0 | 6.0 | 40 | 770 | 4.0 |
|   (*Marie Calllender's* | | | | | | | |
|     Pasta al Dente | | | | | | | |
|     Balsamico), 10.5 oz. | 440 | 24.0 | 46.0 | 18.0 | 85 | 990 | 5.0 |
|   (*Smart Ones*), 10 oz. . | 290 | 20.0 | 40.0 | 6.0 | 60 | 720 | 3.0 |

| Food and Measure | cal. | prot. (gms) | carbo. (gms) | fat (gms) | chol. (mgs) | sod. (mgs) | fiber (gms) |
|---|---|---|---|---|---|---|---|
| and broccoli (*Marie Callender's*), 13 oz. | 650 | 31.0 | 41.0 | 40.0 | 70 | 1150 | 6.0 |
| fettuccine Alfredo: | | | | | | | |
| (*Stouffer's*), 10.5 oz. | 570 | 26.0 | 55.0 | 27.0 | 50 | 850 | 5.0 |
| (*Stouffer's*), 15 oz. | 840 | 31.0 | 94.0 | 38.0 | 75 | 1050 | 5.0 |
| w/broccoli (*Michelina's*), 8.5 oz. | 310 | 15.0 | 38.0 | 10.0 | 45 | 700 | 2.0 |
| fingers (*Banquet*), 7 oz. | 480 | 17.0 | 56.0 | 21.0 | 50 | 700 | 5.0 |
| Florentine: | | | | | | | |
| (*Birds Eye Voila!*), 1 cup* | 230 | 14.0 | 27.0 | 6.0 | 30 | 590 | 3.0 |
| (*Contessa* Micro-Steam), 1 cup* | 340 | 14.0 | 38.0 | 14.0 | 60 | 450 | 2.0 |
| (*Kashi*), 10 oz. | 290 | 22.0 | 31.0 | 9.0 | 45 | 550 | 5.0 |
| (*Lean Cuisine Dinnertime Cuisine*), 13.25 oz. | 410 | 28.0 | 54.0 | 9.0 | 45 | 840 | 6.0 |
| baked (*Lean Cuisine Comfort*), 8 oz. | 200 | 18.0 | 14.0 | 8.0 | 40 | 660 | 3.0 |
| fried: | | | | | | | |
| (*Banquet*), 8 oz. | 440 | 22.0 | 30.0 | 26.0 | 80 | 1140 | 4.0 |
| (*Banquet*), 10 oz. | 350 | 12.0 | 35.0 | 17.0 | 35 | 930 | 5.0 |
| breast (*Stouffer's*), 8.9 oz. | 360 | 20.0 | 30.0 | 18.0 | 45 | 880 | 2.0 |
| breast, gravy, potato (*Michelina's*), 8 oz. | 290 | 11.0 | 30.0 | 15.0 | 40 | 910 | 2.0 |
| fritter, w/potato, 5 oz.: | | | | | | | |
| (*Michelina's* Littles) | 270 | 10.0 | 34.0 | 10.0 | 15 | 950 | 3.0 |
| (*Michelina's* Pop'n) | 290 | 8.0 | 37.0 | 11.0 | 10 | 630 | 3.0 |
| garlic: | | | | | | | |
| (*Birds Eye Voila!*), 1 cup* | 240 | 11.0 | 21.0 | 8.0 | 30 | 940 | 3.0 |
| (*Birds Eye Voila!* Family Skillets), 1 cup* | 240 | 11.0 | 29.0 | 8.0 | 20 | 540 | 3.0 |
| (*Lean Cuisine* Market Creations), 10.5 oz. | 270 | 20.0 | 33.0 | 6.0 | 30 | 670 | 4.0 |
| (*Michelina's* Tuscan-Inspired), 8 oz. | 320 | 15.0 | 46.0 | 7.0 | 30 | 580 | 2.0 |
| (*Stouffer's Easy Express Skillets*), ½ of 23-oz. pkg. | 330 | 24.0 | 45.0 | 6.0 | 40 | 990 | 5.0 |

| Food and Measure | cal. | prot. (gms) | carbo. (gms) | fat (gms) | chol. (mgs) | sod. (mgs) | fiber (gms) |
|---|---|---|---|---|---|---|---|
| **Chicken entree, frozen, garlic** *(cont.)* | | | | | | | |
| balsamic (*Healthy Choice Café Steamers*), 10 oz. .. | 270 | 20.0 | 38.0 | 4.0 | 30 | 540 | 6.0 |
| penne (*Contessa MicroSteam*), 1 cup* | 270 | 13.0 | 34.0 | 9.0 | 25 | 430 | 2.0 |
| spicy (*Wanchai Ferry*), ½ of 24-oz. pkg.* .. | 410 | 12.0 | 60.0 | 14.0 | 20 | 960 | 2.0 |
| General Tso's: | | | | | | | |
| crispy (*Contessa On the Stove*), 9.6 oz. . | 410 | 12.0 | 59.0 | 14.0 | 25 | 480 | 3.0 |
| w/out sauce ...... | 290 | 11.0 | 39.0 | 10.0 | 25 | 160 | 3.0 |
| spicy (*Healthy Choice Café Steamers*), 10.8 oz. ......... | 320 | 15.0 | 53.0 | 3.5 | 30 | 500 | 4.0 |
| ginger: | | | | | | | |
| (*Organic Bistro*), 10 oz. ........... | 360 | 24.0 | 37.0 | 14.0 | 40 | 430 | 7.0 |
| garlic stir-fry w/ (*Lean Cuisine Spa Cuisine*), 9.825 oz. . | 280 | 20.0 | 42.0 | 4.0 | 30 | 550 | 5.0 |
| sweet and sour (*Lean Cuisine* Market Creations), 10.5 oz. | 280 | 21.0 | 43.0 | 2.0 | 30 | 680 | 4.0 |
| glazed: | | | | | | | |
| (*Lean Cuisine* Cafe), 8.5 oz. .......... | 210 | 17.0 | 29.0 | 2.0 | 35 | 400 | 0 |
| (*Michelina's Lean Gourmet*), 8 oz. ... | 250 | 10.0 | 46.0 | 3.0 | 20 | 470 | 1.0 |
| grilled: | | | | | | | |
| (*Lean Cuisine* Cafe Fiesta), 8.5 oz. .... | 260 | 19.0 | 33.0 | 6.0 | 45 | 600 | 4.0 |
| bake (*Marie Callender's*), 13 oz. . | 500 | 31.0 | 34.0 | 26.0 | 80 | 1230 | 4.0 |
| barbecue sauce (*Michelina's Lean Gourmet*), 8 oz. ... | 260 | 11.0 | 36.0 | 9.0 | 35 | 800 | 3.0 |
| basil (*Healthy Choice Café Steamers*), 10.6 oz. ......... | 270 | 20.0 | 34.0 | 6.0 | 35 | 600 | 7.0 |
| Caesar (*Lean Cuisine* Cafe), 8.5 oz. ..... | 260 | 18.0 | 33.0 | 6.0 | 35 | 590 | 3.0 |
| honey Dijon (*Lean Cuisine* Cafe), 8 oz. | 180 | 15.0 | 19.0 | 5.0 | 40 | 630 | 2.0 |

| Food and Measure | cal. | prot. (gms) | carbo. (gms) | fat (gms) | chol. (mgs) | sod. (mgs) | fiber (gms) |
|---|---|---|---|---|---|---|---|
| marinara (*Healthy Choice Café Steamers*), 10 oz. . . | 270 | 21.0 | 35.0 | 4.5 | 30 | 550 | 5.0 |
| mesquite barbecue sauce (*Boston Market*), 10 oz. . . . . . . . . . . | 340 | 22.0 | 37.0 | 11.0 | 65 | 1160 | 3.0 |
| and penne (*Lean Cuisine Dinnertime Cuisine*), 14 oz. . . . | 330 | 18.0 | 53.0 | 5.0 | 30 | 600 | 6.0 |
| w/penne (*Marie Callender's*), 13 oz. . | 390 | 29.0 | 35.0 | 15.0 | 70 | 860 | 6.0 |
| primavera (*Lean Cuisine Spa Cuisine*), 9.375 oz. . . . . . . . . | 200 | 17.0 | 26.0 | 3.0 | 20 | 580 | 5.0 |
| Southwest (*Boston Market* Dinner), 14 oz. . . . . . . . . . . . | 410 | 25.0 | 45.0 | 14.0 | 65 | 1220 | 5.0 |
| and vegetables (*Stouffer's Easy Express Skillets*), ½ of 25-oz. pkg. . . . . . . . | 360 | 26.0 | 43.0 | 9.0 | 40 | 860 | 4.0 |
| herb, country (*Healthy Choice* Complete), 11.35 oz. . . . . . . . . . | 240 | 15.0 | 34.0 | 5.0 | 30 | 600 | 5.0 |
| honey: | | | | | | | |
| balsamic (*Healthy Choice* Steam), 9 oz. . . . . . . . . . . . | 220 | 13.0 | 34.0 | 3.5 | 25 | 540 | 5.0 |
| ginger (*Healthy Choice*), 8.5 oz. . . . | 310 | 14.0 | 53.0 | 4.5 | 25 | 310 | 3.0 |
| mustard (*Banquet*), 9 oz. . . . . . . . . . . . | 360 | 12.0 | 42.0 | 14.0 | 20 | 750 | 4.0 |
| roasted (*Boston Market*), 9.2 oz. . . . | 410 | 20.0 | 46.0 | 17.0 | 50 | 1140 | 2.0 |
| korma (*Ethnic Gourmet*), 10 oz. . . . . | 340 | 21.0 | 44.0 | 9.0 | 40 | 720 | 3.0 |
| kung pao (*Wanchai Ferry*), ½ of 24-oz. pkg.* . . . . | 520 | 25.0 | 72.0 | 15.0 | 40 | 1260 | 3.0 |
| w/lasagna rollatini (*Lean Cuisine Comfort*), 10 oz. . . . . . | 290 | 18.0 | 34.0 | 9.0 | 40 | 560 | 3.0 |
| lemon: | | | | | | | |
| (*Lean Cuisine Spa Cuisine*), 9 oz. . . . . | 260 | 16.0 | 35.0 | 6.0 | 25 | 460 | 5.0 |

| Food and Measure | cal. | prot. (gms) | carbo. (gms) | fat (gms) | chol. (mgs) | sod. (mgs) | fiber (gms) |
|---|---|---|---|---|---|---|---|
| **Chicken entree, frozen, lemon** *(cont.)* | | | | | | | |
| herb (*Healthy Choice* Steam), 8.7 oz. .... | 210 | 15.0 | 29.0 | 3.5 | 25 | 510 | 4.0 |
| lemon garlic shrimp (*Healthy Choice Café Steamers*), 10 oz. .... | 260 | 16.0 | 35.0 | 6.0 | 45 | 600 | 6.0 |
| lemongrass: | | | | | | | |
| (*Lean Cuisine Spa Cuisine*), 9.375 oz. . | 260 | 19.0 | 33.0 | 6.0 | 25 | 550 | 5.0 |
| coconut (*Kashi*), 10 oz. ........... | 300 | 18.0 | 38.0 | 8.0 | 10 | 680 | 7.0 |
| and basil (*Ethnic Gourmet*), 10 oz. .. | 380 | 20.0 | 56.0 | 9.0 | 30 | 310 | 5.0 |
| Margherita: | | | | | | | |
| (*Healthy Choice Café Steamers*), 10 oz. ... | 320 | 18.0 | 45.0 | 7.0 | 35 | 580 | 5.0 |
| (*Lean Cuisine* Market Creations), 10.5 oz. | 300 | 20.0 | 37.0 | 8.0 | 35 | 710 | 4.0 |
| Marsala: | | | | | | | |
| (*Contessa* MicroSteam), 1 cup* | 280 | 15.0 | 33.0 | 9.0 | 40 | 350 | 2.0 |
| (*Lean Cuisine* Café), 8.1 oz. ........... | 250 | 14.0 | 29.0 | 9.0 | 25 | 620 | 2.0 |
| w/broccoli (*Smart Ones*), 9 oz. ...... | 160 | 16.0 | 11.0 | 6.0 | 40 | 590 | 3.0 |
| Mediterranean (*Lean Cuisine Spa Cuisine*), 10.5 oz. ........... | 240 | 19.0 | 32.0 | 4.0 | 40 | 590 | 6.0 |
| Mexicana (*El Monterey* Family), ⅕ of 32-oz. pkg. ..... | 290 | 14.0 | 27.0 | 6.0 | 40 | 640 | 3.0 |
| Moroccan (*Organic Bistro*), 10.75 oz. .... | 340 | 22.0 | 41.0 | 10.0 | 40 | 300 | 7.0 |
| Monterey: | | | | | | | |
| (*Healthy Choice* Complete), 11 oz. .. | 340 | 19.0 | 48.0 | 8.0 | 40 | 600 | 7.0 |
| (*Stouffer's*), 14.5 oz. ... | 530 | 31.0 | 54.0 | 21.0 | 80 | 1300 | 5.0 |
| nuggets meal: | | | | | | | |
| (*Banquet*), 6.75 oz. .... | 320 | 14.0 | 29.0 | 16.0 | 25 | 580 | 4.0 |
| fries (*Banquet*), 5 oz. . | 280 | 10.0 | 31.0 | 13.0 | 15 | 560 | 3.0 |
| orange: | | | | | | | |
| (*Contessa On the Stove*), 9 oz. ...... | 360 | 16.0 | 53.0 | 9.0 | 40 | 720 | 3.0 |
| w/out sauce ....... | 280 | 15.0 | 37.0 | 8.0 | 40 | 210 | 3.0 |

| Food and Measure | cal. | prot. (gms) | carbo. (gms) | fat (gms) | chol. (mgs) | sod. (mgs) | fiber (gms) |
|---|---|---|---|---|---|---|---|
| (*Lean Cuisine* Cafe), 9 oz. | 300 | 14.0 | 46.0 | 7.0 | 25 | 580 | 2.0 |
| (*Wanchai Ferry*), ⅓ of 24-oz. pkg.* | 410 | 11.0 | 61.0 | 14.0 | 20 | 770 | 2.0 |
| peel (*Lean Cuisine Dinnertime Cuisine*), 12 oz. | 380 | 14.0 | 60.0 | 9.0 | 20 | 720 | 4.0 |
| sauce (*Cedarlane*), 10 oz. | 360 | 17.0 | 61.0 | 4.0 | 35 | 650 | 1.0 |
| sesame (*Smart Ones Fruit Inspirations*), 9 oz. | 320 | 14.0 | 48.0 | 8.0 | 20 | 680 | 2.0 |
| zest, sweet and spicy (*Healthy Choice Café Steamers*), 10 oz. | 290 | 17.0 | 46.0 | 4.0 | 30 | 480 | 6.0 |
| Oriental (*Smart Ones*), 9 oz. | 230 | 14.0 | 41.0 | 2.0 | 25 | 700 | 2.0 |
| pad Thai, see "Noodle entree" | | | | | | | |
| Parmesan: | | | | | | | |
| (*Birds Eye Voila!*), 1 cup* | 360 | 14.0 | 50.0 | 11.0 | 15 | 800 | 2.0 |
| (*Boston Market* Dinner), 16 oz. | 620 | 33.0 | 69.0 | 24.0 | 50 | 1580 | 7.0 |
| (*Lean Cuisine* Comfort), 10.9 oz. | 310 | 21.0 | 39.0 | 8.0 | 35 | 660 | 5.0 |
| (*Marie Callender's*), 16 oz. | 620 | 29.0 | 57.0 | 30.0 | 45 | 1040 | 9.0 |
| (*Smart Ones*), 11 oz. | 290 | 26.0 | 35.0 | 5.0 | 40 | 630 | 4.0 |
| creamy (*Michelina's Lean Gourmet*), 8 oz. | 250 | 13.0 | 37.0 | 4.5 | 30 | 580 | 2.0 |
| creamy (*Smart Ones*), 9 oz. | 210 | 18.0 | 24.0 | 5.0 | 30 | 730 | 4.0 |
| and shrimp (*Marie Callender's*), 13 oz. | 420 | 26.0 | 45.0 | 15.0 | 60 | 1200 | 6.0 |
| parmigiana: | | | | | | | |
| (*Banquet*), 9.4 oz. | 360 | 17.0 | 37.0 | 16.0 | 20 | 840 | 7.0 |
| (*Cedarlane*), 10 oz. | 400 | 22.0 | 57.0 | 10.0 | 45 | 520 | 5.0 |
| (*Healthy Choice* Complete), 11.6 oz. | 350 | 16.0 | 49.0 | 10.0 | 25 | 530 | 7.0 |
| (*Stouffer's*), 12 oz. | 410 | 23.0 | 47.0 | 14.0 | 40 | 900 | 4.0 |
| (*Stouffer's*), ¼ of 52.5-oz. pkg. | 460 | 18.0 | 56.0 | 18.0 | 35 | 1060 | 4.0 |

| Food and Measure | cal. | prot. (gms) | carbo. (gms) | fat (gms) | chol. (mgs) | sod. (mgs) | fiber (gms) |
|---|---|---|---|---|---|---|---|
| **Chicken entree, frozen** *(cont.)* | | | | | | | |
| pasta and/and pasta: | | | | | | | |
| (*Kashi* Pomodoro), | | | | | | | |
|   10 oz. . . . . . . . . . . | 280 | 19.0 | 38.0 | 6.0 | 25 | 470 | 6.0 |
| (*Stouffer's Easy* | | | | | | | |
|   *Express* Skillets), | | | | | | | |
|   ½ of 25-oz. pkg. . . . | 480 | 25.0 | 60.0 | 15.0 | 35 | 1200 | 4.0 |
| Alfredo, w/chicken | | | | | | | |
|   broccoli (*Lean* | | | | | | | |
|   *Cuisine*), 10 oz. . . . | 300 | 16.0 | 45.0 | 6.0 | 30 | 660 | 3.0 |
| broccoli bake | | | | | | | |
|   (*Stouffer's* Family), | | | | | | | |
|   ⅛ of 45-oz. pkg. . . . | 300 | 19.0 | 24.0 | 14.0 | 45 | 990 | 1.0 |
| Caesar (*Cedarlane*), | | | | | | | |
|   10 oz. . . . . . . . . . . | 500 | 27.0 | 46.0 | 22.0 | 60 | 790 | 3.0 |
| carbonara (*Marie* | | | | | | | |
|   *Callender's* Pasta al | | | | | | | |
|   Dente), 10 oz. . . . . . | 390 | 22.0 | 45.0 | 13.0 | 45 | 780 | 5.0 |
| Cordon Bleu | | | | | | | |
|   (*Stouffer's* Family), | | | | | | | |
|   ¼ of 37-oz. pkg. . . . | 330 | 20.0 | 28.0 | 15.0 | 35 | 920 | 2.0 |
| cream sauce | | | | | | | |
|   (*Michelina's* | | | | | | | |
|   *Authentico*), 8 oz. . . | 290 | 12.0 | 38.0 | 10.0 | 35 | 800 | 2.0 |
| cream sauce | | | | | | | |
|   (*Michelina's Budget* | | | | | | | |
|   *Gourmet*), 8 oz. . . . | 290 | 11.0 | 37.0 | 9.0 | 30 | 760 | 2.0 |
| marinara (*Banquet*), | | | | | | | |
|   6.5 oz. . . . . . . . . . . | 290 | 12.0 | 29.0 | 14.0 | 15 | 550 | 3.0 |
| Parmesan (*Stouffer's Easy* | | | | | | | |
|   *Express* Skillet), | | | | | | | |
|   ½ of 25-oz. pkg. . . . | 480 | 25.0 | 60.0 | 15.0 | 35 | 1200 | 4.0 |
| peas/carrots | | | | | | | |
|   (*Michelina's* | | | | | | | |
|   *Authentico*), 8 oz. . . | 290 | 13.0 | 36.0 | 13.0 | 40 | 860 | 2.0 |
| patty, w/marinara | | | | | | | |
|   (*Banquet* Family), | | | | | | | |
|   1 pc. w/sauce . . . . . . . | 170 | 9.0 | 15.0 | 9.0 | 15 | 550 | 3.0 |
| peanut sauce (*Lean* | | | | | | | |
|   *Cuisine Spa Cuisine*), | | | | | | | |
|   9 oz. . . . . . . . . . . . . . | 290 | 24.0 | 33.0 | 7.0 | 25 | 570 | 5.0 |
| pecan (*Lean Cuisine* | | | | | | | |
|   *Spa Cuisine*), 9 oz. . . . | 310 | 18.0 | 43.0 | 7.0 | 35 | 580 | 5.0 |

| Food and Measure | cal. | prot. (gms) | carbo. (gms) | fat (gms) | chol. (mgs) | sod. (mgs) | fiber (gms) |
|---|---|---|---|---|---|---|---|
| penne: | | | | | | | |
| (*Michelina's Authentico*), 8.5 oz. | 330 | 14.0 | 48.0 | 9.0 | 35 | 610 | 2.0 |
| creamy tomato (*Birds Eye Voila!*), 1 cup* | 210 | 12.0 | 29.0 | 4.5 | 25 | 520 | 3.0 |
| Modesto (*Marie Callender's* Pasta al Dente), 11 oz. | 410 | 21.0 | 43.0 | 17.0 | 40 | 950 | 5.0 |
| w/vegetables (*Birds Eye Voila!*), 1 cup* | 200 | 13.0 | 28.0 | 3.0 | 25 | 800 | 2.0 |
| vodka (*Contessa On the Stove*), 8.8 oz. | 410 | 17.0 | 47.0 | 16.0 | 55 | 790 | 3.0 |
| w/out sauce | 240 | 15.0 | 39.0 | 2.5 | 25 | 180 | 3.0 |
| pesto: | | | | | | | |
| (*Healthy Choice Café Steamers* Classico), 10.6 oz. | 320 | 19.0 | 39.0 | 9.0 | 35 | 580 | 4.0 |
| w/bow-ties (*Lean Cuisine* Café), 9.5 oz. | 340 | 23.0 | 42.0 | 9.0 | 30 | 550 | 4.0 |
| sun-dried tomato (*Lean Cuisine* Cafe), 8.6 oz. | 270 | 18.0 | 28.0 | 9.0 | 30 | 570 | 4.0 |
| piccata, lemon herb (*Smart Ones*), 9 oz. | 230 | 12.0 | 41.0 | 2.0 | 25 | 540 | 2.0 |
| pie/pot pie, 8 oz., except as noted: | | | | | | | |
| (*Applegate Farms*) | 490 | 15.0 | 58.0 | 23.0 | 25 | 630 | 3.0 |
| (*Banquet*), 7 oz. | 300 | 10.0 | 34.0 | 21.0 | 30 | 1040 | 3.0 |
| (*Bell & Evans*), ½ of 16-oz. pkg. | 520 | 16.0 | 48.0 | 29.0 | 50 | 630 | 2.0 |
| (*Blake's Natural*) | 370 | 15.0 | 40.0 | 17.0 | 25 | 380 | 3.0 |
| (*Blake's* Organic) | 340 | 15.0 | 34.0 | 17.0 | 30 | 470 | 5.0 |
| (*Boston Market*) | 560 | 16.0 | 43.0 | 36.0 | 55 | 930 | 2.0 |
| (*Marie Callender's*), 1 cup | 520 | 14.0 | 45.0 | 31.0 | 30 | 800 | 3.0 |
| (*Pacific* Organic), 1 cup | 400 | 15.0 | 46.0 | 19.0 | 75 | 900 | 7.0 |
| (*Stouffer's*) | 580 | 21.0 | 50.0 | 33.0 | 60 | 890 | 2.0 |
| (*Stouffer's*) 10 oz. | 630 | 21.0 | 57.0 | 35.0 | 55 | 1020 | 2.0 |
| all meat (*Blake's* Natural) | 360 | 16.0 | 34.0 | 18.0 | 25 | 380 | 1.0 |
| all meat (*Blake's* Organic) | 290 | 18.0 | 25.0 | 13.0 | 45 | 650 | 3.0 |

| Food and Measure | cal. | prot. (gms) | carbo. (gms) | fat (gms) | chol. (mgs) | sod. (mgs) | fiber (gms) |
|---|---|---|---|---|---|---|---|
| **Chicken entree, frozen, pie/pot pie** *(cont.)* | | | | | | | |
| w/broccoli (*Banquet*), 7 oz. . . . . . . . . . . | 360 | 9.0 | 34.0 | 20.0 | 30 | 930 | 3.0 |
| cheesy (*Marie Callender's*), 1 cup . | 570 | 16.0 | 44.0 | 36.0 | 35 | 880 | 3.0 |
| honey-roasted (*Marie Callender's*), 1 cup | 520 | 14.0 | 48.0 | 30.0 | 30 | 880 | 4.0 |
| mushroom and (*Marie Callender's*), 1 cup . | 540 | 14.0 | 48.0 | 33.0 | 20 | 780 | 5.0 |
| Parmesan (*Marie Callender's*), 1 cup . | 510 | 17.0 | 44.0 | 29.0 | 20 | 830 | 4.0 |
| pineapple (*Healthy Choice*), 9 oz. . . . . . . . | 380 | 9.0 | 68.0 | 7.0 | 10 | 210 | 5.0 |
| portobello (*Lean Cuisine Dinnertime Cuisine*), 12 oz. . . . . . . | 390 | 32.0 | 48.0 | 8.0 | 55 | 560 | 2.0 |
| primavera: | | | | | | | |
| penne (*Boston Market Dinner*), 16 oz. . . . . | 530 | 34.0 | 58.0 | 16.0 | 90 | 1620 | 5.0 |
| w/spirals (*Michelina's*), 8 oz. . . . . . . . . . . . | 320 | 14.0 | 48.0 | 7.0 | 25 | 630 | 3.0 |
| rice and/and rice: | | | | | | | |
| (*Glutino* Pomodoro), 9.2 oz. . . . . . . . . . | 190 | 11.0 | 33.0 | 2.5 | 15 | 910 | 3.0 |
| (*Glutino* Ranchero), 9.2 oz. . . . . . . . . . | 180 | 14.0 | 30.0 | 2.0 | 20 | 790 | 4.0 |
| (*Stouffer's* Grandma's), ¼ of 36-oz. pkg. . . . | 360 | 19.0 | 37.0 | 15.0 | 70 | 880 | 1.0 |
| (*Stouffer's Easy Express Skillets Savory*), ½ of 24-oz. pkg. . . . | 330 | 18.0 | 50.0 | 6.0 | 30 | 980 | 2.0 |
| and cheese (*Banquet Family*), 1 cup . . . . | 200 | 10.0 | 24.0 | 7.0 | 30 | 940 | 2.0 |
| cheesy (*Marie Callender's*), 13 oz. . | 430 | 33.0 | 38.0 | 16.0 | 85 | 1330 | 4.0 |
| rice, fried, see "Rice entree, frozen" | | | | | | | |
| roast/roasted: | | | | | | | |
| fresca (*Healthy Choice Café Steamers*), 10.6 oz. . . . . . . . . | 230 | 17.0 | 29.0 | 5.0 | 40 | 550 | 6.0 |
| garlic (*Lean Cuisine Cafe*), 8.875 oz. . . . | 170 | 19.0 | 10.0 | 6.0 | 40 | 580 | 0 |

| Food and Measure | cal. | prot. (gms) | carbo. (gms) | fat (gms) | chol. (mgs) | sod. (mgs) | fiber (gms) |
|---|---|---|---|---|---|---|---|
| herb (*Lean Cuisine Comfort*), 8 oz. . . . . | 170 | 16.0 | 20.0 | 3.0 | 35 | 540 | 3.0 |
| herb (*Marie Callender's*), 14 oz. . | 460 | 30.0 | 32.0 | 21.0 | 135 | 940 | 5.0 |
| honey (*Lean Cuisine Spa Cuisine*), 1 pkg. | 280 | 18.0 | 44.0 | 4.0 | 30 | 600 | 5.0 |
| honey (*Marie Callender's*), 14 oz. . | 320 | 19.0 | 38.0 | 10.0 | 45 | 1030 | 7.0 |
| w/lemon pepper fettuccine (*Lean Cuisine*), 8.125 oz. . | 260 | 16.0 | 36.0 | 6.0 | 30 | 650 | 3.0 |
| Marsala (*Healthy Choice Café Steamers*), 10.4 oz. | 250 | 18.0 | 30.0 | 6.0 | 35 | 540 | 4.0 |
| w/mashed potato (*Smart Ones*), 9.5 oz. . . . . . | 180 | 17.0 | 20.0 | 4.0 | 40 | 820 | 2.0 |
| oven (*Boston Market Dinner*), 16 oz. . . . . | 390 | 30.0 | 34.0 | 15.0 | 75 | 1740 | 4.0 |
| oven (*Healthy Choice Complete*), 11.4 oz. . | 260 | 14.0 | 37.0 | 6.0 | 35 | 600 | 5.0 |
| w/stuffing (*Stouffer's*), 9.63 oz. . . . . . . . . | 460 | 26.0 | 34.0 | 24.0 | 80 | 990 | 5.0 |
| verde (*Healthy Choice Steam*), 8.6 oz. . . . . | 240 | 14.0 | 37.0 | 3.5 | 25 | 500 | 3.0 |
| Romano fresca (*Healthy Choice Steam*), 8 oz. . | 230 | 16.0 | 29.0 | 5.0 | 25 | 490 | 4.0 |
| rosemary: | | | | | | | |
| (*Lean Cuisine Spa Cuisine*), 8.25 oz. . . | 230 | 17.0 | 30.0 | 5.0 | 30 | 600 | 5.0 |
| and sweet potatoes (*Healthy Choice Steam*), 9 oz. . . . . . | 170 | 12.0 | 23.0 | 2.5 | 30 | 500 | 5.0 |
| Santa Fe (*Marie Callender's*), 12.5 oz. . | 410 | 24.0 | 55.0 | 11.0 | 65 | 820 | 5.0 |
| sesame: | | | | | | | |
| (*Banquet*), 8 oz. . . . . . | 340 | 10.0 | 40.0 | 16.0 | 15 | 690 | 4.0 |
| (*Contessa On the Stove*), 1/3 pkg.: | | | | | | | |
| w/sauce, 7.4 oz. . . . | 220 | 11.0 | 35.0 | 4.0 | 25 | 610 | 3.0 |
| w/out sauce . . . . . . | 170 | 11.0 | 35.0 | 4.0 | 25 | 200 | 3.0 |
| (*Healthy Choice Complete*), 11.8 oz. . | 330 | 19.0 | 50.0 | 6.0 | 35 | 580 | 5.0 |
| (*Lean Cuisine Cafe*), 9 oz. . . . . . . . . . . . | 330 | 16.0 | 47.0 | 9.0 | 25 | 650 | 2.0 |

| Food and Measure | cal. | prot. (gms) | carbo. (gms) | fat (gms) | chol. (mgs) | sod. (mgs) | fiber (gms) |
|---|---|---|---|---|---|---|---|
| **Chicken entree, frozen, sesame** *(cont.)* | | | | | | | |
| (*Michelina's Lean Gourmet*), 8 oz. . . . | 270 | 11.0 | 51.0 | 2.0 | 15 | 660 | 2.0 |
| (*Stouffer's*), 15 oz. . . . | 590 | 25.0 | 87.0 | 16.0 | 95 | 1210 | 6.0 |
| glazed (*Healthy Choice Steam*), 9 oz. . . . . . | 320 | 14.0 | 55.0 | 4.5 | 25 | 590 | 3.0 |
| stir-fry w/ (*Lean Cuisine Spa Cuisine*), 9.825 oz. . . . . . . . | 300 | 20.0 | 41.0 | 6.0 | 40 | 590 | 5.0 |
| sweet (*Healthy Choice Café Steamers*), 10.3 oz. . . . . . . . . | 330 | 17.0 | 50.0 | 6.0 | 30 | 400 | 6.0 |
| Southwest, whole grains (*Kashi*), 10 oz. . . . . . | 240 | 16.0 | 32.0 | 5.0 | 30 | 680 | 6.0 |
| stir-fry: | | | | | | | |
| (*Contessa On the Stove*), ⅓ pkg.: | | | | | | | |
| w/sauce, 8 oz. . . . . | 170 | 13.0 | 23.0 | 3.0 | 35 | 690 | 4.0 |
| w/out sauce . . . . . . | 110 | 12.0 | 10.0 | 2.5 | 30 | 250 | 4.0 |
| (*Birds Eye Voila!*), 1 cup* . . . . . . . . . . | 200 | 11.0 | 31.0 | 2.5 | 15 | 1040 | 2.0 |
| sweet and sour: | | | | | | | |
| (*Banquet*), 8 oz. . . . . . | 390 | 10.0 | 56.0 | 14.0 | 15 | 570 | 3.0 |
| (*Birds Eye Voila!*), 1 cup* . . . . . . . . . . | 200 | 10.0 | 38.0 | 1.0 | 20 | 580 | 2.0 |
| (*Contessa On the Stove*), 9.5 oz. . . . . | 400 | 13.0 | 61.0 | 12.0 | 35 | 480 | 2.0 |
| w/out sauce . . . . . . | 320 | 12.0 | 41.0 | 12.0 | 35 | 160 | 2.0 |
| (*Healthy Choice Complete*), 12 oz. . . | 440 | 14.0 | 73.0 | 10.0 | 20 | 480 | 6.0 |
| (*Kashi*), 10 oz. . . . . . . | 320 | 18.0 | 55.0 | 3.5 | 35 | 380 | 6.0 |
| (*Lean Cuisine* Cafe), 10 oz. . . . . . . . . . . | 300 | 18.0 | 51.0 | 3.0 | 30 | 560 | 2.0 |
| (*Marie Callender's*), 14 oz. . . . . . . . . . . | 520 | 15.0 | 92.0 | 10.0 | 20 | 620 | 7.0 |
| (*Michelina's Authentico*), 8 oz. . . | 330 | 10.0 | 66.0 | 2.5 | 15 | 620 | 1.0 |
| (*Michelina's Lean Gourmet*), 8 oz. . . . | 330 | 10.0 | 65.0 | 3.0 | 15 | 640 | 1.0 |
| (*Smart Ones*), 9 oz. . . | 210 | 16.0 | 31.0 | 2.0 | 20 | 510 | 2.0 |
| (*Stouffer's Easy Express* Skillets), ½ of 25-oz. pkg. . . . | 380 | 13.0 | 66.0 | 7.0 | 30 | 1220 | 2.0 |

| Food and Measure | cal. | prot. (gms) | carbo. (gms) | fat (gms) | chol. (mgs) | sod. (mgs) | fiber (gms) |
|---|---|---|---|---|---|---|---|
| (*Wanchai Ferry*), ½ of 24-oz. pkg.* | 590 | 14.0 | 87.0 | 21.0 | 25 | 850 | 3.0 |
| Szechuan, w/noodles (*Wanchai Ferry*), ½ of 24-oz. pkg. | 510 | 24.0 | 69.0 | 16.0 | 40 | 1320 | 3.0 |
| tandoori w/spinach (*Ethnic Gourmet*), 10 oz. | 170 | 14.0 | 19.0 | 4.5 | 30 | 840 | 3.0 |
| teriyaki: | | | | | | | |
| (*Birds Eye Voila!*), 1 cup* | 200 | 12.0 | 34.0 | 1.5 | 20 | 890 | 2.0 |
| (*Cedarlane*), 10 oz. | 370 | 14.0 | 54.0 | 8.0 | 35 | 1130 | 2.0 |
| (*Healthy Choice* Complete), 11 oz. | 360 | 18.0 | 58.0 | 6.0 | 35 | 520 | 4.0 |
| (*Stouffer's Easy Express* Skillets), ½ of 25-oz. pkg. | 270 | 18.0 | 41.0 | 4.0 | 40 | 850 | 5.0 |
| stir-fry (*Lean Cuisine*), 9 oz. | 250 | 12.0 | 46.0 | 2.0 | 20 | 570 | 2.0 |
| and vegetables (*Smart Ones*), 9 oz. | 230 | 14.0 | 39.0 | 3.0 | 25 | 620 | 3.0 |
| Thai: | | | | | | | |
| w/rice noodles (*Smart Ones*), 9 oz. | 260 | 15.0 | 42.0 | 4.0 | 25 | 620 | 2.0 |
| style (*Lean Cuisine*), 9 oz. | 260 | 21.0 | 35.0 | 4.0 | 35 | 540 | 0 |
| tikka masala, 10 oz.: | | | | | | | |
| (*Cedarlane*) | 420 | 14.0 | 47.0 | 23.0 | 40 | 710 | 3.0 |
| (*Ethnic Gourmet*) | 260 | 19.0 | 32.0 | 6.0 | 45 | 680 | 3.0 |
| tomato, fire-roasted (*Healthy Choice* Complete), 11.7 oz. | 310 | 19.0 | 46.0 | 5.0 | 35 | 500 | 6.0 |
| Tuscan (*Lean Cuisine Dinnertime Cuisine*), 12 oz. | 280 | 22.0 | 34.0 | 6.0 | 40 | 780 | 4.0 |
| vegetables and: | | | | | | | |
| Chinese style (*Michelina's Budget Gourmet*), 8 oz. | 310 | 8.0 | 57.0 | 5.0 | 5 | 670 | 2.0 |
| Italian style (*Michelina's Budget Gourmet*), 8 oz. | 270 | 11.0 | 44.0 | 5.0 | 10 | 540 | 4.0 |
| Szechuan, spicy (*Smart Ones*), 9 oz. | 240 | 11.0 | 38.0 | 5.0 | 10 | 710 | 4.0 |

| Food and Measure | cal. | prot. (gms) | carbo. (gms) | fat (gms) | chol. (mgs) | sod. (mgs) | fiber (gms) |
|---|---|---|---|---|---|---|---|
| **Chicken entree, frozen, vegetables and** *(cont.)* | | | | | | | |
| Szechuan style | | | | | | | |
| (*Michelina's Budget* | | | | | | | |
| *Gourmet*), 8 oz. ... | 280 | 10.0 | 51.0 | 2.5 | 5 | 880 | 2.0 |
| and vegetables: | | | | | | | |
| (*Lean Cuisine* | | | | | | | |
| Cafe), 10.5 oz. .... | 240 | 20.0 | 29.0 | 5.0 | 30 | 640 | 3.0 |
| pot pie gravy (*Birds* | | | | | | | |
| *Eye Voila!*), 1 cup* . | 290 | 14.0 | 29.0 | 13.0 | 35 | 740 | 4.0 |
| **Chicken entree, microwave,** | | | | | | | |
| 10-oz. cont., | | | | | | | |
| except as noted: | | | | | | | |
| barbecue, sweet | | | | | | | |
| hickory (*Healthy Choice* | | | | | | | |
| *Fresh Mixers*), 7.9 oz. . | 370 | 16.0 | 70.0 | 3.0 | 35 | 600 | 5.0 |
| breast w/gravy: | | | | | | | |
| w/dressing (*Hormel* | | | | | | | |
| *Compleats*) ....... | 270 | 23.0 | 29.0 | 7.0 | 45 | 800 | 2.0 |
| mashed potato | | | | | | | |
| (*Hormel Compleats*) | 200 | 19.0 | 24.0 | 3.0 | 35 | 950 | 2.0 |
| cacciatore (*Healthy* | | | | | | | |
| *Choice Fresh* | | | | | | | |
| *Mixers*), 7.9 oz. ... | 310 | 20.0 | 49.0 | 4.0 | 30 | 600 | 6.0 |
| chipotle (*Chi-Chi's* | | | | | | | |
| *Fiesta Plates*) ....... | 330 | 17.0 | 18.0 | 21.0 | 55 | 890 | 1.0 |
| and dumplings: | | | | | | | |
| (*Dinty Moore* Micro | | | | | | | |
| Cup), 7.5 oz. ..... | 200 | 10.0 | 26.0 | 6.0 | 25 | 890 | 1.0 |
| (*Hormel Compleats*) .. | 260 | 13.0 | 34.0 | 8.0 | 40 | 990 | 1.0 |
| garlic, savory | | | | | | | |
| (*ChiChi's Fiesta Plates*) | 370 | 20.0 | 21.0 | 23.0 | 60 | 970 | 5.0 |
| grilled, pasta (*Hormel* | | | | | | | |
| *Compleats*) ......... | 270 | 17.0 | 28.0 | 10.0 | 40 | 900 | 2.0 |
| marinara (*Hormel* | | | | | | | |
| *Compleats*) ......... | 250 | 20.0 | 33.0 | 4.0 | 30 | 520 | 4.0 |
| mole (*Doña Maria* | | | | | | | |
| *Platillos*) ........... | 350 | 24.0 | 25.0 | 17.0 | 70 | 980 | 3.0 |
| and noodles (*Hormel* | | | | | | | |
| *Compleats*) ......... | 240 | 15.0 | 27.0 | 8.0 | 60 | 990 | 2.0 |
| pasta primavera w/ | | | | | | | |
| (*Hormel Compleats*) .. | 220 | 16.0 | 31.0 | 4.0 | 30 | 590 | 2.0 |
| w/penne, Alfredo | | | | | | | |
| (*Hormel Compleats*) .. | 330 | 15.0 | 28.0 | 18.0 | 50 | 990 | 2.0 |

| Food and Measure | cal. | prot. (gms) | carbo. (gms) | fat (gms) | chol. (mgs) | sod. (mgs) | fiber (gms) |
|---|---|---|---|---|---|---|---|
| and rice (*Hormel Compleats*) ........ | 280 | 11.0 | 34.0 | 11.0 | 45 | 990 | 1.0 |
| salsa (*Chi-Chi's Fiesta Plates*) ............ | 260 | 17.0 | 26.0 | 10.0 | 40 | 720 | 1.0 |
| Santa Fe (*Hormel Compleats*) ........ | 280 | 20.0 | 41.0 | 4.0 | 40 | 550 | 4.0 |
| sesame: | | | | | | | |
| (*Hormel Compleats*) .. | 320 | 22.0 | 41.0 | 8.0 | 50 | 600 | 2.0 |
| teriyaki (*Healthy Choice Fresh Mixers*), 7.9 oz. ... | 380 | 13.0 | 69.0 | 6.0 | 30 | 600 | 3.0 |
| Southwest (*Healthy Choice Fresh Mixers*), 7.9 oz. ...... | 310 | 13.0 | 60.0 | 2.5 | 15 | 550 | 5.0 |
| sweet and sour (*Healthy Choice Fresh Mixers*), 7.9 oz. ...... | 390 | 12.0 | 78.0 | 3.0 | 25 | 400 | 5.0 |
| teriyaki, w/rice (*Hormel Compleats*) ........ | 270 | 13.0 | 50.0 | 1.5 | 20 | 930 | 2.0 |
| Tuscan (*Healthy Choice Fresh Mixers*), 7.4 oz. ...... | 320 | 18.0 | 50.0 | 5.0 | 25 | 540 | 6.0 |
| **"Chicken" entree, vegetarian**, frozen, 1 pkg.: | | | | | | | |
| breast, curry vindaloo sauce (*Yves*), ½ of 10.6-oz. pkg. ....... | 170 | 25.0 | 13.0 | 3.0 | 0 | 700 | 3.0 |
| enchilada (*MorningStar Farms Chik'n*), 9.5 oz. . | 280 | 12.0 | 47.0 | 7.0 | 10 | 520 | 6.0 |
| sesame (*MorningStar Farms Chik'n*), 9.5 oz. . | 310 | 14.0 | 46.0 | 9.0 | 0 | 530 | 4.0 |
| sweet and sour (*MorningStar Farms Chik'n*), 10 oz. ...... | 340 | 14.0 | 56.0 | 6.0 | 0 | 550 | 4.0 |
| **Chicken entree mix**, 1 cup\*, except as noted: | | | | | | | |
| (*Banquet Homestyle Bakes*), 1 serving: | | | | | | | |
| Alfredo, cheesy ...... | 410 | 15.0 | 38.0 | 21.0 | 40 | 950 | 3.0 |
| and biscuits, creamy .. | 350 | 10.0 | 39.0 | 17.0 | 15 | 1080 | 5.0 |
| country ............ | 360 | 10.0 | 43.0 | 17.0 | 20 | 1350 | 4.0 |
| and dumplings ...... | 220 | 11.0 | 30.0 | 6.0 | 20 | 1330 | 5.0 |

| Food and Measure | cal. | prot. (gms) | carbo. (gms) | fat (gms) | chol. (mgs) | sod. (mgs) | fiber (gms) |
|---|---|---|---|---|---|---|---|
| **Chicken entree mix** *(cont.)* | | | | | | | |
| (*Chicken Helper*): | | | | | | | |
| creamy, and noodles .. | 280 | 25.0 | 24.0 | 9.0 | 60 | 750 | <1.0 |
| enchilada, cheesy .... | 330 | 25.0 | 42.0 | 7.0 | 60 | 820 | <1.0 |
| fettuccine Alfredo .... | 280 | 25.0 | 27.0 | 8.0 | 55 | 790 | 1.0 |
| (*Good Earth Restaurant Favorites*): | | | | | | | |
| herb crusted ........ | 300 | 23.0 | 25.0 | 12.0 | 55 | 540 | 1.0 |
| Mediterranean ...... | 290 | 26.0 | 23.0 | 11.0 | 60 | 530 | 2.0 |
| Tuscan ............ | 300 | 24.0 | 26.0 | 11.0 | 55 | 620 | 3.0 |
| (*Helper Complete Meals*): | | | | | | | |
| butter biscuits ....... | 270 | 9.0 | 37.0 | 9.0 | 15 | 940 | 2.0 |
| cheesy ............. | 210 | 10.0 | 32.0 | 5.0 | 15 | 850 | 1.0 |
| cheesy rice, broccoli .. | 230 | 9.0 | 36.0 | 6.0 | 15 | 850 | <1.0 |
| fettuccine Alfredo .... | 210 | 9.0 | 31.0 | 5.0 | 15 | 890 | 1.0 |
| fried rice w/ ........ | 190 | 7.0 | 39.0 | 4.5 | 5 | 840 | 1.0 |
| (*Macaroni Grill Restaurant Favorites*): | | | | | | | |
| Alfredo w/linguine ... | 310 | 26.0 | 27.0 | 11.0 | 70 | 710 | <1.0 |
| basil Parmesan, 1½ cup* ......... | 480 | 29.0 | 42.0 | 21.0 | 100 | 1060 | 4.0 |
| basil Parmesan, creamy, and pasta . | 300 | 26.0 | 26.0 | 11.0 | 70 | 590 | 1.0 |
| Florentine, grilled, 1½ cup* ......... | 560 | 40.0 | 54.0 | 19.0 | 95 | 1110 | 3.0 |
| garlic herb, penne .... | 240 | 21.0 | 22.0 | 7.0 | 45 | 390 | 2.0 |
| Marsala w/linguine ... | 330 | 23.0 | 30.0 | 13.0 | 60 | 450 | <1.0 |
| picatta w/angel hair .. | 280 | 22.0 | 24.0 | 11.0 | 70 | 600 | <1.0 |
| (*Wanchai Ferry Restaurant Favorites*): | | | | | | | |
| cashew ............ | 330 | 21.0 | 38.0 | 10.0 | 45 | 490 | <1.0 |
| kung pao .......... | 320 | 23.0 | 36.0 | 9.0 | 50 | 640 | 1.0 |
| spicy garlic ......... | 280 | 20.0 | 34.0 | 7.0 | 45 | 380 | <1.0 |
| sweet and sour ...... | 300 | 19.0 | 40.0 | 7.0 | 45 | 310 | <1.0 |
| cheddar herb (*Annie's* Organic Skillet Meals) ............ | 450 | 20.0 | 45.0 | 21.5 | 55 | 880 | 1.0 |
| **Chicken fat** (*Empire Kosher*), 1 tbsp. ...... | 120 | 0 | 0 | 13.0 | 10 | 0 | 0 |
| **Chicken giblets**, simmered, chopped, 1 cup ...... | 228 | 37.5 | 1.4 | 6.9 | 570 | 85 | 0 |
| **Chicken gravy**, ¼ cup: | | | | | | | |
| (*Campbell's*) .......... | 40 | 0 | 3.0 | 3.0 | 5 | 260 | 0 |
| (*Campbell's* Nonfat) .... | 15 | 1.0 | 3.0 | 0 | 5 | 310 | 0 |

| Food and Measure | cal. | prot. (gms) | carbo. (gms) | fat (gms) | chol. (mgs) | sod. (mgs) | fiber (gms) |
|---|---|---|---|---|---|---|---|
| (*Franco-American* Slow Roast) . . . . . . . . | 20 | 1.0 | 3.0 | .5 | <5 | 240 | 0 |
| (*Heinz* Home Style Classic) . . . . . . . . . . . | 30 | 0 | 3.0 | 2.0 | <5 | 250 | 0 |
| **Chicken gravy mix** (*McCormick*), 2 tsp. . . | 20 | 0 | 4.0 | .5 | 0 | 340 | 0 |
| **Chicken lunch meat,** breast, 2 oz., except as noted: | | | | | | | |
| (*Black Bear*) . . . . . . . . . | 70 | 11.0 | 1.0 | 2.0 | 30 | 400 | 0 |
| barbecue: | | | | | | | |
| (*Black Bear*) . . . . . . . . | 70 | 11.0 | 1.0 | 2.0 | 30 | 400 | 0 |
| (*Boar's Head* All American) . . . . . . . | 60 | 13.0 | 2.0 | .5 | 35 | 340 | 0 |
| (*Thumann's*) . . . . . . . . | 60 | 13.0 | 0 | 1.0 | 30 | 260 | 0 |
| shaved (*Oscar Mayer* Deli Fresh), 1.8 oz. . . | 50 | 9.0 | 2.0 | 1.0 | 25 | 570 | 0 |
| Buffalo style: | | | | | | | |
| (*Black Bear*) . . . . . . . . | 70 | 11.0 | 1.0 | 2.0 | 30 | 420 | 0 |
| (*Boar's Head* Blazing Buffalo) . . . | 60 | 13.0 | 0 | 1.0 | 35 | 390 | 0 |
| (*Jennie-O*) . . . . . . . . . . | 50 | 12.0 | 1.0 | .5 | 30 | 400 | 0 |
| (*Thumann's*) . . . . . . . . | 60 | 13.0 | 0 | 1.0 | 30 | 260 | 0 |
| Cajun (*Oscar Mayer* Deli Fresh Shaved), ¼ of 8-oz. pkg. . . . . . . | 50 | 9.0 | 2.0 | 1.0 | 25 | 530 | 0 |
| chipotle (*Applegate Farms* Deli) . . . . . . . . . | 60 | 12.0 | 1.0 | .5 | 30 | 400 | 0 |
| lemon pepper (*Boar's Head*) . . . . . . . . . . . . . | 60 | 13.0 | 1.0 | 1.0 | 35 | 360 | 0 |
| mesquite (*Di Lusso*) . . . . | 60 | 12.0 | 0 | 1.0 | 30 | 450 | 0 |
| roast/oven roast: | | | | | | | |
| (*Applegate Farms* Deli Counter) . . . . . | 70 | 12.0 | 1.0 | 1.5 | 30 | 310 | 0 |
| (*Applegate Farms* Organic) . . . . . . . . . | 60 | 10.0 | 1.0 | 1.5 | 30 | 360 | 0 |
| (*Boar's Head* EverRoast) . . . . . . . | 50 | 13.0 | 1.0 | .5 | 30 | 440 | 0 |
| (*Boar's Head* Golden Classic) . . . . . . . . . | 60 | 13.0 | 0 | 1.0 | 35 | 350 | 0 |
| (*Di Lusso*) . . . . . . . . . | 50 | 10.0 | 0 | 1.5 | 20 | 420 | 0 |
| (*Jennie-O*) . . . . . . . . . | 50 | 12.0 | 1.0 | 1.0 | 30 | 450 | 0 |
| (*Oscar Mayer*), ¼ of 10-oz. pkg. . . . . . . . | 90 | 10.0 | 2.0 | 4.0 | 35 | 750 | 0 |

| Food and Measure | cal. | prot. (gms) | carbo. (gms) | fat (gms) | chol. (mgs) | sod. (mgs) | fiber (gms) |
|---|---|---|---|---|---|---|---|
| **Chicken lunch meat, roast/oven roast** *(cont.)* | | | | | | | |
| (*Oscar Mayer* Homestyle), 1 oz. . . | 40 | 5.0 | 1.0 | 2.0 | 15 | 330 | 0 |
| (*Oscar Mayer* Thin Sliced) . . . . . . . . . | 60 | 10.0 | 1.0 | 1.5 | 30 | 710 | 0 |
| (*Oscar Mayer* White), 1 oz. . . . . . . . . . . | 35 | 5.0 | 1.0 | 1.5 | 15 | 330 | 0 |
| (*Thumann's*) . . . . . . . . | 60 | 13.0 | 0 | 1.0 | 30 | 260 | 0 |
| rotisserie style: | | | | | | | |
| (*Black Bear*) . . . . . . . . | 70 | 11.0 | 1.0 | 2.0 | 30 | 400 | 0 |
| (*Boar's Head*) . . . . . . . | 60 | 13.0 | 0 | 1.0 | 35 | 400 | 0 |
| (*Hormel Natural Choice*) . . . . . . . . . | 50 | 11.0 | 0 | 1.0 | 35 | 470 | 0 |
| shaved (*Oscar Mayer* Deli Fresh), 1.8 oz. . | 50 | 9.0 | 2.0 | 1.0 | 25 | 530 | 0 |
| smoked: | | | | | | | |
| (*Applegate Farms* Deli Counter) . . . . . | 70 | 12.0 | 2.0 | 1.5 | 30 | 310 | 0 |
| (*Applegate Farms* Organic) . . . . . . . . . | 60 | 10.0 | 1.0 | 1.5 | 30 | 360 | 0 |
| hickory (*Boar's Head*) . | 60 | 13.0 | 0 | .5 | 35 | 360 | 0 |
| mesquite (*Jennie-O*) . . | 50 | 12.0 | 1.0 | .5 | 30 | 440 | 0 |
| strips, grilled or oven roasted (*Hormel Natural Choice*) . . . . . . | 60 | 12.0 | 0 | 1.5 | 35 | 340 | 0 |
| **Chicken pie**, see "Chicken entree" | | | | | | | |
| **Chicken salad**, fresh, see "Salad blend kit" | | | | | | | |
| **Chicken salad kit**, w/crackers: | | | | | | | |
| (*Bumble Bee*): | | | | | | | |
| 2.9-oz can salad . . . . . | 140 | 8.0 | 10.0 | 8.0 | 25 | 410 | 0 |
| 6 crackers, .6 oz. . . . . | 90 | 2.0 | 12.0 | 4.5 | 0 | 180 | 0 |
| (*Bumble Bee Lunch on the Run* Kit), kit components: | | | | | | | |
| chicken salad . . . . . | 160 | 8.0 | 10.0 | 8.0 | 28 | 420 | 0 |
| crackers, 6 . . . . . . . | 90 | 1.0 | 10.0 | 4.0 | 0 | 115 | 1.0 |
| mixed fruit cup . . . . | 80 | 0 | 19.0 | 0 | 0 | 15 | 1.0 |
| cookie . . . . . . . . . . | 115 | 2.0 | 15.0 | 5.0 | 10 | 80 | 0 |
| kit total, 8.2 oz. . . . . . . | 445 | 11.0 | 54.0 | 17.0 | 38 | 630 | 2.0 |
| (*Tyson* Salad Kit), 3.8-oz. pkg. . . . . . . . . | 240 | 18.0 | 15.0 | 12.0 | 45 | 610 | 1.0 |

| Food and Measure | cal. | prot. (gms) | carbo. (gms) | fat (gms) | chol. (mgs) | sod. (mgs) | fiber (gms) |
|---|---|---|---|---|---|---|---|
| **Chicken sandwich**, see "Panini," "Melts," and "Wrap, filled" | | | | | | | |
| **Chicken sausage**, see "Sausage" and specific listings | | | | | | | |
| **Chicken seasoning**, (see also "Chicken coating mix" and "Rubs"): | | | | | | | |
| (*Grill Mates* Montreal), ¾ tsp. | 5 | 0 | 1.0 | 0 | 0 | 135 | 0 |
| (*Grill Mates* Montreal Grinder), ¼ tsp. | 0 | 0 | 0 | 0 | 0 | 90 | 0 |
| (*McCormick Bag 'n Season*), 2 tsp. | 15 | 0 | 3.0 | 0 | 0 | 380 | 0 |
| (*McCormick Perfect Pinch*), ¼ tsp. | 0 | 0 | 0 | 0 | 0 | 115 | 0 |
| country (*McCormick Bag 'n Season*), 2 tsp. | 20 | 0 | 3.0 | .5 | 0 | 650 | 0 |
| glaze, barbecue, 1 tbsp.: | | | | | | | |
| honey (*McCormick*) | 25 | 0 | 5.0 | 0 | 0 | 480 | 0 |
| honey mustard (*McCormick*) | 25 | <1.0 | 4.0 | .5 | 0 | 500 | 0 |
| herb, Italian (*McCormick* Slow Cookers), 2 tsp. | 15 | 0 | 3.0 | 0 | 0 | 400 | 0 |
| Marsala, w/garlic and basil (*Lawry's* Tuscan), 1 tbsp. | 20 | <1.0 | 5.0 | 0 | 0 | 460 | 0 |
| mushroom casserole (*McCormick* One Dish), 1 tbsp. | 25 | 1.0 | 3.0 | .5 | 0 | 510 | 0 |
| and rice (*A Taste of Thai*), ¼ pkt. | 48 | <1.0 | 4.0 | 2.5 | 0 | 1073 | 0 |
| rice casserole (*McCormick* One Dish), 2 tsp. | 20 | <1.0 | 4.0 | 0 | 0 | 360 | 0 |
| roast (*Kikkoman*), 1 tbsp. | 25 | <1.0 | 4.0 | .5 | 0 | 1710 | 0 |
| rotisserie (*McCormick Perfect Pinch*), ¼ tsp. | 0 | 0 | <1.0 | 0 | 0 | 310 | 0 |
| sun-dried tomato and garlic (*Lawry's* Mediterranean), 2 tsp. | 15 | 0 | 3.0 | 0 | 0 | 370 | 0 |

| Food and Measure | cal. | prot. (gms) | carbo. (gms) | fat (gms) | chol. (mgs) | sod. (mgs) | fiber (gms) |
|---|---|---|---|---|---|---|---|
| **Chicken seasoning** *(cont.)* | | | | | | | |
| wings, Buffalo: | | | | | | | |
| (*McCormick* Original), | | | | | | | |
| 1 tbsp. . . . . . . . . . | 25 | 0 | 6.0 | 0 | 0 | 500 | 0 |
| barbecue, hickory | | | | | | | |
| (*McCormick*), 2 tsp. | 25 | 0 | 6.0 | 0 | 0 | 440 | 0 |
| garlic herb | | | | | | | |
| (*McCormick*), 1 tbsp. | 25 | 0 | 5.0 | 0 | 0 | 500 | 0 |
| **Chicken spread**, white | | | | | | | |
| (*Underwood*), ¼ cup . | 130 | 10.0 | 2.0 | 8.0 | 30 | 350 | 0 |
| **Chicken wontons**, | | | | | | | |
| frozen, Buffalo | | | | | | | |
| (*Original Rangoon*), | | | | | | | |
| 3 pcs., 3 oz. . . . . . . . | 220 | 12.0 | 29.0 | 5.0 | 25 | 580 | <1.0 |
| *Chick-fil-A:* | | | | | | | |
| breakfast: | | | | | | | |
| bagel, chicken/egg/ | | | | | | | |
| cheese . . . . . . . . . | 490 | 29.0 | 49.0 | 20.0 | 240 | 1230 | 3.0 |
| biscuit, plain . . . . . . . | 310 | 5.0 | 41.0 | 14.0 | 0 | 700 | 2.0 |
| biscuit, bacon/egg/ | | | | | | | |
| cheese . . . . . . . . . | 500 | 21.0 | 44.0 | 27.0 | 230 | 1390 | 2.0 |
| biscuit, chicken . . . . . . | 440 | 17.0 | 47.0 | 20.0 | 25 | 1230 | 3.0 |
| biscuit, chicken, | | | | | | | |
| spicy . . . . . . . . . | 450 | 16.0 | 50.0 | 20.0 | 30 | 1300 | 2.0 |
| biscuit, sausage . . . . . | 590 | 16.0 | 43.0 | 39.0 | 45 | 1300 | 2.0 |
| burrito, chicken . . . . . | 450 | 24.0 | 43.0 | 20.0 | 260 | 990 | 2.0 |
| burrito, sausage . . . . . . | 510 | 23.0 | 40.0 | 28.0 | 270 | 990 | 2.0 |
| *Chick-n-Minis* . . . . . . . | 280 | 16.0 | 30.0 | 10.0 | 40 | 650 | 1.0 |
| cinnamon cluster . . . . | 430 | 7.0 | 63.0 | 17.0 | 30 | 240 | 2.0 |
| hash browns . . . . . . . . | 270 | 3.0 | 25.0 | 18.0 | 0 | 440 | 2.0 |
| yogurt parfait . . . . . . . | 230 | 6.0 | 44.0 | 3.0 | 10 | 60 | 0 |
| w/cookie crumbs . . | 240 | 7.0 | 47.0 | 4.5 | 10 | 75 | 0 |
| w/granola . . . . . . . . | 290 | 7.0 | 53.0 | 6.0 | 10 | 85 | 1.0 |
| classics: | | | | | | | |
| *Chick-n-Strips* . . . . . . | 480 | 46.0 | 23.0 | 23.0 | 105 | 1640 | 2.0 |
| nuggets . . . . . . . . . . | 400 | 42.0 | 17.0 | 18.0 | 105 | 1490 | 1.0 |
| classics, sandwich: | | | | | | | |
| chargrilled . . . . . . . . | 290 | 29.0 | 36.0 | 4.0 | 55 | 1030 | 3.0 |
| chargrilled club . . . . . . | 410 | 37.0 | 37.0 | 12.0 | 80 | 1370 | 3.0 |
| chicken . . . . . . . . . . . | 430 | 30.0 | 38.0 | 17.0 | 60 | 1410 | 3.0 |
| chicken, spicy . . . . . . | 480 | 31.0 | 44.0 | 20.0 | 65 | 1660 | 3.0 |
| chicken, spicy, deluxe . | 570 | 36.0 | 46.0 | 27.0 | 80 | 1810 | 4.0 |
| chicken deluxe . . . . . . | 490 | 33.0 | 41.0 | 22.0 | 70 | 1660 | 3.0 |

| Food and Measure | cal. | prot. (gms) | carbo. (gms) | fat (gms) | chol. (mgs) | sod. (mgs) | fiber (gms) |
|---|---|---|---|---|---|---|---|
| chicken salad ....... | 490 | 28.0 | 55.0 | 19.0 | 80 | 1130 | 5.0 |
| *Cool Wrap:* | | | | | | | |
| chargrilled chicken ... | 410 | 33.0 | 50.0 | 12.0 | 55 | 1290 | 9.0 |
| chicken Caesar ...... | 460 | 40.0 | 47.0 | 15.0 | 65 | 1510 | 8.0 |
| spicy chicken ....... | 410 | 35.0 | 48.0 | 12.0 | 60 | 1380 | 8.0 |
| salad, no dressing: | | | | | | | |
| chargrilled & fruit .... | 220 | 22.0 | 22.0 | 6.0 | 55 | 640 | 4.0 |
| chargrilled garden .... | 180 | 23.0 | 11.0 | 6.0 | 55 | 650 | 4.0 |
| *Chick-n-Strips* ..... | 460 | 40.0 | 26.0 | 22.0 | 90 | 1350 | 5.0 |
| Southwest chargrilled . | 240 | 26.0 | 18.0 | 9.0 | 60 | 820 | 5.0 |
| salad add-ons: | | | | | | | |
| croutons ........... | 60 | 1.0 | 9.0 | 2.0 | 0 | 150 | 0 |
| harvest nut granola ... | 60 | 1.0 | 8.0 | 3.0 | 0 | 25 | 1.0 |
| honey roasted | | | | | | | |
| sunflower kernels .. | 90 | 2.0 | 4.0 | 7.0 | 0 | 55 | 1.0 |
| tortilla strips ........ | 80 | 1.0 | 8.0 | 4.0 | 0 | 50 | 1.0 |
| salad dressing: | | | | | | | |
| blue cheese ......... | 160 | 1.0 | 1.0 | 16.0 | 20 | 280 | 0 |
| buttermilk ranch ..... | 160 | 0 | 1.0 | 17.0 | 5 | 280 | 0 |
| Caesar ............ | 160 | 1.0 | 1.0 | 17.0 | 30 | 240 | 0 |
| honey mustard, free .. | 60 | 0 | 14.0 | 0 | 0 | 220 | 1.0 |
| light Italian ......... | 15 | 0 | 2.0 | .5 | 0 | 510 | 0 |
| sauces: | | | | | | | |
| barbecue ........... | 45 | 0 | 11.0 | 0 | 0 | 180 | 0 |
| Buffalo ............ | 10 | 0 | 1.0 | 0 | 0 | 420 | 0 |
| buttermilk ranch ..... | 110 | 0 | 1.0 | 12.0 | 5 | 200 | 0 |
| *Chick-fil-A* .......... | 140 | 0 | 6.0 | 13.0 | 10 | 170 | 0 |
| honey mustard ...... | 45 | 0 | 11.0 | 0 | 0 | 150 | 0 |
| honey roasted BBQ ... | 60 | 0 | 2.0 | 5.0 | 5 | 70 | 0 |
| Polynesian ......... | 110 | 0 | 14.0 | 6.0 | 0 | 210 | 0 |
| sides: | | | | | | | |
| carrot raisin salad .... | 390 | 2.0 | 60.0 | 18.0 | 10 | 240 | 5.0 |
| chicken salad cup .... | 350 | 28.0 | 9.0 | 22.0 | 120 | 1130 | 1.0 |
| cole slaw ........... | 580 | 3.0 | 31.0 | 50.0 | 35 | 450 | 5.0 |
| fruit cup ........... | 110 | 1.0 | 27.0 | 0 | 0 | 5 | 3.0 |
| hearty chicken soup .. | 220 | 12.0 | 30.0 | 6.0 | 40 | 1760 | 3.0 |
| side salad .......... | 70 | 5.0 | 5.0 | 4.5 | 15 | 110 | 2.0 |
| *Waffle Potato Fries* ... | 400 | 5.0 | 48.0 | 21.0 | 0 | 190 | 5.0 |
| desserts: | | | | | | | |
| cheesecake ......... | 310 | 5.0 | 22.0 | 23.0 | 115 | 280 | 1.0 |
| fudge nut brownie ... | 370 | 5.0 | 45.0 | 19.0 | 25 | 180 | 3.0 |
| *Icedream* .......... | 170 | 5.0 | 31.0 | 4.0 | 15 | 115 | 0 |
| lemon pie .......... | 360 | 6.0 | 58.0 | 13.0 | 30 | 290 | 1.0 |

| Food and Measure | cal. | prot. (gms) | carbo. (gms) | fat (gms) | chol. (mgs) | sod. (mgs) | fiber (gms) |
|---|---|---|---|---|---|---|---|
| **Chick-fil-A** *(cont.)* | | | | | | | |
| milkshake: | | | | | | | |
|   chocolate .......... | 750 | 16.0 | 113.0 | 28.0 | 95 | 520 | 1.0 |
|   cookies & cream ..... | 700 | 17.0 | 100.0 | 33.0 | 95 | 550 | 1.0 |
|   peppermint chocolate | | | | | | | |
|     chip ............ | 930 | 16.0 | 149.0 | 31.0 | 95 | 550 | 1.0 |
|   strawberry ......... | 770 | 16.0 | 118.0 | 28.0 | 95 | 530 | 1.0 |
|   vanilla ............. | 660 | 16.0 | 91.0 | 27.0 | 95 | 510 | 0 |
| **Chickpeas**, see | | | | | | | |
|   "Garbanzo beans" | | | | | | | |
| **Chicory, witloof**: | | | | | | | |
| (*Frieda's* Endive), | | | | | | | |
|   2 cups, 3 oz. ........ | 15 | 1.0 | 3.0 | 0 | 0 | 20 | 3.0 |
| 5–7" head, 1.9 oz. ...... | 9 | .5 | 2.1 | .1 | 0 | 1 | 1.6 |
| ½ cup ............... | 8 | .4 | 1.8 | <.1 | 0 | 1 | 1.4 |
| **Chicory greens**: | | | | | | | |
| trimmed, 1 oz. ......... | 7 | .5 | 1.3 | .1 | 0 | 13 | 1.1 |
| chopped, ½ cup ....... | 21 | 1.5 | 4.2 | .3 | 0 | 41 | 3.6 |
| **Chicory root**: | | | | | | | |
| 1 medium, 2.6 oz. ...... | 44 | .8 | 10.5 | .1 | 0 | 30 | n.a. |
| 1" pcs., ½ cup ......... | 33 | .6 | 7.9 | .1 | 0 | 23 | n.a. |
| **Chili**, canned, 1 cup: | | | | | | | |
| w/beans: | | | | | | | |
|   (*Bush's* Chunky) ..... | 260 | 15.0 | 28.0 | 10.0 | 15 | 1250 | 8.0 |
|   (*Bush's* Original) ..... | 250 | 14.0 | 26.0 | 10.0 | 15 | 1250 | 7.0 |
|   (*Campbell's* Chunky | | | | | | | |
|     Roadhouse) ...... | 230 | 15.0 | 25.0 | 8.0 | 25 | 880 | 6.0 |
|   (*Dennison's*) ........ | 360 | 20.0 | 38.0 | 14.0 | 40 | 1030 | 11.0 |
|   (*Dennison's* Chili | | | | | | | |
|     Con Carne) ....... | 350 | 22.0 | 31.0 | 15.0 | 40 | 970 | 11.0 |
|   (*Dennison's* | | | | | | | |
|     Chunky) ......... | 300 | 20.0 | 32.0 | 10.0 | 40 | 1020 | 9.0 |
|   (*Hormel*) ............ | 260 | 16.0 | 33.0 | 7.0 | 30 | 1200 | 3.5 |
|   (*Hormel* Chunky) .... | 260 | 17.0 | 32.0 | 7.0 | 30 | 1160 | 7.0 |
|   (*Hormel* Homestyle) .. | 350 | 16.0 | 28.0 | 19.0 | 40 | 1020 | 5.0 |
|   (*Hormel* Less Salt) ... | 260 | 16.0 | 33.0 | 7.0 | 30 | 880 | 7.0 |
|   (*Stagg* Chunkéro) .... | 320 | 16.0 | 28.0 | 16.0 | 40 | 850 | 6.0 |
|   (*Stagg* Classic) ..... | 330 | 16.0 | 27.0 | 17.0 | 45 | 810 | 6.0 |
|   (*Stagg* Country Brand) | 330 | 15.0 | 28.0 | 17.0 | 35 | 1140 | 6.0 |
|   (*Stagg* Fiesta Grill) ... | 250 | 15.0 | 25.0 | 10.0 | 40 | 950 | 6.0 |
|   (*Stagg* Laredo) ...... | 310 | 15.0 | 25.0 | 17.0 | 40 | 1100 | 7.0 |
|   (*Stagg* Quick Draw) .. | 290 | 18.0 | 26.0 | 13.0 | 45 | 770 | 6.0 |
|   (*Stagg* Steakhouse | | | | | | | |
|     Reserve) ........ | 280 | 21.0 | 24.0 | 11.0 | 45 | 1120 | 5.0 |

| Food and Measure | cal. | prot. (gms) | carbo. (gms) | fat (gms) | chol. (mgs) | sod. (mgs) | fiber (gms) |
|---|---|---|---|---|---|---|---|
| (*Stagg Silverado*) .... | 260 | 17.0 | 30.0 | 8.0 | 30 | 860 | 6.0 |
| (*Wolf*) ............. | 350 | 18.0 | 25.0 | 19.0 | 40 | 960 | 8.0 |
| (*Wolf* Homestyle) .... | 290 | 15.0 | 27.0 | 14.0 | 30 | 870 | 8.0 |
| (*Van Camp's*) ....... | 350 | 17.0 | 31.0 | 18.0 | 35 | 900 | 7.0 |
| 3 bean (*Hormel* Chili Master) ..... | 220 | 13.0 | 26.0 | 7.0 | 25 | 990 | 6.0 |
| hot (*Bush's*) ........ | 250 | 14.0 | 26.0 | 10.0 | 15 | 1260 | 7.0 |
| hot (*Dennison's*) ..... | 350 | 21.0 | 36.0 | 14.0 | 40 | 930 | 11.0 |
| hot (*Dennison's* Chunky) ......... | 300 | 20.0 | 32.0 | 10.0 | 40 | 930 | 9.0 |
| hot (*Hormel*) ........ | 260 | 16.0 | 33.0 | 7.0 | 30 | 1190 | 7.0 |
| hot (*Stagg Dynamite*) . | 340 | 17.0 | 30.0 | 17.0 | 40 | 800 | 8.0 |
| hot/spicy (*Campbell's Chunky* Firehouse) . | 230 | 15.0 | 25.0 | 8.0 | 25 | 870 | 6.0 |
| hot/spicy (*Campbell's Chunky* Firehouse Micro) .......... | 230 | 15.0 | 25.0 | 8.0 | 25 | 860 | 6.0 |
| hot/spicy (*Hormel*) ... | 260 | 16.0 | 33.0 | 7.0 | 25 | 1300 | 9.0 |
| mild (*Wolf*) ......... | 350 | 18.0 | 25.0 | 19.0 | 40 | 1050 | 8.0 |
| steak, grilled (*Campbell's Chunky*) | 200 | 16.0 | 27.0 | 3.0 | 20 | 870 | 7.0 |
| tomato, roasted (*Hormel Chili Master*) .... | 210 | 14.0 | 25.0 | 6.0 | 25 | 990 | 7.0 |
| w/out beans: | | | | | | | |
| (*Bush's* No Bean) .... | 240 | 13.0 | 16.0 | 14.0 | 25 | 1380 | 3.0 |
| (*Campbell's Chunky* Hold the Beans) ... | 240 | 18.0 | 20.0 | 10.0 | 35 | 770 | 5.0 |
| (*Dennison's* Chili Con Carne) ....... | 310 | 21.0 | 20.0 | 16.0 | 55 | 1150 | 3.0 |
| (*Hormel*) ........... | 220 | 16.0 | 18.0 | 9.0 | 40 | 970 | 3.0 |
| (*Hormel* Chunky) .... | 210 | 16.0 | 19.0 | 8.0 | 40 | 1130 | 4.0 |
| (*Hormel* Less Salt) ... | 220 | 16.0 | 18.0 | 9.0 | 40 | 710 | 3.0 |
| (*Stagg Steak House*) .. | 320 | 17.0 | 14.0 | 22.0 | 65 | 1080 | 2.0 |
| (*Wolf*) ............. | 400 | 19.0 | 19.0 | 28.0 | 55 | 950 | 5.0 |
| (*Van Camp's*) ....... | 390 | 20.0 | 20.0 | 26.0 | 50 | 1080 | 6.0 |
| hot (*Hormel*) ........ | 220 | 16.0 | 18.0 | 9.0 | 40 | 970 | 3.0 |
| hot (*Wolf*) .......... | 400 | 19.0 | 19.0 | 28.0 | 55 | 960 | 5.0 |
| hot/spicy (*Hormel*) ... | 220 | 16.0 | 19.0 | 9.0 | 40 | 1030 | 3.0 |
| lean (*Wolf*) ......... | 210 | 23.0 | 17.0 | 6.0 | 65 | 950 | 5.0 |
| mild (*Wolf*) ......... | 400 | 19.0 | 19.0 | 28.0 | 55 | 950 | 5.0 |
| tomato, roasted (*Hormel Chili Master*) .. | 210 | 14.0 | 13.0 | 11.0 | 40 | 990 | 2.0 |
| chicken, w/beans: | | | | | | | |
| (*Stagg* Santa Fe) ..... | 200 | 15.0 | 25.0 | 4.0 | 25 | 900 | 6.0 |

| Food and Measure | cal. | prot. (gms) | carbo. (gms) | fat (gms) | chol. (mgs) | sod. (mgs) | fiber (gms) |
|---|---|---|---|---|---|---|---|
| **Chili, chicken** *(cont.)* | | | | | | | |
| (*Stagg Ranch House*) . | 240 | 17.0 | 26.0 | 8.0 | 55 | 780 | 7.0 |
| chipotle (*Hormel Chili Master*) ..... | 240 | 17.0 | 28.0 | 7.0 | 50 | 970 | 7.0 |
| white (*Hormel Chili Master*) ..... | 220 | 19.0 | 17.0 | 8.0 | 50 | 990 | 4.0 |
| white (*Stagg*) ....... | 260 | 17.0 | 20.0 | 12.0 | 70 | 1010 | 4.0 |
| turkey, w/beans: | | | | | | | |
| (*Hormel*) .......... | 210 | 17.0 | 28.0 | 3.0 | 45 | 1250 | 6.0 |
| (*Stagg Ranchero*) .... | 260 | 20.0 | 34.0 | 5.0 | 35 | 790 | 9.0 |
| (*Wolf*) ............. | 230 | 23.0 | 29.0 | 2.5 | 25 | 1080 | 10.0 |
| turkey, w/out beans: | | | | | | | |
| (*Hormel*) .......... | 190 | 23.0 | 16.0 | 3.0 | 80 | 1230 | 3.0 |
| (*Wolf*) ............. | 180 | 24.0 | 15.0 | 2.5 | 35 | 1270 | 4.0 |
| vegetable/vegetarian: | | | | | | | |
| (*Dennison's*) ........ | 190 | 9.0 | 34.0 | 1.5 | 0 | 800 | 9.0 |
| (*Health Valley* Organic Tame Tomato No Salt) ......... | 210 | 10.0 | 41.0 | 2.5 | 0 | 70 | 8.0 |
| (*Hormel*) .......... | 190 | 11.0 | 35.0 | 1.0 | 0 | 780 | 10.0 |
| (*Worthington*) ....... | 280 | 24.0 | 25.0 | 10.0 | 0 | 1130 | 8.0 |
| 4 bean (*Stagg Vegetable Garden*) . | 200 | 10.0 | 37.0 | 1.0 | 0 | 890 | 8.0 |
| 3 bean chipotle (*Health Valley* Organic) .... | 200 | 11.0 | 37.0 | 3.0 | 0 | 470 | 8.0 |
| great northern bean/ barley (*Eden* Organic) ......... | 200 | 9.0 | 38.0 | 1.0 | 0 | 490 | 8.0 |
| kidney bean/kamut (*Eden* Organic) .... | 240 | 14.0 | 43.0 | 2.0 | 0 | 460 | 11.0 |
| medium (*Amy's* Organic) ......... | 280 | 15.0 | 35.0 | 9.0 | 0 | 680 | 7.0 |
| medium (*Amy's* Organic Light Sodium) ......... | 280 | 15.0 | 35.0 | 9.0 | 0 | 340 | 7.0 |
| medium, w/vegetables (*Amy's* Organic) ... | 190 | 7.0 | 29.0 | 6.0 | 0 | 590 | 8.0 |
| pinto/spelt (*Eden* Organic) ......... | 220 | 11.0 | 42.0 | 1.5 | 0 | 460 | 8.0 |
| spicy (*Amy's* Organic) | 280 | 15.0 | 35.0 | 9.0 | 0 | 680 | 7.0 |
| spicy (*Amy's* Organic Light Sodium) .... | 280 | 15.0 | 35.0 | 9.0 | 0 | 340 | 7.0 |
| spicy (*Health Valley* Organic) ......... | 190 | 10.0 | 36.0 | 3.0 | 0 | 470 | 8.0 |

| Food and Measure | cal. | prot. (gms) | carbo. (gms) | fat (gms) | chol. (mgs) | sod. (mgs) | fiber (gms) |
|---|---|---|---|---|---|---|---|
| white bean (*Health Valley* Organic Santa Fe) ........ | 200 | 10.0 | 39.0 | 3.0 | 0 | 470 | 9.0 |
| vegetarian, black bean: | | | | | | | |
| (*Amy's* Organic) ..... | 200 | 13.0 | 31.0 | 3.0 | 0 | 680 | 13.0 |
| (*Amy's* Organic Southwestern) .... | 240 | 12.0 | 40.0 | 4.0 | 0 | 680 | 10.0 |
| mango (*Health Valley* Organic) ......... | 210 | 9.0 | 41.0 | 3.0 | 0 | 460 | 7.0 |
| mole (*Health Valley* Organic) ......... | 200 | 11.0 | 36.0 | 3.0 | 0 | 470 | 7.0 |
| and quinoa (*Eden* Organic) ......... | 190 | 10.0 | 35.0 | 1.5 | 0 | 460 | 6.0 |
| **Chili, frozen** (see also "Chili entree, frozen"), vegetarian: | | | | | | | |
| (*Tabatchnick*), 7.5 oz. ... | 180 | 12.0 | 28.0 | 3.5 | 0 | 360 | 8.0 |
| 3 bean (*MorningStar Farms*), 1 cup ....... | 170 | 12.0 | 32.0 | 2.5 | 0 | 490 | 10.0 |
| 2 bean (*Moosewood* Organic Texas), 1 cup . | 190 | 9.0 | 31.0 | 4.5 | 0 | 940 | 9.0 |
| **Chili, mix**, vegetarian: | | | | | | | |
| (*Fantastic*), ⅓ cup ... | 140 | 12.0 | 25.0 | 1.0 | 0 | 890 | 6.0 |
| **Chili beans** (see also "Chili starter" and "Mexican beans"), canned, ½ cup: | | | | | | | |
| (*Bush's*) ............. | 120 | 6.0 | 20.0 | 1.0 | 0 | 480 | 6.0 |
| (*S&W* Chili Makin's Original) ........... | 100 | 5.0 | 20.0 | .5 | 0 | 710 | 5.0 |
| chili sauce (*Bush's*) ..... | 100 | 6.0 | 22.0 | .5 | 0 | 480 | 7.0 |
| w/chipotle (*S&W*) ...... | 110 | 7.0 | 23.0 | 1.0 | 0 | 530 | 6.0 |
| w/jalapeño/red pepper (*Eden* Organic) ...... | 130 | 9.0 | 21.0 | 0 | 0 | 250 | 7.0 |
| tomato sauce (*S&W*) ... | 110 | 7.0 | 23.0 | 1.0 | 0 | 620 | 6.0 |
| **Chili entree, frozen**, 1 pkg.: | | | | | | | |
| bean, black: | | | | | | | |
| chipotle w/rice (*Mimi's Gourmet* Organic), 11.5 oz. ......... | 290 | 10.0 | 48.0 | 8.0 | 0 | 700 | 10.0 |
| and corn (*Mimi's Gourmet* Organic), 10.5 oz. ......... | 250 | 10.0 | 40.0 | 6.0 | 0 | 680 | 11.0 |

| Food and Measure | cal. | prot. (gms) | carbo. (gms) | fat (gms) | chol. (mgs) | sod. (mgs) | fiber (gms) |
|---|---|---|---|---|---|---|---|
| **Chili entree, frozen** *(cont.)* | | | | | | | |
| bean, 3: | | | | | | | |
| (*Kettle Cuisine*), 10 oz. | 220 | 11.0 | 36.0 | 3.5 | 0 | 450 | 13.0 |
| w/rice (*Mimi's Gourmet* Organic), 11.5 oz. . . . . . . . . | 250 | 10.0 | 40.0 | 6.0 | 0 | 680 | 11.0 |
| bean, white, and jalapeño (*Mimi's Gourmet* Organic), 10.5 oz. . . . . | 230 | 10.0 | 35.0 | 6.0 | 0 | 660 | 9.0 |
| beef steak, Angus (*Kettle Cuisine*), 10 oz. | 250 | 22.0 | 21.0 | 9.0 | 35 | 540 | 8.0 |
| w/vegetables: | | | | | | | |
| and cornbread (*Amy's*), 10.5 oz. . . | 340 | 11.0 | 59.0 | 6.0 | 10 | 680 | 10.0 |
| and tofu steaks (*Helen's Kitchen* Organic), 10 oz. . . . | 220 | 14.0 | 29.0 | 5.0 | 0 | 340 | 8.0 |
| **Chili entree, microwave**, 1 cont.: | | | | | | | |
| (*Hormel Compleats*), 10 oz.: | | | | | | | |
| w/beans . . . . . . . . . . . | 310 | 18.0 | 20.0 | 18.0 | 65 | 950 | 4.0 |
| chili'n mac . . . . . . . . . | 270 | 17.0 | 34.0 | 7.0 | 30 | 980 | 6.0 |
| chili'n spuds . . . . . . . . | 290 | 13.0 | 33.0 | 12.0 | 30 | 760 | 4.0 |
| (*Hormel* Microcup), 7.375 oz.: | | | | | | | |
| w/beans . . . . . . . . . . . | 220 | 13.0 | 28.0 | 6.0 | 25 | 790 | 6.0 |
| hot . . . . . . . . . . . . . . | 220 | 13.0 | 27.0 | 6.0 | 20 | 900 | 6.0 |
| w/out beans . . . . . . . . | 190 | 14.0 | 16.0 | 8.0 | 35 | 860 | 2.0 |
| **Chili paste** (see also "Curry paste"), 1 tsp.: | | | | | | | |
| green (*Tiger Tiger*) . . . . . | 12 | <1.0 | 3.0 | .4 | 0 | 100 | <1.0 |
| red (*Tiger Tiger*) . . . . . . . | 13 | <1.0 | 3.0 | .4 | 0 | 100 | <1.0 |
| **Chili pepper**, see "Pepper, chili" | | | | | | | |
| **Chili pocket**, frozen, 3-bean (*Aunt Trudy's* Organic), 5-oz. pkg. . . | 260 | 8.0 | 42.0 | 7.0 | 0 | 300 | 5.0 |
| **Chili powder**: | | | | | | | |
| (*McCormick*), ¼ tsp. . . . . | 2 | 0 | 0 | 0 | 0 | 10 | 0 |
| 1 tbsp. . . . . . . . . . . . . . . | 24 | .9 | 4.1 | 1.3 | 0 | 76 | 2.6 |
| 1 tsp. . . . . . . . . . . . . . | 8 | .3 | 1.4 | .4 | 0 | 26 | .9 |
| hot, Mexican style (*McCormick*), 1 tsp. . . | 10 | 0 | 1.0 | 0 | 0 | 50 | <1.0 |

| Food and Measure | cal. | prot. (gms) | carbo. (gms) | fat (gms) | chol. (mgs) | sod. (mgs) | fiber (gms) |
|---|---|---|---|---|---|---|---|
| **Chili sauce, Asian** (see also specific listings), 2 tbsp., except as noted: | | | | | | | |
| (*Heaven and Earth Dragon Fire*), 1 tbsp. | 25 | 0 | 6.0 | 0 | 0 | 50 | 0 |
| (*Kikkoman* Thai) | 70 | 0 | 15.0 | 1.0 | 0 | 240 | 1.0 |
| (*Tiger Tiger* Sriracha Dipping) | 20 | 0 | 5.0 | 0 | 0 | 300 | <1.0 |
| garlic: | | | | | | | |
| (*Roland*), 1 tbsp. | 10 | 0 | 3.0 | 0 | 0 | 680 | 0 |
| pepper (*A Taste of Thai*), 1 tsp. | 5 | 0 | 1.0 | 0 | 0 | 95 | 0 |
| ginger (*Roland*) | 35 | 0 | 8.0 | 0 | 0 | 210 | 0 |
| mango (*Roland*) | 45 | 0 | 11.0 | 0 | 0 | 220 | 0 |
| pineapple (*Roland*) | 40 | 0 | 9.0 | 0 | 0 | 200 | 0 |
| sweet: | | | | | | | |
| (*Ka•Me*), 1 tbsp. | 35 | 0 | 9.0 | 0 | 0 | 240 | 1.0 |
| (*Tiger Tiger* Dipping) | 50 | 0 | 12.0 | 0 | 0 | 200 | 1.0 |
| red (*A Taste of Thai*), 1 tsp. | 5 | 0 | 1.0 | 0 | 0 | 95 | 0 |
| **Chili sauce, Mexican**, red, ¼ cup: | | | | | | | |
| (*La Victoria*) | 20 | 0 | 3.0 | 0 | 0 | 320 | 1.0 |
| (*Las Palmas*) | 20 | 0 | 2.0 | .5 | 0 | 310 | 1.0 |
| **Chili sauce, sweet** (*Frank's RedHot*), 2 tbsp. | 70 | 0 | 17.0 | 0 | 0 | 460 | 0 |
| **Chili sauce, tomato:** | | | | | | | |
| (*Del Monte*), 1 tbsp. | 20 | 0 | 5.0 | 0 | 0 | 480 | 0 |
| (*Heinz*), 1 tbsp. | 20 | 0 | 4.0 | 0 | 0 | 230 | 0 |
| (*Wolf* Hot Dog), 2 tbsp. | 25 | 1.0 | 4.0 | 1.0 | 0 | 120 | 1.0 |
| **Chili seasoning mix:** | | | | | | | |
| (*Adolph's Meal Makers*), 1 tbsp. | 30 | <1.0 | 5.0 | 1.0 | 0 | 290 | 1.0 |
| (*Lawry's*), 1 tsp. | 10 | 0 | 2.0 | 0 | 0 | 500 | 0 |
| (*McCormick*), 1⅓ tbsp. | 30 | 1.0 | 5.0 | .5 | 0 | 310 | 2.0 |
| (*McCormick* Less Sodium), 1 tbsp. | 30 | 1.0 | 5.0 | .5 | 0 | 210 | 1.0 |
| (*McCormick* Slow Cookers), 2 tsp. | 15 | <1.0 | 2.0 | 0 | 0 | 420 | 0 |
| (*Old El Paso*), 2 tsp. | 15 | 0 | 3.0 | 0 | 0 | 630 | 0 |
| (*Ortega*), 1⅓ tbsp. | 30 | 0 | 5.0 | .5 | 0 | 440 | 0 |

| Food and Measure | cal. | prot. (gms) | carbo. (gms) | fat (gms) | chol. (mgs) | sod. (mgs) | fiber (gms) |
|---|---|---|---|---|---|---|---|
| **Chili seasoning mix** *(cont.)* | | | | | | | |
| hot: | | | | | | | |
|   (*McCormick*), 1⅓ tbsp. | .35 | 1.0 | 4.0 | 1.0 | 0 | 370 | 0 |
|   (*Wick Fowler's* 2- | | | | | | | |
|     Alarm Kit), 3 tbsp. | 60 | 2.0 | 10.0 | 1.5 | 0 | 980 | 0 |
| mild (*McCormick*), | | | | | | | |
|   1⅓ tbsp. . . . . . . . . . . | 30 | <1.0 | 5.0 | 0 | 0 | 490 | <1.0 |
| Tex-Mex | | | | | | | |
|   (*McCormick*), 1 tbsp. | 35 | <1.0 | 4.0 | 1.0 | 0 | 360 | 2.0 |
| white chicken | | | | | | | |
|   (*McCormick*), 1 tbsp. | 30 | 0 | 5.0 | .5 | 0 | 450 | 0 |
| **Chili starter** (*Bush's* | | | | | | | |
| *Chili Magic*), canned: | | | | | | | |
| Texas, ½ cup . . . . . . . . . | 120 | 5.0 | 20.0 | 2.0 | 0 | 1130 | 5.0 |
| Texas, 1 cup* . . . . . . . . . | 230 | 22.0 | 15.0 | 9.0 | 55 | 880 | 4.0 |
| traditional, ½ cup . . . . . . | 110 | 5.0 | 19.0 | 1.0 | 0 | 890 | 5.0 |
| traditional, 1 cup* . . . . . . | 220 | 22.0 | 15.0 | 8.0 | 55 | 770 | 3.0 |
| **Chimichanga**, frozen: | | | | | | | |
| beef/bean: | | | | | | | |
|   (*El Monterey* Family | | | | | | | |
|     Pack), 4-oz. pc. . . . | 310 | 9.0 | 33.0 | 15.0 | 15 | 300 | 2.0 |
|   (*El Monterey* 2-Pack), | | | | | | | |
|     4-oz. pc. . . . . . . . . . | 310 | 9.0 | 33.0 | 15.0 | 15 | 400 | 2.0 |
|   spicy (*El Monterey* | | | | | | | |
|     Red Hot XX | | | | | | | |
|     Large!), 10 oz. . . . . | 880 | 22.0 | 79.0 | 53.0 | 35 | 720 | 4.0 |
| chicken/cheese: | | | | | | | |
|   (*José Olé*), 5 oz. . . . . . | 330 | 11.0 | 45.0 | 11.0 | 20 | 540 | 2.0 |
|   mini (*El Monterey*), | | | | | | | |
|     2 pcs., 3 oz. . . . . . . | 190 | 8.0 | 22.0 | 8.0 | 15 | 310 | 0 |
|   Monterey Jack (*El* | | | | | | | |
|     *Monterey* Supreme), | | | | | | | |
|     5 oz. . . . . . . . . . . . | 280 | 12.0 | 37.0 | 10.0 | 20 | 640 | 2.0 |
| jalapeno/cheese, spicy | | | | | | | |
|   (*El Monterey* Family/ | | | | | | | |
|   2-Pack), 4 oz. . . . . . . . | 250 | 8.0 | 34.0 | 9.0 | 5 | 290 | 2.0 |
| nacho cheese/beef, mini | | | | | | | |
|   (*El Monterey*), 2 pcs., | | | | | | | |
|   3 oz. . . . . . . . . . . . . . | 240 | 8.0 | 22.0 | 13.0 | 20 | 330 | 1.0 |
| steak/cheese: | | | | | | | |
|   (*José Olé*), 5 oz. . . . . . | 350 | 12.0 | 41.0 | 14.0 | 20 | 640 | 2.0 |
|   cheddar, mini (*José* | | | | | | | |
|     *Olé*), 3 pcs., 3.8 oz. | 370 | 11.0 | 37.0 | 20.0 | 20 | 680 | 3.0 |

| Food and Measure | cal. | prot. (gms) | carbo. (gms) | fat (gms) | chol. (mgs) | sod. (mgs) | fiber (gms) |
|---|---|---|---|---|---|---|---|
| shredded (*El Monterey* Supreme), 5 oz. | 330 | 12.0 | 35.0 | 15.0 | 30 | 350 | 1.0 |
| **Chipotle**, see "Pepper, chipotle" | | | | | | | |
| **Chipotle dip**: | | | | | | | |
| (*Bison*), 2 tbsp. | 50 | 1.0 | 2.0 | 4.5 | 20 | 190 | 0 |
| (*Margaritaville*), 1 oz. | 120 | 1.0 | 1.0 | 13.0 | 20 | 75 | 0 |
| ***Chipotle Mexican Grill:*** | | | | | | | |
| flour tortilla, burrito, 1 | 290 | 7.0 | 44.0 | 9.0 | 0 | 670 | 2.0 |
| flour tortilla, taco, 1 | 90 | 2.0 | 13.0 | 2.5 | 0 | 200 | <1.0 |
| crispy taco, 1 | 60 | <1.0 | 9.0 | 2.0 | 0 | 10 | 1.0 |
| cilantro-lime rice, 3 oz. | 130 | 2.0 | 23.0 | 3.0 | 0 | 150 | 0 |
| black beans, 4 oz. | 120 | 7.0 | 23.0 | 1.0 | 0 | 250 | 11.0 |
| pinto beans, 4 oz. | 120 | 7.0 | 22.0 | 1.0 | 5 | 330 | 10.0 |
| fajita vegetables, 2.5 oz. | 20 | 1.0 | 4.0 | .5 | 0 | 170 | 1.0 |
| barbacoa, 4 oz. | 170 | 24.0 | 2.0 | 7.0 | 60 | 510 | 0 |
| chicken, 4 oz. | 190 | 32.0 | 1.0 | 6.5 | 115 | 370 | 0 |
| carnitas, 4 oz. | 190 | 27.0 | 1.0 | 8.0 | 70 | 540 | 0 |
| steak, 4 oz. | 190 | 30.0 | 2.0 | 6.5 | 65 | 320 | 0 |
| salsa: | | | | | | | |
| tomato, 3.5 oz. | 20 | 1.0 | 4.0 | 0 | 0 | 470 | <1.0 |
| corn, 3.5 oz. | 80 | 3.0 | 15.0 | 1.5 | 0 | 410 | 3.0 |
| green tomatillo, ¼ cup | 15 | 1.0 | 3.0 | 0 | 0 | 230 | 1.0 |
| red tomatillo, ¼ cup | 40 | 2.0 | 8.0 | 1.0 | 0 | 510 | 4.0 |
| cheese, 1 oz. | 100 | 8.0 | 0 | 8.5 | 30 | 180 | 0 |
| sour cream, 2 oz. | 120 | 2.0 | 2.0 | 10.0 | 40 | 30 | 0 |
| guacamole, 3.5 oz. | 150 | 2.0 | 8.0 | 13.0 | 0 | 190 | 6.0 |
| romaine, salad, 2.5 oz. | 10 | 1.0 | 2.0 | 0 | 0 | 5 | 1.0 |
| romaine, tacos, 1 oz. | 5 | 0 | 1.0 | 0 | 0 | 0 | 1.0 |
| chips, 4 oz. | 570 | 8.0 | 73.0 | 27.0 | 0 | 420 | 8.0 |
| vinaigrette, ¼ cup | 260 | 0 | 12.0 | 24.5 | 0 | 700 | 1.0 |
| **Chitterlings**, pork, simmered, 4 oz. | 344 | 11.6 | 0 | 32.6 | 162 | 44 | 0 |
| **Chives**: | | | | | | | |
| fresh, 1 oz. | 9 | .9 | 1.2 | .2 | 0 | 1 | .9 |
| fresh, chopped, 1 tbsp. | 1 | .1 | .1 | <.1 | 0 | <1 | .1 |
| freeze-dried, 1 tbsp. | 1 | <.1 | .1 | <.1 | 0 | 6 | <1.0 |
| **Chocolate**, see "Candy" | | | | | | | |
| **Chocolate, baking**, .5 oz., except as noted: | | | | | | | |
| (*Nestlé Choco Bake*) | 80 | 1.0 | 4.0 | 8.0 | 0 | 0 | 2.0 |
| bars: | | | | | | | |
| bittersweet (*Baker's*) | 70 | 1.0 | 7.0 | 6.0 | 0 | 0 | 1.0 |
| semisweet (*Baker's*) | 70 | 1.0 | 8.0 | 4.5 | 0 | 0 | 1.0 |

| Food and Measure | cal. | prot. (gms) | carbo. (gms) | fat (gms) | chol. (mgs) | sod. (mgs) | fiber (gms) |
|---|---|---|---|---|---|---|---|
| **Chocolate, baking, bars** *(cont.)* | | | | | | | |
| semisweet (*Hershey's*) | 70 | 1.0 | 9.0 | 4.0 | 0 | 0 | 1.0 |
| semisweet (*Nestlé* | | | | | | | |
| Toll House) ....... | 70 | 0 | 9.0 | 4.0 | 0 | 0 | 0 |
| sweet (*Baker's German*) | 60 | 1.0 | 8.0 | 4.0 | 0 | 0 | 1.0 |
| white (*Baker's*) ...... | 60 | 1.0 | 9.0 | 4.5 | 0 | 10 | 0 |
| bars, unsweetened: | | | | | | | |
| (*Baker's*) ............ | 70 | 2.0 | 4.0 | 7.0 | 0 | 0 | 2.0 |
| (*Hershey's*) .......... | 70 | 2.0 | 4.0 | 7.0 | 0 | 0 | 2.0 |
| chips or morsels: | | | | | | | |
| dark (*Hershey's* | | | | | | | |
| Special Dark*) ..... | 70 | 1.0 | 9.0 | 4.5 | 0 | 5 | 1.0 |
| milk (*Hershey's*) ..... | 70 | 1.0 | 9.0 | 4.5 | 5 | 10 | 1.0 |
| milk (*Hershey's Kisses*), | | | | | | | |
| 11 pcs., .5 oz. .... | 70 | 1.0 | 9.0 | 4.5 | 5 | 20 | 0 |
| milk (*Nestlé Toll* | | | | | | | |
| House) .......... | 70 | 0 | 9.0 | 4.0 | 4 | 5 | 0 |
| mint (*Hershey's*) ..... | 70 | 1.0 | 10.0 | 4.0 | 0 | 0 | 1.0 |
| mini, semisweet or | | | | | | | |
| white (*Nestlé Toll* | | | | | | | |
| House Toppers*) ... | 70 | 0 | 9.0 | 4.0 | 0 | 0 | 0 |
| semisweet (*Hershey's*) | 70 | 1.0 | 10.0 | 4.0 | 0 | 0 | 1.0 |
| semisweet (*Nestlé Toll* | | | | | | | |
| House) .......... | 70 | 0 | 9.0 | 4.0 | 0 | 0 | 0 |
| toffee (*Heath Chips*) .. | 80 | 0 | 9.0 | 5.0 | 5 | 50 | 0 |
| white (*Hershey's*) .... | 80 | 1.0 | 9.0 | 4.0 | 0 | 35 | 0 |
| white (*Nestlé Toll* | | | | | | | |
| House) .......... | 70 | 0 | 9.0 | 4.0 | 0 | 15 | 0 |
| chunks or pieces: | | | | | | | |
| semisweet (*Nestlé* | | | | | | | |
| Toll House*), .4 oz. . | 60 | 0 | 8.0 | 3.5 | 0 | 0 | 0 |
| semisweet (*Baker's*) .. | 70 | 1.0 | 9.0 | 4.5 | 0 | 5 | 1.0 |
| **Chocolate dip**, see | | | | | | | |
| "Fruit dip" | | | | | | | |
| **Chocolate drink mix** | | | | | | | |
| (see also "Cocoa"): | | | | | | | |
| (*Nesquik*), 2 tbsp. ...... | 60 | <1.0 | 14.0 | .5 | 0 | 30 | <1.0 |
| (*Nesquik* No Sugar), | | | | | | | |
| 2 tbsp. ............ | 35 | 1.0 | 7.0 | 1.0 | 0 | 70 | 1.0 |
| (*Ovaltine*), 4 tbsp. ...... | 80 | <1.0 | 19.0 | 0 | 0 | 140 | 0 |
| malt (*Ovaltine*), 4 tbsp. .. | 80 | 1.0 | 18.0 | 0 | 0 | 115 | <1.0 |
| **Chocolate milk**, see | | | | | | | |
| "Milk, flavored" | | | | | | | |

| Food and Measure | cal. | prot. (gms) | carbo. (gms) | fat (gms) | chol. (mgs) | sod. (mgs) | fiber (gms) |
|---|---|---|---|---|---|---|---|
| **Chocolate sprinkles** | | | | | | | |
| (*Hershey's*), 2 tbsp. .. | 90 | 1.0 | 12.0 | 4.0 | 0 | 50 | 1.0 |
| **Chocolate syrup**, 2 tbsp.: | | | | | | | |
| (*Fox's U-Bet*) .......... | 120 | 1.0 | 29.0 | 0 | 0 | 35 | 0 |
| (*Hershey's*) ............ | 100 | 1.0 | 24.0 | 0 | 0 | 15 | 1.0 |
| (*Hershey's* Lite) ........ | 40 | 0 | 11.0 | 0 | 0 | 70 | 1.0 |
| (*Hershey's* Sugar Free) .. | 15 | 1.0 | 5.0 | 0 | 0 | 120 | 1.0 |
| (*Nesquik*) ............. | 100 | 0 | 25.0 | 0 | 0 | 55 | <1.0 |
| (*Santa Cruz Organic*) .... | 110 | 1.0 | 26.0 | 0 | 0 | 15 | 1.0 |
| (*Smucker's Sundae*) .... | 100 | <1.0 | 24.0 | 0 | 0 | 20 | 1.0 |
| (*Smucker's Sundae* Sugar Free) ......... | 90 | 1.0 | 23.0 | .5 | 0 | 35 | 1.0 |
| dark (*Hershey's Special Dark*) ............. | 100 | 1.0 | 24.0 | 0 | 0 | 30 | 1.0 |
| double (*Hershey's* Sundae) | 100 | 1.0 | 25.0 | 0 | 0 | 20 | 1.0 |
| malt (*Whoppers*) ....... | 100 | 0 | 25.0 | 0 | 0 | 45 | 1.0 |
| mint or raspberry (*Santa Cruz Organic*) . | 110 | <1.0 | 26.0 | 0 | 0 | 10 | 1.0 |
| **Chocolate topping**, 2 tbsp.: | | | | | | | |
| (*Hershey's* Shell) ....... | 220 | 1.0 | 16.0 | 18.0 | 0 | 15 | 1.0 |
| (*Smucker's Magic Shell*) . | 210 | 1.0 | 17.0 | 16.0 | 0 | 30 | 1.0 |
| dark (*Smucker's* Special Recipe) ............ | 120 | 1.0 | 24.0 | 1.5 | 0 | 50 | 1.0 |
| fudge: | | | | | | | |
| (*Smucker's*) ........ | 120 | 0 | 26.0 | 1.5 | 0 | 65 | 2.0 |
| (*Smucker's Magic Shell*) | 210 | 1.0 | 17.0 | 16.0 | 0 | 45 | <1.0 |
| fudge, hot: | | | | | | | |
| (*Hershey's*) ......... | 120 | 2.0 | 20.0 | 4.0 | 0 | 90 | 1.0 |
| (*Smucker's*) ........ | 130 | 2.0 | 22.0 | 4.5 | 0 | 50 | <1.0 |
| (*Smucker's* Micro) ... | 130 | 2.0 | 22.0 | 3.5 | 0 | 45 | <1.0 |
| (*Smucker's* Special Recipe) .......... | 130 | 2.0 | 21.0 | 4.5 | 0 | 60 | <1.0 |
| (*Smucker's* Sugar Free) | 90 | 1.0 | 23.0 | .5 | 0 | 40 | 1.0 |
| dark (*Hershey's Special Dark*) ..... | 110 | 1.0 | 19.0 | 4.0 | 0 | 100 | 1.0 |
| milk (*Smucker's* Special Recipe) ............ | 120 | 2.0 | 21.0 | 4.0 | 0 | 80 | 1.0 |
| mint (*Smucker's*) ...... | 120 | 1.0 | 25.0 | 1.5 | 0 | 55 | 1.0 |
| s'mores (*Smucker's Magic Shell*) ........ | 220 | 1.0 | 19.0 | 16.0 | 0 | 35 | 1.0 |
| **Chorizo**: | | | | | | | |
| (*Applegate Farms*), 1 oz. . | 110 | 8.0 | 0 | 8.0 | 30 | 490 | 0 |

| Food and Measure | cal. | prot. (gms) | carbo. (gms) | fat (gms) | chol. (mgs) | sod. (mgs) | fiber (gms) |
|---|---|---|---|---|---|---|---|
| **Chorizo** *(cont.)* | | | | | | | |
| (*Del Oro* Mexican Style), 2 oz. ........ | 160 | 8.0 | 0 | 14.0 | 40 | 360 | 0 |
| (*Johnsonville* Grilling), 3-oz. link .......... | 280 | 16.0 | 3.0 | 22.0 | 55 | 840 | 0 |
| (*Palacios*), 1 oz. ....... | 140 | 7.0 | 0 | 12.0 | 25 | 500 | 0 |
| pork and beef, 2 oz. .... | 255 | 13.5 | 1.0 | 21.4 | 49 | 692 | 0 |
| **Chorizo, vegetarian**: | | | | | | | |
| (*Soyrizo*), 4 tbsp., 1.9 oz. | 120 | 7.0 | 5.0 | 9.0 | 0 | 440 | 3.0 |
| (*Yves*), ⅓ link, 2 oz. .... | 80 | 5.0 | 6.0 | 4.5 | 0 | 260 | 2.0 |
| **Chow chow pickle**: | | | | | | | |
| (*Crosse & Blackwell*), 1 tbsp. ............ | 10 | 0 | 1.0 | 0 | 0 | 200 | <1.0 |
| hot or mild (*Mrs. Renfro's*), 1 tbsp. .... | 10 | 0 | 3.0 | 0 | 0 | 45 | 0 |
| sweet, w/cauliflower, ¼ cup ............ | 74 | .9 | 16.5 | .5 | 0 | 321 | .9 |
| **Chow mein seasoning** | | | | | | | |
| (*Kikkoman*), 1 tbsp. .. | 15 | 1.0 | 3.0 | 0 | 0 | 500 | 0 |
| **Christmas melon** | | | | | | | |
| (*Frieda's Camouflage Melon*), ½ cup, 5 oz. . | 50 | 1.0 | 13.0 | 0 | 0 | 15 | 1.0 |
| **Chrysanthemum garland**, 1" pcs.: | | | | | | | |
| raw, ½ cup ........... | 2 | .2 | .5 | <.1 | 0 | 7 | .4 |
| boiled, drained, ½ cup .. | 10 | .8 | 2.2 | .1 | 0 | 27 | 1.2 |
| **Chutney**, 1 tbsp., except as noted: | | | | | | | |
| apple curry (*Crosse & Blackwell*) ........ | 25 | 0 | 7.0 | 0 | 0 | 25 | 0 |
| apricot chardonnay (*Crosse & Blackwell*) . | 25 | 0 | 6.0 | 0 | 0 | 20 | 0 |
| coriander (*Bombay Authentics*), 2 tbsp. .. | 60 | 0 | 6.0 | 3.0 | 0 | 390 | 1.0 |
| cranberry (*Crosse & Blackwell*) ........ | 40 | 0 | 10.0 | 0 | 0 | 0 | 0 |
| fruits and nuts (*Tiger Tiger*), 2 tbsp. ....... | 70 | 0 | 16.0 | 0 | 0 | 230 | 0 |
| ginger pineapple (*Neera's*) ........... | 31 | 0 | 7.0 | 0 | 0 | 54 | 0 |
| mango: (*Bombay Authentics*), 2 tbsp. .......... | 60 | 1.0 | 11.0 | 1.0 | 0 | 115 | 1.0 |

| Food and Measure | cal. | prot. (gms) | carbo. (gms) | fat (gms) | chol. (mgs) | sod. (mgs) | fiber (gms) |
|---|---|---|---|---|---|---|---|
| (*Crosse & Blackwell* Hot/Major Grey) ... | 60 | 0 | 14.0 | 0 | 0 | 170 | 0 |
| (*London* Pub Major Grey) | 50 | 0 | 13.0 | 0 | 0 | 105 | 0 |
| (*Neera's*) ........... | 20 | 0 | 5.0 | 0 | 0 | 26 | 0 |
| (*Patak's* Major Grey) .. | 50 | 0 | 12.0 | 0 | 0 | 310 | 0 |
| (*Roland* Indian), 2 tbsp. | 100 | 0 | 25.0 | 0 | 0 | 320 | 0 |
| (*Roland* Major Grey), 2 tbsp. ........ | 80 | 0 | 21.0 | 0 | 0 | 80 | 0 |
| all varieties (*Tiger Tiger*), 2 tbsp. .... | 60 | 0 | 16.0 | 0 | 0 | 230 | 0 |
| hot (*Patak's*) ........ | 50 | 0 | 13.0 | 0 | 0 | 310 | 0 |
| mint (*Bombay Authentics*), 2 tbsp. ........... | 70 | 0 | 5.0 | 6.0 | 0 | 190 | 1.0 |
| papaya ginger or lime (*Tiger Tiger*), 2 tbsp. ... | 50 | 0 | 13.0 | 0 | 0 | 180 | 0 |
| peach: | | | | | | | |
| (*Crosse & Blackwell* Zinfandel) ........ | 20 | 0 | 5.0 | 0 | 0 | 15 | 0 |
| (*Neera's*) ........... | 22 | 0 | 6.0 | 0 | 0 | 30 | 0 |
| (*Roland*), 2 tbsp. .... | 60 | 0 | 15.0 | 0 | 0 | 105 | 0 |
| pear cardamom: | | | | | | | |
| (*Crosse & Blackwell*) . | 25 | 5 | 6.0 | 0 | 0 | 10 | 0 |
| (*Neera's*) ........... | 30 | 0 | 7.0 | 0 | 0 | 23 | 1.0 |
| tomato: | | | | | | | |
| (*Roland*), 2 tbsp. .... | 60 | 0 | 16.0 | 0 | 0 | 115 | 0 |
| mint (*Neera's*) ....... | 30 | 1.0 | 5.0 | 2.0 | 0 | 54 | 1.0 |
| vegetable, hot (*Neera's*) . | 21 | 0 | 2.0 | 2.0 | 0 | 49 | 0 |
| **Cilantro**, see "Coriander" | | | | | | | |
| **Cinnamon**, ground, 1 tsp. | 6 | .1 | 2.1 | .1 | 0 | 1 | 1.4 |
| **Cinnamon baking chips** (*Hershey's*), 1 tbsp., .5 oz. ....... | 80 | 1.0 | 9.0 | 4.0 | 0 | 45 | 0 |
| **Cinnamon sugar**, 1 tsp.: | | | | | | | |
| (*McCormick*) .......... | 15 | 0 | 3.0 | 0 | 0 | 0 | 0 |
| (*McCormick* Grinder) ... | 10 | 0 | 2.0 | 0 | 0 | 0 | 0 |
| **Cisco**, meat only: | | | | | | | |
| raw, 4 oz. ........... | 112 | 21.5 | 0 | 2.2 | 57 | 62 | 0 |
| smoked, 4 oz. ......... | 201 | 18.6 | 0 | 13.5 | 36 | 545 | 0 |
| **Citronella root**, see "Lemongrass" | | | | | | | |
| **Citrus drink**, 8 fl. oz., except as noted: | | | | | | | |
| (*Five Alive*) ........... | 120 | 2.0 | 30.0 | 0 | 0 | 15 | 0 |
| (*SoBe Energy*) ......... | 110 | 0 | 27.0 | 0 | 0 | 15 | 0 |

| Food and Measure | cal. | prot. (gms) | carbo. (gms) | fat (gms) | chol. (mgs) | sod. (mgs) | fiber (gms) |
|---|---|---|---|---|---|---|---|
| **Citrus drink** *(cont.)* | | | | | | | |
| punch (*Minute Maid*) ... | 120 | 0 | 32.0 | 0 | 0 | 15 | 0 |
| frozen*: | | | | | | | |
| (*Five Alive*) ......... | 110 | 0 | 27.0 | 0 | 0 | 0 | 0 |
| punch (*Minute Maid*) . | 110 | 0 | 31.0 | 0 | 0 | 0 | 0 |
| **Clam**, meat only: | | | | | | | |
| raw: | | | | | | | |
| 4 oz. ............... | 84 | 14.5 | 2.9 | 1.1 | 39 | 64 | 0 |
| 9 large or 20 small, | | | | | | | |
| 6.3 oz. .......... | 133 | 23.0 | 4.6 | 1.8 | 60 | 100 | 0 |
| boiled, poached, or | | | | | | | |
| steamed, 4 oz. ...... | 168 | 29.0 | 5.8 | 2.2 | 76 | 127 | 0 |
| **Clam, canned**: | | | | | | | |
| whole (*Roland*): | | | | | | | |
| Pacific, ⅓ cup ....... | 45 | 4.0 | 6.0 | 1.0 | 21 | 260 | 0 |
| pink, ½ cup ........ | 70 | 13.0 | 1.0 | 2.0 | 68 | 450 | 0 |
| razor, ½ cup ........ | 60 | 12.0 | 1.0 | 1.0 | 48 | 340 | 1.0 |
| whole, baby, ¼ cup: | | | | | | | |
| (*Bumble Bee*) ....... | 45 | 9.0 | 2.0 | 1.0 | 70 | 290 | 0 |
| (*Chicken of the Sea*) .. | 30 | 6.0 | 1.0 | 0 | 10 | 290 | 0 |
| (*Roland*), ½ cup ..... | 50 | 10.0 | 2.0 | 0 | 48 | 280 | 0 |
| baby, boiled (*Crown* | | | | | | | |
| *Prince*), 3-oz. can .... | 90 | 13.0 | 3.0 | 3.0 | 70 | 450 | 0 |
| chopped/minced, ¼ cup: | | | | | | | |
| (*Bumble Bee*) ....... | 25 | 4.0 | 3.0 | 0 | 5 | 350 | 0 |
| (*Chicken of the Sea*) .. | 30 | 5.0 | 2.0 | 0 | 12 | 370 | 0 |
| (*Roland*), ⅓ cup ..... | 45 | 10.0 | 0 | 0 | 15 | 310 | 0 |
| arctic (*Chincoteague*) . | 15 | 2.0 | 1.0 | 0 | 5 | 240 | 0 |
| ocean (*Chincoteague*) . | 25 | 6.0 | 0 | 0 | 5 | 310 | 0 |
| sea (*Chincoteague*) ... | 25 | 6.0 | <1.0 | 0 | 15 | 260 | 0 |
| **Clam, frozen**: | | | | | | | |
| fried, breaded, 3 oz.: | | | | | | | |
| (*Chincoteague*) ...... | 240 | 8.0 | 26.0 | 12.0 | 10 | 750 | <1.0 |
| (*Mrs. Paul's*), 18 pcs. . | 270 | 8.0 | 31.0 | 12.0 | 10 | 600 | 1.0 |
| strips, breaded, 3 oz.: | | | | | | | |
| (*Blue Horizon*) ...... | 210 | 8.0 | 15.0 | 7.0 | 25 | 210 | 1.0 |
| (*SeaPak* Crunchy) .... | 250 | 7.0 | 24.0 | 14.0 | 15 | 420 | 0 |
| (*Schooner*), 7 pcs. ... | 260 | 6.0 | 36.0 | 10.0 | 0 | 370 | 1.0 |
| stuffed, in shell | | | | | | | |
| (*Matlaw's* Tray Pack), | | | | | | | |
| 2.2-oz. pc. ......... | 110 | 5.0 | 12.0 | 4.5 | 0 | 390 | 1.0 |
| **Clam, smoked**, canned | | | | | | | |
| in oil, drained: | | | | | | | |
| (*Bumble Bee*), 2 oz. ..... | 130 | 11.0 | 1.0 | 9.0 | 40 | 460 | 0 |

| Food and Measure | cal. | prot. (gms) | carbo. (gms) | fat (gms) | chol. (mgs) | sod. (mgs) | fiber (gms) |
|---|---|---|---|---|---|---|---|
| baby: | | | | | | | |
| (*Crown Prince*), ⅓ cup | 90 | 10.0 | 2.0 | 5.0 | 45 | 330 | 0 |
| (*Crown Prince* | | | | | | | |
| *Natural* 3 oz.), 2.3 oz. | 150 | 16.0 | <1.0 | 10.0 | 15 | 340 | 0 |
| (*Roland*), ⅓ cup ..... | 90 | 10.0 | 2.0 | 5.0 | 45 | 330 | 0 |
| **Clam juice**, ½ cup: | | | | | | | |
| ocean (*Chincoteague*) ... | 10 | 2.0 | 1.0 | 0 | 0 | 1490 | 0 |
| sea (*Chincoteague*) ..... | 15 | 1.0 | 0 | 0 | 0 | 590 | 0 |
| **Clam sauce**, canned: | | | | | | | |
| red, ½ cup: | | | | | | | |
| (*Chincoteague*) ...... | 100 | 5.0 | 8.0 | 5.0 | 10 | 550 | <1.0 |
| (*Progresso*) ........ | 60 | 4.0 | 8.0 | 1.0 | 10 | 350 | 1.0 |
| white, ½ cup: | | | | | | | |
| (*Chincoteague*) ...... | 120 | 4.0 | 9.0 | 8.0 | 10 | 490 | 0 |
| (*Progresso*) ........ | 120 | 4.0 | 4.0 | 10.0 | 5 | 880 | 1.0 |
| (*Progresso* Deluxe) ... | 150 | 9.0 | 5.0 | 10.0 | 20 | 710 | 0 |
| **Clementine**, see | | | | | | | |
| "Tangerine" | | | | | | | |
| **Cloves**, ground: | | | | | | | |
| 1 tbsp. ............... | 21 | .4 | 4.0 | 1.3 | 0 | 16 | <1.0 |
| 1 tsp. ............... | 7 | .1 | 1.3 | .4 | 0 | 5 | .2 |
| **Cobbler**, frozen (*Mrs. Smith's*), ⅛ pkg.: | | | | | | | |
| apple crumb ......... | 270 | 2.0 | 45.0 | 9.0 | 0 | 210 | 2.0 |
| blackberry ........... | 250 | 2.0 | 43.0 | 8.0 | 0 | 210 | 1.0 |
| cherry crumb ........ | 270 | 2.0 | 46.0 | 9.0 | 0 | 200 | 1.0 |
| peach .............. | 240 | 2.0 | 40.0 | 8.0 | 0 | 210 | <1.0 |
| **Cocktail mixers**, see specific listings | | | | | | | |
| **Cocktail sauce**, see "Seafood sauce" | | | | | | | |
| **Cocoa**, 1 tbsp.: | | | | | | | |
| (*Hershey's* Natural) ..... | 10 | 1.0 | 3.0 | .5 | 0 | 0 | 2.0 |
| (*Nestlé Toll House*) ..... | 15 | 1.0 | 3.0 | .5 | 0 | 0 | 1.0 |
| (*Roland*) ............. | 15 | 1.0 | 3.0 | 1.0 | 0 | 0 | 1.0 |
| dark (*Hershey's Special Dark*) ....... | 10 | 1.0 | 3.0 | .5 | 0 | 65 | 2.0 |
| **Cocoa mix**, 1 pkt.: | | | | | | | |
| (*Land O Lakes Cocoa Classics*): | | | | | | | |
| all flavors, except arctic white, butter-scotch, Irish crème, vanilla, and mocha . | 140 | 3.0 | 26.0 | 3.5 | 0 | 270 | <1.0 |

| Food and Measure | cal. | prot. (gms) | carbo. (gms) | fat (gms) | chol. (mgs) | sod. (mgs) | fiber (gms) |
|---|---|---|---|---|---|---|---|
| **Cocoa mix (Land O Lakes)** *(cont.)* | | | | | | | |
| arctic white ......... | 160 | 2.0 | 26.0 | 6.0 | 0 | 180 | 0 |
| butterscotch ........ | 140 | 3.0 | 26.0 | 3.5 | 0 | 260 | <1.0 |
| Irish crème .......... | 140 | 3.0 | 26.0 | 3.0 | 0 | 270 | <1.0 |
| mocha ............. | 140 | 4.0 | 25.0 | 3.0 | 0 | 280 | <1.0 |
| (*Swiss Miss*): | | | | | | | |
| breakfast, great start .. | 110 | 1.0 | 23.0 | 2.0 | 0 | 135 | 1.0 |
| breakfast, pick me up . | 110 | 1.0 | 23.0 | 2.0 | 0 | 160 | 1.0 |
| chocolate, indulgent .. | 150 | 2.0 | 26.0 | 3.5 | 0 | 170 | 1.0 |
| chocolate, rich ...... | 110 | 2.0 | 24.0 | 1.5 | 0 | 160 | 1.0 |
| diet ............... | 25 | 2.0 | 4.0 | 0 | 0 | 160 | 1.0 |
| fat free ............ | 50 | 2.0 | 10.0 | 0 | 0 | 180 | <1.0 |
| marshmallow lovers .. | 120 | 1.0 | 23.0 | 2.5 | 0 | 160 | <1.0 |
| marshmallow lovers, | | | | | | | |
| fat free .......... | 70 | 3.0 | 13.0 | 0 | 0 | 180 | <1.0 |
| no sugar added ..... | 60 | 1.0 | 10.0 | 1.0 | 0 | 170 | <1.0 |
| vanilla, French ...... | 115 | 1.0 | 23.0 | 2.0 | 0 | 180 | 0 |
| **Coconut**, fresh, shelled: | | | | | | | |
| (*Dole*), 1.4 oz. ......... | 140 | 1.0 | 6.0 | 14.0 | 0 | 10 | 4.0 |
| (*Frieda's* White/ | | | | | | | |
| Young), ¼ cup, | | | | | | | |
| 1.4 oz. .......... | 140 | 1.0 | 6.0 | 13.0 | 0 | 10 | 4.0 |
| (*Frieda's* Whole), 2 oz. .. | 130 | 0 | 5.0 | 14.0 | 0 | 10 | 2.0 |
| 1 oz. ............... | 100 | .9 | 4.3 | 9.5 | 0 | 6 | 2.6 |
| shredded or grated, | | | | | | | |
| 1 cup not packed .... | 283 | 2.7 | 12.2 | 26.8 | 0 | 16 | 7.2 |
| **Coconut, cream of**, | | | | | | | |
| canned: | | | | | | | |
| (*Coco López*), 2 tbsp. ... | 130 | 0 | 21.0 | 5.0 | 0 | 15 | 0 |
| (*Roland*), 2 tbsp. ...... | 110 | 0 | 19.0 | 3.0 | 0 | 10 | 0 |
| (*Vigo*), 2 tbsp. ......... | 110 | 0 | 17.0 | 10.0 | 0 | 15 | 0 |
| **Coconut, dried**: | | | | | | | |
| flaked, sweetened: | | | | | | | |
| (*Baker's Angel Flake*), | | | | | | | |
| 2 tbsp. .......... | 70 | 1.0 | 6.0 | 5.0 | 0 | 40 | 1.0 |
| (*Mounds*), 2 tbsp. ..... | 80 | 1.0 | 6.0 | 6.0 | 0 | 35 | 1.0 |
| ⅓ cup ............ | 117 | .8 | 11.8 | 7.9 | 0 | 63 | 1.1 |
| toasted, 1 oz. ......... | 168 | 1.5 | 12.6 | 13.4 | 0 | 11 | 1.0 |
| **Coconut flour** (*Bob's Red Mill* Organic), | | | | | | | |
| 2 tbsp. ............ | 60 | 2.0 | 8.0 | 2.0 | 0 | 30 | 5.0 |
| **Coconut milk**, canned: | | | | | | | |
| (*Ka•Me*), ¼ cup ........ | 90 | <1.0 | 1.0 | 9.0 | 0 | 15 | 0 |
| (*Ka•Me* Lite), ¼ cup .... | 40 | 0 | <1.0 | 4.0 | 0 | 10 | 0 |

| Food and Measure | cal. | prot. (gms) | carbo. (gms) | fat (gms) | chol. (mgs) | sod. (mgs) | fiber (gms) |
|---|---|---|---|---|---|---|---|
| (*Roland* Classic), 2 tbsp. | 50 | 0 | 1.0 | 5.0 | 0 | 15 | 1.0 |
| (*Roland* Grade-A), 2 tbsp. | 80 | 0 | 3.0 | 8.0 | 0 | 5 | 1.0 |
| (*Roland* Lite), 2 tbsp. | 25 | 0 | 1.0 | 2.0 | 0 | 25 | 0 |
| (*Roland* Organic), 2 tbsp. | 50 | 1.0 | 1.0 | 5.0 | 0 | 0 | 1.0 |
| (*A Taste of Thai*), ⅓ cup | 120 | 1.0 | 2.0 | 11.0 | 0 | 25 | 0 |
| (*A Taste of Thai* Lite), ⅓ cup | 50 | 1.0 | 2.0 | 4.5 | 0 | 15 | 0 |
| (*Vigo*), ¼ cup | 120 | 0 | 2.0 | 12.0 | 0 | 10 | 0 |
| **Coconut milk beverage** (*So Delicious*), 8 fl. oz.: | | | | | | | |
| original | 80 | 1.0 | 7.0 | 5.0 | 0 | 15 | 0 |
| original, cultured | 70 | 1.0 | 6.0 | 6.0 | 0 | 5 | 3.0 |
| unsweetened | 50 | 1.0 | 1.0 | 5.0 | 0 | 15 | 0 |
| strawberry, cultured | 100 | 0 | 15.0 | 5.0 | 0 | 5 | 2.0 |
| vanilla | 90 | 1.0 | 9.0 | 5.0 | 0 | 15 | 0 |
| vanilla, cultured | 110 | 1.0 | 16.0 | 1.5 | 0 | 10 | 3.0 |
| **Coconut nectar** (*R.W. Knudsen*), 8 fl. oz. | 140 | 1.0 | 27.0 | 5.0 | 0 | 55 | 3.0 |
| **Coconut water**, canned (*Roland*), 11.8 fl. oz. | 130 | 0 | 29.0 | 2.0 | 0 | 55 | 0 |
| **Cod**, meat only: | | | | | | | |
| Atlantic, 4 oz.: | | | | | | | |
| raw | 93 | 20.2 | 0 | .8 | 49 | 62 | 0 |
| baked or broiled | 119 | 25.9 | 0 | 1.0 | 62 | 88 | 0 |
| Pacific, 4 oz.: | | | | | | | |
| raw | 93 | 20.3 | 0 | .7 | 42 | 81 | 0 |
| baked or broiled | 119 | 26.0 | 0 | .9 | 53 | 103 | 0 |
| **Cod, canned**, Atlantic, w/liquid, 4 oz. | 119 | 25.8 | 0 | 1.0 | 62 | 247 | 0 |
| **Cod, dried**, Atlantic, salted, 1 oz. | 81 | 17.6 | 0 | .7 | 42 | 1968 | 0 |
| **Cod, smoked**, Alaskan black, see "Sablefish" | | | | | | | |
| **Cod entree**, frozen, stuffed (*Oven Poppers*), 5-oz. pc.: | | | | | | | |
| au gratin | 220 | 24.0 | 5.0 | 11.0 | 75 | 450 | 1.0 |
| broccoli, cheese | 150 | 20.0 | 4.0 | 6.0 | 55 | 330 | 1.0 |
| **Cod liver, smoked**, canned (*Roland*), ⅓ cup, 2 oz. | 290 | 3.0 | 0 | 30.0 | 120 | 320 | 0 |

| Food and Measure | cal. | prot. (gms) | carbo. (gms) | fat (gms) | chol. (mgs) | sod. (mgs) | fiber (gms) |
|---|---|---|---|---|---|---|---|
| **Cod liver oil**, see "Oil" | | | | | | | |
| **Coffee:** | | | | | | | |
| brewed, 6 fl. oz. . . . . . . . | 4 | .1 | .8 | 0 | 0 | 4 | 0 |
| instant, regular, | | | | | | | |
| 1 rounded tsp. . . . . . . | 4 | .2 | .7 | tr. | 0 | 1 | 0 |
| vanilla or hazelnut | | | | | | | |
| (*Taster's Choice*), 1 tsp. | 5 | 0 | 1.0 | 0 | 0 | 0 | 0 |
| **Coffee, iced**, 8 fl. oz., | | | | | | | |
| except as noted: | | | | | | | |
| (*Starbucks Frappuccino*), | | | | | | | |
| 9.5 fl. oz. . . . . . . . . . | 200 | 6.0 | 37.0 | 3.0 | 15 | 100 | 0 |
| (*Starbucks DoubleShot*) . | 110 | 6.0 | 19.0 | 1.5 | 10 | 90 | 0 |
| café au lait (*Pom×*), | | | | | | | |
| 10.5 oz. . . . . . . . . . . | 170 | 7.0 | 29.0 | 3.0 | 15 | 130 | 0 |
| cappuccino, mocha | | | | | | | |
| (*Bolthouse Farms*) . . . | 180 | 10.0 | 29.0 | 2.5 | 13 | 106 | 0 |
| caramel (*Starbucks* | | | | | | | |
| *Frappuccino*), | | | | | | | |
| 9.5 fl. oz. . . . . . . . . . | 200 | 6.0 | 36.0 | 3.0 | 15 | 100 | 0 |
| chocolate (*Pom×*), | | | | | | | |
| 10.5 oz. . . . . . . . . . . | 190 | 10.0 | 49.0 | 0 | 0 | 160 | 2.0 |
| cinnamon dulce (*Star-* | | | | | | | |
| *bucks Doubleshot* | | | | | | | |
| *Energy+*) . . . . . . . . . . | 110 | 7.0 | 18.0 | 1.5 | 10 | 90 | 0 |
| espresso and cream: | | | | | | | |
| (*Starbucks* | | | | | | | |
| *Doubleshot*) . . . . . . | 170 | 5.0 | 22.0 | 7.0 | 25 | 85 | 0 |
| (*Starbucks* | | | | | | | |
| *Doubleshot* Light) . | 90 | 4.0 | 7.0 | 5.0 | 20 | 60 | 0 |
| latte: | | | | | | | |
| (*Pacific* Organic) . . . . . | 110 | 4.0 | 17.0 | 2.5 | 10 | 190 | 0 |
| mocha or vanilla | | | | | | | |
| (*Health is Wealth* | | | | | | | |
| Nutriccino/Ener-G), | | | | | | | |
| 9.5 fl. oz. . . . . . . . . | 190 | 4.0 | 37.0 | 3.0 | 10 | 260 | 0 |
| vanilla (*Bolthouse* | | | | | | | |
| *Farms*) . . . . . . . . . . | 160 | 10.0 | 22.0 | 3.0 | 10 | 75 | 1.0 |
| mocha: | | | | | | | |
| (*Pacific* Organic) . . . . . | 130 | 4.0 | 23.0 | 2.5 | 10 | 200 | 0 |
| (*Starbucks* | | | | | | | |
| *Doubleshot* Energy+) | 110 | 7.0 | 18.0 | 1.5 | 10 | 85 | 0 |
| (*Starbucks Frap-* | | | | | | | |
| *puccino*), 9.5 fl. oz. | 180 | 7.0 | 33.0 | 3.0 | 15 | 95 | 0 |

| Food and Measure | cal. | prot. (gms) | carbo. (gms) | fat (gms) | chol. (mgs) | sod. (mgs) | fiber (gms) |
|---|---|---|---|---|---|---|---|
| (*Starbucks Frappuccino* Lite), 9.5 fl. oz. .... | 100 | 6.0 | 12.0 | 3.0 | 15 | 95 | 0 |
| dark chocolate (*Starbucks Frappuccino*), 9.5 fl. oz. ........ | 190 | 7.0 | 35.0 | 3.5 | 15 | 190 | 0 |
| vanilla: | | | | | | | |
| (*Pacific* Organic) ..... | 120 | 4.0 | 20.0 | 2.0 | 10 | 190 | 0 |
| (*Starbucks Doubleshot* Energy+) | 110 | 7.0 | 18.0 | 1.5 | 10 | 100 | 0 |
| (*Starbucks Frappuccino*), 9.5 fl. oz. | 200 | 6.0 | 37.0 | 3.0 | 15 | 100 | 0 |
| **Coffee, mix** (*Land O Lakes Cappuccino Classics*), 1 pkt.: | | | | | | | |
| amaretto Italia ......... | 140 | 3.0 | 24.0 | 3.0 | 0 | 135 | 0 |
| mocha, Suisse ........ | 140 | 3.0 | 24.0 | 3.5 | 0 | 95 | <1.0 |
| suprema ............. | 140 | 3.0 | 25.0 | 3.0 | 0 | 120 | 0 |
| vanilla, French ......... | 140 | 3.0 | 25.0 | 3.0 | 0 | 95 | 0 |
| **Coffee creamer**, see "Creamer" | | | | | | | |
| **Coffee substitute** (*Kaffree Roma*), 1 tsp. | 10 | 0 | 2.0 | 0 | 0 | 0 | 0 |
| **Coleslaw**, see "Salad blend kit" | | | | | | | |
| **Coleslaw dressing**, see "Salad dressing" | | | | | | | |
| **Collard greens**, fresh: | | | | | | | |
| raw: | | | | | | | |
| (*Glory*), 2 cups ...... | 25 | 2.0 | 5.0 | 0 | 0 | 15 | 3.0 |
| (*Green Giant* Fresh), 1.3 oz. .......... | 10 | 1.0 | 2.0 | 0 | 0 | 5 | 1.0 |
| chopped, ½ cup ..... | 6 | .3 | 1.3 | <.1 | 0 | 4 | .7 |
| trimmed, 1 oz. ...... | 9 | .4 | 2.0 | .1 | 0 | 6 | 1.0 |
| boiled, drained, chopped, ½ cup ..... | 17 | .9 | 3.9 | .1 | 0 | 10 | 1.3 |
| **Collard greens, canned**, ½ cup: | | | | | | | |
| chopped: | | | | | | | |
| (*Allens* No Salt) ..... | 30 | 1.0 | 5.0 | .5 | 0 | 20 | 3.0 |
| (*Bush's*) ........... | 30 | 2.0 | 4.0 | 0 | 0 | 410 | 2.0 |
| seasoned: | | | | | | | |
| (*Allens*) ............ | 30 | 1.0 | 5.0 | 0 | 0 | 420 | 2.0 |
| (*Glory* Sensibly) ..... | 20 | 2.0 | 4.0 | 0 | 0 | 240 | 2.0 |

| Food and Measure | cal. | prot. (gms) | carbo. (gms) | fat (gms) | chol. (mgs) | sod. (mgs) | fiber (gms) |
|---|---|---|---|---|---|---|---|
| **Collard greens, canned, seasoned** *(cont.)* | | | | | | | |
| (*Glory* Southern) .... | 35 | 2.0 | 5.0 | 0 | 0 | 490 | 2.0 |
| turkey flavor (*Glory*) .... | 25 | 2.0 | 5.0 | 0 | 0 | 580 | 2.0 |
| **Collard greens, frozen,** chopped, ½ cup: | | | | | | | |
| (*McKenzie's*), 1 cup ..... | 30 | 2.0 | 3.0 | 0 | 0 | 30 | 2.0 |
| (*Seabrook Farms*), ½ cup | 30 | 2.0 | 2.0 | 0 | 0 | 20 | 2.0 |
| boiled, drained, ½ cup .. | 31 | 2.5 | 6.1 | .4 | 0 | 42 | n.a. |
| **Conch**, fresh, baked or broiled, 4 oz. ..... | 147 | 29.8 | 1.9 | 1.4 | 74 | 174 | 0 |
| **Conch, canned**, baby, whole, in water (*Roland*), ½ cup ..... | 60 | 13.0 | 1.0 | .5 | 100 | 320 | 0 |
| **Cookie:** | | | | | | | |
| (*Gamesa Marias*), 8 pcs., 1 oz. ........ | 120 | 2.0 | 24.0 | 1.5 | 0 | 160 | <1.0 |
| (*Pepperidge Farm Bordeaux*), 4 pcs., .9 oz. ............. | 130 | 2.0 | 19.0 | 5.0 | 10 | 95 | <1.0 |
| (*Social Tea* Biscuit 12.35 oz.), 1.1 oz. .... | 140 | 2.0 | 24.0 | 4.0 | 0 | 150 | 1.0 |
| (*Social Tea* Biscuit 11 oz.), 1.1 oz. ...... | 140 | 2.0 | 24.0 | 4.0 | 0 | 125 | 1.0 |
| (*TLC* Happy Trail Mix), 1.1-oz. pc. ..... | 140 | 2.0 | 21.0 | 5.0 | 0 | 75 | 4.0 |
| almond (*Alessi* Cantuc- cini), 5 pcs., 1 oz. .... | 115 | 3.0 | 19.0 | 3.0 | 12 | 60 | 0 |
| amaretti (*Roland*), 8 pcs., 1.1 oz. ........ | 130 | 2.0 | 25.0 | 2.0 | 0 | 15 | 1.0 |
| animal: | | | | | | | |
| (*Animalitos*), 14 pcs., 1.1 oz. .......... | 110 | 2.0 | 25.0 | .5 | 0 | 160 | <1.0 |
| (*Barbara's Snackimals* Snickerdoodle), 10 pcs., 1.1 oz. ... | 120 | 2.0 | 19.0 | 4.0 | 0 | 65 | 0 |
| (*Barnum's Animals*), 1 oz. ............. | 120 | 2.0 | 22.0 | 3.5 | 0 | 140 | 1.0 |
| (*Keebler*), 8 pcs., 1 oz. | 130 | 2.0 | 22.0 | 4.0 | 0 | 135 | <1.0 |
| (*Mother's* Circus), 6 pcs., 1 oz. ...... | 150 | <1.0 | 20.0 | 7.0 | 0 | 55 | <1.0 |
| chocolate chip (*Barbara's Snackimals*), 10 pcs., 1.1 oz. ... | 120 | 1.0 | 19.0 | 4.0 | 0 | 80 | 0 |

| Food and Measure | cal. | prot. (gms) | carbo. (gms) | fat (gms) | chol. (mgs) | sod. (mgs) | fiber (gms) |
|---|---|---|---|---|---|---|---|
| frosted (*Keebler*), 8 pcs., 1 oz. | 160 | <1.0 | 22.0 | 7.0 | 0 | 80 | <1.0 |
| iced (*Keebler*), 6 pcs., 1.1 oz. | 140 | 2.0 | 22.0 | 4.5 | 0 | 100 | <1.0 |
| iced (*Nabisco* Classics), 1 oz. | 140 | 1.0 | 21.0 | 6.0 | 0 | 90 | 0 |
| oatmeal (*Barbara's Snackimals*), 10 pcs., 1.1 oz. | 120 | 1.0 | 17.0 | 5.0 | 0 | 85 | <1.0 |
| vanilla (*Barbara's Snackimals*), 10 pcs., 1.1 oz. | 110 | 2.0 | 17.0 | 4.0 | 0 | 65 | 0 |
| apricot raspberry (*Pepperidge Farm Verona*), 3 pcs., .9 oz. | 140 | 2.0 | 22.0 | 5.0 | 10 | 100 | <1.0 |
| arrowroot (*Nabisco*), .2-oz. pc. | 20 | 0 | 4.0 | .5 | 0 | 15 | 0 |
| biscotti: |  |  |  |  |  |  |  |
| (*Nonni's* Original), .7-oz. pc. | 90 | 2.0 | 14.0 | 3.0 | 20 | 65 | 0 |
| almond (*New York Style*), 3 pcs., 1 oz. | 120 | 2.0 | 20.0 | 4.0 | 30 | 45 | 0 |
| chocolate (*New York Style*), 3 pcs., 1 oz. | 120 | 3.0 | 19.0 | 4.0 | 30 | 40 | 1.0 |
| chocolate, dipped (*Nonni's* Decadence), .85-oz. pc. | 110 | 2.0 | 17.0 | 4.5 | 20 | 65 | 1.0 |
| chocolate dipped (*Nonni's* Cioccolati), .85-oz. pc. | 110 | 2.0 | 17.0 | 4.5 | 20 | 70 | 1.0 |
| chocolate dipped, nuts (*Nonni's* Noci Cioccolati), .85-oz. pc. | 110 | 2.0 | 17.0 | 4.5 | 20 | 75 | 0 |
| lemon (*Nonni's*), .85-oz. pc. | 110 | 2.0 | 17.0 | 4.5 | 20 | 75 | 0 |
| toffee almond (*Nonni's*), 1.2-oz. pc. | 130 | 2.0 | 19.0 | 6.0 | 25 | 70 | 1.0 |
| black and white (*Entenmann's* Single), 3-oz. pc. | 360 | 3.0 | 60.0 | 12.0 | 40 | 200 | <1.0 |
| butter/butter flavor: |  |  |  |  |  |  |  |
| (*Entenmann's* Holiday), 3 pcs., .9 oz. | 130 | 1.0 | 16.0 | 7.0 | 15 | 105 | 0 |

| Food and Measure | cal. | prot. (gms) | carbo. (gms) | fat (gms) | chol. (mgs) | sod. (mgs) | fiber (gms) |
|---|---|---|---|---|---|---|---|
| **Cookie, butter/butter flavor** *(cont.)* | | | | | | | |
| (*Murray Cookie Jar Classics*), 8 pcs., 1.1 oz. . . . . . . . . . | 140 | 2.0 | 22.0 | 5.0 | 0 | 130 | <1.0 |
| (*Pepperidge Farm Chessmen*), 3 pcs., .9 oz. . . . . . . . . . . | 120 | 2.0 | 18.0 | 5.0 | 20 | 80 | <1.0 |
| Danish, 4 pcs., 1.1 oz. | 160 | 2.0 | 19.0 | 8.0 | 20 | 80 | 1.0 |
| cheesecake middle (*Fudge Shoppe*), 3 pcs., .9 oz.: | | | | | | | |
| chocolate graham . . . . | 130 | 1.0 | 17.0 | 7.0 | 0 | 85 | <1.0 |
| fudge . . . . . . . . . . . . | 130 | 1.0 | 17.0 | 7.0 | 0 | 65 | <1.0 |
| chocolate: | | | | | | | |
| (*Pepperidge Farm Collection*), 2 pcs. . | 130 | 1.0 | 16.0 | 7.0 | <5 | 70 | <1.0 |
| bites (*Murray Sugar Free*), .75-oz. pouch | 80 | 1.0 | 16.0 | 2.5 | 0 | 125 | 3.0 |
| top (*Lu* Petit Ecolier), 2 pcs. . . . . . . . . . . | 130 | 1.0 | 17.0 | 6.0 | 5 | 50 | 1.0 |
| top (*Pepperidge Farm Geneva*), 3 pcs. . . . | 160 | 2.0 | 19.0 | 9.0 | 0 | 95 | 1.0 |
| wafer (*Famous*), 5 pcs., 1.1 oz. . . . . | 140 | 2.0 | 24.0 | 4.0 | 5 | 230 | 1.0 |
| chocolate cake, Black Forest or mint (*Snack-Well's*), .6-oz. pc. . . | 50 | 1.0 | 12.0 | .5 | 0 | 40 | 0 |
| chocolate chip/chunk: | | | | | | | |
| (*Back to Nature*), .9 oz. . . . . . . . . . . . | 130 | 1.0 | 17.0 | 6.0 | 0 | 70 | 1.0 |
| (*Chips Ahoy!*), 3 pcs., 1.1 oz. . . . . . . . . . | 160 | 2.0 | 21.0 | 8.0 | 0 | 105 | 1.0 |
| (*Chips Ahoy!* 15 oz.), 3 pcs., 1.2 oz. . . . . | 160 | 2.0 | 22.0 | 8.0 | 0 | 110 | 1.0 |
| (*Chips Ahoy!* Bite Size Go-Pak), 14 pcs., 1.1 oz. . . . | 150 | 1.0 | 20.0 | 7.0 | 0 | 110 | 1.0 |
| (*Chips Ahoy!* Candy Blasts), .6-oz. pc. . . | 90 | 1.0 | 11.0 | 4.5 | 0 | 55 | 0 |
| (*Chips Ahoy!* Chewy .9-oz. pc. . . . . . . . | 120 | 1.0 | 18.0 | 6.0 | 0 | 80 | 1.0 |
| (*Chips Ahoy!* Chunky), .6-oz. pc. . . . . . . . | 80 | 1.0 | 11.0 | 4.5 | 0 | 55 | 1.0 |
| (*Chips Ahoy!* Mini), 5 pcs., 1.1 oz. . . . . | 150 | 1.0 | 21.0 | 7.0 | 0 | 105 | 1.0 |

| Food and Measure | cal. | prot. (gms) | carbo. (gms) | fat (gms) | chol. (mgs) | sod. (mgs) | fiber (gms) |
|---|---|---|---|---|---|---|---|
| (*Chips Deluxe Chocolate Lovers*), .6-oz. pc. ........ | 80 | <1.0 | 10.0 | 4.5 | 0 | 65 | <1.0 |
| (*Chips Deluxe* Original), 2 pcs., 1.1 oz. .... | 160 | 2.0 | 19.0 | 8.0 | <5 | 105 | <1.0 |
| (*Chips Deluxe* Soft 'n Chewy), 1.2 oz. . | 150 | 1.0 | 22.0 | 7.0 | 0 | 115 | <1.0 |
| (*Chips Deluxe Gripz*), .9-oz. pkg. ....... | 120 | 1.0 | 18.0 | 5.0 | 0 | 95 | <1.0 |
| (*Dare* Breaktime), 4 pcs., 1.1 oz. .... | 140 | 1.0 | 22.0 | 6.0 | 0 | 200 | 0 |
| (*Entenmann's* Original), 3 pcs., 1.1 oz. .... | 140 | 1.0 | 20.0 | 7.0 | <5 | 80 | <1.0 |
| (*Entenmann's* Soft Baked Chunk), 1.3-oz. pc. ....... | 190 | 2.0 | 25.0 | 9.0 | 15 | 140 | 0 |
| (*Famous Amos*), 4 pcs., 1 oz. ...... | 150 | 1.0 | 20.0 | 7.0 | <5 | 105 | <1.0 |
| (*Glutino*), 4 pcs., 1 oz. | 130 | 1.0 | 20.0 | 5.0 | 5 | 65 | <1.0 |
| (*Grandma's* Big), 1.4-oz. pc. ....... | 190 | 2.0 | 25.0 | 9.0 | 0 | 105 | <1.0 |
| (*Grandma's* Rich 'n Chewy), 1 pkg. .... | 270 | 2.0 | 38.0 | 12.0 | 10 | 105 | 2.0 |
| (*Health Valley* Mini), 4 pcs., 1 oz. ...... | 140 | 1.0 | 18.0 | 6.0 | 5 | 120 | 1.0 |
| (*Keebler* Danish Wedding), 4 pcs., .9 oz. ..... | 130 | 1.0 | 18.0 | 6.0 | 0 | 70 | <1.0 |
| (*Keebler Soft Batch*), .6-oz. pc. ........ | 80 | <1.0 | 11.0 | 3.5 | 0 | 55 | <1.0 |
| (*Keebler Soft Batch*), 2.25-oz. pkg. ..... | 340 | 2.0 | 42.0 | 14.0 | 0 | 220 | 1.0 |
| (*Mother's* 11.5 oz.), 2 pcs., 1.1 oz. .... | 160 | 2.0 | 21.0 | 8.0 | <5 | 125 | <1.0 |
| (*Mother's* 14-oz. Bag), 4 pcs., 1.1 oz. .... | 150 | 2.0 | 20.0 | 7.0 | 10 | 160 | <1.0 |
| (*Murray Sugar Free*), 3 pcs., 1.1 oz. .... | 150 | 2.0 | 20.0 | 9.0 | <5 | 130 | 2.0 |
| (*Murray Cookie Jar Classics*), 8 pcs., 1.1 oz. .......... | 140 | 2.0 | 22.0 | 5.0 | 0 | 130 | <1.0 |
| chocolate (*Health Valley* Mini), 4 pcs., 1 oz. ............. | 140 | 2.0 | 18.0 | 7.0 | 5 | 110 | 1.0 |

| Food and Measure | cal. | prot. (gms) | carbo. (gms) | fat (gms) | chol. (mgs) | sod. (mgs) | fiber (gms) |
|---|---|---|---|---|---|---|---|
| **Cookie, chocolate chip/chunk** *(cont.)* | | | | | | | |
| coconut (*Chips Deluxe*), 2 pcs., 1.1 oz. .... | 160 | 2.0 | 18.0 | 9.0 | 0 | 90 | 1.0 |
| dark (*Pepperidge Farm Nantucket*), .9-oz. pc. ........ | 130 | 1.0 | 18.0 | 6.0 | 10 | 95 | 0 |
| dark (*Pepperidge Farm Nantucket* Soft), 1.1-oz. pc. ....... | 140 | 1.0 | 22.0 | 6.0 | 10 | 75 | 0 |
| dark, brownie (*Pepperidge Farm Captiva* Soft), 1 pc. | 140 | 1.0 | 22.0 | 6.0 | 10 | 75 | 0 |
| dark, double (*Pepperidge Farm Nantucket*), .9-oz. pc. | 140 | 1.0 | 19.0 | 7.0 | 10 | 105 | 0 |
| dark, pecans (*Pepperidge Farm Chesapeake*), .9-oz. pc. ........ | 130 | 1.0 | 17.0 | 6.0 | <5 | 60 | 0 |
| fudge (*Grandma's Big*), 1.4-oz. pc. ... | 170 | 2.0 | 27.0 | 7.0 | 10 | 150 | 1.0 |
| macadamia (*Mauna Loa*), 4 pcs., 1 oz. . | 150 | 1.0 | 17.0 | 9.0 | 0 | 80 | 1.0 |
| milk (*Entenmann's*), 3 pcs., 1.1 oz. .... | 150 | 1.0 | 20.0 | 7.0 | 5 | 90 | 0 |
| milk (*Pepperidge Farm Montauk*), 1 pc. ............ | 130 | 1.0 | 18.0 | 6.0 | 10 | 100 | 0 |
| milk (*Pepperidge Farm Montauk* Soft), 1 pc. ....... | 140 | 1.0 | 22.0 | 6.0 | 10 | 75 | 0 |
| milk, macadamia (*Pepperidge Farm Sausalito*), .9-oz. pc. | 130 | 1.0 | 17.0 | 6.0 | <5 | 60 | 0 |
| milk, macadamia (*Pepperidge Farm Sausalito* Soft), 1 pc. | 140 | 1.0 | 22.0 | 6.0 | 10 | 75 | 0 |
| oatmeal (*Chips Deluxe*), 2 pcs., 1.1 oz. .... | 150 | 2.0 | 20.0 | 7.0 | 0 | 105 | 1.0 |
| peanut butter cups (*Chips Deluxe*), .6-oz. pc. ........ | 80 | 1.0 | 10.0 | 4.5 | 0 | 45 | <1.0 |
| pecan (*Famous Amos*), 4 pcs., 1 oz. ...... | 150 | 2.0 | 18.0 | 8.0 | 0 | 95 | 1.0 |

| Food and Measure | cal. | prot. (gms) | carbo. (gms) | fat (gms) | chol. (mgs) | sod. (mgs) | fiber (gms) |
|---|---|---|---|---|---|---|---|
| pecan (*Murray Sugar Free*), 3 pcs., 1.1 oz. | 160 | 2.0 | 19.0 | 10.0 | <5 | 125 | 2.0 |
| rainbow (*Chips Deluxe*), .6-oz. pc. | 80 | <1.0 | 10.0 | 4.0 | 0 | 55 | <1.0 |
| white, macadamia (*Pepperidge Farm Tahoe*), .9-oz. pc. | 130 | 1.0 | 17.0 | 6.0 | <5 | 60 | 0 |
| white fudge (*Chips Ahoy!* Chewy), .9-oz. pc. | 120 | 1.0 | 18.0 | 5.0 | 0 | 120 | 1.0 |
| white fudge (*Chips Ahoy!* Chunky), .6-oz. pc. | 90 | 1.0 | 11.0 | 4.5 | 0 | 60 | 0 |
| chocolate crème, 2 pcs.: | | | | | | | |
| (*Tim Tam*) | 190 | 2.0 | 24.0 | 10.0 | <5 | 65 | <1.0 |
| caramel (*Tim Tam*) | 190 | 2.0 | 26.0 | 9.0 | 5 | 65 | <1.0 |
| dark (*Tim Tam*) | 190 | 2.0 | 26.0 | 9.0 | 0 | 55 | 0 |
| chocolate sandwich: | | | | | | | |
| (*Back to Nature* Classic), .9 oz. | 130 | 1.0 | 18.0 | 6.0 | 0 | 130 | 1.0 |
| (*Country Choice* Organic), 2 pcs., 1 oz. | 130 | 1.0 | 19.0 | 5.0 | 0 | 100 | <1.0 |
| (*Dare*), 2 pcs., 1.4 oz. | 200 | 2.0 | 27.0 | 10.0 | 0 | 130 | 1.0 |
| (*Emperador*), 2 pcs., .9 oz. | 120 | 1.0 | 19.0 | 4.0 | 0 | 105 | <1.0 |
| (*Famous Amos*), 3 pcs., 1.2 oz. | 160 | 1.0 | 25.0 | 7.0 | 0 | 140 | <1.0 |
| (*Glutino*), 2 pcs., 1 oz. | 140 | 1.0 | 20.0 | 6.0 | 0 | 90 | <1.0 |
| (*Grandma's* Mini), 9 pcs., 1.1 oz. | 150 | 2.0 | 22.0 | 6.0 | 0 | 140 | 1.0 |
| (*Health Valley Cookie Cremes*), 2 pcs. | 130 | 1.0 | 19.0 | 5.0 | 0 | 100 | 0 |
| (*Murray*), 3 pcs. | 140 | 1.0 | 21.0 | 6.0 | 0 | 115 | <1.0 |
| (*Murray Sugar Free*), 3 pcs., 1 oz. | 130 | 1.0 | 18.0 | 7.0 | 0 | 90 | 1.0 |
| (*Oreo*), 3 pcs., 1.2 oz. | 160 | 1.0 | 25.0 | 7.0 | 0 | 160 | 1.0 |
| (*Oreo*), 1.2-oz. pkg. | 160 | 1.0 | 28.0 | 7.0 | 0 | 170 | 1.0 |
| (*Oreo*), 2-oz. pkg. | 270 | 3.0 | 41.0 | 11.0 | 0 | 310 | 2.0 |
| (*Oreo* Mini), 1 oz. | 140 | 1.0 | 21.0 | 6.0 | 0 | 160 | 1.0 |
| (*Oreo* Mini Bite Size), 1 oz. | 130 | 1.0 | 21.0 | 6.0 | 0 | 160 | 1.0 |
| (*Oreo* Mini Fun Size), 9 pcs., 1 oz. | 130 | 1.0 | 20.0 | 6.0 | 0 | 150 | 1.0 |

| Food and Measure | cal. | prot. (gms) | carbo. (gms) | fat (gms) | chol. (mgs) | sod. (mgs) | fiber (gms) |
|---|---|---|---|---|---|---|---|
| **Cookie, chocolate sandwich** *(cont.)* | | | | | | | |
| (*Oreo* Reduced Fat), | | | | | | | |
| 3 pcs., 1.2 oz. .... | 150 | 1.0 | 27.0 | 4.5 | 0 | 160 | 1.0 |
| (*Oreo Double Stuf*), | | | | | | | |
| 1.5-oz. pkg. ...... | 210 | 1.0 | 30.0 | 10.0 | 0 | 180 | 1.0 |
| (*Oreo Double Stuf* | | | | | | | |
| 6 oz.), 1 oz. ...... | 140 | 1.0 | 20.0 | 7.0 | 0 | 120 | 1.0 |
| (*Oreo Double Stuf* | | | | | | | |
| 15 oz.), 1 oz. ..... | 140 | 1.0 | 21.0 | 7.0 | 0 | 120 | 1.0 |
| (*Pepperidge Farm* | | | | | | | |
| *Brussels*), 3 pcs. .. | 150 | 2.0 | 20.0 | 7.0 | 5 | 65 | 1.0 |
| (*Pepperidge Farm* | | | | | | | |
| *Milano*), 3 pcs. .... | 180 | 2.0 | 21.0 | 10.0 | 10 | 80 | <1.0 |
| black and white | | | | | | | |
| (*Pepperidge Farm* | | | | | | | |
| *Milano*), 3 pcs. .... | 180 | 2.0 | 21.0 | 10.0 | <5 | 85 | 1.0 |
| chocolate, mint | | | | | | | |
| (*Pepperidge Farm* | | | | | | | |
| *Milano*), 2 pcs. .... | 130 | 1.0 | 16.0 | 7.0 | <5 | 120 | <1.0 |
| chocolate, raspberry | | | | | | | |
| (*Pepperidge Farm* | | | | | | | |
| *Milano*), 2 pcs. .... | 130 | 1.0 | 16.0 | 7.0 | <5 | 65 | <1.0 |
| chocolate crème (*Country* | | | | | | | |
| *Choice* Organic), | | | | | | | |
| 2 pcs., 1 oz. ...... | 130 | 1.0 | 19.0 | 5.0 | 0 | 100 | <1.0 |
| chocolate crème | | | | | | | |
| (*Oreo Double Stuf*), | | | | | | | |
| 3 pcs., 1.1 oz. .... | 150 | 1.0 | 21.0 | 7.0 | 0 | 110 | 1.0 |
| coconut (*Pepperidge* | | | | | | | |
| *Farm Tahiti*), 2 pcs. | 170 | 2.0 | 17.0 | 10.0 | 5 | 40 | 2.0 |
| dark (*Lu* Petit | | | | | | | |
| Ecolier), 2 pcs., .9 oz. | 130 | 1.0 | 17.0 | 6.0 | 5 | 50 | 1.0 |
| double (*Pepperidge* | | | | | | | |
| *Farm Milano*), 2 pcs. | 140 | 2.0 | 17.0 | 8.0 | 10 | 70 | <1.0 |
| Madeleine (*Lu* Petite), | | | | | | | |
| 2 pcs., 1.1 oz. .... | 150 | 2.0 | 19.0 | 9.0 | 15 | 110 | 1.0 |
| milk (*Pepperidge Farm* | | | | | | | |
| *Milano*), 3 pcs. .... | 170 | 2.0 | 21.0 | 9.0 | 10 | 110 | <1.0 |
| mint (*Pepperidge* | | | | | | | |
| *Farm Milano*), | | | | | | | |
| 2 pcs., .9 oz. ..... | 130 | 1.0 | 16.0 | 7.0 | <5 | 65 | <1.0 |
| mint, chocolate coated | | | | | | | |
| (*Oreo*), 1.3 oz. .... | 180 | 2.0 | 25.0 | 9.0 | 0 | 120 | 1.0 |

| Food and Measure | cal. | prot. (gms) | carbo. (gms) | fat (gms) | chol. (mgs) | sod. (mgs) | fiber (gms) |
|---|---|---|---|---|---|---|---|
| mint/crème (*Oreo* Double Delight), 1 oz. ............ | 140 | 1.0 | 20.0 | 7.0 | 0 | 120 | 1.0 |
| orange (*Pepperidge Farm Milano*), 2 pcs. | 130 | 1.0 | 16.0 | 7.0 | <5 | 65 | <1.0 |
| raspberry or straw- berry (*Pepperidge Farm Milano*), 2 pcs. | 130 | 1.0 | 16.0 | 7.0 | <5 | 40 | <1.0 |
| red crème (*Oreo Winter*), 1-oz. pc. .. | 140 | 1.0 | 20.0 | 7.0 | 0 | 125 | 1.0 |
| and vanilla (*Country Choice* Organic Duplex Cremes), 2 pcs., 1 oz. ...... | 130 | 1.0 | 19.0 | 5.0 | 0 | 110 | <1.0 |
| and vanilla (*Murray* Duplex Cremes), 3 pcs., 1 oz. ...... | 140 | 1.0 | 21.0 | 5.0 | 0 | 105 | <1.0 |
| chocolate/vanilla (*Annie's* Bunnies Gluten Free), 27 pcs., 1.1 oz. . | 120 | 2.0 | 19.0 | 3.5 | 0 | 105 | 1.0 |
| cinnamon: | | | | | | | |
| (*Gamesa Roscas*), 3 pcs., 1 oz. ...... | 130 | 2.0 | 22.0 | 4.0 | 0 | 130 | 1.0 |
| spiced (*Nabisco Classics*), 1.1 oz. .. | 140 | 1.0 | 24.0 | 4.5 | 0 | 105 | 1.0 |
| cocoa crème sandwich (*Nabisco* Classics), .67-oz. pc. ......... | 90 | 1.0 | 14.0 | 3.5 | 0 | 60 | 0 |
| coconut: | | | | | | | |
| (*Dare* Breaktime), 4 pcs., 1.1 oz. .... | 140 | 2.0 | 22.0 | 5.0 | 0 | 105 | 1.0 |
| (*Gamesa Barras de Coco*), 5 pcs., 1 oz. | 120 | 2.0 | 21.0 | 3.5 | 0 | 130 | <1.0 |
| (*Gamesa Hawaianas*), 3 pcs., 1 oz. ...... | 130 | 2.0 | 22.0 | 3.5 | 0 | 115 | <1.0 |
| (*Mother's Cocadas*), 5 pcs., 1.1 oz. .... | 160 | 2.0 | 21.0 | 8.0 | <5 | 140 | <1.0 |
| (*Murray Cookie Jar Classics* Bars), 6 pcs., 1.1 oz. .... | 150 | 2.0 | 24.0 | 5.0 | 0 | 160 | <1.0 |
| crème sandwich (*Dare*), 2 pcs., 1.4 oz. | 210 | 1.0 | 26.0 | 11.0 | 0 | 105 | <1.0 |
| w/fudge (*Fudge Shoppe*), 2 pcs., 1 oz. ...... | 140 | <1.0 | 17.0 | 8.0 | 0 | 55 | <1.0 |

| Food and Measure | cal. | prot. (gms) | carbo. (gms) | fat (gms) | chol. (mgs) | sod. (mgs) | fiber (gms) |
|---|---|---|---|---|---|---|---|
| **Cookie** (cont.) | | | | | | | |
| cranberry pecan granola | | | | | | | |
| (*Back to Nature*), | | | | | | | |
| 1.1 oz. . . . . . . . . . . . . | 130 | 2.0 | 20.0 | 6.0 | 0 | 105 | 2.0 |
| crèmes, assorted | | | | | | | |
| (*Peek Freans*), 1 oz. . . . | 140 | 1.0 | 19.0 | 6.0 | 0 | 50 | 0 |
| devil's food cake | | | | | | | |
| (*SnackWell's Fat Free*), | | | | | | | |
| .6-oz. pc. . . . . . . . . . | 50 | 1.0 | 12.0 | 0 | 0 | 25 | 0 |
| fig filled/bar: | | | | | | | |
| (*Newtons*), 2 pcs., | | | | | | | |
| 1.1 oz. . . . . . . . . . | 110 | 1.0 | 22.0 | 2.0 | 0 | 125 | 1.0 |
| (*Newtons*), 2-oz. pkg. . | 200 | 2.0 | 39.0 | 4.0 | 0 | 230 | 3.0 |
| (*Newtons Fat Free*), | | | | | | | |
| 1 oz. . . . . . . . . . . . | 90 | 1.0 | 22.0 | 0 | 0 | 125 | 1.0 |
| (*Newtons Minis*), | | | | | | | |
| 1.3 oz. . . . . . . . . . | 130 | 2.0 | 26.0 | 3.0 | 0 | 140 | 2.0 |
| (*Newtons Whole* | | | | | | | |
| *Grain*), 1.1 oz. . . . . | 110 | 1.0 | 21.0 | 2.0 | 0 | 115 | 2.0 |
| blueberry (*Barbara's*), | | | | | | | |
| 1.3 oz. . . . . . . . . . | 120 | 1.0 | 27.0 | 1.0 | 0 | 45 | 1.0 |
| multigrain (*Barbara's*), | | | | | | | |
| .66 oz. . . . . . . . . . | 60 | 1.0 | 13.0 | 0 | 0 | 25 | 1.0 |
| raspberry (*Barbara's*), | | | | | | | |
| 1.3 oz. . . . . . . . . . | 120 | 1.0 | 27.0 | 0 | 0 | 50 | 2.0 |
| whole wheat | | | | | | | |
| (*Barbara's*), 1.3 oz. . . | 110 | 1.0 | 25.0 | .5 | 0 | 50 | 2.0 |
| fortune: | | | | | | | |
| (*La Choy*), 5 pcs. . . . . | 130 | 2.0 | 29.0 | 1.0 | 0 | 10 | <1.0 |
| (*Roland*), .3-oz. pc. . . . | 30 | 0 | 7.0 | 0 | 0 | 20 | 0 |
| coconut (*A Taste of* | | | | | | | |
| *Thai*), 5 pcs. . . . . . . | 89 | <1.0 | 13.0 | 4.0 | 3 | 41 | 0 |
| fudge: | | | | | | | |
| double, brownie | | | | | | | |
| (*Country Choice* | | | | | | | |
| *Organic*), .8-oz. pc. . | 90 | 1.0 | 16.0 | 3.0 | 5 | 80 | 1.0 |
| mint (*Back to* | | | | | | | |
| *Nature*), 1.1 oz. . . . | 150 | 1.0 | 21.0 | 7.0 | 0 | 160 | 1.0 |
| fudge stripes, 1.1 oz.: | | | | | | | |
| (*Back to Nature*) . . . . . | 160 | 1.0 | 21.0 | 8.0 | 0 | 150 | 1.0 |
| (*Fudge Shoppe*), 3 pcs. | 150 | 1.0 | 21.0 | 7.0 | 0 | 110 | <1.0 |
| fudge coated, 1 oz.: | | | | | | | |
| (*Fudge Shoppe* | | | | | | | |
| *Grasshopper*), 4 pcs. | 150 | 1.0 | 20.0 | 7.0 | 0 | 75 | <1.0 |

| Food and Measure | cal. | prot. (gms) | carbo. (gms) | fat (gms) | chol. (mgs) | sod. (mgs) | fiber (gms) |
|---|---|---|---|---|---|---|---|
| grahams (*Fudge Shoppe* Deluxe), 3 pcs. .... | 140 | 1.0 | 18.0 | 7.0 | 0 | 70 | <1.0 |
| peanut butter filled (*Fudge Shoppe*), 2 pcs., 1.1 oz. .... | 160 | 2.0 | 17.0 | 9.0 | 0 | 105 | <1.0 |
| fudge sandwich: | | | | | | | |
| (*E. L. Fudge*), .6-oz. pc. ........ | 90 | 1.0 | 13.0 | 3.5 | <5 | 50 | <1.0 |
| (*E. L. Fudge* Double Stuffed), 2 pcs., 1.2 oz. .......... | 180 | 2.0 | 24.0 | 9.0 | <5 | 95 | 1.0 |
| (*Oreo Fudgies*), 1.1 oz. | 140 | 1.0 | 22.0 | 6.0 | 0 | 140 | 1.0 |
| double (*Mother's*), 2 pcs., 1.3 oz. .... | 170 | 2.0 | 27.0 | 7.0 | 0 | 95 | 1.0 |
| fudge coated (*Oreo*), .7-oz. pc. ........ | 100 | 1.0 | 13.0 | 5.0 | 0 | 70 | 1.0 |
| fudge coated, mint (*Oreo*), .6-oz. pc. .. | 90 | 1.0 | 12.0 | 4.5 | 0 | 70 | 1.0 |
| fudge coated, white (*Oreo*), .7-oz. pc. .. | 100 | 1.0 | 13.0 | 5.0 | 0 | 65 | 0 |
| fudge sticks, 3 pcs.: | | | | | | | |
| (*Fudge Shoppe*), 1 oz. | 150 | <1.0 | 21.0 | 7.0 | 0 | 110 | <1.0 |
| peanut butter (*Fudge Shoppe*), 1 oz. .... | 160 | 2.0 | 17.0 | 9.0 | 0 | 40 | <1.0 |
| ginger: | | | | | | | |
| (*Dare* Breaktime), 4 pcs. 1.1 oz. ..... | 130 | 2.0 | 23.0 | 4.0 | 0 | 95 | 0 |
| (*Pepperidge Farm* Ginger Family), 4 pcs. ........... | 160 | 2.0 | 26.0 | 5.0 | <5 | 135 | 1.0 |
| (*Pepperidge Farm* Gingerman), 4 pcs., .9 oz. ........... | 130 | 2.0 | 21.0 | 3.5 | 10 | 90 | <1.0 |
| ginger snaps: | | | | | | | |
| (*Country Choice* Organic), 5 pcs., 1.1 oz. .......... | 140 | 1.0 | 22.0 | 5.0 | 0 | 85 | 0 |
| (*Murray* Old Fashion), 5 pcs., 1.1 oz. .... | 140 | 2.0 | 22.0 | 5.0 | 0 | 160 | <1.0 |
| (*Nabisco*), 4 pcs., 1 oz. ............ | 120 | 1.0 | 23.0 | 2.5 | 0 | 190 | 1.0 |
| ginger lemon crèmes, 2 pcs., 1 oz.: | | | | | | | |
| (*Carr's*) ............ | 130 | 1.0 | 20.0 | 5.0 | 0 | 95 | 0 |

| Food and Measure | cal. | prot. (gms) | carbo. (gms) | fat (gms) | chol. (mgs) | sod. (mgs) | fiber (gms) |
|---|---|---|---|---|---|---|---|
| **Cookie, ginger lemon crèmes** *(cont.)* | | | | | | | |
| (*Country Choice* Organic) ......... | 130 | 1.0 | 19.0 | 5.0 | 0 | 120 | <1.0 |
| golden crème sandwich: | | | | | | | |
| (*Oreo*), 1.8-oz. pkg. .. | 250 | 2.0 | 37.0 | 10.0 | 0 | 190 | 1.0 |
| (*Oreo* Mini), 1 oz. .... | 140 | 1.0 | 21.0 | 6.0 | 0 | 105 | 0 |
| (*Oreo* Original), 1.25 oz. .......... | 170 | 1.0 | 25.0 | 7.0 | 0 | 120 | 0 |
| (*Oreo Double Stuf*), 1.1 oz. .......... | 150 | 1.0 | 21.0 | 7.0 | 0 | 80 | 0 |
| chocolate crème (*Oreo Uh-Oh*), 1.25 oz. .. | 170 | 2.0 | 25.0 | 7.0 | 0 | 135 | 1.0 |
| graham cracker: | | | | | | | |
| (*Annie's* Bunny Friends), 30 pcs., 1.1 oz. .......... | 130 | 2.0 | 21.0 | 4.5 | 0 | 115 | 1.0 |
| (*Annie's* Bunny Friends Family), 27 pcs., 1.1 oz. ... | 130 | 2.0 | 22.0 | 4.5 | 0 | 105 | 2.0 |
| (*Keebler* Original), 8 pcs., 1 oz. ...... | 120 | 2.0 | 22.0 | 3.5 | 0 | 160 | <1.0 |
| (*Nabisco* Original), 1.1 oz. .......... | 130 | 2.0 | 24.0 | 3.0 | 0 | 190 | 1.0 |
| amaranth or oat bran (*Health Valley*), 6 pcs., 1 oz. ...... | 120 | 3.0 | 22.0 | 3.0 | 0 | 80 | 3.0 |
| gingerbread (*Nabisco*), 1.1 oz. .......... | 130 | 2.0 | 24.0 | 3.0 | 0 | 210 | 1.0 |
| rice bran (*Health Valley*), 6 pcs., 1 oz. | 120 | 2.0 | 22.0 | 3.0 | 0 | 40 | 1.0 |
| s'mores, mini (*Nabisco*), 1 oz. ... | 140 | 1.0 | 21.0 | 6.0 | 0 | 120 | 1.0 |
| graham, chocolate: | | | | | | | |
| (*Annie's* Bunny), 27 pcs., 1.1 oz. ... | 130 | 2.0 | 21.0 | 4.5 | 0 | 75 | 2.0 |
| (*Goldfish*), 50 pcs. ... | 130 | 2.0 | 22.0 | 4.0 | 0 | 125 | 2.0 |
| (*Honey Maid*), 1.2 oz. . | 140 | 2.0 | 27.0 | 3.5 | 0 | 220 | 2.0 |
| (*Teddy Grahams*), 24 pcs., 1.1 oz. ... | 130 | 2.0 | 22.0 | 4.5 | 0 | 160 | 1.0 |
| chip (*Annie's* Bunny), 27 pcs., 1.1 oz. ... | 130 | 2.0 | 21.0 | 4.5 | 0 | 95 | 1.0 |
| chip (*Teddy Grahams*), 24 pcs., 1.1 oz. ... | 130 | 1.0 | 23.0 | 4.5 | 0 | 170 | 1.0 |

| Food and Measure | cal. | prot. (gms) | carbo. (gms) | fat (gms) | chol. (mgs) | sod. (mgs) | fiber (gms) |
|---|---|---|---|---|---|---|---|
| graham, cinnamon: | | | | | | | |
| (*Honey Maid*), 1.2 oz. . | 150 | 2.0 | 28.0 | 3.0 | 0 | 190 | 1.0 |
| (*Honey Maid* Low | | | | | | | |
| Fat), 1.2 oz. ...... | 140 | 2.0 | 29.0 | 2.0 | 0 | 210 | 1.0 |
| (*Keebler*), 8 pcs., 1 oz. | 130 | 2.0 | 23.0 | 3.5 | 0 | 140 | 1.0 |
| (*Ricanelas*), 8 pcs., | | | | | | | |
| 1.1 oz. ........... | 140 | 2.0 | 24.0 | 4.0 | 0 | 180 | 2.0 |
| (*Teddy Grahams.*), | | | | | | | |
| .75-oz. pkg. ...... | 90 | 1.0 | 16.0 | 3.0 | 0 | 95 | 1.0 |
| (*Teddy Grahams*), | | | | | | | |
| 1.1 oz. .......... | 130 | 2.0 | 23.0 | 4.0 | 0 | 150 | 1.0 |
| or vanilla (*Goldfish*), | | | | | | | |
| 50 pcs. .......... | 140 | 0 | 22.0 | 5.0 | 0 | 135 | 1.0 |
| graham, fudge dipped | | | | | | | |
| (*Murray Sugar Free*), | | | | | | | |
| 4 pcs., 1.1 oz. ....... | 140 | 2.0 | 19.0 | 8.0 | 0 | 85 | 1.0 |
| graham, honey: | | | | | | | |
| (*Goldfish*), 50 pcs. ... | 140 | 2.0 | 23.0 | 4.5 | 0 | 150 | 1.0 |
| (*Honey Maid*), 1.1 oz. . | 130 | 2.0 | 24.0 | 3.0 | 0 | 190 | 1.0 |
| (*Honey Maid* Low | | | | | | | |
| Fat), 1.1 oz. ...... | 140 | 2.0 | 28.0 | 2.0 | 0 | 220 | 2.0 |
| (*Keebler*), 8 pcs., 1 oz. | 120 | 2.0 | 23.0 | 4.5 | 0 | 135 | <1.0 |
| (*Teddy Grahams*), | | | | | | | |
| 24 pcs., 1.1 oz. ... | 130 | 2.0 | 23.0 | 4.0 | 0 | 150 | 1.0 |
| sticks (*Back to | | | | | | | |
| Nature*), 1.1 oz. ... | 130 | 2.0 | 25.0 | 3.0 | 0 | 190 | 1.0 |
| granola: | | | | | | | |
| dark chocolate (*Nature | | | | | | | |
| Valley* Thins), .6 oz. | 80 | 1.0 | 11.0 | 4.0 | 0 | 75 | <1.0 |
| honey nut (*Back to | | | | | | | |
| Nature*), 1.1 oz. ... | 140 | 3.0 | 18.0 | 7.0 | 0 | 105 | 2.0 |
| peanut butter (*Nature | | | | | | | |
| Valley* Thins), .6 oz. | 90 | 1.0 | 10.0 | 4.5 | 0 | 85 | <1.0 |
| ladyfingers: | | | | | | | |
| (*Alessi* Biscotti | | | | | | | |
| Savoiardi), 4 pcs., | | | | | | | |
| 1.2 oz. .......... | 120 | 2.0 | 25.0 | 1.0 | 35 | 50 | 1.0 |
| (*Roland* Champagne), | | | | | | | |
| 4 pcs., 1 oz. ...... | 110 | 2.0 | 23.0 | 1.0 | 8 | 90 | 0 |
| (*Roland* Italian), | | | | | | | |
| 4 pcs., 1.1 oz. .... | 110 | 3.0 | 22.0 | 1.0 | 45 | 75 | 0 |
| lemon: | | | | | | | |
| (*Pepperidge Farm*), | | | | | | | |
| 4 pcs. ........... | 160 | 2.0 | 21.0 | 8.0 | 5 | 105 | 0 |

| Food and Measure | cal. | prot. (gms) | carbo. (gms) | fat (gms) | chol. (mgs) | sod. (mgs) | fiber (gms) |
|---|---|---|---|---|---|---|---|
| **Cookie, lemon** *(cont.)* | | | | | | | |
| iced (*Mother's* Lemon- | | | | | | | |
| ade), 4 pcs., 1 oz. ... | 150 | 1.0 | 19.0 | 7.0 | <5 | 75 | <1.0 |
| wafers (*Anna's*), | | | | | | | |
| 6 pcs., 1 oz. ...... | 140 | 2.0 | 19.0 | 7.0 | 0 | 140 | 2.0 |
| lemon sandwich: | | | | | | | |
| (*Dare* Crème), 2 pcs., | | | | | | | |
| 1.4 oz. ......... | 200 | 2.0 | 27.0 | 9.0 | 0 | 130 | 0 |
| (*Emperador*), 6 pcs. ... | 270 | 3.0 | 45.0 | 8.0 | 0 | 260 | 1.0 |
| (*Murray* Crèmes), | | | | | | | |
| 3 pcs., 1 oz. ...... | 140 | 1.0 | 21.0 | 5.0 | 0 | 90 | <1.0 |
| (*Murray Sugar Free*), | | | | | | | |
| 3 pcs., 1 oz. ...... | 130 | 1.0 | 19.0 | 7.0 | 0 | 55 | <1.0 |
| (*SnackWell's*), 3 pcs., | | | | | | | |
| 1.1 oz. .......... | 130 | 1.0 | 23.0 | 6.0 | 0 | 135 | 2.0 |
| macaroons (*Mother's*), | | | | | | | |
| 2 pcs., 1.1 oz. ....... | 170 | 2.0 | 17.0 | 11.0 | 0 | 90 | 1.0 |
| macadamia toffee | | | | | | | |
| crunch (*Mauna Loa*), | | | | | | | |
| 4 pcs., 1 oz. ........ | 150 | 1.0 | 17.0 | 9.0 | 0 | 95 | 1.0 |
| Madeleines, 2 pcs.: | | | | | | | |
| butter (*Entenmann's* | | | | | | | |
| Ultimate Petite), | | | | | | | |
| 1.8 oz. .......... | 240 | 2.0 | 26.0 | 14.0 | 80 | 80 | 0 |
| chocolate (*Entenmann's* | | | | | | | |
| Ultimate), 1.5 oz. .. | 200 | 2.0 | 27.0 | 10.0 | 35 | 135 | 0 |
| maple leaf crème | | | | | | | |
| sandwich (*Dare*), | | | | | | | |
| 2 pcs., 1.2 oz. ....... | 170 | 1.0 | 25.0 | 7.0 | 0 | 105 | 0 |
| marshmallow, w/ | | | | | | | |
| chocolate, 2 pcs.: | | | | | | | |
| (*Dare* Whippet), | | | | | | | |
| 2 pcs., 1.2 oz. .... | 150 | 1.0 | 24.0 | 5.0 | 0 | 50 | <1.0 |
| (*Mallomars*), .9 oz. ... | 120 | 1.0 | 18.0 | 5.0 | 0 | 40 | 1.0 |
| (*Twirls*), 1.1 oz. ...... | 130 | 1.0 | 20.0 | 6.0 | 0 | 75 | 0 |
| w/nuts (*Granesa Arcoiris*), | | | | | | | |
| 2 pcs., 1 oz. ...... | 120 | 1.0 | 18.0 | 5.0 | 0 | 50 | <1.0 |
| raspberry (*Dare* Whippet), | | | | | | | |
| 2 pcs., 1.2 oz. .... | 160 | 1.0 | 27.0 | 5.0 | 0 | 50 | <1.0 |
| mint, fudge coated: | | | | | | | |
| (*Fudge Shoppe* | | | | | | | |
| Grasshopper), | | | | | | | |
| 4 pcs., 1 oz. ...... | 150 | 1.0 | 20.0 | 7.0 | 0 | 75 | <1.0 |

| Food and Measure | cal. | prot. (gms) | carbo. (gms) | fat (gms) | chol. (mgs) | sod. (mgs) | fiber (gms) |
|---|---|---|---|---|---|---|---|
| dipped (*Murray Sugar Free*), 4 pcs., .9 oz. | 130 | 2.0 | 17.0 | 7.0 | 0 | 95 | 1.0 |
| mint sandwich (*Country Choice* Organic Crèmes), 2 pcs., 1 oz. | 130 | 1.0 | 19.0 | 5.0 | 0 | 100 | <1.0 |
| oatmeal: | | | | | | | |
| (*Back to Nature* Crispy), .9 oz. | 120 | 1.0 | 18.0 | 5.0 | 0 | 100 | 1.0 |
| (*Country Choice* Old Fashioned Organic), .8-oz. pc. | 100 | 1.0 | 15.0 | 3.0 | 5 | 80 | 1.0 |
| (*Dare* Breaktime), 4 pcs., 1.1 oz. | 130 | 2.0 | 22.0 | 4.0 | 0 | 190 | 1.0 |
| (*Mother's*), 3 pcs., .9 oz. | 130 | 2.0 | 19.0 | 5.0 | 0 | 170 | <1.0 |
| (*Murray Sugar Free*), 3 pcs., 1.1 oz. | 140 | 2.0 | 21.0 | 7.0 | 0 | 130 | 3.0 |
| (*Nabisco* Classics), .7-oz. pc. | 90 | 1.0 | 14.0 | 3.5 | 0 | 100 | 0 |
| (*Pepperidge Farm*), 3 pcs. | 140 | 2.0 | 22.0 | 6.0 | 5 | 85 | <1.0 |
| chocolate, dark (*Pepperidge Farm Catalina* Soft), 1 pc. | 140 | 2.0 | 22.0 | 5.0 | 5 | 70 | 1.0 |
| chocolate, dark (*TLC*), 1.1-oz. pc. | 130 | 2.0 | 20.0 | 5.0 | 5 | 65 | 4.0 |
| chocolate almond cherry (*Pepperidge Farm Sonoma*), 1 pc. | 140 | 2.0 | 21.0 | 6.0 | 5 | 70 | 1.0 |
| chocolate chip (*Chips Ahoy!* Chewy), 1 oz. | 120 | 1.0 | 18.0 | 6.0 | 0 | 80 | 1.0 |
| chocolate chip (*Country Choice* Organic), .8-oz. pc. | 100 | 2.0 | 15.0 | 4.0 | 5 | 60 | 1.0 |
| chocolate chip (*Quaker* Breakfast), 1.7-oz. pc. | 180 | 3.0 | 31.0 | 6.0 | 5 | 190 | 5.0 |
| cranberry (*Country Choice* Organic), .8-oz. pc. | 100 | 1.0 | 16.0 | 3.0 | 5 | 65 | 1.0 |
| iced (*Country Choice* Organic), 4 pcs. | 120 | 1.0 | 21.0 | 4.0 | 0 | 120 | <1.0 |
| iced (*Mother's*), 4 pcs. | 150 | 2.0 | 23.0 | 6.0 | 0 | 160 | <1.0 |

| Food and Measure | cal. | prot. (gms) | carbo. (gms) | fat (gms) | chol. (mgs) | sod. (mgs) | fiber (gms) |
|---|---|---|---|---|---|---|---|
| **Cookie, oatmeal** *(cont.)* | | | | | | | |
| iced (*Nabisco* Classics), .67-oz. pc. ....... | 90 | 1.0 | 14.0 | 3.5 | 0 | 90 | 0 |
| oatmeal raisin: | | | | | | | |
| (*Baker's Treasures*), 2 pcs., 1.1 oz. .... | 130 | 2.0 | 22.0 | 4.5 | <5 | 105 | 1.0 |
| (*Country Choice Organic*), .8-oz. pc. | 100 | 1.0 | 16.0 | 3.0 | 5 | 65 | 1.0 |
| (*Grandma's* Big), 1.2-oz. pc. ....... | 150 | 2.0 | 25.0 | 5.0 | 10 | 200 | 1.0 |
| (*Health Valley* Wheat Free), .8-oz. pc. ... | 90 | 2.0 | 14.0 | 3.5 | 0 | 50 | 1.0 |
| (*Nabisco* Classics Soft), .8-oz. pc. ... | 100 | 1.0 | 17.0 | 3.5 | 0 | 160 | 1.0 |
| (*Pepperidge Farm Santa Cruz* Soft), .9-oz. pc. ........ | 130 | 2.0 | 23.0 | 4.5 | <5 | 90 | 2.0 |
| (*Quaker* Breakfast), 1.7-oz. pc. ....... | 170 | 3.0 | 33.0 | 4.5 | 5 | 190 | 5.0 |
| flax (*TLC*), 1.1-oz. pc. . | 130 | 2.0 | 20.0 | 4.5 | 0 | 70 | 4.0 |
| peanut butter: | | | | | | | |
| (*Grandma's* Big), 1.2-oz. pc. ....... | 270 | 3.0 | 20.0 | 9.0 | 0 | 135 | <1.0 |
| (*Murray Sugar Free*), 3 pcs., 1 oz. ...... | 150 | 3.0 | 16.0 | 9.0 | <5 | 130 | 1.0 |
| chocolate chip (*Chips Ahoy!* Chunky), .6-oz. pc. ........ | 90 | 1.0 | 10.0 | 5.0 | 0 | 75 | 0 |
| peanut butter sandwich: | | | | | | | |
| (*Back to Nature* Crème), .9 oz. .... | 130 | 2.0 | 17.0 | 5.0 | 0 | 95 | 1.0 |
| (*Grandma's*), 5 pcs. .. | 210 | 0 | 28.0 | 10.0 | <5 | 160 | 2.0 |
| (*Nutter Butter*), .9 oz. . | 120 | 2.0 | 17.0 | 5.0 | 0 | 90 | 1.0 |
| (*Nutter Butter* 16 oz.), 1 oz. ............. | 130 | 20 | 20 | 5.0 | 0 | 110 | 1.0 |
| (*Nutter Butter* Bites), 10 pcs., 1.1 oz. ......... | 140 | 2.0 | 21.0 | 6.0 | 0 | 115 | 1.0 |
| (*Nutter Butter* Bites), 1.25-oz. pkg. ..... | 170 | 3.0 | 24.0 | 7.0 | 0 | 135 | 1.0 |
| puff pastry, glazed (*Alessi* Sfogliatine), 3 pcs., 1 oz. ........ | 150 | 2.0 | 18.0 | 8.0 | 8 | 75 | 1.0 |

| Food and Measure | cal. | prot. (gms) | carbo. (gms) | fat (gms) | chol. (mgs) | sod. (mgs) | fiber (gms) |
|---|---|---|---|---|---|---|---|
| raspberry: | | | | | | | |
| (*Newtons*), 2 pcs., | | | | | | | |
| 1 oz. . . . . . . . . . . . . | 100 | 1.0 | 21.0 | 1.5 | 0 | 110 | 0 |
| tart (*Pepperidge Farm* | | | | | | | |
| *Montieri*), 2 pcs. . . . | 120 | 1.0 | 23.0 | 3.0 | 0 | 70 | <1.0 |
| shortbread: | | | | | | | |
| (*Lorna Doone*), 4 pcs., | | | | | | | |
| 1 oz. . . . . . . . . . . . . | 140 | 1.0 | 20.0 | 7.0 | 0 | 150 | 0 |
| (*Murray Sugar Free*), | | | | | | | |
| 8 pcs., 1.1 oz. . . . . | 130 | 2.0 | 21.0 | 5.0 | 0 | 140 | 2.0 |
| (*Pepperidge Farm*), | | | | | | | |
| 2 pcs., .9 oz. . . . . . | 130 | 1.0 | 17.0 | 6.0 | 20 | 105 | <1.0 |
| (*Sandies* Simply | | | | | | | |
| Shortbread), 2 pcs., | | | | | | | |
| 1.1 oz. . . . . . . . . . . | 160 | 2.0 | 19.0 | 9.0 | 15 | 90 | 0 |
| (*Sandies Rite Bites*), | | | | | | | |
| .75-oz. pkg. . . . . . . | 100 | 1.0 | 16.0 | 3.5 | 0 | 90 | <1.0 |
| (*SnackWell's* Sugar | | | | | | | |
| Free), 3 pcs., 1.1 oz. | 130 | 2.0 | 21.0 | 6.0 | 5 | 140 | 2.0 |
| bites (*Murray Sugar* | | | | | | | |
| *Free*), .75-oz. pouch | 80 | 1.0 | 16.0 | 3.5 | 0 | 110 | 3.0 |
| cashew (*Sandies*), | | | | | | | |
| 2 pcs., 1.1 oz. . . . . | 160 | 2.0 | 18.0 | 9.0 | <5 | 110 | <1.0 |
| chocolate chip pecan | | | | | | | |
| (*Sandies*), 2 pcs. . . | 170 | 2.0 | 18.0 | 10.0 | <5 | 95 | <1.0 |
| dark chocolate almond | | | | | | | |
| (*Sandies*), 2 pcs. . . | 160 | 2.0 | 18.0 | 9.0 | <5 | 90 | <1.0 |
| lemon, iced (*Nabisco* | | | | | | | |
| Classics), 1.2 oz. . . | 150 | 2.0 | 26.0 | 4.5 | 0 | 180 | 1.0 |
| pecan (*Sandies*), | | | | | | | |
| 2 pcs., 1.1 oz. . . . . | 160 | 1.0 | 18.0 | 10.0 | <5 | 105 | <1.0 |
| pecan (*Murray Sugar* | | | | | | | |
| *Free*), 3 pcs., 1.1 oz. | 160 | 2.0 | 18.0 | 11.0 | <5 | 110 | 1.0 |
| shortbread w/candy bits | | | | | | | |
| (*Susanna's*), | | | | | | | |
| 3 pcs., 1 oz.: | | | | | | | |
| butterscotch . . . . . . . . | 140 | 2.0 | 19.0 | 6.0 | 20 | 55 | 1.0 |
| lemon . . . . . . . . . . . . . | 140 | 1.0 | 20.0 | 5.0 | 15 | 50 | 0 |
| key lime . . . . . . . . . . . | 140 | 2.0 | 19.0 | 7.0 | 20 | 55 | 1.0 |
| strawberry . . . . . . . . . | 140 | 2.0 | 19.0 | 7.0 | 20 | 50 | 1.0 |
| spice (*Pepperidge Farm* | | | | | | | |
| *Sanibel* Snickerdoodle | | | | | | | |
| Soft), 1 pc. . . . . . . . . | 140 | 2.0 | 22.0 | 5.0 | 10 | 100 | <1.0 |

| Food and Measure | cal. | prot. (gms) | carbo. (gms) | fat (gms) | chol. (mgs) | sod. (mgs) | fiber (gms) |
|---|---|---|---|---|---|---|---|
| **Cookie** *(cont.)* | | | | | | | |
| strawberry: | | | | | | | |
| (*Newtons*), 2 pcs., | | | | | | | |
| 1 oz. ............ | 100 | 1.0 | 21.0 | 1.5 | 0 | 110 | 1.0 |
| (*Newtons* Minis), | | | | | | | |
| 1.3 oz. .......... | 130 | 2.0 | 27.0 | 3.0 | 0 | 140 | 2.0 |
| (*Pepperidge Farm* | | | | | | | |
| *Verona*), 3 pcs. .... | 140 | 2.0 | 22.0 | 5.0 | 10 | 100 | <1.0 |
| crèmes (*Emperador*), | | | | | | | |
| 2 pcs., .9 oz. ..... | 120 | 2.0 | 19.0 | 4.0 | <5 | 65 | <1.0 |
| sugar: | | | | | | | |
| (*Pepperidge Farm*), | | | | | | | |
| 3 pcs., 1.1 oz. .... | 150 | 2.0 | 21.0 | 7.0 | 10 | 65 | <1.0 |
| (*Pepperidge Farm* | | | | | | | |
| *Mystic* Soft), 1 pc. . | 140 | 2.0 | 22.0 | 5.0 | 10 | 90 | 0 |
| sugar wafer (*Gamesa*), | | | | | | | |
| 3 pcs., 1.2 oz.: | | | | | | | |
| chocolate ......... | 160 | 1.0 | 23.0 | 7.0 | 0 | 30 | 0 |
| strawberry ......... | 160 | 1.0 | 24.0 | 6.0 | 0 | 25 | 0 |
| vanilla ............ | 160 | 1.0 | 25.0 | 7.0 | 0 | 25 | 0 |
| tartlettes (*Roland*), | | | | | | | |
| 2 pcs., 1.2 oz.: | | | | | | | |
| apricot filled ........ | 150 | 2.0 | 23.0 | 5.0 | 0 | 65 | 0 |
| chocolate filled ...... | 160 | 2.0 | 21.0 | 8.0 | 0 | 75 | 1.0 |
| lemon filled ......... | 140 | 2.0 | 24.0 | 5.0 | 0 | 75 | 1.0 |
| raspberry filled ...... | 140 | 1.0 | 24.0 | 5.0 | 0 | 65 | 0 |
| strawberry filled ..... | 140 | 2.0 | 24.0 | 5.0 | 0 | 65 | 0 |
| vanilla sandwich: | | | | | | | |
| (*Cameo*), 1 oz. ...... | 130 | 1.0 | 21.0 | 5.0 | 0 | 105 | 0 |
| (*Country Choice* | | | | | | | |
| Organic Crèmes), | | | | | | | |
| 2 pcs., 1 oz. ...... | 130 | 1.0 | 19.0 | 5.0 | 0 | 120 | 0 |
| (*Emperador*), 2 pcs., | | | | | | | |
| .9 oz. ........... | 120 | 2.0 | 19.0 | 3.5 | 0 | 75 | 0 |
| (*Famous Amos*), | | | | | | | |
| 3 pcs., 1.2 oz. .... | 170 | 2.0 | 25.0 | 7.0 | 0 | 100 | 1.0 |
| (*Glutino*), 2 pcs., 1 oz. | 140 | <1.0 | 20.0 | 6.0 | 0 | 60 | 0 |
| (*Grandma's*), 5 pcs. .. | 210 | 2.0 | 30.0 | 9.0 | 0 | 90 | 1.0 |
| (*Grandma's* Mini), | | | | | | | |
| 9 pcs., 1.1 oz. .... | 150 | 2.0 | 22.0 | 7.0 | <5 | 90 | <1.0 |
| (*Health Valley Cookie* | | | | | | | |
| Cremes), 2 pcs. ... | 130 | 1.0 | 20.0 | 5.0 | 0 | 110 | 0 |
| (*Keebler* Crèmes | | | | | | | |
| Snack), 2-oz. pkg. . | 280 | 2.0 | 42.0 | 11.0 | 0 | 190 | <1.0 |

| Food and Measure | cal. | prot. (gms) | carbo. (gms) | fat (gms) | chol. (mgs) | sod. (mgs) | fiber (gms) |
|---|---|---|---|---|---|---|---|
| (*Mother's* English Tea), 2 pcs., 1.3 oz. | 180 | 2.0 | 27.0 | 7.0 | 0 | 100 | <1.0 |
| (*Mother's* Crèmes), 2 pcs., 1.3 oz. .... | 180 | 2.0 | 26.0 | 7.0 | 0 | 105 | <1.0 |
| (*Murray* Crèmes), 3 pcs., 1 oz. ...... | 140 | 1.0 | 21.0 | 5.0 | 0 | 90 | <1.0 |
| (*Murray* Sugar Free), 3 pcs., 1 oz. ...... | 130 | 1.0 | 20.0 | 6.0 | 0 | 55 | <1.0 |
| (*SnackWell's* Crème), .9-oz. pc. ........ | 110 | 1.0 | 20.0 | 3.0 | 0 | 130 | 1.0 |
| (*SnackWell's* Crème), 1.7-oz. pkg. ...... | 210 | 2.0 | 38.0 | 5.0 | 0 | 230 | 1.0 |
| (*Vienna Fingers*), 2 pcs., 1.1 oz. .... | 150 | 1.0 | 22.0 | 6.0 | 0 | 90 | <1.0 |
| chocolate crème (*Vienna Fingers*), 2 pcs., 1.1 oz. .... | 150 | 1.0 | 22.0 | 6.0 | 0 | 95 | <1.0 |
| French (*Nabisco Classics*), .67-oz. pc. | 90 | 1.0 | 14.0 | 3.5 | 0 | 60 | 0 |
| taffy flavor (*Mother's*), 2 pcs., 1.3 oz. .... | 180 | 1.0 | 27.0 | 8.0 | 0 | 125 | <1.0 |
| vanilla wafer: | | | | | | | |
| (*Jack's*), 9 pcs., 1.2 oz. | 140 | 2.0 | 25.0 | 4.0 | 0 | 110 | <1.0 |
| (*Jackson's*), 8 pcs., 1.1 oz. | 140 | 2.0 | 23.0 | 4.5 | <5 | 120 | <1.0 |
| (*Keebler*), 8 pcs., 1.1 oz. | 140 | 1.0 | 22.0 | 5.0 | 0 | 120 | <1.0 |
| (*Murray*), 8 pcs., 1.1 oz. .......... | 140 | 1.0 | 21.0 | 6.0 | 0 | 120 | <1.0 |
| (*Murray* Sugar Free), 9 pcs., 1.1 oz. .... | 130 | 2.0 | 24.0 | 5.0 | 0 | 90 | 2.0 |
| (*Nilla*), 8 pcs., 1.1 oz. . | 140 | 1.0 | 21.0 | 6.0 | 5 | 115 | 0 |
| (*Nilla* Reduced Fat), 8 pcs., 1 oz. ...... | 120 | 1.0 | 24.0 | 2.0 | 0 | 110 | 0 |
| crème (*Murray* Sugar Free*), 4 pcs., 1 oz. . | 130 | <1.0 | 19.0 | 8.0 | 0 | 20 | 4.0 |
| fudge dipped (*Murray Sugar Free*), 4 pcs., 1.1 oz. .... | 150 | 1.0 | 19.0 | 10.0 | 0 | 20 | 4.0 |
| mini (*Back to Nature*), 1.1 oz. ... | 150 | 2.0 | 24.0 | 4.5 | 5 | 180 | 0 |
| mini (*Keebler*), 18 pcs., 1.1 oz. ... | 140 | 1.0 | 21.0 | 6.0 | 0 | 120 | <1.0 |
| mini (*Nilla*), 1.1 oz. ... | 140 | 1.0 | 21.0 | 6.0 | 5 | 115 | 0 |

| Food and Measure | cal. | prot. (gms) | carbo. (gms) | fat (gms) | chol. (mgs) | sod. (mgs) | fiber (gms) |
|---|---|---|---|---|---|---|---|
| **Cookie** *(cont.)* | | | | | | | |
| wafer, rolled, crème filled *(Pepperidge Farm Pirouette)*, 2 pcs., .9 oz.: | | | | | | | |
| chocolate fudge | 120 | 2.0 | 18.0 | 4.0 | 0 | 30 | 1.0 |
| chocolate hazelnut | 120 | 1.0 | 19.0 | 5.0 | 5 | 40 | 1.0 |
| mint chocolate | 120 | 1.0 | 18.0 | 4.5 | <5 | 40 | <1.0 |
| vanilla, French | 120 | 1.0 | 18.0 | 5.0 | <5 | 40 | 0 |
| **Cookie, frozen/chilled,** ready-to-bake, 1 pc., except as noted: | | | | | | | |
| assorted *(Pillsbury Holiday Cookies)* | 120 | 1.0 | 15.0 | 6.0 | 5 | 85 | 0 |
| chocolate chip: | | | | | | | |
| *(Nestlé Toll House)* | 130 | 1.0 | 17.0 | 6.0 | 5 | 90 | 0 |
| *(Nestlé Toll House Jumbo)* | 170 | 2.0 | 23.0 | 9.0 | 10 | 150 | 1.0 |
| *(Nestlé Ultimates Lovers)* | 180 | 2.0 | 23.0 | 9.0 | 15 | 150 | 1.0 |
| *(Pillsbury)*, 2 pcs. | 170 | 2.0 | 23.0 | 8.0 | <5 | 125 | <1.0 |
| *(Pillsbury Slice and Bake)*, 1/16 pkg. | 130 | 1.0 | 18.0 | 6.0 | <5 | 95 | 0 |
| *(Pillsbury Big Deluxe)* | 170 | 2.0 | 23.0 | 8.0 | <5 | 125 | <1.0 |
| *(Pillsbury Simply)* | 150 | 1.0 | 19.0 | 8.0 | 5 | 115 | 0 |
| pecan *(Nestlé Ultimates)* | 190 | 2.0 | 22.0 | 10.0 | 15 | 160 | 1.0 |
| white, macadamia *(Nestlé Ultimates)* | 190 | 2.0 | 22.0 | 10.0 | 10 | 160 | 0 |
| chocolate chip, filled *(Nestlé Ultimates)*: | | | | | | | |
| caramel | 160 | 2.0 | 23.0 | 8.0 | 5 | 125 | 0 |
| chocolate | 160 | 1.0 | 23.0 | 7.0 | 5 | 120 | 0 |
| turtle | 160 | 1.0 | 23.0 | 7.0 | 5 | 120 | 1.0 |
| chocolate chunk: | | | | | | | |
| *(Nestlé Toll House)* | 130 | 1.0 | 17.0 | 6.0 | 5 | 90 | 0 |
| and chip *(Pillsbury)*, 2 pcs. | 170 | 2.0 | 23.0 | 8.0 | <5 | 125 | <1.0 |
| gingerbread *(Pillsbury Slice and Bake)*, 2 balls dough, 1" | 130 | 2.0 | 18.0 | 6.0 | <5 | 105 | 0 |
| oatmeal: | | | | | | | |
| chocolate chip *(Pillsbury)*, 2 pcs. | 160 | 2.0 | 23.0 | 7.0 | <5 | 95 | 1.0 |

| Food and Measure | cal. | prot. (gms) | carbo. (gms) | fat (gms) | chol. (mgs) | sod. (mgs) | fiber (gms) |
|---|---|---|---|---|---|---|---|
| raisin (*Nestlé Toll House*), 2 pcs. | 160 | 2.0 | 24.0 | 6.0 | 15 | 140 | 0 |
| raisin (*Pillsbury Big Deluxe*) | 150 | 2.0 | 24.0 | 6.0 | 0 | 100 | <1.0 |
| peanut butter: | | | | | | | |
| (*Nestlé Ultimates*) | 170 | 2.0 | 23.0 | 8.0 | 15 | 190 | 1.0 |
| (*Pillsbury* Slice and Bake), 1/16 pkg. | 120 | 2.0 | 16.0 | 6.0 | <5 | 135 | 0 |
| (*Pillsbury Reese's Pieces*), 2 pcs. | 170 | 2.0 | 22.0 | 8.0 | 0 | 150 | <1.0 |
| (*Pillsbury Simply*) | 140 | 2.0 | 19.0 | 7.0 | 5 | 150 | <1.0 |
| cup (*Pillsbury Big Deluxe*) | 170 | 2.0 | 22.0 | 8.0 | 0 | 150 | <1.0 |
| cups, chips, chocolate chunks (*Nestlé Ultimates*) | 180 | 2.0 | 23.0 | 9.0 | 15 | 180 | 0 |
| sugar: | | | | | | | |
| (*Nestlé Toll House*), 2 pcs. | 170 | 2.0 | 23.0 | 8.0 | 15 | 120 | 0 |
| (*Pillsbury*), 2 pcs. | 170 | 2.0 | 22.0 | 8.0 | <5 | 100 | 0 |
| (*Pillsbury* Slice and Bake), 1/16 pkg. | 120 | 1.0 | 18.0 | 5.0 | <5 | 95 | 0 |
| turtle (*Pillsbury Big Deluxe* Supreme) | 170 | 2.0 | 22.0 | 8.0 | <5 | 125 | <1.0 |
| white chunk macadamia (*Pillsbury Big Deluxe*) | 170 | 2.0 | 22.0 | 9.0 | 0 | 95 | 0 |
| **Cookie crumbs**: | | | | | | | |
| amaretti (*Roland*), 1.1 oz. | 130 | 2.0 | 24.0 | 2.0 | 0 | 20 | 1.0 |
| graham cracker (*Keebler*), 3 tbsp. | 70 | 1.0 | 13.0 | 1.5 | 0 | 140 | 0 |
| **Cookie mix**: | | | | | | | |
| (*Hodgson Mill* Gluten Free), 1 oz. | 101 | 1.0 | 24.0 | 0 | 0 | 100 | 1.0 |
| (*Pillsbury* Snickerdoodle), 1/18 pkg. | 110 | 1.0 | 23.0 | 1.5 | 0 | 120 | 1.0 |
| (*Pillsbury Funfetti*), 1/18 pkg. | 110 | 1.0 | 23.0 | 2.5 | 0 | 180 | 0 |
| chocolate chip: | | | | | | | |
| (*Arrowhead Mills* Organic), 1/18 pkg. | 80 | 1.0 | 16.0 | 1.5 | 0 | 95 | 0 |
| (*Arrowhead Mills* Organic Gluten Free), 1/18 pkg. | 80 | <1.0 | 16.0 | 1.0 | 0 | 60 | <1.0 |

| Food and Measure | cal. | prot. (gms) | carbo. (gms) | fat (gms) | chol. (mgs) | sod. (mgs) | fiber (gms) |
|---|---|---|---|---|---|---|---|
| **Cookie mix, chocolate chip** *(cont.)* | | | | | | | |
| (*Betty Crocker*), 2 pcs.* | 170 | 1.0 | 22.0 | 8.0 | 25 | 140 | <1.0 |
| (*Betty Crocker* Gluten Free), 2 pcs.* ..... | 150 | 1.0 | 23.0 | 7.0 | 25 | 160 | <1.0 |
| (*Betty Crocker Warm Delights* Micro), 3-oz. bowl ....... | 340 | 4.0 | 58.0 | 11.0 | 0 | 280 | 2.0 |
| (*Dr. Oetker* Organics), 1/12 pkg. ......... | 120 | 1.0 | 24.0 | 2.0 | 0 | 110 | 0 |
| (*Duncan Hines*), 2 pcs.* | 180 | 1.0 | 23.0 | 9.0 | 10 | 85 | 0 |
| (*Duncan Hines* Snack Size), 2 pcs.* ..... | 180 | 2.0 | 24.0 | 9.0 | 35 | 115 | 0 |
| (*"Jiffy"*), 3 tbsp. ..... | 90 | 1.0 | 17.0 | 3.0 | 0 | 125 | 0 |
| fudgy (*Betty Crocker Warm Delights* Micro), 1 bowl .... | 340 | 4.0 | 58.0 | 11.0 | 0 | 280 | 2.0 |
| walnut (*Betty Crocker*), 2 pcs.* .......... | 170 | 2.0 | 21.0 | 9.0 | 25 | 140 | 1.0 |
| chocolate chunk: | | | | | | | |
| dark (*Pillsbury*), 1/18 pkg. | 120 | 1.0 | 21.0 | 3.5 | 0 | 160 | 1.0 |
| double (*Betty Crocker*), 2 pcs.* .......... | 150 | 2.0 | 21.0 | 6.0 | 10 | 105 | 0 |
| chocolate/oatmeal/ caramel (*Betty Crocker* Carmelita), 1/16 pkg.* .. | 190 | 2.0 | 28.0 | 8.0 | 10 | 135 | 1.0 |
| gingerbread (*Pillsbury*), 1/8 pkg. ... | 210 | 2.0 | 38.0 | 5.0 | 0 | 350 | 0 |
| lemon bar (*Betty Crocker Sunkist*), 1/16 pkg.* ... | 140 | 2.0 | 24.0 | 4.0 | 40 | 90 | <1.0 |
| oatmeal: | | | | | | | |
| (*Betty Crocker*), 2 pcs.* | 160 | 2.0 | 22.0 | 7.0 | 25 | 140 | <1.0 |
| (*Dr. Oetker* Organics), 1/12 pkg. ......... | 110 | 1.0 | 24.0 | .5 | 0 | 110 | 0 |
| (*"Jiffy"*), 3 tbsp. ..... | 90 | 2.0 | 18.0 | 1.5 | 0 | 80 | 1.0 |
| chocolate chip (*Betty Crocker*), 2 pcs.* .. | 160 | 2.0 | 21.0 | 8.0 | 25 | 120 | 1.0 |
| chocolate chunk (*Pillsbury*), 1/18 pkg. | 110 | 1.0 | 22.0 | 2.5 | 0 | 110 | 1.0 |
| oatmeal raisin: | | | | | | | |
| (*Arrowhead Mills* Organic), 1/18 pkg. .. | 80 | 1.0 | 16.0 | 0 | 0 | 85 | <1.0 |
| (*Sun•Maid*), 1/4 cup ... | 170 | 2.0 | 35.0 | 2.0 | 0 | 120 | 1.0 |
| peanut butter (*Betty Crocker*), 2 pcs.* .... | 150 | 3.0 | 20.0 | 6.0 | 10 | 150 | 0 |

| Food and Measure | cal. | prot. (gms) | carbo. (gms) | fat (gms) | chol. (mgs) | sod. (mgs) | fiber (gms) |
|---|---|---|---|---|---|---|---|
| peanut butter chip, chocolate (*Betty Crocker*), 2 pcs.* | 160 | 2.0 | 21.0 | 7.0 | 10 | 120 | <1.0 |
| peanut butter bar: |  |  |  |  |  |  |  |
| (*Betty Crocker Reese's*), 1/16 pkg.* | 180 | 2.0 | 20.0 | 10.0 | 10 | 150 | 1.0 |
| chocolate (*Betty Crocker*), 1/16 pkg.* | 180 | 3.0 | 25.0 | 8.0 | 10 | 190 | <1.0 |
| pumpkin spice (*Betty Crocker*), 2 pcs.* | 150 | 2.0 | 22.0 | 6.0 | 25 | 160 | <1.0 |
| rainbow chocolate candy (*Betty Crocker*), 2 pcs.* | 160 | 2.0 | 22.0 | 7.0 | 25 | 140 | 0 |
| sugar: |  |  |  |  |  |  |  |
| (*Arrowhead Mills Organic Bake With Me*), 1/18 pkg. | 90 | 1.0 | 20.0 | .5 | 0 | 45 | 1.0 |
| (*Betty Crocker*), 2 pcs.* | 160 | 2.0 | 21.0 | 8.0 | 25 | 120 | 0 |
| (*"Jiffy"*), 3 tbsp. | 90 | 2.0 | 19.0 | 1.0 | 0 | 80 | 0 |
| turtle bar (*Betty Crocker*), 1/16 pkg.* | 180 | 2.0 | 27.0 | 8.0 | 10 | 160 | 1.0 |
| **Coquito nut** (*Frieda's*), 11 pcs., 1 oz. | 110 | 1.0 | 5.0 | 10.0 | 0 | 5 | 3.0 |
| **Coriander**, fresh, 1/4 cup | 1 | .1 | .1 | <.1 | 0 | 1 | .1 |
| **Coriander, dried:** |  |  |  |  |  |  |  |
| leaf, 1 tsp. | 2 | .1 | .3 | <.1 | 0 | 1 | .1 |
| seed, 1 tsp. | 5 | .2 | 1.0 | .3 | 0 | 1 | .5 |
| **Corkscrew pasta mix** |  |  |  |  |  |  |  |
| cheese, 4 (*Pasta Roni*), 1 cup* | 370 | 11.0 | 49.0 | 15.0 | 10 | 810 | 2.0 |
| **Corn**, fresh: |  |  |  |  |  |  |  |
| baby, .28-oz. ear | 9 | .3 | 2.0 | .1 | 0 | 1 | .2 |
| golden or white: |  |  |  |  |  |  |  |
| raw, 5-oz. ear | 123 | 4.6 | 27.2 | 1.7 | 0 | 21 | 3.9 |
| kernels, boiled, drained, 1/2 cup | 89 | 2.7 | 20.6 | 1.1 | 0 | 14 | 2.3 |
| white, boiled, drained, 2.72-oz. ear | 83 | 2.6 | 19.3 | 1.0 | 0 | 13 | 2.1 |
| **Corn, canned** |  |  |  |  |  |  |  |
| 1/2 cup: |  |  |  |  |  |  |  |
| baby (*Roland*) | 25 | 2.0 | 4.0 | 0 | 0 | 280 | 2.0 |
| kernel, golden: |  |  |  |  |  |  |  |
| (*Del Monte*) | 90 | 2.0 | 18.0 | 1.0 | 0 | 360 | 3.0 |

| Food and Measure | cal. | prot. (gms) | carbo. (gms) | fat (gms) | chol. (mgs) | sod. (mgs) | fiber (gms) |
|---|---|---|---|---|---|---|---|
| **Corn, canned, kernel, golden** *(cont.)* | | | | | | | |
| (*Del Monte* Summer | | | | | | | |
| Crisp Vac Pac) .... | 70 | 2.0 | 13.0 | 1.0 | 0 | 270 | 3.0 |
| (*Freshlike*) ......... | 80 | 3.0 | 17.0 | 1.5 | 0 | 310 | 2.0 |
| (*Green Giant* Whole | | | | | | | |
| Kernel Sweet) ..... | 90 | 2.0 | 20.0 | .5 | 0 | 320 | 1.0 |
| (*Green Giant* Whole | | | | | | | |
| Kernel Sweet 50% | | | | | | | |
| Less Sodium) ..... | 90 | 2.0 | 18.0 | .5 | 0 | 160 | 1.0 |
| (*Green Giant Niblets* | | | | | | | |
| Extra Sweet) ...... | 60 | 2.0 | 12.0 | ·1.0 | 0 | 250 | 2.0 |
| (*Green Giant Niblets* | | | | | | | |
| Vac Pac) ......... | 100 | 2.0 | 20.0 | 1.0 | 0 | 250 | 1.0 |
| (*S&W*) ............ | 60 | 2.0 | 11.0 | 1.0 | 0 | 360 | 3.0 |
| (*S&W* Sweet 'n Crisp) | 70 | 2.0 | 13.0 | 1.0 | 0 | 270 | 3.0 |
| (*Veg-All*) ........... | 80 | 2.0 | 16.0 | 1.0 | 0 | 340 | 2.0 |
| kernel, golden/white: | | | | | | | |
| (*Del Monte*) ........ | 80 | 2.0 | 18.0 | .5 | 0 | 360 | 2.0 |
| (*Green Giant*) ....... | 80 | 2.0 | 17.0 | .5 | 0 | 230 | 2.0 |
| kernel, white: | | | | | | | |
| (*Del Monte*) ........ | 60 | 2.0 | 11.0 | 1.0 | 0 | 360 | 3.0 |
| (*Green Giant* Shoepeg) | 100 | 3.0 | 21.0 | .5 | 0 | 250 | 2.0 |
| cream style: | | | | | | | |
| (*Del Monte*) ........ | 60 | 1.0 | 14.0 | .5 | 0 | 360 | 2.0 |
| (*Freshlike*) ......... | 100 | 2.0 | 21.0 | 1.0 | 0 | 280 | 2.0 |
| (*Green Giant*) ....... | 90 | 2.0 | 19.0 | .5 | 0 | 400 | 1.0 |
| (*S&W*) ............ | 60 | 1.0 | 14.0 | .5 | 0 | 360 | 2.0 |
| (*Veg-All*) ........... | 100 | 2.0 | 21.0 | 1.0 | 0 | 280 | 2.0 |
| seasoned (*Glory*) .... | 80 | 2.0 | 19.0 | .5 | 0 | 490 | 2.0 |
| white (*Del Monte*) .... | 100 | 2.0 | 21.0 | 1.0 | 0 | 360 | 2.0 |
| in butter sauce (*Del | | | | | | | |
| Monte Savory Sides*) . | 90 | 2.0 | 14.0 | 2.5 | 5 | 530 | <1.0 |
| w/chipotle peppers, | | | | | | | |
| white (*Green Giant*) .. | 90 | 2.0 | 19.0 | .5 | 0 | 250 | 2.0 |
| w/diced pepper: | | | | | | | |
| (*Freshlike* Selects) ... | 80 | 2.0 | 16.0 | 1.0 | 0 | 240 | 1.0 |
| (*Green Giant | | | | | | | |
| Mexicorn*) ........ | 90 | 2.0 | 19.0 | .5 | 0 | 270 | 1.0 |
| seasoned (*Del Monte | | | | | | | |
| Fiesta*) ............. | 50 | 2.0 | 12.0 | 1.0 | 0 | 310 | 2.0 |
| w/tomato, black beans | | | | | | | |
| (*Del Monte Savory | | | | | | | |
| Sides* Santa Fe) ...... | 70 | 3.0 | 16.0 | 1.0 | 0 | 510 | 1.0 |

| Food and Measure | cal. | prot. (gms) | carbo. (gms) | fat (gms) | chol. (mgs) | sod. (mgs) | fiber (gms) |
|---|---|---|---|---|---|---|---|
| **Corn, frozen**: | | | | | | | |
| on cob, 1 ear: | | | | | | | |
| (*Allens* 4 Pack) ...... | 160 | 6.0 | 38.0 | 1.5 | 0 | 5 | 4.0 |
| (*Allens* 6/12/24 Pack) . | 80 | 3.0 | 19.0 | .5 | 0 | 0 | 2.0 |
| (*Birds Eye* 4 Pack) ... | 170 | 5.0 | 36.0 | 1.5 | 0 | 0 | 2.0 |
| on cob, mini, 1 ear: | | | | | | | |
| (*Birds Eye*), 3 oz. .... | 90 | 3.0 | 19.0 | 1.0 | 0 | 0 | 1.0 |
| (*Birds Eye* Steamfresh), 3 oz. . | 70 | 2.0 | 13.0 | 1.0 | 0 | 0 | 1.0 |
| (*Green Giant* Extra Sweet), 2.2 oz. .... | 50 | 2.0 | 9.0 | .5 | 0 | 0 | 2.0 |
| (*Green Giant Nibblers*), 2.2 oz. .......... | 70 | 2.0 | 14.0 | .5 | 0 | 5 | 1.0 |
| kernel, golden, ⅔ cup, except as noted: | | | | | | | |
| (*Allens*) ............ | 110 | 3.0 | 21.0 | 1.0 | 0 | 5 | 3.0 |
| (*Allens SteamSupreme* 16 oz.) .......... | 80 | 2.0 | 14.0 | 1.5 | 0 | 10 | 2.0 |
| (*Allens SteamSupreme* 12 oz.) .......... | 100 | 3.0 | 21.0 | 1.0 | 0 | 5 | 2.0 |
| (*Birds Eye/C&W* Petite/Sweet) ..... | 100 | 3.0 | 21.0 | 1.0 | 0 | 0 | 1.0 |
| (*Birds Eye Steamfresh/ Freshlike* Sweet) ... | 70 | 3.0 | 14.0 | 1.0 | 0 | 0 | 2.0 |
| (*Birds Eye Steamfresh* Singles), 3.25-oz. bag ...... | 80 | 3.0 | 14.0 | 1.0 | 0 | 0 | 2.0 |
| (*Cascadian Farm* Organic Super Sweet) | 60 | 2.0 | 11.0 | .5 | 0 | 85 | 2.0 |
| (*Cascadian Farm* Organic Sweet), ¾ cup .... | 90 | 3.0 | 19.0 | 1.0 | 0 | 0 | 2.0 |
| (*C&W Early Harvest* Supersweet) | 70 | 3.0 | 14.0 | 1.0 | 0 | 0 | 2.0 |
| (*Green Giant Niblets Simply Steam*) .... | 70 | 2.0 | 13.0 | 1.0 | 0 | 55 | 2.0 |
| (*Green Giant Niblets Valley Fresh Steamers*) ....... | 90 | 2.0 | 19.0 | 1.0 | 0 | 0 | 2.0 |
| (*Green Giant Niblets Valley Fresh Steamers* Extra Sweet) | 70 | 2.0 | 13.0 | 1.0 | 0 | 0 | 2.0 |
| kernel, golden/white: | | | | | | | |
| (*Birds Eye* Baby/ Freshlike*), ⅔ cup .. | 100 | 3.0 | 20.0 | 1.0 | 0 | 0 | 2.0 |

| Food and Measure | cal. | prot. (gms) | carbo. (gms) | fat (gms) | chol. (mgs) | sod. (mgs) | fiber (gms) |
|---|---|---|---|---|---|---|---|
| **Corn, frozen, kernel, golden/white** *(cont.)* | | | | | | | |
| (*Birds Eye* Steamfresh), ⅔ cup | 80 | 3.0 | 16.0 | 1.0 | 0 | 0 | 2.0 |
| (*C&W* Petite), ⅔ cup . | 100 | 3.0 | 21.0 | 1.0 | 0 | 0 | 1.0 |
| kernel, white, ⅔ cup: | | | | | | | |
| (*Birds Eye* Baby) . . . . . | 90 | 3.0 | 18.0 | 1.0 | 0 | 0 | 3.0 |
| (*C&W* Petite) . . . . . . . | 100 | 3.0 | 21.0 | 1.0 | 0 | 0 | 1.0 |
| (*Freshlike* Tender) . . . . | 80 | 2.0 | 14.0 | 1.5 | 0 | 0 | 2.0 |
| in butter sauce, ¾ cup, except as noted: | | | | | | | |
| (*Allens SteamSupreme*) | 130 | 3.0 | 23.0 | 2.5 | 5 | 130 | 2.0 |
| (*Birds Eye*) . . . . . . . . . | 110 | 2.0 | 21.0 | 1.5 | 0 | 190 | 1.0 |
| (*Birds Eye Steamfresh Lightly Sauced*) . . . | 110 | 3.0 | 21.0 | 1.5 | 0 | 210 | 1.0 |
| (*Green Giant Niblets Bag*), ½ cup cooked | 90 | 3.0 | 15.0 | 1.5 | 0 | 230 | 2.0 |
| (*Green Giant Niblets Box*) . . . . . . . . . . . | 80 | 2.0 | 15.0 | 1.5 | <5 | 270 | 2.0 |
| (*Green Giant Niblets Just for One*), 1 tray | 80 | 2.0 | 15.0 | 1.5 | 0 | 320 | 3.0 |
| (*McKenzie's*), ½ cup . . | 120 | 3.0 | 26.0 | 1.0 | 0 | 500 | 1.0 |
| white (*Green Giant Shoepeg*) . . . . . . . . | 110 | 2.0 | 22.0 | 2.0 | <5 | 340 | 2.0 |
| cream style, ½ cup: | | | | | | | |
| (*Bob Evans* Chilled) . . | 200 | 3.0 | 26.0 | 11.0 | 30 | 290 | 5.0 |
| (*Green Giant*) . . . . . . . | 110 | 2.0 | 24.0 | 1.0 | 0 | 320 | 2.0 |
| white (*McKenzie's*) . . . | 100 | 2.0 | 24.0 | 0 | 0 | 250 | 3.0 |
| yellow (*McKenzie's*) . . | 110 | 2.0 | 25.0 | 0 | 0 | 210 | 2.0 |
| fried (*McKenzie's*), ½ cup . . . . . . . . . . . | 110 | 3.0 | 21.0 | 1.5 | 0 | 280 | 4.0 |
| seasoned (*Birds Eye Steamfresh* Southwestern), ⅔ cup . | 90 | 2.0 | 16.0 | 2.0 | 0 | 260 | 1.0 |
| **Corn, pickled**, baby (*Roland*), ¼ cup . . . . . | 10 | 1.0 | 2.0 | 0 | 0 | 65 | 0 |
| **Corn, roasted** (*Beer Nuts*), 1 oz. . . . . . . . . | 130 | 2.0 | 20.0 | 4.5 | 0 | 120 | 2.0 |
| **Corn, whole-grain**: | | | | | | | |
| 1 oz. . . . . . . . . . . . . . . . | 103 | 2.7 | 21.1 | 1.3 | 0 | 10 | 2.1 |
| 1 cup . . . . . . . . . . . . . . | 605 | 15.6 | 123.3 | 7.9 | 0 | 58 | 12.2 |
| **Corn bran**, crude, 1 cup . | 170 | 6.4 | 65.1 | .7 | 0 | 5 | 64.3 |
| **Corn cake mix**, sweet, dry, ½ cup: | | | | | | | |
| (*Chi-Chi's*) . . . . . . . . . . . | 100 | 1.0 | 23.0 | 0 | 0 | 130 | 0 |

| Food and Measure | cal. | prot. (gms) | carbo. (gms) | fat (gms) | chol. (mgs) | sod. (mgs) | fiber (gms) |
|---|---|---|---|---|---|---|---|
| (*El Torito*) . . . . . . . . . . . | 100 | 1.0 | 22.0 | .5 | 0 | 120 | 0 |
| **Corn chips**, see "Corn crisps/chips" | | | | | | | |
| **Corn combinations**, frozen, baby corn and: | | | | | | | |
| beans and peas | | | | | | | |
| (*Birds Eye*), ¾ cup . . . | 70 | 2.0 | 13.0 | 0 | 0 | 0 | 2.0 |
| vegetables (*Birds Eye/ Freshlike*), ⅔ cup . . . . | 50 | 2.0 | 9.0 | 1.0 | 0 | 10 | 3.0 |
| **Corn crisps/chips** (see also "Snack chips"), 1 oz., except as noted: | | | | | | | |
| (*Bachman* Treasure Puffs) . . . . . . . . . . | 130 | 2.0 | 21.0 | 4.5 | 0 | 260 | <1.0 |
| (*Bugles*), 1.1 oz. . . . . . . . | 160 | 1.0 | 18.0 | 9.0 | 0 | 310 | <1.0 |
| (*Chester's Flamin' Hot* Fries) . . . . . . . . . . | 150 | 2.0 | 17.0 | 8.0 | 0 | 270 | <1.0 |
| (*Chester's Flamin' Hot* Puffcorn) . . . . . . . | 150 | 2.0 | 13.0 | 10.0 | 0 | 320 | 1.0 |
| (*Chipitos* Jumbo) . . . . . . | 150 | 1.0 | 18.0 | 8.0 | 0 | 170 | 2.0 |
| (*Corn Nuts* Original) . . . . | 120 | 3.0 | 20.0 | 4.5 | 0 | 180 | 2.0 |
| (*Corn Nuts* Original 7 oz.) . . . . . . . . . . . . | 130 | 2.0 | 20.0 | 4.5 | 0 | 160 | 1.0 |
| (*Dipsy Doodles*) . . . . . . . | 160 | 1.0 | 16.0 | 10.0 | 0 | 180 | 1.0 |
| (*Fritos* Lightly Salted) . . . | 160 | 2.0 | 16.0 | 10.0 | 0 | 80 | 1.0 |
| (*Fritos* Original) . . . . . . . . | 160 | 2.0 | 15.0 | 10.0 | 0 | 170 | 1.0 |
| (*Fritos Scoops!*) . . . . . . . | 160 | 2.0 | 16.0 | 10.0 | 0 | 110 | 1.0 |
| (*Herr's*), 1.1 oz. . . . . . . . . | 160 | 2.0 | 17.0 | 10.0 | 0 | 170 | 2.0 |
| barbecue: | | | | | | | |
| (*Chipitos*) . . . . . . . . . . | 150 | 2.0 | 16.0 | 8.0 | 0 | 260 | 2.0 |
| (*Corn Nuts*) . . . . . . . . | 130 | 2.0 | 20.0 | 4.5 | 0 | 170 | 2.0 |
| (*Dipsy Doodles*) . . . . . | 160 | 1.0 | 16.0 | 10.0 | 0 | 250 | 1.0 |
| (*Fritos*) . . . . . . . . . . . . | 150 | 2.0 | 16.0 | 10.0 | 0 | 280 | 1.0 |
| honey (*Fritos Flavor Twists*) . . . . . | 150 | 2.0 | 16.0 | 9.0 | 0 | 180 | 1.0 |
| butter flavor (*Chester's* Puffcorn) . . | 160 | 1.0 | 14.0 | 11.0 | 0 | 300 | <1.0 |
| Cajun ranch (*Doritos* Mighty Zingers) . . . . . | 150 | 2.0 | 13.0 | 10.0 | 0 | 290 | 1.0 |
| caramel (*Bugles*), 1.1 oz. | 140 | <1.0 | 17.0 | 8.0 | 0 | 230 | 0 |
| cheddar: | | | | | | | |
| (*Garden of Eatin'* Crunchitos) . . . . . . | 140 | 2.0 | 18.0 | 7.0 | <5 | 310 | 1.0 |

| Food and Measure | cal. | prot. (gms) | carbo. (gms) | fat (gms) | chol. (mgs) | sod. (mgs) | fiber (gms) |
|---|---|---|---|---|---|---|---|
| **Corn crisps/chips, cheddar** *(cont.)* | | | | | | | |
| (*Garden of Eatin'* Puffs) ........... | 150 | 2.0 | 15.0 | 10.0 | <5 | 220 | 1.0 |
| white (*Barbara's* Puffs Bakes) ...... | 160 | 2.0 | 12.0 | 10.0 | 0 | 200 | 1.0 |
| white (*Cheetos* Puffs) . | 150 | 2.0 | 16.0 | 9.0 | 0 | 290 | <1.0 |
| white (*Cheez Doodles* Puffed) .......... | 150 | 2.0 | 15.0 | 9.0 | <5 | 290 | 0 |
| cheddar jalapeño: | | | | | | | |
| (*Cheetos* Crunchy) ... | 170 | 2.0 | 15.0 | 11.0 | <5 | 250 | <1.0 |
| (*Cheez Doodles*) ...... | 150 | 1.0 | 17.0 | 9.0 | 0 | 250 | 0 |
| cheddar salsa (*Doritos* Mighty Zingers) ..... | 150 | 1.0 | 13.0 | 10.0 | 0 | 290 | 0 |
| cheese: | | | | | | | |
| (*Barbara's* Puffs Bakes) .......... | 160 | 2.0 | 14.0 | 10.0 | 0 | 200 | 1.0 |
| (*Barbara's* Puffs Original) ......... | 150 | 2.0 | 15.0 | 10.0 | 0 | 160 | 1.0 |
| (*Cheetos* Crunchy) ... | 160 | 2.0 | 15.0 | 10.0 | <5 | 290 | <1.0 |
| (*Cheetos* Crunchy Baked!) ......... | 130 | 2.0 | 19.0 | 5.0 | 0 | 240 | 0 |
| (*Cheetos* Giant Puffs) . | 150 | 2.0 | 17.0 | 9.0 | 0 | 250 | <1.0 |
| (*Cheetos* Puffs) ...... | 160 | 2.0 | 15.0 | 10.0 | 0 | 370 | <1.0 |
| (*Cheetos* Twisted) .... | 160 | 2.0 | 13.0 | 10.0 | 0 | 350 | 0 |
| (*Cheetos* Flamin' Hot) . | 170 | 2.0 | 15.0 | 11.0 | 0 | 250 | <1.0 |
| (*Cheetos* Flamin' Hot Baked!) ......... | 130 | 3.0 | 19.0 | 5.0 | 0 | 240 | <1.0 |
| (*Cheetos* Flamin' Hot Fantastix!) ..... | 130 | 2.0 | 20.0 | 5.0 | 0 | 210 | 1.0 |
| (*Cheetos* Flamin' Hot Giant Puffs) ... | 150 | 2.0 | 17.0 | 9.0 | 0 | 250 | <1.0 |
| (*Cheetos* Flamin' Hot Limon) ....... | 160 | 1.0 | 15.0 | 11.0 | 0 | 190 | <1.0 |
| (*Cheez Doodles* Crunchy) ........ | 150 | 1.0 | 17.0 | 9.0 | 0 | 220 | 0 |
| (*Cheez Doodles* Puffed) .......... | 150 | 2.0 | 17.0 | 8.0 | 0 | 320 | 0 |
| (*Chester's* Puffcorn) .. | 160 | 2.0 | 14.0 | 11.0 | 0 | 290 | 0 |
| (*Herr's* Crunchy Sticks) .......... | 150 | 1.0 | 17.0 | 9.0 | 0 | 150 | <1.0 |
| (*Herr's* Curls) ....... | 150 | 2.0 | 16.0 | 8.0 | 0 | 350 | 1.0 |
| (*Jax* Baked Curls) .... | 140 | 2.0 | 17.0 | 7.0 | 0 | 300 | 0 |
| (*Jax* Crunchy Twists) . | 160 | 2.0 | 14.0 | 11.0 | 0 | 250 | 0 |

| Food and Measure | cal. | prot. (gms) | carbo. (gms) | fat (gms) | chol. (mgs) | sod. (mgs) | fiber (gms) |
|---|---|---|---|---|---|---|---|
| honey or hot (*Herr's* Curls) ..... | 150 | 2.0 | 16.0 | 8.0 | 0 | 350 | 1.0 |
| honey barbecue (*Cheez Doodles*) ........ | 150 | 1.0 | 17.0 | 9.0 | 0 | 250 | 0 |
| jalapeño (*Barbara's* Puffs) ........... | 150 | 2.0 | 15.0 | 10.0 | 0 | 190 | 1.0 |
| nacho (*Bugles*), 1.1 oz. | 160 | 1.0 | 18.0 | 9.0 | 0 | 310 | 0 |
| nacho (*Corn Nuts*) ... | 130 | 3.0 | 19.0 | 5.0 | 0 | 240 | 2.0 |
| chili cheese: | | | | | | | |
| (*Cheetos* Fantastix!) .. | 130 | 2.0 | 19.0 | 5.0 | 0 | 200 | 1.0 |
| (*Fritos*) ............ | 160 | 2.0 | 15.0 | 10.0 | 0 | 260 | 1.0 |
| (*Herr's*) ............ | 150 | 2.0 | 16.0 | 8.0 | 0 | 360 | 1.0 |
| chili picante (*Corn Nuts*) ............ | 130 | 2.0 | 19.0 | 4.5 | 0 | 290 | 2.0 |
| chocolate peanut butter (*Bugles*), 1.1 oz. ..... | 170 | 2.0 | 20.0 | 9.0 | 0 | 150 | <1.0 |
| chorizo chipotle (*Corn Nuts*) ........ | 130 | 2.0 | 20.0 | 4.5 | 0 | 160 | 1.0 |
| hot (*Fritos Flamin' Hot*) .............. | 160 | 2.0 | 15.0 | 10.0 | 0 | 160 | 1.0 |
| lemon (*Corn Nuts* Limon) ............ | 130 | 2.0 | 20.0 | 4.5 | 0 | 140 | 1.0 |
| onion: | | | | | | | |
| (*Funyuns*) .......... | 140 | 2.0 | 18.0 | 7.0 | 0 | 270 | <1.0 |
| (*Funyuns Flamin' Hot*) ............ | 130 | 2.0 | 16.0 | 7.0 | 0 | 300 | 1.0 |
| (*Herr's* Rings) ....... | 140 | 1.0 | 17.0 | 7.0 | 0 | 400 | 1.0 |
| (*Wise* Rings) ........ | 140 | 0 | 20.0 | 6.0 | 0 | 360 | 0 |
| ranch: | | | | | | | |
| (*Corn Nuts*) ....... | 130 | 2.0 | 20.0 | 4.5 | 0 | 250 | 1.0 |
| (*Corn Nuts* 4 oz.) .... | 130 | 3.0 | 19.0 | 5.0 | 0 | 240 | 2.0 |
| tortilla (see also "Tortilla chips, multigrain"): | | | | | | | |
| (*Bachman* Deli Rounds) ......... | 130 | 2.0 | 20.0 | 6.0 | 0 | 190 | 2.0 |
| (*Bachman* Whole Grain) ........... | 140 | 2.0 | 19.0 | 6.0 | 0 | 50 | 1.5 |
| (*Chi-Chi's* Round/ Authentic) ....... | 140 | 2.0 | 18.0 | 7.0 | 0 | 120 | 1.0 |
| (*Doritos* Tacos at Midnight) ........ | 150 | 2.0 | 17.0 | 8.0 | 0 | 240 | 2.0 |
| (*Doritos* Toasted) .... | 140 | 2.0 | 18.0 | 7.0 | 0 | 120 | 1.0 |
| (*Garden of Eatin'* White Chips) ..... | 140 | 2.0 | 19.0 | 6.0 | 0 | 70 | 2.0 |

| Food and Measure | cal. | prot. (gms) | carbo. (gms) | fat (gms) | chol. (mgs) | sod. (mgs) | fiber (gms) |
|---|---|---|---|---|---|---|---|
| **Corn crisps/chips, tortilla** *(cont.)* | | | | | | | |
| (*Herr's* Restaurant) ... | 140 | 3.0 | 18.0 | 6.0 | 0 | 90 | 2.0 |
| (*Margaritaville*) ...... | 140 | 2.0 | 16.0 | 7.0 | 0 | 90 | 0 |
| (*Mission* Rounds/ | | | | | | | |
| Strips/Triangles) ... | 140 | 2.0 | 17.0 | 7.0 | 0 | 150 | 1.0 |
| (*Mission* Super Thin) . | 140 | 2.0 | 19.0 | 7.0 | 0 | 40 | 2.0 |
| (*Santitas* Restaurant) . | 130 | 2.0 | 19.0 | 6.0 | 0 | 110 | 1.0 |
| (*Snyder's* Restaurant) . | 130 | 2.0 | 20.0 | 5.0 | 0 | 120 | 4.0 |
| (*Snyder's* White) ...... | 140 | 2.0 | 23.0 | 4.5 | 0 | 110 | 2.0 |
| (*Tostitos* Crispy | | | | | | | |
| Rounds) ......... | 140 | 2.0 | 18.0 | 7.0 | 0 | 120 | 2.0 |
| (*Tostitos* Dipping | | | | | | | |
| Strips) .......... | 150 | 2.0 | 19.0 | 7.0 | 0 | 115 | 2.0 |
| (*Tostitos* Restaurant) . | 140 | 2.0 | 19.0 | 7.0 | 0 | 115 | 2.0 |
| (*Tostitos* Scoops!) ... | 140 | 2.0 | 19.0 | 7.0 | 0 | 120 | 2.0 |
| (*Tostitos* Scoops! | | | | | | | |
| Baked!) ......... | 120 | 2.0 | 22.0 | 3.0 | 0 | 125 | 2.0 |
| (*Wise* Restaurant) .... | 150 | 2.0 | 18.0 | 8.0 | 0 | 80 | 1.0 |
| barbecue, Thai | | | | | | | |
| (*Chipitos*) ........ | 130 | 2.0 | 20.0 | 5.0 | 0 | 190 | 2.0 |
| bite size (*Herr's*) ..... | 140 | 3.0 | 18.0 | 6.0 | 0 | 90 | 2.0 |
| bite size (*Tostitos* | | | | | | | |
| Rounds) ......... | 140 | 2.0 | 18.0 | 7.0 | 0 | 110 | 2.0 |
| black bean (*Bachman*) | 140 | 2.0 | 18.0 | 7.0 | 0 | 135 | 3.0 |
| black bean (*Garden* | | | | | | | |
| *of Eatin'*) ........ | 140 | 2.0 | 18.0 | 7.0 | 0 | 70 | 1.0 |
| black bean (*Kettle*) ... | 140 | 3.0 | 18.0 | 7.0 | 0 | 170 | 2.0 |
| black bean chili | | | | | | | |
| (*Garden of Eatin'*) . | 140 | 3.0 | 17.0 | 7.0 | 0 | 130 | 4.0 |
| Buffalo (*Doritos 2nd* | | | | | | | |
| *Degree Burn*) ..... | 150 | 2.0 | 18.0 | 8.0 | 0 | 380 | 1.0 |
| cheese (*Doritos* Spicy | | | | | | | |
| Nacho) .......... | 140 | 2.0 | 18.0 | 7.0 | 0 | 210 | 1.0 |
| cheese (*Doritos Nacho* | | | | | | | |
| *Cheese*) ......... | 150 | 2.0 | 17.0 | 8.0 | 0 | 180 | 1.0 |
| cheese (*Doritos Nacho* | | | | | | | |
| *Cheese* Baked!) ... | 120 | 2.0 | 21.0 | 3.5 | 0 | 230 | 2.0 |
| cheese (*Herr's* | | | | | | | |
| *Nachitas*) ........ | 140 | 2.0 | 18.0 | 6.0 | 0 | 230 | 2.0 |
| cheese, nacho | | | | | | | |
| (*Bravos*) ......... | 150 | 2.0 | 17.0 | 8.0 | 0 | 180 | 1.0 |
| cheese, nacho | | | | | | | |
| (*Chipitos*) ........ | 140 | 2.0 | 19.0 | 6.0 | 0 | 125 | 2.0 |

| Food and Measure | cal. | prot. (gms) | carbo. (gms) | fat (gms) | chol. (mgs) | sod. (mgs) | fiber (gms) |
|---|---|---|---|---|---|---|---|
| cheese, nacho (*Garden of Eatin'*) | 140 | 2.0 | 18.0 | 6.0 | 0 | 140 | 2.0 |
| cheese, nacho (*Guiltless Gourmet* Mucho) | 120 | 2.0 | 22.0 | 3.0 | 0 | 250 | 2.0 |
| cheeseburger (*Doritos* Late Night) | 150 | 2.0 | 17.0 | 8.0 | 0 | 230 | 1.0 |
| cheesy enchilada sour cream (*Doritos Collisions*) | 150 | 2.0 | 17.0 | 8.0 | 0 | 200 | 1.0 |
| chili, spicy sweet (*Doritos*) | 140 | 2.0 | 18.0 | 7.0 | 0 | 270 | 1.0 |
| chili lime (*Garden of Eatin'*) | 140 | 2.0 | 18.0 | 7.0 | 0 | 125 | 2.0 |
| chili lime (*Kettle*) | 140 | 3.0 | 18.0 | 7.0 | 0 | 140 | 2.0 |
| focaccia (*Garden of Eatin'* Bold) | 140 | 2.0 | 19.0 | 6.0 | 0 | 120 | 1.0 |
| guacamole (*Garden of Eatin'*) | 140 | 2.0 | 19.0 | 6.0 | 0 | 170 | 2.0 |
| habanero (*Doritos 3rd Degree Burn*) | 150 | 2.0 | 18.0 | 8.0 | 0 | 220 | 1.0 |
| jalapeño (*Doritos* Late Night Popper) | 150 | 2.0 | 17.0 | 8.0 | 0 | 230 | 2.0 |
| jalapeño (*Doritos 1st Degree Burn*) | 150 | 2.0 | 18.0 | 8.0 | 0 | 240 | 1.0 |
| lime (*Margaritaville Island*) | 130 | 2.0 | 16.0 | 7.0 | 0 | 300 | 0 |
| lime, hint (*Tostitos*) | 150 | 2.0 | 18.0 | 8.0 | 0 | 160 | 1.0 |
| lime, key, jalapeno (*Garden of Eatin'*) | 140 | 2.0 | 18.0 | 7.0 | 0 | 80 | 3.0 |
| mini (*Garden of Eatin'* Rounds) | 140 | 2.0 | 18.0 | 7.0 | 0 | 60 | 2.0 |
| mini (*Garden of Eatin'* Strips) | 140 | 2.0 | 19.0 | 6.0 | 0 | 60 | 2.0 |
| onion (*Garden of Eatin'* Maui) | 140 | 2.0 | 19.0 | 6.0 | 0 | 80 | 1.0 |
| pepper, 3 (*Garden of Eatin'* Bold) | 140 | 2.0 | 18.0 | 7.0 | 0 | 125 | 2.0 |
| pico de gallo (*Garden of Eatin'*) | 140 | 2.0 | 18.0 | 7.0 | 0 | 150 | 3.0 |
| pizza ranch (*Doritos Collisions*) | 150 | 2.0 | 16.0 | 8.0 | 0 | 230 | 2.0 |
| ranch (*Doritos Cool Ranch*) | 150 | 2.0 | 18.0 | 8.0 | 0 | 180 | 2.0 |

| Food and Measure | cal. | prot. (gms) | carbo. (gms) | fat (gms) | chol. (mgs) | sod. (mgs) | fiber (gms) |
|---|---|---|---|---|---|---|---|
| **Corn crisps/chips, tortilla** *(cont.)* | | | | | | | |
| salsa verde (*Doritos*) | 140 | 2.0 | 19.0 | 7.0 | 0 | 210 | 1.0 |
| sea salt (*Garden of Eatin'* Popped) | 110 | 2.0 | 19.0 | 3.0 | 0 | 280 | 3.0 |
| tamari (*Garden of Eatin'*) | 140 | 2.0 | 18.0 | 7.0 | 0 | 160 | 3.0 |
| tortilla, blue corn: | | | | | | | |
| (*Garden of Eatin'*) | 140 | 2.0 | 18.0 | 7.0 | 0 | 10 | 2.0 |
| (*Garden of Eatin' Baked*) | 120 | 3.0 | 20.0 | 3.0 | 0 | 120 | 3.0 |
| (*Garden of Eatin' Popped*) | 120 | 2.0 | 20.0 | 3.0 | 0 | 280 | 3.0 |
| (*Garden of Eatin' Unsalted*) | 140 | 2.0 | 18.0 | 7.0 | 0 | 10 | 2.0 |
| (*Garden of Eatin' Little Soy Blues*) | 140 | 3.0 | 17.0 | 7.0 | 0 | 70 | 2.0 |
| (*Garden of Eatin' Red Hot Blues*) | 140 | 2.0 | 18.0 | 7.0 | 0 | 150 | 2.0 |
| (*Garden of Eatin' Sesame Blues*) | 150 | 3.0 | 16.0 | 8.0 | 0 | 90 | 2.0 |
| (*Garden of Eatin' Sunny Blues*) | 150 | 2.0 | 17.0 | 8.0 | 0 | 70 | 2.0 |
| (*Guiltless Gourmet*) | 120 | 3.0 | 23.0 | 3.0 | 0 | 250 | 2.0 |
| (*Kettle*) | 140 | 3.0 | 18.0 | 7.0 | 0 | 100 | 2.0 |
| (*Tostitos* Natural) | 140 | 2.0 | 19.0 | 6.0 | 0 | 80 | 1.0 |
| (*Tostitos* Restaurant) | 140 | 2.0 | 19.0 | 7.0 | 0 | 115 | 2.0 |
| black bean, spicy (*Guiltless Gourmet*) | 120 | 2.0 | 19.0 | 3.0 | 0 | 250 | 2.0 |
| multigrain (*Garden of Eatin'*) | 130 | 2.0 | 16.0 | 7.0 | 0 | 110 | 2.0 |
| tortilla, red corn: | | | | | | | |
| (*Garden of Eatin'*) | 140 | 2.0 | 18.0 | 7.0 | 0 | 70 | 1.0 |
| (*Garden of Eatin' Salsa Reds*) | 140 | 2.0 | 18.0 | 7.0 | 0 | 170 | 3.0 |
| tortilla, yellow corn: | | | | | | | |
| (*Garden of Eatin'*) | 140 | 2.0 | 18.0 | 7.0 | 0 | 70 | 2.0 |
| (*Garden of Eatin' Baked*) | 120 | 3.0 | 21.0 | 2.0 | 0 | 120 | 3.0 |
| (*Guiltless Gourmet*) | 120 | 2.0 | 19.0 | 3.0 | 0 | 250 | 2.0 |
| (*Kettle*) | 140 | 3.0 | 18.0 | 7.0 | 0 | 100 | 2.0 |
| (*Santitas*) | 140 | 2.0 | 19.0 | 6.0 | 0 | 110 | 2.0 |
| (*Snyder's*) | 140 | 2.0 | 23.0 | 4.5 | 0 | 135 | 2.0 |
| (*Tostitos* Natural) | 140 | 2.0 | 19.0 | 6.0 | 0 | 100 | 1.0 |

| Food and Measure | cal. | prot. (gms) | carbo. (gms) | fat (gms) | chol. (mgs) | sod. (mgs) | fiber (gms) |
|---|---|---|---|---|---|---|---|
| chili lime (*Guiltless Gourmet*) | 120 | 2.0 | 19.0 | 3.0 | 0 | 250 | 2.0 |
| chipotle (*Guiltless Gourmet*) | 123 | 2.0 | 22.0 | 3.0 | 0 | 250 | 2.0 |
| mini (*Garden of Eatin'* Rounds) | 140 | 2.0 | 18.0 | 7.0 | 0 | 60 | 2.0 |
| spinach artichoke Parmesan (*Guiltless Gourmet*) | 110 | 2.0 | 19.0 | 3.0 | 0 | 200 | 2.0 |
| **Corn dish**, frozen: | | | | | | | |
| bites, w/mozzarella (*Veggie Patch/Bistro au Naturel*), 3 pcs. | 150 | 5.0 | 22.0 | 7.0 | 5 | 380 | 4.0 |
| fritters: | | | | | | | |
| (*Delta Pride*), 3 pcs. | 160 | 2.0 | 19.0 | 9.0 | 0 | 85 | 0 |
| (*Lupita's* Texas), 1.3-oz. pc. | 100 | 2.0 | 14.0 | 4.0 | 10 | 200 | 1.0 |
| **Corn dog**, see "Frankfurter, wrapped" | | | | | | | |
| **Corn flake crumbs** (*Kellogg's*), 6 tbsp. | 120 | 2.0 | 29.0 | 0 | 0 | 240 | <1.0 |
| **Corn flour**: | | | | | | | |
| (*Bob's Red Mill* Masa Harina Golden/ Gluten Free), ¼ cup | 100 | 3.0 | 21.0 | 1.0 | 0 | 0 | 2.0 |
| (*Bob's Red Mill* Whole Grain/Stoneground/ Organic), ¼ cup | 110 | 2.0 | 22.0 | 1.0 | 0 | 2 | 4.0 |
| (*Quaker* Masa Harina de Maiz), ¼ cup | 110 | 0 | 24.0 | 1.5 | 0 | 0 | 3.0 |
| whole-grain, 1 cup | 422 | 8.1 | 89.9 | 4.5 | 0 | 6 | 15.7 |
| masa, 1 cup | 416 | 10.7 | 87.0 | 4.3 | 0 | 6 | 10.9 |
| **Corn fritters**, see "Corn dish" | | | | | | | |
| **Corn grits**: | | | | | | | |
| (*Arrowhead Mills* Organic), ¼ cup | 130 | 3.0 | 30.0 | 0 | 0 | 0 | 1.0 |
| (*Quaker* Old Fashioned), ¼ cup | 150 | 4.0 | 32.0 | .5 | 0 | 0 | 1.0 |
| (*Quaker* Quick), ¼ cup | 130 | 3.0 | 29.0 | .5 | 0 | 0 | 2.0 |
| instant (*Quaker*), 1 oz.: | | | | | | | |
| original | 100 | 2.0 | 22.0 | 0 | 0 | 310 | 1.0 |
| bacon flavor, country | 100 | 3.0 | 21.0 | .5 | 0 | 430 | 1.0 |
| butter flavor | 100 | 2.0 | 21.0 | 1.5 | 0 | 340 | 1.0 |

| Food and Measure | cal. | prot. (gms) | carbo. (gms) | fat (gms) | chol. (mgs) | sod. (mgs) | fiber (gms) |
|---|---|---|---|---|---|---|---|
| **Corn grits, instant** *(cont.)* | | | | | | | |
| cheese, cheddar ..... | 100 | 3.0 | 20.0 | 1.5 | 0 | 470 | 1.0 |
| gravy, red-eye, and | | | | | | | |
| country ham ...... | 100 | 3.0 | 21.0 | .5 | 0 | 490 | 1.0 |
| **Corn relish** (*Mrs. Renfro's*), 1 tbsp. .... | 15 | 0 | 4.0 | 0 | 0 | 45 | 0 |
| **Corn soufflé**, frozen (*Stouffer's*), ½ of 12-oz. pkg. ......... | 150 | 5.0 | 22.0 | 5.0 | 65 | 490 | 2.0 |
| **Corn syrup**, 2 tbsp.: | | | | | | | |
| (*Karo* Lite) ............ | 80 | 0 | 20.0 | 0 | 0 | 80 | 0 |
| brown sugar (*Karo*) ..... | 120 | 0 | 29.0 | 0 | 0 | 30 | 0 |
| dark (*Karo*) ........... | 120 | 0 | 31.0 | 0 | 0 | 45 | 0 |
| light (*Karo*) ........... | 120 | 0 | 30.0 | 0 | 0 | 30 | 0 |
| **Cornbread mix** (see also "Corn cake mix" and "Muffin mix"), ⅙ pkg., except as noted: | | | | | | | |
| (*Arrowhead Mills* Organic), ¼ cup ..... | 120 | 4.0 | 25.0 | 1.0 | 0 | 290 | 2.0 |
| (*Aunt Jemima* Easy Mix), ⅛ pkg. ........ | 140 | 2.0 | 24.0 | 4.5 | 0 | 440 | 1.0 |
| (*Betty Crocker* Cornbread & Muffin) . | 110 | 2.0 | 24.0 | 1.0 | 0 | 210 | <1.0 |
| (*Bob's Red Mill* Gluten Free) ........ | 120 | 2.0 | 28.0 | .5 | 0 | 270 | 2.0 |
| (*Glory*), 1.2-oz. sq.* .... | 160 | 2.0 | 24.0 | 4.5 | 35 | 480 | 2.0 |
| (*Hodgson Mill*), ¼ cup .. | 130 | 4.0 | 27.0 | 1.0 | 0 | 340 | 3.0 |
| (*Kentucky Kernel* Sweet), ¼ cup ...... | 120 | 6.0 | 24.0 | 1.5 | 0 | 310 | 0 |
| (*Martha White Cotton Country*), ⅕ pkg. .... | 130 | 2.0 | 24.0 | 3.5 | 0 | 440 | 1.0 |
| buttermilk (*Martha White*), ⅕ pkg. ...... | 130 | 2.0 | 24.0 | 3.0 | 0 | 430 | 1.0 |
| jalapeño (*Hodgson Mill*), ¼ cup ........ | 100 | 4.0 | 21.0 | .5 | 0 | 300 | 1.0 |
| Mexican (*Martha White*) .............. | 110 | 2.0 | 18.0 | 3.0 | 0 | 400 | 1.0 |
| white (*Martha White Family*), 1/18 pkg. ..... | 110 | 2.0 | 21.0 | 2.0 | 0 | 500 | 1.0 |
| yellow (*Martha White*), ⅕ pkg. ............ | 140 | 3.0 | 26.0 | 3.0 | 0 | 470 | 1.0 |
| sweet ............. | 140 | 2.0 | 24.0 | 3.5 | 0 | 250 | 1.0 |

| Food and Measure | cal. | prot. (gms) | carbo. (gms) | fat (gms) | chol. (mgs) | sod. (mgs) | fiber (gms) |
|---|---|---|---|---|---|---|---|
| sweet honey ........ | 130 | 2.0 | 24.0 | 3.5 | 0 | 250 | 2.0 |
| **Cornichon**, see "Pickle" | | | | | | | |
| **Cornish hen**, roasted: | | | | | | | |
| meat w/skin, 4 oz. ...... | 295 | 25.3 | 0 | 20.7 | 149 | 73 | 0 |
| meat only, 4 oz. ........ | 152 | 26.4 | 0 | 4.4 | 120 | 71 | 0 |
| **Cornish hen, frozen,** | | | | | | | |
| whole, raw, 4 oz.: | | | | | | | |
| (*Empire Kosher* | | | | | | | |
| Rock Broiler) ....... | 240 | 21.0 | 0 | 17.0 | 85 | 220 | 0 |
| w/out giblets (*Tyson*) ... | 200 | 19.0 | 0 | 14.0 | 130 | 65 | 0 |
| seasoned (*Perdue* | | | | | | | |
| Oven Ready) ........ | 160 | 16.0 | 1.0 | 10.0 | 75 | 420 | 0 |
| **Cornmeal** (see also | | | | | | | |
| "Corn flour" and | | | | | | | |
| "Polenta"): | | | | | | | |
| all grinds (*Bob's Red* | | | | | | | |
| *Mill* Stoneground/ | | | | | | | |
| Organic), ¼ cup ..... | 110 | 2.0 | 23.0 | 1.0 | 0 | 10 | 5.0 |
| blue: | | | | | | | |
| (*Arrowhead Mills* | | | | | | | |
| Organic), ⅓ cup ... | 130 | 3.0 | 25.0 | 1.5 | 0 | 0 | 5.0 |
| (*Bob's Red Mill* | | | | | | | |
| Stoneground), ¼ cup | 110 | 3.0 | 21.0 | 1.5 | 0 | 0 | 3.0 |
| buttermilk. self-rising | | | | | | | |
| (*Martha White*), | | | | | | | |
| 3 tbsp. .......... | 110 | 3.0 | 22.0 | 1.0 | 0 | 450 | 1.0 |
| white, 3 tbsp.: | | | | | | | |
| (*Martha White*) ...... | 120 | 3.0 | 24.0 | 1.0 | 0 | 0 | 2.0 |
| self-rising (*Martha* | | | | | | | |
| *White*) .......... | 110 | 2.0 | 22.0 | 1.0 | 0 | 440 | 2.0 |
| white or yellow (*Hodgson* | | | | | | | |
| *Mill*), <¼ cup ....... | 100 | 3.0 | 22.0 | 1.0 | 0 | 0 | 3.0 |
| yellow: | | | | | | | |
| (*Arrowhead Mills* | | | | | | | |
| Organic), ⅓ cup ... | 120 | 3.0 | 27.0 | 1.0 | 0 | 0 | 3.0 |
| (*Hodgson Mill* | | | | | | | |
| Organic), <¼ cup .. | 100 | 3.0 | 23.0 | 1.0 | 0 | 0 | 3.0 |
| (*Martha White*), 3 tbsp. | 120 | 3.0 | 25.0 | 1.0 | 0 | 10 | 2.0 |
| self-rising (*Hodgson* | | | | | | | |
| *Mill*), <¼ cup ..... | 90 | 3.0 | 21.0 | 1.0 | 0 | 260 | 3.0 |
| self-rising (*Martha* | | | | | | | |
| *White*), 3 tbsp. .... | 110 | 2.0 | 23.0 | 1.0 | 0 | 460 | 2.0 |
| whole grain, ½ cup ... | 221 | 5.0 | 46.9 | 2.2 | 0 | 21 | 4.5 |

| Food and Measure | cal. | prot. (gms) | carbo. (gms) | fat (gms) | chol. (mgs) | sod. (mgs) | fiber (gms) |
|---|---|---|---|---|---|---|---|
| **Cornstarch**, 1 tbsp. | | | | | | | |
| (*Argo*) | 30 | 0 | 7.0 | 0 | 0 | 0 | 0 |
| (*Hodgson Mill* Pure) | 35 | 0 | 7.0 | 0 | 0 | 0 | 0 |
| **Cosmopolitan drink mixer** (*Stirrings*), 3 fl. oz. | 60 | 0 | 17.0 | 0 | 0 | 0 | 0 |
| **Cottonseed flour**, partially defatted, 1 cup | 337 | 38.5 | 38.1 | 5.8 | 8 | 33 | 2.8 |
| **Cottonseed kernels**, roasted, 1 tbsp. | 51 | 3.3 | 2.2 | 3.6 | 0 | 3 | .6 |
| **Cottonseed meal**, partially defatted, 1 oz. | 104 | 13.9 | 10.9 | 1.4 | 0 | 10 | <1.0 |
| **Country gravy**, see "Gravy, country" and "Gravy mix" | | | | | | | |
| **Couscous**, dry, ¼ cup, except as noted: | | | | | | | |
| (*Fantastic* Organic) | 150 | 5.0 | 31.0 | 0 | 0 | 0 | 2.0 |
| (*Marrakesh Express*) | 220 | 8.0 | 45.0 | 0 | 0 | 10 | 1.0 |
| (*Near East*), ⅓ cup | 220 | 8.0 | 46.0 | 1.0 | 0 | 5 | 2.0 |
| (*Near East* Pearled), ⅓ cup, 2 oz. | 210 | 6.0 | 45.0 | 0 | 0 | 0 | 2.0 |
| (*RiceSelect* Original/ Tri-Color) | 150 | 5.0 | 31.0 | 0 | 0 | 0 | 2.0 |
| (*Roland*), ⅓ cup | 200 | 6.0 | 42.0 | 1.0 | 0 | 50 | 3.0 |
| (*Roland* Isreali), ⅓ cup | 190 | 6.0 | 40.0 | 1.0 | 0 | 1 | 2.0 |
| (*Vigo*), ⅓ cup | 190 | 7.0 | 41.0 | 0 | 0 | 10 | 1.0 |
| toasted (*Marrakesh Express* Grande), 3 scoops | 270 | 10.0 | 57.0 | 0 | 0 | 10 | 2.0 |
| whole wheat: | | | | | | | |
| (*Fantastic*) | 150 | 6.0 | 30.0 | 1.0 | 0 | 40 | 2.0 |
| (*Near East*), ⅓ cup | 180 | 7.0 | 37.0 | 1.5 | 0 | 0 | 3.0 |
| (*RiceSelect* Organic) | 210 | 8.0 | 45.0 | 1.0 | 0 | 0 | 7.0 |
| w/flax and soy (*Hodgson Mill*), ⅓ cup | 230 | 10.0 | 48.0 | 2.0 | 0 | 0 | 6.0 |
| **Couscous dish, mix**, 2 oz., except as noted: | | | | | | | |
| broccoli and cheese (*Near East*) | 190 | 8.0 | 40.0 | 1.0 | 0 | 610 | 3.0 |
| chicken: | | | | | | | |
| (*Near East* Meal Kit Provencal), ¼ pkg. | 100 | 4.0 | 21.0 | 1.0 | 0 | 500 | 1.0 |
| herbed (*Near East*) | 190 | 8.0 | 40.0 | 1.0 | 0 | 510 | 3.0 |

| Food and Measure | cal. | prot. (gms) | carbo. (gms) | fat (gms) | chol. (mgs) | sod. (mgs) | fiber (gms) |
|---|---|---|---|---|---|---|---|
| w/vegetables (*Marrakesh Express*) | 190 | 8.0 | 39.0 | 0 | 0 | 700 | 2.0 |
| curry: | | | | | | | |
| (*Marrakesh Express*) . | 190 | 8.0 | 39.0 | 0 | 0 | 530 | 2.0 |
| (*Near East* Mediterranean) .... | 190 | 8.0 | 40.0 | 1.0 | 0 | 500 | 3.0 |
| garlic and olive oil: | | | | | | | |
| roasted (*Near East*) ... | 200 | 8.0 | 40.0 | 1.5 | 0 | 510 | 2.0 |
| roasted (*Near East* Pearled), 2.5 oz. .... | 250 | 8.0 | 54.0 | .5 | 0 | 690 | 2.0 |
| roasted (*Near East* Whole Grain) ..... | 190 | 7.0 | 37.0 | 2.5 | 0 | 510 | 3.0 |
| herb, Mediterranean (*Near East* Meal Kit), ¼ pkg. ......... | 100 | 4.0 | 20.0 | .5 | 0 | 720 | 1.0 |
| mango salsa (*Marrakesh Express*), 2 oz. ...... | 190 | 7.0 | 40.0 | 0 | 0 | 390 | 1.0 |
| mushroom, wild: | | | | | | | |
| (*Marrakesh Express*) . | 190 | 8.0 | 39.0 | .5 | 0 | 600 | 1.0 |
| and herb (*Near East*) .. | 190 | 8.0 | 40.0 | 1.0 | 0 | 580 | 3.0 |
| Parmesan: | | | | | | | |
| (*Marrakesh Express*) . | 200 | 8.0 | 39.0 | 1.0 | 0 | 800 | 1.0 |
| (*Near East*) ......... | 200 | 8.0 | 39.0 | 2.0 | 5 | 510 | 2.0 |
| pine nut, toasted (*Near East*) ......... | 200 | 8.0 | 39.0 | 2.5 | 0 | 460 | 2.0 |
| sun-dried tomato (*Marrakesh Express*) . | 190 | 8.0 | 39.0 | 0 | 0 | 600 | 2.0 |
| tomato lentil (*Near East*) . | 190 | 8.0 | 40.0 | 1.0 | 0 | 600 | 3.0 |
| whole wheat, w/flax and soy (*Hodgson Mill*), ⅓ cup: | | | | | | | |
| chicken herb ........ | 250 | 11.0 | 52.0 | 1.0 | 0 | 223 | 6.0 |
| garlic basil ......... | 235 | 10.0 | 50.0 | 2.0 | 0 | 625 | 6.0 |
| mushroom, wild ..... | 246 | 11.0 | 52.0 | 1.0 | 0 | 362 | 6.0 |
| Parmesan .......... | 240 | 10.0 | 50.0 | 2.5 | 10 | 482 | 6.0 |
| **Couscous entree**, frozen, (*Moosewood* Organic Moroccan Stew), 10 oz. | 150 | 5.0 | 29.0 | 3.0 | 0 | 400 | 5.0 |
| **Cowpeas** (see also "Black-eyed peas"), fresh, ½ cup: | | | | | | | |
| raw: | | | | | | | |
| immature seeds ..... | 65 | 2.1 | 13.7 | .3 | 0 | 3 | 3.6 |
| leafy tips, chopped ... | 5 | .7 | .9 | <.1 | 0 | 1 | n.a. |

| Food and Measure | cal. | prot. (gms) | carbo. (gms) | fat (gms) | chol. (mgs) | sod. (mgs) | fiber (gms) |
|---|---|---|---|---|---|---|---|
| **Cowpeas, raw** *(cont.)* | | | | | | | |
| pods, w/seeds ...... | 21 | 1.6 | 4.5 | .1 | 0 | 2 | n.a. |
| boiled, drained: | | | | | | | |
| immature seeds ..... | 80 | 2.6 | 16.8 | .3 | 0 | 3 | 4.1 |
| leafy tips, chopped ... | 6 | 1.2 | .7 | 0 | 0 | 2 | n.a. |
| pods, w/seeds · ...... | 16 | 1.2 | 3.3 | .1 | 0 | 1 | n.a. |
| **Cowpeas, canned or frozen,** see "Black-eyed peas" | | | | | | | |
| **Cowpeas, catjang**, see "Catjang" | | | | | | | |
| **Crab**, meat only: | | | | | | | |
| raw, 4 oz.: | | | | | | | |
| Alaska king ......... | 95 | 20.8 | 0 | .7 | 47 | 948 | 0 |
| blue .............. | 99 | 20.5 | .1 | 1.2 | 89 | 332 | 0 |
| Dungeness ......... | 98 | 19.8 | .8 | 1.1 | 67 | 335 | 0 |
| queen ............ | 102 | 21.0 | 0 | 1.4 | 62 | 611 | 0 |
| boiled/steamed, 4 oz.: | | | | | | | |
| Alaska king ......... | 110 | 21.9 | 0 | 1.7 | 60 | 1216 | 0 |
| blue .............. | 116 | 22.9 | 0 | 2.0 | 113 | 316 | 0 |
| Dungeness ......... | 125 | 25.3 | 1.1 | 1.4 | 86 | 429 | 0 |
| queen ............ | 130 | 26.9 | 0 | 1.7 | 81 | 784 | 0 |
| **Crab, canned**, 2 oz.: | | | | | | | |
| (*Chicken of the Sea* Fancy) | 40 | 7.0 | 2.0 | 0 | 50 | 400 | 0 |
| (*Consul*) ............. | 45 | 10.0 | 0 | 0 | 55 | 370 | 0 |
| all varieties: | | | | | | | |
| (*Bumble Bee*) ....... | 40 | 9.0 | 0 | .5 | 60 | 260 | 0 |
| (*Phillips*) ........... | 40 | 10.0 | 0 | 0 | 45 | 180 | 0 |
| leg or white (*Roland*) ... | 45 | 10.0 | 0 | 0 | 55 | 370 | 0 |
| lump or jumbo lump (*Chicken of the Sea*) .. | 35 | 7.0 | 1.0 | .5 | 50 | 400 | 0 |
| white (*Chicken of the Sea*) .............. | 30 | 7.0 | 1.0 | 0 | 50 | 400 | 0 |
| **Crab, frozen**, raw: | | | | | | | |
| all varieties (*Chicken of the Sea*), 3 oz. .... | 70 | 17.0 | 0 | .5 | 110 | 250 | 0 |
| soft-shell, breaded: | | | | | | | |
| (*Handy*), 2 pcs., 4.6 oz. .......... | 170 | 13.0 | 25.0 | 2.0 | 80 | 780 | 3.0 |
| panko (*Handy*), 3.1-oz. pc. ....... | 290 | 8.0 | 24.0 | 18.0 | 30 | 630 | 1.0 |
| **"Crab," imitation**: | | | | | | | |
| all styles (*Louis Kemp Crab Delights*), 3 oz. ... | 90 | 6.0 | 15.0 | 0 | 5 | 340 | 0 |

| Food and Measure | cal. | prot. (gms) | carbo. (gms) | fat (gms) | chol. (mgs) | sod. (mgs) | fiber (gms) |
|---|---|---|---|---|---|---|---|
| stick (*Louis Kemp Crab Snack Delights*), 1.5-oz. pc. ......... | 35 | 4.0 | 5.0 | 0 | <5 | 230 | 0 |
| **Crab apple**, fresh: (*Frieda's*), sliced, 1 cup ............. | 85 | 0 | 22.0 | 0 | 0 | 1 | 0 |
| sliced, ½ cup .......... | 42 | .2 | 11.0 | .2 | 0 | 1 | .6 |
| **Crab cake**, frozen, 3-oz. cake, except as noted: (*Blue Horizon* Gluten Free) ........ | 143 | 15.6 | 5.4 | 6.6 | 53 | 352 | .6 |
| (*Phillips* Boardwalk) .... | 200 | 10.0 | 12.0 | 12.0 | 50 | 590 | 1.0 |
| (*Phillips* Coastal) ....... | 220 | 11.0 | 7.0 | 17.0 | 90 | 380 | 0 |
| (*SeaPak*), w/1 oz. sauce . | 240 | 11.0 | 19.0 | 13.0 | 55 | 830 | 1.0 |
| bites (*Blue Horizon*), 4 pcs., 2 oz. ........ | 180 | 5.0 | 8.0 | 14.0 | 45 | 300 | 1.0 |
| deviled (*Mrs. Paul's*) .... | 220 | 20.0 | 12.0 | 12.0 | 60 | 320 | 3.0 |
| Maryland style: (*Phillips*) ........... | 190 | 11.0 | 6.0 | 13.0 | 75 | 450 | 0 |
| mini (*Phillips*), 4 pcs., 3 oz. ...... | 140 | 11.0 | 6.0 | 8.0 | 70 | 550 | 0 |
| and shrimp (*Phillips*) ... | 170 | 11.0 | 7.0 | 10.0 | 95 | 470 | 1.0 |
| **Crab cake mix** (*Old Bay Crab Cake Classic*), 1 tbsp. ..... | 25 | 1.0 | 3.0 | .5 | 25 | 240 | 0 |
| **Crab dip**, 2 tbsp.: Maryland (*Phillips*) ..... | 70 | 3.0 | 1.0 | 6.0 | 30 | 95 | 1.0 |
| and spinach (*Phillips*) ... | 60 | 3.0 | 1.0 | 4.5 | 20 | 100 | 0 |
| **Crab dish**, frozen (see also "Crab cake"): (*Phillips* Slammers), 5 pcs., 5 oz. ........ | 390 | 15.0 | 31.0 | 23.0 | 105 | 690 | 2.0 |
| pretzel (*Phillips*), 7-oz. pc. ........... | 580 | 20.0 | 63.0 | 27.0 | 75 | 460 | 2.0 |
| wontons (*Original Rangoon*), 3 pcs., 3 oz. | 220 | 12.0 | 29.0 | 5.0 | 25 | 580 | <1.0 |
| **Cracker** (see also "Snack chips" and specific listings): (*Barbara's Rite Lite Rounds*), .5 oz. ...... | 60 | 1.0 | 11.0 | 2.0 | 0 | 200 | 0 |
| (*Bremner* Cracker), 7 pcs., .5 oz. ........ | 60 | 1.0 | 10.0 | 1.5 | 0 | 120 | 0 |

| Food and Measure | cal. | prot. (gms) | carbo. (gms) | fat (gms) | chol. (mgs) | sod. (mgs) | fiber (gms) |
|---|---|---|---|---|---|---|---|
| **Cracker** *(cont.)* | | | | | | | |
| (*Bremner* Wafer), | | | | | | | |
| 7 pcs. .5 oz. ........ | 70 | 2.0 | 11.0 | 1.5 | 0 | 105 | 0 |
| (*Glutino* Original), | | | | | | | |
| 8 pcs., 1.1 oz. ....... | 140 | <1.0 | 22.0 | 5.0 | 5 | 260 | <1.0 |
| (*Goldfish* Colors), | | | | | | | |
| 55 pcs., 1.1 oz. ...... | 140 | 3.0 | 20.0 | 5.0 | <5 | 240 | 1.0 |
| (*Goldfish* Original), | | | | | | | |
| 55 pcs., 1.1 oz. ...... | 150 | 3.0 | 20.0 | 6.0 | 0 | 230 | <1.0 |
| (*Lavosh-Hawaii* Classic/ | | | | | | | |
| Bite Size/Mini-Bite), 1 oz. | 120 | 3.0 | 19.0 | 3.0 | 21 | 290 | 1.0 |
| (*Ritz* Simply Socials), .5 oz. | 70 | 1.0 | 10.0 | 3.0 | 0 | 140 | 0 |
| (*Sabrosas*), 11 pcs., | | | | | | | |
| 1.1 oz. ............ | 150 | 2.0 | 20.0 | 6.0 | 0 | 190 | 0 |
| (*Sociables*), 7 pcs., .5 oz. | 70 | 1.0 | 9.0 | 3.5 | 0 | 140 | 0 |
| almond rice (*Blue* | | | | | | | |
| *Diamond Nut-Thins*), | | | | | | | |
| 16 pcs., 1.1 oz: | | | | | | | |
| original ............ | 130 | 3.0 | 23.0 | 2.5 | 0 | 115 | 1.0 |
| barbecue, 17 pcs. .... | 130 | 2.0 | 23.0 | 3.0 | 0 | 180 | 1.0 |
| cheddar ........... | 130 | 3.0 | 22.0 | 4.0 | 0 | 250 | <1.0 |
| ranch, country ...... | 130 | 3.0 | 22.0 | 3.5 | 0 | 220 | <1.0 |
| sea salt, hint of ..... | 130 | 3.0 | 24.0 | 2.5 | 0 | 80 | 1.0 |
| *Smokehouse* ........ | 130 | 3.0 | 23.0 | 3.0 | 0 | 160 | <1.0 |
| apple honey (*Skinny* | | | | | | | |
| *Dippers*), 2 pcs., .6 oz. | 50 | 2.0 | 10.0 | 1.0 | 0 | 90 | 1.0 |
| asiago, toasted (*TLC*), | | | | | | | |
| 15 pcs., 1.1 oz. .... | 130 | 3.0 | 21.0 | 4.0 | 0 | 200 | 2.0 |
| bruschetta (*TLC* Mediter- | | | | | | | |
| ranean), 4 pcs., 1 oz. . | 120 | 3.0 | 18.0 | 4.0 | 0 | 140 | 3.0 |
| butter/buttery: | | | | | | | |
| (*Annie's* Bunny Organic), | | | | | | | |
| 10 pcs., .5 oz. .... | 70 | 1.0 | 10.0 | 2.5 | 0 | 160 | 0 |
| (*Back to Nature* Clas- | | | | | | | |
| sic Rounds), .5 oz. . | 70 | 1.0 | 11.0 | 2.0 | 0 | 150 | 0 |
| (*Breton* Original), | | | | | | | |
| 4 pcs., .6 oz. ..... | 90 | 2.0 | 11.0 | 4.0 | 0 | 160 | <1.0 |
| (*Breton* Minis), | | | | | | | |
| 15 pcs., .5 oz. .... | 80 | 2.0 | 9.0 | 3.5 | 0 | 130 | <1.0 |
| (*Breton* Reduced Fat/ | | | | | | | |
| Sodium), 7 pcs., | | | | | | | |
| 1.1 oz. ........... | 120 | 4.0 | 22.0 | 2.0 | 0 | 150 | 2.0 |
| (*Cabaret*), 3 pcs., .5 oz. | 70 | <1.0 | 9.0 | 3.5 | 0 | 65 | 0 |

| Food and Measure | cal. | prot. (gms) | carbo. (gms) | fat (gms) | chol. (mgs) | sod. (mgs) | fiber (gms) |
|---|---|---|---|---|---|---|---|
| (*FlipSides* Original), 5 pcs., .6 oz. | 70 | 1.0 | 10.0 | 3.5 | 0 | 190 | <1.0 |
| (*Keebler Club* Original), 4 pcs., .5 oz. | 70 | <1.0 | 9.0 | 3.0 | 0 | 125 | <1.0 |
| (*Keebler Club* Reduced Fat), 5 pcs., .6 oz. | 70 | 1.0 | 12.0 | 2.0 | 0 | 150 | <1.0 |
| (*Keebler Club* Snack Stick), 12 pcs., 1 oz. | 130 | 1.0 | 19.0 | 6.0 | 0 | 320 | <1.0 |
| (*Pepperidge Farm* Golden Butter), 4 pcs., .5 oz. | 70 | 1.0 | 11.0 | 2.5 | <5 | 100 | 0 |
| (*Ritz* Hint of Salt), 5 pcs., .6 oz. | 80 | 1.0 | 10.0 | 4.0 | 0 | 35 | 0 |
| (*Ritz* Original), 5 pcs., .6 oz. | 80 | 1.0 | 10.0 | 4.5 | 0 | 135 | 0 |
| (*Ritz* Reduced Fat), 5 pcs., .5 oz. | 70 | 1.0 | 11.0 | 2.0 | 0 | 160 | 0 |
| (*Ritz* Toasted Chips), 1 oz. | 130 | 2.0 | 21.0 | 4.5 | 0 | 250 | 1.0 |
| (*Ritz* Mini Smilin' Snak-Saks), .5 oz. | 70 | 1.0 | 11.0 | 1.5 | 0 | 160 | 0 |
| (*Roland* Country Style), 4 pcs., .5 oz. | 70 | 1.0 | 9.0 | 2.0 | 0 | 110 | 0 |
| (*Toasteds* Buttercrisp), 5 pcs., .6 oz. | 80 | <1.0 | 10.0 | 4.0 | 0 | 150 | <1.0 |
| (*Town House* Original), 5 pcs., .6 oz. | 80 | <1.0 | 10.0 | 4.5 | 0 | 130 | <1.0 |
| (*Town House* Reduced Fat), 6 pcs., .6 oz. | 60 | 1.0 | 11.0 | 1.5 | 0 | 160 | <1.0 |
| (*Town House* Toppers), 3 pcs., .5 oz. | 70 | 1.0 | 9.0 | 3.0 | 0 | 135 | 0 |
| honey (*Ritz*), .6 oz. | 80 | 1.0 | 10.0 | 4.0 | 0 | 70 | 0 |
| minis (*Keebler Club*), 17 pcs., .5 oz. | 70 | <1.0 | 10.0 | 3.0 | 0 | 150 | 0 |
| caraway (*Bremner* Wafer), 7 pcs., .5 oz. | 70 | 2.0 | 11.0 | 1.5 | 0 | 105 | 1.0 |
| cheddar, 1.1 oz., except as noted: | | | | | | | |
| (*Annie's* Bunnies Original/Organic), 50 pcs. | 150 | 3.0 | 19.0 | 7.0 | 0 | 250 | 0 |
| (*Annie's* Bunny Classic Organic), 9 pcs., .5 oz. | 70 | 1.0 | 9.0 | 3.5 | 0 | 160 | 0 |

| Food and Measure | cal. | prot. (gms) | carbo. (gms) | fat (gms) | chol. (mgs) | sod. (mgs) | fiber (gms) |
|---|---|---|---|---|---|---|---|
| **Cracker, cheddar** (cont.) | | | | | | | |
| (*Back to Nature* Crispy) .......... | 140 | 3.0 | 20.0 | 5.0 | 0 | 320 | 1.0 |
| (*Better Cheddars*), 22 pcs. .......... | 160 | 3.0 | 18.0 | 8.0 | 5 | 360 | 1.0 |
| (*Cheese Nips*) ....... | 150 | 3.0 | 19.0 | 6.0 | 0 | 340 | 1.0 |
| (*Cheese Nips* Reduced Fat) .............. | 130 | 3.0 | 21.0 | 3.5 | 0 | 350 | 1.0 |
| (*Combos*), 1 oz. ..... | 140 | 2.0 | 18.0 | 6.0 | 0 | 290 | 0 |
| (*FlipSides*), 5 pcs., .6 oz. ........... | 70 | 1.0 | 9.0 | 3.5 | 0 | 220 | <1.0 |
| (*Glutino*), 8 pcs. ..... | 140 | 2.0 | 21.0 | 5.0 | 10 | 180 | <1.0 |
| (*Goldfish*), 55 pcs. ... | 140 | 4.0 | 20.0 | 5.0 | <5 | 250 | <1.0 |
| (*Goldfish* Baby), 89 pcs. ........... | 140 | 4.0 | 20.0 | 5.0 | <5 | 250 | <1.0 |
| (*Goldfish* Whole Grain), 55 pcs. ........... | 140 | 4.0 | 19.0 | 5.0 | <5 | 250 | 2.0 |
| (*Goldfish Flavor Blasted* Xtra Bag), 51 pcs. .......... | 140 | <4.0 | 19.0 | 5.0 | <5 | 250 | <1.0 |
| (*Goldfish Flavor Blasted* Xtra Carton), 51 pcs. .......... | 140 | 4.0 | 19.0 | 5.0 | <5 | 320 | <1.0 |
| (*Goldfish World Treasures*), 55 pcs. | 140 | 4.0 | 20.0 | 5.0 | <5 | 250 | <1.0 |
| (*Pepperidge Farm* Crisps), 20 pcs. ... | 140 | 3.0 | 20.0 | 6.0 | <5 | 260 | 2.0 |
| (*Ritz* Toasted Chips), 1 oz. ............ | 130 | 2.0 | 19.0 | 6.0 | 0 | 290 | 0 |
| (*TLC* Country), 18 pcs. | 130 | 3.0 | 20.0 | 4.5 | 0 | 220 | <1.0 |
| garden (*Goldfish*), 56 pcs. ........... | 140 | 3.0 | 20.0 | 5.0 | 5 | 250 | 1.0 |
| garden (*Goldfish Flavor Blasted*), 55 pcs. .. | 140 | 4.0 | 19.0 | 5.0 | 5 | 290 | 1.0 |
| Jack (*Cheez-It*), 25 pcs. | 140 | 3.0 | 17.0 | 7.0 | 0 | 240 | <1.0 |
| sharp, and Parmesan (*Cheez-It Duoz*), 25 pcs. .......... | 150 | 3.0 | 18.0 | 8.0 | 0 | 260 | <1.0 |
| smoked, and Monterey Jack (*Cheez-It Duoz*), 25 pcs. .......... | 150 | 3.0 | 18.0 | 8.0 | 0 | 270 | <1.0 |
| sour cream/onion (*Annie's* Bunnies), 55 pcs. .......... | 140 | 3.0 | 18.0 | 6.0 | 0 | 250 | <1.0 |

| Food and Measure | cal. | prot. (gms) | carbo. (gms) | fat (gms) | chol. (mgs) | sod. (mgs) | fiber (gms) |
|---|---|---|---|---|---|---|---|
| white (*Annie's Bunnies*), 55 pcs. | 140 | 3.0 | 18.0 | 6.0 | 0 | 160 | <1.0 |
| white (*Cheez-It*), 25 pcs. | 150 | 3.0 | 19.0 | 8.0 | 0 | 210 | <1.0 |
| white (*Cheez-It Reduced Fat*), 25 pcs. | 130 | 3.0 | 22.0 | 4.0 | 0 | 240 | <1.0 |
| white (*Melba Snacks*), 4 pcs., .5 oz. | 50 | 2.0 | 10.0 | 1.0 | 0 | 135 | 1.0 |
| white, flax (*Back to Nature*), 1 oz. | 130 | 3.0 | 20.0 | 4.5 | 0 | 140 | 2.0 |
| whole wheat (*Annie's Bunnies*), 50 pcs. | 130 | 3.0 | 17.0 | 6.0 | 0 | 250 | 3.0 |
| cheese: | | | | | | | |
| (*Carr's* Cheese Melts), 3 pcs., .5 oz. | 60 | 2.0 | 7.0 | 2.5 | <5 | 110 | <1.0 |
| (*Cheez-It* Big), 13 pcs., 1.1 oz. | 150 | 3.0 | 17.0 | 8.0 | 0 | 230 | <1.0 |
| (*Cheez-It* Original), 27 pcs., 1.1 oz. | 150 | 3.0 | 17.0 | 8.0 | 0 | 230 | <1.0 |
| (*Cheez-It* Reduced Fat), 29 pcs., 1.1 oz. | 130 | 4.0 | 20.0 | 4.5 | 0 | 250 | <1.0 |
| (*Cheez-It* Whole Grain), 27 pcs., 1.1 oz. | 150 | 3.0 | 17.0 | 8.0 | 0 | 250 | 1.0 |
| (*Cheez-It Gripz*), .9-oz. pkg. | 120 | 3.0 | 15.0 | 6.0 | 0 | 200 | <1.0 |
| (*Ritz* Real Cheese), 1.38-oz. pkg. | 200 | 3.0 | 22.0 | 11.0 | 5 | 400 | 1.0 |
| 4 (*Pepperidge Farm* Crisps), 20 pcs., 1.1 oz. | 140 | 3.0 | 19.0 | 6.0 | <5 | 270 | 1.0 |
| 4, Italian (*Cheez-It*), 25 pcs., 1.1 oz. | 150 | 3.0 | 19.0 | 7.0 | 0 | 250 | <1.0 |
| hot/spicy (*Cheez-It*), 25 pcs., 1.1 oz. | 150 | 2.0 | 18.0 | 8.0 | 0 | 300 | <1.0 |
| cheese sandwich: | | | | | | | |
| (*Cheez Waffies*), 6 pcs., 1 oz. | 140 | 2.0 | 15.0 | 8.0 | <5 | 380 | 0 |
| (*Ritz Bits*), 1 oz. | 150 | 2.0 | 17.0 | 9.0 | 0 | 250 | 0 |
| (*Ritz Bits*), 1.5 oz. | 220 | 3.0 | 24.0 | 13.0 | 5 | 480 | 1.0 |
| bacon chedder (*Cheetos*), 1 pkg. | 190 | 3.0 | 24.0 | 10.0 | 0 | 330 | 1.0 |
| cheddar (*Austin*), 1.4 oz. | 190 | 3.0 | 23.0 | 10.0 | 0 | 350 | <1.0 |

| Food and Measure | cal. | prot. (gms) | carbo. (gms) | fat (gms) | chol. (mgs) | sod. (mgs) | fiber (gms) |
|---|---|---|---|---|---|---|---|
| **Cracker, cheese sandwich** *(cont.)* | | | | | | | |
| cheddar (*Keebler Club*), 1.3 oz. . . . . . . | 130 | 3.0 | 24.0 | 9.0 | 0 | 290 | <1.0 |
| cheddar (*Ritz Crackerfuls*), 1 oz. . | 130 | 2.0 | 17.0 | 7.0 | 5 | 230 | 3.0 |
| cheddar, toast (*Cheetos*), 1 pkg. . . | 200 | 3.0 | 23.0 | 11.0 | <5 | 410 | 1.0 |
| 4 cheese (*Ritz Crackerfuls*), 1 oz. . | 130 | 2.0 | 17.0 | 7.0 | 5 | 220 | 3.0 |
| 4 cheese (*Triscuit Thin Crisps*), 1.1 oz. | 140 | 3.0 | 22.0 | 4.5 | 0 | 160 | 3.0 |
| grilled (*Austin*), 1.4 oz. | 190 | 3.0 | 24.0 | 9.0 | 0 | 350 | <1.0 |
| jalapeño, toast (*Doritos*), 1 pkg. . . . . . . . . . . . | 200 | 3.0 | 23.0 | 11.0 | 0 | 340 | 1.0 |
| pepper jack (*Austin/ Keebler Club*), 1.4 oz. | 190 | 3.0 | 24.0 | 9.0 | 0 | 390 | <1.0 |
| cheeseburger (*Combos*), 1 oz. . . . . . . . . . . . . . | 140 | 2.0 | 18.0 | 6.0 | 0 | 370 | 0 |
| chicken flavor (*Chicken in a Bisket*), 12 pcs., 1.1 oz. . . . . . . . . . . . | 160 | 2.0 | 19.0 | 8.0 | 0 | 310 | 1.0 |
| chipotle (*Skinny Dippers*), 3 pcs., 1 oz. | 70 | 2.0 | 15.0 | 1.0 | 0 | 135 | 1.0 |
| flatbread: | | | | | | | |
| (*Kontos* Cocktail), 2 pcs., .5 oz. . . . . . | 44 | 2.0 | 8.0 | 1.0 | 0 | 100 | 1.0 |
| (*Wasa* Whole Grain), 1 pc., .4 oz. . . . . . . | 40 | 1.0 | 10.0 | 0 | 0 | 50 | 2.0 |
| (*Wasa* Fiber), 1 pc. . . . | 35 | 1.0 | 8.0 | .5 | 0 | 60 | 2.0 |
| (*Wasa* Hearty), 1 pc. . . | 45 | 1.0 | 11.0 | 0 | 0 | 70 | 2.0 |
| everything (*JJ Flats*), 6 pcs., 1 oz. . . . . . | 110 | 4.0 | 16.0 | 4.0 | 0 | 135 | 2.0 |
| garlic (*JJ Flats*), 6 pcs., 1 oz. . . . . . . | 120 | 4.0 | 15.0 | 4.0 | 0 | 135 | 2.0 |
| garlic parsley or Tuscan herb (*Wheat Thins*), .5 oz. . . . . . | 60 | 1.0 | 12.0 | 1.5 | 0 | 125 | 1.0 |
| herb, Italian (*Town House* Crisps), 6 pcs., .6-oz. pc. . . | 70 | 1.0 | 12.0 | 2.0 | 0 | 130 | <1.0 |
| multigrain, 7 (*JJ Flats*), 1 oz. . . . . . . | 100 | 4.0 | 18.0 | 1.0 | 0 | 200 | 1.0 |
| multigrain (*Wasa*), 1 pc., .5 oz. . . . . . . | 45 | 2.0 | 10.0 | 0 | 0 | 80 | 2.0 |

| Food and Measure | cal. | prot. (gms) | carbo. (gms) | fat (gms) | chol. (mgs) | sod. (mgs) | fiber (gms) |
|---|---|---|---|---|---|---|---|
| multigrain flax (*Back to Nature*), 1 oz. ... | 130 | 3.0 | 20.0 | 4.0 | 0 | 120 | 2.0 |
| sea salt/olive oil (*Town House* Crisps), 6 pcs., .6-oz. pc. ........ | 70 | 1.0 | 12.0 | 2.0 | 0 | 150 | <1.0 |
| seeds and spice (*New York Style Crispini*), 6 pcs., 1 oz. ...... | 110 | 4.0 | 16.0 | 4.0 | 0 | 135 | 2.0 |
| sesame (*JJ Flats*), 6 pcs., 1 oz. ...... | 130 | 5.0 | 14.0 | 5.0 | 0 | 135 | 2.0 |
| sesame (*New York Style Crispini*), 6 pcs., 1 oz. ...... | 130 | 5.0 | 14.0 | 5.0 | 0 | 135 | 2.0 |
| sesame garlic (*New York Style Crispini*), 6 pcs., 1 oz. ...... | 120 | 4.0 | 15.0 | 4.0 | 0 | 135 | 2.0 |
| garlic: | | | | | | | |
| buttery (*Keebler Club*), 4 pc., .5 oz. | 70 | <1.0 | 9.0 | 3.0 | 0 | 150 | <1.0 |
| roasted (*Melba Snacks*), 4 pcs., .5 oz. ..... | 50 | 2.0 | 10.0 | 1.0 | 0 | 130 | 1.0 |
| roasted or Parmesan (*Nonni's* Panetini), 5 pcs., 1 oz. ...... | 120 | 4.0 | 19.0 | 4.0 | 0 | 300 | <1.0 |
| flax w/honey (*Skinny Dippers*), 2 pcs., .6 oz. | 50 | 2.0 | 9.0 | 1.0 | 0 | 100 | 1.0 |
| garlic herb: | | | | | | | |
| (*All-Bran*), 18 pcs., 1.1 oz. .......... | 120 | 3.0 | 19.0 | 6.0 | 0 | 250 | 5.0 |
| (*FlipSides*), 5 pcs., .6 oz. .......... | 70 | 1.0 | 9.0 | 3.5 | 0 | 230 | <1.0 |
| (*Town House Toppers*), 3 pcs., .5 oz. ..... | 70 | <1.0 | 10.0 | 3.0 | 0 | 135 | 0 |
| filled (*Ritz Crackerfuls*), 1 oz. | 140 | 2.0 | 17.0 | 7.0 | 5 | 220 | 3.0 |
| graham, see "Cookie" | | | | | | | |
| grain, whole, and seeds (*Dare Grainsfirst*), 4 pcs., .6 oz. ........ | 80 | 2.0 | 11.0 | 3.0 | 0 | 140 | 2.0 |
| hazelnut/rice (*Blue Diamond Nut-Thins*), 16 pcs., 1.1 oz. ...... | 130 | 2.0 | 23.0 | 3.0 | 0 | 115 | <1.0 |

| Food and Measure | cal. | prot. (gms) | carbo. (gms) | fat (gms) | chol. (mgs) | sod. (mgs) | fiber (gms) |
|---|---|---|---|---|---|---|---|
| **Cracker** *(cont.)* | | | | | | | |
| herb: | | | | | | | |
| (*Special K* Savory), | | | | | | | |
| 24 pcs., 1.1 oz. ... | 120 | 3.0 | 22.0 | 3.0 | 0 | 240 | 3.0 |
| garden (*Health Valley* | | | | | | | |
| Organic), 4 pcs., | | | | | | | |
| .5 oz. ........... | 70 | 1.0 | 10.0 | 3.0 | 0 | 170 | 0 |
| matzo (*Manischewitz*): | | | | | | | |
| plain, 1.1 oz. pc. ..... | 120 | 3.0 | 27.0 | 0 | 0 | 0 | 1.0 |
| egg, 1.1 oz pc. ...... | 130 | 3.0 | 28.0 | .5 | 15 | 10 | 1.0 |
| multigrain: | | | | | | | |
| (*All-Bran*), 18 pcs., | | | | | | | |
| 1.1 oz. .......... | 130 | 2.0 | 19.0 | 6.0 | 0 | 230 | 5.0 |
| (*Breton*), 4 pcs., .6 oz. | 70 | 1.0 | 10.0 | 3.5 | 0 | 160 | <1.0 |
| (*Glutino*), 8 pcs., | | | | | | | |
| 1.1 oz. .......... | 140 | <1.0 | 22.0 | 5.0 | 5 | 150 | <1.0 |
| (*Keebler Club*), 4 pcs., | | | | | | | |
| .5 oz. ........... | 70 | 1.0 | 9.0 | 3.0 | 0 | 120 | <1.0 |
| (*Melba Snacks* Whole | | | | | | | |
| Grain), 4 pcs., .5 oz. | 50 | 2.0 | 10.0 | 1.0 | 0 | 125 | 2.0 |
| (*Special K*), 24 pcs., | | | | | | | |
| 1.1 oz. .......... | 120 | 3.0 | 23.0 | 3.0 | 0 | 250 | 3.0 |
| (*Town House Bistro*), | | | | | | | |
| 2 pcs., .6 oz. ..... | 80 | 1.0 | 11.0 | 3.0 | 0 | 130 | <1.0 |
| (*Town House Toppers*), | | | | | | | |
| 3 pcs., .5 oz. ..... | 70 | 1.0 | 10.0 | 2.5 | 0 | 120 | <1.0 |
| (*Vinta* Original), | | | | | | | |
| 3 pcs., .7 oz. ..... | 100 | 2.0 | 12.0 | 4.5 | 0 | 180 | 1.0 |
| (*Vinta* Original Snack), | | | | | | | |
| 6 pcs., .7 oz. ..... | 100 | 2.0 | 13.0 | 5.0 | 0 | 160 | 1.0 |
| (*Wheat Thins*), 1.1 oz. | 140 | 2.0 | 22.0 | 4.5 | 0 | 230 | 2.0 |
| (*Wheat Thins* | | | | | | | |
| Toasted Chips | | | | | | | |
| Great Plains), 1 oz. . | 120 | 2.0 | 20.0 | 4.0 | 0 | 240 | 1.0 |
| 5 (*Wheat Thins* Fiber | | | | | | | |
| Selects), 1.1 oz. ... | 120 | 2.0 | 22.0 | 4.5 | 0 | 260 | 5.0 |
| 7 (*TLC*), 15 pcs., 1.1 oz. | 120 | 3.0 | 21.0 | 3.5 | 0 | 160 | 2.0 |
| 7, stoneground | | | | | | | |
| (*TLC*), 4 pcs., 1 oz. . | 130 | 3.0 | 17.0 | 5.0 | 0 | 140 | 3.0 |
| garlic, roasted, thyme | | | | | | | |
| (*TLC*), 4 pcs., 1 oz. . | 130 | 3.0 | 18.0 | 4.5 | 0 | 140 | 3.0 |
| herb garlic (*Vinta*), | | | | | | | |
| 10 pcs., .7 oz. .... | 100 | 2.0 | 14.0 | 4.5 | 0 | 100 | 1.0 |

| Food and Measure | cal. | prot. (gms) | carbo. (gms) | fat (gms) | chol. (mgs) | sod. (mgs) | fiber (gms) |
|---|---|---|---|---|---|---|---|
| honey (*Skinny Dippers*), 2 pcs., .6 oz. . . . . . | 50 | 2.0 | 10.0 | 1.0 | 0 | 85 | 1.0 |
| honey sesame (*TLC*), 15 pcs., 1.1 oz. . . . | 120 | 3.0 | 22.0 | 3.0 | 0 | 140 | 2.0 |
| roasted red pepper (*Vinta*), 3 pcs., .7 oz. | 90 | 2.0 | 13.0 | 3.5 | 0 | 115 | 1.0 |
| vegetable, fire-roasted (*TLC*), 15 pcs., 1.1 oz. . . . . . . . . | 120 | 3.0 | 21.0 | 3.5 | 0 | 210 | 2.0 |
| onion (*Toasteds*), 5 pcs., .6 oz. . . . . . . . . . . . | 80 | 1.0 | 11.0 | 3.5 | 0 | 160 | <1.0 |
| Parmesan, 1.1 oz.: | | | | | | | |
| (*Goldfish*), 60 pcs. . . . | 130 | 4.0 | 20.0 | 4.0 | 0 | 280 | <1.0 |
| garlic (*Cheez-It*), 25 pcs. . . . . . . . . . | 150 | 3.0 | 19.0 | 8.0 | 0 | 260 | <1.0 |
| garlic (*Triscuit Thin Crisps*) . . . . . . . . . | 140 | 3.0 | 22.0 | 5.0 | 0 | 180 | 3.0 |
| peanut butter sandwich, 1.4-oz. pkg., except as noted: | | | | | | | |
| (*Ritz*) . . . . . . . . . . . . | 190 | 4.0 | 24.0 | 9.0 | 0 | 370 | 1.0 |
| (*Ritz Bits*), 1 oz. . . . . . | 140 | 3.0 | 16.0 | 8.0 | 0 | 240 | 1.0 |
| (*Ritz Bits*), 1.25 oz. . . . | 170 | 4.0 | 20.0 | 10.0 | 0 | 280 | 1.0 |
| cheese (*Austin*) . . . . . . | 190 | 4.0 | 23.0 | 10.0 | 0 | 330 | 1.0 |
| cheese (*Frito-Lay*) . . . . | 190 | 5.0 | 23.0 | 9.0 | 0 | 370 | 2.0 |
| cheese (*Keebler*) . . . . . | 190 | 4.0 | 23.0 | 10.0 | 0 | 330 | 1.0 |
| and jelly (*Keebler* PB'n J) . . . . . . . . . . | 190 | 3.0 | 26.0 | 8.0 | 0 | 230 | <1.0 |
| toast (*Austin*) . . . . . . . | 190 | 4.0 | 23.0 | 9.0 | 0 | 300 | 1.0 |
| toast (*Frito-Lay*) . . . . . | 200 | 4.0 | 23.0 | 10.0 | 0 | 310 | 2.0 |
| pecan/rice (*Blue Diamond Nut-Thins*), 16 pcs., 1.1 oz. . . . . . . | 130 | 2.0 | 23.0 | 3.5 | 0 | 130 | <1.0 |
| pepper, 3, spicy (*Melba Snacks*), 4 pcs., .5 oz. | 50 | 2.0 | 10.0 | 1.0 | 0 | 135 | 1.0 |
| pepper, cracked (*Health Valley* Organic), 4 pcs., .6 oz. . . . . . . . . | 70 | 1.0 | 10.0 | 3.0 | 0 | 190 | 0 |
| pepper jack (*Cheez-It*), 25 pcs., 1.1 oz. . . . . . . | 150 | 3.0 | 19.0 | 8.0 | 0 | 260 | <1.0 |
| pepperoni pizza (*Combos*), 1 oz. . . . . . | 140 | 2.0 | 18.0 | 7.0 | 0 | 280 | 0 |
| pizza flavor, 1.1 oz.: | | | | | | | |
| (*Goldfish*), 55 pcs. . . . | 140 | 3.0 | 20.0 | 5.0 | 0 | 230 | <1.0 |

| Food and Measure | cal. | prot. (gms) | carbo. (gms) | fat (gms) | chol. (mgs) | sod. (mgs) | fiber (gms) |
|---|---|---|---|---|---|---|---|
| **Cracker, pizza flavor** *(cont.)* | | | | | | | |
| (*Goldfish Flavor Blasted* Xplosive), 51 pcs. . . . . . . . . . | 140 | 3.0 | 20.0 | 5.0 | 0 | 280 | 1.0 |
| cheesy (*Goldfish Flavor Blasted* Xtra), 55 pcs. . . . . . . . . . | 140 | 3.0 | 20.0 | 5.0 | 0 | 310 | 1.0 |
| poppy thyme (*Back to Nature*), 1 oz. . . . . . | 130 | 2.0 | 21.0 | 4.0 | 0 | 270 | 1.0 |
| pretzel cracker: | | | | | | | |
| (*Goldfish*), 43 pcs. . . . | 130 | 3.0 | 24.0 | 2.5 | 0 | 430 | <1.0 |
| (*Pepperidge Farm* Pretzel Thins), 11 pcs. . . . . . . . . . | 110 | 2.0 | 21.0 | 0 | 0 | 340 | 1.0 |
| (*Pretzel Crisps* Classic/ Deli Original), 11 pcs. | 110 | 3.0 | 23.0 | 0 | 0 | 330 | 1.0 |
| (*Pretzel Crisps* Supreme), 11 pcs. . . . . . . . . . | 110 | 3.0 | 23.0 | .5 | 0 | 170 | 1.0 |
| (*Snyder's* Chips), 14 pcs. . . . . . . . . . | 110 | 3.0 | 24.0 | .5 | 0 | 310 | 1.0 |
| Buffalo wing (*Pretzel Crisps* Deli), 10 pcs. | 110 | 3.0 | 22.0 | 1.5 | 0 | 540 | 1.0 |
| cheese, 3 (*Pretzel Crisps* Tuscan), 10 pcs. . . . | 110 | 3.0 | 22.0 | 1.5 | 0 | 520 | 1.0 |
| cinnamon toast (*Pretzel Crisps*), 10 pcs. . . . | 110 | 3.0 | 23.0 | 1.5 | 0 | 320 | 1.0 |
| everything (*Pretzel Crisps*), 11 pcs. . . . | 110 | 3.0 | 23.0 | .5 | 0 | 170 | 1.0 |
| garlic Parmesan (*Pretzel Crisps* Deli), 10 pcs. . . . . . . . . . | 110 | 3.0 | 22.0 | 1.5 | 0 | 410 | 1.0 |
| sesame (*Pretzel Crisps* Deli), 11 pcs. . . . . . | 110 | 3.0 | 22.0 | 1.5 | 0 | 220 | 1.0 |
| veggie, garden (*Snyder's* Chips), 15 pcs. . . . . | 130 | 3.0 | 24.0 | .5 | 0 | 340 | 1.0 |
| ranch (*Goldfish Flavor Blasted* Racing), 54 pcs., 1.1 oz. . . . . . . | 130 | 4.0 | 19.0 | 4.5 | <5 | 250 | <1.0 |
| rice, 16 pcs., 1 oz., except as noted: | | | | | | | |
| (*Ka•Me* Original) . . . . . | 110 | 2.0 | 24.0 | 1.0 | 0 | 75 | 0 |
| all varieties, except maki rolls (*Roland Feng Shui*), 1.1 oz. . | 110 | 2.0 | 25.0 | 0 | 0 | 280 | 2.0 |

| Food and Measure | cal. | prot. (gms) | carbo. (gms) | fat (gms) | chol. (mgs) | sod. (mgs) | fiber (gms) |
|---|---|---|---|---|---|---|---|
| cheese (*Ka•Me*) ..... | 110 | 3.0 | 21.0 | 1.5 | <5 | 70 | <1.0 |
| maki rolls (*Roland Feng Shui*), 1.1 oz. . | 110 | 2.0 | 25.0 | 0 | 0 | 190 | 2.0 |
| mini (*Ka•Me*), .75-oz. pkg. ...... | 90 | 1.0 | 16.0 | 1.0 | 0 | 110 | 0 |
| seasoned (*Ka•Me*) ... | 110 | 2.0 | 22.0 | 1.0 | 0 | 90 | <1.0 |
| sesame (*Ka•Me*) ..... | 110 | 2.0 | 22.0 | 2.0 | 0 | 60 | <1.0 |
| sesame, black, and soy (*Ka•Me*) ....... | 100 | 2.0 | 22.0 | .5 | 0 | 170 | <1.0 |
| wasabi (*Ka•Me*) ..... | 110 | 2.0 | 21.0 | 1.5 | <5 | 85 | <1.0 |
| rice, brown: | | | | | | | |
| (*Eden* Organic), 8 pcs., 1.1 oz. .... | 120 | 3.0 | 22.0 | 2.0 | 0 | 230 | 2.0 |
| (*Ka•Me* Crisps), 13 pcs., .9 oz. .... | 110 | 2.0 | 21.0 | 2.0 | 0 | 230 | 1.0 |
| barbecue, Korean (*Ka•Me* Crisps), 13 pcs., .9 oz. .... | 110 | 2.0 | 21.0 | 2.5 | 0 | 150 | 1.0 |
| nori maki (*Eden* Organic), 15 pcs., 1.1 oz. .......... | 110 | 3.0 | 24.0 | 0 | 0 | 160 | 2.0 |
| sesame (*San-J*), 5 pcs., 1 oz. ........ | 140 | 4.0 | 17.0 | 6.0 | 0 | 160 | 1.0 |
| sesame, black (*San-J*), 5 pcs., 1 oz. ........ | 140 | 4.0 | 17.0 | 6.0 | 0 | 170 | 2.0 |
| Szechuan (*Ka•Me* Crisps), 13 pcs., .9 oz. ............ | 110 | 2.0 | 21.0 | 2.0 | 0 | 210 | 1.0 |
| tamari (*San-J*), 6 pcs., 1.1 oz. ....... | 120 | 3.0 | 26.0 | .5 | 0 | 220 | <1.0 |
| teriyaki (*Ka•Me* Crisps), 13 pcs., .9 oz. ............ | 110 | 2.0 | 20.0 | 2.5 | 0 | 240 | 1.0 |
| rosemary (*Carr's*), 4 pcs., .5 oz. ............. | 70 | 2.0 | 11.0 | 2.5 | 0 | 140 | <1.0 |
| rye: | | | | | | | |
| (*Skinny Dippers*), 2 pcs., .6 oz. ..... | 60 | 2.0 | 10.0 | 1.5 | 0 | 160 | 1.0 |
| (*Triscuit*), 1 oz. ...... | 120 | 3.0 | 19.0 | 4.5 | 0 | 150 | 3.0 |
| saltines, 5 pcs., .5 oz., except as noted: | | | | | | | |
| (*Annie's* Bunny Organic), 13 pcs., .5 oz. .... | 70 | 2.0 | 11.0 | 1.5 | 0 | 160 | 0 |
| (*Krispy*) .......... | 60 | 1.0 | 11.0 | 1.5 | 0 | 150 | <1.0 |

| Food and Measure | cal. | prot. (gms) | carbo. (gms) | fat (gms) | chol. (mgs) | sod. (mgs) | fiber (gms) |
|---|---|---|---|---|---|---|---|
| **Cracker, saltines** *(cont.)* | | | | | | | |
| (*Premium* Fat Free) ... | 60 | 2.0 | 13.0 | 0 | 0 | 200 | 0 |
| (*Premium* Low | | | | | | | |
| Sodium) ......... | 60 | 1.0 | 11.0 | 1.5 | 0 | 30 | 0 |
| (*Premium* Original) ... | 60 | 1.0 | 11.0 | 1.5 | 0 | 190 | 0 |
| (*Premium* Original | | | | | | | |
| 8 oz.) ........... | 70 | 1.0 | 11.0 | 1.5 | 0 | 220 | 0 |
| (*Premium* Unsalted | | | | | | | |
| Top) ............ | 60 | 1.0 | 11.0 | 1.5 | 0 | 130 | 0 |
| (*Wheatines*) ........ | 60 | 1.0 | 11.0 | 1.0 | 0 | 80 | 1.0 |
| (*Zesta* Original) ...... | 60 | 1.0 | 11.0 | 1.5 | 0 | 150 | <1.0 |
| minis (*Premium*), | | | | | | | |
| .5 oz. ........... | 70 | 1.0 | 10.0 | 2.5 | 0 | 140 | 0 |
| multigrain (*Premium*) . | 60 | 1.0 | 10.0 | 1.5 | 0 | 170 | 0 |
| whole wheat (*Krispy*) . | 60 | 1.0 | 11.0 | 1.5 | 0 | 230 | <1.0 |
| whole wheat (*Zesta*) .. | 60 | 1.0 | 11.0 | 1.5 | 0 | 230 | <1.0 |
| sea salt (*Melba Snacks*), | | | | | | | |
| 4 pcs., .5 oz. ........ | 50 | 2.0 | 10.0 | 1.0 | 0 | 140 | 1.0 |
| sesame: | | | | | | | |
| (*Bremner* Wafer), | | | | | | | |
| 7 pcs., .5 oz. ..... | 70 | 2.0 | 11.0 | 2.0 | 0 | 105 | 0 |
| (*Breton*), 3 pcs., .5 oz. | 70 | 2.0 | 8.0 | 3.5 | 0 | 110 | <1.0 |
| (*Health Valley* Organic), | | | | | | | |
| 4 pcs., .6 oz. ..... | 70 | 1.0 | 10.0 | 3.0 | 0 | 200 | <1.0 |
| (*Melba Snacks*), | | | | | | | |
| 4 pcs., .5 oz. ..... | 60 | 2.0 | 9.0 | 1.5 | 0 | 135 | 1.0 |
| (*Toasteds*), 5 pcs., | | | | | | | |
| .6 oz. ........... | 80 | 1.0 | 10.0 | 4.0 | 0 | 140 | <1.0 |
| (*Wasa*), .5-oz. pc. .... | 60 | 2.0 | 9.0 | 1.5 | 0 | 85 | <1.0 |
| tarragon (*Back to | | | | | | | |
| Nature*), 1 oz. ..... | 130 | 2.0 | 21.0 | 4.5 | 0 | 270 | 1.0 |
| toasted (*Pepperidge | | | | | | | |
| Farm* Snack Sticks), | | | | | | | |
| 12 pcs., 1.1 oz. ... | 140 | 4.0 | 20.0 | 5.0 | 0 | 290 | 2.0 |
| soda/water: | | | | | | | |
| (*Carr's Table Water*), | | | | | | | |
| 5 pcs., .6 oz. ..... | 70 | 2.0 | 13.0 | 1.5 | 0 | 100 | <1.0 |
| (*Dare* Water Cracker), | | | | | | | |
| 4 pcs., .5 oz. ..... | 60 | 1.0 | 12.0 | 1.0 | 0 | 50 | <1.0 |
| (*Glutino* Table), | | | | | | | |
| 3 pcs., 1.2 oz. .... | 160 | <1.0 | 24.0 | 7.0 | 0 | 270 | 0 |
| (*Jacob's* Biscuits for | | | | | | | |
| Cheese), 3 pcs., | | | | | | | |
| .6 oz. ........... | 70 | 1.0 | 10.0 | 2.5 | 0 | 110 | 1.0 |

| Food and Measure | cal. | prot. (gms) | carbo. (gms) | fat (gms) | chol. (mgs) | sod. (mgs) | fiber (gms) |
|---|---|---|---|---|---|---|---|
| (*Jacob's* Cream), 2 pcs., .5 oz. | 70 | 2.0 | 11.0 | 2.5 | 0 | 80 | 0 |
| (*Keebler* Export Soda), 3 pcs., .5 oz. | 60 | 1.0 | 10.0 | 1.5 | 0 | 85 | <1.0 |
| (*Roland* Classic), 4 pcs., .5 oz. | 60 | 1.0 | 11.0 | 1.0 | 0 | 65 | 0 |
| cracked pepper (*Carr's Table Water*), 5 pcs., .6 oz. | 70 | 2.0 | 13.0 | 1.5 | 0 | 100 | <1.0 |
| cracked pepper (*Dare* Water Cracker), 4 pcs., .5 oz. | 60 | 1.0 | 12.0 | 1.0 | 0 | 45 | <1.0 |
| cracked pepper (*Roland*), 4 pcs., .5 oz. | 60 | 0 | 10.0 | 2.0 | 0 | 65 | 0 |
| garlic, roasted, herb (*Carr's Table Water*), 5 pcs., .6 oz. | 70 | 2.0 | 13.0 | 1.5 | 0 | 120 | <1.0 |
| garlic herb or toasted sesame (*Roland*), 4 pcs., .5 oz. | 60 | 1.0 | 11.0 | 1.0 | 0 | 65 | 0 |
| poppy/sesame (*Carr's*), 4 pcs., .6 oz. | 80 | 2.0 | 9.0 | 5.0 | <5 | 135 | <1.0 |
| sesame, toasted (*Carr's Table Water*), 5 pcs., .6 oz. | 70 | 2.0 | 12.0 | 1.5 | 0 | 100 | <1.0 |
| sesame, toasted (*Dare* Water Cracker), 4 pcs., .5 oz. | 70 | 2.0 | 11.0 | 1.5 | 0 | 45 | <1.0 |
| vegetable (*Roland*), 4 pcs., .5 oz. | 70 | 1.0 | 11.0 | 2.0 | 0 | 130 | 0 |
| whole wheat (*Roland*), 4 pcs., .5 oz. | 60 | 1.0 | 9.0 | 2.0 | 0 | 105 | 1.0 |
| soup/oyster, .5 oz.: | | | | | | | |
| (*Bremner* Oyster), 50 pcs. | 60 | 1.0 | 10.0 | 1.0 | 0 | 130 | 0 |
| (*Bremner* Soup & Chili), 50 pcs. | 60 | 2.0 | 11.0 | 1.5 | 0 | 110 | 0 |
| (*Krispy*), 16 pcs. | 60 | 1.0 | 11.0 | 1.5 | 0 | 230 | <1.0 |
| (*Premium*) | 60 | 1.0 | 11.0 | 1.5 | 0 | 170 | 0 |
| sour cream/onion: | | | | | | | |
| (*Goldfish Flavor Blasted* Slammin'), 57 pcs., 1.1 oz. | 140 | 4.0 | 18.0 | 5.0 | 0 | 270 | <1.0 |

| Food and Measure | cal. | prot. (gms) | carbo. (gms) | fat (gms) | chol. (mgs) | sod. (mgs) | fiber (gms) |
|---|---|---|---|---|---|---|---|
| **Cracker, sour cream/onion** *(cont.)* | | | | | | | |
| (*Ritz* Toasted Chips), 1 oz. . . . . . . . . . . | 130 | 2.0 | 19.0 | 6.0 | 0 | 270 | 0 |
| spelt (*Skinny Dippers* Organic), 3 pcs., 1 oz. | 90 | 3.0 | 15.0 | 1.5 | 0 | 150 | 3.0 |
| sunflower basil (*Back to Nature*), 1 oz. . . . . . | 130 | 2.0 | 21.0 | 4.5 | 0 | 270 | 1.0 |
| toasts, .6 oz., 2 pcs., except as noted: | | | | | | | |
| (*Alessi*) . . . . . . . . . . . . | 50 | 2.0 | 8.0 | 0 | 0 | 70 | 0 |
| (*Melba Toast* Classic), 3 pcs. . . . . . . . . . . | 60 | 2.0 | 13.0 | 0 | 0 | 110 | 1.0 |
| (*Melba Toast* Whole Grain), 3 pcs. . . . . . | 60 | 2.0 | 12.0 | 0 | 0 | 135 | 2.0 |
| (*New York Style Panetini*) . . . . . . . . . | 70 | 1.0 | 8.0 | 3.5 | 0 | 75 | 1.0 |
| cheese, 3 (*New York Style Panetini*) . . . . | 70 | 2.0 | 8.0 | 4.0 | 0 | 160 | 1.0 |
| garlic (*New York Style Panetini*) . . . . . . . . . | 70 | 1.0 | 8.0 | 3.5 | 0 | 170 | 1.0 |
| garlic Parmesan (*New York Style Panetini*) | 70 | 1.0 | 8.0 | 4.0 | 0 | 135 | 1.0 |
| rosemary olive oil (*Melba Toast*), 3 pcs. | 60 | 2.0 | 12.0 | .5 | 0 | 110 | 1.0 |
| rye (*Melba Toast*), 3 pcs. . . . . . . . . . . | 60 | 2.0 | 12.0 | 0 | 0 | 110 | 1.0 |
| sesame (*Melba Toast*), 3 pcs. . . . . . . . . . . | 60 | 2.0 | 11.0 | 1.5 | 0 | 170 | 1.0 |
| sourdough (*Melba Toast*), 3 pcs. . . . . . | 60 | 2.0 | 12.0 | 0 | 0 | 105 | 1.0 |
| wheat (*Melba Toast*), 3 pcs. . . . . . | 60 | 2.0 | 13.0 | 0 | 0 | 110 | 2.0 |
| whole wheat (*Alessi*) . | 70 | 2.0 | 13.0 | 0 | 0 | 70 | 1.0 |
| tomato, sun-dried, basil (*Nonni's* Panetini), 5 pcs., 1 oz. . . . . . . | 120 | 4.0 | 17.0 | 4.0 | 0 | 170 | <1.0 |
| vegetable: | | | | | | | |
| (*Glutino*), 8 pcs., 1.1 oz. | 130 | <1.0 | 22.0 | 4.5 | 5 | 260 | <1.0 |
| (*Vegetable Thins*), 14 pcs., 1.1 oz. . . . | 150 | 2.0 | 20.0 | 7.0 | 0 | 330 | 1.0 |
| (*Vivant*), 3 pcs., .5 oz. . | 60 | 1.0 | 9.0 | 2.5 | 0 | 120 | 0 |
| bruschetta (*Health Valley* Organic), 4 pcs., .6 oz. . . . . . | 70 | 1.0 | 10.0 | 3.0 | 0 | 210 | 0 |

| Food and Measure | cal. | prot. (gms) | carbo. (gms) | fat (gms) | chol. (mgs) | sod. (mgs) | fiber (gms) |
|---|---|---|---|---|---|---|---|
| garden (*Breton*), 4 pcs., .6 oz. | 90 | 1.0 | 12.0 | 3.5 | 0 | 170 | <1.0 |
| garden (*Breton* Minis), 15 pcs., .5 oz. | 80 | 1.0 | 10.0 | 3.5 | 0 | 100 | <1.0 |
| garden (*Wheat Thins* Fiber Select), 1.1 oz. | 120 | 2.0 | 22.0 | 4.0 | 0 | 260 | 5.0 |
| garden valley (*Wheat Thins* Toasted Chips), 1 oz. | 130 | 2.0 | 19.0 | 5.0 | 0 | 290 | 1.0 |
| roasted (*Ritz*), .6 oz. | 80 | 1.0 | 10.0 | 3.5 | 0 | 150 | 0 |
| wheat: | | | | | | | |
| (*Back to Nature* Crispy), 1.1 oz. | 130 | 2.0 | 22.0 | 4.0 | 0 | 290 | 1.0 |
| (*Barbara's Wheatines*), .5 oz. | 60 | 1.0 | 11.0 | 1.0 | 0 | 80 | 1.0 |
| (*Pepperidge Farm* Crisps), 17 pcs. | 140 | 2.0 | 21.0 | 5.0 | 0 | 240 | 2.0 |
| (*Pepperidge Farm* Harvest), 3 pcs., .5 oz. | 80 | 1.0 | 11.0 | 3.5 | 0 | 125 | <1.0 |
| (*Toasteds*), 5 pcs., .6 oz. | 70 | 1.0 | 11.0 | 3.0 | 0 | 140 | <1.0 |
| (*Town House*), 5 pcs., .6 oz. | 80 | 1.0 | 10.0 | 4.0 | 0 | 170 | <1.0 |
| (*Wheat Thins* Big), 11 pcs., 1.1 oz. | 140 | 2.0 | 22.0 | 5.0 | 0 | 240 | 2.0 |
| (*Wheat Thins* Chips), 1 oz. | 130 | 2.0 | 19.0 | 5.0 | 0 | 240 | 1.0 |
| (*Wheat Thins* Hint of Salt), 1.1 oz. | 150 | 2.0 | 23.0 | 5.0 | 0 | 60 | 2.0 |
| (*Wheat Thins* Original), 16 pcs., 1.1 oz. | 140 | 2.0 | 22.0 | 5.0 | 0 | 230 | 2.0 |
| (*Wheat Thins* Original 4 oz.), 1.1 oz. | 140 | 2.0 | 21.0 | 6.0 | 0 | 260 | 1.0 |
| (*Wheat Thins* Reduced Fat), 1.1 oz. | 130 | 2.0 | 22.0 | 3.5 | 0 | 230 | 2.0 |
| (*Wheatables* Original Golden Wheat), 17 pcs., 1.1 oz. | 140 | 2.0 | 20.0 | 6.0 | 0 | 210 | 1.0 |
| almond (*Wheatables* Nut Crisps), 16 pcs., 1.1 oz. | 140 | 3.0 | 20.0 | 6.0 | 0 | 220 | 1.0 |
| cracked (*Bremner*), 7 pcs., .5 oz. | 70 | 2.0 | 11.0 | 1.5 | 0 | 100 | 0 |

| Food and Measure | cal. | prot. (gms) | carbo. (gms) | fat (gms) | chol. (mgs) | sod. (mgs) | fiber (gms) |
|---|---|---|---|---|---|---|---|
| **Cracker, wheat** *(cont.)* | | | | | | | |
| cream cheese/chive (*Wheat Thins*), 1 oz. | 140 | 2.0 | 20.0 | 5.0 | 0 | 260 | 1.0 |
| honey (*Keebler Club Snack Sticks*), 12 pcs., 1 oz. ..... | 130 | 1.0 | 19.0 | 6.0 | 0 | 260 | <1.0 |
| honey, toasted (*Wheatables*), 17 pcs., 1.1 oz. ... | 140 | 2.0 | 20.0 | 6.0 | 0 | 200 | 1.0 |
| Parmesan basil (*Wheat Thins*), 1.1 oz. .... | 140 | 2.0 | 21.0 | 5.0 | 0 | 290 | 1.0 |
| pecan (*Wheatables Nut Crisps*), 16 pcs., 1.1 oz. .......... | 140 | 2.0 | 20.0 | 7.0 | 0 | 200 | 1.0 |
| ranch (*Wheat Thins*), 1 oz. ............. | 140 | 2.0 | 20.0 | 5.0 | 0 | 230 | 1.0 |
| stoned (*Health Valley Organic*), 4 pcs., .6 oz. | 70 | 1.0 | 10.0 | 3.0 | 0 | 170 | <1.0 |
| stoned (*Red Oval Farms*), 2 pcs., .5 oz. | 60 | 1.0 | 10.0 | 1.5 | 0 | 210 | 1.0 |
| stoned (*Red Oval Farms* Lower Sodium), 2 pcs., .5 oz. ..... | 60 | 1.0 | 11.0 | 1.5 | 0 | 70 | 1.0 |
| stoned (*Wheat Thins*), .5 oz. ............ | 60 | 2.0 | 11.0 | 1.5 | 0 | 210 | 1.0 |
| stoned, mini (*Red Oval Farms*), 1.1 oz. | 130 | 3.0 | 22.0 | 3.0 | 0 | 430 | 1.0 |
| stoneground (*Back to Nature* Organic), .6 oz. ........... | 70 | 1.0 | 11.0 | 2.5 | 0 | 135 | 1.0 |
| stoneground (*Wheatsworth*), 5 pcs., .6 oz. | 80 | 2.0 | 10.0 | 3.5 | 0 | 180 | 1.0 |
| toasted (*Pepperidge Farm* Crisps), 17 pcs., 1.1 oz. ... | 140 | 2.0 | 21.0 | 5.0 | 0 | 240 | 2.0 |
| tomato, sun-dried, basil (*Wheat Thins* 9.5 oz.), 1.1 oz. ... | 140 | 2.0 | 21.0 | 5.0 | 0 | 200 | 1.0 |
| tomato, sun-dried, basil (*Wheat Thins* 15 oz.), 1.1 oz. ..... | 140 | 2.0 | 20.0 | 6.0 | 0 | 240 | 1.0 |
| wheat, whole: | | | | | | | |
| (*Back to Nature* Harvest), 1 oz. ..... | 120 | 3.0 | 19.0 | 4.5 | 0 | 180 | 3.0 |

| Food and Measure | cal. | prot. (gms) | carbo. (gms) | fat (gms) | chol. (mgs) | sod. (mgs) | fiber (gms) |
|---|---|---|---|---|---|---|---|
| (*Carr's*), 2 pcs., .6 oz. | 80 | 1.0 | 10.0 | 4.0 | 0 | 100 | 1.0 |
| (*Health Valley* Organic), 4 pcs., .5 oz. | 70 | 2.0 | 9.0 | 3.0 | 0 | 170 | 1.0 |
| (*Heart to Heart*), 7 pcs., 1.1 oz. | 120 | 3.0 | 22.0 | 3.5 | 0 | 85 | 4.0 |
| (*Ritz*), 5 pcs., .5 oz. | 70 | 1.0 | 11.0 | 2.5 | 0 | 120 | 1.0 |
| (*Ritz* Simply Social), .5 oz. | 70 | 1.0 | 10.0 | 3.0 | 0 | 150 | 1.0 |
| (*Skinny Dippers* Organic), 3 pcs., 1 oz. | 70 | 2.0 | 15.0 | 1.0 | 0 | 150 | 2.0 |
| (*Triscuit* Hint of Salt), 1 oz. | 130 | 3.0 | 19.0 | 5.0 | 0 | 50 | 3.0 |
| (*Triscuit* Original), 1 oz. | 120 | 3.0 | 19.0 | 4.5 | 0 | 180 | 3.0 |
| (*Triscuit* Reduced Fat), 1 oz. | 120 | 3.0 | 21.0 | 3.0 | 0 | 160 | 3.0 |
| (*Triscuit* Thin Crisps), 15 pcs., 1.1 oz. | 130 | 3.0 | 21.0 | 5.0 | 0 | 180 | 3.0 |
| (*Wheat Thins* 100%), 1.1 oz. | 140 | 2.0 | 21.0 | 6.0 | 0 | 280 | 2.0 |
| cracked pepper/olive oil (*Triscuit*), 1 oz. | 120 | 3.0 | 20.0 | 4.0 | 0 | 140 | 3.0 |
| garlic, roasted (*Heart to Heart*), 7 pcs., 1.1 oz. | 120 | 3.0 | 22.0 | 3.5 | 0 | 75 | 4.0 |
| garlic, roasted (*Triscuit*), 1 oz. | 120 | 3.0 | 20.0 | 4.5 | 0 | 140 | 3.0 |
| herb, garden (*Triscuit*), 1 oz. | 120 | 3.0 | 20.0 | 4.0 | 0 | 125 | 3.0 |
| rosemary/olive oil (*Triscuit*), 1 oz. | 120 | 3.0 | 20.0 | 4.0 | 0 | 135 | 3.0 |
| toast (*Trois Petits Cochons* Petits), 8 pcs., .6 oz. | 60 | 3.0 | 12.0 | .5 | 0 | 120 | 3.0 |
| tomato, fire-roasted (*Triscuit*), 1 oz. | 120 | 3.0 | 20.0 | 4.0 | 0 | 150 | 3.0 |
| zwieback (*Nabisco*), .3-oz. pc. | 35 | 1.0 | 6.0 | 1.0 | 0 | 10 | 0 |
| **Cracker meal**, ¼ cup: | | | | | | | |
| (*Nabisco*) | 110 | 3.0 | 22.0 | 0 | 0 | 15 | 1.0 |
| matzo (*Manischewitz*) | 110 | 3.0 | 23.0 | 0 | 0 | 0 | 1.0 |
| **Cranberry**, fresh: | | | | | | | |
| (*Dole*), 1 cup, 3.3 oz. | 45 | 0 | 12.0 | 0 | 0 | 0 | 4.0 |
| (*Ocean Spray*), 2 oz. | 30 | 0 | 6.0 | 0 | 0 | 0 | 2.0 |

| Food and Measure | cal. | prot. (gms) | carbo. (gms) | fat (gms) | chol. (mgs) | sod. (mgs) | fiber (gms) |
|---|---|---|---|---|---|---|---|
| **Cranberry** *(cont.)* | | | | | | | |
| whole, ½ cup ......... | 23 | .2 | 6.0 | .1 | 0 | 1 | 2.0 |
| chopped, ½ cup ....... | 27 | .2 | 7.0 | .1 | 0 | 1 | 2.3 |
| **Cranberry, canned**, see "Cranberry sauce" | | | | | | | |
| **Cranberry, dried,** ⅓ cup, 1.4 oz.: | | | | | | | |
| (*Craisins*) ........... | 130 | 0 | 33.0 | 0 | 0 | 0 | 2.0 |
| (*Earthbound Farm* Organic) ........... | 130 | 0 | 34.0 | 0 | 0 | 2 | 2.0 |
| (*Eden* Organic) ........ | 140 | 0 | 33.0 | .5 | 0 | 20 | 2.0 |
| (*Mariani*) ............. | 130 | 0 | 35.0 | 0 | 0 | 0 | 2.0 |
| (*Sun•Maid* Cape Cod) ... | 130 | 0 | 33.0 | 0 | 0 | 0 | 2.0 |
| (*Sunsweet*) ........... | 140 | 0 | 35.0 | 0 | 0 | 0 | 2.0 |
| cherry or orange flavor (*Craisins*) .......... | 130 | 0 | 33.0 | 0 | 0 | 0 | 2.0 |
| concord grape flavor (*Mariani*) ............. | 140 | 1.0 | 35.0 | 0 | 0 | 35 | 1.0 |
| juice infused, all fruits (*Craisins*) .......... | 140 | 0 | 34.0 | 0 | 0 | 0 | 0 |
| **Cranberry bean:** | | | | | | | |
| dry (*Bob's Red Mill*), ¼ cup ............. | 140 | 10.0 | 25.0 | .5 | 0 | 0 | 10.0 |
| boiled, ½ cup ......... | 120 | 8.2 | 21.5 | .4 | 0 | 1 | 3.0 |
| canned, ½ cup ....... | 108 | 7.2 | 19.7 | .4 | 0 | 431 | n.a. |
| **Cranberry drink,** 8 fl. oz.: | | | | | | | |
| (*Apple & Eve* Light) ..... | 40 | 0 | 9.0 | 0 | 0 | 10 | 0 |
| (*Santa Cruz Organic* Nectar) ............ | 110 | <1.0 | 27.0 | 0 | 0 | 25 | 0 |
| cocktail: | | | | | | | |
| (*Apple & Eve*) ....... | 130 | 0 | 32.0 | 0 | 0 | 25 | 0 |
| (*Langers*) ........... | 140 | 0 | 35.0 | 0 | 0 | 10 | 0 |
| (*Nantucket Nectars*) .. | 130 | 0 | 33.0 | 0 | 0 | 25 | 0 |
| (*Ocean Spray*) ....... | 120 | 0 | 30.0 | 0 | 0 | 35 | 0 |
| (*Ocean Spray* Calcium) | 130 | 0 | 31.0 | 0 | 0 | 35 | 0 |
| (*Tropicana*) .......... | 140 | 0 | 35.0 | 0 | 0 | 25 | 0 |
| (*Veryfine*) .......... | 160 | 0 | 41.0 | 0 | 0 | 15 | 0 |
| (*Welch's*) .......... | 130 | 0 | 35.0 | 0 | 0 | 5 | 0 |
| frozen* (*Cascadian Farm* Organic) .... | 120 | 0 | 32.0 | 0 | 0 | 15 | 0 |
| white (*Langers*) ........ | 120 | 0 | 28.0 | 0 | 0 | 10 | 0 |

| Food and Measure | cal. | prot. (gms) | carbo. (gms) | fat (gms) | chol. (mgs) | sod. (mgs) | fiber (gms) |
|---|---|---|---|---|---|---|---|
| **Cranberry drink blend**, 8 fl. oz.: | | | | | | | |
| all varieties (*Ocean Spray* White) | 110 | 0 | 27.0 | 0 | 0 | 50 | 0 |
| apple (*Cran•Apple*) | 130 | 0 | 32.0 | 0 | 0 | 80 | 0 |
| apple raspberry (*Minute Maid*) | 120 | 0 | 33.0 | 0 | 0 | 25 | 0 |
| berry (*Langers*) | 135 | 0 | 34.0 | 0 | 0 | 10 | 0 |
| blackberry (*V8 V-Fusion* Light) | 50 | 0 | 12.0 | 0 | 0 | 70 | 0 |
| cherry (*Cran•Cherry*) | 120 | 0 | 30.0 | 0 | 0 | 35 | 0 |
| grape: | | | | | | | |
| (*Apple & Eve* Light) | 40 | 0 | 9.0 | 0 | 0 | 5 | 0 |
| (*Cran•Grape*) | 120 | 0 | 31.0 | 0 | 0 | 80 | 0 |
| (*Langers*) | 165 | 0 | 41.0 | 0 | 0 | 10 | 0 |
| (*Minute Maid*) | 150 | 0 | 39.0 | 0 | 0 | 20 | 0 |
| frozen* (*Langers*) | 150 | 0 | 37.0 | 0 | 0 | 10 | 0 |
| grapefruit (*SoBe Elixer*) | 100 | 0 | 26.0 | 0 | 0 | 10 | 0 |
| w/lime (*Langers*) | 140 | 0 | 35.0 | 0 | 0 | 10 | 0 |
| pomegranate: | | | | | | | |
| (*Cran•Pomegranate*) | 120 | 0 | 30.0 | 0 | 0 | 35 | 0 |
| raspberry (*Northland*) | 100 | 0 | 26.0 | 0 | 0 | 10 | 0 |
| raspberry: | | | | | | | |
| (*Apple & Eve* Light) | 40 | 0 | 9.0 | 0 | 0 | 10 | 0 |
| (*Cran-Raspberry*) | 110 | 0 | 28.0 | 0 | 0 | 70 | 0 |
| (*Langers*) | 150 | 0 | 36.0 | 0 | 0 | 10 | 0 |
| (*Snapple*) | 100 | 0 | 26.0 | 0 | 0 | 5 | 0 |
| frozen* (*Langers*) | 140 | 0 | 35.0 | 0 | 0 | 10 | 0 |
| white (*Langers*) | 120 | 0 | 28.0 | 0 | 0 | 10 | 0 |
| ruby red (*Florida's Natural* Cocktail) | 130 | 0 | 32.0 | 0 | 0 | 15 | 0 |
| strawberry (*Cran• Strawberry*) | 110 | 0 | 27.0 | 0 | 0 | 80 | 0 |
| tangerine (*Cran• Tangerine*) | 120 | 0 | 30.0 | 0 | 0 | 35 | 0 |
| **Cranberry juice**, 8 fl. oz.: | | | | | | | |
| (*After the Fall* Cape Cod) | 120 | 0 | 30.0 | 0 | 0 | 15 | 0 |
| (*Apple & Eve* & More) | 130 | 0 | 32.0 | 0 | 0 | 25 | 0 |
| (*Apple & Eve* Naturally) | 130 | 1.0 | 32.0 | 0 | 0 | 20 | 0 |
| (*Northland*) | 130 | 0 | 33.0 | 0 | 0 | 35 | 0 |

| Food and Measure | cal. | prot. (gms) | carbo. (gms) | fat (gms) | chol. (mgs) | sod. (mgs) | fiber (gms) |
|---|---|---|---|---|---|---|---|
| **Cranberry juice** *(cont.)* | | | | | | | |
| (*Northland* Organic) .... | 120 | 0 | 31.0 | 0 | 0 | 15 | 0 |
| (*R.W. Knudsen* Nectar) .. | 130 | <1.0 | 31.0 | 0 | 0 | 40 | 0 |
| (*R.W. Knudsen* Organic) . | 140 | 1.0 | 35.0 | 0 | 0 | 15 | 0 |
| (*R.W. Knudsen Just* | | | | | | | |
| *Cranberry*) ......... | 70 | 0 | 18.0 | 0 | 0 | 30 | 0 |
| (*R.W. Knudsen Just* | | | | | | | |
| *Cranberry* Organic) ... | 70 | 0 | 18.0 | 0 | 0 | 10 | 0 |
| cocktail, see "Cranberry drink" | | | | | | | |
| frozen*: | | | | | | | |
| (*Cascadian Farm* | | | | | | | |
| Organic) ......... | 120 | 0 | 32.0 | 0 | 0 | 15 | 0 |
| (*Langers*) .......... | 120 | 0 | 35.0 | 0 | 0 | 10 | 0 |
| sparkling (*R.W.* | | | | | | | |
| *Knudsen*) .......... | 130 | <1.0 | 31.0 | 0 | 0 | 45 | 0 |
| **Cranberry juice blend**, 8 fl. oz.: | | | | | | | |
| (*Ocean Spray* Premium) . | 140 | 0 | 36.0 | 0 | 0 | 35 | 0 |
| (*Simply Nutritious* | | | | | | | |
| *Vita Cranberry*) ...... | 130 | 0 | 31.0 | 0 | 0 | 10 | 0 |
| apple (*Apple & Eve*) .... | 130 | 1.0 | 33.0 | 0 | 0 | 20 | 0 |
| berry, wild, mixed | | | | | | | |
| (*Apple & Eve*) ....... | 130 | 0 | 33.0 | 0 | 0 | 25 | 0 |
| blackberry: | | | | | | | |
| (*Northland*) ......... | 140 | 0 | 35.0 | 0 | 0 | 35 | 0 |
| (*V8 V-Fusion*) ....... | 100 | 0 | 26.0 | 0 | 0 | 90 | 0 |
| blueberry: | | | | | | | |
| (*Northland*) ......... | 140 | 0 | 34.0 | 0 | 0 | 35 | 0 |
| (*Ocean Spray*) ....... | 140 | 0 | 36.0 | 0 | 0 | 35 | 0 |
| (*R.W. Knudsen* | | | | | | | |
| Organic) | 130 | 0 | 33.0 | 0 | 0 | 15 | 0 |
| cherry (*Northland*) ..... | 140 | 0 | 35.0 | 0 | 0 | 35 | 0 |
| goji (*Santa Cruz* | | | | | | | |
| *Organic*) ........... | 120 | 0 | 30.0 | 0 | 0 | 15 | 0 |
| grape: | | | | | | | |
| (*Apple & Eve*) ....... | 140 | 1.0 | 34.0 | 0 | 0 | 25 | 0 |
| (*Northland*) ......... | 140 | 0 | 36.0 | 0 | 0 | 35 | 0 |
| (*Ocean Spray*) ....... | 150 | 0 | 37.0 | 0 | 0 | 35 | 0 |
| peach mango (*Apple* | | | | | | | |
| *& Eve*) ............. | 120 | 0 | 31.0 | 0 | 0 | 20 | 0 |
| pomegranate: | | | | | | | |
| (*Northland*) ......... | 140 | 0 | 34.0 | 0 | 0 | 25 | 0 |
| (*Ocean Spray*) ....... | 140 | 0 | 34.0 | 0 | 0 | 35 | 0 |

| Food and Measure | cal. | prot. (gms) | carbo. (gms) | fat (gms) | chol. (mgs) | sod. (mgs) | fiber (gms) |
|---|---|---|---|---|---|---|---|
| *(R.W. Knudsen* Organic) ......... | 130 | 0 | 32.0 | 0 | 0 | 15 | 0 |
| raspberry: | | | | | | | |
| (*After the Fall*) ....... | 130 | 1.0 | 32.0 | 0 | 0 | 10 | 0 |
| (*Apple & Eve*) ....... | 120 | 1.0 | 30.0 | 0 | 0 | 20 | 0 |
| (*Northland*) ......... | 140 | 0 | 34.0 | 0 | 0 | 35 | 0 |
| (*Ocean Spray*) ....... | 140 | 0 | 34.0 | 0 | 0 | 35 | 0 |
| (*R.W. Knudsen*) ..... | 130 | 0 | 32.0 | 0 | 0 | 20 | 0 |
| strawberry banana (*Ocean Spray* 100% Fruit & Veggie) ...... | 130 | 0 | 31.0 | 0 | 0 | 60 | 0 |
| **Cranberry juice concentrate** (*R.W. Knudsen*), 8 fl. oz.* .. | 45 | 0 | 18.0 | 0 | 0 | 25 | 0 |
| **Cranberry sauce**, can/jar, ¼ cup: | | | | | | | |
| (*R.W. Knudsen*) ........ | 110 | 0 | 27.0 | 0 | 0 | 0 | 0 |
| all styles: | | | | | | | |
| (*Ocean Spray*) ....... | 110 | 0 | 25.0 | 0 | 0 | 10 | 1.0 |
| (*S&W*) ............. | 100 | 0 | 26.0 | 0 | 0 | 35 | 1.0 |
| orange or raspberry blend (*Cran•Fruit*) .... | 120 | 0 | 29.0 | 0 | 0 | 35 | 1.0 |
| **Crayfish**, mixed species: | | | | | | | |
| farmed, meat only: | | | | | | | |
| raw, 4 oz. .......... | 82 | 16.8 | 0 | 1.1 | 122 | 70 | 0 |
| raw, 8 pcs., .95 oz. ... | 19 | 4.0 | 0 | .3 | 29 | 17 | 0 |
| boiled or steamed, 4 oz. ............. | 99 | 19.9 | 0 | 1.5 | 155 | 110 | 0 |
| wild, meat only: | | | | | | | |
| raw, 4 oz. .......... | 87 | 18.1 | 0 | 1.1 | 129 | 66 | 0 |
| raw, 8 pcs., .95 oz. ... | 21 | 4.3 | 0 | .3 | 31 | 16 | 0 |
| boiled or steamed, 4 oz. ............. | 93 | 19.0 | 0 | 1.4 | 151 | 107 | 0 |
| **Cream**: | | | | | | | |
| half-and-half: | | | | | | | |
| 1 cup ............. | 315 | 7.2 | 10.4 | 27.8 | 89 | 98 | 0 |
| 1 tbsp. ............. | 20 | .4 | .6 | 1.7 | 6 | 6 | 0 |
| light, coffee or table: | | | | | | | |
| 1 cup ............. | 469 | 6.5 | 8.8 | 46.3 | 159 | 95 | 0 |
| 1 tbsp. ............. | 29 | .4 | .6 | 2.9 | 10 | 6 | 0 |
| medium (25% fat): | | | | | | | |
| 1 cup ............. | 583 | 5.9 | 8.3 | 59.8 | 209 | 88 | 0 |
| 1 tbsp. ............. | 37 | .4 | .5 | 3.8 | 13 | 6 | 0 |
| sour, see "Cream, sour" | | | | | | | |

| Food and Measure | cal. | prot. (gms) | carbo. (gms) | fat (gms) | chol. (mgs) | sod. (mgs) | fiber (gms) |
|---|---|---|---|---|---|---|---|
| **Cream** (cont.) | | | | | | | |
| whipped topping, see "Cream topping" | | | | | | | |
| whipping[1], light: | | | | | | | |
|   1 cup ............. | 699 | 5.2 | 7.1 | 73.9 | 265 | 82 | 0 |
|   1 tbsp. ............. | 44 | .3 | .4 | 4.6 | 17 | 5 | 0 |
| whipping[1], heavy: | | | | | | | |
|   1 cup ............. | 821 | 4.9 | 6.6 | 88.1 | 326 | 89 | 0 |
|   1 tbsp. ............. | 52 | .3 | .4 | 5.6 | 21 | 6 | 0 |
| **Cream, clotted** (*The Devon Cream Company*), 1 oz. ..... | 140 | 0 | <1.0 | 15.0 | 45 | 5 | 0 |
| **Cream, sour**, 2 tbsp., except as noted: | | | | | | | |
| (*Breakstone's*) ......... | 60 | 1.0 | 1.0 | 5.0 | 20 | 10 | 0 |
| (*Cabot*) ............. | 50 | 1.0 | 1.0 | 5.0 | 15 | 35 | 0 |
| (*Friendship*) ......... | 60 | 1.0 | 1.0 | 5.0 | 20 | 15 | 0 |
| (*Knudsen* Hampshire) ... | 60 | 1.0 | 1.0 | 6.0 | 20 | 10 | 0 |
| 1 cup ............... | 493 | 7.3 | 9.8 | 48.2 | 102 | 123 | 0 |
| light/low fat: | | | | | | | |
|   (*Breakstone's*) ...... | 40 | 1.0 | 2.0 | 3.0 | 15 | 20 | 0 |
|   (*Cabot*) ............. | 35 | 1.0 | 2.0 | 2.5 | 10 | 25 | 0 |
|   (*Friendship*) ........ | 40 | 1.0 | 3.0 | 2.5 | 10 | 25 | 0 |
|   (*Knudsen*) .......... | 30 | 2.0 | 2.0 | 2.0 | 10 | 20 | 0 |
| nonfat: | | | | | | | |
|   (*Breakstone's*) ...... | 30 | 1.0 | 5.0 | 0 | 5 | 25 | 0 |
|   (*Cabot*) ............. | 20 | 1.0 | 3.0 | 0 | 0 | 40 | 0 |
|   (*Knudsen*) .......... | 30 | 2.0 | 5.0 | 0 | 5 | 25 | 0 |
| **"Cream," sour, nondairy** (*Tofutti Sour Supreme*/Non-Hydrogenated), 2 tbsp. | 85 | 1.0 | 9.0 | 5.0 | 0 | 160 | 0 |
| **Cream gravy**, see "Gravy, country" | | | | | | | |
| **Cream sauce**, in jars (*Roland*), 1 tbsp: | | | | | | | |
| porcini ............... | 55 | 1.0 | 0 | 6.0 | 0 | 185 | 0 |
| truffle, black .......... | 20 | 0 | 1.0 | 2.0 | 0 | 100 | 0 |
| truffle, white ......... | 60 | 1.0 | 1.0 | 6.0 | 25 | 10 | 0 |
| walnut porcini ......... | 70 | 0 | 0 | 8.0 | 0 | 120 | 0 |
| **Cream of tartar**, 1 tsp. .. | 7 | 0 | 1.9 | 0 | 0 | 2 | 0 |

---

[1] Unwhipped; volume approximately doubled when whipped.

| Food and Measure | cal. | prot. (gms) | carbo. (gms) | fat (gms) | chol. (mgs) | sod. (mgs) | fiber (gms) |
|---|---|---|---|---|---|---|---|
| **Cream topping**, whipped, 2 tbsp.: | | | | | | | |
| (*Cabot*) . . . . . . . . . . . . . | 15 | 0 | 1.0 | 1.5 | 5 | 5 | 0 |
| (*Cool Whip*) . . . . . . . . . . | 25 | 0 | 2.0 | 1.5 | 0 | 0 | 0 |
| (*Cool Whip* Extra Creamy Can) . . . . . . . | 20 | 0 | 2.0 | 2.0 | 0 | 0 | 0 |
| (*Cool Whip* Extra Creamy Tub) . . . . . . . | 25 | 0 | 2.0 | 2.0 | 0 | 5 | 0 |
| (*Cool Whip* Fat Free) . . . . | 15 | 0 | 3.0 | 0 | 0 | 5 | 0 |
| (*Cool Whip* Lite Can) . . . . | 15 | 0 | 2.0 | 1.0 | 0 | 0 | 0 |
| (*Cool Whip* Lite/ Sugar Free Tub) . . . . . | 20 | 0 | 3.0 | 1.0 | 0 | 0 | 0 |
| (*Reddi Wip* Extra Creamy) | 20 | 0 | <1.0 | 1.5 | 5 | 0 | 0 |
| (*Reddi Wip* Original) . . . . | 15 | 0 | <1.0 | 1.0 | <5 | 0 | 0 |
| chocolate (*Reddi Wip*) . . | 15 | 0 | 1.0 | 1.0 | <5 | 0 | 0 |
| **Cream topping mix** (*Dream Whip*), 2 tbsp.* | 10 | 0 | 2.0 | 0 | 0 | 0 | 0 |
| **Creamer**, flavored (*Bailey's*), 1 tbsp.: | | | | | | | |
| caramel . . . . . . . . . . . . . | 40 | 0 | 6.0 | 1.5 | 5 | 0 | 0 |
| chocolate . . . . . . . . . . . | 40 | 0 | 6.0 | 1.5 | 5 | 15 | 0 |
| crème brulée . . . . . . . . . | 40 | 0 | 6.0 | 1.5 | 5 | 5 | 0 |
| hazelnut . . . . . . . . . . . . . | 35 | 0 | 5.0 | 1.5 | 5 | 5 | 0 |
| original Irish cream . . . . . | 40 | 0 | 6.0 | 1.5 | 5 | 5 | 0 |
| toffee almond cream . . . . | 40 | 0 | 6.0 | 1.5 | 5 | 5 | 0 |
| vanilla, French . . . . . . . . . | 40 | 0 | 6.0 | 1.5 | 5 | 0 | 0 |
| **Creamer, nondairy**: | | | | | | | |
| fluid, 1 tbsp.: | | | | | | | |
| (*Coffee-mate*) . . . . . . . | 20 | 0 | 2.0 | 1.0 | 0 | 0 | 0 |
| (*Coffee-mate* Lowfat) . | 10 | 0 | 2.0 | .5 | 0 | 5 | 0 |
| (*Coffee-mate* Nonfat) . | 10 | 0 | 2.0 | 0 | 0 | 0 | 0 |
| (*Silk*) . . . . . . . . . . . . . | 15 | 0 | 1.0 | 1.0 | 0 | 10 | 0 |
| (*So Delicious* Coconut Milk) . . . . | 10 | 0 | 1.0 | 0 | 0 | 0 | 0 |
| powder, 1 tsp. | | | | | | | |
| (*Coffee-mate*) . . . . . . . | 10 | 0 | 1.0 | .5 | 0 | 0 | 0 |
| (*Coffee-mate* Nonfat) . | 10 | 0 | 2.0 | 0 | 0 | 0 | 0 |
| (*Cremora*) . . . . . . . . . | 10 | 0 | 1.0 | .5 | 0 | 10 | 0 |
| (*Cremora* Lite) . . . . . . | 10 | 0 | 1.0 | 0 | 0 | 5 | 0 |
| **Creamer, nondairy, flavored, powder** (*Coffee-mate*), 4 tsp., except as noted: | | | | | | | |
| all flavors, sugar free, | | | | | | | |

| Food and Measure | cal. | prot. (gms) | carbo. (gms) | fat (gms) | chol. (mgs) | sod. (mgs) | fiber (gms) |
|---|---|---|---|---|---|---|---|
| **Creamer, nondairy, flavored, powder** *(cont.)* | | | | | | | |
| 1 tbsp. | 30 | 0 | 2.0 | 2.5 | 0 | 15 | 0 |
| chocolate, creamy | 60 | 0 | 9.0 | 2.5 | 0 | 30 | 0 |
| chocolate toffee | 60 | 0 | 9.0 | 2.5 | 0 | 15 | 0 |
| cinnamon vanilla | 60 | 0 | 8.0 | 3.0 | 0 | 20 | 0 |
| hazelnut | 60 | 0 | 9.0 | 3.0 | 0 | 15 | 0 |
| peppermint mocha | 60 | 0 | 8.0 | 3.0 | 0 | 15 | 0 |
| vanilla, French | 60 | 0 | 9.0 | 2.5 | 0 | 15 | 0 |
| vanilla, French, nonfat | 50 | 0 | 11.0 | 0 | 0 | 15 | 0 |
| vanilla caramel | 60 | 0 | 9.0 | 3.0 | 0 | 15 | 0 |
| **Crème fraîche** (*Vermont Butter & Cheese*), 1 oz. | 110 | 1.0 | 1.0 | 11.0 | 25 | 20 | 0 |
| **Creole gravy mix**, red (*Zatarain's*), ¼ cup* | 25 | <1.0 | 4.0 | 1.0 | 0 | 230 | 0 |
| **Creole seasoning** (*Zatarain's* Shrimp Creole), 2 tsp. | 25 | <1.0 | 4.0 | .5 | 0 | 480 | 0 |
| **Crepe**, French style (*Frieda's*), .5-oz. pc. | 50 | 1.0 | 9.0 | 1.0 | 6 | 79 | 0 |
| **Crepe dessert**, filled, frozen, 1 pc.: | | | | | | | |
| apple cinnamon (*Lupita's*), 2.5 oz. | 110 | 2.0 | 20.0 | 2.5 | 0 | 60 | 1.0 |
| cheesecake, 2.25 oz.: | | | | | | | |
| blueberry (*Lupita's*) | 140 | 2.0 | 19.0 | 7.0 | 0 | 60 | 1.0 |
| strawberry (*Golden*) | 140 | 2.0 | 19.0 | 7.0 | 0 | 60 | 1.0 |
| chocolate (*Chocolate Lover's Delight*), 1.75 oz. | 170 | 3.0 | 18.0 | 9.0 | <5 | 120 | 0 |
| mango (*Lupita's*), 2.5 oz. | 110 | 2.0 | 20.0 | 2.5 | 0 | 60 | 1.0 |
| **Cress, garden:** | | | | | | | |
| raw, ½ cup | 8 | .7 | 1.4 | .2 | 0 | 4 | .3 |
| boiled, drained, ½ cup | 16 | 1.3 | 2.6 | .4 | 0 | 5 | .5 |
| **Cress, water**, see "Watercress" | | | | | | | |
| **Croaker**, meat only, raw, Atlantic, 4 oz. | 119 | 20.2 | 0 | 3.6 | 69 | 63 | 0 |
| **Croissant:** | | | | | | | |
| butter, 1-oz. pc. | 115 | 2.3 | 13.0 | 6.0 | 19 | 211 | .7 |

| Food and Measure | cal. | prot. (gms) | carbo. (gms) | fat (gms) | chol. (mgs) | sod. (mgs) | fiber (gms) |
|---|---|---|---|---|---|---|---|
| apple, 2-oz. pc. ........ | 144 | 4.2 | 21.0 | 4.9 | 18 | 155 | 1.4 |
| cheese, 1.5-oz. pc. ..... | 174 | 3.9 | 19.7 | 8.8 | 24 | 233 | 1.1 |
| **Croissant, frozen** (*Sara Lee* Petite), | | | | | | | |
| 1-oz. pc. ........... | 120 | 3.0 | 13.0 | 6.0 | 0 | 160 | 0 |
| **Crookneck squash:** (*Frieda's* Baby), | | | | | | | |
| 1 cup, 4.5 oz. ....... | 25 | 1.0 | 5.0 | 0 | 0 | 3 | 3.0 |
| sliced, ½ cup: | | | | | | | |
| raw, ends trimmed ... | 12 | .6 | 2.6 | .2 | 0 | 1 | .7 |
| boiled, drained ...... | 18 | .8 | 3.9 | .3 | 0 | 1 | 1.3 |
| **Crookneck squash, canned**, cut, drained, | | | | | | | |
| no salt, ½ cup ....... | 14 | .7 | 3.2 | .1 | 0 | 5 | 1.1 |
| **Crookneck squash, frozen**, boiled, | | | | | | | |
| sliced, ½ cup ....... | 24 | 1.2 | 5.3 | .2 | 0 | 6 | 1.2 |
| **Croutons** (see also "Salad toppers"), 2 tbsp. or ¼ oz., except as noted: | | | | | | | |
| Caesar: | | | | | | | |
| (*Cardini's*) .......... | 35 | 1.0 | 4.0 | 1.5 | 0 | 50 | 0 |
| (*Chatham Village*) .... | 35 | 1.0 | 4.0 | 1.5 | 0 | 50 | 0 |
| (*Fresh Gourmet*) ..... | 30 | 1.0 | 5.0 | 1.0 | 0 | 80 | 0 |
| (*Fresh Gourmet* Organic) ......... | 30 | 1.0 | 4.0 | 1.5 | 0 | 80 | 0 |
| (*Marzetti*) .......... | 35 | 1.0 | 4.0 | 1.5 | 0 | 50 | 0 |
| (*New York* Texas Toast) ........... | 35 | 1.0 | 4.0 | 1.5 | 0 | 70 | 0 |
| (*Pepperidge Farm* Classic), 6 pcs. .... | 30 | <1.0 | 5.0 | 1.0 | 0 | 60 | 0 |
| garlic (*Fresh Gourmet* Fat Free) . | 30 | 1.0 | 5.0 | 0 | 0 | 55 | 0 |
| Parmesan (*Fresh Gourmet*) ........ | 30 | 1.0 | 4.0 | 0 | 0 | 80 | 0 |
| cheese and garlic: | | | | | | | |
| (*Chatham Village*) .... | 40 | 1.0 | 3.0 | 2.5 | 0 | 60 | 0 |
| (*Fresh Gourmet*) ..... | 30 | 1.0 | 5.0 | 1.0 | 0 | 65 | 0 |
| (*Marzetti*) .......... | 40 | 1.0 | 3.0 | 2.5 | 0 | 60 | 0 |
| (*New York* Texas Toast) ........... | 35 | 1.0 | 4.0 | 1.5 | 0 | 65 | 0 |
| (*Rothbury Farms*) .... | 30 | 1.0 | 5.0 | 1.0 | 0 | 100 | 0 |

| Food and Measure | cal. | prot. (gms) | carbo. (gms) | fat (gms) | chol. (mgs) | sod. (mgs) | fiber (gms) |
|---|---|---|---|---|---|---|---|
| **Croutons, cheese and garlic** *(cont.)* | | | | | | | |
| cheesy (*Fresh Gourmet* Tiny Bites) .......... | 30 | 1.0 | 5.0 | 1.0 | 0 | 75 | 0 |
| cornbread, butter (*Fresh Gourmet*) ..... | 30 | 1.0 | 4.0 | 1.0 | 0 | 60 | 0 |
| garlic (*Cardini's*) ........ | 35 | 1.0 | 4.0 | 1.5 | 0 | 55 | 0 |
| garlic and butter: | | | | | | | |
| (*Chatham Village*) .... | 35 | 1.0 | 4.0 | 1.5 | 0 | 55 | 0 |
| (*Fresh Gourmet*) ..... | 30 | 1.0 | 5.0 | 1.0 | 0 | 65 | 0 |
| (*Marzetti*) .......... | 35 | 1.0 | 4.0 | 1.5 | 0 | 55 | 0 |
| (*New York* Texas Toast) ........... | 35 | 1.0 | 4.0 | 1.5 | 0 | 55 | 0 |
| (*Rothbury Farms*) .... | 30 | 1.0 | 5.0 | 1.0 | 0 | 90 | 0 |
| garlic and onion: | | | | | | | |
| (*Chatham Village*) .... | 30 | 1.0 | 5.0 | 0 | 0 | 85 | 0 |
| (*Marzetti*) .......... | 30 | 1.0 | 5.0 | 0 | 0 | 85 | 0 |
| herb, garden: | | | | | | | |
| (*Chatham Village*) .... | 35 | 1.0 | 4.0 | 1.5 | 0 | 55 | 0 |
| (*Fresh Gourmet*) ..... | 30 | 1.0 | 5.0 | 1.0 | 0 | 90 | 0 |
| Italian seasoned: | | | | | | | |
| (*Cardini's*) .......... | 30 | 1.0 | 4.0 | 1.5 | 0 | 80 | 0 |
| (*Fresh Gourmet*) ..... | 30 | 1.0 | 5.0 | 1.0 | 0 | 80 | 0 |
| (*Pepperidge Farm* Zesty), 6 pcs. ...... | 30 | <1.0 | 5.0 | 1.0 | 0 | 55 | 0 |
| (*Rothbury Farms*) .... | 30 | 1.0 | 5.0 | 1.0 | 0 | 105 | 0 |
| ranch: | | | | | | | |
| (*Fresh Gourmet* Country) ......... | 30 | 1.0 | 4.0 | 1.0 | 0 | 80 | 0 |
| (*Marzetti*) .......... | 35 | 1.0 | 4.0 | 1.5 | 0 | 95 | 0 |
| Parmesan (*Fresh Gourmet* Fat Free) . | 30 | 1.0 | 5.0 | 0 | 0 | 80 | 0 |
| Romano (*Cardini's*) ..... | 40 | 1.0 | 3.0 | 2.5 | 0 | 60 | 0 |
| sea salt and pepper: | | | | | | | |
| (*Chatham Village*) .... | 35 | 1.0 | 4.0 | 1.5 | 0 | 105 | 0 |
| (*Marzetti*) .......... | 35 | 1.0 | 4.0 | 1.5 | 0 | 105 | 0 |
| (*New York* Texas Toast) ........... | 35 | 1.0 | 4.0 | 1.5 | 0 | 105 | 0 |
| seasoned: | | | | | | | |
| (*Fresh Gourmet* Organic) ......... | 30 | 0 | 4.0 | 1.5 | 0 | 70 | 0 |
| (*New York* Texas Toast) ........... | 35 | 1.0 | 4.0 | 1.5 | 0 | 95 | 1.0 |
| (*Pepperidge Farm*) ... | 30 | <1.0 | 5.0 | 1.0 | 0 | 75 | 0 |

| Food and Measure | cal. | prot. (gms) | carbo. (gms) | fat (gms) | chol. (mgs) | sod. (mgs) | fiber (gms) |
|---|---|---|---|---|---|---|---|
| (*Rothbury Farms*) .... | 30 | 1.0 | 5.0 | 1.0 | 0 | 105 | 0 |
| (*Rothbury Farms* Fat Free) ......... | 25 | 1.0 | 5.0 | 0 | 0 | 100 | 0 |
| (*Rothbury Farms* Organic) ......... | 30 | 1.0 | 4.0 | 1.0 | 0 | 65 | 1.0 |
| (*Rothbury Farms* Texas Toast), 3 pcs. | 30 | 1.0 | 5.0 | 1.0 | 0 | 105 | 0 |
| whole grain (*Marzetti*) ... | 35 | 1.0 | 4.0 | 2.0 | 0 | 95 | 1.0 |
| **Crowder peas**, see "Peas, crowder" | | | | | | | |
| **Cucumber**, w/peel: | | | | | | | |
| (*Frieda's* Hothouse), ⅔ cup, 3 oz. ........ | 10 | 1.0 | 2.0 | 0 | 0 | 0 | 1.0 |
| (*Frieda's* Japanese), sliced, ½ cup ....... | 10 | 0 | 2.0 | 0 | 0 | 6 | 0 |
| 1 medium, 8¼" long .... | 38 | 2.1 | 8.3 | .4 | 0 | 6 | 2.4 |
| sliced, ½ cup .......... | 7 | .4 | 1.4 | .1 | 0 | 1 | .4 |
| **Cucumber, pickled**, see "Pickles" | | | | | | | |
| **Cucuzza squash** (*Frieda's*), sliced, 1 cup, 4 oz. ......... | 16 | 1.0 | 4.0 | 0 | 0 | 2 | 0 |
| **Cumin**, ground, 1 tsp. ... | 8 | .4 | .9 | .5 | 0 | 4 | .2 |
| **Cupcake**, see "Cake, snack" | | | | | | | |
| **Cupcake topping**, (*Smucker's Magic Shell*), 2 tbsp. ....... | 220 | 1.0 | 17.0 | 16.0 | 5 | 50 | 0 |
| **Curacao, blue**, non-alcoholic (*Angostura*), 1 fl. oz. ... | 55 | 0 | 13.0 | 0 | 0 | 5 | 0 |
| **Currant juice**, see "Black currant juice" | | | | | | | |
| **Currants**, fresh: | | | | | | | |
| black, Europe, ½ cup ... | 36 | .8 | 8.6 | .2 | 0 | 1 | 3.0 |
| red (*Frieda's*), 1 cup .... | 63 | 1.0 | 15.0 | 0 | 0 | 1 | 5.0 |
| red or white, ½ cup ..... | 31 | .8 | 7.7 | .1 | 0 | 1 | 2.4 |
| **Currants, dried**, Zante: | | | | | | | |
| (*Sun•Maid*), ¼ cup ..... | 120 | 1.0 | 30.0 | 0 | 0 | 10 | 2.0 |
| ½ cup ............... | 204 | 2.9 | 53.3 | .2 | 0 | 6 | 4.9 |
| **Curry, vegetable**, see "Vegetable dish" | | | | | | | |

| Food and Measure | cal. | prot. (gms) | carbo. (gms) | fat (gms) | chol. (mgs) | sod. (mgs) | fiber (gms) |
|---|---|---|---|---|---|---|---|
| **Curry paste**, 2 tbsp., except as noted: | | | | | | | |
| (*Tiger Tiger* Balti) ...... | 65 | 1.0 | 5.0 | 5.0 | 0 | 650 | 1.0 |
| (*Tiger Tiger* Kashmiri) ... | 120 | 2.0 | 9.0 | 10.0 | 0 | 910 | 4.0 |
| biryani (*Patak's*) ....... | 90 | 1.0 | 6.0 | 6.0 | 0 | 470 | 3.0 |
| green: | | | | | | | |
| (*Roland*), 1 tbsp. .... | 25 | 0 | 3.0 | 2.0 | 0 | 390 | 1.0 |
| (*A Taste of Thai*), 1 tsp. | 5 | 0 | 1.0 | 0 | 0 | 250 | 1.0 |
| (*Tiger Tiger*), 1 tbsp. .. | 10 | 0 | 3.0 | 0 | 0 | 490 | 0 |
| hot or mild (*Patak's*) .... | 110 | 2.0 | 7.0 | 9.0 | 0 | 480 | 4.0 |
| Madras (*Tiger Tiger*) .... | 120 | 1.0 | 7.0 | 11.0 | 0 | 790 | 3.0 |
| Panang (*A Taste of Thai*), 1 tsp. ........ | 10 | <1.0 | 2.0 | 0 | 0 | 150 | 0 |
| red: | | | | | | | |
| (*Roland*), 1 tbsp. .... | 40 | 0 | 3.0 | 2.0 | 0 | 580 | 1.0 |
| (*A Taste of Thai*), 1 tsp. | 10 | 0 | 2.0 | 0 | 0 | 340 | 0 |
| (*Tiger Tiger*), 1 tbsp. ... | 15 | 1.0 | 3.0 | 0 | 0 | 550 | <1.0 |
| tandoori: | | | | | | | |
| (*Neera's* Grilling), 2 tsp. | 19 | 0 | 3.0 | 2.0 | 0 | 155 | 1.0 |
| (*Patak's*) ........... | 40 | 1.0 | 7.0 | 1.0 | 0 | 1200 | 1.0 |
| (*Tiger Tiger*) ........ | 25 | 1.0 | 5.0 | 1.0 | 0 | 710 | 2.0 |
| tikka: | | | | | | | |
| (*Patak's*) ........... | 50 | 1.0 | 6.0 | 2.5 | 0 | 830 | 2.0 |
| (*Tiger Tiger*) ........ | 70 | 1.0 | 6.0 | 8.0 | 0 | 670 | 3.0 |
| vindaloo: | | | | | | | |
| (*Neera's*), 2 tsp. ..... | 48 | 0 | 3.0 | 4.0 | 0 | 118 | 1.0 |
| (*Tiger Tiger*) ........ | 115 | 1.0 | 6.0 | 11.0 | 0 | 790 | 3.0 |
| yellow: | | | | | | | |
| (*Roland*), 1 tbsp. .... | 30 | 0 | 3.0 | 2.0 | 0 | 450 | 0 |
| (*A Taste of Thai*), 1 tsp. | 5 | 0 | 1.0 | 0 | 0 | 230 | 0 |
| **Curry powder**: | | | | | | | |
| 1 tbsp. ............... | 20 | .8 | 3.7 | .9 | 0 | 3 | 1.0 |
| 1 tsp. ................ | 6 | .3 | 1.2 | .3 | 0 | 1 | .3 |
| Masala: | | | | | | | |
| (*Neera's*), 2 tsp. ..... | 13 | 1.0 | 3.0 | 1.0 | 0 | 167 | 1.0 |
| (*Neera's* Garam), ¼ tsp. | 2 | 0 | 0 | 0 | 0 | 0 | 0 |
| **Curry sauce**, simmer, jar/pouch, ½ cup, except as noted: | | | | | | | |
| (*Ethnic Gourmet* Bombay), 4 oz. ...... | 70 | 2.0 | 10.0 | 1.5 | 0 | 540 | 2.0 |
| butter chicken: | | | | | | | |
| (*Devya* Organic) ..... | 80 | 3.0 | 14.0 | 1.5 | 0 | 150 | 3.0 |
| (*Tiger Tiger* Punjabi) .. | 302 | 1.4 | 13.9 | 26.6 | 22 | 480 | 1.0 |

| Food and Measure | cal. | prot. (gms) | carbo. (gms) | fat (gms) | chol. (mgs) | sod. (mgs) | fiber (gms) |
|---|---|---|---|---|---|---|---|
| coconut (*Maya Kaimal*) .. | 130 | 2.0 | 13.0 | 9.0 | 0 | 640 | 2.0 |
| Dopiaza (*Patak's*) ...... | 110 | 2.0 | 11.0 | 7.0 | 0 | 390 | 3.0 |
| Jalfrezi: | | | | | | | |
|   (*Bombay Authentics*) . | 90 | 1.0 | 7.0 | 7.0 | 0 | 360 | 1.0 |
|   (*Patak's*) ........... | 160 | 2.0 | 14.0 | 10.0 | 0 | 390 | 4.0 |
|   (*Seeds of Change* | | | | | | | |
|     Organic), ⅓ cup ... | 90 | 1.0 | 9.0 | 6.0 | 0 | 270 | 2.0 |
| korma: | | | | | | | |
|   (*Bombay Authentics*), | | | | | | | |
|     ¼ cup ........... | 110 | 2.0 | 7.0 | 8.0 | 0 | 240 | 1.0 |
|   (*Maya Kaimal*) ...... | 130 | 3.0 | 11.0 | 9.0 | 10 | 670 | 2.0 |
|   (*Patak's*) ........... | 190 | 2.0 | 13.0 | 14.0 | 10 | 390 | 3.0 |
|   (*Seeds of Change* | | | | | | | |
|     Organic), ⅓ cup ... | 140 | 1.0 | 9.0 | 11.0 | 10 | 290 | 1.0 |
|   (*Tasty Bite* Good), | | | | | | | |
|     ½ of 7-oz. pouch .. | 110 | 1.0 | 7.0 | 9.0 | 0 | 10 | 1.0 |
|   mild (*Tiger Tiger* | | | | | | | |
|     Kashmiri) ........ | 372 | 1.9 | 13.0 | 34.6 | 19 | 480 | .7 |
| Madras: | | | | | | | |
|   (*Maya Kaimal*), ⅓ cup | 100 | 1.0 | 6.0 | 8.0 | 0 | 370 | 1.0 |
|   (*Neera's*), 4 oz. ...... | 110 | 1.0 | 6.0 | 9.0 | 0 | 530 | 1.0 |
|   (*Seeds of Change* | | | | | | | |
|     Organic), ⅓ cup ... | 60 | 1.0 | 8.0 | 4.0 | 0 | 240 | 1.0 |
| Masala: | | | | | | | |
|   (*Ethnic Gourmet* | | | | | | | |
|     Calcutta), 4 oz. .... | 90 | 2.0 | 10.0 | 4.5 | 5 | 500 | 1.0 |
|   (*Maya Kaimal* Butter), | | | | | | | |
|     ⅓ cup ........... | 120 | 2.0 | 7.0 | 10.0 | 20 | 440 | 1.0 |
|   channa (*Devya* Organic) | 140 | 3.0 | 18.0 | 6.0 | 0 | 430 | 3.0 |
| Rogan Josh: | | | | | | | |
|   (*Bombay Authentics*), | | | | | | | |
|     ¼ cup ........... | 100 | 2.0 | 6.0 | 7.0 | 0 | 300 | 1.0 |
|   (*Patak's*) ........... | 90 | 2.0 | 11.0 | 4.0 | 0 | 400 | 4.0 |
|   (*Tasty Bite*), ½ of | | | | | | | |
|     7-oz. pouch ...... | 110 | 1.0 | 9.0 | 8.0 | 0 | 15 | 2.0 |
|   (*Tiger Tiger* Lahori) ... | 206 | 1.2 | 12.5 | 16.7 | 21 | 480 | 1.0 |
| satay (*Tiger Tiger*) ...... | 303 | 4.0 | 38.0 | 15.0 | 0 | 814 | <1.0 |
| spinach (*Ethnic Gourmet* | | | | | | | |
|   Punjab Saag), 4 oz. .. | 60 | 2.0 | 6.0 | 3.0 | 5 | 500 | 1.0 |
| tamarind (*Maya Kaimal*) . | 140 | 2.0 | 10.0 | 9.0 | 0 | 640 | 3.0 |
| tandoori chicken | | | | | | | |
|   (*Devya* Organic) ...... | 140 | 3.0 | 17.0 | 7.0 | 0 | 480 | 3.0 |
| Thai curry: | | | | | | | |
|   green (*Tiger Tiger*) ... | 163 | 2.5 | 9.9 | 12.5 | 0 | 580 | 1.0 |

| Food and Measure | cal. | prot. (gms) | carbo. (gms) | fat (gms) | chol. (mgs) | sod. (mgs) | fiber (gms) |
|---|---|---|---|---|---|---|---|
| **Curry sauce** *(cont.)* | | | | | | | |
| red (*Kikkoman*), ¼ cup | 90 | 1.0 | 7.0 | 6.0 | 0 | 500 | 0 |
| red (*Tiger Tiger*) ..... | 172 | 2.5 | 10.5 | 13.3 | 0 | 620 | 1.0 |
| yellow (*Kikkoman*), | | | | | | | |
| ¼ cup ........... | 90 | 1.0 | 6.0 | 6.0 | 0 | 510 | 0 |
| tikka (*Neera's*), 4 oz. .... | 130 | 3.0 | 10.0 | 10.0 | 10 | 410 | 2.0 |
| tikka Masala: | | | | | | | |
| (*Kikkoman*), ¼ cup ... | 70 | 1.0 | 6.0 | 3.0 | 5 | 500 | 1.0 |
| (*Maya Kaimal* Jar | | | | | | | |
| 12.5 oz.), ⅓ cup ... | 90 | 2.0 | 6.0 | 7.0 | 10 | 340 | <1.0 |
| (*Maya Kaimal* 15 oz.) . | 160 | 3.0 | 9.0 | 13.0 | 25 | 390 | 2.0 |
| (*Patak's*) ........... | 160 | 2.0 | 14.0 | 10.0 | 0 | 390 | 4.0 |
| (*Seeds of Change*), | | | | | | | |
| ⅓ cup ........... | 90 | 1.0 | 8.0 | 7.0 | 10 | 280 | 2.0 |
| (*Tasty Bite*), ½ of | | | | | | | |
| 7-oz. pouch ...... | 120 | 1.0 | 9.0 | 10.0 | 0 | 20 | 2.0 |
| (*Tiger Tiger* Peshwari) | 221 | 1.7 | 15.0 | 17.0 | 28 | 600 | 1.2 |
| vegetable (*Devya* | | | | | | | |
| Organic) ........... | 130 | 4.0 | 16.0 | 6.0 | 0 | 420 | 3.0 |
| vindaloo: | | | | | | | |
| (*Bombay Authentics*), | | | | | | | |
| ¼ cup ........... | 100 | 2.0 | 6.0 | 8.0 | 0 | 300 | 1.0 |
| (*Maya Kaimal*) ...... | 130 | 2.0 | 10.0 | 9.0 | 0 | 720 | 3.0 |
| (*Neera's*), 4 oz. ...... | 140 | 2.0 | 14.0 | 9.0 | 0 | 590 | 2.0 |
| **Cusk**, meat only: | | | | | | | |
| raw, 4 oz. ............ | 99 | 21.6 | 0 | .8 | 47 | 36 | 0 |
| baked, broiled, or | | | | | | | |
| microwaved, 4 oz. ... | 127 | 27.6 | 0 | 1.0 | 60 | 45 | 0 |
| **Custard apple**, | | | | | | | |
| trimmed, 1 oz. ...... | 29 | .5 | 7.1 | .2 | 0 | 1 | 1.0 |
| **Custard marrow**, see | | | | | | | |
| "Chayote" | | | | | | | |
| **Cuttlefish**, meat only | | | | | | | |
| raw, 4 oz. ............ | 90 | 18.4 | .9 | .8 | 127 | 422 | 0 |
| boiled or steamed, 4 oz. . | 179 | 36.8 | 1.9 | 1.6 | 254 | 844 | 0 |
| **Cuttlefish, canned**, in | | | | | | | |
| ink sauce, 2 oz.: | | | | | | | |
| (*Roland* Calamares) .... | 110 | 7.0 | 0 | 9.0 | 40 | 380 | 0 |
| (*Vigo* Squid) .......... | 130 | 9.0 | 2.0 | 10.0 | 44 | 250 | 0 |
| **Cuttlefish, dried** | | | | | | | |
| (*Roland* Saki Ika) .5 oz.: | | | | | | | |
| seasoned, flat ......... | 44 | 8.0 | 3.0 | 0 | 54 | 273 | 0 |
| seasoned, strips ....... | 44 | 8.0 | 1.0 | 0 | 54 | 273 | 0 |
| shredded, hot ......... | 44 | 8.0 | 1.0 | 0 | 54 | 283 | 0 |

# D

| Food and Measure | cal. | prot. (gms) | carbo. (gms) | fat (gms) | chol. (mgs) | sod. (mgs) | fiber (gms) |
|---|---|---|---|---|---|---|---|
| **Daikon**, see "Radish, Oriental" | | | | | | | |
| **Daiquiri drink mixer:** | | | | | | | |
| peach or strawberry, frozen (*Bacardi*), | | | | | | | |
| 2 fl. oz. .......... | 120 | 0 | 32.0 | 0 | 0 | 0 | 0 |
| strawberry (*Angostura*), | | | | | | | |
| 8 fl. oz. .......... | 120 | 0 | 31.0 | 0 | 0 | 240 | 0 |
| ***Dairy Queen/Brazier:*** | | | | | | | |
| burgers, original: | | | | | | | |
| cheeseburger ....... | 400 | 19.0 | 34.0 | 18.0 | 65 | 920 | 1.0 |
| double .......... | 640 | 34.0 | 34.0 | 34.0 | 125 | 1230 | 1.0 |
| double, bacon .... | 730 | 41.0 | 35.0 | 41.0 | 150 | 1550 | 1.0 |
| hamburger ......... | 350 | 17.0 | 33.0 | 14.0 | 50 | 680 | 1.0 |
| hamburger, double ... | 540 | 29.0 | 33.0 | 26.0 | 100 | 740 | 1.0 |
| *Grillburger:* | | | | | | | |
| ¼ lb. ............. | 490 | 26.0 | 43.0 | 24.0 | 65 | 690 | 2.0 |
| ¼ lb., w/cheese ..... | 540 | 28.0 | 43.0 | 28.0 | 80 | 940 | 2.0 |
| ¼ lb. *FlameThrower* .. | 740 | 35.0 | 41.0 | 49.0 | 115 | 1230 | 2.0 |
| ½ lb. ............. | 710 | 44.0 | 43.0 | 41.0 | 130 | 770 | 2.0 |
| ½ lb., w/cheese ..... | 810 | 51.0 | 44.0 | 49.0 | 155 | 1080 | 2.0 |
| ½ lb. *FlameThrower* .. | 1010 | 56.0 | 41.0 | 70.0 | 190 | 1540 | 2.0 |
| bacon cheese ....... | 630 | 35.0 | 44.0 | 35.0 | 100 | 1260 | 2.0 |
| mushroom Swiss .... | 620 | 29.0 | 39.0 | 37.0 | 75 | 910 | 2.0 |
| hot dog: | | | | | | | |
| plain ............. | 290 | 11.0 | 22.0 | 17.0 | 35 | 900 | 1.0 |
| cheese ........... | 340 | 14.0 | 21.0 | 22.0 | 50 | 830 | 1.0 |
| chili ............. | 330 | 13.0 | 24.0 | 20.0 | 40 | 1050 | 1.0 |
| chili cheese ........ | 380 | 16.0 | 23.0 | 24.0 | 55 | 980 | 1.0 |
| foot long .......... | 560 | 20.0 | 39.0 | 35.0 | 65 | 1600 | 2.0 |
| foot long, chili cheese .......... | 670 | 28.0 | 41.0 | 43.0 | 95 | 1720 | 2.0 |

| Food and Measure | cal. | prot. (gms) | carbo. (gms) | fat (gms) | chol. (mgs) | sod. (mgs) | fiber (gms) |
|---|---|---|---|---|---|---|---|
| ***Dairy Queen/Brazier*** *(cont.)* | | | | | | | |
| sandwich, chicken: | | | | | | | |
| crispy ............. | 560 | 20.0 | 48.0 | 28.0 | 35 | 1020 | 3.0 |
| crispy, w/cheese ..... | 610 | 22.0 | 48.0 | 32.0 | 45 | 1260 | 3.0 |
| crispy, wrap ........ | 290 | 11.0 | 17.0 | 17.0 | 30 | 620 | 2.0 |
| crispy, *FlameThrower* . | 860 | 30.0 | 51.0 | 55.0 | 75 | 1850 | 3.0 |
| crispy, *FlameThrower* | | | | | | | |
| wrap ............ | 300 | 11.0 | 17.0 | 18.0 | 35 | 620 | 2.0 |
| grilled ............. | 370 | 24.0 | 32.0 | 16.0 | 55 | 810 | 1.0 |
| grilled, wrap ........ | 200 | 12.0 | 9.0 | 13.0 | 35 | 450 | 1.0 |
| grilled, *FlameThrower* . | 590 | 34.0 | 34.0 | 36.0 | 100 | 1570 | 1.0 |
| sandwich, iron grill: | | | | | | | |
| BLT supreme ....... | 590 | 26.0 | 42.0 | 33.0 | 75 | 1560 | 2.0 |
| classic club ......... | 570 | 32.0 | 42.0 | 29.0 | 75 | 1750 | 2.0 |
| turkey ............. | 520 | 29.0 | 42.0 | 25.0 | 65 | 1560 | 2.0 |
| chicken salad, crispy .... | 460 | 29.0 | 31.0 | 19.0 | 70 | 1230 | 6.0 |
| chicken salad, grilled .... | 280 | 31.0 | 14.0 | 11.0 | 75 | 890 | 4.0 |
| *Chicken Strip Basket*: | | | | | | | |
| 4 pc., country gravy .. | 1190 | 41.0 | 121.0 | 48.0 | 70 | 3030 | 9.0 |
| 6 pc., country gravy .. | 1410 | 54.0 | 125.0 | 59.0 | 110 | 3760 | 10.0 |
| shrimp basket ......... | 1000 | 19.0 | 116.0 | 49.0 | 125 | 3650 | 8.0 |
| quesadilla basket: | | | | | | | |
| chicken ............ | 1200 | 47.0 | 115.0 | 60.0 | 125 | 2740 | 9.0 |
| veggie ............. | 1030 | 28.0 | 114.0 | 50.0 | 65 | 2270 | 9.0 |
| regional sandwiches: | | | | | | | |
| barbecued beef ...... | 270 | 16.0 | 41.0 | 6.0 | 30 | 970 | 1.0 |
| barbecued pork ...... | 310 | 17.0 | 41.0 | 9.0 | 50 | 830 | 2.0 |
| fish fillet ........... | 430 | 16.0 | 51.0 | 18.0 | 30 | 1160 | 2.0 |
| fish fillet, w/cheese ... | 480 | 18.0 | 52.0 | 22.0 | 40 | 1400 | 2.0 |
| grilled cheese ....... | 290 | 13.0 | 30.0 | 13.0 | 40 | 1020 | 1.0 |
| sides: | | | | | | | |
| fries, large ......... | 500 | 6.0 | 70.0 | 21.0 | 0 | 1040 | 5.0 |
| fries, regular ........ | 310 | 4.0 | 43.0 | 13.0 | 0 | 640 | 3.0 |
| onion rings ......... | 360 | 6.0 | 47.0 | 16.0 | 0 | 840 | 2.0 |
| side salad .......... | 50 | 2.0 | 11.0 | 0 | 0 | 50 | 3.0 |
| *Arctic Rush*, medium ... | 310 | 0 | 63.0 | 0 | 0 | 0 | 0 |
| *Blizzard*, medium: | | | | | | | |
| banana split ........ | 570 | 13.0 | 93.0 | 16.0 | 55 | 230 | 1.0 |
| brownie batter ...... | 950 | 18.0 | 126.0 | 44.0 | 65 | 550 | 6.0 |
| *Butterfinger* ........ | 740 | 16.0 | 114.0 | 26.0 | 55 | 350 | 0 |
| cappuccino *Heath* .... | 690 | 15.0 | 92.0 | 28.0 | 105 | 390 | 0 |
| choco cherry love .... | 650 | 14.0 | 96.0 | 24.0 | 55 | 240 | 1.0 |
| chocolate xtreme .... | 970 | 17.0 | 75.0 | 45.0 | 75 | 600 | 5.0 |
| cookie dough ....... | 1020 | 18.0 | 148.0 | 40.0 | 75 | 580 | 2.0 |

| Food and Measure | cal. | prot. (gms) | carbo. (gms) | fat (gms) | chol. (mgs) | sod. (mgs) | fiber (gms) |
|---|---|---|---|---|---|---|---|
| Hawaiian | 600 | 13.0 | 92.0 | 21.0 | 50 | 240 | 3.0 |
| *M&M's* | 840 | 16.0 | 127.0 | 30.0 | 65 | 270 | 2.0 |
| *Oreo* cookies | 680 | 14.0 | 100.0 | 25.0 | 50 | 530 | 1.0 |
| raspberry truffle | 860 | 17.0 | 129.0 | 33.0 | 70 | 260 | 5.0 |
| *Reese's* cups | 760 | 18.0 | 101.0 | 31.0 | 60 | 380 | 2.0 |
| *Snicker's* | 850 | 18.0 | 123.0 | 33.0 | 60 | 400 | 2.0 |
| tropical | 770 | 16.0 | 86.0 | 42.0 | 50 | 340 | 5.0 |
| *DQ* cone, medium: | | | | | | | |
| chocolate | 340 | 9.0 | 54.0 | 10.0 | 30 | 160 | 0 |
| chocolate, dipped | 470 | 9.0 | 61.0 | 22.0 | 30 | 150 | 1.0 |
| vanilla | 330 | 9.0 | 53.0 | 10.0 | 30 | 140 | 0 |
| waffle, w/soft-serve | 420 | 10.0 | 67.0 | 13.0 | 35 | 135 | 0 |
| *DQ* sundae, medium: | | | | | | | |
| banana | 330 | 8.0 | 53.0 | 10.0 | 30 | 130 | 1.0 |
| caramel | 430 | 9.0 | 74.0 | 11.0 | 35 | 210 | 0 |
| cherry | 350 | 8.0 | 57.0 | 10.0 | 30 | 140 | 0 |
| chocolate | 400 | 8.0 | 70.0 | 12.0 | 30 | 170 | 1.0 |
| hot fudge | 440 | 9.0 | 67.0 | 15.0 | 35 | 200 | 1.0 |
| marshmallow | 410 | 8.0 | 74.0 | 10.0 | 30 | 150 | 0 |
| pineapple | 340 | 8.0 | 54.0 | 10.0 | 30 | 140 | 0 |
| strawberry | 350 | 8.0 | 56.0 | 10.0 | 30 | 140 | 0 |
| *MooLatté*, 16 oz.: | | | | | | | |
| cappuccino | 500 | 8.0 | 71.0 | 18.0 | 35 | 170 | 0 |
| caramel | 630 | 9.0 | 100.0 | 19.0 | 40 | 230 | 0 |
| mocha | 580 | 9.0 | 83.0 | 23.0 | 35 | 200 | 0 |
| vanilla, French | 560 | 8.0 | 88.0 | 18.0 | 35 | 160 | 0 |
| shakes, medium: | | | | | | | |
| caramel | 850 | 19.0 | 138.0 | 24.0 | 80 | 430 | 0 |
| chocolate | 780 | 19.0 | 131.0 | 26.0 | 70 | 340 | 2.0 |
| hot fudge | 850 | 20.0 | 124.0 | 31.0 | 70 | 410 | 1.0 |
| strawberry | 650 | 18.0 | 97.0 | 21.0 | 70 | 290 | 1.0 |
| **Dandelion greens**: | | | | | | | |
| raw (*Frieda's*), 2 cups, 3 oz. | 40 | 2.0 | 8.0 | 0 | 0 | 65 | 3.0 |
| raw, chopped, ½ cup | 13 | .8 | 2.6 | .2 | 0 | 22 | 1.0 |
| boiled, drained, chopped, ½ cup | 17 | 1.0 | 3.3 | .3 | 0 | 23 | 1.5 |
| **Danish**, see "Cake" and "Cake, snack" | | | | | | | |
| **Dasheen**, see "Taro" | | | | | | | |
| **Date**, dried, 1.4 oz., except as noted: | | | | | | | |
| (*Dole*), 5–6 pcs. | 110 | <1.0 | 30.0 | 0 | 0 | 0 | 3.0 |

| Food and Measure | cal. | prot. (gms) | carbo. (gms) | fat (gms) | chol. (mgs) | sod. (mgs) | fiber (gms) |
|---|---|---|---|---|---|---|---|
| **Date** *(cont.)* | | | | | | | |
| (*Earthbound Farm* Organic) .......... | 120 | 1.0 | 31.0 | 0 | 0 | 0 | 3.0 |
| (*Frieda's* Medjool), 2–3 pcs. .......... | 120 | 1.0 | 31.0 | 0 | 0 | 0 | 3.0 |
| (*Mariani* Calavo), 5–6 pcs. .......... | 120 | 1.0 | 31.0 | 0 | 0 | 0 | 3.0 |
| (*Sun•Maid*), ¼ cup ..... | 110 | 1.0 | 30.0 | 0 | 0 | 0 | 4.0 |
| (*Sunsweet*), 5–6 pcs. ... | 120 | 1.0 | 30.0 | 0 | 0 | 0 | 3.0 |
| 10 pcs. , 2.9 oz. ....... | 228 | 1.6 | 61.0 | .4 | 0 | 2 | 6.2 |
| pitted, ½ cup .......... | 245 | 1.8 | 65.4 | .5 | 0 | 3 | 6.7 |
| chopped: | | | | | | | |
| (*Dole*), ¼ cup ....... | 120 | 1.0 | 31.0 | 0 | 0 | 0 | 3.0 |
| (*Sun•Maid*), ¼ cup ... | 120 | 1.0 | 33.0 | 0 | 0 | 5 | 3.0 |
| (*Sunsweet*) ......... | 120 | 1.0 | 31.0 | 0 | 0 | 0 | 3.0 |
| **Date, Indian**, see "Tamarindo" | | | | | | | |
| **Deli dressing** (*Thumann's*), 1 tsp. .. | 100 | 0 | 0 | 11.0 | 0 | 50 | 0 |
| **Delicata squash** (*Frieda's*), ¾ cup, 3 oz. .............. | 30 | 1.0 | 7.0 | 0 | 0 | 0 | 1.0 |
| **Dill dip**, 2 tbsp.: | | | | | | | |
| (*Marzetti*) ........... | 120 | 1.0 | 2.0 | 13.0 | 20 | 200 | 0 |
| (*Marzetti* Light) ...... | 60 | 0 | 2.0 | 5.0 | 5 | 230 | 0 |
| (*Marzetti* Nonfat) ...... | 30 | 1.0 | 6.0 | 0 | 0 | 300 | 0 |
| creamy (*Marie's*) ...... | 100 | 1.0 | 2.0 | 10.0 | 15 | 140 | 0 |
| **Dill seed**, 1 tsp. ...... | 6 | .3 | 1.2 | .3 | 0 | <1 | .4 |
| **Dill weed**, fresh: | | | | | | | |
| 5 sprigs .............. | <1 | <1.0 | .1 | <.1 | 0 | 1 | <.1 |
| 1 cup ................ | 4 | .3 | .6 | .1 | 0 | 5 | .2 |
| **Dill weed, dried**, 1 tsp. . | 3 | .2 | .6 | <.1 | 0 | 2 | .1 |
| **Dip**, see specific listings | | | | | | | |
| **Dipping sauce**, see specific listings | | | | | | | |
| **Dock:** | | | | | | | |
| raw, chopped, 1 cup .... | 29 | 2.6 | 4.3 | .9 | 9 | 5 | 3.9 |
| boiled, drained, 4 oz. .............. | 23 | 2.1 | 3.3 | .7 | 0 | 3 | <1.0 |
| **Dolphin fish**, see "Mahi mahi" | | | | | | | |
| ***Domino's Pizza:*** | | | | | | | |
| small, entire pizza: | | | | | | | |
| hand-tossed crust .... | 820 | 25.0 | 139.0 | 19.0 | 0 | 930 | 5.0 |

| Food and Measure | cal. | prot. (gms) | carbo. (gms) | fat (gms) | chol. (mgs) | sod. (mgs) | fiber (gms) |
|---|---|---|---|---|---|---|---|
| thin crust | 490 | 12.0 | 67.0 | 19.0 | 5 | 85 | 3.0 |
| sauce, entire pizza: | | | | | | | |
| BBQ | 80 | 1.0 | 17.0 | 0 | 0 | 310 | 1.0 |
| garlic Parm | 190 | 1.0 | 2.0 | 20.0 | 10 | 340 | 0 |
| hearty marinara | 50 | 2.0 | 8.0 | 1.5 | 5 | 530 | 1.0 |
| new pizza sauce | 50 | 2.0 | 10.0 | 0 | 0 | 450 | 2.0 |
| cheese, entire pizza: | | | | | | | |
| regular | 260 | 16.0 | 5.0 | 20.0 | 75 | 870 | 1.0 |
| cheese only/extra | 380 | 23.0 | 8.0 | 28.0 | 105 | 1250 | 1.0 |
| toppings, entire pizza: | | | | | | | |
| anchovies | 60 | 6.0 | 0 | 4.0 | 25 | 1660 | 0 |
| bacon | 270 | 16.0 | 5.0 | 20.0 | 65 | 1010 | 0 |
| banana peppers | 15 | 1.0 | 2.0 | 0 | 0 | 200 | 1.0 |
| beef | 220 | 11.0 | 0 | 18.0 | 50 | 400 | 0 |
| cheese, American | 210 | 11.0 | 2.0 | 17.0 | 50 | 1020 | 0 |
| cheese, cheddar | 110 | 7.0 | 0 | 9.0 | 30 | 180 | 0 |
| cheese, feta | 60 | 5.0 | 1.0 | 4.0 | 10 | 260 | 0 |
| cheese, Parmesan | 110 | 9.0 | 1.0 | 8.0 | 20 | 310 | 0 |
| cheese, provolone | 100 | 6.0 | 0 | 8.0 | 30 | 240 | 0 |
| chicken | 100 | 16.0 | 2.0 | 3.0 | 40 | 520 | 0 |
| chorizo | 60 | 9.0 | 1.0 | 3.0 | 20 | 430 | 0 |
| garlic | 30 | 1.0 | 7.0 | 0 | 0 | 0 | 0 |
| green chili pepper | 10 | 0 | 2.0 | 0 | 0 | 5 | 1.0 |
| green pepper | 10 | 0 | 2.0 | 0 | 0 | 0 | 1.0 |
| ham | 60 | 7.0 | 0 | 3.0 | 20 | 680 | 0 |
| jalapeños | 15 | 1.0 | 3.0 | 0 | 0 | 720 | 1.0 |
| mushrooms | 15 | 2.0 | 2.0 | 0 | 0 | 15 | 1.0 |
| olives, black | 70 | 0 | 1.0 | 7.0 | 0 | 310 | 1.0 |
| olives, green | 70 | 0 | 1.0 | 7.0 | 0 | 940 | 1.0 |
| onions | 10 | 0 | 3.0 | 0 | 0 | 5 | 0 |
| pepperoni | 160 | 7.0 | 0 | 14.0 | 35 | 680 | 0 |
| pepperoni, large | 180 | 7.0 | 1.0 | 16.0 | 35 | 630 | 0 |
| Philly steak | 70 | 10.0 | 1.0 | 2.5 | 25 | 400 | 0 |
| pineapple | 45 | 0 | 11.0 | 0 | 0 | 5 | 1.0 |
| roasted red pepper | 10 | 0 | 2.0 | 0 | 0 | 70 | 0 |
| salami | 150 | 9.0 | 1.0 | 12.0 | 35 | 630 | 0 |
| sausage, Italian | 250 | 9.0 | 6.0 | 21.0 | 40 | 740 | 0 |
| sausage, sliced | 180 | 9.0 | 0 | 15.0 | 35 | 420 | 0 |
| spinach | 10 | 1.0 | 2.0 | 0 | 0 | 35 | 1.0 |
| tomato | 15 | 1.0 | 4.0 | 0 | 0 | 220 | 1.0 |
| wing sauce | 10 | 0 | 2.0 | 0 | 0 | 920 | 1.0 |
| medium, entire pizza: | | | | | | | |
| deep dish crust | 1290 | 34.0 | 199.0 | 43.0 | 0 | 2020 | 23.0 |
| hand-tossed crust | 1060 | 33.0 | 181.0 | 23.0 | 0 | 1190 | 6.0 |

| Food and Measure | cal. | prot. (gms) | carbo. (gms) | fat (gms) | chol. (mgs) | sod. (mgs) | fiber (gms) |
|---|---|---|---|---|---|---|---|
| ***Domino's Pizza*, medium** *(cont.)* | | | | | | | |
| thin crust | 670 | 17.0 | 93.0 | 26.0 | 5 | 120 | 5.0 |
| sauce, entire pizza: | | | | | | | |
| BBQ | 130 | 1.0 | 29.0 | 0 | 0 | 510 | 1.0 |
| garlic Parm | 390 | 3.0 | 4.0 | 40.0 | 20 | 680 | 0 |
| hearty marinara | 80 | 2.0 | 12.0 | 2.5 | 5 | 800 | 2.0 |
| new pizza sauce | 70 | 2.0 | 13.0 | 0 | 0 | 630 | 3.0 |
| cheese, entire pizza: | | | | | | | |
| regular | 380 | 23.0 | 8.0 | 28.0 | 105 | 1250 | 1.0 |
| cheese only/extra | 560 | 34.0 | 12.0 | 42.0 | 155 | 1870 | 2.0 |
| toppings, entire pizza: | | | | | | | |
| anchovies | 110 | 13.0 | 0 | 8.0 | 45 | 3310 | 0 |
| bacon | 340 | 20.0 | 6.0 | 26.0 | 80 | 1260 | 0 |
| banana peppers | 15 | 1.0 | 3.0 | 0 | 0 | 270 | 21.0 |
| beef | 300 | 16.0 | 0 | 26.0 | 65 | 570 | 1.0 |
| cheese, American | 310 | 16.0 | 3.0 | 26.0 | 80 | 1530 | 0 |
| cheese, cheddar | 230 | 140 | 1.0 | 19.0 | 60 | 350 | 0 |
| cheese, feta | 90 | 7.0 | 1.0 | 6.0 | 15 | 380 | 0 |
| cheese, Parmesan | 170 | 13.0 | 1.0 | 12.0 | 35 | 460 | 0 |
| cheese, provolone | 200 | 12.0 | 1.0 | 16.0 | 60 | 470 | 0 |
| chicken | 140 | 22.0 | 3.0 | 4.5 | 60 | 730 | 0 |
| chorizo | 90 | 12.0 | 1.0 | 4.0 | 30 | 600 | 0 |
| garlic | 40 | 2.0 | 9.0 | 0 | 0 | 0 | 0 |
| green chili pepper | 10 | 1.0 | 3.0 | 0 | 0 | 10 | 2.0 |
| green pepper | 10 | 0 | 3.0 | 0 | 0 | 0 | 1.0 |
| ham | 90 | 11.0 | 0 | 4.5 | 35 | 1020 | 0 |
| jalapeños | 15 | 1.0 | 3.0 | 0 | 0 | 960 | 2.0 |
| mushrooms | 20 | 3.0 | 2.0 | 0 | 0 | 25 | 1.0 |
| olives, black | 100 | 1.0 | 2.0 | 10.0 | 0 | 410 | 2.0 |
| olives, green | 100 | 1.0 | 2.0 | 10.0 | 0 | 1250 | 2.0 |
| onions | 15 | 1.0 | 4.0 | 0 | 0 | 5 | 1.0 |
| pepperoni | 240 | 11.0 | 0 | 21.0 | 50 | 1020 | 0 |
| pepperoni, large | 270 | 11.0 | 1.0 | 25.0 | 55 | 960 | 0 |
| Philly steak | 90 | 12.0 | 2.0 | 3.0 | 30 | 500 | 0 |
| pineapple | 60 | 0 | 16.0 | 0 | 0 | 10 | 1.0 |
| roasted red pepper | 10 | 1.0 | 2.0 | 0 | 0 | 95 | 1.0 |
| salami | 220 | 13.0 | 1.0 | 18.0 | 55 | 950 | 0 |
| sausage, Italian | 350 | 12.0 | 9.0 | 30.0 | 55 | 1030 | 0 |
| sausage, sliced | 290 | 15.0 | 0 | 26.0 | 60 | 710 | 0 |
| spinach | 10 | 1.0 | 2.0 | 0 | 0 | 35 | 1.0 |
| tomato | 20 | 1.0 | 5.0 | 0 | 0 | 310 | 2.0 |
| wing sauce | 10 | 0 | 2.0 | 0 | 0 | 920 | 1.0 |
| large, entire pizza: | | | | | | | |
| Brooklyn crust | 750 | 25.0 | 138.0 | 11.0 | 0 | 780 | 5.0 |

| Food and Measure | cal. | prot. (gms) | carbo. (gms) | fat (gms) | chol. (mgs) | sod. (mgs) | fiber (gms) |
|---|---|---|---|---|---|---|---|
| deep dish crust ....... | 1700 | 46.0 | 268.0 | 53.0 | 0 | 2600 | 29.0 |
| hand-tossed crust .... | 1420 | 45.0 | 244.0 | 31.0 | 0 | 1600 | 8.0 |
| thin crust .......... | 920 | 23.0 | 127.0 | 36.0 | 5 | 160 | 7.0 |
| sauce, entire pizza: | | | | | | | |
| BBQ ............ | 180 | 1.0 | 40.0 | 0 | 0 | 720 | 1.0 |
| garlic Parm ...... | 510 | 4.0 | 5.0 | 53.0 | 30 | 910 | 1.0 |
| hearty marinara ... | 100 | 3.0 | 15.0 | 3.0 | 5 | 1060 | 3.0 |
| new pizza sauce ... | 100 | 3.0 | 10.0 | 0 | 0 | 890 | 4.0 |
| cheese, entire pizza: | | | | | | | |
| regular .......... | 530 | 32.0 | 11.0 | 39.0 | 145 | 1750 | 2.0 |
| cheese only/extra .. | 790 | 48.0 | 16.0 | 59.0 | 220 | 2620 | 3.0 |
| toppings, entire pizza: | | | | | | | |
| anchovies ........ | 110 | 13.0 | 0 | 8.0 | 45 | 3310 | 0 |
| bacon ........... | 470 | 29.0 | 9.0 | 36.0 | 110 | 1770 | 0 |
| banana peppers ... | 25 | 1.0 | 5.0 | 0 | 0 | 410 | 3.0 |
| beef ............. | 430 | 22.0 | 0 | 37.0 | 95 | 810 | 1.0 |
| cheese, American .. | 360 | 19.0 | 3.0 | 30.0 | 90 | 1780 | 0 |
| cheese, cheddar ... | 290 | 18.0 | 1.0 | 23.0 | 75 | 440 | 0 |
| cheese, feta ...... | 120 | 10.0 | 1.0 | 8.0 | 20 | 510 | 0 |
| cheese, Parmesan . | 220 | 17.0 | 2.0 | 16.0 | 45 | 610 | 0 |
| cheese, provolone . | 250 | 15.0 | 1.0 | 20.0 | 75 | 590 | 0 |
| chicken .......... | 200 | 31.0 | 5.0 | 6.0 | 80 | 1040 | 0 |
| chorizo .......... | 130 | 17.0 | 1.0 | 6.0 | 45 | 850 | 0 |
| garlic ........... | 50 | 2.0 | 12.0 | 0 | 0 | 5 | 0 |
| green chili pepper . | 15 | 1.0 | 4.0 | 0 | 0 | 15 | 3.0 |
| green pepper ..... | 15 | 1.0 | 4.0 | 0 | 0 | 0 | 1.0 |
| ham ............. | 120 | 15.0 | 0 | 6.0 | 45 | 1360 | 0 |
| jalapeños ........ | 25 | 1.0 | 5.0 | .5 | 0 | 1440 | 2.0 |
| mushrooms ...... | 30 | 4.0 | 3.0 | 0 | 0 | 35 | 1.0 |
| olives, black ...... | 150 | 1.0 | 3.0 | 15.0 | 0 | 620 | 3.0 |
| olives, green ...... | 150 | 1.0 | 3.0 | 15.0 | 0 | 1870 | 3.0 |
| onions .......... | 25 | 1.0 | 5.0 | 0 | 0 | 10 | 1.0 |
| pepperoni ........ | 320 | 15.0 | 0 | 28.0 | 65 | 1370 | 0 |
| pepperoni, large ... | 360 | 15.0 | 1.0 | 33.0 | 70 | 1270 | 0 |
| Philly steak ....... | 120 | 17.0 | 3.0 | 4.5 | 45 | 690 | 0 |
| pineapple ........ | 90 | 1.0 | 23.0 | 0 | 0 | 15 | 1.0 |
| roasted red pepper . | 15 | 1.0 | 3.0 | 0 | 0 | 140 | 1.0 |
| salami .......... | 290 | 18.0 | 2.0 | 24.0 | 70 | 1270 | 0 |
| sausage, Italian ... | 500 | 17.0 | 13.0 | 42.0 | 80 | 1470 | 0 |
| sausage, sliced .... | 390 | 20.0 | 0 | 34.0 | 85 | 940 | 0 |
| spinach ......... | 15 | 2.0 | 2.0 | 0 | 0 | 45 | 1.0 |
| tomato .......... | 30 | 1.0 | 7.0 | 0 | 0 | 450 | 3.0 |
| wing sauce ....... | 15 | 0 | 3.0 | 0 | 0 | 1380 | 1.0 |

| Food and Measure | cal. | prot. (gms) | carbo. (gms) | fat (gms) | chol. (mgs) | sod. (mgs) | fiber (gms) |
|---|---|---|---|---|---|---|---|
| ***Domino's Pizza*** *(cont.)* | | | | | | | |
| pasta, ½ breadbowl: | | | | | | | |
|   chicken Alfredo ...... | 700 | 25.0 | 93.0 | 26.0 | 50 | 1040 | 3.0 |
|   chicken carbonara ... | 740 | 28.0 | 94.0 | 28.0 | 55 | 1110 | 3.0 |
|   mac-n-cheese ....... | 730 | 27.0 | 95.0 | 28.0 | 55 | 1390 | 3.0 |
|   pasta primavera ..... | 670 | 20.0 | 94.0 | 24.0 | 35 | 880 | 4.0 |
|   sausage marinara .... | 730 | 26.0 | 97.0 | 27.0 | 35 | 1380 | 4.0 |
| pasta, dish, 1 bowl: | | | | | | | |
|   chicken Alfredo ...... | 600 | 27.0 | 58.0 | 29.0 | 100 | 1080 | 2.0 |
|   chicken carbonara ... | 670 | 32.0 | 59.0 | 35.0 | 115 | 1220 | 2.0 |
|   mac-n-cheese ....... | 670 | 30.0 | 61.0 | 34.0 | 105 | 1770 | 2.0 |
|   pasta primavera ..... | 540 | 16.0 | 59.0 | 27.0 | 65 | 770 | 3.0 |
|   sausage marinara .... | 670 | 28.0 | 66.0 | 32.0 | 65 | 1760 | 5.0 |
| sandwich, 1 pc.: | | | | | | | |
|   Buffalo chicken ...... | 830 | 42.0 | 74.0 | 41.0 | 115 | 2690 | 3.0 |
|   chicken bacon ranch .. | 870 | 45.0 | 72.0 | 45.0 | 125 | 2380 | 2.0 |
|   chicken Parm ....... | 750 | 47.0 | 73.0 | 30.0 | 120 | 2200 | 3.0 |
|   chicken habanero .... | 800 | 46.0 | 83.0 | 32.0 | 125 | 2170 | 3.0 |
|   Italian ............. | 820 | 41.0 | 70.0 | 41.0 | 130 | 2700 | 3.0 |
|   Philly cheesesteak ... | 690 | 39.0 | 70.0 | 28.0 | 105 | 2120 | 3.0 |
|   sausage and peppers . | 860 | 40.0 | 74.0 | 45.0 | 125 | 2260 | 4.0 |
|   veggie, Mediterranean | 680 | 32.0 | 72.0 | 29.0 | 85 | 2050 | 4.0 |
| salad, no dressing: | | | | | | | |
|   chicken Caesar, ½ .... | 90 | 9.0 | 5.0 | 3.5 | 20 | 290 | 2.0 |
|   garden fresh, ½ ..... | 70 | 4.0 | 5.0 | 3.5 | 10 | 80 | 2.0 |
|   croutons ........... | 90 | 2.0 | 11.0 | 3.5 | 0 | 140 | 0 |
|   dressings: | | | | | | | |
|     blue cheese ...... | 230 | 2.0 | 2.0 | 24.0 | 25 | 440 | 0 |
|     buttermilk ranch ... | 230 | 1.0 | 2.0 | 24.0 | 10 | 390 | 0 |
|     Caesar, creamy .... | 210 | 1.0 | 2.0 | 21.0 | 10 | 520 | 0 |
|     Italian, golden ..... | 210 | 0 | 2.0 | 22.0 | 0 | 360 | 0 |
|     Italian, light ...... | 20 | 0 | 3.0 | 1.0 | 0 | 770 | 0 |
| sides, 1 serving: | | | | | | | |
|   bread, cheesy ....... | 120 | 4.0 | 11.0 | 6.0 | 5 | 140 | 0 |
|   breadstick .......... | 110 | 2.0 | 11.0 | 6.0 | 0 | 100 | 0 |
|   *Buffalo Chicken Kickers* | 100 | 9.0 | 7.0 | 4.5 | 20 | 280 | 0 |
|   Buffalo wings, plain .. | 200 | 16.0 | 1.0 | 14.0 | 50 | 320 | 0 |
|     barbecue ........ | 230 | 17.0 | 6.0 | 14.0 | 50 | 410 | 0 |
|     hot ............. | 200 | 16.0 | 2.0 | 14.0 | 50 | 690 | 0 |
|   dipping cup: | | | | | | | |
|     blue cheese ...... | 240 | 1.0 | 2.0 | 25.0 | 20 | 310 | 0 |
|     garlic ........... | 250 | 0 | 0 | 28.0 | 0 | 160 | 0 |
|     hot ............. | 50 | 0 | 3.0 | 4.5 | 0 | 1480 | 0 |
|     Italian ........... | 220 | 0 | 1.0 | 24.0 | 0 | 460 | 0 |

| Food and Measure | cal. | prot. (gms) | carbo. (gms) | fat (gms) | chol. (mgs) | sod. (mgs) | fiber (gms) |
|---|---|---|---|---|---|---|---|
| marinara ......... | 25 | 1.0 | 5.0 | 0 | 0 | 270 | 0 |
| Parmesan peppercorn | 310 | 2.0 | 3.0 | 33.0 | 15 | 510 | 0 |
| ranch ........... | 200 | 0 | 2.0 | 21.0 | 10 | 340 | 0 |
| dessert: | | | | | | | |
| chocolate lava cake ... | 350 | 4.0 | 47.0 | 17.0 | 65 | 170 | 1.0 |
| *Cinna Stix* .......... | 120 | 2.0 | 14.0 | 6.0 | 0 | 85 | 1.0 |
| dipping icing ..... | 250 | 0 | 57.0 | 2.5 | 0 | 0 | 0 |
| **Donuts** (*Entenmann's*): | | | | | | | |
| plain, 1.75-oz. pc. ..... | 220 | 2.0 | 24.0 | 13.0 | 15 | 230 | <1.0 |
| chocolate frosted: | | | | | | | |
| rich, 2.1-oz. pc. ..... | 300 | 2.0 | 30.0 | 20.0 | 10 | 190 | 1.0 |
| *Pop'ems*, 4 pcs., 2.1 oz. | 320 | 2.0 | 28.0 | 23.0 | 10 | 180 | 1.0 |
| *Softees*, 4 pcs., 2 oz. . | 230 | 2.0 | 24.0 | 14.0 | 20 | 240 | <1.0 |
| crullers, 2 pcs. ........ | 210 | 1.0 | 25.0 | 12.0 | 10 | 140 | 0 |
| crumb, 2.1-oz. pc. ...... | 250 | 2.0 | 36.0 | 12.0 | 10 | 210 | <1.0 |
| devil's food, 1 pc.: | | | | | | | |
| crumb, 2.1 oz. ...... | 250 | 2.0 | 35.0 | 12.0 | 10 | 200 | 1.0 |
| frosted, 2.4 oz. ...... | 310 | 3.0 | 36.0 | 18.0 | 10 | 170 | 2.0 |
| frosted, rich, 2.1 oz. .. | 290 | 2.0 | 30.0 | 19.0 | 10 | 190 | 1.0 |
| glazed, 2.1-oz. pc. ...... | 260 | 2.0 | 34.0 | 13.0 | 15 | 220 | <1.0 |
| *Pop'ems*, 4 pcs., 1.8 oz. | 220 | 2.0 | 30.0 | 10.0 | 0 | 170 | 0 |
| buttermilk, 2.25-oz. pc. | 270 | 2.0 | 37.0 | 13.0 | 15 | 230 | <1.0 |
| powdered sugar, *Softees*, | | | | | | | |
| 4 pcs., 2 oz. ...... | 250 | 3.0 | 32.0 | 12.0 | 25 | 290 | <1.0 |
| **Donuts, gluten free** | | | | | | | |
| (*Glutino*), 2-oz. pc.: | | | | | | | |
| glazed, original ........ | 180 | 3.0 | 26.0 | 7.0 | 30 | 190 | 0 |
| glazed chocolate ....... | 180 | 3.0 | 25.0 | 8.0 | 20 | 180 | 2.0 |
| **Dow gok**, see | | | | | | | |
| "Yard-long bean" | | | | | | | |
| **Dragon fruit** | | | | | | | |
| (*Frieda's*), 3.5 oz. .... | 60 | 2.0 | 0 | 1.5 | 0 | 60 | 0 |
| **Dragon fruit drink**: | | | | | | | |
| (*Snapple* Antioxidant | | | | | | | |
| Water), 8 fl. oz. ....... | 50 | 0 | 12.0 | 0 | 0 | 0 | 0 |
| yumberry (*Apple &* | | | | | | | |
| *Eve*), 8 fl. oz. ......... | 120 | 0 | 28.0 | 0 | 0 | 15 | 0 |
| **Drum**, freshwater, | | | | | | | |
| meat only: | | | | | | | |
| raw, 4 oz. ............ | 135 | 19.9 | 0 | 5.6 | 73 | 85 | 0 |
| baked or broiled, 4 oz. .. | 173 | 25.5 | 0 | 7.2 | 93 | 109 | 0 |
| **Duck**, domesticated, | | | | | | | |
| roasted, 4 oz.: | | | | | | | |
| meat w/skin ........... | 382 | 21.5 | 0 | 32.1 | 95 | 67 | 0 |

| Food and Measure | cal. | prot. (gms) | carbo. (gms) | fat (gms) | chol. (mgs) | sod. (mgs) | fiber (gms) |
|---|---|---|---|---|---|---|---|
| **Duck** *(cont.)* | | | | | | | |
| meat only ........... | 228 | 26.6 | 0 | 12.7 | 101 | 74 | 0 |
| young, Peking: | | | | | | | |
|   breast, meat w/skin .. | 229 | 27.8 | 0 | 12.3 | 154 | 95 | 0 |
|   leg, meat w/skin ..... | 246 | 30.3 | 0 | 12.9 | 129 | 125 | 0 |
| **Duck, frozen**, raw: | | | | | | | |
| breast fillet: | | | | | | | |
|   (*Bell & Evans*), 3 oz. .. | 150 | 22.0 | 1.0 | 7.0 | 115 | 65 | 0 |
|   honey orange (*Bell* | | | | | | | |
|     *& Evans*), 3 oz. ..... | 160 | 18.0 | 3.0 | 8.0 | 100 | 390 | 0 |
|   l'orange (*Maple Leaf* | | | | | | | |
|     *Farms*), 4 oz. ...... | 260 | 15.0 | 3.0 | 21.0 | 95 | 320 | 0 |
| leg quarter (*Maple Leaf* | | | | | | | |
|   *Farms*), 4 oz. ....... | 330 | 16.0 | 0 | 29.0 | 85 | 85 | 0 |
| **Duck, wild**, raw: | | | | | | | |
| meat w/skin, 4 oz. ...... | 239 | 19.8 | 0 | 17.2 | 91 | 64 | 0 |
| breast meat, 4 oz. ...... | 139 | 22.5 | 0 | 4.8 | 87 | 65 | 0 |
| **Duck fat**, 1 tbsp. ....... | 115 | 0 | 0 | 12.8 | 13 | 0 | 0 |
| **Duck sauce**, see "Sweet and sour sauce" | | | | | | | |
| **Duck seasoning mix**, Asian (*Lobo*), ¼ pkt. .. | 30 | 0 | 8.0 | 0 | 0 | 1260 | 0 |
| **Dulce de leche**, spread/ topping, see "Caramel" | | | | | | | |
| **Dumpling, sweet**, frozen (*Pepperidge Farm*): | | | | | | | |
| apple, 1 pc. ........... | 250 | 3.0 | 29.0 | 11.0 | 0 | 300 | 1.0 |
| peach, 1 pc. .......... | 320 | 3.0 | 34.0 | 11.0 | 0 | 220 | 4.0 |
| **Dumpling squash**, see "Sweet dumpling squash" | | | | | | | |
| **Dunkin' Donuts:** | | | | | | | |
| breakfast/sandwiches: | | | | | | | |
|   bacon/egg/cheese: | | | | | | | |
|     bagel ........... | 530 | 24.0 | 66.0 | 19.0 | 205 | 1340 | 5.0 |
|     biscuit .......... | 490 | 18.0 | 35.0 | 30.0 | 205 | 1300 | 1.0 |
|     croissant ........ | 530 | 20.0 | 38.0 | 33.0 | 205 | 1030 | 2.0 |
|     English muffin .... | 370 | 18.0 | 34.0 | 18.0 | 205 | 1030 | 1.0 |
|   chicken biscuit ...... | 500 | 20.0 | 48.0 | 25.0 | 35 | 1260 | 2.0 |
|   egg/cheese: | | | | | | | |
|     bagel ........... | 480 | 20.0 | 66.0 | 15.0 | 200 | 1130 | 5.0 |
|     biscuit .......... | 440 | 14.0 | 35.0 | 27.0 | 200 | 1090 | 1.0 |
|     croissant ........ | 480 | 16.0 | 38.0 | 29.0 | 200 | 820 | 2.0 |
|     English muffin .... | 320 | 14.0 | 34.0 | 15.0 | 200 | 820 | 1.0 |

| Food and Measure | cal. | prot. (gms) | carbo. (gms) | fat (gms) | chol. (mgs) | sod. (mgs) | fiber (gms) |
|---|---|---|---|---|---|---|---|
| ham/egg/cheese: | | | | | | | |
|   bagel | 510 | 26.0 | 66.0 | 16.0 | 215 | 1390 | 5.0 |
|   biscuit | 480 | 19.0 | 35.0 | 28.0 | 215 | 1350 | 1.0 |
|   croissant | 510 | 21.0 | 38.0 | 31.0 | 215 | 1080 | 2.0 |
|   English muffin | 360 | 20.0 | 34.0 | 16.0 | 215 | 1080 | 1.0 |
| sausage biscuit | 450 | 12.0 | 33.0 | 28.0 | 45 | 1020 | 1.0 |
| sausage/egg/cheese: | | | | | | | |
|   bagel | 680 | 29.0 | 67.0 | 32.0 | 250 | 1590 | 5.0 |
|   biscuit | 640 | 22.0 | 36.0 | 44.0 | 250 | 1550 | 1.0 |
|   croissant | 680 | 24.0 | 39.0 | 46.0 | 250 | 1280 | 2.0 |
|   English muffin | 520 | 23.0 | 34.0 | 31.0 | 250 | 1280 | 1.0 |
| hash browns, 9 pc. | 200 | 2.0 | 22.0 | 11.0 | 0 | 730 | 3.0 |
| *Wake-Up Wrap:* | | | | | | | |
|   bacon/egg/cheese | 210 | 10.0 | 14.0 | 12.0 | 105 | 580 | 1.0 |
|   egg/cheese | 180 | 8.0 | 14.0 | 11.0 | 105 | 470 | 1.0 |
|   egg white, cheese | 150 | 8.0 | 13.0 | 7.0 | 10 | 480 | 1.0 |
|   egg white, turkey | 150 | 11.0 | 14.0 | 5.0 | 15 | 400 | 1.0 |
|   egg white, veggies | 150 | 10.0 | 14.0 | 6.0 | 15 | 340 | 1.0 |
|   ham/egg/cheese | 200 | 11.0 | 14.0 | 11.0 | 115 | 600 | 1.0 |
|   sausage/egg/cheese | 280 | 12.0 | 14.0 | 19.0 | 130 | 700 | 1.0 |
| flatbread sandwich: | | | | | | | |
|   cheese, grilled | 380 | 16.0 | 35.0 | 18.0 | 45 | 850 | 1.0 |
|   egg white/turkey | 280 | 19.0 | 32.0 | 8.0 | 15 | 770 | 3.0 |
|   egg white/veggie | 280 | 16.0 | 32.0 | 10.0 | 20 | 690 | 3.0 |
|   ham/cheese | 320 | 20.0 | 34.0 | 11.0 | 40 | 960 | 2.0 |
|   turkey/cheddar/bacon | 410 | 21.0 | 36.0 | 20.0 | 50 | 1110 | 1.0 |
| bagel, plain | 320 | 11.0 | 63.0 | 2.5 | 0 | 660 | 5.0 |
|   blueberry | 330 | 11.0 | 65.0 | 3.0 | 0 | 620 | 5.0 |
|   cinnamon raisin | 330 | 11.0 | 65.0 | 3.5 | 0 | 450 | 5.0 |
|   everything | 350 | 13.0 | 66.0 | 4.5 | 0 | 660 | 5.0 |
|   garlic | 340 | 12.0 | 68.0 | 2.5 | 0 | 660 | 6.0 |
|   multigrain | 390 | 14.0 | 65.0 | 8.0 | 0 | 560 | 9.0 |
|   onion | 310 | 11.0 | 63.0 | 2.0 | 0 | 380 | 3.0 |
|   poppy seed | 350 | 13.0 | 64.0 | 6.0 | 0 | 660 | 5.0 |
|   salt | 320 | 11.0 | 63.0 | 2.5 | 0 | 3420 | 5.0 |
|   sesame | 360 | 13.0 | 63.0 | 6.0 | 0 | 660 | 5.0 |
|   twist, cheddar | 400 | 17.0 | 63.0 | 9.0 | 20 | 800 | 5.0 |
|   twist, chocolate chip | 340 | 10.0 | 66.0 | 4.0 | 0 | 530 | 4.0 |
|   twist, cinnamon | 350 | 11.0 | 72.0 | 3.5 | 0 | 460 | 5.0 |
|   wheat | 320 | 12.0 | 61.0 | 3.5 | 0 | 550 | 5.0 |
| biscuit | 280 | 5.0 | 32.0 | 14.0 | 0 | 620 | 1.0 |
| brownie | 440 | 3.0 | 58.0 | 23.0 | 55 | 250 | 1.0 |
| croissant, plain | 310 | 7.0 | 35.0 | 16.0 | 0 | 350 | 1.0 |

| Food and Measure | cal. | prot. (gms) | carbo. (gms) | fat (gms) | chol. (mgs) | sod. (mgs) | fiber (gms) |
|---|---|---|---|---|---|---|---|
| **Dunkin' Donuts** (cont.) | | | | | | | |
| cookie, chocolate chunk: | | | | | | | |
|   reverse | 380 | 5.0 | 50.0 | 18.0 | 40 | 320 | 2.0 |
|   triple | 360 | 5.0 | 53.0 | 15.0 | 35 | 380 | 2.0 |
| cookie, oatmeal raisin | 320 | 5.0 | 54.0 | 9.0 | 30 | 210 | 3.0 |
| Danish: | | | | | | | |
|   apple cheese | 330 | 4.0 | 41.0 | 16.0 | 0 | 270 | 1.0 |
|   cheese | 330 | 5.0 | 39.0 | 17.0 | 5 | 270 | 1.0 |
|   strawberry cheese | 320 | 4.0 | 40.0 | 16.0 | 0 | 260 | 1.0 |
| donuts/sticks: | | | | | | | |
|   apple crumb | 490 | 4.0 | 80.0 | 18.0 | 0 | 350 | 2.0 |
|   apple 'n spice | 270 | 3.0 | 32.0 | 14.0 | 0 | 350 | 1.0 |
|   Bavarian Kreme | 270 | 4.0 | 31.0 | 15.0 | 0 | 350 | 1.0 |
|   banana, chocolate dip | 290 | 5.0 | 41.0 | 12.0 | 0 | 260 | 2.0 |
|   blueberry cake | 340 | 4.0 | 44.0 | 17.0 | 30 | 570 | 1.0 |
|   blueberry crumb | 500 | 4.0 | 84.0 | 18.0 | 0 | 350 | 2.0 |
|   Boston Kreme | 310 | 3.0 | 39.0 | 16.0 | 0 | 370 | 1.0 |
|   Boston Kreme, cocoa | 280 | 5.0 | 39.0 | 13.0 | 0 | 270 | 2.0 |
|   bow tie | 310 | 4.0 | 39.0 | 15.0 | 0 | 400 | 1.0 |
|   chocolate cake, double | 380 | 4.0 | 36.0 | 25.0 | 0 | 410 | 2.0 |
|   chocolate coconut | 550 | 5.0 | 47.0 | 39.0 | 0 | 390 | 2.0 |
|   chocolate frosted | 270 | 3.0 | 31.0 | 15.0 | 0 | 340 | 1.0 |
|   chocolate frosted cake | 370 | 4.0 | 45.0 | 23.0 | 25 | 320 | 1.0 |
|   chocolate frosted cocoa | 250 | 4.0 | 32.0 | 11.0 | 0 | 260 | 2.0 |
|   chocolate frosted | | | | | | | |
|     coffee roll | 410 | 7.0 | 53.0 | 19.0 | 0 | 420 | 3.0 |
|   chocolate glazed cake | 370 | 3.0 | 35.0 | 24.0 | 0 | 390 | 1.0 |
|   chocolate Kreme fill | 370 | 4.0 | 42.0 | 21.0 | 0 | 370 | 1.0 |
|   cinnamon cake | 340 | 3.0 | 38.0 | 22.0 | 25 | 300 | 1.0 |
|   cinnamon cake stick | 350 | 4.0 | 44.0 | 18.0 | 35 | 420 | 2.0 |
|   cocoa butternut | 260 | 4.0 | 36.0 | 11.0 | 0 | 250 | 2.0 |
|   cocoa coconut | 260 | 5.0 | 33.0 | 13.0 | 0 | 260 | 2.0 |
|   cocoa coffee roll | 310 | 5.0 | 44.0 | 14.0 | 0 | 360 | 3.0 |
|   cocoa confetti | 270 | 4.0 | 35.0 | 12.0 | 0 | 260 | 2.0 |
|   cocoa glazed | 240 | 4.0 | 32.0 | 11.0 | 0 | 240 | 2.0 |
|   cocoa Kreme puff | 300 | 4.0 | 34.0 | 16.0 | 0 | 260 | 2.0 |
|   coffee roll | 400 | 7.0 | 53.0 | 18.0 | 0 | 400 | 3.0 |
|   dulce de chocolate | 350 | 4.0 | 45.0 | 17.0 | 5 | 360 | 2.0 |
|   dulce de leche | 290 | 4.0 | 31.0 | 16.0 | 0 | 340 | 1.0 |
|   eclair | 390 | 5.0 | 52.0 | 19.0 | 0 | 360 | 2.0 |
|   French crueller | 250 | 2.0 | 18.0 | 20.0 | 35 | 105 | 0 |
|   glazed | 260 | 3.0 | 31.0 | 14.0 | 0 | 330 | 1.0 |
|   glazed cake | 360 | 3.0 | 44.0 | 22.0 | 25 | 300 | 1.0 |

| Food and Measure | cal. | prot. (gms) | carbo. (gms) | fat (gms) | chol. (mgs) | sod. (mgs) | fiber (gms) |
|---|---|---|---|---|---|---|---|
| glazed cake stick ..... | 370 | 4.0 | 48.0 | 18.0 | 35 | 420 | 1.0 |
| glazed cake stick, | | | | | | | |
| chocolate ........ | 390 | 3.0 | 40.0 | 25.0 | 0 | 540 | 2.0 |
| jelly, cocoa ......... | 300 | 5.0 | 45.0 | 12.0 | 0 | 260 | 2.0 |
| jelly filled .......... | 290 | 3.0 | 36.0 | 14.0 | 0 | 340 | 1.0 |
| jelly stick ........... | 420 | 4.0 | 60.0 | 18.0 | 35 | 440 | 1.0 |
| lemon filled ......... | 270 | 4.0 | 31.0 | 15.0 | 0 | 350 | 1.0 |
| maple frosted ....... | 270 | 3.0 | 32.0 | 15.0 | 0 | 340 | 1.0 |
| maple frosted cocoa .. | 250 | 4.0 | 33.0 | 11.0 | 0 | 250 | 2.0 |
| marble frosted ...... | 270 | 3.0 | 32.0 | 15.0 | 0 | 340 | 1.0 |
| old fashioned cake ... | 320 | 3.0 | 33.0 | 22.0 | 25 | 300 | 1.0 |
| piña boom ......... | 270 | 4.0 | 32.0 | 15.0 | 0 | 350 | 1.0 |
| piña colada ......... | 330 | 4.0 | 42.0 | 17.0 | 0 | 380 | 1.0 |
| powdered cake ...... | 340 | 4.0 | 38.0 | 22.0 | 25 | 300 | 1.0 |
| powdered cake stick .. | 360 | 5.0 | 43.0 | 18.0 | 35 | 420 | 2.0 |
| powdered cocoa ..... | 220 | 5.0 | 25.0 | 11.0 | 0 | 240 | 2.0 |
| strawberry frosted ... | 280 | 3.0 | 32.0 | 15.0 | 0 | 340 | 1.0 |
| stick, plain ......... | 330 | 4.0 | 36.0 | 18.0 | 35 | 420 | 1.0 |
| sugar raised ........ | 230 | 3.0 | 22.0 | 14.0 | 0 | 330 | 1.0 |
| sugared cocoa ...... | 200 | 4.0 | 23.0 | 11.0 | 0 | 240 | 2.0 |
| triple cocoa ......... | 260 | 5.0 | 35.0 | 12.0 | 0 | 260 | 2.0 |
| vanilla Kreme filled ... | 380 | 4.0 | 42.0 | 23.0 | 0 | 370 | 1.0 |
| fritters: | | | | | | | |
| apple .............. | 410 | 6.0 | 60.0 | 17.0 | 0 | 380 | 2.0 |
| cocoa, double ....... | 430 | 5.0 | 62.0 | 19.0 | 0 | 430 | 3.0 |
| glazed ............. | 410 | 6.0 | 60.0 | 17.0 | 0 | 380 | 2.0 |
| vanilla cocoa ........ | 440 | 5.0 | 63.0 | 20.0 | 0 | 420 | 2.0 |
| *Munchkins*, 1 pc.: | | | | | | | |
| cake, plain ......... | 60 | 1.0 | 6.0 | 3.5 | 5 | 65 | 0 |
| cake, glazed ........ | 70 | 1.0 | 8.0 | 3.5 | 5 | 65 | 0 |
| cake, powdered ..... | 60 | 1.0 | 7.0 | 3.5 | 5 | 65 | 0 |
| chocolate cake glazed . | 70 | 1.0 | 8.0 | 3.5 | 0 | 85 | 0 |
| cinnamon cake ...... | 60 | 1.0 | 6.0 | 3.5 | 5 | 65 | 0 |
| cocoa Kreme puff .... | 50 | 1.0 | 7.0 | 2.5 | 0 | 45 | 0 |
| glazed ............. | 70 | 1.0 | 7.0 | 4.0 | 0 | 80 | 0 |
| glazed, cocoa ....... | 35 | 1.0 | 6.0 | 3.5 | 5 | 65 | 0 |
| jelly filled .......... | 80 | 1.0 | 9.0 | 4.0 | 0 | 85 | 0 |
| sugared ........... | 60 | 1.0 | 6.0 | 3.5 | 5 | 65 | 0 |
| muffin, English ........ | 160 | 5.0 | 31.0 | 2.0 | 0 | 350 | 1.0 |
| muffins: | | | | | | | |
| blueberry .......... | 480 | 6.0 | 81.0 | 15.0 | 65 | 470 | 2.0 |
| blueberry, reduced fat . | 430 | 6.0 | 80.0 | 9.0 | 65 | 650 | 2.0 |
| chocolate, triple ..... | 630 | 7.0 | 80.0 | 31.0 | 10 | 440 | 4.0 |

| Food and Measure | cal. | prot. (gms) | carbo. (gms) | fat (gms) | chol. (mgs) | sod. (mgs) | fiber (gms) |
|---|---|---|---|---|---|---|---|
| **Dunkin' Donuts, muffins** (cont.) | | | | | | | |
| chocolate chip ...... | 590 | 7.0 | 92.0 | 22.0 | 70 | 490 | 3.0 |
| coffee cake muffin ... | 630 | 7.0 | 95.0 | 25.0 | 70 | 510 | 1.0 |
| corn ............. | 490 | 6.0 | 80.0 | 16.0 | 75 | 820 | 1.0 |
| coffee, hot, 10 fl. oz.: | | | | | | | |
| plain ............. | 5 | 0 | 1.0 | 0 | 0 | 5 | 0 |
| w/cream ......... | 60 | 1.0 | 2.0 | 6.0 | 20 | 20 | 0 |
| w/cream, sugar ... | 120 | 1.0 | 19.0 | 6.0 | 20 | 20 | 0 |
| w/milk .......... | 25 | 1.0 | 2.0 | 1.0 | 5 | 20 | 0 |
| w/milk, sugar ..... | 80 | 1.0 | 20.0 | 1.0 | 5 | 20 | 0 |
| blueberry, cinnamon, | | | | | | | |
| or raspberry ...... | 15 | 0 | 2.0 | 0 | 0 | 5 | 0 |
| caramel ........... | 10 | 0 | 2.0 | 0 | 0 | 5 | 0 |
| coconut, hazelnut, | | | | | | | |
| or French vanilla ... | 10 | 0 | 1.0 | 0 | 0 | 5 | 0 |
| mocha ............ | 110 | 1.0 | 26.0 | 0 | 0 | 20 | 1.0 |
| w/cream ......... | 170 | 2.0 | 27.0 | 6.0 | 20 | 30 | 1.0 |
| coffee, iced, 16 fl. oz.: | | | | | | | |
| plain ............. | 10 | 1.0 | 2.0 | 0 | 0 | 5 | 0 |
| w/cream ......... | 70 | 1.0 | 3.0 | 6.0 | 20 | 20 | 0 |
| w/cream, sugar ... | 120 | 1.0 | 20.0 | 6.0 | 20 | 20 | 0 |
| w/milk .......... | 30 | 2.0 | 3.0 | 1.0 | 5 | 20 | 0 |
| w/milk, sugar ..... | 90 | 2.0 | 21.0 | 1.0 | 5 | 20 | 0 |
| *Dunkin' Dark* roast | | | | | | | |
| w/cream, sugar ... | 130 | 1.0 | 20.0 | 6.0 | 20 | 20 | 0 |
| mocha, w/cream ..... | 180 | 2.0 | 28.0 | 6.0 | 20 | 35 | 1.0 |
| *Coolatta*, 16 fl. oz.: | | | | | | | |
| coffee, w/cream ..... | 400 | 3.0 | 49.0 | 23.0 | 80 | 75 | 0 |
| coffee, w/milk ....... | 240 | 4.0 | 50.0 | 4.0 | 15 | 90 | 0 |
| coffee, w/skim milk ... | 210 | 4.0 | 51.0 | 0 | 0 | 90 | 0 |
| orange, *Tropicana* .... | 230 | 1.0 | 57.0 | 0 | 0 | 40 | 0 |
| strawberry fruit ...... | 310 | 0 | 75.0 | 0 | 0 | 45 | 0 |
| vanilla bean ......... | 430 | 3.0 | 91.0 | 6.0 | 20 | 170 | 0 |
| espresso drinks, hot: | | | | | | | |
| cappuccino, small .... | 80 | 4.0 | 7.0 | 4.0 | 15 | 70 | 0 |
| w/sugar ......... | 140 | 4.0 | 24.0 | 4.0 | 15 | 70 | 0 |
| espresso ........... | 5 | 0 | 1.0 | 0 | 0 | 5 | 0 |
| w/sugar ......... | 30 | 0 | 7.0 | 0 | 0 | 5 | 0 |
| latte, 10 fl. oz.: | | | | | | | |
| caramel swirl ..... | 220 | 8.0 | 35.0 | 6.0 | 25 | 150 | 0 |
| lite latte ........ | 80 | 7.0 | 13.0 | 0 | 0 | 110 | 0 |
| mocha raspberry .. | 230 | 7.0 | 36.0 | 6.0 | 25 | 110 | 1.0 |
| mocha spice ...... | 220 | 7.0 | 35.0 | 6.0 | 25 | 95 | 1.0 |
| vanilla lite ........ | 90 | 7.0 | 14.0 | 0 | 0 | 110 | 0 |

| Food and Measure | cal. | prot. (gms) | carbo. (gms) | fat (gms) | chol. (mgs) | sod. (mgs) | fiber (gms) |
|---|---|---|---|---|---|---|---|
| *Turbo Shot*, large .... | 10 | 0 | 2.0 | 0 | 0 | 15 | 0 |
| latte, iced, 16 fl. oz.: | | | | | | | |
| w/milk ............. | 120 | 6.0 | 10.0 | 6.0 | 25 | 105 | 0 |
| w/milk, sugar ....... | 170 | 6.0 | 27.0 | 6.0 | 25 | 100 | 0 |
| w/skim milk ........ | 70 | 7.0 | 11.0 | 0 | 0 | 110 | 0 |
| w/skim milk, sugar ... | 130 | 7.0 | 28.0 | 0 | 0 | 110 | 0 |
| caramel swirl ....... | 220 | 8.0 | 35.0 | 6.0 | 25 | 150 | 0 |
| w/skim milk ...... | 180 | 9.0 | 36.0 | 0 | 5 | 150 | 0 |
| mocha raspberry .... | 230 | 7.0 | 36.0 | 6.0 | 25 | 110 | 1.0 |
| mocha spice ........ | 220 | 7.0 | 35.0 | 6.0 | 25 | 95 | 1.0 |
| mocha swirl ........ | 220 | 7.0 | 35.0 | 6.0 | 25 | 115 | 1.0 |
| vanilla lite .......... | 90 | 7.0 | 14.0 | 0 | 0 | 110 | 0 |
| drinks, other: | | | | | | | |
| *Dunkaccino*, small ... | 230 | 2.0 | 35.0 | 11.0 | 10 | 5 | 0 |
| hot chocolate, small .. | 220 | 2.0 | 39.0 | 7.0 | 0 | 270 | 2.0 |
| caramel, small .... | 230 | 2.0 | 40.0 | 7.0 | 0 | 270 | 2.0 |
| white, small ...... | 230 | 2.0 | 38.0 | 8.0 | 5 | 310 | 1.0 |
| vanilla chai, 14 fl. oz. . | 330 | 11.0 | 53.0 | 8.0 | 10 | 180 | 1.0 |
| **Durian,** fresh: | | | | | | | |
| ½ of 1.3-lb. fruit ....... | 442 | 4.4 | 81.5 | 16.0 | 0 | 3 | 11.4 |
| chopped, ½ cup ....... | 179 | 1.8 | 32.9 | 6.5 | 0 | 2 | 4.6 |
| **Durian, frozen** | | | | | | | |
| (*Frieda's*), chopped, | | | | | | | |
| 1 cup, 8.6 oz. ....... | 357 | 4.0 | 66.0 | 13.0 | 0 | 5 | 10.0 |

# E

| Food and Measure | cal. | prot. (gms) | carbo. (gms) | fat (gms) | chol. (mgs) | sod. (mgs) | fiber (gms) |
|---|---|---|---|---|---|---|---|
| **Eclair**, fresh (*Entenmann's*), 3.6-oz. pc. .. | 260 | 3.0 | 46.0 | 9.0 | 65 | 190 | 3.0 |
| **Eclair, frozen**: | | | | | | | |
| (*Smart Ones*), 2-oz. pc. ... | 140 | 3.0 | 24.0 | 4.0 | 30 | 180 | 1.0 |
| mini (*Roland*), 6 pcs.: | | | | | | | |
| w/chocolate ........ | 260 | 4.0 | 23.0 | 17.0 | 85 | 70 | 1.0 |
| w/out chocolate ..... | 220 | 3.0 | 19.0 | 14.0 | 90 | 70 | 0 |
| **Edamame** (see also "Soybean"), fresh (*Frieda's*), ½ cup in pod or 1 cup shelled .. | 100 | 8.0 | 10.0 | 3.0 | 0 | 10 | 3.0 |
| **Edamame, frozen**: | | | | | | | |
| in pod: | | | | | | | |
| (*Cascadian Farm* Organic), ⅔ cup edible ..... | 120 | 10.0 | 9.0 | 5.0 | 0 | 10 | 3.0 |
| (*C&W* Soybeans), 1 cup in pod ...... | 110 | 9.0 | 12.0 | 3.5 | 0 | 0 | 9.0 |
| shelled: | | | | | | | |
| (*Cascadian Farm* Organic), ⅔ cup ... | 120 | 10.0 | 9.0 | 5.0 | 0 | 10 | 3.0 |
| (*C&W* Soybeans), ½ cup ........... | 100 | 10.0 | 7.0 | 3.5 | 0 | 5 | 7.0 |
| (*Seapoint Farms* Regular/ Organic), ½ cup ... | 100 | 8.0 | 9.0 | 3.0 | 0 | 30 | 4.0 |
| (*Seapoint Farms* Salted), ½ cup ........... | 100 | 8.0 | 9.0 | 3.0 | 0 | 260 | 4.0 |
| **Edamame combinations** (*Seapoint Farms* Veggie Blends), frozen: | | | | | | | |
| Eat Your Greens, 3 oz. ... | 60 | 5.0 | 7.0 | 1.5 | 0 | 30 | 3.0 |
| garden blend, ¾ cup .... | 60 | 4.0 | 7.0 | 1.5 | 0 | 25 | 3.0 |
| oriental blend, ¾ cup ... | 60 | 4.0 | 8.0 | 1.0 | 0 | 20 | 3.0 |

| Food and Measure | cal. | prot. (gms) | carbo. (gms) | fat (gms) | chol. (mgs) | sod. (mgs) | fiber (gms) |
|---|---|---|---|---|---|---|---|
| **Edamame snack:** | | | | | | | |
| dry-roasted (*Seapoint Farms*): | | | | | | | |
| goji blend, 1 oz. ..... | 120 | 11.0 | 15.0 | 3.0 | 0 | 140 | 7.0 |
| lightly salted, ¼ cup .. | 130 | 14.0 | 10.0 | 4.0 | 0 | 150 | 8.0 |
| wasabi, ¼ cup ...... | 130 | 14.0 | 9.0 | 4.5 | 0 | 130 | 7.0 |
| roasted (*Roland Feng Shui*), ¼ cup ...... | 130 | 13.0 | 9.0 | 4.0 | 0 | 230 | 7.0 |
| **Edamame dip,** 2 tbsp.: | | | | | | | |
| (*Emerald Valley*) ....... | 70 | 2.0 | 3.0 | 6.0 | 0 | 190 | 1.0 |
| ginger wasabi (*Emerald Valley*) ............ | 70 | 2.0 | 4.0 | 5.0 | 0 | 180 | <1.0 |
| **Eel,** meat only: | | | | | | | |
| raw, 4 oz. ............ | 209 | 20.9 | 0 | 3.2 | 143 | 58 | 0 |
| baked or broiled, 4 oz. .. | 268 | 26.8 | 0 | 17.0 | 183 | 74 | 0 |
| **Eel, smoked,** canned in oil (*Roland*), ⅓ cup, 2 oz. ........ | 230 | 8.0 | 0 | 22.0 | 30 | 355 | 0 |
| **Egg, chicken:** | | | | | | | |
| raw, 1 large: | | | | | | | |
| whole ............. | 75 | 6.3 | .6 | 5.0 | 213 | 63 | 0 |
| white only ......... | 17 | 3.5 | .3 | 0 | 0 | 55 | 0 |
| yolk only (w/small portion white) .... | 59 | 2.8 | .3 | 5.1 | 213 | 7 | 0 |
| raw, white only: | | | | | | | |
| (*All Whites*), ¼ cup ... | 30 | 6.0 | 1.0 | 0 | 0 | 95 | 0 |
| (*Egg Beaters*), 3 tbsp. . | 25 | 5.0 | 1.0 | 0 | 0 | 75 | 0 |
| (*Organic Valley*), ¼ cup ............ | 25 | 5.0 | 1.0 | 0 | 0 | 90 | 0 |
| hard-boiled, chopped, 1 cup ............. | 210 | 17.1 | 1.5 | 14.4 | 578 | 169 | 0 |
| **Egg, chicken, dried:** | | | | | | | |
| whole: | | | | | | | |
| 1 oz. .............. | 168 | 13.0 | 1.4 | 11.9 | 544 | 148 | 0 |
| stabilized, 1 oz. ...... | 174 | 13.7 | .7 | 12.5 | 572 | 155 | 0 |
| white, flakes, 1 oz. ..... | 100 | 21.8 | 1.2 | <.1 | 0 | 328 | 0 |
| yolk, 1 oz. ......... | 195 | 8.7 | .1 | 17.4 | 830 | 26 | 0 |
| **Egg, duck,** 1 egg ...... | 130 | 9.0 | 1.0 | 9.6 | 619 | 102 | 0 |
| **Egg, goose,** 1 egg ...... | 267 | 20.0 | 1.9 | 19.1 | 1227 | 199 | 0 |
| **Egg, quail,** | | | | | | | |
| fresh, 1 egg ............ | 14 | 1.2 | <.1 | 1.0 | 76 | 13 | 0 |
| canned (*Roland*), 6 eggs . | 80 | 6.0 | 1.0 | 6.0 | 110 | 90 | 0 |
| **Egg, substitute,** ¼ cup: | | | | | | | |
| (*Better'n Eggs*) ........ | 30 | 6.0 | 1.0 | 0 | 0 | 120 | 0 |

| Food and Measure | cal. | prot. (gms) | carbo. (gms) | fat (gms) | chol. (mgs) | sod. (mgs) | fiber (gms) |
|---|---|---|---|---|---|---|---|
| **Egg, substitute** *(cont.)* | | | | | | | |
| (*Better'n Eggs* Plus) .... | 35 | 6.0 | 1.0 | 0 | 0 | 105 | 0 |
| (*Egg Beaters*) ......... | 30 | 6.0 | 1.0 | 0 | 0 | 115 | 0 |
| cheese/chive (*Egg Beaters*) ........... | 35 | 5.0 | 1.0 | 1.0 | <5 | 210 | 0 |
| Southwest (*Egg Beaters*) ........... | 30 | 5.0 | 1.0 | 0 | 0 | 180 | 0 |
| vegetable, garden (*Egg Beaters*) ....... | 30 | 5.0 | 1.0 | 0 | 0 | 160 | 0 |
| **Egg, turkey**, 1 egg ..... | 135 | 10.8 | .9 | 9.4 | 737 | 119 | 0 |
| **Egg breakfast**, frozen (see also "Breakfast sandwich" and specific listings), 1 pkg., except as noted: | | | | | | | |
| omelet: | | | | | | | |
| cheese, 3 (*Jimmy Dean*), ½ of 8.6-oz. pkg. ...... | 290 | 16.0 | 4.0 | 23.0 | 305 | 830 | 1.0 |
| ham/cheese (*Aunt Jemima*), 5.2 oz. .. | 240 | 12.0 | 17.0 | 14.0 | 195 | 710 | 2.0 |
| ham/cheese (*Jimmy Dean*), ½ of 8.6-oz. pkg. ...... | 250 | 16.0 | 4.0 | 19.0 | 295 | 770 | 0 |
| sausage/cheese (*Jimmy Dean*), ½ of 8.6-oz. pkg. ...... | 270 | 15.0 | 5.0 | 22.0 | 295 | 570 | 0 |
| omelet, egg white (*Cedarlane*): | | | | | | | |
| green chili/cheese/ ranchero, 8.5 oz. .. | 240 | 18.0 | 21.0 | 10.0 | 30 | 700 | 2.0 |
| spinach/mushroom, 8 oz. ............ | 270 | 23.0 | 18.0 | 12.0 | 30 | 670 | 2.0 |
| turkey bacon/vegetable/ cheese, 8 oz. ..... | 300 | 24.0 | 21.0 | 13.0 | 45 | 640 | 1.0 |
| scrambled, w/potatoes: | | | | | | | |
| bacon (*Jimmy Dean* Bowl), 8 oz. ...... | 520 | 30.0 | 22.0 | 34.0 | 395 | 1490 | 3.0 |
| cheesy (*Smart Ones*), 6.5 oz. .......... | 210 | 15.0 | 18.0 | 9.0 | 70 | 510 | 3.0 |
| ham (*Aunt Jemima*), 6.8 oz. .......... | 260 | 16.0 | 21.0 | 13.0 | 195 | 920 | 2.0 |
| ham (*Jimmy Dean* Bowl), 8 oz. ...... | 390 | 24.0 | 23.0 | 23.0 | 360 | 1170 | 3.0 |

| Food and Measure | cal. | prot. (gms) | carbo. (gms) | fat (gms) | chol. (mgs) | sod. (mgs) | fiber (gms) |
|---|---|---|---|---|---|---|---|
| ham/cheese (*Smart Ones*), 6.5 oz. . . . . . | 220 | 21.0 | 13.0 | 9.0 | 65 | 610 | 2.0 |
| sausage (*Aunt Jemima*), 6.8 oz. . . . . . . . . . | 300 | 15.0 | 21.0 | 18.0 | 200 | 890 | 2.0 |
| sausage (*Jimmy Dean* Bowl), 8.6 oz. . . . . . | 710 | 12.0 | 91.0 | 34.0 | 265 | 1000 | 2.0 |
| sausage/gravy (*Jimmy Dean* Bowl), 9.8 oz. | 380 | 15.0 | 29.0 | 23.0 | 270 | 1020 | 3.0 |
| turkey bacon (*Jimmy Dean D-lights* Bowl), 8.5 oz. . . . . . | 240 | 19.0 | 20.0 | 9.0 | 25 | 760 | 2.0 |
| turkey sausage (*Jimmy Dean D-lights* Bowl), 7 oz. . . . . . . | 230 | 23.0 | 19.0 | 7.0 | 20 | 700 | 2.0 |
| scrambled, hash browns: | | | | | | | |
| bacon (*Aunt Jemima*), 5.25 oz. . . . . . . . . | 300 | 15.0 | 14.0 | 20.0 | 340 | 910 | 1.0 |
| bacon/cheese (*Jimmy Dean*), 8 oz. . . . . . . | 390 | 16.0 | 36.0 | 19.0 | 345 | 860 | 3.0 |
| sausage (*Aunt Jemima*), 6.25 oz. . . . . . . . . | 360 | 16.0 | 15.0 | 26.0 | 385 | 940 | 1.0 |
| sausage/cheese (*Jimmy Dean*), 8 oz. . . . . . . | 390 | 15.0 | 36.0 | 20.0 | 320 | 820 | 3.0 |
| **Egg roll** (see also "Spring roll"): | | | | | | | |
| (*Empire Kosher* Mini), 4 pcs., 3 oz. . . . . . . . . | 110 | 3.0 | 15.0 | 4.5 | 0 | 470 | 2.0 |
| chicken (*Michelina's*), 6 pcs., 3 oz. . . . . . . . . | 170 | 5.0 | 22.0 | 7.0 | 5 | 440 | 1.0 |
| shrimp (*Michelina's*), 6 pcs., 3 oz. . . . . . . . . | 170 | 4.0 | 23.0 | 7.0 | 5 | 360 | 1.0 |
| spinach (*Health is Wealth*), 3-oz. pc. . . . . | 170 | 8.0 | 18.0 | 8.0 | 0 | 310 | 3.0 |
| vegetable (*Health is Wealth*), 3-oz. pc. . . . . | 130 | 4.0 | 21.0 | 4.0 | 0 | 550 | 3.0 |
| **Egg roll entree**, frozen, vegetable (*Lean Cuisine*), 9-oz. pkg. . . . | 320 | 8.0 | 62.0 | 4.0 | 0 | 630 | 2.0 |
| **Egg roll wrapper** (see also "Wrappers"): | | | | | | | |
| (*Frieda's*), 2 pcs. . . . . . . . | 120 | 3.0 | 27.0 | 1.0 | 5 | 240 | 1.0 |
| (*Nasoya*), 3 pcs. . . . . . . . | 170 | 7.0 | 35.0 | .5 | 10 | 410 | 1.0 |
| **Eggnog**, chilled, ½ cup: | | | | | | | |
| (*Hood* Golden) . . . . . . . . | 180 | 4.0 | 22.0 | 9.0 | 65 | 95 | 0 |

| Food and Measure | cal. | prot. (gms) | carbo. (gms) | fat (gms) | chol. (mgs) | sod. (mgs) | fiber (gms) |
|---|---|---|---|---|---|---|---|
| **Eggnog** *(cont.)* | | | | | | | |
| (*Hood* Light) . . . . . . . . . | 140 | 4.0 | 22.0 | 4.0 | 45 | 95 | 0 |
| (*Turkey Hill*) . . . . . . . . . | 190 | 5.0 | 23.0 | 9.0 | 65 | 90 | 0 |
| cinnamon (*Hood*) . . . . . . | 180 | 4.0 | 21.0 | 9.0 | 60 | 115 | 0 |
| sugar cookie (*Hood*) . . . . | 180 | 4.0 | 22.0 | 9.0 | 65 | 110 | 0 |
| vanilla: | | | | | | | |
| (*Hood*) . . . . . . . . . . . . | 180 | 4.0 | 22.0 | 9.0 | 65 | 95 | 0 |
| (*Turkey Hill* Light) . . . . | 150 | 5.0 | 23.0 | 4.5 | 45 | 95 | 0 |
| **"Eggnog," nondairy**, | | | | | | | |
| soy (*Silk* Nog), ½ cup . | 90 | 3.0 | 15.0 | 2.0 | 0 | 75 | 0 |
| **Eggplant,** fresh: | | | | | | | |
| raw (*Frieda's* Chinese/ | | | | | | | |
| Japanese), cubed, | | | | | | | |
| 1 cup . . . . . . . . . . . . | 20 | 1.0 | 5.0 | 0 | 0 | 2 | 3.0 |
| raw, 1" pcs., ½ cup . . . . . | 11 | .4 | 2.5 | .1 | 0 | 1 | 1.0 |
| boiled, drained, 1" | | | | | | | |
| cubes, ½ cup . . . . . . . | 13 | .4 | 3.2 | .1 | 0 | 2 | 1.2 |
| **Eggplant, canned**, | | | | | | | |
| roasted, pulp (*Roland*), | | | | | | | |
| 2 tbsp. . . . . . . . . . . . | 5 | 1.0 | 1.0 | 0 | 0 | 115 | 0 |
| **Eggplant dip/appetizer**: | | | | | | | |
| (*Sabra* Turkish | | | | | | | |
| Salad), 2 tbsp. . . . . . . | 35 | 1.0 | 3.0 | 2.0 | 0 | 150 | <1.0 |
| baba ghanoush, 2 tbsp.: | | | | | | | |
| (*Peloponnese*) . . . . . . | 40 | 1.0 | 2.0 | 3.0 | 0 | 250 | 1.0 |
| (*Sabra* Classic) . . . . . . | 70 | 0 | 2.0 | 7.0 | 5 | 160 | 0 |
| caponata: | | | | | | | |
| (*Alessi* Can), ⅓ cup . . | 140 | 2.0 | 7.0 | 7.0 | 0 | 310 | 4.0 |
| (*Alessi* Jar), ⅓ cup . . . | 140 | 2.0 | 6.0 | 12.0 | 0 | 430 | 6.0 |
| (*Roland* Can), ⅓ cup . . | 140 | 2.0 | 11.0 | 10.0 | 0 | 630 | 4.0 |
| (*Roland* Jar), ⅓ cup . . | 150 | 2.0 | 6.0 | 13.0 | 0 | 470 | 7.0 |
| (*Sabra*), 2 tbsp. . . . . . | 55 | 2.0 | 2.0 | 4.5 | 0 | 65 | <1.0 |
| grilled: | | | | | | | |
| (*Roland*), 3 pcs., | | | | | | | |
| 1.3 oz. . . . . . . . . . | 45 | 1.0 | 4.0 | 3.0 | 0 | 170 | 2.0 |
| (*Sabra*), 2 tbsp. . . . . . | 20 | 1.0 | 3.0 | .5 | 0 | 180 | 0 |
| hummus, see "Hummus" | | | | | | | |
| ratatouille (*Sabra*) | | | | | | | |
| 2 tbsp. . . . . . . . . . . . | 35 | 0 | 2.0 | 3.0 | 0 | 80 | 0 |
| roasted, 2 tbsp.: | | | | | | | |
| meze (*Peloponnese*) . . | 20 | 1.0 | 3.0 | 1.0 | 0 | 200 | 0 |
| spread (*Peloponnese*) . | 30 | 0 | 3.0 | 2.5 | 0 | 240 | 0 |
| stuffed, rolled (*Roland*), | | | | | | | |
| 3.5-oz. pc. . . . . . . . . . | 80 | 1.0 | 11.0 | 4.0 | 0 | 300 | 4.0 |

| Food and Measure | cal. | prot. (gms) | carbo. (gms) | fat (gms) | chol. (mgs) | sod. (mgs) | fiber (gms) |
|---|---|---|---|---|---|---|---|
| **Eggplant entree, frozen**, 1 pkg., except as noted: | | | | | | | |
| (*Ethnic Gourmet* Bhartha), 11 oz. ..... | 300 | 8.0 | 47.0 | 9.0 | 0 | 650 | 10.0 |
| baked, stacked (*Cedarlane*), 9 oz. .............. | 280 | 17.0 | 31.0 | 11.0 | 35 | 570 | 3.0 |
| moussaka (*Cedarlane* Eggplant Mediterranean), 10 oz. | 230 | 13.0 | 22.0 | 10.0 | 20 | 590 | 6.0 |
| Parmesan (*Cedarlane*), ½ of 10-oz. pkg. ..... | 160 | 7.0 | 16.0 | 8.0 | 15 | 390 | 3.0 |
| parmigiana: | | | | | | | |
| (*Celentano*), 10 oz. ... | 450 | 12.0 | 35.0 | 30.0 | 35 | 730 | 7.0 |
| (*Celentano*), ½ of 14-oz. pkg. ....... | 320 | 8.0 | 25.0 | 21.0 | 25 | 490 | 5.0 |
| (*Celentano*), ⅓ of 25-oz. pkg. ....... | 360 | 10.0 | 28.0 | 24.0 | 30 | 580 | 6.0 |
| (*Celentano* Vegan), 10 oz. ........... | 410 | 12.0 | 41.0 | 22.0 | 0 | 460 | 8.0 |
| and red pepper pie (*The Fillo Factory*), ½ of 10-oz. pkg. ..... | 230 | 4.0 | 35.0 | 9.0 | 0 | 310 | 3.0 |
| rollettes, 10 oz.: | | | | | | | |
| (*Celentano*) ......... | 380 | 11.0 | 33.0 | 23.0 | 30 | 770 | 7.0 |
| (*Celentano* Vegan) ... | 360 | 13.0 | 36.0 | 17.0 | 0 | 520 | 8.0 |
| **Eggplant entree, microwave** (*TastyBite* Punjab), ½ of 10-oz. pkg. ..... | 140 | 4.0 | 13.0 | 9.0 | 0 | 510 | 2.0 |
| **Eggplant pocket**, frozen, and roasted peppers (*Aunt Trudy's* Organic), 5-oz. pc. ........... | 210 | 4.0 | 34.0 | 7.0 | 0 | 310 | 3.0 |
| **Eggplant relish**, Indian (*Tiger Tiger* Brinjal), 1 tbsp. ............ | 70 | 0 | 16.0 | .5 | 0 | 120 | <1.0 |
| **Eight ball squash** (*Frieda's*), 1 cup, 4.4 oz. ............ | 18 | 2.0 | 4.0 | 0 | 0 | 4 | 1.0 |
| **Elderberries**, ½ cup .... | 53 | .5 | 13.3 | .4 | 0 | 4 | 5.1 |
| **Elk**, meat only, roasted, 4 oz. ....... | 166 | 34.2 | 0 | 2.2 | 83 | 69 | 0 |

| Food and Measure | cal. | prot. (gms) | carbo. (gms) | fat (gms) | chol. (mgs) | sod. (mgs) | fiber (gms) |
|---|---|---|---|---|---|---|---|
| **Empanadas**, frozen, chicken/cheese (*José Olé*), 2 pcs., 4 oz. .... | 320 | 10.0 | 37.0 | 14.0 | 35 | 730 | 1.0 |
| **Emu**, ground, pan-broiled, 4 oz. .... | 185 | 32.2 | 0 | 5.3 | 99 | 74 | 0 |
| **Enchilada entree**, frozen, 1 pkg., except as noted: | | | | | | | |
| (*Amy's* Bowls Santa Fe), 10 oz. .......... | 350 | 16.0 | 47.0 | 11.0 | 5 | 780 | 9.0 |
| bake (*Michelina's Lean Gourmet*), 8.5 oz. .... | 300 | 11.0 | 47.0 | 8.0 | 15 | 750 | 6.0 |
| beef, spicy (*El Monterey* Family), ⅕ of 40-oz. pkg. ..... | 290 | 10.0 | 40.0 | 12.0 | 20 | 820 | 2.0 |
| beef and tamale combo (*Banquet*), 8.5 oz. .... | 310 | 10.0 | 44.0 | 10.0 | 10 | 930 | 11.0 |
| black bean: | | | | | | | |
| (*Amy's* Light Sodium), ½ of 9.5-oz. pkg. .. | 160 | 5.0 | 22.0 | 6.0 | 0 | 190 | 3.0 |
| (*Amy's* Whole Meal), 10 oz. .......... | 330 | 9.0 | 53.0 | 8.0 | 0 | 740 | 9.0 |
| and cheese (*Amy's* Light & Lean), 8 oz. | 240 | 8.0 | 44.0 | 4.5 | 5 | 480 | 4.0 |
| and tofu (*Cedarlane* Meal Organic), 9 oz. | 220 | 10.0 | 42.0 | 3.0 | 0 | 390 | 6.0 |
| and vegetable (*Amy's*), ½ of 9.5-oz. pkg. .. | 160 | 5.0 | 22.0 | 6.0 | 0 | 390 | 3.0 |
| cheese: | | | | | | | |
| (*Amy's*), ½ of 9.5-oz. pkg. ............ | 240 | 10.0 | 18.0 | 14.0 | 35 | 440 | 2.0 |
| (*Amy's* Whole Meal), 9 oz. ............ | 370 | 17.0 | 41.0 | 15.0 | 30 | 680 | 9.0 |
| (*El Monterey* Family), ⅕ of 40-oz. pkg. .... | 320 | 10.0 | 29.0 | 18.0 | 40 | 1530 | 1.0 |
| w/tofu steaks (*Helen's Kitchen* Organic), ½ of 10-oz. pkg. .... | 210 | 9.0 | 20.0 | 11.0 | 20 | 390 | 3.0 |
| chicken: | | | | | | | |
| (*Banquet*), 8.5 oz. .... | 280 | 7.0 | 44.0 | 9.0 | 10 | 870 | 5.0 |
| (*Cedarlane*), 9 oz. .... | 370 | 22.0 | 42.0 | 14.0 | 50 | 790 | 6.0 |
| (*El Monterey* Family), ⅕ of 40-oz. pkg. .... | 320 | 6.0 | 56.0 | 7.0 | 5 | 650 | 2.0 |

| Food and Measure | cal. | prot. (gms) | carbo. (gms) | fat (gms) | chol. (mgs) | sod. (mgs) | fiber (gms) |
|---|---|---|---|---|---|---|---|
| (*Stouffer's* Party), | | | | | | | |
| ⅛ of 57-oz. pkg. .... | 280 | 12.0 | 30.0 | 12.0 | 40 | 720 | 3.0 |
| Monterey (*Smart* | | | | | | | |
| *Ones*), 9.5 oz. ..... | 310 | 12.0 | 41.0 | 10.0 | 25 | 730 | 5.0 |
| chicken Suiza, 9 oz.: | | | | | | | |
| (*Lean Cuisine*) ...... | 280 | 10.0 | 48.0 | 5.0 | 20 | 600 | 3.0 |
| (*Smart Ones*) ....... | 290 | 11.0 | 48.0 | 5.0 | 25 | 640 | 3.0 |
| pie, 3-layer (*Cedarlane* | | | | | | | |
| Organic), ½ of | | | | | | | |
| 11-oz. pkg. ......... | 215 | 13.0 | 27.0 | 7.0 | 15 | 595 | 3.0 |
| spinach/cheese (*Amy's* | | | | | | | |
| Verde Whole Meal), | | | | | | | |
| 10 oz. ............. | 390 | 15.0 | 54.0 | 13.0 | 30 | 690 | 8.0 |
| vegetable (*Cedarlane* | | | | | | | |
| Organic Lowfat), | | | | | | | |
| ½ of 9-oz. pkg. ...... | 140 | 9.0 | 20.0 | 3.0 | 10 | 310 | 3.0 |
| **Enchilada entree kit** | | | | | | | |
| (*Old El Paso* Dinner): | | | | | | | |
| ¼ pkg. mix ........... | 150 | 3.0 | 27.0 | 4.0 | 0 | 1390 | 2.0 |
| ¼ pkg.* .............. | 390 | 34.0 | 28.0 | 17.0 | 90 | 1610 | 2.0 |
| **Enchilada sauce,** | | | | | | | |
| ¼ cup: | | | | | | | |
| (*Ortega*) ............. | 10 | <1.0 | 4.0 | .5 | 0 | 340 | <1.0 |
| (*Rosarita*) ............ | 20 | 0 | 3.0 | 1.0 | 0 | 430 | 1.0 |
| green: | | | | | | | |
| (*Las Palmas*) ....... | 25 | 0 | 3.0 | 1.5 | 0 | 340 | 0 |
| mild (*La Victoria*) .... | 20 | 0 | 4.0 | 0 | 0 | 330 | 0 |
| mild (*Old El Paso*) .... | 25 | 0 | 4.0 | 1.5 | 0 | 280 | 0 |
| hot (*Las Palmas*) ....... | 15 | 0 | 2.0 | .5 | 0 | 330 | 0 |
| hot, medium, or mild | | | | | | | |
| (*Old El Paso*) ....... | 20 | 0 | 3.0 | 0 | 0 | 360 | 0 |
| medium (*Las Palmas*) ... | 15 | 0 | 2.0 | .5 | 0 | 310 | 1.0 |
| mild (*Las Palmas*) ...... | 20 | 0 | 2.0 | .5 | 0 | 310 | 1.0 |
| red, mild or hot (*La* | | | | | | | |
| *Victoria*) ............ | 25 | 0 | 3.0 | 1.5 | 0 | 400 | 0 |
| tomato (*Las Palmas*) .... | 20 | <1.0 | 5.0 | 0 | 0 | 290 | <1.0 |
| **Enchilada sauce mix:** | | | | | | | |
| (*Lawry's*), 2 tsp. ....... | 20 | <1.0 | 4.0 | 0 | 0 | 260 | 0 |
| (*McCormick*), 2 tsp. .... | 15 | 0 | 3.0 | 0 | 0 | 300 | 0 |
| **Endive**, chopped, ½ cup . | 4 | .3 | .8 | .1 | 0 | 6 | .8 |
| **Endive, Belgian**, see | | | | | | | |
| "Chicory, witloof" | | | | | | | |
| **Epazote**, raw, 2 sprigs .. | 1 | 0 | .3 | 0 | 0 | 172 | .2 |

| Food and Measure | cal. | prot. (gms) | carbo. (gms) | fat (gms) | chol. (mgs) | sod. (mgs) | fiber (gms) |
|---|---|---|---|---|---|---|---|
| **Eppaw**, raw, ½ cup ..... | 75 | 2.3 | 15.8 | .9 | 0 | 6 | n.a. |
| **Escargot**, see "Snail, canned" | | | | | | | |
| **Escarole**, see "Endive" | | | | | | | |
| **Etouffee sauce base** (*Zatarain's*), 1⅓ tbsp. . | 35 | 1.0 | 7.0 | 0 | 0 | 440 | 1.0 |

# F

| Food and Measure | cal. | prot. (gms) | carbo. (gms) | fat (gms) | chol. (mgs) | sod. (mgs) | fiber (gms) |
|---|---|---|---|---|---|---|---|
| **Fajita entree kit** (*Old El Paso* Dinner): | | | | | | | |
| ⅛ pkg. mix only | 190 | 4.0 | 33.0 | 5.0 | 0 | 1010 | 1.0 |
| ⅛ pkg., 2 tortillas* | 330 | 25.0 | 34.0 | 10.0 | 55 | 1230 | 2.0 |
| **Fajita seasoning mix:** | | | | | | | |
| (*Chi-Chi's*), ¼ pkg. | 35 | 0 | 7.0 | 1.0 | 0 | 520 | 0 |
| (*Lawry's*), 2 tsp. | 10 | 0 | 3.0 | 0 | 0 | 400 | 0 |
| (*McCormick*), 2 tsp. | 15 | 0 | 3.0 | 0 | 0 | 260 | 0 |
| (*Old El Paso*), 2 tsp. | 15 | 0 | 3.0 | 0 | 0 | 370 | 0 |
| (*Ortega*), 1½ tsp. | 15 | 0 | 3.0 | 0 | 0 | 430 | 0 |
| chicken (*Lawry's*), 1 tsp. | 10 | 0 | 2.0 | 0 | 0 | 320 | 0 |
| **Falafel**, frozen: | | | | | | | |
| balls (*Veggie Patch*), 4 pcs., 3 oz. | 180 | 5.0 | 21.0 | 9.0 | 0 | 380 | 6.0 |
| flats (*Dr. Praeger's*), 3 pcs., 1.8 oz. | 110 | 5.0 | 14.0 | 4.5 | 0 | 135 | 4.0 |
| **Falafel mix:** | | | | | | | |
| (*Fantastic*), ¼ cup | 130 | 8.0 | 20.0 | 2.0 | 0 | 280 | 5.0 |
| (*Near East*), ¼ cup | 100 | 10.0 | 18.0 | 1.0 | 0 | 560 | 5.0 |
| **Farfalle entree**, frozen, basil pesto/tofu (*Helen's Kitchen Organic*), 10-oz. pkg. | 590 | 26.0 | 61.0 | 27.0 | 15 | 420 | 6.0 |
| **Farina**, whole-grain: | | | | | | | |
| dry, 1 oz. | 105 | 3.0 | 22.1 | .1 | 0 | 1 | .8 |
| cooked, 1 cup | 116 | 3.4 | 24.6 | .2 | 0 | 1 | 3.3 |
| **Farro** (see also "Spelt") (*Roland*), dry, ¼ cup | 170 | 7.0 | 33.0 | 0 | 0 | 30 | 3.0 |
| **Fava**, see "Broad bean" | | | | | | | |
| **Fava flour** (see also "Garbanzo flour") | | | | | | | |

| Food and Measure | cal. | prot. (gms) | carbo. (gms) | fat (gms) | chol. (mgs) | sod. (mgs) | fiber (gms) |
|---|---|---|---|---|---|---|---|
| **Fava flour** *(cont.)* | | | | | | | |
| (*Bob's Red Mill*), | | | | | | | |
| ¼ cup . . . . . . . . . . . . | 110 | 9.0 | 19.0 | .5 | 0 | 0 | 8.0 |
| **Feijoa**, raw: | | | | | | | |
| (*Frieda's*), 1.76-oz. pc. . . | 25 | 1.0 | 5.0 | 0 | 0 | 2 | 0 |
| w/skin, 2.3-oz. pc. . . . . . | 25 | .6 | 5.3 | .4 | 0 | 2 | 0 |
| pureed, ½ cup . . . . . . . . | 60 | 1.5 | 12.9 | 1.0 | 0 | 4 | 0 |
| **Fennel**, bulb, raw: | | | | | | | |
| 8.3-oz. bulb . . . . . . . . . . | 72 | 2.9 | 17.1 | .5 | 0 | 122 | 7.3 |
| sliced: | | | | | | | |
| (*Frieda's*), 1 cup . . . . . | 25 | 1.0 | 6.0 | 0 | 0 | 45 | 3.0 |
| 1 cup, 3 oz. . . . . . . . . | 27 | 1.1 | 6.3 | .2 | 0 | 45 | 2.7 |
| **Fennel seed**, 1 tsp. . . . . | 7 | .3 | 1.1 | .3 | 0 | 2 | <1.0 |
| **Fenugreek seed**, 1 tsp. . . | 12 | .9 | 2.2 | .2 | 0 | 2 | <1.0 |
| **Fettuccine**, see "Pasta" | | | | | | | |
| **Fettuccine dish mix**, | | | | | | | |
| 1 cup*: | | | | | | | |
| Alfredo (*Pasta Roni*) . . . . | 450 | 11.0 | 44.0 | 24.0 | 5 | 1050 | 2.0 |
| curly, white cheddar | | | | | | | |
| broccoli sauce | | | | | | | |
| (*Annie's*) . . . . . . . . . . . | 270 | 10.0 | 39.0 | 9.5 | 25 | 510 | 2.0 |
| **Fettuccine entree**, | | | | | | | |
| frozen, 1 pkg.: | | | | | | | |
| Alfredo: | | | | | | | |
| (*Banquet*), 8 oz. . . . . . | 280 | 10.0 | 35.0 | 11.0 | 20 | 700 | 3.0 |
| (*Lean Cuisine*), | | | | | | | |
| 9.25 oz. . . . . . . . . . | 330 | 12.0 | 54.0 | 7.0 | 15 | 600 | 3.0 |
| (*Marie Callender's*), | | | | | | | |
| 13 oz. . . . . . . . . . . . | 650 | 24.0 | 61.0 | 34.0 | 65 | 1220 | 5.0 |
| (*Michelina's* | | | | | | | |
| *Authentico*), 8.5 oz. | 330 | 12.0 | 45.0 | 11.0 | 35 | 670 | 2.0 |
| (*Michelina's Budget* | | | | | | | |
| *Gourmet*), 7.5 oz. . . | 290 | 10.0 | 41.0 | 9.0 | 25 | 590 | 2.0 |
| (*Smart Ones*), 9.25 oz. | 240 | 12.0 | 41.0 | 4.0 | 5 | 570 | 4.0 |
| (*Stouffer's*), 11.5 oz. . . | 630 | 15.0 | 63.0 | 35.0 | 50 | 840 | 3.0 |
| w/chicken, see "Chicken | | | | | | | |
| entree, frozen" | | | | | | | |
| **Fiddlehead fern**, fresh, | | | | | | | |
| raw, 4 oz. . . . . . . . . . | 39 | 5.2 | 6.3 | .5 | 0 | 1 | n.a. |
| **Fig**, fresh: | | | | | | | |
| 1 large, 2.3 oz. . . . . . . . | 47 | .5 | 12.3 | .2 | 0 | 1 | 2.1 |
| 1 medium, 1.8 oz. . . . . . | 37 | .4 | 9.6 | .2 | 0 | 1 | 1.7 |
| **Fig, canned**, in light syrup | | | | | | | |
| (*Roland* Katoda), ½ cup | 120 | 1.0 | 28.0 | 0 | 0 | 0 | 1.0 |

| Food and Measure | cal. | prot. (gms) | carbo. (gms) | fat (gms) | chol. (mgs) | sod. (mgs) | fiber (gms) |
|---|---|---|---|---|---|---|---|
| **Fig, dried**: | | | | | | | |
| (*Jenny* Kalamata), 4 pcs. . | 120 | 1.0 | 28.0 | 0 | 0 | 5 | 5.0 |
| (*Sun•Maid* Mission/ | | | | | | | |
| Calimyrna), ¼ cup, | | | | | | | |
| 1.4 oz. . . . . . . . . . . . . | 120 | 1.0 | 28.0 | 0 | 0 | 0 | 5.0 |
| 10 figs, 6.6 oz. . . . . . . . . | 477 | 5.7 | 122.2 | 2.2 | 0 | 20 | 17.4 |
| **Filberts**, see "Hazelnuts" | | | | | | | |
| **Fillo dough**, frozen: | | | | | | | |
| sheets: | | | | | | | |
| (*Apollo*), 3 sheets, | | | | | | | |
| 1.7 oz. . . . . . . . . . . | 130 | 3.0 | 27.0 | 1.0 | 0 | 330 | 1.0 |
| (*Athens*), 2 oz. . . . . . . | 180 | 4.0 | 37.0 | 1.5 | 0 | 230 | 1.0 |
| (*The Fillo Factory* | | | | | | | |
| 12" x 17"), 2.3 oz. . . | 180 | 6.0 | 40.0 | 1.5 | 0 | 310 | 1.0 |
| (*The Fillo Factory* | | | | | | | |
| 14" x 18"), 2 oz. . . . | 160 | 5.0 | 35.0 | 1.0 | 0 | 270 | 1.0 |
| (*The Fillo Factory* | | | | | | | |
| Organic 13" x 18"), | | | | | | | |
| 1.6 oz. . . . . . . . . . . | 130 | 4.0 | 28.0 | 1.0 | 0 | 160 | 1.0 |
| (*Kontos*), .3 oz. . . . . . . | 30 | 1.0 | 6.0 | 0 | 0 | 70 | 0 |
| extra thick (*Apollo* | | | | | | | |
| Horiatiko), 2 oz. . . . | 200 | 4.0 | 34.0 | 4.5 | 0 | 470 | 1.0 |
| extra thick (*The Fillo* | | | | | | | |
| *Factory*), 2 oz. . . . . | 160 | 1.0 | 35.0 | 1.0 | 0 | 270 | 1.0 |
| whole wheat (*The* | | | | | | | |
| *Fillo* Factory Organic | | | | | | | |
| 13" x 18"), ⅛ pkg. . . | 140 | 4.0 | 30.0 | 1.0 | 0 | 200 | 2.0 |
| shells: | | | | | | | |
| (*The Fillo Factory* | | | | | | | |
| Organic), .7-oz. pc. | 80 | 2.0 | 13.0 | 2.0 | 0 | 55 | 0 |
| mini (*Athens*), 2 pcs., | | | | | | | |
| .3 oz. . . . . . . . . . . . | 35 | 0 | 4.0 | 2.0 | 0 | 25 | 0 |
| mini (*The Fillo* | | | | | | | |
| *Factory* Organic), | | | | | | | |
| 3 pcs., .4 oz. . . . . . | 45 | 1.0 | 7.0 | 1.5 | 0 | 30 | 0 |
| shredded (kataifi): | | | | | | | |
| (*Athens/Apollo*), 2 oz. . | 120 | 3.0 | 22.0 | 1.5 | 0 | 115 | <1.0 |
| (*Kontos*), 1 oz. . . . . . . | 90 | 2.0 | 20.0 | 1.0 | 0 | 170 | 0 |
| (*The Fillo Factory*), | | | | | | | |
| 2 oz. . . . . . . . . . . . . | 180 | 5.0 | 35.0 | 2.0 | 0 | 140 | 4.0 |
| **Finishing sauce** | | | | | | | |
| (*Roland*), 1 tbsp.: | | | | | | | |
| chipotle . . . . . . . . . . . . . | 60 | 0 | 2.0 | 6.0 | 0 | 360 | 0 |
| cranberry horseradish . . . | 70 | 0 | 4.0 | 6.0 | 0 | 160 | 0 |

| Food and Measure | cal. | prot. (gms) | carbo. (gms) | fat (gms) | chol. (mgs) | sod. (mgs) | fiber (gms) |
|---|---|---|---|---|---|---|---|
| **Finishing sauce** *(cont.)* | | | | | | | |
| kalamata feta .......... | 60 | 0 | 1.0 | 6.0 | 0 | 200 | 0 |
| wasabi .............. | 60 | 0 | 1.0 | 6.0 | 0 | 380 | 0 |
| yellow pepper ......... | 50 | 0 | 1.0 | 5.0 | 0 | 210 | 0 |
| **Finocchiona sausage** | | | | | | | |
| *(Applegate Farms)*, | | | | | | | |
| 1 oz. .............. | 110 | 8.0 | 0 | 8.0 | 30 | 460 | 0 |
| **Fireweed**, leaves, | | | | | | | |
| fresh, 1 cup ........ | 24 | 1.1 | 4.4 | .7 | 0 | 8 | 2.4 |
| **Fish**, see specific | | | | | | | |
| listings | | | | | | | |
| **Fish, canned** (see | | | | | | | |
| also specific fish), | | | | | | | |
| steaks, 1 can: | | | | | | | |
| w/green chili *(Crown* | | | | | | | |
| *Prince)*, 4.25 oz., | | | | | | | |
| drained ............ | 200 | 22.0 | 0 | 12.0 | 55 | 170 | <1.0 |
| in hot sauce: | | | | | | | |
| *(Chicken of the Sea)*, | | | | | | | |
| 3.75 oz. ......... | 70 | 9.0 | 1.0 | 3.0 | 50 | 430 | 1.0 |
| *(Crown* Prince), | | | | | | | |
| 4.25 oz. ......... | 230 | 24.0 | 0 | 15.0 | 65 | 190 | <1.0 |
| in mustard *(Crown* | | | | | | | |
| *Prince)*, 4.25 oz. ..... | 190 | 21.0 | 5.0 | 9.0 | 55 | 730 | 0 |
| **Fish, frozen** (see also | | | | | | | |
| "Fish entree"): | | | | | | | |
| bites, and chips | | | | | | | |
| *(Blue Horizon)*, | | | | | | | |
| 4 pcs., 2 oz. ........ | 110 | 7.0 | 5.0 | 7.0 | 70 | 230 | 0 |
| fillet, battered, 2 pcs.: | | | | | | | |
| *(Gorton's* Crispy), | | | | | | | |
| 3.8 oz. .......... | 230 | 8.0 | 22.0 | 12.0 | 25 | 650 | 3.0 |
| beer *(Gorton's)*, | | | | | | | |
| 3.6 oz. .......... | 250 | 7.0 | 16.0 | 18.0 | 25 | 550 | 1.0 |
| beer *(Mrs. Paul's/Van* | | | | | | | |
| *de Kamp's)*, 3.8 oz. | 240 | 11.0 | 18.0 | 13.0 | 40 | 920 | 0 |
| lemon pepper | | | | | | | |
| *(Gorton's)*, 3.7 oz. | 270 | 8.0 | 20.0 | 18.0 | 20 | 580 | 1.0 |
| fillet, breaded, 2 pcs.: | | | | | | | |
| *(Gorton's* Crunchy | | | | | | | |
| Golden), 3.8 oz. ... | 240 | 9.0 | 23.0 | 12.0 | 30 | 500 | 0 |
| *(Mrs. Paul's* Crispy), | | | | | | | |
| 4.5 oz. .......... | 290 | 14.0 | 27.0 | 14.0 | 45 | 1010 | <1.0 |

| Food and Measure | cal. | prot. (gms) | carbo. (gms) | fat (gms) | chol. (mgs) | sod. (mgs) | fiber (gms) |
|---|---|---|---|---|---|---|---|
| (*Mrs. Paul's/Van de Kamp's* Crunchy 6 Pc.), 3.8 oz. | 250 | 13.0 | 23.0 | 12.0 | 40 | 490 | <1.0 |
| (*Van de Kamp's* Crispy 10 Pc.), 3.9 oz. | 230 | 8.0 | 21.0 | 13.0 | 20 | 440 | <1.0 |
| (*Van de Kamp's* Crispy 6 Pc.), 3.5 oz. | 230 | 11.0 | 21.0 | 11.0 | 35 | 790 | <1.0 |
| (*Van de Kamp's* Crunchy), 3.5 oz. | 220 | 11.0 | 20.0 | 10.0 | 35 | 420 | <1.0 |
| (*Van de Kamp's Healthy Selects*), 3.7 oz. | 180 | 12.0 | 24.0 | 1.0 | 40 | 490 | <1.0 |
| garlic herb (*Gorton's*), 3.7 oz. | 230 | 9.0 | 22.0 | 12.0 | 30 | 770 | 0 |
| lemon herb (*Gorton's*), 3.7 oz. | 240 | 9.0 | 21.0 | 13.0 | 25 | 720 | 0 |
| potato crunch (*Gorton's*), 3.7 oz. | 240 | 9.0 | 20.0 | 14.0 | 25 | 790 | 2.0 |
| fillet, grilled (*Gorton's*), 3.8-oz. pc.: | | | | | | | |
| Cajun blackened | 100 | 17.0 | 1.0 | 3.0 | 60 | 330 | 0 |
| garlic butter | 100 | 17.0 | 1.0 | 3.0 | 70 | 290 | 0 |
| Italian herb | 100 | 16.0 | 1.0 | 3.0 | 60 | 300 | 0 |
| lemon butter | 100 | 17.0 | 1.0 | 3.0 | 75 | 320 | 0 |
| lemon pepper | 100 | 17.0 | 1.0 | 3.0 | 70 | 290 | 0 |
| nuggets, fish shape: | | | | | | | |
| (*Dr. Praeger's*), 3 pcs., 1.55 oz. | 90 | 4.0 | 9.0 | 4.0 | 10 | 210 | 0 |
| (*Mrs. Paul's*), 4 pcs., 4.25 oz. | 280 | 14.0 | 25.0 | 13.0 | 45 | 530 | <1.0 |
| nuggets, wild Alaskan (*Blue Horizon*), 6 pcs., 3 oz. | 230 | 10.0 | 23.0 | 10.0 | 35 | 440 | 1.0 |
| popcorn, 8 pcs.: | | | | | | | |
| (*Mrs. Paul's*), 4.1 oz. | 280 | 14.0 | 27.0 | 13.0 | 40 | 580 | 1.0 |
| (*Van de Kamp's*), 4.1 oz. | 270 | 14.0 | 25.0 | 13.0 | 40 | 510 | <1.0 |
| (*SeaPak*), 3 oz. | 190 | 9.0 | 18.0 | 9.0 | 30 | 370 | 1.0 |
| portions, breaded (*Van de Kamp's* Crispy), 2 pcs., 4.5 oz. | 320 | 12.0 | 29.0 | 16.0 | 35 | 770 | <1.0 |

| Food and Measure | cal. | prot. (gms) | carbo. (gms) | fat (gms) | chol. (mgs) | sod. (mgs) | fiber (gms) |
|---|---|---|---|---|---|---|---|
| **Fish, frozen** *(cont.)* | | | | | | | |
| sticks, breaded: | | | | | | | |
| (*Dr. Praeger's* Fillet), 3 pcs., 2.9 oz. . . . . | 150 | 7.0 | 16.0 | 6.0 | 15 | 290 | <1.0 |
| (*Dr. Praeger's* Minced), 3 pcs., 1.7 oz. . . . . . . . . | 110 | 5.0 | 10.0 | 6.0 | 15 | 170 | <1.0 |
| (*Mrs. Paul's/Van de Kamp's* Crunchy), 6 pcs., 3.4 oz. . . . . | 220 | 11.0 | 20.0 | 10.0 | 35 | 420 | <1.0 |
| (*Mrs. Paul's/Van de Kamp's* Crunchy Xtra Large), 4 pcs., 3 oz. . . . . . . . . . . . | 190 | 10.0 | 18.0 | 9.0 | 30 | 370 | <1.0 |
| (*Mrs. Paul's/Van de Kamp's Healthy Selects*), 6 pcs., 3.6 oz. . . . . | 160 | 9.0 | 26.0 | 2.0 | 25 | 430 | <1.0 |
| sticks, gluten free (*Blue Horizon*), 4½ pcs., 3.1 oz. . . . . . | 240 | 9.0 | 26.0 | 10.0 | 40 | 370 | 3.0 |
| tenders, 3 pcs.: | | | | | | | |
| (*Gorton's* Extra Crunchy), 3.2 oz. . . | 190 | 8.0 | 22.0 | 10.0 | 30 | 610 | 0 |
| (*Gorton* Original Batter), 3.6 oz. . . . . | 230 | 8.0 | 12.0 | 12.0 | 20 | 660 | 1.0 |
| (*Mrs. Paul's/Van de Kamp's*), 3.6 oz. . . . | 230 | 11.0 | 21.0 | 11.0 | 35 | 800 | <1.0 |
| beer batter (*Gorton's*), 3.3 oz. . . . . . . . . . | 230 | 7.0 | 18.0 | 14.0 | 20 | 650 | 2.0 |
| **Fish cake**, see specific fish listings | | | | | | | |
| **Fish coating**, see "Seafood coating mix" | | | | | | | |
| **Fish entree**, frozen (see also "Fish, frozen" and specific fish listings), 1 pkg.: | | | | | | | |
| fillet, crusted: | | | | | | | |
| Parmesan (*Lean Cuisine*), 9 oz. . . . . | 290 | 15.0 | 40.0 | 8.0 | 30 | 650 | 4.0 |
| tortilla (*Lean Cuisine*), 8 oz. . . . . . . . . . . | 290 | 13.0 | 40.0 | 9.0 | 35 | 540 | 2.0 |
| fillet, golden (*Marie Callender's*), 12 oz. . . . | 400 | 20.0 | 50.0 | 13.0 | 45 | 1310 | 4.0 |

| Food and Measure | cal. | prot. (gms) | carbo. (gms) | fat (gms) | chol. (mgs) | sod. (mgs) | fiber (gms) |
|---|---|---|---|---|---|---|---|
| lemon pepper: | | | | | | | |
| (*Healthy Choice* Complete), 10.7 oz. | 310 | 14.0 | 50.0 | 5.0 | 25 | 450 | 5.0 |
| (*Lean Cuisine* Cafe), 9 oz. . . . . . . . . . . . | 290 | 15.0 | 40.0 | 8.0 | 25 | 520 | 2.0 |
| sticks, breaded (*Banquet* Meal), 7.3 oz. . . . . . . . | 310 | 11.0 | 44.0 | 10.0 | 25 | 540 | 4.0 |
| **Fish sauce**, Asian, 1 tbsp.: | | | | | | | |
| (*Golden Boy*) . . . . . . . . . | 10 | 2.0 | 1.0 | 0 | 0 | 1370 | 0 |
| (*Ka•Me*) . . . . . . . . . . . . | 5 | 0 | 0 | 0 | 0 | 380 | 0 |
| (*Roland*) . . . . . . . . . . . . | 10 | 2.0 | 1.0 | 0 | 0 | 1180 | 0 |
| (*A Taste of Thai*) . . . . . . | 15 | 2.0 | 1.0 | 0 | 0 | 1187 | 0 |
| **Fish seasoning**, see "Seafood coating mix" | | | | | | | |
| *Five Guys:* | | | | | | | |
| burgers: | | | | | | | |
| hamburger . . . . . . . . | 700 | 39.0 | 39.0 | 43.0 | 125 | 430 | 2.0 |
| cheeseburger . . . . . . . | 840 | 47.0 | 40.0 | 55.0 | 165 | 1050 | 2.0 |
| bacon burger . . . . . . . | 780 | 43.0 | 39.0 | 50.0 | 140 | 690 | 2.0 |
| bacon cheeseburger . . | 920 | 61.0 | 40.0 | 62.0 | 180 | 1310 | 2.0 |
| little burgers: | | | | | | | |
| hamburger . . . . . . . . | 480 | 23.0 | 39.0 | 26.0 | 65 | 380 | 2.0 |
| cheeseburger . . . . . . . | 550 | 27.0 | 39.5 | 32.0 | 85 | 690 | 2.0 |
| bacon burger . . . . . . . | 560 | 27.0 | 39.0 | 33.0 | 80 | 640 | 2.0 |
| bacon cheeseburger . . | 630 | 31.0 | 39.5 | 39.0 | 100 | 950 | 2.0 |
| dogs: | | | | | | | |
| hot dog . . . . . . . . . . . . | 545 | 18.0 | 40.0 | 35.0 | 61 | 1130 | 2.0 |
| cheese dog . . . . . . . . . | 615 | 22.0 | 40.5 | 41.0 | 81 | 1440 | 2.0 |
| bacon dog . . . . . . . . . | 625 | 22.0 | 40.0 | 42.0 | 76 | 1390 | 2.0 |
| bacon cheese dog . . . . | 695 | 26.0 | 40.5 | 48.0 | 96 | 1700 | 2.0 |
| other sandwiches: | | | | | | | |
| veggie . . . . . . . . . . . . . | 440 | 16.0 | 60.0 | 15.0 | 25 | 1040 | 2.0 |
| grilled cheese . . . . . . . | 470 | 11.0 | 41.0 | 26.0 | 35 | 715 | 2.5 |
| fries: | | | | | | | |
| regular . . . . . . . . . . . . | 620 | 10.0 | 78.0 | 30.0 | n.a. | 90 | 6.0 |
| regular, ½ serving . . . | 310 | 8.0 | 39.0 | 15.0 | n.a. | 45 | 3.0 |
| large . . . . . . . . . . . . . . | 1474 | 24.0 | 184.0 | 71.0 | n.a. | 213 | 14.0 |
| toppings, 1 serving: | | | | | | | |
| cheese . . . . . . . . . . . | 70 | 4.0 | <1.0 | 6.0 | 20 | 310 | 0 |
| bacon . . . . . . . . . . . . | 80 | 4.0 | 0 | 7.0 | 15 | 260 | 0 |
| mushrooms . . . . . . . . | 10 | 1.0 | 1.0 | 0 | 0 | 100 | <1.0 |
| green pepper . . . . . . . | 5 | 0 | 2.0 | 0 | 0 | 1 | <1.0 |
| onions . . . . . . . . . . . . | 10 | 0 | 3.0 | 0 | 0 | 1 | <1.0 |

| Food and Measure | cal. | prot. (gms) | carbo. (gms) | fat (gms) | chol. (mgs) | sod. (mgs) | fiber (gms) |
|---|---|---|---|---|---|---|---|
| **Five Guys, toppings** (cont.) | | | | | | | |
| jalapeños . . . . . . . . . . | 3 | 0 | <1.0 | 0 | 0 | 184 | 0 |
| lettuce . . . . . . . . . . . . | 4 | 0 | 1.0 | 0 | 0 | 3 | <1.0 |
| tomato . . . . . . . . . . . . | 9 | <1.0 | 2.0 | 0 | 0 | 3 | <1.0 |
| mayonnaise . . . . . . . . | 100 | 0 | n.a. | 11.0 | 10 | 75 | n.a. |
| *A.1.* sauce . . . . . . . . . . | 15 | 0 | 3.0 | 0 | 0 | 280 | 0 |
| BBQ sauce . . . . . . . . . | 60 | 0 | 16.0 | 0 | 0 | 400 | 0 |
| mustard . . . . . . . . . . . | 0 | 0 | 0 | 0 | 0 | 55 | 0 |
| relish . . . . . . . . . . . . | 15 | 0 | 4.0 | 0 | 0 | 85 | 0 |
| pickle chips . . . . . . . . | 5 | 0 | 1.0 | 0 | 0 | 265 | 0 |
| **Flagelot beans**, dry: | | | | | | | |
| (*Bob's Red Mill*), ¼ cup . | 150 | 10.0 | 27.0 | .5 | 0 | 5 | 11.0 |
| (*Roland*), ¼ cup . . . . . . . | 120 | 8.0 | 21.0 | 0 | 0 | 10 | 9.0 |
| **Flageolet beans**, canned | | | | | | | |
| (*Roland*), ½ cup . . . . | 130 | 7.0 | 23.0 | 1.0 | 0 | 390 | 6.0 |
| **Flan**, see "Pudding" | | | | | | | |
| **Flatbread**, see "Bread" | | | | | | | |
| and "Cracker" | | | | | | | |
| **Flatbread melts**, see | | | | | | | |
| "Melts" | | | | | | | |
| **Flatfish**, meat only: | | | | | | | |
| raw, 4 oz. . . . . . . . . . . | 104 | 21.4 | 0 | 1.4 | 54 | 92 | 0 |
| baked or broiled, 4 oz. . . | 133 | 27.4 | 0 | 1.7 | 77 | 119 | 0 |
| **Flax seed**: | | | | | | | |
| (*Arrowhead Mills* | | | | | | | |
| Organic), 3 tbsp. . . . . . | 140 | 6.0 | 9.0 | 9.0 | 0 | 0 | 7.0 |
| (*Hodgson Mill* Travel | | | | | | | |
| Milled Flax/Organic | | | | | | | |
| Golden), 1 pkt. . . . . . . | 30 | 1.0 | 2.0 | 2.0 | 0 | 0 | 2.0 |
| brown: | | | | | | | |
| (*Bob's Red Mill* | | | | | | | |
| Organic), 2 tbsp. . . | 90 | 4.0 | 7.0 | 8.0 | 0 | 5 | 6.0 |
| (*Nature's Path* | | | | | | | |
| *FlaxPlus* Organic), | | | | | | | |
| 2 tbsp. . . . . . . . . . . | 110 | 4.0 | 6.0 | 8.0 | 0 | 5 | 5.0 |
| milled (*Hodgson* | | | | | | | |
| *Mill*), 2 tbsp. . . . . . . | 60 | 3.0 | 4.0 | 5.0 | 0 | 0 | 4.0 |
| whole grain (*Hodgson* | | | | | | | |
| *Mill*), 3 tbsp. . . . . . . | 160 | 6.0 | 9.0 | 11.0 | 0 | 9 | 9.0 |
| golden: | | | | | | | |
| (*Arrowhead Mills* | | | | | | | |
| Organic), 3 tbsp. . . | 160 | 8.0 | 10.0 | 10.0 | 0 | 10 | 9.0 |
| (*Bob's Red Mill*), | | | | | | | |
| 3 tbsp. . . . . . . . . . | 160 | 6.0 | 11.0 | 11.0 | 0 | 10 | 9.0 |

| Food and Measure | cal. | prot. (gms) | carbo. (gms) | fat (gms) | chol. (mgs) | sod. (mgs) | fiber (gms) |
|---|---|---|---|---|---|---|---|
| (*Bob's Red Mill* Organic), 2 tbsp. . . | 90 | 4.0 | 7.0 | 8.0 | 0 | 5 | 6.0 |
| (*Hodgson Mill* Milled Organic), 2 tbsp. . . | 65 | 3.0 | 4.0 | 4.0 | 0 | 0 | 4.0 |
| **Flax seed meal**, 2 tbsp: | | | | | | | |
| (*Arrowhead Mills* Organic) . . . . . . . . . . . | 80 | 3.0 | 5.0 | 4.5 | 0 | 0 | 4.0 |
| (*Bob's Red Mill* Regular/Organic) . . . . | 60 | 3.0 | 4.0 | 4.5 | 0 | 0 | 4.0 |
| (*Nature's Path* *FlaxPlus* Organic) . . . . | 80 | 3.0 | 4.0 | 6.0 | 0 | 0 | 4.0 |
| **Flounder**, fresh, see "Flatfish" | | | | | | | |
| **Flounder, frozen**: | | | | | | | |
| breaded (*Mrs. Paul's*), 2.7-oz. pc. . . . . . . . . | 160 | 11.0 | 11.0 | 7.0 | 25 | 150 | 0 |
| garlic encrusted (*SeaPak*), 6 oz., w/sauce . . . . . . . | 300 | 19.0 | 40.0 | 7.0 | 40 | 1010 | 1.0 |
| stuffed (*Oven Poppers*), 5-oz. pc. | | | | | | | |
| au gratin . . . . . . . . . . . | 220 | 24.0 | 5.0 | 11.0 | 75 | 450 | 1.0 |
| broccoli/cheese . . . . . | 150 | 20.0 | 4.0 | 6.0 | 55 | 330 | 1.0 |
| crab . . . . . . . . . . . . . . | 240 | 17.0 | 15.0 | 13.0 | 35 | 400 | 0 |
| garlic/shrimp/almonds | 260 | 16.0 | 16.0 | 14.0 | 40 | 380 | 0 |
| stuffed, crab (*Oven Poppers Qwickies*), 3 oz. . | 150 | 10.0 | 9.0 | 8.0 | 20 | 250 | 0 |
| **Flour**, see "Wheat flour" and specific listings | | | | | | | |
| **Flour, gluten free** (see also specific flours), all purpose: | | | | | | | |
| (*Glutino*), 1 oz. . . . . . . . . | 90 | 1.0 | 26.0 | 0 | 0 | 115 | <1.0 |
| (*Bob's Red Mill*), ¼ cup . | 100 | 3.0 | 22.0 | 1.0 | 0 | 0 | 3.0 |
| **Focaccia, stuffed**, frozen (*Cedarlane*), ⅓ of 12-oz. pkg.: | | | | | | | |
| Mediterranean . . . . . . . . . | 296 | 13.0 | 37.0 | 10.0 | 22 | 485 | 1.0 |
| tomato and basil . . . . . . . | 275 | 14.0 | 33.0 | 9.0 | 14 | 528 | 2.0 |
| **Focaccia sticks** (*New York Style*), 3 pcs., .5 oz.: | | | | | | | |
| quattro formaggio . . . . . . | 70 | 1.0 | 7.0 | 4.0 | 0 | 150 | 0 |
| roasted garlic herb . . . . . | 70 | 1.0 | 7.0 | 4.0 | 0 | 170 | 0 |
| rosemary sea salt . . . . . . | 70 | 1.0 | 7.0 | 4.0 | 0 | 200 | 0 |

| Food and Measure | cal. | prot. (gms) | carbo. (gms) | fat (gms) | chol. (mgs) | sod. (mgs) | fiber (gms) |
|---|---|---|---|---|---|---|---|
| **Foie gras**, see "Pâté, liver" | | | | | | | |
| **Foo qua**, see "Balsam pear" | | | | | | | |
| **Frankfurter**, 1 link, 1.6 oz., except as noted: | | | | | | | |
| (*Ball Park* Bun Size/ Franks), 2 oz. . . . . . . . | 180 | 5.0 | 5.0 | 15.0 | 40 | 480 | 0 |
| (*Ball Park* Fat Free), 1.76 oz. . . . . . . . . . . | 50 | 6.0 | 6.0 | 0 | 10 | 430 | 0 |
| (*Ball Park* Lite), 1.76 oz. . . . . . . . . . . | 100 | 5.0 | 4.0 | 7.0 | 30 | 410 | 0 |
| (*Ball Park* Singles) . . . . . | 140 | 5.0 | 3.0 | 12.0 | 35 | 430 | 0 |
| (*Black Bear* Deli), 2 oz. . . | 170 | 7.0 | 2.0 | 15.0 | 25 | 490 | 0 |
| (*Boar's Head*), 2 oz. . . . . . | 150 | 7.0 | 0 | 14.0 | 25 | 460 | 0 |
| (*Oscar Mayer* Bun Length), 2 oz. . . . . . . . | 170 | 6.0 | 1.0 | 16.0 | 45 | 680 | 0 |
| (*Oscar Mayer* Premium), 2 oz. . . . . . . . . . . . . . | 160 | 7.0 | 1.0 | 14.0 | 45 | 470 | 0 |
| (*Oscar Mayer* Wieners) . . | 130 | 5.0 | 1.0 | 12.0 | 35 | 540 | 0 |
| (*Oscar Mayer* Wieners Light) . . . . . . . . . . . . | 90 | 5.0 | 1.0 | 6.0 | 30 | 380 | 0 |
| beef: | | | | | | | |
| (*Applegate Farms*), 1.5 oz. . . . . . . . . . | 80 | 5.0 | 0 | 6.0 | 20 | 380 | 0 |
| (*Applegate Farms* Big Apple), 2 oz. . . . | 100 | 9.0 | 1.0 | 6.0 | 20 | 640 | 0 |
| (*Applegate Farms* Organic), 1.5 oz. . . | 70 | 6.0 | 1.0 | 4.6 | 20 | 430 | 0 |
| (*Applegate Farms* Organic Stadium-style), 2 oz. . . . . . . . . . . . | 110 | 7.0 | 0 | 8.0 | 30 | 330 | 0 |
| (*Applegate Farms* The Great Organic), 2 oz. . . . . . . . . . . . | 110 | 7.0 | 0 | 8.0 | 30 | 330 | 0 |
| (*Ball Park* Angus), 2 oz. . . . . . . . . . . . . | 170 | 7.0 | 3.0 | 15.0 | 35 | 520 | 0 |
| (*Ball Park* Angus Lower Fat), 1.9 oz. . | 130 | 6.0 | 2.0 | 10.0 | 30 | 510 | 0 |
| (*Ball Park* Bun Size), 2 oz. . . . . . . . . . . . | 190 | 7.0 | 4.0 | 16.0 | 35 | 550 | 0 |
| (*Ball Park* Fat Free), 1.76 oz. . . . . . . . . | 50 | 5.0 | 7.0 | 0 | 10 | 430 | 0 |

| Food and Measure | cal. | prot. (gms) | carbo. (gms) | fat (gms) | chol. (mgs) | sod. (mgs) | fiber (gms) |
|---|---|---|---|---|---|---|---|
| (*Ball Park* Franks), 2 oz. ........... | 190 | 7.0 | 4.0 | 16.0 | 35 | 550 | 0 |
| (*Ball Park* Jumbo), 2.5 oz. .......... | 240 | 9.0 | 5.0 | 20.0 | 45 | 670 | 0 |
| (*Ball Park* Lite), 1.76 oz. ......... | 110 | 5.0 | 5.0 | 7.0 | 20 | 420 | 0 |
| (*Ball Park Grillmaster* Deli), 2.9 oz. ........ | 250 | 9.0 | 3.0 | 21.0 | 45 | 750 | 0 |
| (*Ball Park Singles*) ... | 150 | 5.0 | 3.0 | 13.0 | 25 | 430 | 0 |
| (*Black Bear* Fat Free), 1.8 oz. .......... | 40 | 6.0 | 4.0 | 0 | 15 | 390 | 0 |
| (*Black Bear* Gourmet Lite), 2 oz. ....... | 60 | 8.0 | 3.0 | 1.5 | 15 | 390 | 0 |
| (*Black Bear* New York), 2 oz. ........ | 150 | 7.0 | 2.0 | 13.0 | 30 | 480 | 0 |
| (*Black Bear* Wieners), 2.3 oz. ........... | 180 | 8.0 | 0 | 16.0 | 30 | 480 | 0 |
| (*Boar's Head* Lite) .... | 90 | 7.0 | 0 | 6.0 | 25 | 270 | 0 |
| (*Boar's Head* Natural Casing), 2 oz. ..... | 160 | 7.0 | 1.0 | 14.0 | 30 | 440 | 0 |
| (*Boar's Head* Skinless) | 120 | 6.0 | 0 | 11.0 | 20 | 350 | 0 |
| (*Hebrew National*), 1.7 oz. ........... | 150 | 6.0 | 1.0 | 14.0 | 25 | 460 | 0 |
| (*Hebrew National* Jumbo), 3 oz. ..... | 270 | 10.0 | 2.0 | 25.0 | 45 | 810 | 0 |
| (*Hebrew National* 97% Fat Free), 1.7 oz. ........... | 40 | 6.0 | 3.0 | 1.0 | 10 | 520 | 0 |
| (*Hebrew National* ¼ Pound), 4 oz. ... | 360 | 13.0 | 3.0 | 33.0 | 60 | 1070 | 0 |
| (*Hebrew National* Reduced Fat), 1.7 oz. | 110 | 5.0 | 2.0 | 9.0 | 20 | 490 | 0 |
| (*Oscar Mayer*), 2 oz. ... | 180 | 7.0 | 2.0 | 16.0 | 35 | 420 | 0 |
| (*Oscar Mayer*) ....... | 130 | 5.0 | 1.0 | 12.0 | 30 | 470 | 0 |
| (*Oscar Mayer* Light) .. | 90 | 5.0 | 2.0 | 7.0 | 20 | 380 | 0 |
| (*Oscar Mayer XXL*), 2.7 oz. ........... | 230 | 9.0 | 1.0 | 22.0 | 50 | 740 | 0 |
| (*Wranglers*), 2 oz. .... | 170 | 7.0 | 1.0 | 15.0 | 35 | 560 | 0 |
| beef/cheddar (*Oscar Mayer*), 2 oz. ....... | 170 | 7.0 | 2.0 | 15.0 | 35 | 600 | 0 |
| cheese: | | | | | | | |
| (*Ball Park*), 2 oz. ..... | 190 | 6.0 | 5.0 | 16.0 | 40 | 550 | 0 |
| (*Oscar Mayer* Dogs) .. | 140 | 5.0 | 1.0 | 13.0 | 35 | 540 | 0 |
| (*Wranglers*), 2 oz. .... | 170 | 7.0 | 1.0 | 15.0 | 35 | 610 | 0 |

| Food and Measure | cal. | prot. (gms) | carbo. (gms) | fat (gms) | chol. (mgs) | sod. (mgs) | fiber (gms) |
|---|---|---|---|---|---|---|---|
| **Frankfurter** *(cont.)* | | | | | | | |
| chicken: | | | | | | | |
| (*Applegate Farms*), | | | | | | | |
| 1.5 oz. . . . . . . . . . | 60 | 7.0 | 0 | 3.0 | 35 | 380 | 0 |
| (*Applegate Farms* | | | | | | | |
| Organic), 1.5 oz. . . | 70 | 7.0 | 0 | 4.5 | 30 | 430 | 0 |
| (*Empire Kosher*), 2 oz. | 110 | 6.0 | 0 | 7.0 | 50 | 550 | 0 |
| (*Foster Farms*), 2 oz. . | 140 | 7.0 | 1.0 | 12.0 | 30 | 550 | 0 |
| cocktail, beef: | | | | | | | |
| (*Boar's Head*), 5 pcs. . | 170 | 8.0 | 0 | 15.0 | 30 | 430 | 0 |
| (*Hebrew National*), | | | | | | | |
| 5 pcs. . . . . . . . . . . | 180 | 7.0 | 1.0 | 16.0 | 30 | 540 | 0 |
| (*Hillshire Farm Lit'l* | | | | | | | |
| *Beef Franks*), 6 pcs. | 170 | 6.0 | 2.0 | 15.0 | 30 | 560 | 0 |
| cocktail, pork | | | | | | | |
| (*Applegate Farms* | | | | | | | |
| Organic Smokey), 7 pcs. | 120 | 8.0 | 1.0 | 9.0 | 35 | 390 | 0 |
| jalapeño/cheddar | | | | | | | |
| (*Oscar Mayer*), 2 oz. . . | 160 | 8.0 | 2.0 | 14.0 | 35 | 480 | 0 |
| salmon (*A&B Famous*), | | | | | | | |
| 2 links, 2.6 oz. . . . . . | 170 | 9.0 | 4.0 | 14.0 | 30 | 510 | 0 |
| smoked: | | | | | | | |
| (*Hormel* Smokies), | | | | | | | |
| 1 oz. . . . . . . . . . . . | 80 | 4.0 | 1.0 | 7.0 | 20 | 290 | 0 |
| (*Wranglers*), 2 oz. . . . . | 170 | 7.0 | 1.0 | 15.0 | 35 | 560 | 0 |
| w/cheese (*Hormel* | | | | | | | |
| Smokies), 1 oz. . . . | 80 | 4.0 | 1.0 | 7.0 | 20 | 310 | 0 |
| turkey: | | | | | | | |
| (*Applegate Farms*), | | | | | | | |
| 1.5 oz. . . . . . . . . . | 40 | 6.0 | 0 | 2.0 | 25 | 260 | 0 |
| (*Applegate Farms* | | | | | | | |
| Organic), 1.5 oz. . . | 50 | 6.0 | 0 | 2.5 | 20 | 320 | 0 |
| (*Ball Park*), 2 oz. . . . . . | 110 | 6.0 | 6.0 | 7.0 | 30 | 580 | 0 |
| (*Empire Kosher*), 2 oz. | 100 | 6.0 | 0 | 8.0 | 45 | 540 | 0 |
| (*Foster Farms*), 2 oz. . | 140 | 7.0 | 1.0 | 12.0 | 25 | 560 | 0 |
| (*Jennie-O*), 1.2 oz. . . . | 70 | 4.0 | 1.0 | 5.0 | 25 | 370 | 0 |
| (*Jennie-O* Jumbo), | | | | | | | |
| 2 oz. . . . . . . . . . . . | 120 | 7.0 | 2.0 | 9.0 | 45 | 610 | 0 |
| (*Oscar Mayer*) . . . . . . . | 100 | 5.0 | 2.0 | 8.0 | 30 | 510 | 0 |
| (*Oscar Mayer* Bun | | | | | | | |
| Length), 2 oz. . . . . . | 120 | 6.0 | 3.0 | 10.0 | 35 | 640 | 0 |
| cheese (*Oscar Mayer*) . | 90 | 6.0 | 2.0 | 7.0 | 40 | 490 | 1.0 |
| smoked, white (*Ball* | | | | | | | |
| *Park*), 1.76 oz. . . . . | 45 | 6.0 | 5.0 | 0 | 10 | 420 | 0 |

| Food and Measure | cal. | prot. (gms) | carbo. (gms) | fat (gms) | chol. (mgs) | sod. (mgs) | fiber (gms) |
|---|---|---|---|---|---|---|---|
| **"Frankfurter," vegetarian, canned**, 1 link: | | | | | | | |
| (*Loma Linda* Big), 1.8 oz. | 110 | 11.0 | 3.0 | 6.0 | 0 | 220 | 2.0 |
| (*Loma Linda* Big Low Fat), 1.8 oz. ..... | 80 | 12.0 | 3.0 | 2.5 | 0 | 240 | 2.0 |
| (*Loma Linda* Protein Links), 1.2 oz. ....... | 70 | 7.0 | 1.0 | 4.0 | 0 | 160 | 1.0 |
| (Worthington Super-Links), 1.7 oz. ....... | 110 | 7.0 | 2.0 | 8.0 | 0 | 350 | 1.0 |
| (*Worthington Veja-Links*), 1.1 oz. ... | 50 | 5.0 | 1.0 | 3.0 | 0 | 180 | 0 |
| **"Frankfurter," vegetarian, frozen/chilled**, 1 link, 1.6 oz., except as noted: | | | | | | | |
| (*Tofurky*) ............. | 80 | 11.0 | 5.0 | 2.0 | 0 | 390 | 3.0 |
| (*Veggie Patch Veggie Dogs*) ............. | 90 | 7.0 | 3.0 | 5.0 | 0 | 310 | 0 |
| (*Worthington Leanies*), 1.4 oz. | 100 | 8.0 | 2.0 | 7.0 | 0 | 430 | 1.0 |
| (*Yves* Hot Dogs) ....... | 50 | 10.0 | 2.0 | .5 | 0 | 400 | 0 |
| (*Yves* Hot Dogs Jumbo), 2.7 oz. ..... | 110 | 16.0 | 5.0 | 3.0 | 0 | 460 | 0 |
| (*Yves* The Good Dog) ... | 70 | 8.0 | 1.0 | 3.5 | 0 | 430 | 0 |
| (*Yves* Tofu Dogs), 1.3 oz. ............ | 45 | 8.0 | 2.0 | 1.0 | 0 | 300 | 0 |
| cocktail, in pastry (*Health is Wealth*), 3 pcs., 2.4 oz. ....... | 220 | 8.0 | 16.0 | 16.0 | 0 | 200 | 3.0 |
| **Frankfurter, wrapped**: | | | | | | | |
| (*Hebrew National* Franks in a Blanket), 5 pcs., 2.9 oz. ....... | 290 | 8.0 | 12.0 | 23.0 | 25 | 570 | 1.0 |
| corn dogs (*Foster Farms*), 1 pc., except as noted: | | | | | | | |
| cheese, 2.6 oz. ...... | 200 | 6.0 | 22.0 | 10.0 | 20 | 650 | 0 |
| chili cheese, 2.6 oz. .. | 190 | 7.0 | 21.0 | 9.0 | 25 | 670 | 1.0 |
| honey crunch, 2.6 oz. . | 180 | 7.0 | 19.0 | 9.0 | 25 | 540 | 0 |
| honey crunch, jumbo, 4 oz. ............. | 280 | 10.0 | 26.0 | 15.0 | 45 | 830 | 1.0 |
| honey crunch, mini 4 pcs., 2.6 oz. .... | 210 | 7.0 | 18.0 | 12.0 | 45 | 490 | 1.0 |

| Food and Measure | cal. | prot. (gms) | carbo. (gms) | fat (gms) | chol. (mgs) | sod. (mgs) | fiber (gms) |
|---|---|---|---|---|---|---|---|
| **French toast**, frozen: | | | | | | | |
| (*Aunt Jemima* | | | | | | | |
|   Homestyle), 2 pcs. ... | 220 | 8.0 | 37.0 | 4.5 | 75 | 350 | 1.0 |
| cinnamon (*Aunt* | | | | | | | |
|   *Jemima*), 2 pcs. ...... | 220 | 7.0 | 37.0 | 4.5 | 75 | 360 | 1.0 |
| cinnamon sticks (*Aunt* | | | | | | | |
|   *Jemima*), 4 pcs. ...... | 280 | 5.0 | 45.0 | 9.0 | 0 | 310 | 2.0 |
| sticks, toaster, 2 pcs.: | | | | | | | |
|   (*Van's* Natural) ...... | 190 | 3.0 | 33.0 | 5.0 | 0 | 400 | 1.0 |
|   cinnamon (*Van's* | | | | | | | |
|     Wheat Free) ...... | 190 | 2.0 | 39.0 | 3.5 | 0 | 310 | 1.0 |
| whole grain (*Aunt* | | | | | | | |
|   *Jemima*), 2 pcs. ...... | 210 | 9.0 | 34.0 | 5.0 | 75 | 330 | 3.0 |
| **French toast breakfast** | | | | | | | |
|   (see also "Breakfast | | | | | | | |
|   sandwich"), w/ | | | | | | | |
|   sausage, frozen: | | | | | | | |
| (*Aunt Jemima*), 5.5 oz. ... | 290 | 14.0 | 40.0 | 8.0 | 100 | 610 | 1.0 |
| sticks (*Jimmy D's* | | | | | | | |
|   Duos), 2 sticks, | | | | | | | |
|   2 sausage links ...... | 210 | 12.0 | 19.0 | 10.0 | 105 | 440 | 1.0 |
| **Frog's legs**, raw, 2 oz. ... | 41 | 9.2 | 0 | .2 | 28 | 32 | 0 |
| **Frosting**, ready-to- | | | | | | | |
|   spread, 2 tbsp., | | | | | | | |
|   except as noted: | | | | | | | |
| buttercream: | | | | | | | |
|   (*Betty Crocker*) ...... | 140 | 0 | 23.0 | 5.0 | 0 | 70 | 0 |
|   (*Betty Crocker* | | | | | | | |
|     Whipped) ........ | 100 | 0 | 10.0 | 5.0 | 0 | 25 | 0 |
|   (*Duncan Hines*) ...... | 140 | 0 | 23.0 | 6.0 | 0 | 70 | 0 |
|   (*Pillsbury Creamy* | | | | | | | |
|     Supreme) ........ | 150 | 0 | 24.0 | 6.0 | 0 | 70 | 0 |
| caramel (*Duncan Hines*) . | 140 | 0 | 23.0 | 6.0 | 0 | 70 | 0 |
| cherry (*Betty Crocker*) ... | 140 | 0 | 23.0 | 5.0 | 0 | 70 | 0 |
| chocolate: | | | | | | | |
|   (*Betty Crocker*) ...... | 130 | 0 | 21.0 | 5.0 | 0 | 95 | <1.0 |
|   (*Betty Crocker* | | | | | | | |
|     Whipped) ........ | 90 | <1.0 | 14.0 | 4.5 | 0 | 60 | <1.0 |
|   (*Duncan Hines*) ...... | 140 | 0 | 22.0 | 6.0 | 0 | 95 | <1.0 |
|   (*Duncan Hines* | | | | | | | |
|     Whipped), 3 tbsp. . | 140 | <1.0 | 20.0 | 7.0 | 0 | 70 | <1.0 |
|   (*Pillsbury Creamy* | | | | | | | |
|     Supreme) ........ | 140 | 0 | 21.0 | 6.0 | 0 | 90 | 0 |

| Food and Measure | cal. | prot. (gms) | carbo. (gms) | fat (gms) | chol. (mgs) | sod. (mgs) | fiber (gms) |
|---|---|---|---|---|---|---|---|
| buttercream (*Duncan Hines*) .......... | 140 | 0 | 22.0 | 6.0 | 0 | 90 | <1.0 |
| dark (*Betty Crocker*) .. | 130 | <1.0 | 20.0 | 5.0 | 0 | 105 | <1.0 |
| dark (*Pillsbury Creamy Supreme*) . | 140 | 0 | 21.0 | 6.0 | 0 | 125 | 1.0 |
| milk (*Betty Crocker*) .. | 130 | 0 | 21.0 | 5.0 | 0 | 90 | 0 |
| milk (*Betty Crocker* Whipped) ........ | 100 | 0 | 14.0 | 4.5 | 0 | 55 | <1.0 |
| milk (*Duncan Hines*) .. | 140 | 0 | 22.0 | 6.0 | 0 | 90 | <1.0 |
| milk (*Pillsbury Creamy Supreme*) . | 140 | 0 | 21.0 | 6.0 | 0 | 55 | <1.0 |
| milk (*Pillsbury Whipped Supreme*) ........ | 100 | 0 | 14.0 | 4.5 | 0 | 45 | 0 |
| chocolate fudge: | | | | | | | |
| (*Pillsbury Creamy Supreme*) ........ | 140 | 0 | 21.0 | 6.0 | 0 | 90 | 0 |
| (*Pillsbury Creamy Supreme* No Sugar) | 90 | 0 | 16.0 | 6.0 | 0 | 85 | 3.0 |
| (*Pillsbury Creamy Supreme* Reduced Sugar) .......... | 100 | 0 | 17.0 | 6.0 | 0 | 95 | 4.0 |
| (*Pillsbury Easy Frost*) . | 140 | 0 | 21.0 | 6.0 | 0 | 125 | <1.0 |
| (*Pillsbury Funfetti*) ... | 150 | 0 | 23.0 | 6.0 | 0 | 95 | <1.0 |
| dark (*Duncan Hines*) .. | 130 | <1.0 | 21.0 | 6.0 | 0 | 120 | <1.0 |
| chocolate fudge chip, triple (*Betty Crocker*) . | 140 | <1.0 | 22.0 | 5.0 | 0 | 90 | <1.0 |
| coconut pecan: | | | | | | | |
| (*Betty Crocker*) ...... | 140 | 0 | 19.0 | 7.0 | 0 | 55 | <1.0 |
| (*Duncan Hines*) ...... | 150 | 0 | 18.0 | 9.0 | 0 | 75 | <1.0 |
| (*Pillsbury Creamy Supreme*) ........ | 160 | 1.0 | 17.0 | 10.0 | 0 | 60 | <1.0 |
| confetti (*Pillsbury Funfetti*) ........... | 150 | 0 | 25.0 | 6.0 | 0 | 70 | 0 |
| cream cheese: | | | | | | | |
| (*Betty Crocker*) ...... | 140 | 0 | 23.0 | 5.0 | 0 | 70 | 0 |
| (*Betty Crocker* Whipped) ........ | 100 | 0 | 15.0 | 5.0 | 0 | 45 | 0 |
| (*Duncan Hines*) ...... | 140 | 0 | 23.0 | 6.0 | 0 | 70 | 0 |
| (*Duncan Hines* Whipped), 3 tbsp. . | 160 | 0 | 22.0 | 8.0 | 0 | 70 | 0 |
| (*Pillsbury Creamy Supreme*) ........ | 150 | 0 | 24.0 | 6.0 | 0 | 70 | 0 |
| (*Pillsbury Easy Frost*) . | 150 | 0 | 24.0 | 6.0 | 0 | 80 | 0 |

| Food and Measure | cal. | prot. (gms) | carbo. (gms) | fat (gms) | chol. (mgs) | sod. (mgs) | fiber (gms) |
|---|---|---|---|---|---|---|---|
| **Frosting, cream cheese** *(cont.)* | | | | | | | |
| (*Pillsbury Whipped* | | | | | | | |
| *Supreme*) ........ | 100 | 0 | 15.0 | 5.0 | 0 | 20 | 0 |
| lemon: | | | | | | | |
| (*Betty Crocker*) ...... | 140 | 0 | 23.0 | 5.0 | 0 | 70 | 0 |
| (*Duncan Hines*) ...... | 150 | 0 | 24.0 | 6.0 | 0 | 70 | 0 |
| (*Pillsbury Creamy* | | | | | | | |
| *Supreme*) ........ | 150 | 0 | 23.0 | 6.0 | 0 | 70 | 0 |
| rainbow chip (*Betty* | | | | | | | |
| *Crocker*) ........... | 140 | 0 | 23.0 | 5.0 | 0 | 70 | 0 |
| strawberry: | | | | | | | |
| (*Betty Crocker* | | | | | | | |
| *Whipped Mist*) .... | 100 | 0 | 15.0 | 5.0 | 0 | 25 | 0 |
| (*Pillsbury Creamy* | | | | | | | |
| *Supreme*) ........ | 150 | 0 | 24.0 | 6.0 | 0 | 70 | 0 |
| (*Pillsbury Whipped* | | | | | | | |
| *Supreme*) ........ | 110 | 0 | 15.0 | 5.0 | 0 | 20 | 0 |
| cream (*Duncan Hines*) | 140 | 0 | 23.0 | 6,0 | 0 | 70 | 0 |
| vanilla: | | | | | | | |
| (*Betty Crocker* | | | | | | | |
| *Whipped*) ........ | 100 | 0 | 15.0 | 5.0 | 0 | 25 | 0 |
| (*Duncan Hines*) ...... | 140 | 0 | 23.0 | 6.0 | 0 | 70 | 0 |
| (*Duncan Hines* | | | | | | | |
| *Whipped*), 3 tbsp. . | 150 | 0 | 22.0 | 7.0 | 0 | 60 | 0 |
| (*Pillsbury Creamy* | | | | | | | |
| *Supreme*) ........ | 150 | 0 | 24.0 | 6.0 | 0 | 70 | 0 |
| (*Pillsbury Creamy* | | | | | | | |
| *Supreme* Reduced | | | | | | | |
| Sugar) .......... | 120 | 0 | 18.0 | 7.0 | 0 | 60 | 3.0 |
| (*Pillsbury Creamy* | | | | | | | |
| *Supreme* No Sugar) | 100 | 0 | 17.0 | 6.0 | 0 | 55 | 3.0 |
| (*Pillsbury Easy Frost*) . | 150 | 0 | 24.0 | 6.0 | 0 | 70 | 0 |
| (*Pillsbury Funfetti*) ... | 150 | 0 | 25.0 | 6.0 | 0 | 70 | 0 |
| (*Pillsbury/Pillsbury* | | | | | | | |
| *Funfetti Whipped* | | | | | | | |
| *Supreme*) ........ | 100 | 0 | 15.0 | 5.0 | 0 | 20 | 0 |
| pink (*Pillsbury* | | | | | | | |
| *Funfetti*) .......... | 140 | 0 | 23.0 | 5.0 | 0 | 65 | 0 |
| vanilla or white: | | | | | | | |
| (*Betty Crocker*) ...... | 140 | 0 | 23.0 | 5.0 | 0 | 70 | 0 |
| or whipped cream | | | | | | | |
| (*Betty Crocker* | | | | | | | |
| *Whipped*) ........ | 100 | 0 | 15.0 | 5.0 | 0 | 25 | 0 |

| Food and Measure | cal. | prot. (gms) | carbo. (gms) | fat (gms) | chol. (mgs) | sod. (mgs) | fiber (gms) |
|---|---|---|---|---|---|---|---|
| white: | | | | | | | |
| (*Duncan Hines* | | | | | | | |
| Whipped), 3 tbsp. | 150 | 0 | 22.0 | 7.0 | 0 | 60 | 0 |
| (*Pillsbury Creamy* | | | | | | | |
| *Supreme* Classic) | 150 | 0 | 24.0 | 6.0 | 0 | 70 | 0 |
| (*Pillsbury Whipped* | | | | | | | |
| *Supreme*) | 100 | 0 | 15.0 | 5.0 | 0 | 20 | 0 |
| **Frosting mix:** | | | | | | | |
| chocolate (*Dr. Oetker* | | | | | | | |
| Organics), 1/12 pkg. | 110 | 0 | 26.0 | 0 | 0 | 65 | 0 |
| fudge ("*Jiffy*"), 1/4 pkg. | 150 | <1.0 | 28.0 | 4.0 | 0 | 130 | <1.0 |
| vanilla (*Dr. Oetker* | | | | | | | |
| Organics), 1/12 pkg. | 110 | 0 | 27.0 | 0 | 0 | 65 | 0 |
| white: | | | | | | | |
| (*Betty Crocker* | | | | | | | |
| Fluffy), 6 tbsp.* | 100 | <1.0 | 24.0 | 0 | 0 | 55 | 0 |
| ("*Jiffy*"), 1/4 pkg. | 150 | 0 | 28.0 | 4.0 | 0 | 140 | 0 |
| **Fruit**, see specific | | | | | | | |
| listings | | | | | | | |
| **Fruit, mixed**, can/jar | | | | | | | |
| (see also "Fruit | | | | | | | |
| cocktail"), 1/2 cup, | | | | | | | |
| except as noted: | | | | | | | |
| in juice: | | | | | | | |
| (*Del Monte*), 4 oz. | 50 | 0 | 13.0 | 0 | 0 | 10 | <1.0 |
| (*Del Monte* Cherry Bowl) | 70 | 0 | 17.0 | 0 | 0 | <20 | 2.0 |
| (*Del Monte Fruit* | | | | | | | |
| *Naturals* Cherry) | 70 | <1.0 | 17.0 | 0 | 0 | 10 | <1.0 |
| (*Del Monte Orchard* | | | | | | | |
| *Select*) | 80 | <1.0 | 19.0 | 0 | 0 | 10 | <1.0 |
| chunky (*Del Monte*) | 60 | 0 | 15.0 | 0 | 0 | 10 | 1.0 |
| chunky (*S&W* | | | | | | | |
| Natural Style) | 80 | <1.0 | 19.0 | 0 | 0 | 20 | 3.0 |
| citrus (*Del Monte* | | | | | | | |
| Salad Bowl) | 60 | 1.0 | 16.0 | 0 | 0 | 10 | 2.0 |
| citrus (*Del Monte* | | | | | | | |
| *Fruit Naturals* | | | | | | | |
| Salad) | 70 | 0 | 20.0 | 0 | 0 | 20 | 0 |
| in juice, tropical: | | | | | | | |
| (*Del Monte*) | 60 | 0 | 16.0 | 0 | 0 | 15 | 1.0 |
| (*Del Monte*), 4 oz. | 70 | <1.0 | 18.0 | 0 | 0 | 5 | <1.0 |
| (*Del Monte Fruit* | | | | | | | |
| *Naturals* Hawaiian | | | | | | | |
| Style Medley) | 70 | 1.0 | 18.0 | 0 | 0 | 10 | 3.0 |

| Food and Measure | cal. | prot. (gms) | carbo. (gms) | fat (gms) | chol. (mgs) | sod. (mgs) | fiber (gms) |
|---|---|---|---|---|---|---|---|
| **Fruit, mixed, in juice, tropical** *(cont.)* | | | | | | | |
| (*Del Monte Fruit Naturals* Medley) .. | 70 | <1.0 | 18.0 | 0 | 0 | 5 | <1.0 |
| (*Dole* Can) ......... | 90 | 0 | 21.0 | 0 | 0 | 0 | 1.0 |
| mango/passion fruit juice (*Del Monte Superfruit*), 6 oz. .. | 120 | 2.0 | 29.0 | 0 | 0 | 25 | 3.0 |
| in extra light syrup: | | | | | | | |
| (*Del Monte* Lite), 4-oz. can ........ | 50 | 0 | 13.0 | 0 | 0 | 10 | <1.0 |
| chunky (*Del Monte* Lite) ............ | 60 | 0 | 15.0 | 0 | 0 | 10 | 1.0 |
| citrus (*Del Monte/ SunFresh* Salad) ... | 70 | 0 | 20.0 | 0 | 0 | 20 | 0 |
| in light syrup: | | | | | | | |
| (*Del Monte*), 4-oz. cup | 70 | <1.0 | 18.0 | 0 | 0 | 10 | <1.0 |
| (*Del Monte*), 4-oz. can | 80 | 0 | 20.0 | 0 | 0 | 10 | <1.0 |
| (*Dole* bowl), 4 oz. ..... | 80 | 0 | 19.0 | 0 | 0 | 0 | 1.0 |
| (*Dole* jar) .......... | 80 | 0 | 21.0 | 0 | 0 | 0 | 1.0 |
| (*Del Monte* Cherry), 4-oz. cup ........ | 70 | <1.0 | 18.0 | 0 | 0 | 10 | <1.0 |
| (*Del Monte* Cherry/ Very Cherry) ...... | 90 | <1.0 | 22.0 | 0 | 0 | 10 | <1.0 |
| citrus (*Del Monte*) ... | 80 | 0 | 20.0 | 0 | 0 | 20 | 0 |
| in light syrup, tropical: | | | | | | | |
| (*Del Monte*) ........ | 80 | 0 | 21.0 | 0 | 0 | 10 | 1.0 |
| (*Del Monte SunFresh* Salad) ... | 80 | 1.0 | 20.0 | 0 | 0 | 10 | 0 |
| (*Dole* Bowl), 4 oz. ..... | 80 | <1.0 | 19.0 | 0 | 0 | 0 | 1.0 |
| (*Dole* Jar) .......... | 90 | 1.0 | 22.0 | 0 | 0 | 10 | 1.0 |
| w/passion fruit juice (*Del Monte SunFresh*) ....... | 70 | 0 | 18.0 | 0 | 0 | 10 | 1.0 |
| w/passion fruit juice (*Roland*) .... | 100 | 1.0 | 23.0 | 0 | 0 | 0 | 2.0 |
| in heavy syrup, chunky (*Del Monte*) ........ | 100 | 0 | 24.0 | 0 | 0 | 10 | 1.0 |
| in gelatin: | | | | | | | |
| cherry (*Del Monte*), 4.5-oz. cup ....... | 90 | 0 | 23.0 | 0 | 0 | 40 | 0 |
| cherry (*Dole* Sugar Free), 4.3-oz. cup .. | 60 | 0 | 14.0 | 0 | 0 | 45 | 1.0 |
| cherry or peach (*Dole*), 4.3-oz. cup . | 100 | 0 | 24.0 | 0 | 0 | 25 | 1.0 |

| Food and Measure | cal. | prot. (gms) | carbo. (gms) | fat (gms) | chol. (mgs) | sod. (mgs) | fiber (gms) |
|---|---|---|---|---|---|---|---|
| **Fruit, mixed, candied,** | | | | | | | |
| 1 oz. .............. | 91 | .1 | 23.4 | 0 | 0 | 28 | .5 |
| **Fruit, mixed, dried,** | | | | | | | |
| 1.4 oz., ¼ cup, | | | | | | | |
| except as noted: | | | | | | | |
| (*Mariani*) ............. | 100 | 2.0 | 27.0 | 0 | 0 | 25 | 3.0 |
| (*Sun•Maid*) ........... | 100 | 1.0 | 26.0 | 0 | 0 | 35 | 3.0 |
| (*Sun•Maid* Bits) ........ | 120 | 1.0 | 29.0 | 0 | 0 | 20 | 2.0 |
| (*Sunsweet* Orchard) .... | 100 | 1.0 | 25.0 | 0 | 0 | 60 | 3.0 |
| all varieties (*Annie's* | | | | | | | |
| Snacks), .8-oz. pkg. .. | 70 | 0 | 18.0 | 0 | 0 | 45 | 0 |
| tropical mix: | | | | | | | |
| (*Mariani* Island) ..... | 140 | 1.0 | 33.0 | 0 | 0 | 100 | 2.0 |
| (*Mariani* Medley), | | | | | | | |
| ⅓ cup ........... | 130 | 1.0 | 31.0 | 0 | 0 | 40 | 3.0 |
| (*Sun•Maid* Trio) ..... | 140 | 0 | 34.0 | 0 | 0 | 75 | 1.0 |
| **Fruit, mixed, frozen:** | | | | | | | |
| (*Birds Eye*), 1⅓ cup .... | 60 | 1.0 | 14.0 | 0 | 0 | 0 | 3.0 |
| (*C&W Ultimate*), ⅔ cup .. | 50 | 1.0 | 13.0 | 0 | 0 | 5 | 2.0 |
| (*Dole Wildly Nutritious*), | | | | | | | |
| ¾ cup ............. | 60 | 0 | 16.0 | 0 | 0 | 5 | 2.0 |
| tropical (*Dole Wildly* | | | | | | | |
| *Nutritious*), ¾ cup ... | 70 | 0 | 17.0 | 0 | 0 | 0 | 3.0 |
| **Fruit bar**, frozen | | | | | | | |
| (see also "Ice bar," | | | | | | | |
| and "Iced confection | | | | | | | |
| bar,"), 1 bar: | | | | | | | |
| all varieties: | | | | | | | |
| (*Breyers Pure Fruit*) .. | 40 | 0 | 10.0 | 0 | 0 | 0 | 0 |
| (*Breyers Pure Fruit* | | | | | | | |
| No Sugar) ....... | 25 | 0 | 5.0 | 0 | 0 | 0 | 0 |
| (*Dreyer's/Edy's* | | | | | | | |
| Variety No Sugar) .. | 30 | 0 | 8.0 | 0 | 0 | 0 | 1.0 |
| (*Minute Maid*) ....... | 60 | 0 | 15.0 | 0 | 0 | 10 | 0 |
| and cream (*Dreyer's/ | | | | | | | |
| Edy's* Variety | | | | | | | |
| Snack Size) ...... | 45 | 0 | 9.0 | 0 | 0 | 15 | 0 |
| acai blueberry (*Dreyer's/ | | | | | | | |
| Edy's*) ............. | 60 | 0 | 16.0 | 0 | 0 | 0 | 0 |
| banana and cream | | | | | | | |
| (*FrozFruit*) .......... | 160 | 1.0 | 27.0 | 6.0 | 25 | 15 | 1.0 |
| cherry: | | | | | | | |
| (*Dreyer's/Edy's* Variety | | | | | | | |
| Snack Size) ...... | 50 | 0 | 13.0 | 0 | 0 | 0 | 0 |

| Food and Measure | cal. | prot. (gms) | carbo. (gms) | fat (gms) | chol. (mgs) | sod. (mgs) | fiber (gms) |
|---|---|---|---|---|---|---|---|
| **Fruit bar, cherry** *(cont.)* | | | | | | | |
| (*Minute Maid* Juice) .. | 60 | 0 | 15.0 | 0 | 0 | 10 | 0 |
| coconut: | | | | | | | |
| (*Dreyer's/Edy's*) ..... | 120 | 3.0 | 21.0 | 3.0 | 0 | 40 | 1.0 |
| (*FrozFruit*) .......... | 200 | 2.0 | 19.0 | 14.0 | 35 | 25 | <1.0 |
| (*FrozFruit* 6 Pack) .... | 150 | 1.0 | 14.0 | 10.0 | 25 | 20 | <1.0 |
| (*Palapa Azul*) ....... | 80 | 0 | 10.0 | 4.0 | 0 | 10 | 0 |
| (*Whole Fruit*) ....... | 140 | 2.0 | 18.0 | 7.0 | 15 | 40 | 1.0 |
| cucumber chile | | | | | | | |
| (*Palapa Azul*) ....... | 40 | 0 | 10.0 | 0 | 0 | 180 | 1.0 |
| grape: | | | | | | | |
| (*Dreyer's/Edy's*) ..... | 80 | 0 | 20.0 | 0 | 0 | 0 | 0 |
| (*Dreyer's/Edy's* Variety Snack Size) ...... | 50 | 0 | 13.0 | 0 | 0 | 0 | 0 |
| (*Minute Maid* Juice) .. | 60 | 0 | 15.0 | 0 | 0 | 15 | 0 |
| lemon lime (*Whole Fruit* No Sugar) ...... | 45 | 0 | 15.0 | 0 | 0 | 10 | 0 |
| lemonade (*Dreyer's/ Edy's*) ............. | 80 | 0 | 20.0 | 0 | 0 | 0 | 0 |
| lime: | | | | | | | |
| (*Dreyer's/Edy's*) ..... | 80 | 0 | 20.0 | 0 | 0 | 0 | 0 |
| (*Dreyer's/Edy's* Variety Pack) ..... | 60 | 0 | 13.0 | 0 | 0 | 0 | 0 |
| (*Whole Fruit*) ....... | 70 | 0 | 17.0 | 0 | 0 | 5 | 0 |
| double (*FrozFruit*) .... | 120 | 0 | 32.0 | 0 | 0 | 15 | 0 |
| mango: | | | | | | | |
| (*Palapa Azul*) ....... | 70 | 0 | 18.0 | 0 | 0 | 0 | 0 |
| (*Whole Fruit*) ....... | 60 | 0 | 16.0 | 0 | 0 | 5 | <1.0 |
| chunky (*FrozFruit*) ... | 140 | 0 | 35.0 | 0 | 0 | 15 | 0 |
| mango chile (*Palapa Azul*) .............. | 70 | 0 | 17.0 | 0 | 0 | 290 | 0 |
| mango raspberry (*Sweet Nothings*) .......... | 100 | 1.0 | 23.0 | 0 | 0 | 10 | 0 |
| orange (*Minute Maid* Juice) | 60 | 0 | 15.0 | 0 | 0 | 10 | 0 |
| orange and cream (*Dreyer's/Edy's*) ..... | 80 | 1.0 | 16.0 | 1.5 | 5 | 30 | 0 |
| papaya (*Palapa Azul* Mexican) ............ | 60 | 0 | 14.0 | 0 | 0 | 0 | 1.0 |
| piña colada, creamy (*FrozFruit*) .......... | 190 | 2.0 | 37.0 | 3.5 | 5 | 25 | <1.0 |
| pineapple: | | | | | | | |
| (*Dreyer's/Edy's*) ..... | 80 | 0 | 19.0 | 0 | 0 | 0 | 0 |
| (*Palapa Azul*) ....... | 60 | 0 | 15.0 | 0 | 0 | 0 | 1.0 |
| chunky (*FrozFruit*) ... | 120 | 0 | 30.0 | 0 | 0 | 10 | 0 |

| Food and Measure | cal. | prot. (gms) | carbo. (gms) | fat (gms) | chol. (mgs) | sod. (mgs) | fiber (gms) |
|---|---|---|---|---|---|---|---|
| pomegranate: | | | | | | | |
| (*Dreyer's/Edy's*) ..... | 70 | 0 | 17.0 | 0 | 0 | 0 | 0 |
| cherry (*FrozFruit*) .... | 140 | 0 | 35.0 | 0 | 0 | 15 | 0 |
| strawberries and cream | | | | | | | |
| (*FrozFruit*) .......... | 160 | <1.0 | 27.0 | 5.0 | 20 | 25 | <1.0 |
| strawberry: | | | | | | | |
| (*Dreyer's/Edy's*) ..... | 80 | 0 | 21.0 | 0 | 0 | 0 | 0 |
| (*Dreyer's/Edy's* | | | | | | | |
| Variety Pack) ..... | 60 | 0 | 13.0 | 0 | 0 | 0 | 0 |
| (*Palapa Azul*) ....... | 50 | 0 | 13.0 | 0 | 0 | 0 | 1.0 |
| (*Whole Fruit*) ....... | 70 | 0 | 17.0 | 0 | 0 | 5 | <1.0 |
| (*Whole Fruit* No Sugar) | 50 | 0 | 16.0 | 0 | 0 | 10 | <1.0 |
| chunky (*FrozFruit*) ... | 130 | 0 | 33.0 | 0 | 0 | 15 | <1.0 |
| chunky (*FrozFruit* | | | | | | | |
| 6 Pack) .......... | 100 | 0 | 25.0 | 0 | 0 | 10 | <1.0 |
| chunky (*FrozFruit* No | | | | | | | |
| Sugar 6 Pack) .... | 35 | 0 | 15.0 | 0 | 0 | 10 | 3.0 |
| tangerine (*Dreyer's/* | | | | | | | |
| *Edy's*) ............. | 80 | 0 | 19.0 | 0 | 0 | 0 | 0 |
| tropical: | | | | | | | |
| (*Dreyer's/Edy's* Variety | | | | | | | |
| Snack Size) ...... | 50 | 0 | 13.0 | 0 | 0 | 0 | 0 |
| all flavors (*Minute* | | | | | | | |
| *Maid* Juice) ...... | 60 | 0 | 15.0 | 0 | 0 | 10 | 0 |
| watermelon (*Palapa* | | | | | | | |
| *Azul* Sandia) ........ | 50 | 0 | 14.0 | 0 | 0 | 0 | 0 |
| wildberry (*Dreyer's/Edy's* | | | | | | | |
| Variety Pack) ....... | 60 | 0 | 13.0 | 0 | 0 | 0 | 0 |
| **Fruit cocktail**, can/jar, | | | | | | | |
| ½ cup: | | | | | | | |
| (*Del Monte Carb* | | | | | | | |
| *Clever*) ............. | 40 | 0 | 11.0 | 0 | 0 | 10 | <1.0 |
| in juice: | | | | | | | |
| (*Del Monte* 100%) ... | 60 | 0 | 15.0 | 0 | 0 | 10 | 1.0 |
| (*S&W* Natural Style) .. | 80 | 0 | 20.0 | 0 | 0 | 20 | 2.0 |
| w/liquid ............ | 55 | .6 | 14.1 | 0 | 0 | 5 | 1.2 |
| in extra light syrup | | | | | | | |
| (*Del Monte* Lite) ..... | 60 | 0 | 15.0 | 0 | 0 | 10 | 1.0 |
| in light syrup: | | | | | | | |
| (*S&W*) ............. | 70 | 0 | 18.0 | 0 | 0 | 15 | 1.0 |
| w/liquid ............ | 72 | .5 | 18.8 | .1 | 0 | 7 | 1.4 |
| in heavy syrup: | | | | | | | |
| (*Del Monte*) ........ | 100 | 0 | 24.0 | 0 | 0 | 10 | 1.0 |
| w/liquid ............ | 91 | .5 | 23.4 | .1 | 0 | 7 | 1.2 |

| Food and Measure | cal. | prot. (gms) | carbo. (gms) | fat (gms) | chol. (mgs) | sod. (mgs) | fiber (gms) |
|---|---|---|---|---|---|---|---|
| **Fruit dip**, 2 tbsp., except as noted: | | | | | | | |
| caramel: | | | | | | | |
| (*Litehouse* Nonfat) ... | 110 | 1.0 | 27.0 | 0 | 0 | 140 | 0 |
| (*Litehouse* Original) .. | 110 | 1.0 | 25.0 | 1.5 | 0 | 125 | 0 |
| (*Marzetti* Apple Dip Fat Free) ......... | 100 | 0 | 25.0 | 0 | 0 | 105 | 0 |
| (*Marzetti* Apple Dip Light) ........... | 100 | 1.0 | 26.0 | 1.5 | 5 | 75 | 0 |
| (*Marzetti* Apple Dip Old Fashioned) .... | 140 | 0 | 22.0 | 6.0 | 5 | 75 | 0 |
| chocolate (*Litehouse*) . | 120 | 1.0 | 23.0 | 3.0 | 0 | 120 | 0 |
| cinnamon (*Litehouse*) . | 120 | 1.0 | 26.0 | 1.0 | 0 | 100 | 0 |
| cinnamon (*Marzetti* Apple Dip) ....... | 90 | 0 | 22.0 | 1.0 | 5 | 60 | 0 |
| chocolate: | | | | | | | |
| (*Litehouse*), 1.4 oz. ... | 100 | 0 | 25.0 | 1.5 | 0 | 45 | 4.0 |
| (*Marzetti*) .......... | 110 | 1.0 | 23.0 | 2.0 | 0 | 85 | 1.0 |
| milk (*Baker's* Real) ... | 80 | 1.0 | 9.0 | 5.0 | 0 | 10 | 0 |
| semisweet, dark (*Baker's* Real) ..... | 70 | 1.0 | 9.0 | 4.5 | 0 | 5 | 1.0 |
| cream cheese: | | | | | | | |
| (*Litehouse*) ......... | 80 | 1.0 | 10.0 | 4.0 | 5 | 105 | 0 |
| (*Marzetti*) .......... | 70 | 0 | 10.0 | 3.0 | 15 | 85 | 0 |
| strawberry (*Marzetti*) ........ | 70 | 0 | 9.0 | 3.5 | 15 | 90 | 0 |
| honey vanilla cream (*Marie's*) ........... | 60 | 1.0 | 5.0 | 4.5 | 15 | 20 | 0 |
| peanut butter caramel (*Marzetti* Apple Dip) .............. | 120 | 2.0 | 17.0 | 5.0 | 0 | 160 | 1.0 |
| yogurt: | | | | | | | |
| strawberry (*Litehouse*) | 50 | 1.0 | 10.0 | 1.5 | 0 | 45 | 0 |
| vanilla (*Litehouse*) ... | 60 | 1.0 | 10.0 | 1.5 | 0 | 50 | 0 |
| vanilla (*Litehouse* Single), 2 oz. ...... | 110 | 2.0 | 19.0 | 3.0 | 0 | 70 | 0 |
| vanilla, French (*Marzetti* Light) ... | 45 | 0 | 10.0 | 0 | 0 | 45 | 0 |
| **Fruit drink blend** (see also specific listings), 8 fl. oz., except as noted: | | | | | | | |
| (*Odwalla Heart Health* Smoothie) .......... | 130 | 1.0 | 30.0 | 0 | 0 | 20 | 0 |

| Food and Measure | cal. | prot. (gms) | carbo. (gms) | fat (gms) | chol. (mgs) | sod. (mgs) | fiber (gms) |
|---|---|---|---|---|---|---|---|
| (*Odwalla Mo'Beta* Antioxidant Smoothie) | 150 | 1.0 | 37.0 | 0 | 0 | 15 | 1.0 |
| (*Odwalla Super Protein*) ......... | 190 | 10.0 | 35.0 | 1.0 | 0 | 180 | 1.0 |
| (*Odwalla Superfood Pink Poetry* Smoothie) ......... | 140 | 2.0 | 32.0 | 0 | 0 | 15 | 0 |
| (*V8 Splash* Medley) ..... | 70 | 0 | 18.0 | 0 | 0 | 50 | 0 |
| citrus (*Odwalla C Monster* Smoothie) .. | 150 | 2.0 | 36.0 | 0 | 0 | 15 | 0 |
| punch: | | | | | | | |
| (*Apple & Eve*) ....... | 120 | 0 | 29.0 | 0 | 0 | 20 | 0 |
| (*AriZona*) .......... | 100 | 0 | 26.0 | 0 | 0 | 25 | 0 |
| (*Lipton Brisk*) ....... | 110 | 0 | 29.0 | 0 | 0 | 55 | 0 |
| (*Minute Maid*), 12 fl. oz. ......... | 160 | 0 | 44.0 | 0 | 0 | 110 | 0 |
| (*Minute Maid* 3%) ... | 110 | 0 | 30.0 | 0 | 0 | 75 | 0 |
| (*Minute Maid* 5%) ... | 120 | 0 | 31.0 | 0 | 0 | 15 | 0 |
| (*Minute Maid* Coolers), 6.75 fl. oz. ....... | 100 | 0 | 26.0 | 0 | 0 | 15 | 0 |
| (*Snapple*) .......... | 110 | 0 | 27.0 | 0 | 0 | 5 | 0 |
| (*SoBe Power*) ....... | 110 | 0 | 27.0 | 0 | 0 | 15 | 0 |
| (*Tropicana*) ......... | 130 | 0 | 32.0 | 0 | 0 | 25 | 0 |
| (*Tropicana* Light) .... | 10 | 0 | 2.0 | 0 | 0 | 25 | 0 |
| (*Turkey Hill*) ........ | 100 | 0 | 25.0 | 0 | 0 | 10 | 0 |
| (*Veryfine*) .......... | 80 | 0 | 20.0 | 0 | 0 | 14 | 0 |
| (*Veryfine*), 10 fl. oz. .. | 100 | 0 | 25.0 | 0 | 0 | 17 | 0 |
| (*Welch's*) .......... | 130 | 0 | 31.0 | 0 | 0 | 20 | 0 |
| frozen* (*Minute Maid*) | 110 | 0 | 30.0 | 0 | 0 | 0 | 0 |
| w/yumberry and goji berry (*Honest Ade* Organic) ......... | 48 | 0 | 12.0 | 0 | 0 | 5 | 0 |
| tropical: | | | | | | | |
| (*Bolthouse Farms C-Boost Smoothie*) | 152 | 1.0 | 36.0 | 0 | 0 | 15 | <1.0 |
| (*Minute Maid*) ....... | 110 | 0 | 30.0 | 0 | 0 | 15 | 0 |
| (*Minute Maid* Coolers), 6.75 fl. oz. ....... | 100 | 0 | 26.0 | 0 | 0 | 15 | 0 |
| (*Odwalla Serious Energy*) ......... | 160 | 1.0 | 39.0 | 0 | 0 | 20 | 0 |
| (*Odwalla Wholly Grain!* Tropical Medley Smoothie) . | 200 | 3.0 | 45.0 | 1.0 | 0 | 25 | 3.0 |

| Food and Measure | cal. | prot. (gms) | carbo. (gms) | fat (gms) | chol. (mgs) | sod. (mgs) | fiber (gms) |
|---|---|---|---|---|---|---|---|
| **Fruit drink blend, tropical** *(cont.)* | | | | | | | |
| (*Santa Cruz Organic* | | | | | | | |
| Box) . . . . . . . . . . . . | 110 | 0 | 27.0 | 0 | 0 | 5 | 0 |
| (*Tropicana*) . . . . . . . . | 120 | 0 | 31.0 | 0 | 0 | 25 | 0 |
| (*Tropicana Twister* | | | | | | | |
| Fury) . . . . . . . . . . . | 140 | 0 | 35.0 | 0 | 0 | 25 | 0. |
| (*V8 Splash*) . . . . . . . . | 70 | 0 | 18.0 | 0 | 0 | 50 | 0 |
| colada (*V8 Splash* | | | | | | | |
| Smoothies) . . . . . . | 100 | 3.0 | 21.0 | 0 | 0 | 50 | 1.0 |
| frozen* (*Minute Maid*) | 100 | 0 | 28.0 | 0 | 0 | 0 | 0 |
| **Fruit glaze**, see | | | | | | | |
| specific fruits | | | | | | | |
| **Fruit juice blend** | | | | | | | |
| (see also specific | | | | | | | |
| listings), 8 fl. oz., | | | | | | | |
| except as noted: | | | | | | | |
| (*Bolthouse Farms* | | | | | | | |
| *Green Goodness* | | | | | | | |
| Smoothie) . . . . . . . . . . | 140 | 2.0 | 33.0 | 0 | 0 | 25 | 1.0 |
| (*Ceres* Medley) . . . . . . . . | 130 | 0 | 31.0 | 0 | 0 | 10 | 2.0 |
| (*Langers* Autumn/ | | | | | | | |
| Spring/Winter) . . . . . . | 120 | 0 | 30.0 | 0 | 0 | 10 | 0 |
| (*Langers* Summer) . . . . . | 120 | 0 | 31.0 | 0 | 0 | 10 | 0 |
| (*Odwalla Superfood* | | | | | | | |
| Smoothie) . . . . . . . . . . | 130 | 1.0 | 30.0 | .5 | 0 | 10 | 0 |
| (*Odwalla Superfood* | | | | | | | |
| Red Rhapsody | | | | | | | |
| Smoothie) . . . . . . . . . . | 110 | 1.0 | 26.0 | 0 | 0 | 15 | 0 |
| (*R.W. Knudsen* | | | | | | | |
| Razzleberry) . . . . . . . . | 120 | 0 | 30.0 | 0 | 0 | 15 | 0 |
| (*R.W. Knudsen* | | | | | | | |
| Razzleberry Box) . . . . | 120 | <1.0 | 28.0 | 0 | 0 | 15 | 0 |
| (*Simply Nutritious* | | | | | | | |
| *Mega Antioxidant*) . . . | 120 | 0 | 29.0 | 0 | 0 | 20 | 0 |
| (*Simply Nutritious* | | | | | | | |
| *Mega C*) . . . . . . . . . . . | 140 | 0 | 34.0 | 0 | 0 | 15 | 0 |
| (*Simply Nutritious* | | | | | | | |
| *Mega Green*) . . . . . . . . | 130 | 1.0 | 31.0 | 0 | 0 | 35 | 0 |
| (*Simply Nutritious* | | | | | | | |
| *Morning Blend*) . . . . . | 130 | 1.0 | 30.0 | 0 | 0 | 25 | 0 |
| (*Simply Nutritious* | | | | | | | |
| *Plum Boost*) . . . . . . . . | 120 | 1.0 | 33.0 | 0 | 0 | 10 | 0 |
| (*Simply Nutritious* | | | | | | | |
| *Vita Juice*) . . . . . . . . . . | 120 | 1.0 | 31.0 | 0 | 0 | 40 | <1.0 |

| Food and Measure | cal. | prot. (gms) | carbo. (gms) | fat (gms) | chol. (mgs) | sod. (mgs) | fiber (gms) |
|---|---|---|---|---|---|---|---|
| punch: | | | | | | | |
| (*Apple & Eve*), | | | | | | | |
| 6.75 fl. oz. ....... | 100 | 1.0 | 24.0 | 0 | 0 | 25 | 0 |
| (*Snapple*), 11.5 fl. oz. . | 170 | 0 | 42.0 | 0 | 0 | 15 | 0 |
| (*Tropicana*), 10 fl. oz. . | 170 | 1.0 | 40.0 | 0 | 0 | 30 | 0 |
| (*Veryfine*), 11.5 fl. oz. . | 190 | 0 | 47.0 | 0 | 0 | 60 | 0 |
| tropical: | | | | | | | |
| (*Dole* Paradise) ...... | 120 | <1.0 | 29.0 | 0 | 0 | 40 | 0 |
| (*R.W. Knudsen* Box) .. | 120 | <1.0 | 29.0 | 0 | 0 | 15 | 0 |
| **Fruit pectin** (*Sure•* | | | | | | | |
| *Jell*), ⅛ tsp ......... | 0 | 0 | 0 | 0 | 0 | 5 | 0 |
| **Fruit sauce**, Asian, | | | | | | | |
| four (*Heaven and* | | | | | | | |
| *Earth*), 1 tbsp. ....... | 20 | <1.0 | 9.0 | <1.0 | 0 | 10 | 0 |
| **Fruit spread** (see also | | | | | | | |
| "Jam and preserves" | | | | | | | |
| and specific listings), | | | | | | | |
| all fruits, 1 tbsp.: | | | | | | | |
| (*Cascadian Farm* | | | | | | | |
| Organic) ......... | 40 | 0 | 10.0 | 0 | 0 | 0 | 0 |
| (*Smucker's Simply Fruit*) | 40 | 0 | 10.0 | 0 | 0 | 0 | 0 |
| (*Sorrell Ridge*) ...... | 36 | 0 | 9.0 | 0 | 0 | 0 | 0 |
| except blackberry | | | | | | | |
| (*Polaner Fancy* | | | | | | | |
| *Fruit* w/Fiber) ..... | 30 | 0 | 10.0 | 0 | 0 | 0 | 3.0 |
| apricot: | | | | | | | |
| (*Polaner All Fruit* | | | | | | | |
| w/Fiber) ......... | 30 | 0 | 9.0 | 0 | 0 | 0 | 3.0 |
| (*Roland*) ........... | 45 | 0 | 12.0 | 0 | 0 | 0 | 0 |
| blackberry: | | | | | | | |
| (*Polaner All Fruit* | | | | | | | |
| w/Fiber) ......... | 30 | 0 | 10.0 | 0 | 0 | 0 | 3.0 |
| (*Polaner Fancy Fruit* | | | | | | | |
| w/Fiber) ......... | 30 | 0 | 9.0 | 0 | 0 | 0 | 3.0 |
| blueberry or peach | | | | | | | |
| (*Polaner All* | | | | | | | |
| *Fruit* w/Fiber) ...... | 30 | 0 | 9.0 | 0 | 0 | 0 | 3.0 |
| cherry (*Roland*) ........ | 40 | 0 | 10.0 | 0 | 0 | 0 | 0 |
| peach (*Roland*) ........ | 50 | 0 | 12.0 | 0 | 0 | 0 | 0 |
| raspberry or mixed | | | | | | | |
| berry (*Roland*) ...... | 30 | 0 | 7.0 | 0 | 0 | 0 | 0 |
| raspberry or strawberry: | | | | | | | |
| (*Polaner All Fruit* | | | | | | | |
| w/Fiber) ......... | 35 | 0 | 10.0 | 0 | 0 | 0 | 3.0 |

| Food and Measure | cal. | prot. (gms) | carbo. (gms) | fat (gms) | chol. (mgs) | sod. (mgs) | fiber (gms) |
|---|---|---|---|---|---|---|---|
| **Fruit spread, raspberry or strawberry** *(cont.)* | | | | | | | |
| seedless (*Polaner All Fruit* w/Fiber) ..... | 30 | 0 | 9.0 | 0 | 0 | 0 | 3.0 |
| strawberry (*Roland*) .... | 35 | 0 | 9.0 | 0 | 0 | 0 | 0 |
| **Fruit syrup** (see also specific fruit listings), all fruits (*Smucker's*), ¼ cup .. | 200 | 0 | 51.0 | 0 | 0 | 0 | 0 |
| **Fruit and nut mix**, see "Trail mix" | | | | | | | |
| **Fudge topping**, see "Chocolate topping" | | | | | | | |
| **Fuki**, see "Butterbur" | | | | | | | |
| **Fung quat**, see "Arrowroot" | | | | | | | |
| **Fuzzy melon**, see "Wax gourd" | | | | | | | |
| **Fuzzy navel**, drink mixer, frozen (*Bacardi*), 2 fl. oz. ..... | 120 | 0 | 33.0 | 0 | 0 | 0 | 0 |

# G

| Food and Measure | cal. | prot. (gms) | carbo. (gms) | fat (gms) | chol. (mgs) | sod. (mgs) | fiber (gms) |
|---|---|---|---|---|---|---|---|
| **Gai choy**, see "Cabbage, mustard" | | | | | | | |
| **Gai lan**, see "Kale, Chinese" | | | | | | | |
| **Galanga**, see "Ginger" | | | | | | | |
| **Garbanzo bean**: | | | | | | | |
| dry, ¼ cup: | | | | | | | |
| (*Arrowhead Mills* Organic Chickpeas) | 160 | 9.0 | 27.0 | 2.5 | 0 | 10 | 8.0 |
| (*Bob's Red Mill*) ..... | 150 | 8.0 | 25.0 | 2.5 | 0 | 10 | 7.0 |
| (*Eden* Organic) ...... | 170 | 9.0 | 28.0 | 2.0 | 0 | 10 | 12.0 |
| (*Roland* Ceci) ....... | 160 | 10.0 | 23.0 | 3.0 | 0 | 5 | 7.0 |
| baby, split (*Bob's Red Mill* Chana Dal) .... | 170 | 9.0 | 29.0 | 3.0 | 0 | 10 | 8.0 |
| boiled, ½ cup ........ | 134 | 7.3 | 22.5 | 2.1 | 0 | 6 | 2.9 |
| pre-soaked (*Frieda's*), ⅓ cup, 3 oz. ........ | 150 | 7.0 | 23.0 | 3.0 | 0 | 230 | 22.0 |
| **Garbanzo bean, canned**, ½ cup: | | | | | | | |
| (*Allens/East Texas Fair* Chick Peas) ..... | 120 | 5.0 | 19.0 | 2.5 | 0 | 330 | 8.0 |
| (*Bush's*) ............. | 105 | 6.0 | 20.0 | 2.0 | 0 | 470 | 5.0 |
| (*Bush's* Reduced Sodium) ........... | 105 | 6.0 | 20.0 | 2.0 | 0 | 230 | 5.0 |
| (*Eden* Organic) ........ | 130 | 7.0 | 23.0 | 1.0 | 0 | 30 | 5.0 |
| (*Progresso* Chick Peas) . | 100 | 5.0 | 17.0 | 1.5 | 0 | 280 | 4.0 |
| (*Roland*) ............. | 110 | 7.0 | 20.0 | 1.0 | 0 | 350 | 7.0 |
| (*S&W*) .............. | 110 | 7.0 | 15.0 | 2.5 | 0 | 460 | 6.0 |
| (*S&W* Less Salt) ...... | 110 | 7.0 | 15.0 | 2.5 | 0 | 220 | 3.0 |
| (*S&W* Organic) ........ | 120 | 6.0 | 15.0 | 2.0 | 0 | 390 | 3.0 |
| **Garbanzo dish**, 1 pkg., except as noted: | | | | | | | |
| (*Devya* Organic Channa/ Dhal Tadka), 3.5 oz. .. | 280 | 7.0 | 55.0 | 3.7 | 0 | 1550 | 10.0 |

| Food and Measure | cal. | prot. (gms) | carbo. (gms) | fat (gms) | chol. (mgs) | sod. (mgs) | fiber (gms) |
|---|---|---|---|---|---|---|---|
| **Garbanzo dish** *(cont.)* | | | | | | | |
| (*Tamarind Tree* Au | | | | | | | |
| Chole), 9.25 oz. . . . . . | 350 | 12.0 | 63.0 | 6.0 | 0 | 620 | 9.0 |
| (*Tasty Bite* Channa Masala), | | | | | | | |
| ½ of 10-oz. pkg. . . . . . | 180 | 6.0 | 20.0 | 8.0 | 0 | 400 | 6.0 |
| (*Tasty Bite* Chickpeas), | | | | | | | |
| ½ of 8-oz. pkg. . . . . . . | 210 | 9.0 | 30.0 | 7.0 | 0 | 350 | 10.0 |
| **Garbanzo entree**, | | | | | | | |
| frozen, channa masala | | | | | | | |
| (*Kashi*), 9.5-oz. pkg. . . | 310 | 11.0 | 44.0 | 9.0 | 0 | 690 | 8.0 |
| **Garbanzo flour**, | | | | | | | |
| stoneground, ¼ cup: | | | | | | | |
| (*Bob's Red Mill*) . . . . . . . | 110 | 6.0 | 18.0 | 2.0 | 0 | 5 | 5.0 |
| and fava flour (*Bob's* | | | | | | | |
| *Red Mill* Gluten Free) . | 110 | 6.0 | 18.0 | 1.5 | 0 | 5 | 6.0 |
| **Garlic**, fresh: | | | | | | | |
| (*Frieda's* Black), .63 oz. . . | 40 | 2.0 | 8.0 | 0 | 0 | 0 | 3.0 |
| (*Frieda's* Elephant), | | | | | | | |
| chopped, 1 tbsp. . . . . . | 5 | 0 | 1.0 | 0 | 0 | 0 | 0 |
| trimmed, 1 oz. . . . . . . . . | 42 | 1.8 | 9.4 | .1 | 0 | 5 | .6 |
| 1 clove, .1 oz. . . . . . . . . | 4 | .2 | 1.0 | <.1 | 0 | 1 | .1 |
| granulated/minced, | | | | | | | |
| 1 tsp. . . . . . . . . . . . . | 13 | .7 | 2.9 | 0 | 0 | 1 | 0 |
| **Garlic, in jars**, 1 tsp., | | | | | | | |
| except as noted: | | | | | | | |
| cloves, w/herbs, in | | | | | | | |
| water (*Roland*), 2 tbsp. | 10 | 0 | 2.0 | 0 | 0 | 270 | 0 |
| crushed (*McCormick* | | | | | | | |
| California) . . . . . . . . . . | 10 | 0 | 0 | 0 | 0 | 0 | 0 |
| minced (*McCormick* | | | | | | | |
| California) . . . . . . . . . . | 15 | <1.0 | 0 | .5 | 0 | 0 | 0 |
| paste, minced (*Tiger* | | | | | | | |
| *Tiger*) . . . . . . . . . . . . . | 16 | <1.0 | 2.0 | .4 | 0 | 100 | <1.0 |
| roasted (*McCormick*) . . . | 5 | 0 | 0 | 0 | 0 | 0 | 0 |
| **Garlic bread**, see "Bread, | | | | | | | |
| frozen/chilled" | | | | | | | |
| **Garlic bread sprinkle** | | | | | | | |
| (*McCormick*), ½ tsp. . | 10 | 0 | <1.0 | 0 | 0 | 65 | 0 |
| **Garlic jelly** (*Campagna*), | | | | | | | |
| 1 tbsp. . . . . . . . . . . . . | 45 | 0 | 12.0 | 0 | 0 | 0 | 0 |
| **Garlic oil**, olive oil | | | | | | | |
| (*McCormick*), 1 tsp. . . | 10 | 0 | 0 | .5 | 0 | 0 | 0 |
| **Garlic Parmesan dip** | | | | | | | |
| (*Heluva Good*), 2 tbsp. | 60 | 1.0 | 2.0 | 5.0 | 20 | 160 | 0 |

| Food and Measure | cal. | prot. (gms) | carbo. (gms) | fat (gms) | chol. (mgs) | sod. (mgs) | fiber (gms) |
|---|---|---|---|---|---|---|---|
| **Garlic pepper**, ¼ tsp., except as noted: | | | | | | | |
| (*Lawry's*) ............. | 0 | 0 | 1.0 | 0 | 0 | 0 | 0 |
| (*McCormick* Grinder) ... | 0 | 0 | 0 | 0 | 0 | 75 | 0 |
| 1 tsp. ................ | 8 | .3 | 1.8 | 0 | 0 | 360 | .3 |
| w/red bell and black (*McCormick* California Style) ..... | 0 | 0 | 0 | 0 | 0 | 105 | 0 |
| **Garlic powder**, 1 tsp. ... | 10 | .5 | 2.3 | 0 | 0 | 1 | 0 |
| **Garlic puree** (*Frieda's* Delight), 1 tbsp.: | | | | | | | |
| chipotle flavor ......... | 117 | 0 | 1.0 | 11.0 | 0 | 55 | 0 |
| green olive ........... | 115 | 0 | 1.0 | 12.0 | 0 | 61 | 0 |
| original ............. | 122 | 0 | 1.0 | 13.0 | 0 | 34 | 0 |
| sun-dried tomato ...... | 116 | 0 | 2.0 | 12.0 | 0 | 56 | 0 |
| **Garlic salt**, ¼ tsp.: | | | | | | | |
| (*Lawry's*) ............. | 0 | 0 | 0 | 0 | 0 | 240 | 0 |
| (*McCormick*) .......... | 0 | 0 | 0 | 0 | 0 | 490 | 0 |
| w/parsley (*McCormick*) .. | 0 | 0 | 0 | 0 | 0 | 220 | 0 |
| sea salt (*McCormick* Grinder) ............ | 0 | 0 | 0 | 0 | 0 | 125 | 0 |
| **Garlic sauce**, Asian (*Dai Day*), 2 tbsp. .... | 96 | 0 | 24.0 | 0 | 0 | 500 | 0 |
| **Garlic seasoning blend** (see also specific listings): | | | | | | | |
| and herbs: | | | | | | | |
| (*McCormick*), ¼ tsp. . | 0 | 0 | 0 | 0 | 0 | 50 | 0 |
| Italian (*McCormick*), 1 tsp. ........... | 5 | 0 | <1.0 | 0 | 0 | 0 | 0 |
| onion medley (*Grill Mates*), ¼ tsp. ...... | 0 | 0 | 0 | 0 | 0 | 125 | 0 |
| roasted, and, ¼ tsp.: | | | | | | | |
| bell pepper (*McCormick Perfect Pinch*) .... | 0 | 0 | 0 | 0 | 0 | 75 | 0 |
| herbs (*Grill Mates*) ... | 0 | 0 | 0 | 0 | 0 | 170 | 0 |
| **Garlic spread**, 1 tsp.: | | | | | | | |
| (*Lawry's*) ............. | 25 | 0 | 0 | 2.5 | 0 | 50 | 0 |
| puree or roasted (*Alessi*) ............. | 8 | 0 | 0 | 1.0 | 0 | 25 | 0 |
| **Gefilte fish**, in jars, drained, 1 pc.: | | | | | | | |
| (*Mother's* Old Fashioned), 2 oz. .... | 60 | 6.0 | 3.0 | 2.5 | 20 | 220 | 1.0 |

| Food and Measure | cal. | prot. (gms) | carbo. (gms) | fat (gms) | chol. (mgs) | sod. (mgs) | fiber (gms) |
|---|---|---|---|---|---|---|---|
| **Gefilte fish** *(cont.)* | | | | | | | |
| (*Rokeach*), 2 oz. . . . . . . . | 60 | 6.0 | 3.0 | 3.0 | 35 | 290 | 0 |
| (*Yehuda*), 1.8 oz. . . . . . . | 42 | 3.0 | 6.0 | 1.0 | 10 | 255 | .5 |
| **Gefilte fish, frozen** | | | | | | | |
| (*A&B Famous* Old | | | | | | | |
| Fashioned), 2 oz.: | | | | | | | |
| homemade or sweet . . . . | 80 | 6.0 | 7.0 | 3.5 | 50 | 220 | 1.0 |
| pike and white . . . . . . . . . | 70 | 7.0 | 5.0 | 2.0 | 65 | 290 | 2.0 |
| precooked . . . . . . . . . . . . | 80 | 6.2 | 9.0 | 2.5 | 40 | 170 | 1.0 |
| salmon . . . . . . . . . . . . . . | 140 | 12.0 | 4.0 | 8.0 | 20 | 260 | <1.0 |
| **Gelatin**, unflavored | | | | | | | |
| (*Knox*), ¼ pkt. . . . . . . . | 5 | 2.0 | 0 | 0 | 0 | 0 | 0 |
| **Gelatin dessert**, | | | | | | | |
| ready-to-eat, 3.5 oz.: | | | | | | | |
| all fruit flavors: | | | | | | | |
| (*Jell-O*) . . . . . . . . . . . . | 70 | 1.0 | 17.0 | 0 | 0 | 40 | 0 |
| (*Jell-O* No Sugar) . . . . | 10 | 1.0 | 0 | 0 | 0 | 45 | 0 |
| cherry blue raspberry | | | | | | | |
| (*Jell-O X-Treme*) . . . . . | 70 | 0 | 17.0 | 0 | 0 | 40 | 0 |
| cherry (*Hunt's Snack* | | | | | | | |
| *Pack* No Sugar) . . . . . | 10 | 0 | 2.0 | 0 | 0 | 65 | <1.0 |
| w/fruit, see specific | | | | | | | |
| fruit listings | | | | | | | |
| strawberry (*Hunt's* | | | | | | | |
| *Snack Pack*) . . . . . . . . | 100 | 0 | 25.0 | 0 | 0 | 40 | 0 |
| strawberry/orange: | | | | | | | |
| (*Hunt's Snack Pack*) . . | 100 | 0 | 25.0 | 0 | 0 | 45 | 0 |
| (*Hunt's Snack Pack* | | | | | | | |
| No Sugar) . . . . . . . | 5 | 0 | 1.0 | 0 | 0 | 45 | <1.0 |
| watermelon/green apple | | | | | | | |
| (*Jell-O X-Treme*) . . . . | 100 | 0 | 24.0 | 0 | 0 | 45 | 0 |
| **Gelatin dessert mix** | | | | | | | |
| (*Jell-O*), ½ cup*: | | | | | | | |
| all fruit flavors: | | | | | | | |
| regular . . . . . . . . . . . . | 80 | 2.0 | 19.0 | 0 | 0 | —[1] | 0 |
| sugar free . . . . . . . . . | 10 | 1.0 | 0 | 0 | 0 | —[2] | 0 |
| Margarita or piña colada . | 80 | 1.0 | 19.0 | 0 | 0 | 95 | 0 |
| **Gelatin substitute**, | | | | | | | |
| unflavored (*Lieber's*), | | | | | | | |
| ¼ pkt, ½ cup* . . . . . . | 80 | 0 | 21.0 | 0 | 0 | 45 | 0 |

---

[1] Sodium values vary between 75 and 120 mgs. according to flavor.
[2] Sodium values vary between 45 and 80 mgs. according to flavor.

| Food and Measure | cal. | prot. (gms) | carbo. (gms) | fat (gms) | chol. (mgs) | sod. (mgs) | fiber (gms) |
|---|---|---|---|---|---|---|---|
| **Giardiniera**, see "Vegetables, mixed, pickled" | | | | | | | |
| **Ginger**, trimmed root: | | | | | | | |
| (*Frieda's* Galanga), | | | | | | | |
| 1 tbsp. . . . . . . . . . . | 10 | 0 | 1.0 | 0 | 0 | 1 | 0 |
| 1 oz. . . . . . . . . . . . . . | 20 | .5 | 4.3 | .2 | 0 | 4 | .6 |
| sliced, ¼ cup . . . . . . . . | 17 | .4 | 3.6 | .2 | 0 | 3 | .5 |
| **Ginger, candied or crystallized**, 1.1 oz.: | | | | | | | |
| (*Frieda's*), 9 pcs. . . . . . . | 100 | 0 | 26.0 | 0 | 0 | 10 | 0 |
| slices (*Roland*), 5 pcs. . . | 100 | 0 | 25.0 | 0 | 0 | 25 | 1.0 |
| **Ginger, ground**, 1 tsp. . . | 6 | .2 | 1.3 | .1 | 0 | 1 | .2 |
| **Ginger, pickled**: | | | | | | | |
| Japanese, 1 oz. . . . . . . . | 10 | .1 | 2.1 | <.1 | 0 | 105 | 0 |
| sliced, w/shiso leaves (*Eden* Organic), | | | | | | | |
| 1 tbsp., .5 oz. . . . . . . . | 20 | 0 | 4.0 | 0 | 0 | 100 | <1.0 |
| sushi (*Roland* Shoga), | | | | | | | |
| 1 tbsp. . . . . . . . . . . | 0 | 0 | 0 | 0 | 0 | 70 | 0 |
| **Ginger, in syrup**, in jars (*Roland*), 4 pcs. . . | 80 | 0 | 21.0 | 0 | 0 | 5 | 0 |
| **Ginger paste**, minced (*Tiger Tiger*), 1 tsp. . . . | 12 | <1.0 | 3.0 | .4 | 0 | 100 | <1.0 |
| **Ginger sauce**, mint, Asian (*Heaven and Earth*), 1 tbsp. . . . . . . . | 35 | 0 | 9.0 | 0 | 0 | 10 | 1.0 |
| **Ginkgo nut**, shelled: | | | | | | | |
| raw, 1 oz. . . . . . . . . . . . | 52 | 1.2 | 10.7 | .5 | 0 | 2 | <1.0 |
| canned, drained, 1 oz. . . . | 32 | .6 | 6.3 | .5 | 0 | 87 | 2.6 |
| dried, 1 oz. . . . . . . . . . | 99 | 2.9 | 20.6 | .8 | 0 | 4 | n.a. |
| **Glacé**, see "Fruit, mixed, candied" | | | | | | | |
| **Glaze**, see specific listings | | | | | | | |
| **Gluten**, see "Wheat gluten" | | | | | | | |
| **Gnocchi, frozen/ chilled**, potato: | | | | | | | |
| (*Italian Village*), 1 cup . . . | 240 | 7.0 | 51.0 | 1.0 | 15 | 970 | 3.0 |
| garlic basil (*Rising Moon Organics*), ½ cup | 220 | 6.0 | 48.0 | 0 | 0 | 650 | 3.0 |
| **Gnocchi, pkg.**, potato: | | | | | | | |
| (*Alessi*), ¾ cup . . . . . . . | 170 | 4.0 | 35.0 | 1.0 | 0 | 660 | 3.0 |
| (*Vigo*), 2 oz. . . . . . . . . . | 80 | 2.0 | 18.0 | 0 | 0 | 253 | 0 |

| Food and Measure | cal. | prot. (gms) | carbo. (gms) | fat (gms) | chol. (mgs) | sod. (mgs) | fiber (gms) |
|---|---|---|---|---|---|---|---|
| **Goat**, meat only, | | | | | | | |
| roasted, 4 oz. . . . . . . . | 162 | 30.7 | 0 | 3.4 | 85 | 98 | 0 |
| **Gobo root**, see | | | | | | | |
| "Burdock root" | | | | | | | |
| **Gochujang sauce** (*Annie* | | | | | | | |
| *Chun's*), 1 tbsp. . . . . . | 45 | <1.0 | 10.0 | .5 | 0 | 350 | <1.0 |
| **Goji berries**, dried | | | | | | | |
| (*Frieda's*), ⅓ pkg., 1 oz. | 101 | 3.0 | 20.0 | 1.0 | 2 | 121 | 6.0 |
| **Goji drink blend**, | | | | | | | |
| 8 fl. oz.: | | | | | | | |
| peach (*Apple & Eve*) . . . . | 120 | 0 | 28.0 | 0 | 0 | 15 | 0 |
| melon (*SoBe Lifewater*) . | 40 | 0 | 17.0 | 0 | 0 | 20 | 0 |
| raspberry (*V8 V-Fusion*) . | 110 | 0 | 27.0 | 0 | 0 | 120 | 0 |
| **Goji juice**, 8 fl. oz.: | | | | | | | |
| (*Bossa Nova*) . . . . . . . . | 85 | 1.0 | 21.0 | 0 | 0 | 25 | 0 |
| (*R.W. Knudsen* Organic) . | 150 | 1.0 | 37.0 | 0 | 0 | 15 | <1.0 |
| **Golden nugget squash** | | | | | | | |
| (*Frieda's*), 3 oz. . . . . . . | 30 | 1.0 | 7.0 | 0 | 0 | 0 | 1.0 |
| **Goose**, roasted: | | | | | | | |
| meat w/skin, 4 oz. . . . . . . | 346 | 28.5 | 0 | 24.9 | 103 | 79 | 0 |
| meat only, 4 oz. . . . . . . . . | 270 | 32.9 | 0 | 14.4 | 109 | 86 | 0 |
| **Goose fat**, 1 tbsp. . . . . . . | 115 | 0 | 0 | 12.8 | 13 | 0 | 0 |
| **Goose liver**, see | | | | | | | |
| "Liver" and "Pâté" | | | | | | | |
| **Gooseberries**, fresh: | | | | | | | |
| (*Frieda's*), 1 cup . . . . . . | 66 | 1.0 | 15.0 | 1.0 | 0 | 0 | 6.0 |
| ½ cup . . . . . . . . . . . . . . | 34 | .7 | 7.6 | .4 | 0 | 1 | 3.2 |
| **Gourd**, boiled, ½ cup: | | | | | | | |
| dishcloth, 1" slices . . . . . | 50 | .6 | 12.8 | .3 | 0 | 18 | <1.0 |
| white-flower, 1" cubes . . . | 11 | .4 | 2.7 | <.1 | 0 | 1 | <1.0 |
| **Gourd, dried**, see | | | | | | | |
| "Kanpyo" | | | | | | | |
| **Grains**, see specific | | | | | | | |
| listings | | | | | | | |
| **Grains, mixed** | | | | | | | |
| (*RiceSelect Royal* | | | | | | | |
| *Blend*), ¼ cup: | | | | | | | |
| w/brown/wild rice . . . . . . | 160 | 5.0 | 34.0 | 1.5 | 0 | 5 | 2.0 |
| w/brown/red rice . . . . . . | 160 | 4.0 | 33.0 | 1.5 | 0 | 5 | 2.0 |
| **Grains, mixed, dish, mix**, | | | | | | | |
| 2 oz., except as noted: | | | | | | | |
| brown rice/wheat (*Near East*): | | | | | | | |
| barley, chicken herb | | | | | | | |
| 2.5 oz. . . . . . . . . . | 250 | 7.0 | 52.0 | 2.0 | 0 | 710 | 5.0 |

| Food and Measure | cal. | prot. (gms) | carbo. (gms) | fat (gms) | chol. (mgs) | sod. (mgs) | fiber (gms) |
|---|---|---|---|---|---|---|---|
| bulgur, roasted garlic . | 190 | 6.0 | 41.0 | 2.0 | 0 | 510 | 5.0 |
| pecan and garlic . . . . . | 220 | 6.0 | 38.0 | 5.0 | 0 | 480 | 4.0 |
| 7-grain pilaf (*Kashi*), | | | | | | | |
| ½ cup* . . . . . . . . . . . . | 170 | 6.0 | 33.0 | 2.5 | 0 | 0 | 6.0 |
| wheat pilaf, w/orzo | | | | | | | |
| (*Near East*) . . . . . . . . . | 170 | 7.0 | 40.0 | 1.0 | 0 | 640 | 8.0 |
| white rice/wheat, | | | | | | | |
| creamy Parmesan | | | | | | | |
| (*Near East*), 2.5 oz. . . . | 240 | 7.0 | 49.0 | 3.0 | 5 | 690 | 3.0 |
| **Grains, mixed, entree**, | | | | | | | |
| frozen, seven grain, | | | | | | | |
| (*Kashi*), 10-oz. pkg.: | | | | | | | |
| black bean mango . . . . . . | 340 | 8.0 | 58.0 | 8.0 | 0 | 380 | 7.0 |
| Mayan harvest bake . . . . | 340 | 9.0 | 58.0 | 9.0 | 0 | 380 | 8.0 |
| **Granadilla**, see | | | | | | | |
| "Passion fruit" | | | | | | | |
| **Granola**, see "Cereal" | | | | | | | |
| **Granola/cereal bar** | | | | | | | |
| (see also "Toaster | | | | | | | |
| pastry"), 1 bar, except | | | | | | | |
| as noted: | | | | | | | |
| (*Mariani* Honey Bar) . . . . | 160 | 4.0 | 25.0 | 6.0 | 0 | 15 | 2.0 |
| (*Odwalla Bar! Super* | | | | | | | |
| *Protein*) . . . . . . . . . . . | 210 | 14.0 | 30.0 | 4.5 | 0 | 150 | 4.0 |
| (*Odwalla Bar!* | | | | | | | |
| *Superfood*) . . . . . . . . . | 200 | 4.0 | 39.0 | 3.5 | 0 | 85 | 3.0 |
| almond: | | | | | | | |
| (*Nature Valley* Sweet | | | | | | | |
| & Salty Granola) . . . | 160 | 3.0 | 22.0 | 7.0 | 0 | 150 | 2.0 |
| (*Odwalla Bar!* Sweet | | | | | | | |
| & Salty) . . . . . . . . . | 220 | 7.0 | 22.0 | 11.0 | 0 | 65 | 6.0 |
| crunch (*TLC* Crunchy | | | | | | | |
| Granola), 2 bars . . . | 170 | 6.0 | 26.0 | 6.0 | 0 | 150 | 4.0 |
| roasted (*Nature Valley* | | | | | | | |
| Crunch Bar) . . . . . . | 190 | 6.0 | 13.0 | 13.0 | 0 | 180 | 2.0 |
| roasted (*Nature Valley* | | | | | | | |
| Granola), 2 bars . . . | 190 | 4.0 | 28.0 | 8.0 | 0 | 170 | 2.0 |
| apple: | | | | | | | |
| baked, spice (*TLC* | | | | | | | |
| Cereal) . . . . . . . . . | 110 | 2.0 | 21.0 | 3.0 | 0 | 105 | 3.0 |
| or blueberry (*Glutino*) . | 130 | 2.0 | 28.0 | 2.0 | 0 | 5 | 3.0 |
| cobbler (*Health Valley* | | | | | | | |
| Organic Cereal) . . . | 130 | 2.0 | 27.0 | 2.5 | 0 | 85 | 3.0 |

| Food and Measure | cal. | prot. (gms) | carbo. (gms) | fat (gms) | chol. (mgs) | sod. (mgs) | fiber (gms) |
|---|---|---|---|---|---|---|---|
| **Granola/cereal bar, apple** *(cont.)* | | | | | | | |
| Dutch (*Health Valley* Organic Chewy Granola) ......... | 110 | 1.0 | 23.0 | 2.0 | 0 | 15 | 3.0 |
| apple cinnamon: | | | | | | | |
| (*Barbara's Nature's Choice* Cereal) .... | 140 | 2.0 | 28.0 | 2.0 | 0 | 80 | 1.0 |
| (*Country Choice* Organic Cereal) ... | 220 | 5.0 | 40.0 | 3.0 | 0 | 180 | 4.0 |
| (*Entenmann's*) ....... | 140 | 1.0 | 28.0 | 3.0 | 0 | 105 | 1.0 |
| (*Nutri-Grain*) ........ | 120 | 2.0 | 24.0 | 3.0 | 0 | 110 | 3.0 |
| (*Quaker* Oatmeal to Go) ........... | 220 | 4.0 | 44.0 | 4.0 | 15 | 210 | 5.0 |
| baked (*Kellogg's Cinnabon*) ....... | 150 | 1.0 | 26.0 | 4.5 | 0 | 100 | <1.0 |
| apple crisp (*Nature Valley* Granola), 2 bars ............. | 160 | 3.0 | 26.0 | 6.0 | 0 | 140 | 2.0 |
| banana bread (*Quaker* Oatmeal To Go) ...... | 220 | 4.0 | 43.0 | 4.0 | 15 | 220 | 5.0 |
| banana nut: | | | | | | | |
| (*Nature's Path Optimum ReBound Energy Organic*) ... | 190 | 10.0 | 33.0 | 4.0 | 0 | 140 | 4.0 |
| (*Odwalla Bar!*) ...... | 220 | 4.0 | 39.0 | 5.0 | 0 | 105 | 5.0 |
| berry: | | | | | | | |
| (*Odwalla Bar! Berries GoMega*) ........ | 210 | 5.0 | 36.0 | 6.0 | 0 | 210 | 5.0 |
| harvest (*Cascadian Farm* Organic Granola) ......... | 130 | 2.0 | 26.0 | 2.0 | 0 | 115 | 1.0 |
| mixed (*Genisoy* Organic) | 160 | 8.0 | 26.0 | 3.0 | 0 | 85 | 2.0 |
| mixed (*Nature Valley* Trail Mix) ......... | 140 | 2.0 | 26.0 | 3.5 | 0 | 90 | 1.0 |
| mixed (*Nutri-Grain*) .. | 120 | 2.0 | 24.0 | 3.0 | 0 | 110 | 3.0 |
| strawberry (*Nature's Path* Organic Granola) ......... | 140 | 2.0 | 25.0 | 3.5 | 0 | 80 | 2.0 |
| triple (*Barbara's Nature's Choice* Cereal) .... | 150 | 2.0 | 29.0 | 2.0 | 0 | 85 | 2.0 |
| blackberry: | | | | | | | |
| (*Nutri-Grain*) ........ | 120 | 2.0 | 24.0 | 3.0 | 0 | 135 | 3.0 |
| graham (*TLC* Cereal) . | 110 | 2.0 | 21.0 | 3.0 | 0 | 125 | 3.0 |

| Food and Measure | cal. | prot. (gms) | carbo. (gms) | fat (gms) | chol. (mgs) | sod. (mgs) | fiber (gms) |
|---|---|---|---|---|---|---|---|
| blueberry: | | | | | | | |
| (*Barbara's Nature's Choice* Cereal) .... | 150 | 2.0 | 29.0 | 2.0 | 0 | 85 | <2.0 |
| (*Health Valley* Organic Chewy Granola) ... | 110 | 1.0 | 23.0 | 2.0 | 0 | 15 | 3.0 |
| (*Nutri-Grain*) ........ | 120 | 2.0 | 24.0 | 3.0 | 0 | 110 | 3.0 |
| (*Special K*) ......... | 90 | 1.0 | 18.0 | 1.5 | 0 | 90 | <1.0 |
| (*Special K* Fruit Crisps), 2 bars ............ | 100 | 1.0 | 20.0 | 2.0 | 0 | 80 | <1.0 |
| cobbler (*Health Valley* Organic Cereal) ... | 130 | 2.0 | 27.0 | 2.5 | 0 | 85 | 3.0 |
| flax and soy (*Nature's Path Optimum Energy Organic*) ... | 200 | 6.0 | 38.0 | 3.0 | 0 | 100 | 5.0 |
| brown sugar cinnamon (*Quaker* Oatmeal to Go) ............. | 220 | 4.0 | 43.0 | 4.0 | 15 | 230 | 5.0 |
| caramel: | | | | | | | |
| nut (*Quaker Chewy Dipps*) .......... | 140 | 2.0 | 21.0 | 6.0 | 0 | 65 | 1.0 |
| peanut (*GoLean* Roll!) | 190 | 12.0 | 27.0 | 5.0 | 0 | 220 | 6.0 |
| cashew (*Nature Valley* Sweet & Salty) ...... | 160 | 2.0 | 23.0 | 7.0 | 0 | 135 | 1.0 |
| cherry: | | | | | | | |
| (*Barbara's Nature's Choice* Cereal) .... | 140 | 2.0 | 28.0 | 2.0 | 0 | 80 | 1.0 |
| (*Nutri-Grain*) ........ | 120 | 2.0 | 24.0 | 3.0 | 0 | 110 | 3.0 |
| dark chocolate (*TLC* Chewy Granola) ... | 120 | 5.0 | 24.0 | 2.0 | 0 | 65 | 4.0 |
| or strawberry (*Glutino*) | 160 | 3.0 | 30.0 | 3.0 | 0 | 50 | 3.0 |
| cherry pomegranate (*Nutri-Grain Superfruit Fusion*) . | 130 | 2.0 | 26.0 | 3.0 | 0 | 95 | 3.0 |
| chocolate: | | | | | | | |
| (*Fiber One* Chewy) ... | 90 | 1.0 | 17.0 | 2.0 | 0 | 95 | 5.0 |
| (*Genisoy* Organic Rich) | 160 | 9.0 | 25.0 | 3.0 | 0 | 85 | 3.0 |
| (*Kudos M&M's* Granola) .......... | 100 | 1.0 | 17.0 | 3.0 | 0 | 80 | 1.0 |
| (*Kudos Snickers* Granola) .......... | 100 | 1.0 | 16.0 | 3.0 | 0 | 70 | 1.0 |
| (*Odwalla Bar! Choco-walla*) ..... | 210 | 4.0 | 39.0 | 5.0 | 0 | 75 | 5.0 |
| (*Quaker* Granola Bites), .75-oz. bag . | 90 | 2.0 | 14.0 | 3.5 | 0 | 30 | 2.0 |

| Food and Measure | cal. | prot. (gms) | carbo. (gms) | fat (gms) | chol. (mgs) | sod. (mgs) | fiber (gms) |
|---|---|---|---|---|---|---|---|
| **Granola/cereal bar, chocolate** *(cont.)* | | | | | | | |
| (*South Beach Living* Cereal) ......... | 140 | 8.0 | 17.0 | 5.0 | 0 | 125 | 3.0 |
| (*Special K* Chocolatey Drizzle) .......... | 90 | 1.0 | 17.0 | 1.5 | 0 | 105 | <1.0 |
| (*Special K* Protein Snack Delight) .... | 110 | 4.0 | 16.0 | 3.0 | 0 | 85 | <1.0 |
| almond (*Genisoy* Triple Layer) ...... | 230 | 10.0 | 30.0 | 8.0 | 0 | 170 | 2.0 |
| almond (*GoLean* Crunchy!) ......... | 170 | 8.0 | 27.0 | 5.0 | 0 | 210 | 5.0 |
| almond toffee (*GoLean* Chewy) .. | 290 | 13.0 | 45.0 | 6.0 | 0 | 250 | 6.0 |
| banana (*Glutino* Organic) ......... | 100 | 1.0 | 21.0 | 1.5 | 0 | 35 | 1.0 |
| caramel (*Genisoy* Triple Layer) ...... | 220 | 10.0 | 32.0 | 6.0 | 0 | 220 | 1.0 |
| caramel (*GoLean* Crunchy!) ........ | 150 | 8.0 | 28.0 | 3.0 | 0 | 220 | 6.0 |
| coconut (*Nature's Path* Organic Granola Chococonut) ..... | 140 | 2.0 | 24.0 | 4.5 | 0 | 35 | 2.0 |
| dark, almond (*Cascadian Farm* Organic Granola) .. | 130 | 2.0 | 25.0 | 3.5 | 0 | 105 | 5.0 |
| dark, almond (*FiberPlus*) ....... | 130 | 2.0 | 24.0 | 5.0 | 0 | 50 | 9.0 |
| dark, cherry (*Quaker* Chewy Granola) ... | 90 | 1.0 | 19.0 | 2.0 | 0 | 75 | 1.0 |
| dark, mocha hazelnut (*Quaker True Delights* Café Squares) .... | 120 | 2.0 | 20.0 | 4.0 | 0 | 35 | 3.0 |
| dark, and nut (*Nature Valley* Trail Mix) ... | 140 | 2.0 | 25.0 | 4.0 | 0 | 75 | 1.0 |
| dark, raspberry almond (*Quaker True Delights* Granola) .. | 140 | 2.0 | 23.0 | 4.5 | 0 | 55 | 3.0 |
| double (*Special K* Protein Meal) ...... | 170 | 10.0 | 26.0 | 4.5 | 0 | 200 | 5.0 |
| fudge brownie (*Genisoy*) | 240 | 14.0 | 32.0 | 7.0 | 0 | 200 | 2.0 |
| mint (*Quaker Chewy* Granola) ......... | 90 | 1.0 | 19.0 | 2.0 | 0 | 80 | 1.0 |
| mint (*South Beach Living* Snack Bar) .. | 100 | 6.0 | 15.0 | 4.0 | 0 | 150 | 5.0 |

| Food and Measure | cal. | prot. (gms) | carbo. (gms) | fat (gms) | chol. (mgs) | sod. (mgs) | fiber (gms) |
|---|---|---|---|---|---|---|---|
| mint, crispy (*Genisoy*) | 240 | 14.0 | 33.0 | 6.0 | 0 | 200 | 2.0 |
| mocha (*Fiber One* Chewy) | 140 | 2.0 | 29.0 | 4.0 | 0 | 90 | 9.0 |
| peanut (*GoLean* Crunchy!*) | 180 | 9.0 | 30.0 | 5.0 | 0 | 250 | 6.0 |
| peanut (*GoLean* Roll!) | 190 | 12.0 | 27.0 | 5.0 | 0 | 240 | 6.0 |
| peanut (*Special K* Protein Snack) | 110 | 4.0 | 15.0 | 3.5 | 0 | 70 | 1.0 |
| peanut butter (*Fiber One* Chewy) | 90 | 1.0 | 17.0 | 2.5 | 0 | 95 | 5.0 |
| peanut butter (*Glutino* Organic) | 110 | 2.0 | 19.0 | 3.0 | 0 | 50 | 1.0 |
| peanut butter (*Special K* Protein Meal) | 180 | 10.0 | 25.0 | 6.0 | 0 | 250 | 5.0 |
| pretzel (*GoLean* Crunchy!) | 160 | 11.0 | 28.0 | 3.0 | 0 | 250 | 5.0 |
| raspberry (*South Beach Living* Snack Bar) | 100 | 5.0 | 16.0 | 3.0 | 0 | 125 | 5.0 |
| swirl (*Quaker Chewy* Granola) | 90 | 1.0 | 19.0 | 2.0 | 0 | 80 | 1.0 |
| turtle (*GoLean* Roll!) | 190 | 12.0 | 27.0 | 5.0 | 0 | 240 | 6.0 |
| chocolate chip/chunk: | | | | | | | |
| (*Cascadian Farm* Organic Granola) | 140 | 2.0 | 25.0 | 3.5 | 0 | 100 | 1.0 |
| (*Entenmann's* Chewy) | 150 | 2.0 | 25.0 | 6.0 | 5 | 110 | 2.0 |
| (*FiberPlus*) | 120 | 2.0 | 26.0 | 4.0 | 0 | 55 | 9.0 |
| (*Health Valley* Organic Chewy Granola) | 110 | 1.0 | 22.0 | 3.0 | 0 | 15 | 3.0 |
| (*Kudos* Granola) | 120 | 1.0 | 20.0 | 3.5 | 0 | 70 | 1.0 |
| (*Odwalla Bar!* Trail Mix) | 200 | 5.0 | 28.0 | 7.0 | 0 | 90 | 2.0 |
| (*Quaker Chewy* Granola 25% Less Sugar) | 100 | 1.0 | 18.0 | 3.0 | 0 | 75 | 1.0 |
| (*Quaker Chewy* Granola Chip) | 100 | 1.0 | 18.0 | 3.0 | 0 | 75 | 1.0 |
| (*Quaker Chewy* Granola Chunk) | 90 | 1.0 | 19.0 | 2.0 | 0 | 80 | 1.0 |
| (*Quaker Chewy* Dipps) | 140 | 2.0 | 22.0 | 6.0 | 0 | 80 | 1.0 |
| (*Special K* Protein Meal) | 170 | 10.0 | 26.0 | 4.5 | 0 | 180 | 5.0 |
| dark (*Quaker Chewy* Granola w/Fiber/ Omega-3) | 150 | 2.0 | 26.0 | 4.0 | 0 | 35 | 9.0 |

| Food and Measure | cal. | prot. (gms) | carbo. (gms) | fat (gms) | chol. (mgs) | sod. (mgs) | fiber (gms) |
|---|---|---|---|---|---|---|---|
| **Granola/cereal bar** *(cont.)* | | | | | | | |
| dark (*Quaker Simple* | | | | | | | |
| *Harvest* Granola) .. | 150 | 2.0 | 26.0 | 4.5 | 0 | 95 | 2.0 |
| double (*Health Valley* | | | | | | | |
| Organic Chewy | | | | | | | |
| Granola) ......... | 110 | 1.0 | 23.0 | 2.0 | 0 | 15 | 3.0 |
| peanut (*Odwalla Bar!*) . | 230 | 7.0 | 33.0 | 8.0 | 0 | 170 | 4.0 |
| cinnamon: | | | | | | | |
| (*Kellogg's Cinnabon*) . | 150 | 1.0 | 26.0 | 4.5 | 0 | 130 | <1.0 |
| (*Nature Valley* | | | | | | | |
| Granola), 2 bars ... | 160 | 4.0 | 29.0 | 6.0 | 0 | 170 | 2.0 |
| (*Quaker* Granola | | | | | | | |
| Bites), .75-oz. bag . | 90 | 2.0 | 14.0 | 3.5 | 0 | 30 | 2.0 |
| coffee cake (*GoLean* | | | | | | | |
| Crunchy!) ........ | 160 | 8.0 | 26.0 | 4.5 | 0 | 240 | 5.0 |
| Danish (*Health Valley* | | | | | | | |
| Care Creations) ... | 130 | 2.0 | 27.0 | 2.5 | 0 | 80 | 2.0 |
| coconut, dark chocolate | | | | | | | |
| (*TLC* Fruit & Grain) ... | 120 | 4.0 | 21.0 | 3.5 | 0 | 50 | 4.0 |
| coconut banana | | | | | | | |
| macadamia (*Quaker* | | | | | | | |
| *True Delights* Granola) | 140 | 2.0 | 23.0 | 5.0 | 0 | 95 | 3.0 |
| cookies and cream: | | | | | | | |
| (*Genisoy*) .......... | 240 | 14.0 | 32.0 | 6.0 | 0 | 310 | 2.0 |
| (*GoLean* Chewy) ..... | 290 | 13.0 | 50.0 | 6.0 | 0 | 200 | 6.0 |
| (*Quaker Chewy* Granola | | | | | | | |
| 25% Less Sugar) .. | 90 | 1.0 | 18.0 | 2.5 | 0 | 85 | 2.0 |
| cranberry: | | | | | | | |
| almond (*South Beach* | | | | | | | |
| *Living* Cereal) ..... | 140 | 8.0 | 18.0 | 5.0 | 0 | 85 | 3.0 |
| pomegranate (*Nature* | | | | | | | |
| *Valley* Trail Mix) ..... | 120 | 2.0 | 24.0 | 3.0 | 0 | 90 | 1.0 |
| walnut (*TLC* Fruit & | | | | | | | |
| Grain) ........... | 120 | 4.0 | 22.0 | 3.0 | 0 | 50 | 4.0 |
| fruit and nut: | | | | | | | |
| (*Cascadian Farm* | | | | | | | |
| Organic Granola) .. | 140 | 2.0 | 24.0 | 4.0 | 0 | 100 | 1.0 |
| (*Nature Valley* | | | | | | | |
| Trail Mix) ........ | 140 | 3.0 | 25.0 | 4.0 | 0 | 100 | 1.0 |
| fudge sundae (*GoLean* | | | | | | | |
| Roll!) ............. | 190 | 12.0 | 27.0 | 5.0 | 0 | 260 | 6.0 |
| honey almond: | | | | | | | |
| (*Special K* Protein | | | | | | | |
| Meal) .......... | 180 | 10.0 | 23.0 | 6.0 | 0 | 160 | 5.0 |

| Food and Measure | cal. | prot. (gms) | carbo. (gms) | fat (gms) | chol. (mgs) | sod. (mgs) | fiber (gms) |
|---|---|---|---|---|---|---|---|
| flax (*TLC* Chewy) .... | 140 | 7.0 | 19.0 | 5.0 | 0 | 105 | 4.0 |
| honey graham (*Quaker Chewy* Granola 25% Less Sugar) .... | 90 | 1.0 | 18.0 | 2.0 | 0 | 80 | 2.0 |
| honey nut: | | | | | | | |
| (*Cheerios* Milk 'n Cereal) .......... | 160 | 3.0 | 28.0 | 4.0 | 0 | 120 | 1.0 |
| (*Special K*) .......... | 90 | 2.0 | 16.0 | 2.0 | 0 | 110 | <1.0 |
| honey-roasted cashew mixed berry (*Quaker True Delights*) ....... | 130 | 3.0 | 24.0 | 3.5 | 0 | 100 | 3.0 |
| honey toasted, 7 grain (*TLC* Crunchy Granola), 2 bars ..... | 170 | 6.0 | 26.0 | 5.0 | 0 | 150 | 4.0 |
| malted chocolate crisp (*GoLean* Chewy) ..... | 290 | 13.0 | 49.0 | 6.0 | 0 | 200 | 6.0 |
| maple: | | | | | | | |
| (*Country Choice* Organic Cereal) ... | 210 | 5.0 | 41.0 | 3.0 | 0 | 140 | 4.0 |
| brown sugar (*Nature Valley* Granola), 2 bars ... | 190 | 4.0 | 29.0 | 7.0 | 0 | 160 | 2.0 |
| brown sugar (*Quaker* Oatmeal to Go High Fiber) ....... | 210 | 4.0 | 43.0 | 4.0 | 15 | 230 | 10.0 |
| nut (*South Beach Living* Cereal) ..... | 140 | 8.0 | 17.0 | 5.0 | 5 | 140 | 3.0 |
| pecan (*Nature's Path* Organic Granola) .. | 150 | 2.0 | 22.0 | 6.0 | 0 | 105 | 2.0 |
| marshmallow: | | | | | | | |
| (*Rice Krispies Treats*) . | 90 | <1.0 | 17.0 | 2.5 | 0 | 105 | 0 |
| mini (*Rice Krispies Treats*), 4 bars .... | 180 | 1.0 | 34.0 | 4.5 | 0 | 210 | 0 |
| mocha: | | | | | | | |
| (*Odwalla Bar! Mocha-walla*) ..... | 210 | 4.0 | 38.0 | 4.0 | 0 | 90 | 3.0 |
| (*Special K Bliss*) ..... | 90 | 1.0 | 17.0 | 2.0 | 0 | 80 | <1.0 |
| dark, almond (*TLC* Chewy Granola) ... | 130 | 6.0 | 21.0 | 3.5 | 0 | 90 | 4.0 |
| fudge, cafe (*Genisoy*) . | 240 | 15.0 | 31.0 | 6.0 | 0 | 180 | 1.0 |
| nut, mixed: | | | | | | | |
| (*Cascadian Farm* Organic Granola) .. | 160 | 3.0 | 20.0 | 8.0 | 0 | 125 | 1.0 |
| roasted (*Nature Valley* Sweet & Salty) .... | 160 | 3.0 | 21.0 | 8.0 | 0 | 140 | 1.0 |

| Food and Measure | cal. | prot. (gms) | carbo. (gms) | fat (gms) | chol. (mgs) | sod. (mgs) | fiber (gms) |
|---|---|---|---|---|---|---|---|
| **Granola/cereal bar** *(cont.)* | | | | | | | |
| oatmeal raisin: | | | | | | | |
| (*Country Choice* Organic Cereal) ... | 230 | 5.0 | 42.0 | 3.0 | 0 | 180 | 4.0 |
| (*Quaker* Chewy Granola) ......... | 90 | 1.0 | 19.0 | 1.5 | 0 | 80 | 1.0 |
| (*Quaker* Oatmeal to Go) .......... | 220 | 4.0 | 43.0 | 4.0 | 15 | 230 | 5.0 |
| cookie (*GoLean*) ..... | 280 | 13.0 | 49.0 | 5.0 | 0 | 140 | 6.0 |
| oatmeal walnut (*GoLean* Roll!) ............. | 190 | 12.0 | 27.0 | 5.0 | 0 | 250 | 6.0 |
| oats and: | | | | | | | |
| apple streusel (*Fiber One* Chewy) ...... | 130 | 2.0 | 31.0 | 2.0 | 0 | 120 | 9.0 |
| caramel (*Fiber One* Chewy) .......... | 140 | 2.0 | 30.0 | 3.5 | 0 | 105 | 9.0 |
| chocolate (*Fiber One* Chewy) ...... | 140 | 2.0 | 29.0 | 4.0 | 0 | 95 | 9.0 |
| dark chocolate (*Nature Valley* Granola), 2 bars ........... | 190 | 4.0 | 28.0 | 8.0 | 0 | 140 | 3.0 |
| honey (*Barbara's* Crunchy Organic Granola), 2 bars ... | 190 | 4.0 | 27.0 | 8.0 | 0 | 60 | 3.0 |
| honey (*Nature Valley* Granola), 2 bars ... | 190 | 4.0 | 29.0 | 6.0 | 0 | 160 | 2.0 |
| peanut butter (*Fiber One* Chewy) ...... | 150 | 3.0 | 28.0 | 4.5 | 0 | 105 | 9.0 |
| strawberry, w/almond (*Fiber One* Chewy) . | 140 | 2.0 | 29.0 | 3.0 | 0 | 90 | 9.0 |
| orange chocolate (*Nature's Path Optimum* Energy Organic) ..... | 220 | 5.0 | 37.0 | 6.0 | 0 | 120 | 4.0 |
| peaches and berries (*Special K*) ......... | 90 | 1.0 | 18.0 | 2.0 | 0 | 85 | <1.0 |
| peanut: | | | | | | | |
| (*Nature Valley* Sweet & Salty Granola) ... | 170 | 4.0 | 19.0 | 9.0 | 0 | 150 | 2.0 |
| (*Odwalla Bar!* Sweet & Salty) ......... | 190 | 5.0 | 28.0 | 6.0 | 0 | 180 | 2.0 |
| chocolate (*Nature's Path* Organic Granola) .. | 150 | 3.0 | 22.0 | 6.0 | 0 | 125 | 2.0 |

| Food and Measure | cal. | prot. (gms) | carbo. (gms) | fat (gms) | chol. (mgs) | sod. (mgs) | fiber (gms) |
|---|---|---|---|---|---|---|---|
| crunch (*Health Valley* Organic Chewy Granola) ......... | 110 | 2.0 | 21.0 | 3.0 | 0 | 75 | 3.0 |
| pretzel (*Cascadian Farm* Organic Granola Sweet & Salty) .... | 160 | 3.0 | 22.0 | 7.0 | 0 | 180 | 1.0 |
| roasted (*Nature Valley* Crunch Bar) ...... | 190 | 6.0 | 13.0 | 13.0 | 0 | 180 | 2.0 |
| peanut butter: | | | | | | | |
| (*Barbara's* Crunchy Organic Granola), 2 bars ........... | 200 | 4.0 | 26.0 | 9.0 | 0 | 55 | 3.0 |
| (*FiberPlus*) ......... | 130 | 3.0 | 24.0 | 5.0 | 0 | 95 | 9.0 |
| (*Kudos* Granola) ..... | 130 | 2.0 | 18.0 | 6.0 | 0 | 75 | 1.0 |
| (*Nature Valley* Granola), 2 bars ... | 190 | 5.0 | 28.0 | 7.0 | 0 | 180 | 2.0 |
| (*Nature's Path* Organic Granola) .. | 140 | 3.0 | 22.0 | 5.0 | 0 | 90 | 2.0 |
| (*Nature's Path Optimum* Energy Organic) ... | 230 | 7.0 | 33.0 | 8.0 | 0 | 200 | 4.0 |
| (*Pomₓ Bar*) ......... | 200 | 4.0 | 26.0 | 9.0 | 0 | 65 | 4.0 |
| (*Quaker* Granola Bites), .75-oz. bag . | 90 | 2.0 | 14.0 | 3.5 | 0 | 40 | 2.0 |
| (*Quaker Chewy* Granola) | 90 | 2.0 | 18.0 | 2.0 | 0 | 115 | 1.0 |
| (*Quaker Chewy Dipps*) | 150 | 3.0 | 19.0 | 7.0 | 0 | 100 | 1.0 |
| (*Reese's* Snack Barz) . | 280 | 6.0 | 36.0 | 13.0 | 0 | 230 | 1.0 |
| (*Reese's* Sweet/Salty) . | 240 | 7.0 | 26.0 | 13.0 | 0 | 260 | 2.0 |
| (*South Beach Living* Cereal) .......... | 140 | 8.0 | 17.0 | 5.0 | 0 | 120 | 3.0 |
| chip (*Cascadian Farm* Organic Granola) .. | 140 | 2.0 | 25.0 | 4.0 | 0 | 130 | 1.0 |
| and chocolate (*GoLean* Chewy) .......... | 290 | 13.0 | 48.0 | 6.0 | 0 | 280 | 6.0 |
| and chocolate (*Quaker Chewy* Granola w/Fiber/Omega-3) . | 150 | 3.0 | 25.0 | 5.0 | 0 | 35 | 9.0 |
| and chocolate (*Quaker Chewy* Granola w/Protein) ....... | 110 | 5.0 | 18.0 | 3.0 | 0 | 150 | 1.0 |
| w/chocolate (*Reese's* Sweet/Salty) ...... | 160 | 4.0 | 18.0 | 9.0 | 0 | 170 | 1.0 |
| chocolate chip (*Genisoy* Organic) . | 170 | 6.0 | 26.0 | 5.0 | 0 | 190 | 4.0 |

| Food and Measure | cal. | prot. (gms) | carbo. (gms) | fat (gms) | chol. (mgs) | sod. (mgs) | fiber (gms) |
|---|---|---|---|---|---|---|---|
| **Granola/cereal bar, peanut butter** *(cont.)* | | | | | | | |
| chocolate chip (*Quaker Chewy* Granola) ... | 100 | 2.0 | 17.0 | 3.0 | 0 | 95 | 1.0 |
| chocolate chip (*Quaker Chewy* Granola 25% Less Sugar) .. | 100 | 1.0 | 18.0 | 3.0 | 0 | 75 | 1.0 |
| chocolate chip (*South Beach Living*) ..... | 100 | 3.0 | 18.0 | 3.0 | 0 | 160 | 3.0 |
| fudge (*Genisoy*) ..... | 240 | 15.0 | 31.0 | 7.0 | 0 | 220 | 2.0 |
| nutty (*Quaker Chewy* Granola w/Protein) . | 110 | 5.0 | 17.0 | 3.0 | 0 | 160 | 1.0 |
| peanut (*TLC* Chewy Granola) ......... | 140 | 7.0 | 19.0 | 5.0 | 0 | 85 | 4.0 |
| pecan crunch (*Nature Valley* Granola), 2 bars ............ | 190 | 4.0 | 28.0 | 7.0 | 0 | 160 | 2.0 |
| pomegranate: | | | | | | | |
| (*Pomₓ Bar*) ......... | 200 | 3.0 | 30.0 | 8.0 | 0 | 10 | 4.0 |
| cherry (*Nature's Path Optimum* Energy Organic) ......... | 230 | 4.0 | 39.0 | 5.0 | 0 | 140 | 4.0 |
| pretzel, chocolately (*Special K*) ......... | 90 | 1.0 | 17.0 | 2.0 | 0 | 120 | <1.0 |
| pumpkin flax spice (*TLC* Crunchy Granola), 2 bars ..... | 170 | 6.0 | 26.0 | 6.0 | 0 | 140 | 4.0 |
| pumpkin pecan (*TLC* Fruit & Grain) ....... | 120 | 4.0 | 22.0 | 3.0 | 0 | 50 | 4.0 |
| raspberry: | | | | | | | |
| (*Barbara's Nature's Choice* Cereal) .... | 150 | 2.0 | 29.0 | 2.0 | 0 | 85 | 2.0 |
| (*Nutri-Grain*) ........ | 120 | 2.0 | 24.0 | 3.0 | 0 | 110 | 3.0 |
| (*Special K Bliss*) ..... | 90 | 1.0 | 17.0 | 2.0 | 0 | 70 | <1.0 |
| chocolate (*TLC* Fruit & Grain) ..... | 120 | 4.0 | 21.0 | 3.0 | 0 | 50 | 4.0 |
| mocha (*Quaker True Delights Café Squares*) | 120 | 2.0 | 20.0 | 4.0 | 0 | 35 | 3.0 |
| streusel (*Quaker Oatmeal to Go*) .... | 220 | 4.0 | 43.0 | 4.0 | 15 | 220 | 5.0 |
| s'mores (*Quaker Chewy Dipps*/Granola) ...... | 100 | 1.0 | 19.0 | 2.0 | 0 | 80 | 1.0 |
| strawberry: | | | | | | | |
| (*Barbara's Nature's Choice* Cereal) .... | 150 | 2.0 | 29.0 | 2.0 | 0 | 85 | 2.0 |

| Food and Measure | cal. | prot. (gms) | carbo. (gms) | fat (gms) | chol. (mgs) | sod. (mgs) | fiber (gms) |
|---|---|---|---|---|---|---|---|
| (*Entenmann's*) ...... | 140 | 1.0 | 28.0 | 3.0 | 0 | 105 | 1.0 |
| (*Nutri-Grain*) ........ | 120 | 2.0 | 24.0 | 3.0 | 0 | 125 | 3.0 |
| (*Special K*) ......... | 90 | 1.0 | 18.0 | 1.5 | 0 | 95 | <1.0 |
| (*Special K* Fruit Crisps), 2 bars ........... | 100 | 1.0 | 20.0 | 2.0 | 0 | 80 | <1.0 |
| (*Special K* Protein Meal) ........... | 170 | 10.0 | 25.0 | 5.0 | 0 | 160 | 5.0 |
| cobbler (*Health Valley* Organic Cereal) | 130 | 2.0 | 27.0 | 2.5 | 0 | 85 | 3.0 |
| strawberry acai (*NutriGrain Superfruit Fusion*) ... | 130 | 2.0 | 26.0 | 3.0 | 0 | 105 | 3.0 |
| strawberry pomegranate (*Odwalla Bar!*) ...... | 200 | 3.0 | 42.0 | 2.0 | 0 | 95 | 3.0 |
| strawberry vanilla (*Quaker* Chewy Granola) | 90 | 1.0 | 19.0 | 1.5 | 0 | 75 | 1.0 |
| trail mix bar: (*Quaker Simple Harvest* Granola) .. | 150 | 3.0 | 25.0 | 5.0 | 0 | 95 | 2.0 |
| (*TLC* Chewy Granola) . | 140 | 6.0 | 20.0 | 5.0 | 0 | 95 | 4.0 |
| vanilla: chip (*Cascadian Farm* Organic Granola) . | 140 | 2.0 | 26.0 | 3.0 | 0 | 95 | 1.0 |
| crisp (*Special K*) ..... | 90 | 2.0 | 17.0 | 1.5 | 0 | 100 | <1.0 |
| wildberry, organic: (*Glutino*) ........... | 100 | 1.0 | 21.0 | 1.0 | 0 | 65 | 1.0 |
| (*Health Valley* Chewy Granola) ......... | 110 | 1.0 | 23.0 | 2.0 | 0 | 15 | 3.0 |
| yogurt: all varieties (*Nature Valley* Granola) .... | 140 | 2.0 | 26.0 | 4.0 | 0 | 95 | 1.0 |
| blueberry apple (*Barbara's* Fruit & Yogurt) .......... | 150 | 3.0 | 29.0 | 3.0 | 0 | 125 | 1.0 |
| peanut (*Genisoy*) .... | 250 | 14.0 | 31.0 | 8.0 | 0 | 140 | 1.0 |
| strawberry (*Nutri-Grain*) | 130 | 2.0 | 25.0 | 3.5 | 0 | 110 | 3.0 |
| strawberry apple (*Barbara's* Fruit & Yogurt) .......... | 150 | 3.0 | 28.0 | 3.0 | 0 | 125 | 1.0 |
| **Granola clusters** (*Nature Valley*), 1 oz.: | | | | | | | |
| cashew, roasted ....... | 140 | 4.0 | 18.0 | 7.0 | 0 | 160 | 1.0 |
| nut lovers ............ | 150 | 4.0 | 14.0 | 9.0 | 0 | 105 | 1.0 |
| peanut, honey-roasted .. | 160 | 5.0 | 17.0 | 7.0 | 0 | 160 | 1.0 |

| Food and Measure | cal. | prot. (gms) | carbo. (gms) | fat (gms) | chol. (mgs) | sod. (mgs) | fiber (gms) |
|---|---|---|---|---|---|---|---|
| **Grape**, fresh: | | | | | | | |
| (*Chiquita*), 1 cup ....... | 62 | 1.0 | 16.0 | 0 | 0 | 2.0 | 1.0 |
| (*Dole*), 26 pcs., ¾ cup .. | 90 | <1.0 | 23.0 | 0 | 0 | 0 | 1.0 |
| (*Frieda's* Champagne), | | | | | | | |
| ½ cup, 3 oz. ........ | 50 | 1.0 | 15.0 | 0 | 0 | 0 | 1.0 |
| American type | | | | | | | |
| (slipskin): | | | | | | | |
| 10 medium ......... | 15 | .2 | 4.1 | .1 | 0 | tr. | .3 |
| peeled, seeded, ½ cup | 29 | .3 | 7.9 | .2 | 0 | 1 | .6 |
| European type | | | | | | | |
| (adherent skin): | | | | | | | |
| seeded, 1 lb. ........ | 287 | 2.7 | 72.0 | 2.3 | 0 | 7 | 2.7 |
| seedless, 10 medium . | 36 | .3 | 8.9 | .3 | 0 | 1 | .3 |
| seedless/seeded, ½ cup | 57 | .5 | 14.2 | .5 | 0 | 2 | .5 |
| **Grape, canned**, seedless, | | | | | | | |
| in heavy syrup, | | | | | | | |
| w/liquid, ½ cup ...... | 94 | .6 | 25.1 | .1 | 0 | 6 | .5 |
| **Grape drink**, 8 fl. oz.: | | | | | | | |
| (*Apple & Eve* Concord) ... | 130 | 0 | 35.0 | 0 | 0 | 10 | 0 |
| (*Nantucket Nectars* | | | | | | | |
| Organic Concord) .... | 130 | 0 | 31.0 | 0 | 0 | 35 | 0 |
| (*Newman's Own* | | | | | | | |
| Gorilla Grape) ....... | 140 | 0 | 34.0 | 0 | 0 | 140 | 0 |
| (*Santa Cruz Organic* | | | | | | | |
| Box) .............. | 100 | 0 | 23.0 | 0 | 0 | 10 | 0 |
| (*Tropicana*) ........... | 150 | <1.0 | 38.0 | 0 | 0 | 25 | 0 |
| (*Welch's* Concord | | | | | | | |
| Cocktail) .......... | 150 | 0 | 37.0 | 0 | 0 | 20 | 0 |
| (*Welch's* Concord | | | | | | | |
| Cocktail Chilled) ..... | 140 | 0 | 34.0 | 0 | 0 | 20 | 0 |
| frozen* (*Minute Maid* | | | | | | | |
| Cocktail) ........... | 120 | 0 | 33.0 | 0 | 0 | 5 | 0 |
| grapeade: | | | | | | | |
| (*AriZona*) .......... | 100 | 0 | 27.0 | 0 | 0 | 10 | 0 |
| (*Nantucket Nectars*) .. | 140 | 0 | 33.0 | 0 | 0 | 25 | 0 |
| (*Snapple*) .......... | 100 | 0 | 26.0 | 0 | 0 | 5 | 0 |
| punch: | | | | | | | |
| (*Minute Maid*) ....... | 120 | 0 | 32.0 | 0 | 0 | 15 | 0 |
| (*Tropicana*) .......... | 120 | 0 | 29.0 | 0 | 0 | 25 | 0 |
| **Grape drink blend**, | | | | | | | |
| 8 fl. oz.: | | | | | | | |
| cranberry (*Welch's* | | | | | | | |
| Cocktail) ........... | 150 | 0 | 37.0 | 0 | 0 | 20 | 0 |

| Food and Measure | cal. | prot. (gms) | carbo. (gms) | fat (gms) | chol. (mgs) | sod. (mgs) | fiber (gms) |
|---|---|---|---|---|---|---|---|
| pomegranate (*Snapple* Antioxidant Water) ... | 50 | 0 | 13.0 | 0 | 0 | 0 | 0 |
| raspberry (*V8 V-Fusion* Light Concord) ...... | 140 | 0 | 35.0 | 0 | 0 | 125 | 0 |
| red or white, sparkling (*Welch's* Cocktail) .... | 160 | 0 | 40.0 | 0 | 0 | 45 | 0 |
| white grape: | | | | | | | |
| peach (*Welch's*) ..... | 150 | 0 | 36.0 | 0 | 0 | 5 | 0 |
| peach mango (*Welch's*) | 150 | 0 | 37.0 | 0 | 0 | 20 | 0 |
| **Grape juice**, 8 fl. oz., except as noted: | | | | | | | |
| (*Apple & Eve*), 6.75 fl. oz. ......... | 110 | 0 | 29.0 | 0 | 0 | 20 | 0 |
| (*Apple & Eve Organics* Vintage Concord) .... | 160 | 0 | 40.0 | 0 | 0 | 15 | 0 |
| (*Dole*) ............... | 160 | <1.0 | 39.0 | 0 | 0 | 15 | 0 |
| (*Eden* Organic Concord) . | 150 | <1.0 | 37.0 | 0 | 0 | 35 | <1.0 |
| (*Fragile Planet* Organic) .......... | 160 | 0 | 40.0 | 0 | 0 | 15 | 0 |
| (*Langers* Red) ......... | 160 | 0 | 40.0 | 0 | 0 | 15 | 0 |
| (*Minute Maid*), 10 fl. oz. ........... | 150 | 0 | 39.0 | 0 | 0 | 25 | 0 |
| (*R.W. Knudsen*) ........ | 150 | 1.0 | 37.0 | 0 | 0 | 15 | 0 |
| (*R.W. Knudsen* Concord/Kosher/ Organic Concord) .... | 160 | <1.0 | 40.0 | 0 | 0 | 15 | 0 |
| (*R.W. Knudsen* Juice Box) .......... | 130 | 1.0 | 32.0 | 0 | 0 | 15 | 0 |
| (*R.W. Knudsen Just Concord Grape*) ..... | 160 | <1.0 | 40.0 | 0 | 0 | 15 | 0 |
| (*Santa Cruz Organic* Concord) .......... | 160 | <1.0 | 40.0 | 0 | 0 | 15 | 0 |
| (*Snapple*), 11.5 fl. oz. ... | 170 | 0 | 43.0 | 0 | 0 | 15 | 0 |
| (*Tropicana*), 12 fl. oz. ... | 240 | 1.0 | 60.0 | 0 | 0 | 25 | 0 |
| (*Veryfine*) ............ | 160 | 0 | 41.0 | 0 | 0 | 25 | 0 |
| (*Veryfine*), 10 fl. oz. .... | 200 | 0 | 51.0 | 0 | 0 | 30 | 0 |
| (*Welch's*) ............. | 140 | 0 | 38.0 | 0 | 0 | 15 | 0 |
| (*Welch's* Concord) ..... | 170 | 0 | 42.0 | 0 | 0 | 20 | 0 |
| frozen*: | | | | | | | |
| (*Cascadian Farm* Organic) ......... | 150 | 0 | 38.0 | 0 | 0 | 5 | 0 |
| (*Welch's*) .......... | 160 | 0 | 41.0 | 0 | 0 | 0 | 0 |
| sweetened ......... | 128 | .5 | 31.9 | .2 | 0 | 5 | .3 |
| red grape (*Welch's*) ..... | 170 | 0 | 44.0 | 0 | 0 | 20 | 0 |

| Food and Measure | cal. | prot. (gms) | carbo. (gms) | fat (gms) | chol. (mgs) | sod. (mgs) | fiber (gms) |
|---|---|---|---|---|---|---|---|
| **Grape juice** *(cont.)* | | | | | | | |
| sparkling (*R.W. Knudsen*) | 160 | <1.0 | 40.0 | 0 | 0 | 15 | 0 |
| white grape: | | | | | | | |
| (*Langers*) .......... | 160 | 0 | 40.0 | 0 | 0 | 15 | 0 |
| (*Santa Cruz Organic*) . | 160 | <1.0 | 39.0 | 0 | 0 | 10 | 0 |
| (*Welch's*) .......... | 160 | 0 | 39.0 | 0 | 0 | 20 | 0 |
| **Grape juice blend**, | | | | | | | |
|   8 fl. oz., except | | | | | | | |
|   as noted: | | | | | | | |
| all blends, frozen* | | | | | | | |
| (*Welch's*) .......... | 160 | 0 | 41.0 | 0 | 0 | 0 | 0 |
| apple, carrot (*Mott's* | | | | | | | |
|   Medleys) .......... | 140 | 0 | 33.0 | 0 | 0 | 80 | 0 |
| blueberry pomegranate | | | | | | | |
| (*Welch's*) .......... | 160 | 0 | 40.0 | 0 | 0 | 20 | 0 |
| cherry, black (*Welch's*) .. | 170 | 0 | 42.0 | 0 | 0 | 20 | 0 |
| raspberry (*V8 V-Fusion* | | | | | | | |
|   Concord) .......... | 140 | 0 | 35.0 | 0 | 0 | 125 | 0 |
| white grape: | | | | | | | |
| cherry (*Welch's*) ..... | 140 | 0 | 35.0 | 0 | 0 | 15 | 0 |
| mango orange (Welch's) | 150 | 0 | 38.0 | 0 | 0 | 40 | 0 |
| peach (*Welch's*) ..... | 160 | 0 | 39.0 | 0 | 0 | 15 | 0 |
| raspberry (*Apple &* | | | | | | | |
|   *Eve*), 6.75 fl. oz. ... | 100 | 0 | 21.0 | 0 | 0 | 15 | 0 |
| **Grape leaves**, fresh: | | | | | | | |
| 1 cup ................ | 13 | .8 | 2.4 | .3 | 0 | 1 | 1.5 |
| 1 leaf ................ | 3 | .2 | .5 | <.1 | 0 | <1 | .3 |
| **Grape leaves, in jar**: | | | | | | | |
| (*Peloponnese*), .25 oz. .. | 5 | 0 | 1.0 | 0 | 0 | 120 | 0 |
| (*Roland*), 3 pcs., .5 oz. .. | 10 | 1.0 | 2.0 | 0 | 0 | 430 | 0 |
| **Grape leaves, stuffed**: | | | | | | | |
| (*Peloponnese* Dolmas), | | | | | | | |
|   6 pcs. ............. | 180 | 3.0 | 20.0 | 8.0 | 0 | 650 | 1.0 |
| (*Roland*), 5 pcs., 4.7 oz. | 210 | 3.0 | 19.0 | 14.0 | 5 | 510 | 3.0 |
| **Grapefruit**, fresh: | | | | | | | |
| (*Frieda's* Cocktail), | | | | | | | |
|   ½ medium ......... | 65 | 1.0 | 16.0 | 0 | 0 | 0 | 2.0 |
| all areas/varieties: | | | | | | | |
| ½ large, 4.7 oz. ...... | 53 | 1.1 | 13.4 | .2 | 0 | 0 | 1.8 |
| sections, 1 cup ...... | 74 | 1.5 | 18.6 | .2 | 0 | 0 | 2.5 |
| all areas, pink/red: | | | | | | | |
| ½ medium, 3¾" ..... | 37 | .7 | 9.5 | .1 | 0 | 0 | n.a. |
| sections, 1 cup ...... | 69 | 1.3 | 17.7 | .2 | 0 | 0 | n.a. |

| Food and Measure | cal. | prot. (gms) | carbo. (gms) | fat (gms) | chol. (mgs) | sod. (mgs) | fiber (gms) |
|---|---|---|---|---|---|---|---|
| all areas, white: | | | | | | | |
| ½ medium, 3¾" ..... | 39 | .8 | 9.9 | .1 | 0 | 0 | 1.3 |
| sections, 1 cup ...... | 76 | 1.3 | 17.7 | .2 | 0 | 0 | 2.5 |
| California/Arizona: | | | | | | | |
| pink/red, ½ | | | | | | | |
| medium, 3¾" ..... | 46 | .6 | 11.9 | .1 | 0 | 1 | 1.4 |
| pink/red, sections | | | | | | | |
| w/juice, 1 cup ..... | 85 | 1.2 | 22.3 | .2 | 0 | 2 | 2.6 |
| white, ½ medium, | | | | | | | |
| 3¾" ............ | 43 | 1.0 | 10.7 | .1 | 0 | 0 | 1.3 |
| white, sections, | | | | | | | |
| w/juice, 1 cup ..... | 85 | 2.0 | 20.9 | .2 | 0 | 0 | 2.6 |
| Florida: | | | | | | | |
| pink/red, ½ | | | | | | | |
| medium, 3¾" ..... | 37 | .7 | 9.2 | .1 | 0 | 0 | 1.4 |
| pink/red, sections | | | | | | | |
| w/juice, 1 cup ..... | 69 | 1.3 | 17.3 | .2 | 0 | 0 | 2.5 |
| white, ½ medium, | | | | | | | |
| 3¾" ............ | 38 | .7 | 9.7 | .1 | 0 | 0 | .2 |
| white, sections | | | | | | | |
| w/juice, 1 cup ..... | 74 | 1.5 | 18.8 | .2 | 0 | 0 | .4 |
| **Grapefruit, can/jar**, | | | | | | | |
| ½ cup, except | | | | | | | |
| as noted: | | | | | | | |
| in juice: | | | | | | | |
| (*Del Monte* Duo | | | | | | | |
| Bowl) ........... | 60 | 1.0 | 16.0 | 0 | 0 | 10 | 1.0 |
| (*Del Monte SunFresh*) | 45 | 1.0 | 9.0 | 0 | 0 | 15 | 2.0 |
| red (*Del Monte* | | | | | | | |
| Bowl) ........... | 60 | 1.0 | 14.0 | 0 | 0 | 15 | <1.0 |
| red (*Del Monte Fruit* | | | | | | | |
| *Naturals*) ........ | 60 | 0 | 16.0 | 0 | 0 | 15 | <1.0 |
| red (*Del Monte Fruit* | | | | | | | |
| *Naturals* No Sugar) | 40 | <1.0 | 10.0 | 0 | 0 | 15 | .5 |
| red (*Del Monte* | | | | | | | |
| *SunFresh*) ....... | 60 | 1.0 | 14.0 | 0 | 0 | 15 | <1.0 |
| red (*Del Monte* | | | | | | | |
| *SunFresh* No Sugar) | 40 | <1.0 | 10.0 | 0 | 0 | 15 | .5 |
| in light syrup: | | | | | | | |
| (*Roland*), ⅔ cup ..... | 100 | 0 | 24.0 | 0 | 0 | 25 | 0 |
| red (*Del Monte*) ..... | 90 | 1.0 | 21.0 | 0 | 0 | 0 | 1.0 |
| w/liquid ............. | 76 | .7 | 19.6 | .1 | 0 | 3 | .5 |
| in water (*Roland*), | | | | | | | |
| ⅔ cup ............. | 50 | 0 | 14.0 | 0 | 0 | 25 | 0 |

| Food and Measure | cal. | prot. (gms) | carbo. (gms) | fat (gms) | chol. (mgs) | sod. (mgs) | fiber (gms) |
|---|---|---|---|---|---|---|---|
| **Grapefruit, can/jar** *(cont.)* | | | | | | | |
| and orange sections, in | | | | | | | |
| syrup (*Roland*), | | | | | | | |
| ⅔ cup .............. | 100 | 0 | 24.0 | 0 | 0 | 25 | 0 |
| **Grapefruit, Chinese**, | | | | | | | |
| see "Pummelo" | | | | | | | |
| **Grapefruit drink**, | | | | | | | |
| ruby red, 8 fl. oz.: | | | | | | | |
| (*Apple & Eve*) ......... | 130 | 0 | 32.0 | 0 | 0 | 10 | 0 |
| (*Langers*) ............ | 130 | 0 | 33.0 | 0 | 0 | 10 | 0 |
| (*Minute Maid*) ......... | 130 | 0 | 34.0 | 0 | 0 | 20 | 0 |
| (*Ocean Spray* Cocktail) .. | 110 | 0 | 28.0 | 0 | 0 | 65 | 0 |
| (*Ocean Spray Light* | | | | | | | |
| *Ruby*) ............. | 40 | 0 | 10.0 | 0 | 0 | 65 | 0 |
| (*Tropicana*) ........... | 130 | 1.0 | 31.0 | 0 | 0 | 15 | 0 |
| frozen* (*Langers*) ...... | 120 | 0 | 33.0 | 0 | 0 | 10 | 0 |
| **Grapefruit drink blend**, | | | | | | | |
| 8 fl. oz.: | | | | | | | |
| (*Ocean Spray Ruby* | | | | | | | |
| *Pomegranate*) ....... | 120 | 0 | 29.0 | 0 | 0 | 35 | 0 |
| (*Ocean Spray Ruby* | | | | | | | |
| *Tangerine*) ......... | 110 | 0 | 28.0 | 0 | 0 | 65 | 0 |
| **Grapefruit juice**, | | | | | | | |
| 8 fl. oz., except | | | | | | | |
| as noted: | | | | | | | |
| (*Ocean* Spray White) .... | 90 | 0 | 21.0 | 0 | 0 | 35 | 0 |
| (*R.W. Knudsen*) ........ | 100 | 1.0 | 24.0 | 0 | 0 | 10 | 0 |
| (*R.W. Knudsen* | | | | | | | |
| Organic) ........... | 100 | 1.0 | 23.0 | 0 | 0 | 5 | 0 |
| (*Simply Grapefruit*) ..... | 90 | 1.0 | 21.0 | 0 | 0 | 10 | 0 |
| (*Tropicana* Shelf) ...... | 90 | 1.0 | 27.0 | 0 | 0 | 15 | 0 |
| (*Tropicana Pure* Indian | | | | | | | |
| River) ............. | 110 | 2.0 | 25.0 | 0 | 0 | 0 | 0 |
| (*Tropicana Pure* | | | | | | | |
| *Premium* Golden) .... | 90 | 1.0 | 22.0 | 0 | 0 | 0 | 0 |
| (*Veryfine*) ............ | 100 | 0 | 25.0 | 0 | 0 | 20 | 0 |
| (*Veryfine*), 10 fl. oz. .... | 120 | 0 | 31.0 | 0 | 0 | 25 | 0 |
| pink (*Ocean Spray* Blend) | 100 | 0 | 23.0 | 0 | 0 | 35 | 0 |
| ruby red: | | | | | | | |
| (*Dole*) .............. | 140 | 1.0 | 33.0 | 0 | 0 | 15 | 0 |
| (*Florida's Natural*) .... | 90 | 1.0 | 22.0 | 0 | 0 | 0 | 0 |
| (*Ocean Spray* Blend) .. | 110 | 0 | 26.0 | 0 | 0 | 35 | 0 |
| (*R.W. Knudsen* Rio) .. | 140 | 1.0 | 35.0 | 0 | 0 | 15 | 0 |
| (*Tropicana*), 10 fl. oz. . | 170 | 0 | 42.0 | 0 | 0 | 20 | 0 |

| Food and Measure | cal. | prot. (gms) | carbo. (gms) | fat (gms) | chol. (mgs) | sod. (mgs) | fiber (gms) |
|---|---|---|---|---|---|---|---|
| (*Tropicana Pure Premium*) ........ | 90 | 1.0 | 22.0 | 0 | 0 | 0 | 0 |
| canned, unsweetened ... | 94 | 1.3 | 22.1 | .3 | 0 | 3 | .3 |
| fresh, pink or white ..... | 96 | 1.2 | 22.7 | .3 | 0 | 3 | .3 |
| frozen*: | | | | | | | |
| (*Minute Maid*) ....... | 100 | 0 | 25.0 | 0 | 0 | 0 | 0 |
| unsweetened ....... | 101 | 1.4 | 24.0 | .3 | 0 | 3 | .3 |
| **Gravlax**, see "Salmon, marinated" | | | | | | | |
| **Gravy**, see specific listings | | | | | | | |
| **Gravy, country**, canned, sausage (*Campbell's*), ¼ cup ............. | 70 | 2.0 | 4.0 | 5.0 | 5 | 270 | 0 |
| **Gravy mix** (see also specific gravy listings), ¼ cup*: | | | | | | | |
| country style: | | | | | | | |
| (*McCormick* Original) . | 40 | <1.0 | 5.0 | 2.0 | 0 | 270 | 0 |
| peppered (*McCormick*) | 40 | <1.0 | 5.0 | 2.0 | 0 | 260 | 0 |
| sausage (*McCormick*) . | 40 | <1.0 | 5.0 | 1.5 | 0 | 300 | 0 |
| homestyle (*McCormick*) . | 25 | 0 | 4.0 | 1.0 | 0 | 320 | 0 |
| **Great northern bean**: | | | | | | | |
| dry (*Bob's Red Mill*), ¼ cup ............. | 140 | 9.0 | 26.0 | 0 | 0 | 5 | 8.0 |
| boiled, ½ cup ......... | 104 | 7.3 | 18.6 | .4 | 0 | 2 | 6.2 |
| **Great northern bean, canned**, ½ cup: | | | | | | | |
| (*Allens*) .............. | 100 | 6.0 | 19.0 | .5 | 0 | 310 | 7.0 |
| (*Bush's*) ............. | 80 | 6.0 | 17.0 | 0 | 0 | 460 | 6.0 |
| (*Eden* Organic) ........ | 110 | 5.0 | 20.0 | 1.0 | 0 | 45 | 8.0 |
| w/sausage (*Trappey's*) .. | 100 | 6.0 | 18.0 | 1.0 | 0 | 460 | 7.0 |
| seasoned (*Glory*) ...... | 90 | 6.0 | 17.0 | 0 | 0 | 570 | 5.0 |
| **Greek salad**, marinated, w/feta (*Roland*), 7.76-oz. cont. ....... | 610 | 3.0 | 7.0 | 63.0 | 5 | 620 | 5.0 |
| **Green bean, fresh**: | | | | | | | |
| raw: | | | | | | | |
| (*Frieda's* Snap Beans), 3 oz. ..... | 25 | 2.0 | 6.0 | 0 | 0 | 5 | 3.0 |
| (*Green Giant*), ¾ cup . | 20 | 1.0 | 5.0 | 0 | 0 | 0 | 3.0 |
| w/garlic butter (*Green Giant*), 1 cup ..... | 110 | 2.0 | 8.0 | 8.0 | 20 | 190 | 3.0 |
| boiled, drained, ½ cup .. | 22 | 1.2 | 4.9 | .2 | 0 | 2 | 2.0 |

| Food and Measure | cal. | prot. (gms) | carbo. (gms) | fat (gms) | chol. (mgs) | sod. (mgs) | fiber (gms) |
|---|---|---|---|---|---|---|---|
| **Green bean, can/jar,** | | | | | | | |
| ½ cup: | | | | | | | |
| whole: | | | | | | | |
| (*Allens*) . . . . . . . . . . . . | 30 | 1.0 | 6.0 | 0 | 0 | 460 | 3.0 |
| (*Freshlike* Selects) . . . | 35 | 2.0 | 7.0 | 0 | 0 | 380 | 3.0 |
| whole, cut, or French: | | | | | | | |
| (*Del Monte*) . . . . . . . . | 20 | 1.0 | 4.0 | 0 | 0 | 390 | 2.0 |
| (*S&W*) . . . . . . . . . . . . | 20 | 1.0 | 4.0 | 0 | 0 | 390 | 2.0 |
| cut: | | | | | | | |
| (*Allens* No Salt) . . . . . | 15 | 0 | 3.0 | 0 | 0 | 10 | 2.0 |
| (*Allens*) . . . . . . . . . . . . | 30 | 0 | 6.0 | 0 | 0 | 320 | 3.0 |
| (*Bush's*) . . . . . . . . . . . | 20 | 1.0 | 5.0 | 0 | 0 | 400 | 2.0 |
| (*Freshlike*) . . . . . . . . . | 35 | 2.0 | 7.0 | 0 | 0 | 380 | 3.0 |
| (*Freshlike* No Salt) . . . | 25 | 2.0 | 4.0 | 0 | 0 | 0 | 2.0 |
| (*Green Giant* Low | | | | | | | |
| Sodium) . . . . . . . . . | 20 | 1.0 | 4.0 | 0 | 0 | 200 | 1.0 |
| (*Green Giant/Green* | | | | | | | |
| *Giant* Kitchen | | | | | | | |
| *Sliced*) . . . . . . . . . . | 20 | 1.0 | 4.0 | 0 | 0 | 400 | 1.0 |
| (*Veg-All*) . . . . . . . . . . . | 20 | <1.0 | 4.0 | 0 | 0 | 400 | 2.0 |
| dilled (*S&W*), 1 oz. . . . | 20 | 0 | 5.0 | 0 | 0 | 125 | 1.0 |
| w/liquid . . . . . . . . . . . | 18 | 1.0 | 4.2 | .1 | 0 | 311 | 1.8 |
| French style: | | | | | | | |
| (*Allens/Sunshine*) . . . . | 25 | 1.0 | 4.0 | 0 | 0 | 300 | 2.0 |
| (*Freshlike*) . . . . . . . . . | 20 | 1.0 | 3.0 | 0 | 0 | 380 | 3.0 |
| (*Freshlike* No Salt) . . . | 20 | 1.0 | 4.0 | 0 | 0 | 0 | 2.0 |
| (*Green Giant*) . . . . . . . | 20 | 1.0 | 4.0 | 0 | 0 | 390 | 1.0 |
| (*Veg-All*) . . . . . . . . . . . | 20 | <1.0 | 4.0 | 0 | 0 | 400 | 2.0 |
| Italian cut: | | | | | | | |
| (*Allens* Kentucky | | | | | | | |
| Wonder/ | | | | | | | |
| *Sunshine*) . . . . . . . . | 35 | 1.0 | 7.0 | 0 | 0 | 320 | 3.0 |
| (*Allens* Shellouts) . . . . | 50 | 3.0 | 9.0 | 0 | 0 | 320 | 3.0 |
| (*Del Monte*) . . . . . . . . | 30 | 1.0 | 6.0 | 0 | 0 | 390 | 3.0 |
| (*Freshlike* Selects) . . . | 30 | 2.0 | 5.0 | 0 | 0 | 270 | 2.0 |
| seasoned (*Allens* | | | | | | | |
| Kentucky Wonder/ | | | | | | | |
| *Sunshine*) . . . . . . . . | 45 | 2.0 | 8.0 | 0 | 0 | 370 | 3.0 |
| seasoned: | | | | | | | |
| (*Glory* Sensibly) . . . . . | 25 | 1.0 | 5.0 | 0 | 0 | 160 | 2.0 |
| (*Glory* String Beans) . . | 25 | 1.0 | 5.0 | 0 | 0 | 380 | 2.0 |
| w/red pepper (*Del* | | | | | | | |
| *Monte*) . . . . . . . . . . | 20 | 1.0 | 4.0 | 0 | 0 | 360 | 2.0 |

| Food and Measure | cal. | prot. (gms) | carbo. (gms) | fat (gms) | chol. (mgs) | sod. (mgs) | fiber (gms) |
|---|---|---|---|---|---|---|---|
| **Green bean, frozen:** | | | | | | | |
| whole, 1 cup: | | | | | | | |
| (*Birds Eye/Birds Eye Steamfresh/C&W* Petite) . . . . . . . . . | 35 | 1.0 | 5.0 | 0 | 0 | 0 | 2.0 |
| (*Cascadian Farm* Organic Petite) . . . . | 25 | 1.0 | 5.0 | 0 | 0 | 95 | 2.0 |
| (*Green Giant Valley Fresh Steamers*) . . . | 25 | 1.0 | 6.0 | 0 | 0 | 0 | 1.0 |
| cut: | | | | | | | |
| (*Allens SteamSupreme*), ⅔ cup . . . . . . . . . | 30 | 1.0 | 6.0 | 0 | 0 | 0 | 2.0 |
| (*Birds Eye/Freshlike*), ⅔ cup . . . . . . . . . | 30 | 1.0 | 5.0 | 0 | 0 | 0 | 2.0 |
| (*Birds Eye Steamfresh*), 1 cup . . . . . . . . . | 30 | 1.0 | 5.0 | 0 | 0 | 0 | 2.0 |
| (*Cascadian Farm* Organic), ¾ cup . . . | 30 | 1.0 | 6.0 | 0 | 0 | 0 | 2.0 |
| (*C&W*), ¾ cup . . . . . . | 35 | 1.0 | 5.0 | 0 | 0 | 0 | 2.0 |
| (*Green Giant Valley Fresh Steamers*), ¾ cup . . . . . . . . . | 30 | 1.0 | 6.0 | 0 | 0 | 0 | 2.0 |
| French cut: | | | | | | | |
| (*Birds Eye*), ⅔ cup . . . | 30 | 1.0 | 5.0 | 0 | 0 | 0 | 2.0 |
| (*C&W/Freshlike*), 1 cup . . . . . . . . . | 30 | 1.0 | 5.0 | 0 | 0 | 0 | 2.0 |
| Italian cut, ¾ cup: | | | | | | | |
| (*Allens SteamSupreme*) | 40 | 1.0 | 8.0 | 0 | 0 | 0 | 3.0 |
| (*C&W*) . . . . . . . . . . | 35 | 1.0 | 5.0 | 0 | 0 | 0 | 2.0 |
| boiled, drained, ½ cup . . | 19 | 1.0 | 4.4 | .1 | 0 | 6 | 2.0 |
| **Green bean combinations**, fresh, and carrots (*Green Giant* Fresh), 3 oz. . . . . . . . . | 30 | 2.0 | 7.0 | 0 | 0 | 20 | 3.0 |
| **Green bean combinations, canned**, ½ cup: | | | | | | | |
| and potatoes: | | | | | | | |
| (*Allens/Sunshine*) . . . . | 50 | 2.0 | 10.0 | 0 | 0 | 160 | 2.0 |
| (*Glory* Southern) . . . . | 35 | 2.0 | 8.0 | 0 | 0 | 420 | 2.0 |
| ham style flavor (*Del Monte*) . . . . . . . . . | 30 | 1.0 | 6.0 | 0 | 0 | 330 | <1.0 |
| and shelly beans (*Bush's*) . . . . . . . . . . | 45 | 3.0 | 7.0 | 0 | 0 | 400 | 3.0 |

| Food and Measure | cal. | prot. (gms) | carbo. (gms) | fat (gms) | chol. (mgs) | sod. (mgs) | fiber (gms) |
|---|---|---|---|---|---|---|---|
| **Green bean combinations, frozen/chilled**: | | | | | | | |
| w/almonds: | | | | | | | |
| (*C&W*), 1 cup ....... | 80 | 3.0 | 12.0 | 2.0 | 0 | 270 | 4.0 |
| (*Green Giant Simply Steam*), ⅔ cup .... | 50 | 2.0 | 5.0 | 3.0 | 0 | 95 | 2.0 |
| toasted (*Cascadian Farm Organic*), ⅔ cup | 70 | 3.0 | 10.0 | 3.0 | 0 | 115 | 4.0 |
| toasted, lightly (*Birds Eye*), ¾ cup . | 80 | 3.0 | 8.0 | 3.5 | 0 | 410 | 3.0 |
| baby, and carrots (*Birds Eye/Freshlike*), 1 cup . | 35 | 1.0 | 6.0 | 0 | 0 | 20 | 2.0 |
| casserole: | | | | | | | |
| (*Bob Evans*), ½ cup .. | 100 | 3.0 | 12.0 | 5.0 | 5 | 520 | 2.0 |
| (*Green Giant*), ⅔ cup . | 110 | 2.0 | 9.0 | 8.0 | 0 | 450 | 1.0 |
| and spaetzle, in sauce (*Birds Eye* Bavarian), 1 cup ............ | 150 | 5.0 | 16.0 | 7.0 | 30 | 390 | 3.0 |
| stir-fry (*Birds Eye* Crisp), 1 cup cooked ....... | 90 | 3.0 | 17.0 | 0 | 0 | 30 | 2.0 |
| **Green pea flour** (*Bob's Red Mill*), 1½ tbsp. .... | 50 | 4.0 | 9.0 | 0 | 0 | 2 | 4.0 |
| **Green peas**, see "Peas, green" | | | | | | | |
| **Green pepper**, see "Pepper, sweet" | | | | | | | |
| **Greens**, see specific listings | | | | | | | |
| **Greens, mixed**, fresh, see "Salad blend" | | | | | | | |
| **Greens, mixed, canned**: | | | | | | | |
| (*Bush's*), ½ cup ........ | 25 | 2.0 | 3.0 | 0 | 0 | 300 | 2.0 |
| seasoned, ½ cup: | | | | | | | |
| (*Allens*) ............ | 30 | 2.0 | 4.0 | 0 | 0 | 400 | 2.0 |
| (*Allens* No Salt) ..... | 30 | 1.0 | 8.0 | .5 | 0 | 10 | 4.0 |
| (*Glory*) ............ | 35 | 1.0 | 4.0 | 0 | 0 | 490 | 2.0 |
| (*Glory* Sensibly) ..... | 20 | 1.0 | 4.0 | 0 | 0 | 240 | 2.0 |
| (*Sunshine*) ......... | 45 | 4.0 | 6.0 | .5 | 0 | 830 | 1.0 |
| **Grenadine**: | | | | | | | |
| (*Angostura*), 1 tsp. ..... | 10 | 0 | 3.0 | 0 | 0 | 5 | 0 |
| (*Roland*), 1 tbsp. ....... | 40 | 0 | 9.0 | 0 | 0 | 0 | 0 |
| **Griddle cakes**, see "Pancake" and "Breakfast sandwich" | | | | | | | |

| Food and Measure | cal. | prot. (gms) | carbo. (gms) | fat (gms) | chol. (mgs) | sod. (mgs) | fiber (gms) |
|---|---|---|---|---|---|---|---|
| **Grilling sauce** (see also "Barbecue sauce," "Marinade," and specific listings), 1 tbsp.: | | | | | | | |
| (*Hibachi Grill Hunan Smokehut*) . . . . . . . . | 40 | 0 | 8.0 | .5 | 0 | 410 | 0 |
| apricot ginger (*Campagna* Grill/Glaze) | 25 | 0 | 6.0 | 0 | 0 | 0 | 0 |
| balsamic mustard (*Campagna* Grill/Glaze) | 30 | 1.0 | 3.0 | 1.5 | 0 | 115 | 0 |
| cranberry chipotle (*Campagna* Grill/Glaze) | 5 | 0 | 1.0 | 0 | 0 | 0 | 0 |
| ginger sesame, sweet (*Hibachi Grill*) . . . . . . . | 40 | 0 | 8.0 | 1.0 | 0 | 410 | 0 |
| Kobe steak (*Hibachi Grill*) . . . . . . . . . . . . . | 50 | 0 | 3.0 | 4.0 | 0 | 600 | 0 |
| peanut, Thai (*Hibachi Grill*) | 50 | 1.0 | 5.0 | 3.0 | 0 | 270 | 0 |
| teriyaki (*Hibachi Grill*) . . . | 40 | 0 | 10.0 | 0 | 0 | 520 | 0 |
| **Grits**, see "Corn grits" | | | | | | | |
| **Ground cherry**, ½ cup . . . | 37 | 1.3 | 7.8 | .5 | 0 | n.a. | 2.0 |
| **Grouper**, meat only: | | | | | | | |
| raw, 4 oz. . . . . . . . . . . . | 104 | 22.0 | 0 | 1.2 | 42 | 60 | 0 |
| baked or broiled, 4 oz. . . | 134 | 28.2 | 0 | 1.5 | 53 | 60 | 0 |
| **Guacamole**, 2 tbsp.: | | | | | | | |
| (*Calavo* Authentic) . . . . . . | 50 | 1.0 | 2.0 | 5.0 | 0 | 95 | 1.0 |
| (*Calavo* Authentic Frozen) . . . . . . . . . . . . | 50 | 1.0 | 7.0 | 2.5 | 0 | 120 | 1.0 |
| (*Calavo* Fiesta) . . . . . . . . | 60 | 1.0 | 2.0 | 5.0 | 0 | 140 | 2.0 |
| (*Calavo* Mexican) . . . . . . | 70 | <1.0 | 3.0 | 7.0 | 0 | 120 | 1.0 |
| (*Calavo* Original) . . . . . . . | 60 | <1.0 | 6.0 | 4.0 | 0 | 120 | 1.0 |
| (*Kraft*) . . . . . . . . . . . . . . | 50 | 1.0 | 3.0 | 4.5 | 0 | 240 | 0 |
| (*Marie's* Dip) . . . . . . . . . . | 40 | 1.0 | 3.0 | 3.0 | 5 | 140 | 1.0 |
| (*Marzetti* Dip) . . . . . . . . . | 130 | 0 | 2.0 | 13.0 | 15 | 240 | 0 |
| (*Mission*) . . . . . . . . . . . . | 40 | 0 | 3.0 | 3.0 | 0 | 150 | 0 |
| (*Ortega* Dip) . . . . . . . . . | 45 | 1.0 | 4.0 | 3.0 | 0 | 190 | 0 |
| (*Santa Barbara*) . . . . . . . | 40 | <1.0 | 3.0 | 4.0 | 0 | 100 | 0 |
| (*Tofutti Sour Supreme*) . . | 85 | 1.0 | 9.0 | 5.0 | 0 | 160 | 0 |
| caliente (*Calavo*) . . . . . . . | 40 | <1.0 | 2.0 | 3.5 | 0 | 105 | 1.0 |
| garlic: | | | | | | | |
| mild (*Margaritaville* Island) . . . . . . . . . . | 45 | <1.0 | 3.0 | 4.0 | 0 | 105 | 2.0 |

| Food and Measure | cal. | prot. (gms) | carbo. (gms) | fat (gms) | chol. (mgs) | sod. (mgs) | fiber (gms) |
|---|---|---|---|---|---|---|---|
| **Guacamole, in garlic** *(cont.)* | | | | | | | |
| zesty (*Margaritaville* | | | | | | | |
| Island) .......... | 40 | <1.0 | 3.0 | 3.5 | 0 | 100 | 2.0 |
| hot/spicy (*Calavo*) ...... | 80 | <1.0 | 3.0 | 7.0 | 0 | 150 | 1.0 |
| mild (*Calavo*) .......... | 70 | <1.0 | 4.0 | 5.0 | 0 | 125 | 1.0 |
| pico de gallo (*Calavo*) ... | 40 | <1.0 | 2.0 | 3.5 | 0 | 100 | 1.0 |
| spicy (*Calavo*) ........ | 45 | <1.0 | 4.0 | 3.0 | 0 | 110 | 1.0 |
| Western (*Calavo*) ...... | 50 | 0 | 6.0 | 3.0 | 0 | 110 | 1.0 |
| **Guacamole seasoning**: | | | | | | | |
| (*Lawry's*), ½ tsp. ...... | 0 | 0 | 1.0 | 0 | 0 | 130 | 0 |
| (*McCormick*), 1 tsp. .... | 10 | 0 | 1.0 | 0 | 0 | 80 | 0 |
| (*Ortega*), ½ tsp. ....... | 5 | 0 | 1.0 | 0 | 0 | 80 | 0 |
| **Guava** (see also | | | | | | | |
| "Feijoas"), fresh: | | | | | | | |
| (*Frieda's*), 3-oz. pc. ..... | 45 | 1.0 | 10.0 | .5 | 0 | 0 | 5.0 |
| 1 medium, 4 oz. ....... | 45 | .7 | 10.7 | .5 | 0 | 2 | 4.9 |
| ½ cup .............. | 42 | .7 | 9.8 | .5 | 0 | 2 | 4.5 |
| strawberry, ½ cup ...... | 85 | .7 | 21.2 | .7 | 0 | 45 | 7.8 |
| **Guava, canned**, whole, | | | | | | | |
| in syrup (*Herdez*), | | | | | | | |
| 4 pcs., 4.5 oz. ....... | 190 | 0 | 32.0 | 0 | 0 | 10 | 5.0 |
| **Guava drink blend**, | | | | | | | |
| 8 fl. oz.: | | | | | | | |
| (*Nantucket Nectars*) .... | 130 | 0 | 33.0 | 0 | 0 | 25 | 0 |
| pineapple (*Welch's*) ..... | 140 | 0 | 35.0 | 0 | 0 | 5 | 0 |
| **Guava juice** (*Ceres*), | | | | | | | |
| 8 fl. oz. ............. | 120 | 0 | 30.0 | 0 | 0 | 10 | 2.0 |
| **Guava sauce**, ½ cup .... | 43 | .4 | 11.3 | .2 | 0 | 4 | 4.3 |
| **Guavadilla**, see | | | | | | | |
| "Passionfruit" | | | | | | | |
| **Guinea hen**, raw: | | | | | | | |
| meat w/skin, 4 oz. ...... | 179 | 26.5 | 0 | 7.3 | 84 | 86 | 0 |
| meat only, 4 oz. ........ | 125 | 23.4 | 0 | 2.8 | 71 | 78 | 0 |
| **Gumbo mix**: | | | | | | | |
| seasoning (*Zatarain's*), | | | | | | | |
| 1½ tbsp. ........... | 45 | 1.0 | 9.0 | 0 | 0 | 800 | <1.0 |
| w/rice (*Zatarain's*), | | | | | | | |
| 1 cup* ............ | 70 | 2.0 | 16.0 | 0 | 0 | 690 | <1.0 |

# H

| Food and Measure | cal. | prot. (gms) | carbo. (gms) | fat (gms) | chol. (mgs) | sod. (mgs) | fiber (gms) |
|---|---|---|---|---|---|---|---|
| **Habas**, see "Broad bean, mature" | | | | | | | |
| **Haddock**, meat only: | | | | | | | |
| raw, 4 oz. | 99 | 21.5 | 0 | .8 | 65 | 78 | 0 |
| baked or broiled, 4 oz. | 127 | 27.5 | 0 | 1.1 | 84 | 99 | 0 |
| smoked, 4 oz. | 132 | 28.6 | 0 | 1.1 | 87 | 865 | 0 |
| **Haddock, frozen**, fillet, breaded: | | | | | | | |
| (*Mrs. Paul's*), 4-oz. pc. | 230 | 16.0 | 17.0 | 10.0 | 40 | 210 | <1.0 |
| (*Van de Kamp's*), 2 pcs., 3.7 oz. | 240 | 12.0 | 22.0 | 11.0 | 30 | 610 | <1.0 |
| **Hake**, see "Whiting" | | | | | | | |
| **Halibut**, meat only: | | | | | | | |
| Atlantic/Pacific, 4 oz.: | | | | | | | |
| raw | 124 | 23.6 | 0 | 2.6 | 37 | 61 | 0 |
| baked or broiled | 159 | 30.3 | 0 | 3.3 | 46 | 78 | 0 |
| Greenland, 4 oz. | | | | | | | |
| raw | 211 | 16.3 | 0 | 15.7 | 52 | 91 | 0 |
| baked or broiled | 271 | 20.9 | 0 | 20.1 | 67 | 117 | 0 |
| **Halibut, frozen**, fillets, battered (*Van de Kamp's*), 3 pcs., 4 oz. | 280 | 14.0 | 24.0 | 13.0 | 15 | 660 | <1.0 |
| **Halvah**, 1 oz. | 150 | 4.0 | 13.0 | 9.0 | 0 | 30 | 0 |
| **Ham**, fresh, meat only, 4 oz., except as noted: | | | | | | | |
| whole leg, roasted: | | | | | | | |
| lean w/fat | 310 | 30.4 | 0 | 20.0 | 107 | 68 | 0 |
| lean w/fat, diced, 1 cup | 369 | 36.2 | 0 | 23.8 | 127 | 81 | 0 |
| lean only | 239 | 33.4 | 0 | 10.7 | 107 | 73 | 0 |
| lean only, diced, 1 cup | 285 | 39.7 | 0 | 12.7 | 127 | 86 | 0 |

| Food and Measure | cal. | prot. (gms) | carbo. (gms) | fat (gms) | chol. (mgs) | sod. (mgs) | fiber (gms) |
|---|---|---|---|---|---|---|---|
| **Ham** *(cont.)* | | | | | | | |
| rump half, roasted: | | | | | | | |
|   lean w/fat .......... | 286 | 32.7 | 0 | 16.2 | 109 | 70 | 0 |
|   lean only .......... | 235 | 35.1 | 0 | 9.2 | 109 | 74 | 0 |
| shank half, roasted: | | | | | | | |
|   lean w/fat .......... | 328 | 28.7 | 0 | 22.7 | 104 | 67 | 0 |
|   lean only .......... | 244 | 32.0 | 0 | 11.9 | 104 | 73 | 0 |
| **Ham, cured**: | | | | | | | |
| whole leg, lean w/fat: | | | | | | | |
|   unheated, 4 oz. ...... | 279 | 21.0 | .1 | 21.0 | 64 | 1456 | 0 |
|   unheated, chopped | | | | | | | |
|     or diced, 1 cup .... | 344 | 25.9 | .1 | 25.9 | 78 | 1798 | 0 |
|   roasted, 4 oz. ....... | 276 | 24.5 | 0 | 19.0 | 70 | 1346 | 0 |
|   roasted, chopped | | | | | | | |
|     or diced, 1 cup .... | 341 | 30.2 | 0 | 23.5 | 86 | 1661 | 0 |
| whole leg, lean only: | | | | | | | |
|   unheated, 4 oz. ...... | 167 | 25.3 | .1 | 6.5 | 59 | 1719 | 0 |
|   unheated, chopped | | | | | | | |
|     or diced, 1 cup .... | 206 | 31.3 | 0 | 8.0 | 73 | 2122 | 0 |
|   roasted, 4 oz. ....... | 178 | 28.4 | 0 | 6.2 | 62 | 1505 | 0 |
|   roasted, chopped | | | | | | | |
|     or diced, 1 cup .... | 219 | 35.1 | 0 | 7.7 | 77 | 1858 | 0 |
| boneless (11% fat): | | | | | | | |
|   unheated, 4 oz. ...... | 206 | 19.9 | 3.5 | 12.0 | 65 | 1493 | 0 |
|   roasted, 4 oz. ....... | 202 | 25.7 | 0 | 10.2 | 67 | 1701 | 0 |
|   roasted, chopped or | | | | | | | |
|     diced, 1 cup ...... | 249 | 31.7 | 0 | 12.6 | 83 | 2100 | 0 |
| boneless, extra lean | | | | | | | |
|   (5% fat): | | | | | | | |
|   unheated, 4 oz. ...... | 149 | 21.9 | 1.1 | 5.6 | 53 | 1620 | 0 |
|   roasted, 4 oz. ....... | 164 | 23.7 | 1.7 | 6.3 | 60 | 1364 | 0 |
|   roasted, chopped or | | | | | | | |
|     diced, 1 cup ...... | 203 | 29.3 | 2.1 | 7.7 | 74 | 1684 | 0 |
| **Ham, chilled/canned**, | | | | | | | |
|   3 oz., except as | | | | | | | |
|   noted: | | | | | | | |
| (*Black Bear* European | | | | | | | |
|   Classic) ............ | 110 | 14.0 | 1.0 | 5.0 | 40 | 720 | 0 |
| (*Black Label* Can) ...... | 100 | 14.0 | 1.0 | 4.0 | 40 | 1050 | 0 |
| (*Cure 81*) ............. | 100 | 15.0 | 0 | 4.5 | 45 | 890 | 0 |
| (*Curemaster*) .......... | 80 | 14.0 | 0 | 2.5 | 40 | 950 | 0 |
| (*Spiral Cure 81*) ....... | 130 | 16.0 | 1.0 | 7.0 | 50 | 820 | 0 |
| boneless: | | | | | | | |
|   (*Farmland* Bavarian) .. | 130 | 13.0 | 1.0 | 7.0 | 50 | 1070 | 0 |

| Food and Measure | cal. | prot. (gms) | carbo. (gms) | fat (gms) | chol. (mgs) | sod. (mgs) | fiber (gms) |
|---|---|---|---|---|---|---|---|
| (*Farmland* Classic Cure Half) | 90 | 15.0 | 2.0 | 2.0 | 50 | 930 | 0 |
| (*Farmland* Traditional) | 110 | 13.0 | 2.0 | 6.0 | 40 | 1110 | 0 |
| brown sugar (*Cure 81*) | 110 | 15.0 | 2.0 | 4.5 | 45 | 890 | 0 |
| chunk (*Hormel*), 2 oz. | 90 | 9.0 | 0 | 6.0 | 30 | 620 | 0 |
| cubed (*Farmland*), 2 oz. | 50 | 9.0 | 3.0 | .5 | 25 | 530 | 0 |
| diced (*Hormel Pillow Pack*), 2 oz. | 60 | 10.0 | 1.0 | 2.0 | 30 | 580 | 0 |
| honey (*Black Bear*) | 110 | 15.0 | 3.0 | 3.0 | 45 | 680 | 0 |
| maple brown sugar glazed (*Tyson*), 5 oz. | 180 | 21.0 | 14.0 | 4.5 | 60 | 730 | 0 |
| patty, 2-oz. pc.: | | | | | | | |
| (*Hormel*) | 180 | 7.0 | 1.0 | 16.0 | 40 | 620 | 0 |
| and cheese (*Hormel*) | 180 | 7.0 | 0 | 17.0 | 40 | 520 | 0 |
| roast (*Farmland* Steamship) | 140 | 16.0 | 2.0 | 7.0 | 60 | 850 | 0 |
| semi-boneless (*Black Bear*) | 130 | 14.0 | 1.0 | 8.0 | 45 | 720 | 0 |
| smoked, bone-in: | | | | | | | |
| (*Farmland* Picnic), 4.5 oz. | 250 | 17.2 | .9 | 20.2 | 74 | 1700 | 0 |
| (*Thumann's*) | 120 | 11.0 | 1.0 | 5.0 | 45 | 635 | 0 |
| hickory, spiral slice (*Farmland* All Natural) | 100 | 12.0 | 3.0 | 4.0 | 40 | 520 | 0 |
| hickory, spiral slice (*Farmland* Half) | 170 | 15.0 | 1.0 | 11.0 | 60 | 820 | 0 |
| hickory, spiral slice (*Farmland* Quarter) | 140 | 17.0 | 2.0 | 7.0 | 60 | 1040 | 0 |
| honey, spiral slice (*Farmland* Half) | 130 | 16.0 | 5.0 | 5.0 | 45 | 1000 | 0 |
| honey, spiral slice (*Farmland* Quarter) | 160 | 16.0 | 2.0 | 10.0 | 60 | 880 | 0 |
| smoked, boneless: | | | | | | | |
| (*Farmland*) | 90 | 13.0 | 1.0 | 4.0 | 40 | 1080 | 0 |
| (*Farmland* Center Cut) | 120 | 17.0 | 1.0 | 4.5 | 55 | 850 | 0 |
| (*Farmland* Maple River) | 120 | 13.0 | 1.0 | 8.0 | 45 | 1110 | 0 |
| (*Farmland* Old Fashioned Pit) | 130 | 13.0 | 1.0 | 8.0 | 75 | 680 | 0 |
| (*Farmland* Pit Style) | 110 | 13.0 | 2.0 | 5.0 | 45 | 1040 | 0 |
| (*Farmland* Traditional) | 110 | 13.0 | 2.0 | 6.0 | 40 | 1110 | 0 |
| brown sugar, hickory, spiral (*Farmland*) | 140 | 17.0 | 5.0 | 6.0 | 55 | 880 | 0 |

| Food and Measure | cal. | prot. (gms) | carbo. (gms) | fat (gms) | chol. (mgs) | sod. (mgs) | fiber (gms) |
|---|---|---|---|---|---|---|---|
| **Ham, smoked, boneless** *(cont.)* | | | | | | | |
| hickory (*Farmland* Original) ......... | 130 | 15.0 | 2.0 | 6.0 | 50 | 1020 | 0 |
| hickory (*Farmland* Original Sliced) ... | 130 | 14.0 | 2.0 | 7.0 | 50 | 830 | 0 |
| honey, hickory (*Farmland* Original) | 140 | 15.0 | 5.0 | 6.0 | 50 | 1020 | 0 |
| peppered, hickory (*Farmland* Original) | 130 | 15.0 | 2.0 | 6.0 | 50 | 1020 | 0 |
| honey, spiral sliced (*Farmland* Natural Juice) ........... | 115 | 15.0 | 4.0 | 2.0 | 50 | 850 | 0 |
| spiral sliced (*Black Bear*) ........... | 130 | 14.0 | 1.0 | 8.0 | 45 | 720 | 0 |
| steak, boneless: | | | | | | | |
| (*Black Bear* Kitchen Classics) ........ | 90 | 14.0 | 2.0 | 3.0 | 40 | 690 | 0 |
| (*Farmland* Special Select Thick), 4 oz. . | 120 | 19.0 | 3.0 | 3.5 | 60 | 1480 | 0 |
| (*Farmland* Special Select Traditional), 2.3-oz. slice ...... | 70 | 11.0 | 2.0 | 2.0 | 35 | 840 | 0 |
| **Ham and cheese sandwich**, frozen (*Oscar Mayer Deli Creations*), 1 pc.: | | | | | | | |
| cheddar .............. | 460 | 29.0 | 51.0 | 16.0 | 60 | 1410 | 3.0 |
| honey, and Swiss ...... | 440 | 28.0 | 50.0 | 15.0 | 60 | 1410 | 3.0 |
| provolone/focaccia ..... | 370 | 24.0 | 45.0 | 11.0 | 40 | 1300 | 2.0 |
| **Ham and cheese snack** (*Michelina's Lean Gourmet*), 4 pcs., 3.1 oz. ....... | 230 | 10.0 | 32.0 | 7.0 | 20 | 640 | 1.0 |
| **Ham glaze**: | | | | | | | |
| (*Ah-So*), 2 tbsp. ....... | 50 | 0 | 13.0 | 0 | 0 | 15 | 0 |
| (*Crosse & Blackwell*), 1 tbsp. ............. | 30 | 0 | 7.0 | 0 | 0 | 25 | 0 |
| (*Saucy Susan*), 2 tbsp. .. | 80 | 0 | 19.0 | 0 | 0 | 260 | 1.0 |
| brown sugar/spice (*Boar's Head*), 2 tbsp. . | 120 | 0 | 30.0 | 0 | 0 | 95 | 0 |
| **Ham lunch meat** (see also "Capocola/Coppa" and "Proscuitto"), 2 oz., except as noted: | | | | | | | |

| Food and Measure | cal. | prot. (gms) | carbo. (gms) | fat (gms) | chol. (mgs) | sod. (mgs) | fiber (gms) |
|---|---|---|---|---|---|---|---|
| (*Boar's Head* Deluxe) ... | 60 | 9.0 | 2.0 | 1.0 | 25 | 590 | 0 |
| (*Boar's Head* Lower | | | | | | | |
| Sodium) ........... | 60 | 10.0 | 2.0 | 1.0 | 25 | 460 | 0 |
| (*Di Lusso* Deluxe Deli) .. | 50 | 9.0 | 2.0 | 1.0 | 25 | 670 | 0 |
| baked (*Oscar Mayer* | | | | | | | |
| 96% Fat Free), 2.2 oz. . | 60 | 10.0 | 1.0 | 2.0 | 30 | 760 | 0 |
| Black Forest: | | | | | | | |
| (*Applegate Farms*) ... | 50 | 10.0 | 0 | 1.5 | 35 | 480 | 0 |
| (*Applegate Farms* | | | | | | | |
| Deli Counter) ..... | 60 | 9.0 | 0 | 2.5 | 30 | 320 | 0 |
| (*Boar's Head*) ....... | 60 | 10.0 | 2.0 | 1.0 | 30 | 580 | 0 |
| (*Di Lusso*) .......... | 60 | 10.0 | 1.0 | 2.0 | 30 | 580 | 0 |
| (*Oscar Mayer* Deli | | | | | | | |
| Fresh), 1.8 oz. ..... | 45 | 9.0 | 0 | 1.0 | 25 | 640 | 0 |
| (*Thumann's*) ........ | 60 | 10.0 | <1.0 | 1.0 | 21 | 510 | 0 |
| boiled (*Oscar Mayer*), | | | | | | | |
| 2.2 oz. ........... | 60 | 10.0 | 1.0 | 2.0 | 30 | 820 | 0 |
| brown sugar: | | | | | | | |
| (*Di Lusso*) .......... | 80 | 10.0 | 5.0 | 2.0 | 25 | 560 | 0 |
| (*Hormel Natural | | | | | | | |
| Choice*) .......... | 70 | 10.0 | 3.0 | 1.5 | 30 | 570 | 0 |
| (*Oscar Mayer* Deli | | | | | | | |
| Fresh Thin Sliced) . | 70 | 10.0 | 4.0 | 1.0 | 25 | 830 | 0 |
| cured (*Thumann's*) ... | 60 | 10.0 | <1.0 | 1.0 | 21 | 510 | 0 |
| chopped: | | | | | | | |
| (*Black Bear*) ........ | 100 | 9.0 | 1.0 | 6.0 | 35 | 530 | 0 |
| (*Hormel Black Label*) . | 140 | 7.0 | 3.0 | 11.0 | 30 | 690 | 0 |
| (*Oscar Mayer*), 1 oz. .. | 50 | 4.0 | 2.0 | 2.5 | 15 | 290 | 0 |
| cooked: | | | | | | | |
| (*Applegate Farms*) ... | 60 | 11.0 | 0 | 1.5 | 35 | 400 | 0 |
| (*Applegate Farms* | | | | | | | |
| Deli Counter) ..... | 60 | 11.0 | 0 | 1.5 | 35 | 480 | 0 |
| (*Black Bear*) ........ | 60 | 9.0 | 2.0 | 1.0 | 30 | 600 | 0 |
| (*Hormel Natural | | | | | | | |
| Choice*) .......... | 60 | 10.0 | 1.0 | 1.5 | 30 | 520 | 0 |
| (*Oscar Mayer* Deli | | | | | | | |
| Fresh), 1 oz. ...... | 30 | 5.0 | 1.0 | 1.0 | 15 | 240 | 0 |
| (*Thumann's* Deluxe) .. | 60 | 10.0 | <1.0 | 1.0 | 21 | 510 | 0 |
| (*Thumann's* Deluxe | | | | | | | |
| Lower Sodium) ... | 60 | 10.0 | <1.0 | 1.0 | 21 | 400 | 0 |
| fresh ham, see "Pork | | | | | | | |
| lunch meat" | | | | | | | |
| honey/honey cured: | | | | | | | |
| (*Applegate Farms*) ... | 70 | 10.0 | 3.0 | 1.5 | 30 | 450 | 0 |

| Food and Measure | cal. | prot. (gms) | carbo. (gms) | fat (gms) | chol. (mgs) | sod. (mgs) | fiber (gms) |
|---|---|---|---|---|---|---|---|
| **Ham lunch meat, honey/honey cured** *(cont.)* | | | | | | | |
| (*Black Bear*) ........ | 70 | 10.0 | 4.0 | 1.5 | 30 | 540 | 0 |
| (*Hormel Natural Choice*) .......... | 70 | 10.0 | 3.0 | 1.5 | 30 | 520 | 0 |
| (*Oscar Mayer* 96% Fat Free) ......... | 60 | 10.0 | 2.0 | 2.0 | 30 | 460 | 0 |
| (*Oscar Mayer* Deli Fresh), 1.8 oz. .... | 50 | 9.0 | 2.0 | 1.0 | 25 | 650 | 0 |
| (*Oscar Mayer* Thin Sliced) .......... | 60 | 10.0 | 2.0 | 1.0 | 30 | 730 | 0 |
| baked (*Thumann's*) ... | 100 | 10.0 | <1.0 | 2.0 | 21 | 510 | 0 |
| chopped (*Oscar Mayer*), 1 oz. ............. | 60 | 4.0 | 4.0 | 3.5 | 15 | 320 | 0 |
| smoked (*Di Lusso*) ... | 70 | 10.0 | 3.0 | 2.0 | 25 | 600 | 0 |
| honey maple (*Di Lusso*) . | 60 | 10.0 | 2.0 | 2.0 | 30 | 570 | 0 |
| hot (*Thumann's* Deluxe) . | 60 | 10.0 | <1.0 | 1.0 | 21 | 510 | 0 |
| maple/maple glaze: | | | | | | | |
| (*Applegate Farms* Deli Counter) ..... | 60 | 10.0 | 2.0 | 1.5 | 35 | 520 | 0 |
| (*Boar's Head Honey Coat*) ........... | 60 | 10.0 | 3.0 | 1.0 | 20 | 570 | 0 |
| smoked (*Thumann's*) . | 60 | 14.0 | <1.0 | 1.0 | 21 | 510 | 0 |
| pepper (*Boar's Head*) ... | 60 | 10.0 | 2.0 | 1.0 | 20 | 560 | 0 |
| pesto Parmesan (*Boar's Head*) ............. | 70 | 12.0 | 1.0 | 2.5 | 30 | 550 | 0 |
| prosciuttini: | | | | | | | |
| (*Black Bear*) ........ | 50 | 9.0 | 1.0 | 1.5 | 25 | 590 | 0 |
| (*Thumann's*) ........ | 60 | 10.0 | <1.0 | 1.0 | 21 | 510 | 0 |
| rosemary: | | | | | | | |
| (*Black Bear*) ........ | 70 | 11.0 | 1.0 | 2.5 | 30 | 520 | 0 |
| sun-dried tomato (*Boar's Head*) ..... | 70 | 10.0 | 2.0 | 2.5 | 10 | 590 | 0 |
| smoked: | | | | | | | |
| (*Boar's Head Sweet Slice*), 3 oz. ...... | 100 | 15.0 | 1.0 | 3.5 | 30 | 780 | 0 |
| (*Hormel Natural Choice*) .......... | 60 | 10.0 | 1.0 | 1.5 | 30 | 520 | 0 |
| (*Oscar Mayer* 96% Fat Free), 2.2 oz. .. | 70 | 11.0 | 0 | 2.0 | 30 | 820 | 0 |
| (*Oscar Mayer* 98% Fat Free), 2.2 oz. .. | 50 | 10.0 | 0 | 1.0 | 15 | 730 | 0 |
| (*Oscar Mayer* Deli Fresh Thin Sliced) . | 50 | 10.0 | 0 | 1.5 | 25 | 720 | 0 |

| Food and Measure | cal. | prot. (gms) | carbo. (gms) | fat (gms) | chol. (mgs) | sod. (mgs) | fiber (gms) |
|---|---|---|---|---|---|---|---|
| (*Thumann's* Chef's Slice/Deluxe Flat) .. | 60 | 10.0 | 0 | 1.0 | 21 | 510 | 0 |
| double (*Di Lusso*) .... | 70 | 11.0 | 1.0 | 2.0 | 30 | 550 | 0 |
| natural (*Oscar Mayer*), ¼ of 8-oz. pkg. ........ | 60 | 12.0 | 1.0 | 1.0 | 35 | 490 | 0 |
| uncured (*Boar's Head* All Natural) ....... | 60 | 12.0 | <1.0 | 1.5 | 35 | 320 | 0 |
| spiced, see "Lunch meat" | | | | | | | |
| tavern: | | | | | | | |
| (*Black Bear*) ........ | 60 | 10.0 | 1.0 | 1.5 | 30 | 590 | 0 |
| (*Boar's Head*) ....... | 60 | 10.0 | 2.0 | 1.0 | 30 | 580 | 0 |
| honey (*Black Bear*) ... | 60 | 10.0 | 1.0 | 1.5 | 30 | 620 | 0 |
| tomato basil (*Black Bear*) .............. | 70 | 11.0 | 1.0 | 2.5 | 30 | 520 | 0 |
| uncured: | | | | | | | |
| (*Applegate Farms* Organic) ......... | 50 | 10.0 | 0 | 1.5 | 35 | 530 | 0 |
| (*Boar's Head*) ....... | 70 | 12.0 | 1.0 | 1.0 | 35 | 340 | 0 |
| Virginia: | | | | | | | |
| (*Applegate Farms* Deli Counter) ..... | 50 | 9.0 | 1.0 | 1.5 | 30 | 480 | 0 |
| (*Black Bear*) ........ | 60 | 9.0 | 3.0 | 1.0 | 25 | 560 | 0 |
| (*Black Bear* Lite) ..... | 60 | 9.0 | 3.0 | 1.0 | 25 | 460 | 0 |
| (*Oscar Mayer* Shaved), ⅛ of 9-oz. pkg. .... | 50 | 9.0 | 1.0 | 1.5 | 25 | 570 | 0 |
| (*Thumann's*) ......... | 60 | 10.0 | <1.0 | 1.0 | 21 | 510 | 0 |
| smoked (*Boar's Head*) | 60 | 9.0 | 2.0 | 1.0 | 25 | 590 | 0 |
| sugar glaze (*Boar's Head*) ............ | 60 | 9.0 | 3.0 | 1.0 | 25 | 590 | 0 |
| **"Ham" lunch meat, vegetarian** (*Yves*), 4 slices, 2.2 oz. ...... | 100 | 15.0 | 5.0 | 2.0 | 0 | 480 | 0 |
| **Ham patties**, see "Ham, chilled/canned" | | | | | | | |
| **Ham spread**, deviled: | | | | | | | |
| (*Hormel Cure 81*), 4 tbsp., 2 oz. ........ | 150 | 9.0 | 2.0 | 12.0 | 40 | 430 | 0 |
| (*Underwood*), ¼ cup .... | 180 | 8.0 | 1.0 | 15.0 | 35 | 480 | 0 |
| **Hamburger**, see "Beef" | | | | | | | |
| **"Hamburger," vegetarian**, see "Burger, vegetarian" | | | | | | | |

| Food and Measure | cal. | prot. (gms) | carbo. (gms) | fat (gms) | chol. (mgs) | sod. (mgs) | fiber (gms) |
|---|---|---|---|---|---|---|---|
| **Hamburger entree** | | | | | | | |
| **mix**, 1 cup*: | | | | | | | |
| (*Annie's* Organic | | | | | | | |
| Skillet Meal): | | | | | | | |
| cheeseburger, macaroni | 400 | 23.0 | 26.0 | 22.5 | 75 | 600 | 1.0 |
| lasagna, cheesy ..... | 440 | 25.0 | 32.0 | 24.0 | 80 | 830 | 1.0 |
| Stroganoff ......... | 360 | 18.0 | 32.0 | 18.5 | 60 | 760 | 1.0 |
| (*Hamburger Helper*): | | | | | | | |
| cheeseburger: | | | | | | | |
| macaroni ........ | 310 | 22.0 | 27.0 | 12.0 | 60 | 910 | <1.0 |
| macaroni, double .. | 320 | 22.0 | 29.0 | 13.0 | 60 | 730 | 0 |
| hash browns, cheesy . | 400 | 20.0 | 38.0 | 19.0 | 55 | 990 | 2.0 |
| jambalaya, cheesy ... | 320 | 22.0 | 29.0 | 13.0 | 55 | 670 | 1.0 |
| lasagna ............ | 280 | 19.0 | 27.0 | 11.0 | 55 | 860 | <1.0 |
| nacho, cheesy ....... | 330 | 21.0 | 35.0 | 12.0 | 55 | 720 | <1.0 |
| pasta, beef ......... | 280 | 21.0 | 23.0 | 11.0 | 55 | 760 | 1.0 |
| penne, tomato basil .. | 300 | 20.0 | 31.0 | 11.0 | 55 | 710 | 1.0 |
| Philly cheesesteak ... | 320 | 22.0 | 28.0 | 13.0 | 55 | 750 | 1.0 |
| potato, baked, cheesy . | 310 | 20.0 | 31.0 | 12.0 | 60 | 830 | 1.0 |
| potatoes, Stroganoff .. | 290 | 21.0 | 26.0 | 12.0 | 60 | 790 | 1.0 |
| Salisbury .......... | 280 | 20.0 | 25.0 | 11.0 | 55 | 830 | <1.0 |
| spaghetti ........... | 290 | 20.0 | 27.0 | 11.0 | 55 | 810 | 1.0 |
| taco, crunchy ....... | 340 | 20.0 | 33.0 | 14.0 | 55 | 870 | 1.0 |
| (*Helper Complete Meals*): | | | | | | | |
| Stroganoff ......... | 230 | 9.0 | 32.0 | 8.0 | 25 | 800 | 2.0 |
| taco, cheesy ........ | 230 | 8.0 | 37.0 | 5.0 | 20 | 1080 | 1.0 |
| **Hard sauce** (*Crosse* | | | | | | | |
| *& Blackwell*), | | | | | | | |
| 2 tbsp. ............ | 180 | 0 | 25.0 | 8.0 | 20 | 70 | 0 |
| *Hardee's*, 1 serving: | | | | | | | |
| breakfast: | | | | | | | |
| burrito, loaded ...... | 760 | 39.0 | 39.0 | 49.0 | 445 | 1700 | 1.0 |
| *Frisco Sandwich* ..... | 420 | 25.0 | 39.0 | 16.0 | 215 | 1250 | 2.0 |
| *Hardee* platter ....... | 860 | 19.0 | 9.0 | 55.0 | 200 | 1860 | 3.0 |
| *Hash Rounds* medium | 390 | 3.0 | 36.0 | 26.0 | 0 | 490 | 4.0 |
| grits ............... | 110 | 2.0 | 16.0 | 5.0 | 0 | 490 | 1.0 |
| *Low Carb Breakfast* | | | | | | | |
| *Bowl* ........... | 620 | 36.0 | 6.0 | 50.0 | 325 | 1380 | 2.0 |
| pancakes, plain, 3 .... | 300 | 8.0 | 55.0 | 5.0 | 25 | 830 | 2.0 |
| *Sunrise Croissant*, | | | | | | | |
| w/ham .......... | 400 | 21.0 | 27.0 | 23.0 | 225 | 1070 | 1.0 |
| Texas toast sandwich, | | | | | | | |
| w/sausage ....... | 480 | 20.0 | 32.0 | 30.0 | 245 | 960 | 2.0 |

| Food and Measure | cal. | prot. (gms) | carbo. (gms) | fat (gms) | chol. (mgs) | sod. (mgs) | fiber (gms) |
|---|---|---|---|---|---|---|---|
| breakfast biscuit: | | | | | | | |
| *Made From Scratch* | | | | | | | |
| Biscuit . . . . . . . . . . | 370 | 5.0 | 35.0 | 23.0 | 0 | 890 | 0 |
| bacon/egg/cheese . . . . | 530 | 15.0 | 36.0 | 36.0 | 195 | 1390 | 0 |
| *Biscuit 'n' Gravy* . . . . . | 530 | 9.0 | 48.0 | 33.0 | 10 | 1510 | 1.0 |
| chicken fillet . . . . . . . . | 620 | 24.0 | 47.0 | 37.0 | 50 | 1560 | 1.0 |
| *Cinnamon 'n' Raisin* . . | 300 | 3.0 | 40.0 | 15.0 | 0 | 680 | 1.0 |
| ham, country . . . . . . . | 440 | 14.0 | 36.0 | 26.0 | 35 | 1710 | 0 |
| ham/egg/cheese . . . . . | 540 | 23.0 | 36.0 | 33.0 | 220 | 1830 | 0 |
| jelly biscuit . . . . . . . . . | 520 | 5.0 | 44.0 | 34.0 | 0 | 1020 | 0 |
| *Monster Biscuit* . . . . . | 770 | 29.0 | 37.0 | 55.0 | 250 | 2310 | 0 |
| omelet, loaded . . . . . . | 610 | 20.0 | 36.0 | 42.0 | 220 | 1540 | 0 |
| pork chop, breaded . . . | 640 | 25.0 | 46.0 | 39.0 | 35 | 1270 | 1.0 |
| pork chop, gravy . . . . . | 660 | 26.0 | 48.0 | 42.0 | 35 | 1400 | 1.0 |
| sausage . . . . . . . . . . | 530 | 11.0 | 36.0 | 38.0 | 30 | 1240 | 0 |
| sausage, smoked . . . . | 620 | 14.0 | 37.0 | 46.0 | 40 | 1680 | 0 |
| w/egg/cheese . . . . . | 750 | 23.0 | 38.0 | 56.0 | 255 | 1960 | 0 |
| sausage/egg . . . . . . . | 590 | 16.0 | 36.0 | 42.0 | 210 | 1300 | 0 |
| steak, country . . . . . . . | 590 | 13.0 | 43.0 | 40.0 | 25 | 1290 | 1.0 |
| burgers: | | | | | | | |
| *Big Shef*/regular . . . . . | 660 | 26.0 | 36.0 | 46.0 | 90 | 930 | 1.0 |
| cheeseburger . . . . . . . | 350 | 16.0 | 32.0 | 19.0 | 45 | 730 | 1.0 |
| cheeseburger, double . | 530 | 27.0 | 34.0 | 32.0 | 90 | 1070 | 1.0 |
| *Thickburger*, ⅓ lb.: | | | | | | | |
| original . . . . . . . . . . . | 860 | 35.0 | 52.0 | 58.0 | 105 | 1630 | 4.0 |
| bacon/cheese . . . . . . | 850 | 38.0 | 49.0 | 57.0 | 105 | 1650 | 3.0 |
| cheeseburger . . . . . . . | 620 | 35.0 | 51.0 | 33.0 | 80 | 1580 | 3.0 |
| *Frisco* . . . . . . . . . . . . | 930 | 44.0 | 42.0 | 64.0 | 125 | 1840 | 2.0 |
| low carb . . . . . . . . . . | 420 | 30.0 | 5.0 | 32.0 | 115 | 1010 | 2.0 |
| mushroom/Swiss . . . . | 650 | 39.0 | 47.0 | 36.0 | 90 | 1620 | 3.0 |
| *Thickburger*, ⅔ lb.: | | | | | | | |
| double . . . . . . . . . . . | 1150 | 62.0 | 53.0 | 76.0 | 180 | 2410 | 4.0 |
| double bacon/cheese . | 1200 | 65.0 | 50.0 | 84.0 | 185 | 2450 | 3.0 |
| *Monster* . . . . . . . . . . | 1320 | 70.0 | 46.0 | 95.0 | 210 | 3020 | 2.0 |
| *Little Thickburger* . . . . . | 570 | 24.0 | 35.0 | 39.0 | 80 | 1140 | 3.0 |
| *Six Dollar Thickburger* . . | 930 | 46.0 | 57.0 | 59.0 | 130 | 1960 | 4.0 |
| sandwiches: | | | | | | | |
| *Big Hot Ham 'n'* | | | | | | | |
| *Cheese* . . . . . . . . . . | 460 | 36.0 | 40.0 | 20.0 | 75 | 2040 | 2.0 |
| *Big Roast Beef* . . . . . . | 400 | 25.0 | 28.0 | 21.0 | 60 | 1180 | 1.0 |
| chicken, charbroiled: | | | | | | | |
| BBQ . . . . . . . . . . . | 400 | 27.0 | 62.0 | 6.0 | 45 | 1370 | 5.0 |
| club . . . . . . . . . . . . | 630 | 32.0 | 54.0 | 32.0 | 80 | 1730 | 4.0 |
| club, low carb . . . . | 360 | 24.0 | 14.0 | 23.0 | 75 | 1290 | 1.0 |

| Food and Measure | cal. | prot. (gms) | carbo. (gms) | fat (gms) | chol. (mgs) | sod. (mgs) | fiber (gms) |
|---|---|---|---|---|---|---|---|
| **Hardee's, sandwiches** *(cont.)* | | | | | | | |
| chicken fillet ........ | 710 | 33.0 | 62.0 | 30.0 | 55 | 1610 | 5.0 |
| chili dog, jumbo ..... | 400 | 16.0 | 25.0 | 26.0 | 55 | 1170 | 1.0 |
| fish supreme ........ | 630 | 22.0 | 51.0 | 38.0 | 40 | 1310 | 3.0 |
| roast beef .......... | 310 | 17.0 | 28.0 | 15.0 | 40 | 840 | 1.0 |
| chicken *Tenders*: | | | | | | | |
| 3 pc. .............. | 260 | 25.0 | 13.0 | 13.0 | 70 | 770 | 2.0 |
| 5 pc. .............. | 440 | 41.0 | 21.0 | 21.0 | 115 | 1290 | 3.0 |
| *Tender* wrappers: | | | | | | | |
| BBQ .............. | 250 | 14.0 | 24.0 | 12.0 | 35 | 660 | 1.0 |
| honey mustard ...... | 280 | 14.0 | 22.0 | 16.0 | 40 | 640 | 1.0 |
| ranch hand ........ | 270 | 14.0 | 21.0 | 15.0 | 40 | 660 | 1.0 |
| fish 'n' chips basket .... | 1150 | 28.0 | 80.0 | 80.0 | 65 | 2320 | 4.0 |
| sauces: | | | | | | | |
| BBQ .............. | 60 | 0 | 17.0 | 0 | 0 | 270 | 0 |
| Buffalo, creamy ..... | 120 | 1.0 | 3.0 | 13.0 | 10 | 330 | 1.0 |
| buttermilk ranch ..... | 140 | 0 | 3.0 | 14.0 | 15 | 300 | 0 |
| honey mustard ...... | 180 | 0 | 6.0 | 18.0 | 10 | 190 | 0 |
| sides: | | | | | | | |
| fries, medium ....... | 430 | 5.0 | 60.0 | 19.0 | 5 | 960 | 4.0 |
| onion rings ......... | 410 | 3.0 | 45.0 | 24.0 | 0 | 470 | 3.0 |
| side salad .......... | 120 | 7.0 | 7.0 | 7.0 | 20 | 160 | 2.0 |
| *Hand-Scooped Malt*: | | | | | | | |
| chocolate .......... | 780 | 17.0 | 97.0 | 35.0 | 105 | 355 | 2.0 |
| strawberry ......... | 775 | 17.0 | 98.0 | 35.0 | 105 | 310 | 1.0 |
| vanilla ............ | 710 | 17.0 | 97.0 | 35.0 | 105 | 320 | 1.0 |
| *Hand-Scooped Shake*: | | | | | | | |
| chocolate .......... | 700 | 15.0 | 85.0 | 34.0 | 100 | 290 | 1.0 |
| strawberry ......... | 700 | 14.0 | 86.0 | 33.0 | 100 | 240 | 0 |
| vanilla ............ | 710 | 14.0 | 87.0 | 33.0 | 100 | 240 | 0 |
| apple turnover ......... | 270 | 3.0 | 35.0 | 13.0 | 5 | 260 | 1.0 |
| **Hazelnut,** shelled: | | | | | | | |
| all styles (*Diamond*), | | | | | | | |
| ¼ cup, 1.1 oz. ....... | 190 | 4.0 | 5.0 | 18.0 | 0 | 0 | 3.0 |
| dried, 1 oz. .......... | 179 | 3.7 | 4.4 | 17.8 | 0 | 1 | 1.7 |
| dried, chopped, 1 cup ... | 727 | 15.0 | 17.6 | 72.0 | 0 | 3 | 7.0 |
| dry-roasted, salted, 1 oz. | 188 | 2.8 | 5.1 | 18.8 | 0 | 221 | <2.0 |
| oil-roasted, salted, 1 oz. . | 187 | 4.1 | 5.4 | 18.1 | 0 | 223 | 1.8 |
| chopped (*Planters*), | | | | | | | |
| 2-oz. pkg. .......... | 350 | 7.0 | 9.0 | 35.0 | 0 | 0 | 5.0 |
| **Hazelnut beverage** | | | | | | | |
| (*Pacific*), 8 fl. oz.: | | | | | | | |
| chocolate ........... | 120 | 2.0 | 19.0 | 5.0 | 0 | 140 | 1.0 |
| original ............. | 110 | 2.0 | 18.0 | 3.5 | 0 | 120 | 1.0 |

| Food and Measure | cal. | prot. (gms) | carbo. (gms) | fat (gms) | chol. (mgs) | sod. (mgs) | fiber (gms) |
|---|---|---|---|---|---|---|---|
| **Hazelnut butter**, 1 oz. or 2 tbsp.: | | | | | | | |
| (*Kettle Roaster Fresh*) ... | 180 | 4.0 | 5.0 | 17.0 | 0 | 0 | 3.0 |
| (*Nutella*) ............. | 200 | 3.0 | 22.0 | 11.0 | 0 | 15 | 1.0 |
| **Hazelnut meal/flour** (*Bob's Red Mill*), ¼ cup ............. | 180 | 4.0 | 5.0 | 17.0 | 0 | 0 | 3.0 |
| **Head cheese**: | | | | | | | |
| (*Boar's Head*), 2 oz. ...... | 90 | 10.0 | 1.0 | 5.0 | 65 | 420 | 0 |
| (*Thumann's*), 2 oz. ..... | 100 | 12.0 | <1.0 | 2.0 | 21 | 460 | 0 |
| pork, 2 oz. ............ | 88 | 7.7 | 0 | 6.1 | 39 | 465 | 0 |
| **Heart**, braised or simmered, 4 oz.: | | | | | | | |
| beef ................. | 199 | 32.6 | .5 | 6.4 | 219 | 71 | 0 |
| chicken, broiler-fryer .... | 210 | 30.0 | .1 | 9.0 | 274 | 54 | 0 |
| lamb ................ | 210 | 28.3 | 2.2 | 9.0 | 282 | 71 | 0 |
| pork ................ | 168 | 26.8 | .5 | 5.7 | 251 | 40 | 0 |
| turkey .............. | 201 | 30.3 | 2.3 | 6.9 | 256 | 62 | 0 |
| veal ................ | 211 | 33.0 | .1 | 7.7 | 200 | 66 | 0 |
| **Hemp beverage**, 8 fl. oz.: | | | | | | | |
| (*Hemp Dream*): | | | | | | | |
| original ............ | 100 | 4.0 | 8.0 | 6.0 | 0 | 5 | <1.0 |
| vanilla ............ | 110 | 4.0 | 11.0 | 6.0 | 0 | 5 | <1.0 |
| (*Pacific* Hemp Milk): | | | | | | | |
| original ............ | 140 | 4.0 | 20.0 | 5.0 | 0 | 130 | 1.0 |
| chocolate ......... | 190 | 3.0 | 35.0 | 5.0 | 0 | 150 | 2.0 |
| vanilla ............ | 160 | 4.0 | 24.0 | 5.0 | 0 | 135 | 1.0 |
| **Herb gravy mix** (*McCormick*), 2 tsp. .. | 30 | 1.0 | 4.0 | 1.0 | 0 | 250 | 0 |
| **Herbs**, see specific listings | | | | | | | |
| **Herbs, mixed**, ¼ tsp.: | | | | | | | |
| Italian (*McCormick* Grinder) .......... | 0 | 0 | 0 | 0 | 0 | 15 | 0 |
| Mediterranean (*McCormick Perfect Pinch*) ....... | 0 | 0 | 0 | 0 | 0 | 65 | 0 |
| Parmesan (*McCormick Perfect Pinch*) ....... | 0 | 0 | 0 | 0 | 0 | 25 | 0 |
| **Herring**, fresh: | | | | | | | |
| Atlantic, meat only: | | | | | | | |
| raw, 4 oz. .......... | 180 | 20.4 | 0 | 10.3 | 68 | 102 | 0 |
| baked or broiled, 4 oz. | 230 | 26.1 | 0 | 13.1 | 87 | 130 | 0 |

| Food and Measure | cal. | prot. (gms) | carbo. (gms) | fat (gms) | chol. (mgs) | sod. (mgs) | fiber (gms) |
|---|---|---|---|---|---|---|---|
| **Herring, fresh, Atlantic** *(cont.)* | | | | | | | |
| kippered, 4 oz. ...... | 246 | 27.9 | 0 | 14.0 | 93 | 1041 | 0 |
| pickled, 4 oz. ....... | 297 | 16.1 | 10.9 | 20.4 | 15 | 987 | 0 |
| lake, see "Cisco" | | | | | | | |
| Pacific, meat only: | | | | | | | |
| raw, 4 oz. .......... | 224 | 18.6 | 0 | 15.8 | 87 | 84 | 0 |
| baked or broiled, 4 oz. | 284 | 23.8 | 0 | 20.2 | 112 | 108 | 0 |
| **Herring, canned** (see also "Herring, pickled" and "Sardine"): | | | | | | | |
| horseradish sauce (*Roland*), ¼ cup ..... | 120 | 7.0 | 2.0 | 9.0 | 45 | 200 | 0 |
| hot sauce (*Brunswick* Snacks Louisiana), 3.5 oz. ........... | 140 | 16.0 | 2.0 | 8.0 | 70 | 450 | 0 |
| kippered snack, smoked: | | | | | | | |
| (*Bar Harbor*), ¼ cup .. | 110 | 11.0 | 0 | 8.0 | 35 | 230 | 0 |
| (*Brunswick*), 3 oz. ... | 130 | 16.0 | 0 | 8.0 | 65 | 460 | 0 |
| (*Crown* Prince), 3.25 oz. ........ | 190 | 19.0 | 0 | 13.0 | 60 | 390 | 0 |
| (*Roland*), 3.25 oz. .... | 190 | 19.0 | 0 | 13.0 | 60 | 390 | 0 |
| lemon, cracked pepper (*Brunswick* Snacks), 3 oz. .............. | 130 | 15.0 | 0 | 8.0 | 60 | 250 | 0 |
| mushroom sauce (*Roland*), ¼ cup ..... | 80 | 8.0 | 2.0 | 4.0 | 45 | 240 | 0 |
| paprika sauce (*Roland*), ¼ cup ..... | 100 | 7.0 | 3.0 | 6.0 | 45 | 250 | 0 |
| smoked: | | | | | | | |
| (*Roland*), ⅓ cup ..... | 110 | 11.0 | 0 | 8.0 | 35 | 230 | 0 |
| golden (*Brunswick* Snacks 3.25 oz.), 2.8 oz. .......... | 130 | 16.0 | 0 | 8.0 | 60 | 240 | 0 |
| teriyaki (*Brunswick* Snacks), 3.5 oz. ..... | 160 | 16.0 | 5.0 | 8.0 | 70 | 800 | 0 |
| tomato sauce: | | | | | | | |
| (*Roland*), ¼ cup ..... | 100 | 7.0 | 2.0 | 7.0 | 15 | 250 | 0 |
| basil (*Brunswick* Snacks), 3.5 oz. ... | 140 | 16.0 | 2.0 | 8.0 | 70 | 420 | 0 |
| wine sauce (*Roland*), ¼ cup .............. | 100 | 8.0 | 2.0 | 7.0 | 45 | 230 | 0 |
| **Herring, kippered,** see "Herring" and "Herring, canned" | | | | | | | |

| Food and Measure | cal. | prot. (gms) | carbo. (gms) | fat (gms) | chol. (mgs) | sod. (mgs) | fiber (gms) |
|---|---|---|---|---|---|---|---|
| **Herring, pickled**, in jars, ¼ cup, except as noted: | | | | | | | |
| (*Vita* Homestyle) | 100 | 7.0 | 8.0 | 4.5 | 40 | 670 | 0 |
| (*Vita* Tastee Bits) | 100 | 7.0 | 10.0 | 3.5 | 25 | 460 | 0 |
| (*Vita* Lunch) | 110 | 7.0 | 8.0 | 4.5 | 40 | 670 | 0 |
| roll mops (*Vita*) | 110 | 7.0 | 12.0 | 4.0 | 40 | 470 | 0 |
| in sour cream: | | | | | | | |
| (*Elf*) | 100 | 6.0 | 6.0 | 6.0 | 20 | 620 | 0 |
| (*Nathan's* Snacks) | 120 | 6.0 | 11.0 | 6.0 | 40 | 680 | 0 |
| (*Vita*) | 110 | 7.0 | 5.0 | 7.0 | 35 | 600 | 0 |
| in wine sauce: | | | | | | | |
| (*Elf*) | 100 | 8.0 | 9.0 | 3.5 | 25 | 540 | 0 |
| (*Skansen* Tidbits), 2 oz. | 85 | 8.0 | 7.0 | 3.0 | 18 | 550 | <1.0 |
| (*Vita*) | 80 | 6.0 | 11.0 | 2.0 | 10 | 440 | 0 |
| **Herring oil**, see "Oil" | | | | | | | |
| **Hickory nut**, dried, shelled, 1 oz. | 187 | 3.6 | 5.2 | 18.3 | 0 | tr. | 1.8 |
| **Hiziki**, see "Seaweed" | | | | | | | |
| **Hoisin sauce**: | | | | | | | |
| (*House of Tsang*), 1 tsp. | 15 | 0 | 3.0 | 0 | 0 | 120 | 0 |
| (*Ka•Me*), 1 tbsp. | 25 | 0 | 6.0 | 0 | 0 | 230 | 0 |
| (*Kikkoman*), 2 tbsp. | 80 | 1.0 | 17.0 | 1.5 | 0 | 460 | 0 |
| (*Mee Tu*), 2 tbsp. | 80 | 0 | 19.0 | 0 | 0 | 260 | 1.0 |
| (*Roland*), 1 tbsp. | 50 | 0 | 10.0 | 0 | 0 | 410 | 0 |
| (*Sun Luck*), 1 tbsp. | 35 | 1.0 | 9.0 | 0 | 0 | 240 | 0 |
| raspberry (*Heaven and Earth*), 1 tbsp. | 20 | 0 | 4.0 | 0 | 0 | 140 | 0 |
| **Hoki**, frozen, raw (*Seamazz*), 4 oz. | 80 | 23.0 | 0 | .5 | 40 | 95 | 0 |
| **Hollandaise sauce**, in jars (*Reese*), 2 tbsp. | 90 | 1.0 | 1.0 | 9.0 | 75 | 380 | 0 |
| **Hollandaise sauce mix** (*McCormick*), 2 tsp. | 15 | 0 | 1.0 | 0 | 15 | 110 | 0 |
| **Hominy, canned:** | | | | | | | |
| golden, ½ cup: | | | | | | | |
| (*Allens/Allens* Pepi) | 120 | 2.0 | 27.0 | .5 | 0 | 340 | 4.0 |
| (*Bush's*) | 60 | 1.0 | 13.0 | 0 | 0 | 550 | 3.0 |
| white, ½ cup: | | | | | | | |
| (*Allens*) | 100 | 2.0 | 22.0 | .5 | 0 | 340 | 4.0 |
| (*Bush's*) | 70 | 1.0 | 14.0 | 1.0 | 0 | 530 | 4.0 |

| Food and Measure | cal. | prot. (gms) | carbo. (gms) | fat (gms) | chol. (mgs) | sod. (mgs) | fiber (gms) |
|---|---|---|---|---|---|---|---|
| **Hominy grits**, see "Corn grits" | | | | | | | |
| **Honey**, 1 tbsp. . . . . . . . | 60 | 0 | 17.0 | 0 | 0 | 0 | 0 |
| **Honey bun**, see "Bun, sweet" | | | | | | | |
| **Honey mustard**, see "Mustard blends" | | | | | | | |
| **Honey mustard dipping sauce** (*French's*), 2 tbsp. . . . . . . . . . . . | 60 | <1.0 | 12.0 | .5 | 0 | 250 | <1.0 |
| **Honey roll sausage**, beef, 1 oz. . . . . . . . . . | 52 | 5.3 | .6 | 3.0 | 14 | 375 | 0 |
| **Honeycomb** (*Frieda's*), ½ cup, 3 oz. . . . . . . . | 260 | 0 | 70.0 | 0 | 0 | 0 | 0 |
| **Honeydew melon**: | | | | | | | |
| (*Chiquita*), 1 cup, 6.25 oz. . . . . . . . . . . | 64 | 1.0 | 16.0 | 0 | 0 | 32 | 1.0 |
| (*Dole*), ¹⁄₁₀ melon . . . . . . . | 50 | <1.0 | 12.0 | 0 | 0 | 25 | 1.0 |
| (*Earthbound Farm Organic*), ¹⁄₁₀ melon, 4.8 oz. . . . . . . . . . . . | 50 | 1.0 | 13.0 | 0 | 0 | 35 | 1.0 |
| ¹⁄₁₀ melon, 7" x 2" . . . . . . | 46 | .6 | 11.8 | .1 | 0 | 13 | .8 |
| cubed, 1 cup . . . . . . . . . | 60 | .8 | 15.6 | .2 | 0 | 17 | 1.0 |
| **Horned melon** (*Frieda's Kiwano*), 3.5-oz. melon . . . . . . . | 25 | 1.0 | 3.0 | 0 | 0 | 0 | 1.0 |
| **Horseradish**, fresh: | | | | | | | |
| leafy tips, ½ cup: | | | | | | | |
| raw, chopped . . . . . . . | 6 | .9 | .8 | .1 | 0 | 1 | .2 |
| boiled, drained, chopped . . . . . . . . . | 13 | 1.1 | 2.3 | .2 | 0 | 2 | .4 |
| pods, ½ cup: | | | | | | | |
| raw, sliced . . . . . . . . . | 19 | 1.1 | 4.3 | .1 | 0 | 21 | 1.6 |
| boiled, drained, sliced . . . . . . . . . . | 21 | 1.2 | 4.8 | .1 | 0 | 25 | 2.5 |
| **Horseradish, prepared**: | | | | | | | |
| (*Boar's Head*), 1 tsp. . . . . | 0 | 0 | 0 | 0 | 0 | 30 | 0 |
| (*Zatarain's*), 1 tbsp. . . . . . | 15 | 0 | 2.0 | 0 | 0 | 90 | 0 |
| **Horseradish dip** (*Marzetti* Veggie), 2 tbsp. . . . . . . . . . . . | 110 | 1.0 | 3.0 | 11.0 | 15 | 190 | 0 |
| **Horseradish mustard**, see "Mustard blend" | | | | | | | |

| Food and Measure | cal. | prot. (gms) | carbo. (gms) | fat (gms) | chol. (mgs) | sod. (mgs) | fiber (gms) |
|---|---|---|---|---|---|---|---|
| **Horseradish sauce**: | | | | | | | |
| (*Boar's Head* Pub Style), 1 tsp. | 15 | 0 | 1.0 | 1.5 | 5 | 15 | 0 |
| (*Di Lusso*), 1 tsp. | 15 | 0 | 1.0 | 1.0 | 0 | 40 | 0 |
| (*Gold's*), 1 tsp. | 15 | 0 | 1.0 | 1.5 | 0 | 15 | 0 |
| (*Heinz*), 1 tsp. | 25 | 0 | 1.0 | 2.0 | 0 | 35 | 0 |
| **Hot dog**, see "Frankfurter" | | | | | | | |
| **Hot dog sauce**, see "Chili sauce" | | | | | | | |
| **Hot sauce** (see also specific listings), 1 tsp.: | | | | | | | |
| (*Bruce's*) | 0 | 0 | 0 | 0 | 0 | 240 | 0 |
| (*Búfalo* Especial) | 0 | 0 | 0 | 0 | 0 | 140 | 0 |
| (*Búfalo* Salsa Picante) | 0 | 0 | 0 | 0 | 0 | 210 | 0 |
| (*Cajun Chef* Green/ Louisiana) | 0 | 0 | 0 | 0 | 0 | 140 | 0 |
| (*Crystal*) | 0 | 0 | 0 | 0 | 0 | 135 | 0 |
| (*Frank's RedHot* Original/Extra Hot) | 0 | 0 | 0 | 0 | 0 | 190 | 0 |
| (*Glory* Louisiana) | 0 | 0 | 0 | 0 | 0 | 95 | 0 |
| (*Justin Wilson*) | 0 | 0 | 2.0 | 0 | 0 | 120 | 0 |
| (*Louisiana*) | 0 | 0 | 0 | 0 | 0 | 135 | 0 |
| (*Pickapeppa*) | 5 | 0 | 1.0 | 0 | 0 | 40 | 0 |
| (*Tabasco*) | 0 | 0 | 0 | 0 | 0 | 30 | 0 |
| (*Tabasco* Green) | 0 | 0 | 0 | 0 | 0 | 140 | 0 |
| (*Taco Bell*) | 0 | 0 | 0 | 0 | 0 | 50 | 0 |
| (*TryMe* Cajun Sunshine) | 5 | 0 | 0 | 0 | 0 | 120 | 0 |
| (*TryMe* Oyster/Shrimp) | 10 | 0 | 2.0 | 0 | 0 | 100 | 0 |
| (*TryMe* Tiger Sauce) | 10 | 0 | 2.0 | 0 | 0 | 140 | 0 |
| (*TryMe* Yucatan Sunshine) | 5 | 0 | 0 | 0 | 0 | 135 | 0 |
| chipotle (*Búfalo*) | 0 | 0 | 0 | 0 | 0 | 150 | 0 |
| chili: | | | | | | | |
| (*Roland* Hot) | 5 | 0 | 1.0 | 0 | 0 | 190 | 0 |
| (*Roland* Sriracha) | 5 | 0 | 1.0 | 0 | 0 | 60 | 0 |
| (*Sun Luck*) | 0 | 0 | <1.0 | 0 | 0 | 125 | 0 |
| sweet (*Roland* Thai) | 10 | 0 | 3.0 | 0 | 0 | 60 | 0 |
| chili lime (*Frank's RedHot*) | 0 | 0 | 0 | 0 | 0 | 200 | 0 |
| garlic: | | | | | | | |
| (*Roland* Piri-Piri) | 0 | 0 | 0 | 0 | 1 | 60 | 0 |
| (*Sun Luck*) | 5 | 0 | 1.0 | 0 | 0 | 150 | 0 |

| Food and Measure | cal. | prot. (gms) | carbo. (gms) | fat (gms) | chol. (mgs) | sod. (mgs) | fiber (gms) |
|---|---|---|---|---|---|---|---|
| **Hot sauce** *(cont.)* | | | | | | | |
| green pepper (*Emeril's* Kicked Up) ......... | 0 | 0 | 0 | 0 | 0 | 140 | 0 |
| hickory (*Glory*) ........ | 5 | 0 | 2.0 | 0 | 0 | 35 | 0 |
| lemon (*Roland* Piri-Piri) . | 0 | 0 | 0 | 0 | 1 | 70 | 0 |
| jalapeño (*Búfalo*) ....... | 0 | 0 | 0 | 0 | 0 | 115 | 0 |
| mild (*Taco Bell*) ........ | 0 | 0 | 0 | 0 | 0 | 40 | 0 |
| red or wing sauce (*Emeril's*) ......... | 0 | 0 | 0 | 0 | 0 | 140 | 0 |
| Sriracha (*Tuong Ot*) ..... | 5 | 0 | 1.0 | 0 | 0 | 100 | 0 |
| **Hubbard squash**: | | | | | | | |
| raw (*Frieda's*), ¾ cup, 3 oz. .............. | 35 | 2.0 | 7.0 | 0 | 0 | 5 | 2.0 |
| raw, 1 cup ............. | 46 | 2.3 | 10.1 | .6 | 0 | 8 | 2.7 |
| baked, cubed, ½ cup .... | 51 | 2.5 | 11.0 | .6 | 0 | 8 | 2.9 |
| boiled, drained, mashed, ½ cup ...... | 35 | 1.8 | 7.6 | .4 | 0 | 6 | 3.4 |
| **Hummus**, 2 tbsp., 1 oz.: | | | | | | | |
| (*Athenos* Original) ...... | 50 | 1.0 | 5.0 | 3.0 | 0 | 160 | 1.0 |
| (*Athenos Neo Classic* Original) .......... | 80 | 2.0 | 5.0 | 5.0 | 0 | 180 | 1.0 |
| (*Emerald Valley* Organic) ........... | 60 | 2.0 | 5.0 | 4.0 | 0 | 110 | 0 |
| (*Joseph's* Original) ..... | 60 | 2.0 | 5.0 | 4.0 | 0 | 85 | 1.0 |
| (*Margaritaville*) ........ | 70 | 2.0 | 4.0 | 5.0 | 0 | 150 | 1.0 |
| (*Marzetti*) ............ | 70 | 2.0 | 4.0 | 6.0 | 0 | 110 | 1.0 |
| (*Nasoya* Super) ........ | 50 | 4.0 | 2.0 | 3.0 | 0 | 120 | 1.0 |
| (*Sabra* Abu-Goush) ..... | 70 | 1.0 | 3.0 | 7.0 | 0 | 130 | <1.0 |
| (*Sabra* Classic) ........ | 70 | 2.0 | 4.0 | 6.0 | 0 | 120 | 1.0 |
| (*Sabra* Tahini) ........ | 80 | 2.0 | 4.0 | 6.0 | 0 | 120 | 1.0 |
| (*Tribe/Tribe* Organic) .... | 60 | 2.0 | 4.0 | 3.5 | 0 | 130 | 1.0 |
| (*Tribe Origins*) ........ | 70 | 2.0 | 4.0 | 6.0 | 0 | 130 | 1.0 |
| artichoke garlic (*Athenos*) .......... | 50 | 1.0 | 4.0 | 3.0 | 0 | 210 | 1.0 |
| black bean (*Marzetti*) ... | 70 | 0 | 5.0 | 5.0 | 0 | 150 | 2.0 |
| chili, cracked (*Tribe*) .... | 60 | 2.0 | 4.0 | 3.5 | 0 | 135 | 1.0 |
| chipotle: | | | | | | | |
| (*Sabra*) ............. | 70 | 2.0 | 4.0 | 6.0 | 0 | 135 | <1.0 |
| Southwest (*Marzetti*) . | 70 | 1.0 | 5.0 | 4.5 | 0 | 160 | 2.0 |
| spicy (*Tribe*) ........ | 60 | 2.0 | 4.0 | 3.5 | 0 | 130 | 1.0 |
| cilantro jalapeño (*Margaritaville*) ...... | 70 | 2.0 | 4.0 | 5.0 | 0 | 150 | 1.0 |
| cucumber dill (*Athenos*) . | 50 | 1.0 | 5.0 | 3.0 | 0 | 160 | 1.0 |
| dill, savory (*Tribe*) ...... | 60 | 2.0 | 4.0 | 3.5 | 0 | 120 | 1.0 |

| Food and Measure | cal. | prot. (gms) | carbo. (gms) | fat (gms) | chol. (mgs) | sod. (mgs) | fiber (gms) |
|---|---|---|---|---|---|---|---|
| eggplant, roasted: | | | | | | | |
| (*Athenos*) .......... | 45 | 1.0 | 5.0 | 2.0 | 0 | 160 | 1.0 |
| (*Tribe*) ............. | 45 | 2.0 | 3.0 | 3.0 | 0 | 150 | 1.0 |
| garlic (*Margaritaville* | | | | | | | |
| Garlic Lover's) ...... | 70 | 2.0 | 4.0 | 6.0 | 0 | 105 | 1.0 |
| garlic, roasted: | | | | | | | |
| (*Athenos*) .......... | 50 | 1.0 | 5.0 | 3.0 | 0 | 230 | 1.0 |
| (*Athenos Neo Classic*) | 80 | 2.0 | 5.0 | 5.0 | 0 | 200 | 1.0 |
| (*Marzetti*) .......... | 70 | 2.0 | 4.0 | 6.0 | 0 | 110 | 1.0 |
| (*Tribe/Tribe* Organic) .. | 60 | 2.0 | 4.0 | 3.5 | 0 | 130 | 1.0 |
| (*Sabra*) ............. | 70 | 2.0 | 1.0 | 6.0 | 0 | 120 | 1.0 |
| herbs, sea salt (*Sabra*) .. | 25 | 3.0 | 1.0 | 1.0 | 5 | 150 | 0 |
| horseradish (*Tribe*) ..... | 50 | 2.0 | 4.0 | 3.0 | 0 | 125 | 1.0 |
| jalapeño: | | | | | | | |
| (*Sabra*) ............. | 70 | 1.0 | 3.0 | 6.0 | 0 | 170 | <1.0 |
| (*Tribe*) ............. | 60 | 2.0 | 4.0 | 3.5 | 0 | 130 | 1.0 |
| smoked, and garlic | | | | | | | |
| (*Emerald Valley* | | | | | | | |
| Organic) ......... | 60 | 1.0 | 5.0 | 4.0 | 0 | 135 | 0 |
| lemon: | | | | | | | |
| (*Margaritaville*) ...... | 70 | 1.0 | 4.0 | 6.0 | 0 | 105 | 1.0 |
| (*Sabra* Luscious) .... | 70 | 2.0 | 2.0 | 6.0 | 0 | 120 | 1.0 |
| (*Tribe* Zesty) ........ | 60 | 2.0 | 4.0 | 3.5 | 0 | 125 | <1.0 |
| lemon garlic oregano | | | | | | | |
| (*Athenos* Greek) ..... | 50 | 1.0 | 5.0 | 3.0 | 0 | 160 | 1.0 |
| olive: | | | | | | | |
| black (*Athenos*) ..... | 50 | 1.0 | 4.0 | 3.0 | 0 | 170 | 1.0 |
| Calamata (*Tribe*) ..... | 60 | 2.0 | 4.0 | 4.0 | 0 | 150 | <1.0 |
| Greek (*Sabra*) ........ | 70 | 2.0 | 4.0 | 6.0 | 0 | 130 | 1.0 |
| Greek, and roasted | | | | | | | |
| garlic (*Emerald* | | | | | | | |
| *Valley* Organic) .... | 50 | 2.0 | 5.0 | 3.5 | 0 | 140 | 0 |
| pepper, red, roasted: | | | | | | | |
| (*Athenos*) .......... | 50 | 1.0 | 5.0 | 3.0 | 0 | 150 | 1.0 |
| (*Athenos Neo Classic*) | 80 | 2.0 | 5.0 | 6.0 | 0 | 135 | 1.0 |
| (*Emerald Valley* | | | | | | | |
| Organic) ......... | 60 | 1.0 | 4.0 | 4.0 | 0 | 100 | 0 |
| (*Margaritaville*) ...... | 70 | 1.0 | 4.0 | 5.0 | 0 | 105 | 1.0 |
| (*Marzetti*) .......... | 70 | 2.0 | 4.0 | 5.0 | 0 | 150 | 1.0 |
| (*Sabra*) ............. | 70 | 2.0 | 4.0 | 6.0 | 0 | 120 | 1.0 |
| (*Tribe/Tribe* Organic) .. | 50 | 2.0 | 4.0 | 3.0 | 0 | 125 | 1.0 |
| pepper, red, spicy | | | | | | | |
| (*Tribe Origins*) ...... | 70 | 2.0 | 4.0 | 6.0 | 0 | 140 | 1.0 |

| Food and Measure | cal. | prot. (gms) | carbo. (gms) | fat (gms) | chol. (mgs) | sod. (mgs) | fiber (gms) |
|---|---|---|---|---|---|---|---|
| **Hummus** *(cont.)* | | | | | | | |
| pepper, 3, spicy | | | | | | | |
|   *(Athenos)* .......... | 50 | 1.0 | 5.0 | 3.0 | 0 | 230 | 1.0 |
| pesto *(Athenos)* ....... | 50 | 1.0 | 5.0 | 3.0 | 0 | 160 | 1.0 |
| w/salsa *(Sabra)* ........ | 60 | 1.0 | 3.0 | 5.0 | 0 | 135 | <1.0 |
| scallion: | | | | | | | |
|   *(Athenos)* .......... | 50 | 1.0 | 5.0 | 3.0 | 0 | 190 | 1.0 |
|   *(Tribe)* ............. | 60 | 2.0 | 4.0 | 3.5 | 0 | 120 | 1.0 |
| sesame seed, parsley | | | | | | | |
|   *(Athenos Neo Classic)* | 80 | 2.0 | 5.0 | 6.0 | 0 | 160 | 1.0 |
| spice and garlic | | | | | | | |
|   *(Tribe Origins)* ...... | 70 | 2.0 | 4.0 | 6.0 | 0 | 130 | 1.0 |
| spices: | | | | | | | |
|   forty *(Tribe)* ........ | 60 | 2.0 | 4.0 | 3.5 | 0 | 135 | 1.0 |
|   Meditarranean | | | | | | | |
|     *(Tribe* Organic) .... | 60 | 2.0 | 4.0 | 3.5 | 0 | 135 | 1.0 |
| spicy *(Sabra* Supremely) . | 70 | 2.0 | 4.0 | 6.0 | 0 | 130 | <1.0 |
| spinach *(Nasoya* Super) . | 50 | 4.0 | 2.0 | 3.0 | 0 | 120 | <1.0 |
| tomato, sun-dried, and | | | | | | | |
|   basil *(Tribe)* ........ | 60 | 2.0 | 4.0 | 3.5 | 0 | 130 | 1.0 |
| tomato veggie *(Tribe* | | | | | | | |
|   *Origins)* ........... | 70 | 2.0 | 4.0 | 6.0 | 0 | 140 | 1.0 |
| vegetable, garden | | | | | | | |
|   *(Marzetti)* .......... | 70 | 0 | 5.0 | 4.5 | 0 | 170 | 1.0 |
| **Hummus mix** | | | | | | | |
|   *(Fantastic),* dry, .5 oz. . | 45 | 3.0 | 7.0 | 2.0 | 0 | 200 | 2.0 |
| **Hush puppies**, frozen: | | | | | | | |
| *(Delta Pride),* 3 pcs. .... | 140 | 2.0 | 21.0 | 5.0 | 0 | 470 | n.a. |
| *(McKenzie's Gold* | | | | | | | |
|   *King),* 4 pcs., 2 oz. ... | 150 | 2.0 | 25.0 | 4.5 | 0 | 570 | 2.0 |
| jalapeño *(Delta Pride),* | | | | | | | |
|   3 pcs. .............. | 130 | 2.0 | 20.0 | 5.0 | 0 | 470 | n.a. |
| **Hush puppy mix**: | | | | | | | |
| *(Golden Dipt* Corn | | | | | | | |
|   Meal Mix), ¼ cup .... | 120 | 2.0 | 26.0 | 0 | 0 | 540 | 0 |
| *(Martha White),* ¼ cup .. | 120 | 3.0 | 27.0 | .5 | 0 | 610 | 1.0 |
| *(Zatarain's),* 3 tbsp. ..... | 100 | 2.0 | 23.0 | .5 | 0 | 320 | <1.0 |
| **Hyacinth bean**, boiled, | | | | | | | |
|   drained, ½ cup ...... | 22 | 1.3 | 4.1 | .1 | 0 | 1 | n.a. |
| **Hyacinth bean, dried**, | | | | | | | |
|   boiled, ½ cup ....... | 114 | 7.9 | 20.1 | .6 | 0 | 7 | n.a. |

# I

| Food and Measure | cal. | prot. (gms) | carbo. (gms) | fat (gms) | chol. (mgs) | sod. (mgs) | fiber (gms) |
|---|---|---|---|---|---|---|---|
| **Ice**, Italian, 6 fl. oz., except as noted: | | | | | | | |
| cherry: | | | | | | | |
| (*Lindy's Homemade*) | 100 | 0 | 27.0 | 0 | 0 | 10 | 0 |
| (*Luigi's*) | 100 | 0 | 26.0 | 0 | 0 | 10 | <1.0 |
| (*Luigi's* No Sugar) | 60 | 0 | 20.0 | 0 | 0 | 10 | 0 |
| cherry lemon (*Turkey Hill Venice*), ½ cup | 100 | 0 | 24.0 | 0 | 0 | 0 | 0 |
| lemon: | | | | | | | |
| (*Lindy's Homemade*) | 100 | 0 | 26.0 | 0 | 0 | 15 | 0 |
| (*Luigi's*) | 100 | 0 | 26.0 | 0 | 0 | 10 | 0 |
| (*Luigi's* No Sugar) | 60 | 0 | 20.0 | 0 | 0 | 10 | 0 |
| lemon and strawberry (*Luigi's*) | 100 | 0 | 26.0 | 0 | 0 | 10 | 0 |
| lemonade (*Luigi's Blue Razzin' Lemonade*) | 150 | 0 | 39.0 | 0 | 0 | 10 | 0 |
| mango: | | | | | | | |
| (*Luigi's*) | 100 | 0 | 26.0 | 0 | 0 | 10 | 0 |
| (*Turkey Hill Venice*), ½ cup | 100 | 0 | 23.0 | 0 | 0 | 30 | 0 |
| orange (*Lindy's Homemade*) | 100 | 0 | 26.0 | 0 | 0 | 10 | 0 |
| pomegranate blueberry w/acai (*Turkey Hill Venice*), ½ cup | 110 | 0 | 28.0 | 0 | 0 | 5 | 0 |
| raspberry (*Turkey Hill Venice*), ½ cup | 100 | 0 | 24.0 | 0 | 0 | 0 | 0 |
| root beer, strawberry or watermelon (*Lindy's Homemade*) | 100 | 0 | 25.0 | 0 | 0 | 10 | 0 |
| strawberry banana (*Luigi's Blast*) | 150 | 0 | 37.0 | 0 | 0 | 10 | 0 |

| Food and Measure | cal. | prot. (gms) | carbo. (gms) | fat (gms) | chol. (mgs) | sod. (mgs) | fiber (gms) |
|---|---|---|---|---|---|---|---|
| **Ice** *(cont.)* | | | | | | | |
| watermelon or blue raspberry (*Luigi's*) ... | 160 | 0 | 39.0 | 0 | 0 | 15 | 0 |
| **Ice, w/soft-serve ice cream** (*Turkey Hill Duetto*), ½ cup: | | | | | | | |
| banana/strawberry ice ... | 120 | 1.0 | 23.0 | 3.0 | 10 | 30 | 1.0 |
| caramel/apple ice ...... | 120 | 1.0 | 23.0 | 3.0 | 10 | 35 | 0 |
| vanilla, all ice varieties, except mango ....... | 120 | 1.0 | 21.0 | 3.0 | 10 | 35 | 0 |
| vanilla/mango ice ...... | 120 | 1.0 | 20.0 | 3.0 | 10 | 50 | 1.0 |
| **Ice bar** (see also "Fruit bar, frozen" and "Iced confection bar"), 1 pc.: | | | | | | | |
| (*Blue Bunny* Twin Pops) | 70 | 0 | 18.0 | 0 | 0 | 10 | 0 |
| (*Blue Bunny Bomb Pop* Fruit Burst/ Sour Power) ........ | 40 | 0 | 10.0 | 0 | 0 | 10 | 0 |
| (*Blue Bunny Bomb Pop* Sugar Free) ..... | 20 | 0 | 7.0 | 0 | 0 | 10 | 1.0 |
| (*Popsicle* Firecracker) ... | 35 | 0 | 9.0 | 0 | 0 | 0 | 0 |
| (*Popsicle Mega Missle*) .. | 100 | 0 | 24.0 | 0 | 0 | 15 | 0 |
| all flavors: | | | | | | | |
| (*Popsicle* Rainbow) .. | 45 | 0 | 11.0 | 0 | 0 | 5 | 0 |
| (*Popsicle Super Twin*) | 60 | 0 | 14.0 | 0 | 0 | 5 | 0 |
| cherry pineapple: | | | | | | | |
| (*Popsicle Big Stick*) .. | 70 | 0 | 17.0 | 0 | 0 | 0 | 0 |
| (*Popsicle Big Stick* Single) .......... | 60 | 0 | 15.0 | 0 | 0 | 5 | 0 |
| sour (*Popsicle Lick-A-Color* Single) .. | 90 | 0 | 22.0 | 0 | 0 | 10 | 0 |
| spicy: | | | | | | | |
| (*Lucas Chamoy*) ..... | 60 | 0 | 16.0 | 0 | 0 | 480 | 0 |
| (*Lucas Pelucas*) ..... | 70 | 0 | 17.0 | 0 | 0 | 580 | 0 |
| **Ice cream**, ½ cup: | | | | | | | |
| (*Ben & Jerry's* Bonnaroo Buzz) ..... | 280 | 4.0 | 33.0 | 14.0 | 60 | 115 | 0 |
| (*Ben & Jerry's* Late Night Snack) ........ | 270 | 4.0 | 31.0 | 15.0 | 60 | 170 | 0 |
| (*Ben & Jerry's* Chubby Hubby) ............ | 330 | 7.0 | 31.0 | 20.0 | 55 | 150 | 1.0 |
| (*Ben & Jerry's* Dave Matthews Band Magic Brownies) ..... | 240 | 4.0 | 29.0 | 12.0 | 60 | 80 | 0 |

| Food and Measure | cal. | prot. (gms) | carbo. (gms) | fat (gms) | chol. (mgs) | sod. (mgs) | fiber (gms) |
|---|---|---|---|---|---|---|---|
| (*Ben & Jerry's Dublin Mudslide*) .......... | 260 | 4.0 | 29.0 | 15.0 | 60 | 80 | 1.0 |
| (*Ben & Jerry's Everything But The ...*) | 300 | 5.0 | 31.0 | 19.0 | 50 | 80 | 1.0 |
| (*Ben & Jerry's Fossil Fuel*) .............. | 300 | 4.0 | 32.0 | 18.0 | 55 | 85 | 1.0 |
| (*Ben & Jerry's Half Baked*) ............ | 270 | 4.0 | 33.0 | 13.0 | 45 | 85 | 1.0 |
| (*Ben & Jerry's Imagined Whirled Peace*) ...... | 270 | 4.0 | 28.0 | 16.0 | 65 | 105 | 0 |
| (*Ben & Jerry's Karamel Sutra*) ...... | 270 | 4.0 | 32.0 | 14.0 | 50 | 75 | 1.0 |
| (*Ben & Jerry's Phish Food*) ............ | 270 | 4.0 | 37.0 | 12.0 | 30 | 80 | 1.0 |
| (*Ben & Jerry's Stephen Colbert's AmeriCone Dream*) ... | 280 | 4.0 | 32.0 | 15.0 | 60 | 100 | 0 |
| (*Ben & Jerry's Turtle Soup*) ........ | 280 | 4.0 | 30.0 | 15.0 | 60 | 100 | 1.0 |
| (*Dreyer's/Edy's Butterfinger*) ........ | 160 | 2.0 | 22.0 | 7.0 | 10 | 90 | 0 |
| (*Dreyer's/Edy's Slow Churned French Silk*) .............. | 130 | 3.0 | 19.0 | 4.0 | 20 | 65 | 1.0 |
| almond (*Ben & Jerry's Mission to Marzipan*) . | 260 | 4.0 | 32.0 | 13.0 | 60 | 115 | 0 |
| amaretto almond crunch (*Häagen-Dazs*) ...... | 270 | 4.0 | 24.0 | 17.0 | 80 | 80 | 0 |
| apple pie, caramel (*Häagen-Dazs*) ...... | 250 | 3.0 | 28.0 | 14.0 | 65 | 110 | 0 |
| banana fudge walnut (*Ben & Jerry's Chunky Monkey*) ............ | 290 | 4.0 | 30.0 | 17.0 | 55 | 45 | 1.0 |
| banana split: | | | | | | | |
| (*Ben & Jerry's*) ...... | 270 | 4.0 | 30.0 | 15.0 | 60 | 55 | 1.0 |
| (*Häagen-Dazs*) ...... | 280 | 4.0 | 31.0 | 16.0 | 90 | 70 | 0 |
| (*Turkey Hill*) ........ | 150 | 2.0 | 19.0 | 7.0 | 25 | 40 | 1.0 |
| (*Turkey Hill* Light) .... | 110 | 3.0 | 19.0 | 2.5 | 5 | 50 | 1.0 |
| bananas Foster (*Häagen-Dazs*) ...... | 240 | 4.0 | 27.0 | 13.0 | 70 | 75 | 0 |
| black raspberry: | | | | | | | |
| (*Turkey Hill*) ........ | 130 | 2.0 | 16.0 | 7.0 | 25 | 40 | 0 |
| chocolate (*Breyers All Natural*) ........ | 150 | 2.0 | 21.0 | 7.0 | 15 | 45 | <1.0 |

| Food and Measure | cal. | prot. (gms) | carbo. (gms) | fat (gms) | chol. (mgs) | sod. (mgs) | fiber (gms) |
|---|---|---|---|---|---|---|---|
| **Ice cream** *(cont.)* | | | | | | | |
| Boston cream pie | | | | | | | |
| (*Ben & Jerry's*) ...... | 250 | 3.0 | 29.0 | 13.0 | 90 | 105 | 0 |
| brownie, fudge: | | | | | | | |
| (*Ben & Jerry's Chocolate* | | | | | | | |
| *Fudge Brownie*) ... | 250 | 3.0 | 30.0 | 13.0 | 50 | 65 | 2.0 |
| (*Ben & Jerry's Chocolate* | | | | | | | |
| *Fudge Brownie* | | | | | | | |
| Pint) ............ | 250 | 4.0 | 31.0 | 12.0 | 35 | 75 | 2.0 |
| (*Breyers* Smooth & | | | | | | | |
| Dreamy Fat Free) .. | 110 | 3.0 | 26.0 | 0 | 0 | 75 | 4.0 |
| (*Breyers* Smooth & | | | | | | | |
| Dreamy No Sugar) . | 90 | 3.0 | 20.0 | 1.5 | <5 | 85 | 4.0 |
| double (*Dreyer's/Edy's*) | 150 | 2.0 | 23.0 | 5.0 | 15 | 60 | 1.0 |
| double (*Dreyer's/Edy's* | | | | | | | |
| *Slow Churned*) .... | 120 | 3.0 | 17.0 | 4.0 | 20 | 35 | 1.0 |
| brownie batter (*Ben* | | | | | | | |
| *& Jerry's*) .......... | 300 | 5.0 | 33.0 | 17.0 | 65 | 115 | 1.0 |
| brownie mud pie | | | | | | | |
| (*Breyers* Overload!) .. | 130 | 2.0 | 23.0 | 3.5 | 5 | 95 | 1.0 |
| butter almond (*Breyers* | | | | | | | |
| All Natural) ........ | 150 | 3.0 | 15.0 | 9.0 | 20 | 105 | 0 |
| butter pecan: | | | | | | | |
| (*Breyers* All Natural) .. | 150 | 2.0 | 14.0 | 10.0 | 20 | 110 | 0 |
| (*Breyers* Smooth & | | | | | | | |
| Dreamy ½ Fat) .... | 130 | 3.0 | 16.0 | 5.0 | 10 | 115 | 0 |
| (*Breyers* Smooth & | | | | | | | |
| Dreamy Fat Free) .. | 110 | 2.0 | 15.0 | 0 | 10 | 100 | 4.0 |
| (*Dreyer's/Edy's*) ...... | 130 | 1.0 | 17.0 | 6.0 | 10 | 115 | 1.0 |
| (*Dreyer's/Edy's Slow* | | | | | | | |
| *Churned*) ......... | 120 | 3.0 | 16.0 | 5.0 | 20 | 80 | 0 |
| (*Dreyer's/Edy's Slow* | | | | | | | |
| *Churned* No Sugar) | 120 | 3.0 | 15.0 | 5.0 | 10 | 80 | 2.0 |
| (*Häagen-Dazs*) ...... | 310 | 5.0 | 21.0 | 23.0 | 110 | 110 | <1.0 |
| (*Turkey Hill*) ........ | 160 | 2.0 | 15.0 | 10.0 | 25 | 95 | 0 |
| cake flavor: | | | | | | | |
| (*Dreyer's/Edy's Slow* | | | | | | | |
| *Churned* Take the | | | | | | | |
| Cake) ........... | 120 | 3.0 | 18.0 | 4.0 | 20 | 45 | 0 |
| (*Turkey Hill* Party) .... | 160 | 2.0 | 20.0 | 8.0 | 25 | 50 | 0 |
| batter (*Ben & Jerry's*) . | 280 | 4.0 | 28.0 | 17.0 | 60 | 75 | 1.0 |
| caramel: | | | | | | | |
| (*Dreyer's/Edy's Slow* | | | | | | | |
| *Churned* Delight) .. | 120 | 3.0 | 19.0 | 3.5 | 20 | 50 | 0 |

| Food and Measure | cal. | prot. (gms) | carbo. (gms) | fat (gms) | chol. (mgs) | sod. (mgs) | fiber (gms) |
|---|---|---|---|---|---|---|---|
| (*Häagen-Dazs Five*) ... | 240 | 5.0 | 29.0 | 11.0 | 75 | 55 | 0 |
| (*Papaya Azul*) ....... | 250 | 4.0 | 37.0 | 10.0 | 35 | 105 | 0 |
| chunk, triple (*Ben & Jerry's*) | 280 | 3.0 | 32.0 | 16.0 | 65 | 85 | 0 |
| cone (*Häagen-Dazs*) .. | 320 | 4.0 | 32.0 | 19.0 | 100 | 190 | 0 |
| pecan (*Dove*) ....... | 300 | 4.0 | 30.0 | 18.0 | 50 | 95 | 1.0 |
| praline crunch (*Breyer's All Natural*) | 160 | 2.0 | 22.0 | 7.0 | 15 | 85 | 0 |
| swirl chunk (*Breyers Snicker's*) ........ | 170 | 3.0 | 20.0 | 8.0 | 20 | 80 | 0 |
| tracks (*Breyers Smooth & Dreamy*) | 140 | 2.0 | 22.0 | 4.5 | 10 | 100 | 0 |
| chai latte, sweet (*Häagen-Dazs*) ...... | 250 | 4.0 | 23.0 | 16.0 | 80 | 45 | 0 |
| cheesecake brownie (*Ben & Jerry's*) ...... | 250 | 4.0 | 26.0 | 15.0 | 70 | 90 | 0 |
| cherry, black (*Turkey Hill*) .............. | 130 | 2.0 | 18.0 | 6.0 | 25 | 40 | 0 |
| cherry chocolate chip: |  |  |  |  |  |  |  |
| (*Ben & Jerry's Cherry Garcia*) .......... | 250 | 4.0 | 28.0 | 13.0 | 65 | 35 | <1.0 |
| (*Ben & Jerry's Cherry Garcia Pint*) ............ | 240 | 4.0 | 28.0 | 13.0 | 60 | 35 | <1.0 |
| (*Breyers Very*) ...... | 120 | 2.0 | 21.0 | 3.0 | 5 | 50 | 1.0 |
| (*Dove Courtship*) .... | 270 | 4.0 | 27.0 | 16.0 | 45 | 55 | 1.0 |
| (*Dreyer's/Edy's*) ..... | 130 | 1.0 | 21.0 | 5.0 | 10 | 65 | 0 |
| cherry fudge ripple (*Turkey Hill* No Sugar/Fat) .......... | 80 | 3.0 | 22.0 | 0 | 0 | 70 | 4.0 |
| cherry vanilla: |  |  |  |  |  |  |  |
| (*Breyers All Natural*) .. | 130 | 2.0 | 18.0 | 6.0 | 15 | 55 | 0 |
| (*Häagen-Dazs*) ...... | 240 | 4.0 | 23.0 | 15.0 | 100 | 60 | 0 |
| (*Turkey Hill* All Natural Recipe) ... | 150 | 3.0 | 19.0 | 7.0 | 30 | 60 | 0 |
| chocolate: |  |  |  |  |  |  |  |
| (*Ben & Jerry's*) ...... | 250 | 4.0 | 25.0 | 15.0 | 40 | 50 | 2.0 |
| (*Breyers All Natural*) .. | 140 | 2.0 | 17.0 | 7.0 | 20 | 45 | 1.0 |
| (*Breyers Smooth & Dreamy Creamy*) .. | 110 | 3.0 | 17.0 | 3.5 | 10 | 55 | 1.0 |
| (*Breyers Smooth & Dreamy Fat Free*) .. | 90 | 3.0 | 22.0 | 0 | 0 | 55 | 4.0 |
| (*Breyers CarbSmart*) .. | 90 | 2.0 | 13.0 | 6.0 | 15 | 75 | 4.0 |

| Food and Measure | cal. | prot. (gms) | carbo. (gms) | fat (gms) | chol. (mgs) | sod. (mgs) | fiber (gms) |
|---|---|---|---|---|---|---|---|
| **Ice cream, chocolate** *(cont.)* | | | | | | | |
| (*Ciao Bella* Belgian Gelato) . . . . . . . . . . | 230 | 4.0 | 23.0 | 14.0 | 45 | 70 | 0 |
| (*Dove Unconditional*) . | 290 | 4.0 | 31.0 | 17.0 | 40 | 65 | 2.0 |
| (*Dreyer's/Edy's* Grand) | 150 | 3.0 | 17.0 | 8.0 | 25 | 35 | 1.0 |
| (*Dreyer's/Edy's Slow Churned*) . . . . . . . . | 100 | 3.0 | 15.0 | 4.0 | 20 | 30 | 0 |
| (*Häagen-Dazs*) . . . . . . | 270 | 5.0 | 22.0 | 18.0 | 115 | 60 | 1.0 |
| (*Palapa Azul*) . . . . . . . | 280 | 4.0 | 42.0 | 13.0 | 30 | 45 | 2.0 |
| (*Stonyfield* Organic After Dark) . . . . . . . | 240 | 3.0 | 22.0 | 16.0 | 60 | 35 | 1.0 |
| (*Turkey Hill* All Natural Recipe) . . . | 150 | 3.0 | 18.0 | 8.0 | 30 | 45 | 6.0 |
| (*Turkey Hill* Dutch No Sugar/Fat) . . . . . | 70 | 3.0 | 20.0 | 0 | 0 | 75 | 6.0 |
| (*Turkey Hill/Turkey Hill* Dutch) . . . . . . . | 150 | 2.0 | 19.0 | 7.0 | 25 | 45 | 1.0 |
| dark (*Breyers* Smooth & Dreamy Velvet) . . | 110 | 3.0 | 18.0 | 3.5 | 10 | 90 | 1.0 |
| dark (*Häagen-Dazs*) . . | 160 | 5.0 | 21.0 | 17.0 | 90 | 70 | 2.0 |
| dark (*SheerBliss*) . . . . | 290 | 3.0 | 32.0 | 19.0 | 65 | 65 | 0 |
| hot (*Starbucks*) . . . . . . | 203 | 3.0 | 25.0 | 13.0 | 50 | 60 | 1.0 |
| milk (*Häagen-Dazs Five*) . . . . . . . . . . . | 220 | 6.0 | 22.0 | 12.0 | 75 | 75 | <1.0 |
| chocolate, nutty, w/fudge (*Turkey Hill Moose Tracks*) . . . . . . | 140 | 3.0 | 20.0 | 5.0 | 5 | 60 | 2.0 |
| chocolate, triple: | | | | | | | |
| (*Breyers* All Natural) . . | 140 | 2.0 | 17.0 | 7.0 | 20 | 65 | 1.0 |
| (*Breyers* Smooth & Dreamy Creamy No Sugar) . . . . . . . | 100 | 2.0 | 18.0 | 5.0 | 10 | 45 | 3.0 |
| (*Dreyer's/Edy's Slow Churned* No Sugar) | 110 | 3.0 | 17.0 | 3.5 | 10 | 65 | 2.0 |
| chocolate chip/chunk: | | | | | | | |
| (*Breyers* All Natural) . . | 160 | 2.0 | 18.0 | 8.0 | 20 | 45 | 1.0 |
| (*Dreyer's/Edy's* Grand) | 160 | 2.0 | 18.0 | 9.0 | 25 | 45 | 0 |
| (*Dreyer's/Edy's Slow Churned*) . . . . . . . . | 120 | 3.0 | 17.0 | 4.5 | 20 | 50 | 0 |
| chocolate (*Breyers* Smooth & Dreamy) | 140 | 3.0 | 21.0 | 5.0 | 10 | 55 | 1.0 |
| chocolate (*Häagen-Dazs*) . . . . . . . . . . . | 300 | 5.0 | 26.0 | 20.0 | 105 | 55 | 2.0 |

| Food and Measure | cal. | prot. (gms) | carbo. (gms) | fat (gms) | chol. (mgs) | sod. (mgs) | fiber (gms) |
|---|---|---|---|---|---|---|---|
| mint brownie (*Dreyer's/Edy's Nestlé Toll House*) | 140 | 1.0 | 21.0 | 6.0 | 15 | 60 | 0 |
| chocolate chip cookie dough: | | | | | | | |
| (*Ben & Jerry's*) | 260 | 4.0 | 30.0 | 14.0 | 60 | 70 | <1.0 |
| (*Ben & Jerry's* Pint) | 270 | 4.0 | 32.0 | 14.0 | 65 | 80 | 0 |
| (*Breyers* All Natural) | 160 | 2.0 | 20.0 | 8.0 | 15 | 60 | 0 |
| (*Dreyer's/Edy's Nestlé Toll House*) | 150 | 2.0 | 23.0 | 6.0 | 15 | 65 | 0 |
| (*Dreyer's/Edy's Slow Churned*) | 130 | 3.0 | 20.0 | 4.5 | 20 | 60 | 0 |
| (*Häagen-Dazs*) | 310 | 4.0 | 29.0 | 20.0 | 95 | 125 | 0 |
| (*Turkey Hill*) | 160 | 2.0 | 20.0 | 9.0 | 25 | 65 | 0 |
| (*Turkey Hill* Light) | 120 | 3.0 | 20.0 | 3.5 | 10 | 85 | 1.0 |
| chocolate fudge chunk: | | | | | | | |
| (*Dreyer's/Edy's Slow Churned*) | 120 | 3.0 | 18.0 | 4.5 | 20 | 50 | 0 |
| nuts (*Ben & Jerry's New York Super Fudge Chunk*) | 300 | 5.0 | 29.0 | 19.0 | 35 | 55 | 2.0 |
| chocolate hazelnut (*Ciao Bella* Gelato) | 240 | 4.0 | 22.0 | 16.0 | 45 | 60 | 0 |
| chocolate jalapeño (*Ciao Bella* Gelato) | 230 | 4.0 | 23.0 | 14.0 | 45 | 65 | 1.0 |
| chocolate macadamia (*Ben & Jerry's*) | 270 | 4.0 | 25.0 | 18.0 | 50 | 65 | 1.0 |
| chocolate marshmallow (*Turkey Hill*) | 160 | 2.0 | 24.0 | 6.0 | 20 | 100 | 1.0 |
| chocolate mint, dark (*Häagen-Dazs*) | 250 | 5.0 | 19.0 | 17.0 | 90 | 60 | 1.0 |
| chocolate peanut butter: | | | | | | | |
| (*Häagen-Dazs*) | 360 | 8.0 | 27.0 | 24.0 | 100 | 100 | 2.0 |
| cup (*Dreyer's/Edy's*) | 170 | 3.0 | 21.0 | 8.0 | 15 | 85 | 1.0 |
| cup (*Turkey Hill*) | 180 | 3.0 | 18.0 | 11.0 | 25 | 75 | 1.0 |
| cinnamon: | | | | | | | |
| (*Turtle Hill Stuff'd South of Border*) | 120 | 2.0 | 20.0 | 3.5 | 10 | 75 | 1.0 |
| buns (*Ben & Jerry's*) | 290 | 4.0 | 36.0 | 15.0 | 60 | 120 | 0 |
| coconut almond fudge (*Turkey Hill* Light) | 130 | 3.0 | 21.0 | 4.0 | 5 | 100 | 1.0 |
| coffee: | | | | | | | |
| (*Breyers* All Natural) | 130 | 3.0 | 15.0 | 7.0 | 20 | 40 | 0 |
| (*Dreyer's/Edy's* Grand) | 130 | 2.0 | 15.0 | 7.0 | 25 | 35 | 0 |

| Food and Measure | cal. | prot. (gms) | carbo. (gms) | fat (gms) | chol. (mgs) | sod. (mgs) | fiber (gms) |
|---|---|---|---|---|---|---|---|
| **Ice cream, coffee** *(cont.)* | | | | | | | |
| (*Dreyer's/Edy's* Slow Churned) | 105 | 3.0 | 15.0 | 3.5 | 20 | 45 | 0 |
| (*Häagen-Dazs*) | 270 | 5.0 | 21.0 | 18.0 | 120 | 70 | 0 |
| (*Häagen-Dazs Five*) | 220 | 5.0 | 23.0 | 12.0 | 70 | 50 | 0 |
| (*SheerBliss*) | 260 | 3.0 | 25.0 | 18.0 | 65 | 65 | 0 |
| (*Starbucks*) | 210 | 3.0 | 21.0 | 13.0 | 65 | 55 | 0 |
| (*Stonyfield* Organic Gotta Have Java) | 250 | 3.0 | 22.0 | 16.0 | 60 | 45 | 0 |
| (*Turkey Hill* All Natural Recipe) | 140 | 3.0 | 16.0 | 8.0 | 30 | 50 | 0 |
| (*Turkey Hill* Colombian) | 140 | 2.0 | 16.0 | 7.0 | 25 | 45 | 0 |
| caramel (*Starbucks* Macchiato) | 240 | 3.0 | 27.0 | 13.0 | 60 | 105 | 0 |
| chocolate chip (*Starbucks* Java Chip) | 250 | 4.0 | 25.0 | 15.0 | 60 | 50 | <1.0 |
| crunch (*Ben & Jerry's Heath* Bar) | 280 | 4.0 | 29.0 | 16.0 | 60 | 115 | 0 |
| espresso (*Turkey Hill* Light Bavarian) | 120 | 2.0 | 22.0 | 3.0 | 5 | 60 | 1.0 |
| espresso, triple (*Ciao Bella* Gelato) | 220 | 3.0 | 23.0 | 13.0 | 50 | 60 | 0 |
| fudge (*Breyers* Smooth & Dreamy) | 130 | 3.0 | 21.0 | 4.0 | 10 | 65 | <1.0 |
| cookie dough, see "chocolate chip cookie dough," above | | | | | | | |
| cookies and cream: | | | | | | | |
| (*Ben & Jerry's* Milk & Cookies) | 270 | 4.0 | 30.0 | 15.0 | 60 | 105 | <1.0 |
| (*Breyers* All Natural) | 150 | 2.0 | 19.0 | 7.0 | 15 | 90 | 0 |
| (*Breyers Oreo*) | 140 | 2.0 | 21.0 | 5.0 | 15 | 85 | 0 |
| (*Breyers* Smooth & Dreamy ½ Fat) | 130 | 3.0 | 20.0 | 4.0 | 10 | 90 | 0 |
| (*Dreyer's/Edy's*) | 130 | 1.0 | 20.0 | 4.0 | 10 | 80 | 0 |
| (*Dreyer's/Edy's* Slow Churned) | 120 | 3.0 | 18.0 | 4.0 | 20 | 60 | 0 |
| (*Häagen-Dazs*) | 270 | 5.0 | 23.0 | 17.0 | 105 | 95 | 0 |
| (*Stonyfield* Organic) | 270 | 3.0 | 27.0 | 17.0 | 55 | 100 | 0 |
| (*Turkey Hill*) | 150 | 2.0 | 19.0 | 8.0 | 25 | 60 | 0 |
| (*Turkey Hill* Light) | 120 | 2.0 | 20.0 | 3.0 | 5 | 80 | 1.0 |

| Food and Measure | cal. | prot. (gms) | carbo. (gms) | fat (gms) | chol. (mgs) | sod. (mgs) | fiber (gms) |
|---|---|---|---|---|---|---|---|
| (*Turkey Hill* Light Extreme) ........ | 140 | 3.0 | 22.0 | 5.0 | 5 | 80 | 1.0 |
| chocolate (*Breyers* Smooth & Dreamy Fat Free) ........ | 110 | 3.0 | 25.0 | 0 | 0 | 70 | 3.0 |
| chocolate (*Häagen-Dazs* Midnight) .... | 290 | 5.0 | 30.0 | 17.0 | 75 | 95 | 1.0 |
| corn, sweet (*Palapa Azul*) ............. | 160 | 3.0 | 19.0 | 9.0 | 25 | 45 | 0 |
| crème brulée: | | | | | | | |
| (*Ben & Jerry's*) ...... | 310 | 4.0 | 36.0 | 17.0 | 90 | 90 | 0 |
| (*Häagen-Dazs*) ...... | 280 | 4.0 | 23.0 | 19.0 | 120 | 75 | 0 |
| crème caramel (*Stonyfield* Organic) .. | 260 | 3.0 | 28.0 | 14.0 | 55 | 85 | 0 |
| dulce de leche: | | | | | | | |
| (*Ben & Jerry's* Dulce Delish) ..... | 240 | 4.0 | 29.0 | 12.0 | 60 | 65 | 0 |
| (*Breyers* All Natural) .. | 150 | 2.0 | 21.0 | 6.0 | 15 | 105 | 0 |
| (*Ciao Bella* Gelato) ... | 230 | 4.0 | 27.0 | 12.0 | 45 | 85 | 0 |
| (*Dreyer's/Edy's*) ...... | 130 | 1.0 | 22.0 | 4.0 | 10 | 70 | 0 |
| (*Häagen-Dazs*) ...... | 290 | 5.0 | 28.0 | 17.0 | 100 | 95 | 0 |
| espresso, see "coffee," above | | | | | | | |
| flan (*Palapa Azul*) ...... | 200 | 4.0 | 24.0 | 11.0 | 90 | 45 | 0 |
| fried (*Breyers*) ......... | 140 | 2.0 | 23.0 | 4.5 | 10 | 95 | 0 |
| fudge: | | | | | | | |
| ripple (*Turkey Hill*) ... | 140 | 2.0 | 20.0 | 6.0 | 25 | 55 | 0 |
| tracks (*Dreyer's/Edy's* Slow Churned) .... | 120 | 3.0 | 18.0 | 4.5 | 20 | 50 | 0 |
| tracks (*Dreyer's/Edy's* Slow Churned No Sugar) ......... | 110 | 3.0 | 16.0 | 4.0 | 10 | 75 | 2.0 |
| ginger (*Häagen-Dazs Five*) .............. | 230 | 5.0 | 25.0 | 12.0 | 75 | 50 | 0 |
| green tea: | | | | | | | |
| (*Ciao Bella* Matcha Gelato) .......... | 210 | 3.0 | 21.0 | 12.0 | 45 | 70 | 0 |
| (*Häagen-Dazs*) ...... | 250 | 5.0 | 20.0 | 17.0 | 105 | 50 | 0 |
| hazelnut, roasted (*Ciao Bella* Gelato) ... | 230 | 4.0 | 21.0 | 15.0 | 45 | 65 | 0 |
| lemon: | | | | | | | |
| (*Häagen-Dazs Five*) ... | 210 | 5.0 | 26.0 | 10.0 | 60 | 50 | 0 |
| pie (*Turkey Hill*) ..... | 160 | 2.0 | 22.0 | 7.0 | 25 | 105 | 0 |

| Food and Measure | cal. | prot. (gms) | carbo. (gms) | fat (gms) | chol. (mgs) | sod. (mgs) | fiber (gms) |
|---|---|---|---|---|---|---|---|
| **Ice cream** *(cont.)* | | | | | | | |
| lime, Key, graham | | | | | | | |
| (*Ciao Bella* Gelato) ... | 270 | 2.0 | 35.0 | 14.0 | 25 | 130 | 0 |
| malted milk ball | | | | | | | |
| (*Ciao Bella* Gelato) ... | 240 | 4.0 | 29.0 | 13.0 | 40 | 70 | 0 |
| mango: | | | | | | | |
| (*Dreyer's/Edy's*) ..... | 110 | 1.0 | 19.0 | 4.0 | 10 | 50 | 0 |
| (*Häagen-Dazs*) ...... | 250 | 4.0 | 28.0 | 14.0 | 85 | 50 | <1.0 |
| maple brownie (*Ben &* | | | | | | | |
| *Jerry's* Maple Blondie) | 240 | 4.0 | 32.0 | 11.0 | 65 | 90 | 0 |
| maple ginger snap | | | | | | | |
| (*Ciao Bella* Gelato) ... | 210 | 3.0 | 29.0 | 12.0 | 45 | 80 | 0 |
| mint (*Häagen-Dazs Five*) . | 220 | 5.0 | 24.0 | 12.0 | 70 | 50 | 0 |
| mint chocolate chip: | | | | | | | |
| (*Ben & Jerry's Mint* | | | | | | | |
| *Chocolate Chunk*) .. | 270 | 4.0 | 26.0 | 17.0 | 65 | 55 | 1.0 |
| (*Breyers* All Natural) .. | 150 | 2.0 | 18.0 | 8.0 | 15 | 45 | <1.0 |
| (*Breyers* Smooth & | | | | | | | |
| Dreamy ½ Fat) .... | 130 | 3.0 | 18.0 | 4.5 | 10 | 55 | 0 |
| (*Ciao Bella* Gelato) ... | 240 | 3.0 | 25.0 | 14.0 | 40 | 60 | 1.0 |
| (*Dreyer's/Edy's* Grand) | 160 | 2.0 | 18.0 | 9.0 | 25 | 45 | 0 |
| (*Dreyer's/Edy's* Slow | | | | | | | |
| *Churned*) ........ | 120 | 3.0 | 17.0 | 4.5 | 20 | 50 | 0 |
| (*Dreyer's/Edy's* Slow | | | | | | | |
| *Churned* No Sugar) | 110 | 3.0 | 15.0 | 4.5 | 10 | 65 | 2.0 |
| (*Häagen-Dazs*) ...... | 300 | 5.0 | 26.0 | 19.0 | 105 | 85 | <1.0 |
| (*Turkey Hill* All | | | | | | | |
| Natural Recipe) ... | 160 | 3.0 | 18.0 | 9.0 | 25 | 45 | 0 |
| (*Turkey Hill* Choco) ... | 160 | 2.0 | 17.0 | 9.0 | 25 | 45 | 1.0 |
| w/chocolate cookie | | | | | | | |
| (*Turkey Hill Skinny* | | | | | | | |
| *Minty* Light) ...... | 140 | 3.0 | 20.0 | 5.0 | 5 | 80 | 1.0 |
| mint cookie: | | | | | | | |
| (*Ben & Jerry's*) ...... | 250 | 4.0 | 26.0 | 14.0 | 60 | 100 | 0 |
| (*Dreyer's/Edy's* Slow | | | | | | | |
| *Churned*) ........ | 120 | 3.0 | 19.0 | 4.0 | 20 | 65 | 0 |
| mocha: | | | | | | | |
| (*Starbucks* | | | | | | | |
| *Frappuccino*) ..... | 220 | 3.0 | 23.0 | 13.0 | 55 | 65 | <1.0 |
| w/cookie swirl | | | | | | | |
| (*Turkey Hill Stuff'd* | | | | | | | |
| Double Dunker) ... | 140 | 3.0 | 22.0 | 5.0 | 5 | 100 | 1.0 |
| mocha almond fudge: | | | | | | | |
| (*Dreyer's/Edy's*) ..... | 140 | 2.0 | 20.0 | 6.0 | 15 | 65 | 1.0 |

| Food and Measure | cal. | prot. (gms) | carbo. (gms) | fat (gms) | chol. (mgs) | sod. (mgs) | fiber (gms) |
|---|---|---|---|---|---|---|---|
| (*Edy's Slow Churned*) | 120 | 3.0 | 16.0 | 4.5 | 20 | 45 | 0 |
| mud pie (*Ben & Jerry's*) | 270 | 4.0 | 29.0 | 16.0 | 55 | 75 | 1.0 |
| Neapolitan: | | | | | | | |
| (*Ben & Jerry's Neapolitan Dynamite*) | 230 | 4.0 | 30.0 | 11.0 | 45 | 50 | 1.0 |
| (*Dreyer's/Edy's* Grand) | 140 | 2.0 | 16.0 | 7.0 | 25 | 35 | 0 |
| (*Dreyer's/Edy's Slow Churned* No Sugar) | 90 | 3.0 | 13.0 | 3.0 | 10 | 65 | 2.0 |
| (*Dreyer's/Edy's Slow Churned*) | 100 | 3.0 | 15.0 | 3.0 | 20 | 35 | 0 |
| (*Turkey Hill*) | 140 | 2.0 | 17.0 | 7.0 | 25 | 40 | 0 |
| nutty (*Turkey Hill* All Natural) | 150 | 3.0 | 17.0 | 8.0 | 30 | 70 | 0 |
| oatmeal cookie chunk (*Ben & Jerry's*) | 260 | 4.0 | 30.0 | 14.0 | 55 | 115 | 1.0 |
| passion fruit (*Häagen-Dazs Five*) | 220 | 4.0 | 25.0 | 11.0 | 70 | 45 | 0 |
| peach: | | | | | | | |
| (*Breyers* All Natural) | 120 | 2.0 | 17.0 | 4.5 | 15 | 30 | 0 |
| (*Ben & Jerry's Willy Nelson's Peach Cobbler*) | 220 | 3.0 | 28.0 | 11.0 | 50 | 55 | 0 |
| peanut brittle: | | | | | | | |
| (*Ben & Jerry's*) | 260 | 4.0 | 29.0 | 16.0 | 60 | 140 | 0 |
| ripple (*Turkey Hill*) | 170 | 3.0 | 16.0 | 11.0 | 25 | 90 | 1.0 |
| swirl (*Breyers* Overload! Tracks) | 160 | 4.0 | 19.0 | 8.0 | 5 | 95 | 1.0 |
| peanut butter cup: | | | | | | | |
| (*Ben & Jerry's Peanut Butter Cup*) | 340 | 6.0 | 28.0 | 24.0 | 55 | 125 | 1.0 |
| (*Breyers Reese's*) | 160 | 3.0 | 25.0 | 6.0 | 10 | 110 | 1.0 |
| (*Dreyer's/Edy's Slow Churned*) | 130 | 3.0 | 17.0 | 6.0 | 20 | 65 | 0 |
| pecan, honey toasted (*Ciao Bella* Gelato) | 240 | 4.0 | 23.0 | 16.0 | 45 | 70 | 0 |
| peppermint, w/ chocolate (*Häagen-Dazs* Bark) | 280 | 4.0 | 31.0 | 16.0 | 90 | 45 | 0 |
| pineapple coconut (*Häagen-Dazs*) | 230 | 4.0 | 25.0 | 13.0 | 90 | 55 | 0 |
| pistachio: | | | | | | | |
| (*Ben & Jerry's Pistachio Pistachio*) | 250 | 5.0 | 22.0 | 16.0 | 65 | 55 | 1.0 |

| Food and Measure | cal. | prot. (gms) | carbo. (gms) | fat (gms) | chol. (mgs) | sod. (mgs) | fiber (gms) |
|---|---|---|---|---|---|---|---|
| **Ice cream, pistachio** *(cont.)* | | | | | | | |
| (*Ciao Bella* Gelato) ... | 250 | 5.0 | 23.0 | 16.0 | 45 | 95 | 1.0 |
| (*Häagen-Dazs*) ...... | 290 | 5.0 | 22.0 | 20.0 | 110 | 80 | <1.0 |
| pomegranate: | | | | | | | |
| (*SheerBliss*) ........ | 290 | 3.0 | 32.0 | 16.0 | 55 | 60 | 0 |
| w/dark chocolate | | | | | | | |
| (*SheerBliss*) ...... | 320 | 4.0 | 35.0 | 19.0 | 65 | 70 | 0 |
| praline pecan (*Turkey Hill Stuff'd* Paradise) .. | 120 | 2.0 | 20.0 | 3.5 | 5 | 95 | 1.0 |
| pretzel, chocolate | | | | | | | |
| (*Turkey Hill Snyder's*) . | 130 | 3.0 | 21.0 | 3.5 | 10 | 120 | 1.0 |
| rocky road: | | | | | | | |
| (*Breyers* All Natural) .. | 160 | 2.0 | 21.0 | 7.0 | 15 | 40 | <1.0 |
| (*Breyers* Smooth & Dreamy ½ Fat) .... | 140 | 3.0 | 23.0 | 4.5 | 10 | 55 | 1.0 |
| (*Dreyer's/Edy's* Grand) | 190 | 3.0 | 19.0 | 11.0 | 30 | 35 | 1.0 |
| (*Dreyer's/Edy's* Slow Churned) ........ | 120 | 3.0 | 17.0 | 4.0 | 15 | 30 | 0 |
| (*Häagen-Dazs*) ...... | 300 | 5.0 | 29.0 | 18.0 | 90 | 75 | 1.0 |
| (*Turkey Hill*) ........ | 170 | 3.0 | 23.0 | 8.0 | 20 | 125 | 1.0 |
| rum raisin: | | | | | | | |
| (*Häagen-Dazs*) ...... | 270 | 4.0 | 22.0 | 17.0 | 110 | 60 | 0 |
| (*Turkey Hill*) ........ | 140 | 2.0 | 19.0 | 6.0 | 25 | 55 | 0 |
| s'mores (*Ben & Jerry's*) ............ | 290 | 4.0 | 33.0 | 16.0 | 30 | 65 | 1.0 |
| spumoni (*Dreyer's/ Edy's*) ............. | 120 | 1.0 | 19.0 | 4.0 | 15 | 60 | 0 |
| strawberries and cream: | | | | | | | |
| (*Starbucks Frappuccino* Crème) | 190 | 3.0 | 23.0 | 10.0 | 50 | 30 | 0 |
| (*Turkey Hill*) ........ | 120 | 2.0 | 16.0 | 6.0 | 20 | 35 | 1.0 |
| strawberry: | | | | | | | |
| (*Breyers* All Natural) .. | 110 | 2.0 | 16.0 | 5.0 | 15 | 40 | 0 |
| (*Breyers* Smooth & Dreamy Fat Free) .. | 90 | 3.0 | 21.0 | 0 | 0 | 40 | 3.0 |
| (*Ciao Bella* Gelato) ... | 190 | 2.0 | 26.0 | 9.0 | 35 | 50 | 1.0 |
| (*Dreyer's/Edy's* Grand Real) ........... | 130 | 2.0 | 16.0 | 6.0 | 20 | 30 | 0 |
| (*Dreyer's/Edys* Slow Churned) | 110 | 2.0 | 18.0 | 3.0 | 15 | 40 | 0 |
| (*Häagen-Dazs*) ...... | 250 | 4.0 | 23.0 | 16.0 | 95 | 65 | <1.0 |
| (*Häagen-Dazs Five*) ... | 210 | 4.0 | 24.0 | 11.0 | 65 | 40 | 0 |
| strawberry cheesecake: | | | | | | | |
| (*Ben & Jerry's*) ...... | 240 | 3.0 | 30.0 | 14.0 | 50 | 45 | 0 |

| Food and Measure | cal. | prot. (gms) | carbo. (gms) | fat (gms) | chol. (mgs) | sod. (mgs) | fiber (gms) |
|---|---|---|---|---|---|---|---|
| (*Breyers* Smooth & Dreamy) ....... | 120 | 3.0 | 20.0 | 3.5 | 10 | 60 | 0 |
| (*Turkey Hill* Light) .... | 120 | 2.0 | 20.0 | 3.5 | 10 | 105 | 0 |
| (*Turkey Hill Stuff'd*) .. | 120 | 2.0 | 20.0 | 3.0 | 10 | 95 | 1.0 |
| sundae cone (*Dreyer's/ Edy's Nestlé Drumstick*) ....... | 160 | 2.0 | 21.0 | 7.0 | 10 | 60 | 0 |
| tin roof sundae (*Turkey Hill*) ........ | 150 | 2.0 | 19.0 | 8.0 | 25 | 60 | 0 |
| toffee (*Breyers Heath*) ... | 160 | 2.0 | 25.0 | 6.0 | 10 | 130 | 0 |
| vanilla: | | | | | | | |
| (*Ben & Jerry's*) ...... | 230 | 4.0 | 22.0 | 14.0 | 70 | 60 | 0 |
| (*Breyers* All Natural) .. | 130 | 3.0 | 14.0 | 7.0 | 20 | 35 | 0 |
| (*Breyers* All Natural Extra Creamy) .... | 140 | 2.0 | 16.0 | 7.0 | 20 | 50 | 0 |
| (*Breyers* All Natural Homemade) ...... | 140 | 3.0 | 16.0 | 7.0 | 35 | 50 | 0 |
| (*Breyers* All Natural Lactose Free) ..... | 130 | 2.0 | 14.0 | 7.0 | 20 | 35 | 0 |
| (*Breyers CarbSmart*) .. | 90 | 2.0 | 13.0 | 6.0 | 15 | 45 | 4.0 |
| (*Breyers* Smooth & Dreamy Creamy) .. | 110 | 3.0 | 16.0 | 3.5 | 10 | 50 | 0 |
| (*Breyers* Smooth & Dreamy Creamy Fat Free) ......... | 90 | 3.0 | 21.0 | 0 | <5 | 45 | 3.0 |
| (*Breyers* Smooth & Dreamy Creamy No Sugar) ....... | 90 | 2.0 | 15.0 | 4.0 | 10 | 45 | 4.0 |
| (*Ciao Bella* Tahitian Gelato) ......... | 220 | 3.0 | 25.0 | 12.0 | 45 | 70 | 0 |
| (*Dove Beyond Vanilla*) | 240 | 4.0 | 23.0 | 15.0 | 50 | 60 | 2.0 |
| (*Dreyer's/Edy's* Grand) | 140 | 2.0 | 15.0 | 8.0 | 25 | 35 | 0 |
| (*Dreyer's/Edy's* Slow Churned*) ........ | 100 | 3.0 | 15.0 | 3.5 | 20 | 45 | 0 |
| (*Dreyer's/Edy's* Slow Churned* No Sugar) | 90 | 3.0 | 13.0 | 3.0 | 10 | 70 | 2.0 |
| (*Häagen-Dazs*) ...... | 270 | 5.0 | 21.0 | 18.0 | 120 | 70 | 0 |
| (*Land O Lakes*) ...... | 150 | 2.0 | 17.0 | 8.0 | 30 | 40 | 0 |
| (*Land O Lakes* Light) . | 100 | 3.0 | 17.0 | 3.0 | 15 | 30 | 0 |
| (*SheerBliss*) ........ | 300 | 6.0 | 29.0 | 19.0 | 65 | 65 | 0 |
| (*Stonyfield* Organic Gotta Have) ...... | 250 | 3.0 | 21.0 | 16.0 | 60 | 45 | 0 |
| (*Turkey Hill* Original) .. | 140 | 2.0 | 16.0 | 7.0 | 30 | 45 | 0 |

| Food and Measure | cal. | prot. (gms) | carbo. (gms) | fat (gms) | chol. (mgs) | sod. (mgs) | fiber (gms) |
|---|---|---|---|---|---|---|---|
| **Ice cream, vanilla** *(cont.)* | | | | | | | |
| double (*Dreyer's/ Edy's* Grand) ..... | 140 | 3.0 | 16.0 | 7.0 | 35 | 40 | 0 |
| vanilla, French: | | | | | | | |
| (*Breyers* All Natural) .. | 140 | 3.0 | 14.0 | 7.0 | 45 | 40 | 0 |
| (*Breyers* Smooth & Dreamy Creamy No Sugar) ....... | 90 | 2.0 | 15.0 | 4.5 | 30 | 45 | 4.0 |
| (*Dreyer's/Edy's* Grand) | 150 | 2.0 | 16.0 | 9.0 | 50 | 35 | 0 |
| (*Dreyer's/Edy's Slow Churned*) ........ | 100 | 3.0 | 15.0 | 3.5 | 30 | 45 | 0 |
| (*Dreyer's/Edy's Slow Churned* No Sugar) | 100 | 3.0 | 15.0 | 3.0 | 30 | 35 | 2.0 |
| (*Turkey Hill*) ......... | 140 | 2.0 | 16.0 | 7.0 | 50 | 45 | 0 |
| vanilla bean: | | | | | | | |
| (*Breyers* Smooth & Dreamy) ......... | 110 | 3.0 | 16.0 | 3.5 | 10 | 50 | 0 |
| (*Dreyer's/Edy's* Grand) | 140 | 2.0 | 15.0 | 8.0 | 25 | 35 | 0 |
| (*Dreyer's/Edy's Slow Churned*) ........ | 100 | 3.0 | 15.0 | 3.5 | 20 | 45 | 0 |
| (*Dreyer's/Edy's Slow Churned* No Sugar) | 90 | 3.0 | 13.0 | 3.0 | 10 | 70 | 2.0 |
| (*Häagen-Dazs*) ...... | 290 | 5.0 | 26.0 | 18.0 | 105 | 75 | 0 |
| (*Häagen-Dazs Five*) ... | 220 | 5.0 | 24.0 | 11.0 | 70 | 50 | 0 |
| (*Starbucks Frappuccino*) | 200 | 4.0 | 22.0 | 11.0 | 55 | 35 | 0 |
| (*Turkey Hill*) ........ | 140 | 2.0 | 16.0 | 7.0 | 30 | 45 | 0 |
| (*Turkey Hill* All Natural Recipe) ... | 140 | 2.0 | 16.0 | 8.0 | 30 | 50 | 0 |
| (*Turkey Hill* Light) .... | 100 | 3.0 | 16.0 | 2.5 | 10 | 65 | 1.0 |
| (*Turkey Hill* No Sugar/Fat) ....... | 70 | 3.0 | 19.0 | 0 | 0 | 75 | 5.0 |
| vanilla brownie chocolate chunk (*Dove*) | 300 | 4.0 | 31.0 | 19.0 | 50 | 65 | 1.0 |
| vanilla caramel: | | | | | | | |
| (*Breyers* All Natural) .. | 130 | 2.0 | 17.0 | 6.0 | 20 | 50 | 0 |
| fudge (*Ben & Jerry's*) . | 270 | 4.0 | 31.0 | 14.0 | 65 | 100 | 0 |
| vanilla chai (*Stoneyfield* Organic) . | 240 | 3.0 | 21.0 | 16.0 | 60 | 45 | 0 |
| vanilla and chocolate: | | | | | | | |
| (*Breyers* All Natural) .. | 130 | 3.0 | 16.0 | 7.0 | 20 | 45 | 0 |
| (*Dreyer's/Edy's* Grand) | 150 | 3.0 | 16.0 | 8.0 | 25 | 30 | 0 |
| (*Turkey Hill*) ........ | 140 | 2.0 | 17.0 | 7.0 | 25 | 45 | 0 |
| crisps (*Breyers* All Natural Crackle) ... | 160 | 3.0 | 15.0 | 10.0 | 15 | 35 | 0 |

| Food and Measure | cal. | prot. (gms) | carbo. (gms) | fat (gms) | chol. (mgs) | sod. (mgs) | fiber (gms) |
|---|---|---|---|---|---|---|---|
| vanilla and chocolate and strawberry: | | | | | | | |
| (*Breyers* All Natural) .. | 130 | 2.0 | 15.0 | 6.0 | 20 | 35 | 0 |
| (*Breyers* Smooth & Dreamy ½ Fat) .... | 110 | 3.0 | 17.0 | 3.0 | 10 | 50 | 0 |
| (*Breyers* Smooth & Dreamy Creamy No Sugar) ....... | 90 | 2.0 | 15.0 | 4.0 | 10 | 45 | 3.0 |
| vanilla chocolate chip (*Häagen-Dazs*) ...... | 310 | 5.0 | 26.0 | 20.0 | 105 | 75 | <1.0 |
| vanilla chocolate raspberry truffle (*Häagen-Dazs*) ...... | 310 | 5.0 | 32.0 | 18.0 | 105 | 65 | 1.0 |
| vanilla fudge brownie (*Breyers* All Natural) .. | 150 | 2.0 | 20.0 | 7.0 | 15 | 50 | <1.0 |
| vanilla fudge twirl: | | | | | | | |
| (*Breyers* All Natural) .. | 130 | 2.0 | 17.0 | 6.0 | 15 | 55 | 0 |
| (*Dreyer's* Grand) ..... | 150 | 2.0 | 19.0 | 7.0 | 20 | 35 | 0 |
| vanilla honey (*Häagen-Dazs* Honey Bee) .... | 270 | 5.0 | 23.0 | 17.0 | 110 | 50 | 0 |
| vanilla and orange sherbet, see "Sherbet" | | | | | | | |
| vanilla w/peanut butter chips, fudge: | | | | | | | |
| (*Turkey Hill Moose Tracks* Light) ..... | 130 | 3.0 | 19.0 | 6.0 | 10 | 75 | 1.0 |
| (*Turkey Hill Moose Tracks* No Sugar) .. | 120 | 4.0 | 22.0 | 5.0 | 0 | 85 | 5.0 |
| (*Turkey Hill Moose Tracks* Stuff'd) .... | 140 | 3.0 | 20.0 | 6.0 | 5 | 65 | 1.0 |
| vanilla w/peanut butter, chunky (*Turkey Hill*) .. | 180 | 4.0 | 17.0 | 11.0 | 25 | 100 | 1.0 |
| vanilla w/pomegranate: | | | | | | | |
| (*SheerBliss*) ........ | 300 | 3.0 | 33.0 | 17.0 | 60 | 65 | 0 |
| and blueberry (*SheerBliss* Freedom) | 290 | 3.0 | 32.0 | 16.0 | 65 | 60 | 0 |
| vanilla sandwich (*Dreyer's/Edy's Nestle*) | 120 | 1.0 | 21.0 | 4.0 | 10 | 80 | 0 |
| vanilla Swiss almond (*Häagen-Dazs*) ...... | 300 | 5.0 | 24.0 | 20.0 | 105 | 75 | <1.0 |
| vanilla toffee (*Ben & Jerry's Heath Bar Crunch*) ... | 290 | 4.0 | 29.0 | 17.0 | 65 | 110 | 0 |
| waffle cone (*Breyers* Overload!*) ......... | 130 | 2.0 | 22.0 | 3.0 | 5 | 95 | 0 |

| Food and Measure | cal. | prot. (gms) | carbo. (gms) | fat (gms) | chol. (mgs) | sod. (mgs) | fiber (gms) |
|---|---|---|---|---|---|---|---|
| **"Ice cream," nondairy**, ½ cup: | | | | | | | |
| almond pecan (*It's So Delicious*) ....... | 140 | 2.0 | 24.0 | 4.5 | 0 | 175 | 3.0 |
| banana (*Purely Decadent Swinging Anna*) ..... | 230 | 2.0 | 31.0 | 13.0 | 0 | 15 | 5.0 |
| berry, wild (*Tofutti Supreme*) .......... | 190 | 2.0 | 24.0 | 9.0 | 0 | 190 | 0 |
| blueberry cheesecake (*Purely Decadent*) .... | 180 | 1.0 | 33.0 | 6.0 | 0 | 50 | 5.0 |
| "butter" pecan: | | | | | | | |
| (*Organic So Delicious*) ........ | 160 | 2.0 | 22.0 | 7.0 | 0 | 90 | 3.0 |
| (*Soy Dream*) ........ | 190 | 1.0 | 23.0 | 11.0 | 0 | 140 | 1.0 |
| (*Tofutti Better Pecan*) . | 210 | 1.0 | 21.0 | 13.0 | 0 | 220 | 0 |
| carob almond (*Rice Dream*) ........... | 180 | 0 | 26.0 | 10.0 | 0 | 70 | 2.0 |
| carob peppermint (*It's Soy Delicious*) ...... | 115 | 2.0 | 24.0 | 1.5 | 0 | 130 | 2.0 |
| chai (*It's Soy Delicious*) . | 110 | 2.0 | 25.0 | 1.5 | 0 | 160 | 2.0 |
| cherry (*Purely Decadent Nirvana*) .......... | 190 | 1.0 | 32.0 | 9.0 | 0 | 15 | 5.0 |
| chocolate: | | | | | | | |
| (*It's Soy Delicious Awesome*) ....... | 115 | 2.0 | 24.0 | 1.5 | 0 | 130 | 2.0 |
| (*Organic So Delicious Velvet*) .......... | 130 | 2.0 | 23.0 | 3.5 | 0 | 50 | 1.0 |
| (*Purely Decadent Coconut Milk*) .... | 150 | 1.0 | 20.0 | 9.0 | 0 | 5 | 6.0 |
| (*Purely Decadent Obsession*) ........ | 210 | 2.0 | 36.0 | 9.0 | 0 | 15 | 5.0 |
| (*Tofutti* Supreme) .... | 180 | 3.0 | 18.0 | 11.0 | 0 | 180 | 0 |
| Belgian (*Purely Decadent*) ........ | 180 | 1.0 | 30.0 | 7.0 | 0 | 15 | 4.0 |
| chocolate almond: | | | | | | | |
| (*It's Soy Delicious*) ... | 140 | 3.0 | 23.0 | 4.5 | 0 | 165 | 3.0 |
| brownie (*Purely Decadent*) ........ | 210 | 3.0 | 34.0 | 10.0 | 0 | 75 | 6.0 |
| chocolate coffee (*It's Soy Delicious* Black Leopard*) .......... | 110 | 1.0 | 25.0 | 1.5 | 0 | 105 | 2.0 |
| chocolate cookie crunch (*Tofutti*) .......... | 210 | 3.0 | 26.0 | 11.0 | 0 | 100 | 0 |

| Food and Measure | cal. | prot. (gms) | carbo. (gms) | fat (gms) | chol. (mgs) | sod. (mgs) | fiber (gms) |
|---|---|---|---|---|---|---|---|
| chocolate fudge brownie | | | | | | | |
| (*Soy Dream*) ........ | 170 | <1.0 | 21.0 | 9.0 | 0 | 150 | 1.0 |
| chocolate peanut butter: | | | | | | | |
| (*It's Soy Delicious*) ... | 135 | 3.0 | 24.0 | 3.5 | 0 | 155 | 3.0 |
| (*Organic So* | | | | | | | |
| *Delicious*) ........ | 140 | 2.0 | 23.0 | 4.5 | 0 | 60 | 2.0 |
| swirl (*Purely Decadent* | | | | | | | |
| Coconut Milk) .... | 210 | 3.0 | 21.0 | 13.0 | 0 | 40 | 6.0 |
| cinnamon (*Purely Decadent* | | | | | | | |
| Snickerdoodle) ...... | 190 | 1.0 | 34.0 | 6.0 | 0 | 65 | 5.0 |
| cocoa marble fudge | | | | | | | |
| (*Rice Dream*) ....... | 170 | <1.0 | 31.0 | 6.0 | 0 | 90 | 1.0 |
| coconut: | | | | | | | |
| (*Purely Decadent* | | | | | | | |
| Craze) ........... | 240 | 3.0 | 31.0 | 12.0 | 0 | 60 | 6.0 |
| (*Purely Decadent* | | | | | | | |
| Coconut Milk) .... | 170 | 1.0 | 19.0 | 10.0 | 0 | 5 | 6.0 |
| cookie: | | | | | | | |
| (*Purely Decadent* | | | | | | | |
| Avalanche) ....... | 200 | 2.0 | 34.0 | 9.0 | 0 | 70 | 5.0 |
| (*Rice Dream* Cookies | | | | | | | |
| n' Dream) ........ | 170 | 0 | 27.0 | 8.0 | 0 | 75 | 2.0 |
| dough (*Purely Decadent* | | | | | | | |
| Coconut Milk | | | | | | | |
| Gluten Free) ...... | 190 | 1.0 | 24.0 | 9.0 | 0 | 30 | 5.0 |
| dough (*Purely Decadent* | | | | | | | |
| Gluten Free) ...... | 230 | 1.0 | 36.0 | 8.0 | 0 | 75 | 5.0 |
| cookies and "cream" | | | | | | | |
| (*Organic So Delicious*) | 150 | 2.0 | 26.0 | 4.0 | 0 | 80 | 3.0 |
| dulce de leche: | | | | | | | |
| (*Organic So* | | | | | | | |
| *Delicious*) ........ | 140 | 1.0 | 26.0 | 3.0 | 0 | 130 | 2.0 |
| (*Purely Decadent*) .... | 170 | 1.0 | 34.0 | 6.0 | 0 | 90 | 5.0 |
| espresso (*It's Soy* | | | | | | | |
| *Delicious*) .......... | 115 | 2.0 | 23.0 | 1.5 | 0 | 130 | 2.0 |
| green tea: | | | | | | | |
| (*It's Soy Delicious*) ... | 110 | 2.0 | 24.0 | 1.5 | 0 | 130 | 2.0 |
| (*Soy Dream*) ........ | 170 | <1.0 | 21.0 | 9.0 | 0 | 150 | 1.0 |
| lime pie, key (*Purely* | | | | | | | |
| *Decadent*) .......... | 190 | 1.0 | 34.0 | 7.0 | 0 | 75 | 5.0 |
| mango (*Purely* | | | | | | | |
| *Decadent* Coconut | | | | | | | |
| Milk Passionate) ..... | 150 | 1.0 | 19.0 | 7.0 | 0 | 10 | 5.0 |

| Food and Measure | cal. | prot. (gms) | carbo. (gms) | fat (gms) | chol. (mgs) | sod. (mgs) | fiber (gms) |
|---|---|---|---|---|---|---|---|
| **"Ice cream," nondairy** *(cont.)* | | | | | | | |
| mango raspberry | | | | | | | |
| (*It's Soy Delicious*) . . . | 110 | 1.0 | 25.0 | 1.5 | 0 | 105 | 2.0 |
| mint, chunky (*Purely* | | | | | | | |
| *Decadent* Madness) . . | 200 | 2.0 | 35.0 | 8.0 | 0 | 30 | 6.0 |
| mint carob chip | | | | | | | |
| (*Rice Dream*) . . . . . . . | 180 | 0 | 28.0 | 7.0 | 0 | 85 | 0 |
| mint chocolate chip: | | | | | | | |
| (*Purely Decadent*) . . . . | 190 | 1.0 | 27.0 | 8.0 | 0 | 45 | 5.0 |
| (*Purely Decadent* | | | | | | | |
| Coconut Milk) . . . . | 170 | 1.0 | 20.0 | 9.0 | 0 | 5 | 6.0 |
| mint fudge, marble | | | | | | | |
| (*Organic So* | | | | | | | |
| *Delicious*) . . . . . . . . . | 140 | 1.0 | 27.0 | 3.0 | 0 | 55 | 2.0 |
| mocha fudge: | | | | | | | |
| (*Organic So Delicious*) | 130 | 2.0 | 26.0 | 3.0 | 0 | 85 | 3.0 |
| (*Soy Dream*) . . . . . . . . | 140 | 1.0 | 21.0 | 7.0 | 0 | 120 | <1.0 |
| almond (*Purely* | | | | | | | |
| *Decadent*) . . . . . . . . | 200 | 3.0 | 32.0 | 9.0 | 0 | 45 | 6.0 |
| almond (*Purely Decadent* | | | | | | | |
| Coconut Milk) . . . . | 180 | 2.0 | 21.0 | 9.0 | 0 | 30 | 5.0 |
| Neapolitan: | | | | | | | |
| (*Organic So Delicious*) | 120 | 2.0 | 23.0 | 3.5 | 0 | 55 | 2.0 |
| (*Rice Dream*) . . . . . . . | 160 | 0 | 26.0 | 6.0 | 0 | 80 | >1.0 |
| orange vanilla swirl | | | | | | | |
| (*Rice Dream*) . . . . . . . | 160 | 0 | 26.0 | 6.0 | 0 | 85 | 0 |
| peanut butter: | | | | | | | |
| (*Organic So Delicious*) | 150 | 3.0 | 23.0 | 6.0 | 0 | 80 | 3.0 |
| (*Purely Decadent* | | | | | | | |
| Zig Zag) . . . . . . . . . | 230 | 3.0 | 32.0 | 13.0 | 0 | 50 | 5.0 |
| pistachio almond | | | | | | | |
| (*It's Soy Delicious*) . . . | 130 | 3.0 | 23.0 | 4.5 | 0 | 200 | 3.0 |
| pomegranate chip | | | | | | | |
| (*Purely Decadent*) . . . . | 200 | 1.0 | 33.0 | 8.0 | 0 | 40 | 5.0 |
| praline pecan (*Purely* | | | | | | | |
| *Decadent*) . . . . . . . . . | 210 | 2.0 | 33.0 | 10.0 | 0 | 50 | 5.0 |
| raspberry: | | | | | | | |
| (*It's Soy Delicious*) . . . | 115 | 1.0 | 25.0 | 1.5 | 0 | 120 | 2.0 |
| à la mode (*Purely* | | | | | | | |
| *Decadent*) . . . . . . . . | 200 | 2.0 | 34.0 | 7.0 | 0 | 70 | 5.0 |
| rocky road (*Purely* | | | | | | | |
| *Decadent*) . . . . . . . . . | 190 | 2.0 | 31.0 | 8.0 | 0 | 85 | 5.0 |
| strawberry: | | | | | | | |
| (*Organic So Delicious*) | 120 | 1.0 | 23.0 | 3.0 | 0 | 55 | 3.0 |

| Food and Measure | cal. | prot. (gms) | carbo. (gms) | fat (gms) | chol. (mgs) | sod. (mgs) | fiber (gms) |
|---|---|---|---|---|---|---|---|
| (*Purely Decadent*) .... | 170 | 1.0 | 33.0 | 4.5 | 0 | 30 | 4.0 |
| (*Rice Dream*) ....... | 160 | 0 | 25.0 | 8.0 | 0 | 70 | 2.0 |
| cheesecake (*Tofutti*) .. | 200 | 2.0 | 20.0 | 12.0 | 0 | 200 | 0 |
| turtle (*Purely Decadent* Trails) ... | 200 | 1.0 | 31.0 | 8.0 | 0 | 85 | 5.0 |
| vanilla: | | | | | | | |
| (*It's Soy Delicious*) ... | 110 | 2.0 | 24.0 | 1.5 | 0 | 130 | 2.0 |
| (*Purely Decadent* Purely) .......... | 170 | 1.0 | 29.0 | 8.0 | 0 | 20 | 6.0 |
| (*Rice Dream*) ....... | 160 | 0 | 26.0 | 8.0 | 0 | 75 | 2.0 |
| (*Soy Dream*) ........ | 140 | 1.0 | 17.0 | 8.0 | 0 | 125 | <1.0 |
| (*Tofutti*) ........... | 210 | 2.0 | 21.0 | 13.0 | 0 | 130 | 0 |
| bean (*Purely Decadent* Coconut Milk) .... | 150 | 1.0 | 19.0 | 8.0 | 0 | 5 | 6.0 |
| creamy (*Organic So Delicious*) ........ | 130 | 1.0 | 24.0 | 3.0 | 0 | 55 | 3.0 |
| French (*Soy Dream*) .. | 140 | 1.0 | 17.0 | 8.0 | 0 | 125 | <1.0 |
| vanilla almond: | | | | | | | |
| bark (*Tofutti*) ........ | 240 | 2.0 | 24.0 | 15.0 | 0 | 210 | 0 |
| Swiss (*Purely Decadent*) ........ | 200 | 2.0 | 31.0 | 9.0 | 0 | 90 | 6.0 |
| Swiss (*Rice Dream*) .. | 180 | 1.0 | 27.0 | 9.0 | 0 | 70 | 2.0 |
| vanilla fudge: | | | | | | | |
| (*Tofutti*) ........... | 190 | 2.0 | 25.0 | 9.0 | 0 | 130 | 0 |
| swirl (*Soy Dream*) ... | 170 | <1.0 | 20.0 | 9.0 | 0 | 150 | 1.0 |
| vanilla orange (*Organic So Delicious* Twisted) . | 120 | 2.0 | 24.0 | 2.0 | 0 | 40 | 3.0 |
| **Ice cream bar** (see also "Iced confection bar"), 1 pc., except as noted: | | | | | | | |
| (*Ben & Jerry's Half Baked*) ............ | 360 | 5.0 | 46.0 | 18.0 | 50 | 150 | 2.0 |
| almond, toasted: | | | | | | | |
| (*Good Humor* Single) . | 240 | 2.0 | 30.0 | 12.0 | 10 | 40 | 1.0 |
| (*Good Humor* 6 Pack) . | 180 | 2.0 | 22.0 | 10.0 | 10 | 30 | 1.0 |
| brownie, fudge (*Ben & Jerry's*) ...... | 350 | 4.0 | 38.0 | 20.0 | 35 | 75 | 2.0 |
| candy center crunch (*Good Humor*) ...... | 300 | 3.0 | 27.0 | 21.0 | 10 | 75 | <1.0 |
| caramel, w/chocolate: | | | | | | | |
| (*Skinny Cow* Truffle) .. | 100 | 3.0 | 19.0 | 2.0 | 5 | 50 | 3.0 |
| pretzel chips (*Klondike*) ........ | 260 | 3.0 | 29.0 | 15.0 | 10 | 170 | 1.0 |

| Food and Measure | cal. | prot. (gms) | carbo. (gms) | fat (gms) | chol. (mgs) | sod. (mgs) | fiber (gms) |
|---|---|---|---|---|---|---|---|
| **Ice cream bar** *(cont.)* | | | | | | | |
| caramel cookie (*Twix* Single) .......... | 280 | 3.0 | 31.0 | 16.0 | 20 | 85 | 0 |
| cherry, w/chocolate: | | | | | | | |
| (*Ben & Jerry's* Cherry Garcia) .... | 270 | 4.0 | 28.0 | 19.0 | 35 | 35 | 1.0 |
| (*Klondike* Whitehouse) ...... | 250 | 3.0 | 31.0 | 14.0 | 10 | 75 | 1.0 |
| chocolate, w/chocolate: | | | | | | | |
| (*Klondike* Double) .... | 240 | 3.0 | 27.0 | 14.0 | 10 | 75 | 1.0 |
| dark (*Dove*) ......... | 330 | 2.0 | 33.0 | 21.0 | 30 | 40 | 3.0 |
| dark (*Häagen-Dazs*) .. | 290 | 4.0 | 24.0 | 20.0 | 65 | 30 | 2.0 |
| triple, chip (*Breyers* Smooth & Dreamy) | 130 | 2.0 | 17.0 | 6.0 | <5 | 45 | 1.0 |
| chocolate éclair: | | | | | | | |
| (*Good Humor* Single) . | 220 | 2.0 | 30.0 | 11.0 | 10 | 55 | 1.0 |
| (*Good Humor* 6 Pack) . | 160 | 2.0 | 21.0 | 8.0 | 5 | 35 | 1.0 |
| coffee, almond crunch (*Häagen-Dazs* Snack Size) ......... | 190 | 3.0 | 15.0 | 13.0 | 40 | 35 | <1.0 |
| cookie, *Oreo:* | | | | | | | |
| (*Good Humor* Single) . | 250 | 2.0 | 28.0 | 15.0 | 15 | 150 | 1.0 |
| (*Good Humor* 6 Pack) . | 190 | 2.0 | 21.0 | 11.0 | 10 | 75 | 1.0 |
| (*Klondike*) ........... | 250 | 3.0 | 29.0 | 15.0 | 10 | 115 | 1.0 |
| cookies and cream (*Good Humor* Single) . | 90 | 2.0 | 18.0 | 1.5 | 5 | 55 | 2.0 |
| mint, white, w/ chocolate (*Skinny Cow* Truffle) ........ | 100 | 3.0 | 19.0 | 2.0 | 5 | 45 | 3.0 |
| Neapolitan, w/ chocolate (*Klondike*) .. | 250 | 3.0 | 29.0 | 14.0 | 10 | 75 | 1.0 |
| peanut butter, *Reese's:* | | | | | | | |
| (*Good Humor*) ...... | 310 | 4.0 | 27.0 | 21.0 | 15 | 85 | 1.0 |
| (*Klondike*) .......... | 260 | 3.0 | 26.0 | 16.0 | 10 | 90 | 1.0 |
| strawberry, w/chocolate (*Breyers* Smooth & Dreamy) .......... | 120 | 2.0 | 17.0 | 4.5 | <5 | 45 | 0 |
| strawberry shortcake: | | | | | | | |
| (*Good Humor* Single) . | 230 | 2.0 | 31.0 | 12.0 | 10 | 55 | 1.0 |
| (*Good Humor* 6 Pack) . | 170 | 1.0 | 21.0 | 9.0 | 5 | 40 | 0 |
| toffee w/chocolate (*Klondike* Heath) ..... | 230 | 2.0 | 25.0 | 15.0 | 10 | 80 | <1.0 |
| vanilla w/chocolate: | | | | | | | |
| (*Breyers CarbSmart*) .. | 170 | 2.0 | 9.0 | 15.0 | 15 | 45 | 2.0 |

| Food and Measure | cal. | prot. (gms) | carbo. (gms) | fat (gms) | chol. (mgs) | sod. (mgs) | fiber (gms) |
|---|---|---|---|---|---|---|---|
| (*Good Humor*) ...... | 160 | 2.0 | 17.0 | 10.0 | 5 | 40 | 0 |
| (*Klondike* No Sugar) .. | 170 | 4.0 | 21.0 | 9.0 | 5 | 65 | 4.0 |
| (*Klondike* Original) ... | 250 | 3.0 | 29.0 | 14.0 | 10 | 55 | 1.0 |
| (*Klondike* Original | | | | | | | |
| Single) .......... | 290 | 3.0 | 35.0 | 17.0 | 15 | 85 | <1.0 |
| (*Klondike* 100 Calorie) | 100 | 1.0 | 11.0 | 6.0 | 5 | 20 | 2.0 |
| (*Skinny Cow* Truffle) .. | 100 | 3.0 | 19.0 | 2.0 | 5 | 50 | 3.0 |
| almonds (*Dove*) ..... | 340 | 6.0 | 28.0 | 23.0 | 35 | 135 | 1.0 |
| almonds (*Breyers* | | | | | | | |
| CarbSmart*) ....... | 180 | 3.0 | 9.0 | 15.0 | 15 | 40 | 2.0 |
| almonds (*Häagen-Dazs*) | 310 | 5.0 | 22.0 | 22.0 | 65 | 40 | <1.0 |
| almonds (*Häagen-* | | | | | | | |
| *Dazs* Snack Size) .. | 190 | 3.0 | 14.0 | 14.0 | 35 | 25 | <1.0 |
| caramel chip (*Breyers* | | | | | | | |
| Smooth & Dreamy) | 130 | 2.0 | 18.0 | 6.0 | 5 | 55 | 0 |
| dark (*Dove*) ......... | 330 | 4.0 | 31.0 | 21.0 | 35 | 40 | 2.0 |
| dark (*Häagen-Dazs*) .. | 300 | 4.0 | 23.0 | 21.0 | 70 | 45 | <1.0 |
| dark (*Klondike*) ...... | 250 | 3.0 | 29.0 | 14.0 | 10 | 55 | 1.0 |
| dark (*Turkey Hill*) .... | 320 | 3.0 | 26.0 | 23.0 | 25 | 40 | 2.0 |
| dark and milk (*Good* | | | | | | | |
| *Humor* 6 Pack) .... | 180 | 2.0 | 15.0 | 13.0 | 15 | 30 | 1.0 |
| milk (*Ben & Jerry's*) .. | 310 | 4.0 | 26.0 | 21.0 | 45 | 60 | 1.0 |
| milk (*Dove*) ......... | 330 | 4.0 | 31.0 | 21.0 | 35 | 40 | 2.0 |
| milk (*Häagen-Dazs*) .. | 290 | 4.0 | 22.0 | 21.0 | 75 | 55 | 0 |
| vanilla, chocolate crisps: | | | | | | | |
| (*Klondike* Krunch) .... | 250 | 3.0 | 30.0 | 14.0 | 10 | 55 | 1.0 |
| (*Klondike* Krunch | | | | | | | |
| No Sugar) ....... | 170 | 4.0 | 22.0 | 10.0 | 5 | 85 | 4.0 |
| (*Klondike* Krunch | | | | | | | |
| on a Stick) ....... | 250 | 3.0 | 27.0 | 15.0 | 10 | 75 | <1.0 |
| vanilla, French (*Skinny* | | | | | | | |
| *Cow* Truffle) ........ | 100 | 3.0 | 18.0 | 2.0 | 20 | 45 | 3.0 |
| vanilla or chocolate, | | | | | | | |
| chocolate coated | | | | | | | |
| (*Good Humor* Snack | | | | | | | |
| Pop 12 Pack), 2 pcs. . | 210 | 2.0 | 23.0 | 13.0 | 5 | 60 | 0 |
| **"Ice cream" bar, non-** | | | | | | | |
| **dairy** (see also | | | | | | | |
| "Iced confection | | | | | | | |
| bar"), 1 pc.: | | | | | | | |
| coconut almond (*So* | | | | | | | |
| *Delicious* Coconut | | | | | | | |
| Milk Minis) ......... | 170 | 0 | 15.0 | 10.0 | 0 | 10 | 3.0 |
| fudge (*Sweet Nothings*) . | 100 | 1.0 | 23.0 | 0 | 0 | 5 | 0 |

| Food and Measure | cal. | prot. (gms) | carbo. (gms) | fat (gms) | chol. (mgs) | sod. (mgs) | fiber (gms) |
|---|---|---|---|---|---|---|---|
| **"Ice cream" bar, nondairy** *(cont.)* | | | | | | | |
| mint (*Tofutti* Mint | | | | | | | |
| by Mintz!) . . . . . . . . . | 170 | 2.0 | 7.0 | 7.0 | 0 | 80 | 0 |
| vanilla, w/chocolate: | | | | | | | |
| (*Rice Dream*) . . . . . . . | 230 | 1.0 | 24.0 | 15.0 | 0 | 70 | <1.0 |
| (*So Delicious* | | | | | | | |
| Coconut Milk Minis) | 150 | 1.0 | 14.0 | 7.0 | 0 | 10 | 3.0 |
| (*Tofutti* Hooray | | | | | | | |
| Hooray No Sugar) . | 150 | 2.0 | 10.0 | 0 | 0 | 85 | 0 |
| (*Tofutti Marry Me*) . . . | 168 | 2.0 | 22.0 | 8.0 | 0 | 105 | 0 |
| w/nuts (*Rice Dream* | | | | | | | |
| Nutty Bar) . . . . . . . | 320 | 5.0 | 27.0 | 24.0 | 0 | 65 | 2.0 |
| **Ice cream bites**, | | | | | | | |
| chocolate coated: | | | | | | | |
| (*Dreyer's/Edy's* | | | | | | | |
| Dibs), 26 pcs.: | | | | | | | |
| chocolate . . . . . . . . . | 360 | 3.0 | 30.0 | 25.0 | 15 | 85 | 2.0 |
| mint . . . . . . . . . . . . . | 340 | 2.0 | 30.0 | 24.0 | 15 | 75 | 1.0 |
| *Nestlé Crunch* . . . . . . | 340 | 2.0 | 30.0 | 24.0 | 15 | 80 | 1.0 |
| *Nestlé Drumstick* . . . . | 350 | 2.0 | 30.0 | 25.0 | 15 | 75 | 0 |
| vanilla . . . . . . . . . . . . | 340 | 2.0 | 30.0 | 24.0 | 15 | 70 | 1.0 |
| all varieties (*BlissBites*), | | | | | | | |
| 2 pcs., 1.1 oz. . . . . . . | 100 | 1.0 | 9.0 | 7.0 | 10 | 15 | 0 |
| **"Ice cream" bites,** | | | | | | | |
| **nondairy**, vanilla, | | | | | | | |
| chocolate coated | | | | | | | |
| (*Rice Dream*), 15 pcs. . | 220 | 1.0 | 23.0 | 15.0 | 0 | 40 | 1.0 |
| **Ice cream cake** | | | | | | | |
| (*Turkey Hill*): | | | | | | | |
| 8" round, 1/12 cake . . . . . . | 270 | 3.0 | 30.0 | 16.0 | 25 | 130 | 0 |
| 6" round, 1/8 cake . . . . . . . | 300 | 3.0 | 31.0 | 18.0 | 30 | 150 | 0 |
| sheet, 1/16 cake . . . . . . . . . | 270 | 3.0 | 30.0 | 16.0 | 20 | 130 | 0 |
| **Ice cream cone**, filled, | | | | | | | |
| 1 pc.: | | | | | | | |
| (*Good Humor King* | | | | | | | |
| *Cone* Single) . . . . . . . . | 250 | 4.0 | 30.0 | 13.0 | 15 | 100 | 1.0 |
| caramel swirl | | | | | | | |
| (*Drumstick Lil' Drums*) | 110 | 1.0 | 16.0 | 5.0 | 5 | 60 | 0 |
| chocolate: | | | | | | | |
| chocolate swirl (*Drum-* | | | | | | | |
| *stick Lil' Drums*) . . . | 140 | 2.0 | 17.0 | 7.0 | 10 | 60 | 0 |
| w/fudge (*Skinny Cow*) | 150 | 4.0 | 29.0 | 3.0 | 5 | 95 | 3.0 |
| chocolate, triple: | | | | | | | |
| (*Drumstick King*) . . . . | 390 | 5.0 | 46.0 | 21.0 | 40 | 140 | 2.0 |

| Food and Measure | cal. | prot. (gms) | carbo. (gms) | fat (gms) | chol. (mgs) | sod. (mgs) | fiber (gms) |
|---|---|---|---|---|---|---|---|
| brownie (*Good Humor King Cone*) . | 420 | 6.0 | 58.0 | 19.0 | 30 | 110 | 2.0 |
| chocolate fudge brownie (*Drumstick Lil' Drums*) . . . . . . . . . . . | 140 | 1.0 | 18.0 | 7.0 | 5 | 60 | 0 |
| chocolate sundae (*Drumstick* Classic) . . | 310 | 5.0 | 34.0 | 17.0 | 15 | 115 | 2.0 |
| cookie dough (*Drumstick Lil' Drums*) | 140 | 1.0 | 18.0 | 7.0 | 5 | 60 | 0 |
| cookies and cream (*Drumstick Simply Dipped*) . . . . . . . . . . . | 300 | 3.0 | 39.0 | 14.0 | 15 | 115 | 1.0 |
| mint: (*Drumstick Simply Dipped*) . . . . . . . . . | 290 | 3.0 | 38.0 | 14.0 | 15 | 115 | 0 |
| w/fudge (*Skinny Cow*) | 150 | 4.0 | 29.0 | 3.0 | 5 | 90 | 3.0 |
| s'mores (*Drumstick Lil' Drums*) . . . . . . . | 110 | 1.0 | 16.0 | 5.0 | 5 | 60 | 0 |
| sundae (*Good Humor King Cone*) . . . . . . . . . | 260 | 4.0 | 29.0 | 15.0 | 15 | 80 | 1.0 |
| vanilla, w/caramel (*Skinny Cow*) . . . . . . . | 150 | 4.0 | 29.0 | 3.0 | 5 | 80 | 3.0 |
| vanilla, w/chocolate: (*Drumstick Simply Dipped*) | 270 | 2.0 | 37.0 | 13.0 | 15 | 115 | 1.0 |
| swirls (*Drumstick King*) . . . . . . . . . . | 390 | 4.0 | 45.0 | 21.0 | 20 | 140 | 1.0 |
| swirls (*Drumstick Lil' Drums*) . . . . . . . | 140 | 2.0 | 17.0 | 7.0 | 10 | 60 | 1.0 |
| vanilla chocolate (*Good Humor King Cone*) . . . | 390 | 7.0 | 44.0 | 31.0 | 30 | 135 | 1.0 |
| vanilla sundae: (*Drumstick* Classic) . . | 290 | 4.0 | 33.0 | 16.0 | 15 | 100 | 2.0 |
| caramel (*Drumstick*) . . | 320 | 4.0 | 37.0 | 17.0 | 15 | 125 | 2.0 |
| fudge (*Drumstick*) . . . | 310 | 5.0 | 37.0 | 16.0 | 15 | 100 | 2.0 |
| fudge (*Turkey Hill*) . . . | 320 | 6.0 | 33.0 | 18.0 | 20 | 120 | 2.0 |
| **Ice cream cone/cup**, unfilled, 1 pc.: | | | | | | | |
| bowl or cone, waffle (*Keebler*) . . . . . . . . . . | 50 | <1.0 | 10.0 | 1.0 | 0 | 25 | 0 |
| cone: chocolate (*Oreo*) . . . . . | 60 | 1.0 | 12.0 | .5 | 0 | 75 | 0 |
| sugar (*Comet*) . . . . . . | 50 | 1.0 | 11.0 | 0 | 0 | 20 | 0 |
| sugar (*Keebler*) . . . . . . | 50 | 1.0 | 10.0 | .5 | 0 | 55 | 0 |

| Food and Measure | cal. | prot. (gms) | carbo. (gms) | fat (gms) | chol. (mgs) | sod. (mgs) | fiber (gms) |
|---|---|---|---|---|---|---|---|
| **Ice cream cone/cup** *(cont.)* | | | | | | | |
| cup: | | | | | | | |
| (*Comet*) .......... | 20 | 0 | 4.0 | 0 | 0 | 10 | 0 |
| (*Keebler*) .......... | 15 | 0 | 4.0 | 0 | 0 | 20 | 0 |
| fudge dipped (*Keebler* | | | | | | | |
| *Fudge Shoppe*) .... | 40 | 0 | 6.0 | 1.5 | 0 | 10 | 0 |
| rainbow (*Comet*) .... | 20 | 0 | 4.0 | 0 | 1 | 10 | 0 |
| **Ice cream dessert** | | | | | | | |
| (*Smart Ones*), | | | | | | | |
| 1 serving: | | | | | | | |
| brownie à la mode ...... | 200 | 5.0 | 36.0 | 4.0 | 25 | 160 | 3.0 |
| sundae: | | | | | | | |
| chocolate chip cookie | | | | | | | |
| dough ........... | 170 | 3.0 | 32.0 | 3.0 | 5 | 100 | 1.0 |
| mint chocolate chip .. | 150 | 4.0 | 28.0 | 3.0 | 5 | 130 | 1.0 |
| mocha fudge ....... | 160 | 3.0 | 27.0 | 4.0 | 5 | 85 | 1.0 |
| peanut butter cup .... | 170 | 4.0 | 28.0 | 5.0 | 5 | 90 | 3.0 |
| **Ice cream pie**, see | | | | | | | |
| "Ice cream sandwich" | | | | | | | |
| **Ice cream sandwich**, | | | | | | | |
| w/chocolate wafers, | | | | | | | |
| except as noted, | | | | | | | |
| 1 pc: | | | | | | | |
| (*Klondike Choco Taco*) .. | 290 | 4.0 | 36.0 | 15.0 | 10 | 120 | 1.0 |
| brownie sandwich: | | | | | | | |
| chocolate caramel | | | | | | | |
| (*Breyers* Smooth | | | | | | | |
| & Dreamy) ....... | 160 | 3.0 | 30.0 | 4.0 | <5 | 160 | 3.0 |
| vanilla fudge | | | | | | | |
| (*Breyers* Smooth & | | | | | | | |
| Dreamy) ......... | 160 | 3.0 | 30.0 | 4.0 | <5 | 150 | 4.0 |
| chocolate (*Klondike*) .... | 100 | 2.0 | 21.0 | 1.5 | 0 | 65 | 3.0 |
| chocolate chip: | | | | | | | |
| (*Klondike Oreo*) ..... | 200 | 3.0 | 34.0 | 7.0 | 5 | 250 | <1.0 |
| (*Klondike Oreo* | | | | | | | |
| Single) .......... | 220 | 4.0 | 37.0 | 7.0 | 5 | 260 | 2.0 |
| chocolate chip cookie: | | | | | | | |
| (*Breyers* Smooth & | | | | | | | |
| Dreamy) ......... | 160 | 3.0 | 30.0 | 4.0 | <5 | 115 | 1.0 |
| (*Good Humor*) ....... | 270 | 3.0 | 44.0 | 10.0 | 5 | 200 | 1.0 |
| (*Good Humor* Variety | | | | | | | |
| Pack) ........... | 130 | 2.0 | 26.0 | 2.0 | 5 | 90 | 1.0 |
| (*Klondike Mrs.* | | | | | | | |
| *Field's*) .......... | 220 | 3.0 | 35.0 | 8.0 | 5 | 150 | <1.0 |

| Food and Measure | cal. | prot. (gms) | carbo. (gms) | fat (gms) | chol. (mgs) | sod. (mgs) | fiber (gms) |
|---|---|---|---|---|---|---|---|
| cookies and cream | | | | | | | |
| (*Skinny Cow*) ....... | 150 | 4.0 | 31.0 | 2.0 | 3 | 105 | 3.0 |
| mint (*Skinny Cow*) ..... | 140 | 4.0 | 30.0 | 2.0 | 1 | 95 | 3.0 |
| Neapolitan (*Good* | | | | | | | |
| *Humor* Giant) ....... | 250 | 4.0 | 38.0 | 9.0 | 20 | 130 | 1.0 |
| peanut butter: | | | | | | | |
| chocolate (*Klondike*) .. | 210 | 4.0 | 33.0 | 7.0 | 5 | 170 | 1.0 |
| chocolate (*Skinny* | | | | | | | |
| *Cow*) ........... | 150 | 3.0 | 30.0 | 2.0 | 5 | 100 | 3.0 |
| strawberry cheesecake, | | | | | | | |
| vanilla wafer (*Turkey* | | | | | | | |
| *Hill*) .............. | 190 | 3.0 | 30.0 | 7.0 | 20 | 130 | 1.0 |
| strawberry shortcake, | | | | | | | |
| vanilla wafer (*Skinny* | | | | | | | |
| *Cow*) ............. | 150 | 4.0 | 30.0 | 2.0 | 5 | 120 | 3.0 |
| vanilla: | | | | | | | |
| (*Good Humor*) ...... | 160 | 2.0 | 26.0 | 5.0 | 10 | 90 | 0 |
| (*Good Humor* Giant) .. | 250 | 4.0 | 38.0 | 9.0 | 20 | 125 | 1.0 |
| (*Good Humor* Low Fat) | 130 | 2.0 | 26.0 | 2.0 | 5 | 80 | 2.0 |
| (*Healthy Choice*) ..... | 150 | 4.0 | 30.0 | 1.5 | 5 | 120 | 0 |
| (*Klondike* Classic) .... | 180 | 3.0 | 31.0 | 4.5 | 10 | 150 | <1.0 |
| (*Klondike* Classic | | | | | | | |
| Single) .......... | 260 | 5.0 | 50.0 | 5.0 | 10 | 170 | 1.0 |
| (*Klondike* No Sugar) .. | 100 | 3.0 | 20.0 | 2.0 | <5 | 90 | 2.0 |
| (*Skinny Cow*) ....... | 140 | 4.0 | 30.0 | 2.0 | 1 | 95 | 3.0 |
| (*Skinny Cow* No Sugar) | 140 | 4.0 | 30.0 | 2.0 | 15 | 115 | 3.0 |
| (*Turkey Hill* Single) ... | 240 | 3.0 | 33.0 | 11.0 | 30 | 30 | 0 |
| bean (*Turkey Hill*) .... | 190 | 3.0 | 29.0 | 7.0 | 20 | 95 | 1.0 |
| bean (*Turkey Hill* | | | | | | | |
| Light) ........... | 160 | 3.0 | 32.0 | 3.0 | 10 | 95 | 3.0 |
| vanilla, w/cookies (*Turkey* | | | | | | | |
| *Hill* Moose Tracks) ... | 320 | 4.0 | 41.0 | 17.0 | 30 | 150 | 2.0 |
| vanilla and chocolate: | | | | | | | |
| (*Skinny Cow*) ....... | 140 | 4.0 | 30.0 | 2.0 | 5 | 135 | 3.0 |
| (*Turkey Hill* Double | | | | | | | |
| Decker) .......... | 190 | 3.0 | 30.0 | 7.0 | 20 | 105 | 1.0 |
| **"Ice cream" sandwich,** | | | | | | | |
| **nondairy**, w/chocolate | | | | | | | |
| wafers, except as noted, | | | | | | | |
| 1 pc.: | | | | | | | |
| banana split (*So* | | | | | | | |
| *Delicious* Coconut | | | | | | | |
| Milk Minis) .......... | 100 | 1.0 | 15.0 | 3.5 | 0 | 50 | 2.0 |

| Food and Measure | cal. | prot. (gms) | carbo. (gms) | fat (gms) | chol. (mgs) | sod. (mgs) | fiber (gms) |
|---|---|---|---|---|---|---|---|
| **"Ice cream" sandwich, nondairy** *(cont.)* | | | | | | | |
| berry, wild (*Tofutti Cuties*) | 130 | 2.0 | 17.0 | 5.0 | 0 | 121 | 0 |
| chocolate: | | | | | | | |
| (*Organic So Delicious* Low Fat) . . . . . . . . | 160 | 3.0 | 27.0 | 3.0 | 0 | 105 | 2.0 |
| (*Rice Dream* Pie) . . . . | 330 | 3.0 | 40.0 | 19.0 | 0 | 50 | 2.0 |
| (*So Delicious*) . . . . . . . | 150 | 3.0 | 27.0 | 3.0 | 0 | 105 | 2.0 |
| (*So Delicious* Mini) . . . | 90 | 2.0 | 17.0 | 2.0 | 0 | 70 | 1.0 |
| (*Tofutti Cuties*) . . . . . . | 130 | 2.0 | 16.0 | 6.0 | 0 | 110 | 0 |
| chocolate chip, milk (*Tofutti Cuties*) . . . . . . | 130 | 2.0 | 19.0 | 6.0 | 0 | 110 | 0 |
| coconut (*So Delicious* Coconut Milk Minis) . . | 100 | 1.0 | 15.0 | 3.5 | 0 | 50 | 2.0 |
| coffee (*Tofutti Cuties* Coffee Break*) . . . . . . . | 130 | 2.0 | 16.0 | 6.0 | 0 | 110 | 0 |
| cookies and cream (*Tofutti Cuties*) . . . . . . | 130 | 1.0 | 11.0 | 6.0 | 0 | 860 | 0 |
| lime pie, Key (*Tofutti Cuties*) . . . . . . | 130 | 2.0 | 17.0 | 6.0 | 0 | 121 | 0 |
| mint: | | | | | | | |
| (*Organic So Delicious*) | 150 | 3.0 | 28.0 | 3.0 | 0 | 125 | 2.0 |
| (*Rice Dream* Pie) . . . . | 330 | 3.0 | 40.0 | 19.0 | 0 | 50 | 2.0 |
| mocha (*Rice Dream* Pie) . | 330 | 3.0 | 40.0 | 18.0 | 0 | 50 | 2.0 |
| Neapolitan: | | | | | | | |
| (*Organic So Delicious*) | 150 | 3.0 | 28.0 | 3.0 | 0 | 110 | 2.0 |
| (*Organic So Delicious* Mini) . . . . . . . . . . | 90 | 2.0 | 18.0 | 2.0 | 0 | 70 | 2.0 |
| peanut butter (*Tofutti Cuties*) . . . . . . . . . . . . | 130 | 3.0 | 20.0 | 8.0 | 0 | 135 | 0 |
| pomegranate (*So Delicious* Minis) . . . . . | 90 | 2.0 | 18.0 | 2.0 | 0 | 75 | 1.0 |
| strawberry (*Tofutti Cuties* Wave) . . . . . . . | 140 | 2.0 | 20.0 | 6.0 | 0 | 130 | 0 |
| vanilla: | | | | | | | |
| (*Organic So Delicious*) | 150 | 3.0 | 28.0 | 3.0 | 0 | 105 | 2.0 |
| (*Rice Dream* Pie) . . . . | 320 | 3.0 | 40.0 | 17.0 | 0 | 80 | 1.0 |
| (*So Delicious*) . . . . . . . | 150 | 3.0 | 28.0 | 3.0 | 0 | 105 | 2.0 |
| (*So Delicious* Mini) . . . | 90 | 2.0 | 17.0 | 2.0 | 0 | 70 | 1.0 |
| (*Soy Dream* Li'l Dreamers) . . . . . . . | 100 | 1.0 | 15.0 | 4.0 | 0 | 60 | 0 |
| (*Tofutti Cuties*) . . . . . . | 130 | 2.0 | 17.0 | 6.0 | 0 | 121 | 0 |
| **Ice cream and sherbet or sorbet**, see "Sherbet" and "Sorbet bar" | | | | | | | |

| Food and Measure | cal. | prot. (gms) | carbo. (gms) | fat (gms) | chol. (mgs) | sod. (mgs) | fiber (gms) |
|---|---|---|---|---|---|---|---|
| **Ice cream topping**, see specific flavors | | | | | | | |
| **Iced confection bar**, dairy (see also "'Ice cream' bar, nondairy" and "Fruit bar, frozen"), 1 pc., except as noted: | | | | | | | |
| coffee (*Tofutti Coffee Break Treats*) . . . . . . . | 30 | 1.0 | 6.0 | 0 | 0 | 85 | 0 |
| fudge: | | | | | | | |
| (*Breyers CarbSmart*) . . | 100 | 2.0 | 9.0 | 7.0 | 20 | 50 | 1.0 |
| (*Fudgsicle* 2.5 oz.) . . . | 100 | 2.0 | 19.0 | 2.5 | 0 | 80 | 1.0 |
| (*Fudgsicle* Fat Free) . . | 60 | 2.0 | 13.0 | 0 | 0 | 60 | 1.0 |
| (*Fudgsicle* Low Fat) . | 60 | 1.0 | 12.0 | 1.5 | 0 | 55 | 0 |
| (*Fudgsicle* No Sugar) . | 40 | 2.0 | 10.0 | 1.0 | 0 | 50 | 2.0 |
| (*Healthy Choice*) . . . . . | 80 | 3.0 | 13.0 | 1.5 | 5 | 65 | 4.0 |
| (*Skinny Cow*) . . . . . . . | 100 | 4.0 | 22.0 | 1.0 | 3 | 45 | 4.0 |
| (*Tofutti* Totally) . . . . . . | 95 | 1.0 | 19.0 | 1.5 | 0 | 53 | 0 |
| (*Tofutti* Treats) . . . . . . | 30 | 1.0 | 6.0 | 1.5 | 0 | 86 | 0 |
| mini (*Skinny Cow* Pops), 2 pcs. . . . . . | 100 | 3.0 | 19.0 | 2.0 | 5 | 35 | 1.0 |
| triple (*Fudgsicle* Low Fat) . . . . . . . . . . . . . | 60 | 1.0 | 11.0 | 1.5 | 0 | 60 | 0 |
| orange sherbet: | | | | | | | |
| (*Cool Tubes*) . . . . . . . . | 110 | 0 | 24.0 | 1.0 | 5 | 30 | 0 |
| (*Popsicle Pop-Ups*) . . | 90 | 1.0 | 18.0 | 1.0 | 5 | 20 | 0 |
| orange sherbet/vanilla ice cream: | | | | | | | |
| (*Creamsicle* 2.5 oz.) . . | 110 | 1.0 | 21.0 | 2.0 | 5 | 40 | 0 |
| (*Creamsicle* Low Fat) . | 70 | <1.0 | 13.0 | 1.0 | <5 | 20 | 0 |
| (*Creamsicle* No Sugar), 2 pcs. . . . . . . . . . . | 40 | 1.0 | 10.0 | 2.0 | 0 | 5 | 6.0 |
| **Icing**, see "Frosting" | | | | | | | |
| ***In-N-Out Burger:*** | | | | | | | |
| hamburger w/onion . . . . . | 390 | 16.0 | 39.0 | 19.0 | 40 | 650 | 3.0 |
| w/mustard/ketchup . . . | 310 | 16.0 | 41.0 | 10.0 | 35 | 730 | 3.0 |
| protein, w/lettuce . . . . | 240 | 13.0 | 11.0 | 17.0 | 40 | 370 | 3.0 |
| cheeseburger w/onion . . | 480 | 22.0 | 39.0 | 27.0 | 60 | 1000 | 3.0 |
| w/mustard/ketchup . . . | 400 | 22.0 | 41.0 | 18.0 | 60 | 1080 | 3.0 |
| protein, w/lettuce . . . . | 330 | 18.0 | 11.0 | 25.0 | 60 | 720 | 3.0 |
| double-double w/onion . . | 670 | 37.0 | 39.0 | 41.0 | 120 | 1440 | 3.0 |
| w/mustard/ketchup . . . | 590 | 37.0 | 41.0 | 32.0 | 115 | 1520 | 3.0 |
| protein, w/lettuce . . . . | 520 | 33.0 | 11.0 | 39.0 | 40 | 1160 | 3.0 |

| Food and Measure | cal. | prot. (gms) | carbo. (gms) | fat (gms) | chol. (mgs) | sod. (mgs) | fiber (gms) |
|---|---|---|---|---|---|---|---|
| **In-N-Out Burger** (cont.) | | | | | | | |
| fries ................ | 395 | 7.0 | 54.0 | 18.0 | 0 | 245 | 2.0 |
| shake, chocolate ....... | 590 | 10.0 | 72.0 | 29.0 | 15 | 320 | 0 |
| shake, strawberry ...... | 590 | 8.0 | 81.0 | 27.0 | 15 | 270 | 0 |
| shake, vanilla ......... | 580 | 10.0 | 67.0 | 31.0 | 20 | 300 | 0 |
| **Italian sub**, frozen (*Stouffer's Corner Bistro* Zesty), 6 oz. ... | 470 | 20.0 | 40.0 | 25.0 | 50 | 980 | 3.0 |

# J

| Food and Measure | cal. | prot. (gms) | carbo. (gms) | fat (gms) | chol. (mgs) | sod. (mgs) | fiber (gms) |
|---|---|---|---|---|---|---|---|
| **Jackfruit**, fresh, trimmed, 1 oz. | 27 | .4 | 6.8 | .1 | 0 | 1 | .5 |
| **Jackfruit, canned**, in syrup, ½ cup | 82 | .3 | 21.3 | .1 | 0 | 10 | .8 |
| **Jalapeño**, see "Pepper, jalapeno" | | | | | | | |
| **Jalapeño raspberry sauce** (*Fiesta*), 2 tbsp. | 20 | 4.0 | 3.0 | 1.0 | 0 | 220 | 6.0 |
| **Jalapeño spread**, see "Pepper spread" | | | | | | | |
| **Jam and preserves** (see also "Fruit spreads"), 1 tbsp.: | | | | | | | |
| all fruits: | | | | | | | |
| (*Knott's Berry Farm*) | 50 | 0 | 13.0 | 0 | 0 | 0 | 0 |
| (*Knott's Berry Farm* Light) | 20 | 0 | 5.0 | 0 | 0 | 0 | 0 |
| (*Polaner*) | 50 | 0 | 13.0 | 0 | 0 | 0 | 0 |
| (*Smucker's*) | 50 | 0 | 13.0 | 0 | 0 | 0 | 0 |
| (*Smucker's* Low Sugar) | 25 | 0 | 6.0 | 0 | 0 | 0 | 0 |
| (*Smucker's* No Sugar) | 10 | 0 | 5.0 | 0 | 0 | 0 | 0 |
| blackberry guava daiquiri (*Campagna*) | 45 | 0 | 11.0 | 0 | 0 | 0 | 0 |
| grape: | | | | | | | |
| (*Welch's*) | 50 | 0 | 13.0 | 0 | 0 | 10 | 0 |
| (*Welch's* Less Sugar) | 20 | 0 | 5.0 | 0 | 0 | 15 | 0 |
| orange marmalade (*Crosse & Blackwell*) | 50 | 0 | 13.0 | 0 | 0 | 5 | 0 |
| raspberry, brandied (*Campagna*) | 40 | 0 | 10.0 | 0 | 0 | 0 | 0 |

| Food and Measure | cal. | prot. (gms) | carbo. (gms) | fat (gms) | chol. (mgs) | sod. (mgs) | fiber (gms) |
|---|---|---|---|---|---|---|---|
| **Jambalaya entree**, frozen, 1 pkg., except as noted: (*Contessa On the Stove*), ⅓ pkg.: | | | | | | | |
| w/sauce, 8 oz. ....... | 240 | 15.0 | 29.0 | 7.0 | 45 | 900 | 3.0 |
| w/out sauce, 6 oz. ... | 190 | 14.0 | 25.0 | 4.0 | 45 | 370 | 2.0 |
| chicken flavor (*Zatarain's*), 12 oz. ... | 400 | 18.0 | 69.0 | 5.0 | 30 | 1440 | 2.0 |
| pasta, w/chicken and sausage (*Zatarain's*), 10.5 oz. ........... | 380 | 16.0 | 56.0 | 10.0 | 25 | 930 | 4.0 |
| sausage flavor (*Zatarain's*), 12 oz. ... | 500 | 13.0 | 79.0 | 14.0 | 25 | 1020 | 3.0 |
| shrimp, turkey sausage (*Cedarlane*), 10 oz. ... | 290 | 15.0 | 38.0 | 7.0 | 85 | 700 | 2.0 |
| **Java plum**: | | | | | | | |
| 3 medium, .4 oz. ....... | 5 | .1 | 1.4 | <.1 | 0 | 1 | <1.0 |
| seeded, ½ cup ......... | 41 | .5 | 10.5 | .2 | 0 | 9 | <1.0 |
| **Jelly**, fruit, 1 tbsp.: all fruits: | | | | | | | |
| (*Polaner*) .......... | 50 | 0 | 13.0 | 0 | 0 | 5 | 0 |
| (*Smucker's*) ........ | 50 | 0 | 13.0 | 0 | 0 | 0 | 0 |
| apple mint or guava (*Crosse & Blackwell*) . | 50 | 0 | 13.0 | 0 | 0 | 0 | 0 |
| currant, red (*Crosse & Blackwell*) ........ | 50 | 0 | 13.0 | 0 | 0 | 5 | 0 |
| **Jelly, hot pepper** (*Campagna*), 1 tbsp. ... | 50 | 0 | 13.0 | 0 | 0 | 0 | 0 |
| **Jelly, wine**: all wines (*Campagna*), 1 tbsp. ............ | 40 | 0 | 10.0 | 0 | 0 | 0 | 0 |
| balsamic (*Roland*), 1 oz. . | 61 | 0 | 12.8 | .0 | 0 | 0 | 0 |
| Chardonnay or Marsala (*Roland*), 1 oz. ...... | 64 | 0 | 15.6 | 0 | 0 | 0 | 0 |
| Chianti or Merlot (*Roland*), 1 oz. ...... | 62 | 0 | 13.0 | 0 | 0 | 0 | 0 |
| **Jerk sauce**, see "Barbecue sauce" and "Marinade" | | | | | | | |
| **Jerk spice paste** (*Neera's* Jamaican), 2 tsp. ............. | 15 | 1.0 | 4.0 | 0 | 0 | 290 | 1.0 |

| Food and Measure | cal. | prot. (gms) | carbo. (gms) | fat (gms) | chol. (mgs) | sod. (mgs) | fiber (gms) |
|---|---|---|---|---|---|---|---|
| **Jerusalem artichoke**: | | | | | | | |
| (*Frieda's Sunchoke*), | | | | | | | |
| ½ cup, 2.6 oz. ....... | 55 | 2.0 | 13.0 | 0 | 0 | 3 | 1.0 |
| sliced, ½ cup ......... | 57 | 1.5 | 13.1 | <.1 | 0 | 3 | 1.2 |
| **Jew's ear**, see "Pepeao" | | | | | | | |
| **Jicama**, see "Yam | | | | | | | |
| bean" | | | | | | | |
| ***Jimmy John's:*** | | | | | | | |
| 8" sub sandwich: | | | | | | | |
| #1 *Pepe* ........... | 617 | 27.9 | 50.1 | 30.8 | 55 | 1262 | .9 |
| #2 *Big John* ........ | 533 | 25.9 | 48.6 | 23.9 | 49 | 1014 | .9 |
| #3 *Totally Tuna* ...... | 648 | 32.9 | 54.1 | 30.8 | 57 | 1592 | 2.8 |
| #4 *Turkey Tom* ...... | 515 | 24.4 | 50.3 | 21.3 | 38 | 1094 | 1.3 |
| #5 *Vito* ............ | 600 | 30.0 | 51.7 | 28.4 | 64 | 1377 | 1.2 |
| #6 vegetarian ........ | 578 | 19.3 | 52.5 | 30.1 | 50 | 873 | 1.6 |
| *J.J.B.L.T.* ............. | 634 | 25.4 | 48.6 | 35.2 | 40 | 1329 | .9 |
| giant club sandwich: | | | | | | | |
| #7 gourmet smoked | | | | | | | |
| ham club ........ | 775 | 41.5 | 68.8 | 32.4 | 82 | 1877 | .9 |
| #8 *Billy Club* ....... | 799 | 47.0 | 68.2 | 34.1 | 95 | 1958 | 1.1 |
| #9 *Italian Night Club* .. | 951 | 43.6 | 70.4 | 51.0 | 100 | 2166 | 1.2 |
| #10 *Hunter's Club* .... | 807 | 51.7 | 66.7 | 34.8 | 108 | 1781 | .9 |
| #11 *Country Club* .... | 768 | 44.4 | 68.8 | 31.3 | 84 | 1908 | .9 |
| #12 *Beach Club* ..... | 729 | 35.8 | 71.2 | 30.7 | 78 | 1519 | 1.6 |
| #13 *Gourmet Veggie* | | | | | | | |
| *Club* ............ | 773 | 30.4 | 70.6 | 38.1 | 70 | 1235 | 1.6 |
| #14 *Bootlegger Club* .. | 684 | 42.3 | 67.3 | 24.5 | 77 | 1660 | .9 |
| #15 *Club Tuna* ...... | 843 | 44.0 | 72.2 | 38.8 | 77 | 1954 | 2.8 |
| #16 *Club Lulu* ....... | 755 | 39.6 | 67.3 | 33.3 | 63 | 1855 | .9 |
| #17 *Ultimate Porker* .. | 763 | 36.9 | 67.2 | 39.3 | 61 | 1751 | 5.9 |
| plain slims: | | | | | | | |
| 1: ham & cheese ..... | 508 | 31.3 | 65.5 | 9.6 | 46 | 1244 | 0 |
| 2: roast beef ........ | 424 | 29.4 | 64.0 | 2.8 | 39 | 996 | 0 |
| 3: tuna salad ........ | 722 | 35.4 | 67.8 | 30.5 | 57 | 1746 | 1.2 |
| 4: turkey breast ...... | 401 | 27.2 | 65.1 | .6 | 28 | 1075 | 0 |
| 5: salami, capicola, | | | | | | | |
| cheese .......... | 599 | 33.2 | 65.6 | 19.8 | 64 | 1450 | 0 |
| 6: double provolone .. | 545 | 28.8 | 65.0 | 16.0 | 40 | 991 | 0 |
| *The J.J. Gargantuan* .... | 991 | 66.5 | 53.8 | 54.3 | 167 | 2893 | 1.2 |
| real potato chips: | | | | | | | |
| regular, 1.1 oz. ...... | 160 | 2.0 | 18.0 | 8.0 | 0 | 80 | 0 |
| BBQ, 1.1 oz. ........ | 160 | 2.0 | 17.0 | 9.0 | 0 | 90 | 0 |
| jalapeño, 1.1 oz. ..... | 150 | 2.0 | 18.0 | 7.0 | 0 | 290 | .5 |

| Food and Measure | cal. | prot. (gms) | carbo. (gms) | fat (gms) | chol. (mgs) | sod. (mgs) | fiber (gms) |
|---|---|---|---|---|---|---|---|
| ***Jimmy John's*, real potato chips** *(cont.)* | | | | | | | |
| sea salt vinegar, 1.1 oz. | 140 | 2.0 | 16.0 | 8.0 | 0 | 280 | 0 |
| skinny chips, 1 oz. ... | 130 | 2.0 | 19.0 | 5.0 | 0 | 105 | 2.0 |
| pickle, whole .......... | 22 | 1.1 | 4.4 | 0 | 0 | 2314 | 4.4 |
| cookie: | | | | | | | |
| chocolate chunk ..... | 421 | 5.1 | 62.3 | 17.8 | 51 | 427 | 1.4 |
| raisin oatmeal ....... | 421 | 7.0 | 65.0 | 15.8 | 66 | 471 | 3.9 |
| **Jujube**: | | | | | | | |
| raw, seeded, 1 oz. ...... | 22 | .3 | 5.7 | .1 | 0 | 1 | n.a. |
| dried, 1 oz. ........... | 81 | 1.0 | 20.1 | .3 | 0 | 3 | n.a. |
| **Jute**, potherb, ½ cup: | | | | | | | |
| raw ................. | 5 | .7 | .8 | <.1 | 0 | 1 | n.a. |
| boiled, drained ........ | 16 | 1.6 | 3.1 | .1 | 0 | 5 | .9 |

# K

| Food and Measure | cal. | prot. (gms) | carbo. (gms) | fat (gms) | chol. (mgs) | sod. (mgs) | fiber (gms) |
|---|---|---|---|---|---|---|---|
| **Kabocha squash** | | | | | | | |
| (*Frieda's*), 3 oz. ...... | 30 | 1.0 | 7.0 | 0 | 0 | 0 | 1.0 |
| **Kale**, fresh: | | | | | | | |
| (*Glory*), ⅕ pkg., | | | | | | | |
|   2.8 oz. ............ | 40 | 3.0 | 8.0 | .5 | 0 | 35 | 2.0 |
| raw, chopped, ½ cup ... | 17 | 1.1 | 3.4 | .2 | 0 | 15 | .7 |
| boiled, drained, | | | | | | | |
|   chopped, ½ cup ..... | 18 | 1.2 | 3.7 | .3 | 0 | 5 | 3.6 |
| **Kale, canned**, ½ cup: | | | | | | | |
| (*Allens* No Salt) ........ | 30 | 2.0 | 3.0 | .5 | 0 | 20 | 2.0 |
| chopped (*Bush's*) ...... | 30 | 2.0 | 4.0 | 0 | 0 | 330 | 2.0 |
| seasoned, Southern: | | | | | | | |
|   (*Allens*) ............ | 30 | 2.0 | 5.0 | 0 | 0 | 380 | 3.0 |
|   (*Glory*) ............ | 35 | 2.0 | 5.0 | .5 | 5 | 490 | 1.0 |
|   (*Sunshine*) ........ | 35 | 3.0 | 5.0 | .5 | 0 | 830 | 1.0 |
| **Kale, frozen**, boiled, | | | | | | | |
|   drained, chopped, | | | | | | | |
|   ½ cup ............. | 20 | 1.9 | 3.4 | .3 | 0 | 10 | 1.3 |
| **Kale, Chinese**, fresh: | | | | | | | |
| (*Frieda's* Chinese | | | | | | | |
|   Broccoli), chopped, | | | | | | | |
|   1 cup, 3 oz. ......... | 15 | 2.0 | 3.0 | .5 | 0 | 14 | 2.0 |
| cooked, 1 cup ........ | 19 | 1.0 | 3.3 | .6 | 0 | 6 | 2.2 |
| **Kale, Scotch**, ½ cup: | | | | | | | |
| raw, chopped ........ | 14 | 1.0 | 2.8 | .2 | 0 | 24 | .6 |
| boiled, drained, | | | | | | | |
|   chopped ........... | 18 | 1.2 | 3.7 | .3 | 0 | 29 | .8 |
| **Kamranga**, see | | | | | | | |
|   "Carambola" | | | | | | | |
| **Kamut berries** (*Bob's* | | | | | | | |
|   *Red Mill* Organic), | | | | | | | |
|   ¼ cup ............. | 160 | 7.0 | 32.0 | 1.0 | 0 | 0 | 4.0 |

| Food and Measure | cal. | prot. (gms) | carbo. (gms) | fat (gms) | chol. (mgs) | sod. (mgs) | fiber (gms) |
|---|---|---|---|---|---|---|---|
| **Kamut flakes** (see also "Cereal") (*Eden* Organic), ½ cup | 180 | 8.0 | 34.0 | 1.0 | 0 | 0 | 4.0 |
| **Kamut flour**, organic: | | | | | | | |
| (*Arrowhead Mills*), ⅓ cup | 130 | 5.0 | 25.0 | 1.0 | 0 | 0 | 4.0 |
| (*Bob's Red Mill*), ¼ cup | 94 | 3.0 | 21.0 | .5 | 0 | 0 | 3.0 |
| **Kanpo**, dried: | | | | | | | |
| .2-oz. strip | 16 | .5 | 4.1 | <.1 | 0 | 1 | n.a. |
| ½ cup | 70 | 2.3 | 15.6 | .1 | 0 | 4 | n.a. |
| **Kasha**, see "Buckwheat groats" | | | | | | | |
| **Katsu sauce** (*Kikkoman*), 1 tbsp. | 20 | 0 | 5.0 | 0 | 0 | 290 | 0 |
| **Kefir** (*Lifeway*), plain, 8 fl. oz.: | | | | | | | |
| original | 150 | 8.0 | 12.0 | 8.0 | 30 | 125 | 0 |
| Greek style | 210 | 8.0 | 12.0 | 14.0 | 55 | 120 | 0 |
| low fat | 110 | 11.0 | 12.0 | 2.0 | 10 | 125 | 3.0 |
| low fat, organic | 110 | 11.0 | 12.0 | 2.5 | 10 | 125 | 3.0 |
| whole milk, organic | 160 | 10.0 | 12.0 | 8.0 | 30 | 125 | 0 |
| **Ketchup**, 1 tbsp.: | | | | | | | |
| (*Annie's Naturals* Organic) | 15 | 0 | 3.0 | 0 | 0 | 150 | 0 |
| (*Del Monte*) | 15 | 0 | 4.0 | 0 | 0 | 190 | 0 |
| (*Heinz*) | 15 | 0 | 4.0 | 0 | 0 | 190 | 0 |
| (*Hunt's*) | 20 | 0 | 5.0 | 0 | 0 | 190 | 0 |
| (*Hunt's* No Salt) | 25 | 0 | 6.0 | 0 | 0 | 0 | 0 |
| (*Muir Glen* Organic) | 20 | 0 | 4.0 | 0 | 0 | 230 | 0 |
| spicy (*Maya Kaimal*) | 10 | 0 | 2.0 | 0 | 0 | 100 | 0 |
| **KFC**, 1 serving: | | | | | | | |
| *Extra Crispy:* | | | | | | | |
| breast | 510 | 39.0 | 16.0 | 33.0 | 110 | 1100 | 0 |
| drumstick | 150 | 12.0 | 5.0 | 10.0 | 55 | 360 | 0 |
| thigh | 340 | 20.0 | 10.0 | 24.0 | 80 | 780 | 0 |
| whole wing | 190 | 12.0 | 6.0 | 13.0 | 55 | 410 | 1.0 |
| grilled: | | | | | | | |
| breast | 210 | 34.0 | 0 | 8.0 | 105 | 460 | 0 |
| drumstick | 80 | 11.0 | 0 | 4.0 | 55 | 230 | 0 |
| thigh | 160 | 16.0 | 0 | 11.0 | 85 | 420 | 0 |
| whole wing | 80 | 9.0 | 1.0 | 5.0 | 40 | 250 | 0 |
| *Original Recipe:* | | | | | | | |
| breast | 360 | 34.0 | 11.0 | 21.0 | 110 | 1080 | 0 |
| no skin/breading | 160 | 31.0 | 2.0 | 3.5 | 85 | 580 | 0 |

| Food and Measure | cal. | prot. (gms) | carbo. (gms) | fat (gms) | chol. (mgs) | sod. (mgs) | fiber (gms) |
|---|---|---|---|---|---|---|---|
| drumstick .......... | 120 | 11.0 | 3.0 | 7.0 | 45 | 310 | 0 |
| thigh ............... | 250 | 17.0 | 7.0 | 17.0 | 80 | 730 | 0 |
| whole wing ......... | 120 | 11.0 | 3.0 | 7.0 | 50 | 380 | 0 |
| spicy crispy: | | | | | | | |
| breast ............. | 420 | 38.0 | 12.0 | 25.0 | 110 | 1250 | 1.0 |
| drumstick .......... | 160 | 11.0 | 5.0 | 10.0 | 50 | 440 | 0 |
| thigh .............. | 360 | 17.0 | 13.0 | 27.0 | 85 | 1010 | 1.0 |
| whole wing ......... | 170 | 11.0 | 6.0 | 12.0 | 45 | 470 | 1.0 |
| *KFC* fillet: | | | | | | | |
| grilled ............. | 140 | 26.0 | 1.0 | 3.0 | 70 | 560 | 0 |
| *Original Recipe* ...... | 200 | 22.0 | 8.0 | 9.0 | 55 | 670 | 1.0 |
| crispy strips, 3 ........ | 340 | 33.0 | 27.0 | 11.0 | 70 | 1280 | 3.0 |
| crispy strips, 2 ........ | 230 | 22.0 | 18.0 | 7.0 | 50 | 850 | 2.0 |
| popcorn chicken: | | | | | | | |
| large .............. | 560 | 32.0 | 26.0 | 37.0 | 65 | 1480 | 2.0 |
| individual .......... | 400 | 22.0 | 18.0 | 26.0 | 45 | 1040 | 1.0 |
| *Hot Wings*, 1 pc.: | | | | | | | |
| honey BBQ ......... | 80 | 4.0 | 8.0 | 4.0 | 20 | 240 | 0 |
| hot ............... | 70 | 4.0 | 4.0 | 4.0 | 20 | 140 | 0 |
| fiery Buffalo ....... | 70 | 4.0 | 5.0 | 4.0 | 20 | 270 | 0 |
| bowls/pie: | | | | | | | |
| chicken pot pie ...... | 790 | 29.0 | 66.0 | 45.0 | 75 | 1970 | 3.0 |
| *KFC Famous Bowls* potato/ gravy ........... | 680 | 26.0 | 74.0 | 31.0 | 45 | 2130 | 6.0 |
| snack size bowl ..... | 310 | 12.0 | 33.0 | 14.0 | 25 | 930 | 3.0 |
| sandwiches: | | | | | | | |
| double down, grilled .. | 480 | 60.0 | 4.0 | 25.0 | 175 | 1770 | 0 |
| *Original Recipe* .... | 610 | 52.0 | 18.0 | 37.0 | 150 | 1990 | 1.0 |
| *Doublicious*, grilled ... | 380 | 35.0 | 35.0 | 11.0 | 85 | 950 | 2.0 |
| grilled, no sauce ... | 340 | 35.0 | 32.0 | 8.0 | 80 | 880 | 2.0 |
| *Original Recipe* .... | 520 | 32.0 | 40.0 | 25.0 | 85 | 1300 | 2.0 |
| honey BBQ ......... | 320 | 24.0 | 47.0 | 3.5 | 70 | 770 | 3.0 |
| *KFC Snacker* ........ | 290 | 15.0 | 33.0 | 11.0 | 30 | 730 | 3.0 |
| w/out sauce ...... | 240 | 15.0 | 33.0 | 6.0 | 25 | 600 | 2.0 |
| Buffalo .......... | 250 | 15.0 | 35.0 | 6.0 | 25 | 770 | 3.0 |
| cheese, ultimate ... | 270 | 16.0 | 34.0 | 8.0 | 25 | 750 | 2.0 |
| honey BBQ ....... | 210 | 13.0 | 32.0 | 3.5 | 35 | 470 | 2.0 |
| salad, w/out dressing: | | | | | | | |
| Caesar: | | | | | | | |
| grilled ........... | 220 | 33.0 | 6.0 | 7.0 | 85 | 740 | 3.0 |
| crispy ........... | 310 | 29.0 | 23.0 | 11.0 | 60 | 1030 | 5.0 |
| side salad ........ | 40 | 3.0 | 2.0 | 2.0 | 5 | 90 | 1.0 |

| Food and Measure | cal. | prot. (gms) | carbo. (gms) | fat (gms) | chol. (mgs) | sod. (mgs) | fiber (gms) |
|---|---|---|---|---|---|---|---|
| **KFC, salad** *(cont.)* | | | | | | | |
| BLT: | | | | | | | |
|   grilled .......... | 230 | 35.0 | 8.0 | 8.0 | 90 | 920 | 4.0 |
|   crispy .......... | 320 | 31.0 | 25.0 | 12.0 | 65 | 1220 | 5.0 |
| house side salad ..... | 15 | 1.0 | 3.0 | 0 | 0 | 10 | 1.0 |
| salad dressing: | | | | | | | |
| buttermilk ranch ...... | 160 | 0 | 1.0 | 17.0 | 10 | 220 | 0 |
| *Hidden Valley* nonfat .. | 35 | 1.0 | 8.0 | 0 | 0 | 410 | 0 |
| light Italian ......... | 15 | 0 | 2.0 | .5 | 0 | 510 | 0 |
| *KFC* Caesar ......... | 260 | 2.0 | 4.0 | 26.0 | 15.0 | 540 | 0 |
| croutons ........... | 70 | 1.0 | 8.0 | 3.0 | 0 | 160 | 0 |
| sides, individual: | | | | | | | |
| BBQ baked beans .... | 210 | 8.0 | 41.0 | 1.5 | 0 | 780 | 8.0 |
| biscuit ............. | 180 | 4.0 | 23.0 | 8.0 | 0 | 530 | 1.0 |
| coleslaw ........... | 180 | 1.0 | 20.0 | 10.0 | 5 | 150 | 2.0 |
| corn, kernel ........ | 100 | 3.0 | 21.0 | .5 | 0 | 0 | 2.0 |
| corn on cob, 3" .... | 70 | 2.0 | 16.0 | .5 | 0 | 0 | 2.0 |
| corn on cob, 5.5" .... | 140 | 5.0 | 33.0 | 1.0 | 0 | 5 | 4.0 |
| green beans ........ | 20 | 1.0 | 3.0 | 0 | 0 | 290 | 1.0 |
| *KFC* corn muffin ..... | 210 | 3.0 | 28.0 | 9.0 | 35 | 240 | 0 |
| macaroni and cheese . | 160 | 5.0 | 19.0 | 7.0 | 5 | 720 | 1.0 |
| macaroni salad ...... | 190 | 4.0 | 22.0 | 10.0 | 5 | 430 | 1.0 |
| potato salad ........ | 210 | 2.0 | 26.0 | 11.0 | 10 | 560 | 3.0 |
| potato wedges ....... | 310 | 4.0 | 32.0 | 18.0 | 0 | 870 | 4.0 |
| potatoes, mashed .... | 90 | 2.0 | 15.0 | 3.0 | 0 | 320 | 1.0 |
|   w/gravy ......... | 120 | 2.0 | 19.0 | 4.0 | 0 | 530 | 1.0 |
| sauces/spread: | | | | | | | |
| buttery spread ...... | 30 | 0 | 0 | 3.5 | 0 | 30 | 0 |
| honey sauce pkt. ..... | 30 | 0 | 8.0 | 0 | 0 | 0 | 0 |
| dipping sauce: | | | | | | | |
|   chipotle, spicy .... | 70 | 0 | 8.0 | 3.5 | 10 | 220 | 1.0 |
|   creamy ranch ..... | 140 | 0 | 1.0 | 15.0 | 10 | 230 | 0 |
|   honey BBQ ....... | 40 | 0 | 9.0 | 0 | 0 | 310 | 0 |
|   honey mustard .... | 120 | 0 | 6.0 | 10.0 | 5 | 110 | 0 |
|   *KFC* ............ | 70 | 0 | 5.0 | 5.0 | 10 | 135 | 0 |
|   sweet & sour ..... | 45 | 0 | 12.0 | 0 | 0 | 95 | 0 |
| dessert: | | | | | | | |
| apple turnover ...... | 250 | 2.0 | 33.0 | 12.0 | 0 | 160 | 2.0 |
| chocolate chip cake .. | 300 | 4.0 | 39.0 | 15.0 | 50 | 260 | 1.0 |
| *Littlebucket* Parfait: | | | | | | | |
|   chocolate crème ... | 280 | 2.0 | 37.0 | 13.0 | 0 | 240 | 1.0 |
|   lemon crème ..... | 400 | 7.0 | 65.0 | 13.0 | 5 | 220 | 2.0 |
|   strawberry shortcake | 200 | 2.0 | 35.0 | 7.0 | 20 | 140 | 2.0 |
| *Oreo* crème pie ...... | 290 | 3.0 | 34.0 | 16.0 | 5 | 210 | 1.0 |

| Food and Measure | cal. | prot. (gms) | carbo. (gms) | fat (gms) | chol. (mgs) | sod. (mgs) | fiber (gms) |
|---|---|---|---|---|---|---|---|
| *Reese's* pie ........ | 310 | 5.0 | 31.0 | 19.0 | 5 | 200 | 1.0 |
| *Sweet Life* cookie: | | | | | | | |
| chocolate chip .... | 160 | 2.0 | 21.0 | 8.0 | 10 | 85 | 1.0 |
| oatmeal raisin .... | 150 | 2.0 | 22.0 | 6.0 | 10 | 90 | 1.0 |
| **Kidney beans**: | | | | | | | |
| dry, ¼ cup: | | | | | | | |
| dark (*Eden* Organic) .. | 150 | 10.0 | 26.0 | 1.0 | 0 | 10 | 13.0 |
| red (*Bob's Red Mill*) .. | 140 | 9.0 | 25.0 | 0 | 0 | 5 | 6.0 |
| white (*Bob's Red Mill* | | | | | | | |
| Cannellini) ....... | 150 | 11.0 | 26.0 | 0 | 0 | 10 | 7.0 |
| boiled, ½ cup ........ | 112 | 7.6 | 20.1 | .4 | 0 | 2 | 6.5 |
| **Kidney beans, canned**, | | | | | | | |
| ½ cup: | | | | | | | |
| green, see "Flageolets" | | | | | | | |
| red: | | | | | | | |
| (*Eden* Organic) ...... | 100 | 8.0 | 18.0 | 0 | 0 | 15 | 10.0 |
| (*Progresso*) ........ | 110 | 7.0 | 20.0 | .5 | 0 | 280 | 8.0 |
| (*Roland*) ........ | 110 | 9.0 | 18.0 | 0 | 0 | 430 | 7.0 |
| (*S&W*) ........... | 120 | 7.0 | 20.0 | 1.0 | 0 | 380 | 6.0 |
| (*S&W* Organic) ...... | 120 | 7.0 | 20.0 | 1.0 | 0 | 380 | 5.0 |
| (*Van Camp's* New | | | | | | | |
| Orleans Style) .... | 90 | 6.0 | 19.0 | 0 | 0 | 450 | 6.0 |
| red, dark: | | | | | | | |
| (*Allens*) ........... | 130 | 8.0 | 22.0 | .5 | 0 | 310 | 8.0 |
| (*Bush's*) ........... | 105 | 7.0 | 22.0 | 0 | 0 | 260 | 8.0 |
| (*Bush's* Reduced | | | | | | | |
| Sodium) ........ | 105 | 7.0 | 22.0 | 0 | 0 | 130 | 8.0 |
| (*Progresso*) ........ | 110 | 8.0 | 20.0 | 0 | 0 | 340 | 6.0 |
| (*Trappey's*) ........ | 120 | 1.0 | 28.0 | 0 | 0 | 470 | 5.0 |
| (*Van Camp's*) ........ | 90 | 7.0 | 19.0 | 0 | 0 | 730 | 6.0 |
| seasoned (*Bush's*) ... | 110 | 8.0 | 22.0 | 0 | 0 | 450 | 8.0 |
| red, light: | | | | | | | |
| (*Allens/Trappey's*) .... | 120 | 6.0 | 22.0 | .5 | 0 | 340 | 8.0 |
| (*Bush's*) ........... | 100 | 7.0 | 22.0 | 0 | 0 | 260 | 7.0 |
| jalapeño (*Trappey's*) .. | 110 | 6.0 | 19.0 | 1.0 | 0 | 420 | 6.0 |
| white, cannellini: | | | | | | | |
| (*Bush's*) ........... | 110 | 7.0 | 18.0 | .5 | 0 | 300 | 6.0 |
| (*Eden* Organic) ...... | 100 | 6.0 | 17.0 | 1.0 | 0 | 40 | 5.0 |
| (*Progresso*) ........ | 110 | 8.0 | 20.0 | 0 | 0 | 340 | 6.0 |
| (*S&W*) ........... | 110 | 6.0 | 21.0 | 0 | 0 | 200 | 6.0 |
| **Kidney beans,** | | | | | | | |
| **sprouted**, raw, ½ cup | 27 | 3.9 | 3.8 | .5 | 0 | 6 | <1.0 |
| **Kidneys**, braised: | | | | | | | |
| beef, 4 oz. ........... | 163 | 28.9 | 1.1 | 3.9 | 439 | 152 | 0 |

| Food and Measure | cal. | prot. (gms) | carbo. (gms) | fat (gms) | chol. (mgs) | sod. (mgs) | fiber (gms) |
|---|---|---|---|---|---|---|---|
| **Kidneys** *(cont.)* | | | | | | | |
| lamb, 4 oz. ........... | 155 | 26.8 | 1.1 | 4.1 | 641 | 171 | 0 |
| pork, 4 oz. ............ | 171 | 28.8 | 0 | 5.3 | 544 | 91 | 0 |
| pork, chopped, 1 cup ... | 211 | 35.6 | 0 | 6.6 | 673 | 111 | 0 |
| veal, 4 oz. ............ | 185 | 29.8 | 0 | 6.4 | 897 | 125 | 0 |
| **Kielbasa**, 2 oz., | | | | | | | |
| except as noted: | | | | | | | |
| (*Applegate Farms* | | | | | | | |
| Organic), 3-oz. link ... | 190 | 12.0 | 2.0 | 14.0 | 50 | 600 | 0 |
| (*Black Bear* Polska) ..... | 150 | 8.0 | 2.0 | 12.0 | 30 | 420 | 0 |
| (*Boar's Head*) ......... | 120 | 9.0 | 0 | 10.0 | 50 | 440 | 0 |
| (*Hillshire Farm* | | | | | | | |
| Polska) ............ | 190 | 7.0 | 3.0 | 16.0 | 35 | 480 | <1.0 |
| (*Hillshire Farm* | | | | | | | |
| Polska Lite) ......... | 110 | 9.0 | 0 | 8.0 | 35 | 490 | 0 |
| (*Thumann's* Ring) ...... | 150 | 7.0 | 1.0 | 13.0 | 28 | 470 | 0 |
| beef (*Hillshire Farm* | | | | | | | |
| Polska) ............ | 170 | 7.0 | 3.0 | 15.0 | 35 | 520 | <1.0 |
| turkey: | | | | | | | |
| (*Hillshire Farm* | | | | | | | |
| Polska) .......... | 90 | 9.0 | 3.0 | 5.0 | 35 | 490 | 0 |
| (*Jennie-O*) ......... | 100 | 8.0 | 3.0 | 5.0 | 40 | 490 | 0 |
| (*Oscar Mayer* Polska) . | 80 | 9.0 | 1.0 | 6.0 | 40 | 770 | 0 |
| **"Kielbasa," vegetarian** | | | | | | | |
| (*Tofurky*), 3.5 oz. .... | 240 | 26.0 | 12.0 | 12.0 | 0 | 660 | 8.0 |
| **Kim chee** (*Frieda's*), | | | | | | | |
| ¼ cup, 2 oz. ........ | 15 | 1.0 | 2.0 | 0 | 0 | 340 | 1.0 |
| **Kippers**, see "Herring" | | | | | | | |
| **Kiwi**, fresh: | | | | | | | |
| (*Chiquita*), 2.7-oz. pc. ... | 46 | 1.0 | 11.0 | 0 | 0 | 2 | 2.0 |
| all varieties | | | | | | | |
| (*Frieda's*), 5 oz. ...... | 90 | 1.0 | 21.0 | .5 | 0 | 5 | 5.0 |
| 1 large, 3.7 oz. ....... | 55 | .9 | 13.5 | .4 | 0 | 4 | 3.1 |
| 1 medium, 3.1 oz. ...... | 46 | .8 | 11.3 | .3 | 0 | 4 | 2.6 |
| **Kiwi, canned**, in syrup | | | | | | | |
| (*Roland*), ½ cup ..... | 150 | 0 | 38.0 | 0 | 0 | 35 | 4.0 |
| **Kiwi drink blend**, | | | | | | | |
| 8 fl. oz.: | | | | | | | |
| berry (*Nantucket* | | | | | | | |
| *Nectars*) ........... | 120 | 0 | 29.0 | 0 | 0 | 25 | 0 |
| pear (*Snapple*) ........ | 15 | 0 | 2.0 | 0 | 0 | 5 | 0 |
| raspberry or | | | | | | | |
| strawberry (*Langers*) . | 120 | 0 | 29.0 | 0 | 0 | 0 | 0 |

| Food and Measure | cal. | prot. (gms) | carbo. (gms) | fat (gms) | chol. (mgs) | sod. (mgs) | fiber (gms) |
|---|---|---|---|---|---|---|---|
| strawberry: | | | | | | | |
| (*AriZona*) . . . . . . . . . | 120 | 0 | 29.0 | 0 | 0 | 10 | 0 |
| (*Snapple*) . . . . . . . . . | 110 | 0 | 27.0 | 0 | 0 | 10 | 0 |
| frozen* (*Langers*) . . . . | 120 | 0 | 30.0 | 0 | 0 | 15 | 0 |
| **Kiwi juice blend**: | | | | | | | |
| (*Veryfine* Krazy) | | | | | | | |
| 11.5 fl. oz. . . . . . . . . . | 200 | 0 | 49.0 | 0 | 0 | 40 | 0 |
| strawberry (*R.W.* | | | | | | | |
| *Knudsen*), 8 fl. oz. . . . | 120 | 0 | 29.0 | 0 | 0 | 15 | 0 |
| **Knockwurst, 1 link**: | | | | | | | |
| (*Black Bear*), 3.2 oz. . . . . | 240 | 11.0 | 0 | 21.0 | 40 | 650 | 0 |
| (*Thumann's*), 4 oz. . . . . . | 300 | 13.0 | 2.0 | 27.0 | 55 | 960 | 0 |
| beef: | | | | | | | |
| (*Boar's Head*), 4 oz. . . | 310 | 15.0 | 1.0 | 27.0 | 70 | 950 | 0 |
| (*Hebrew National*), | | | | | | | |
| 3 oz. . . . . . . . . . . . | 270 | 10.0 | 2.0 | 25.0 | 45 | 810 | 0 |
| **Kohlrabi**: | | | | | | | |
| raw (*Frieda's*), ⅔ cup, | | | | | | | |
| 3 oz. . . . . . . . . . . . . . | 25 | 1.0 | 5.0 | 0 | 0 | 15 | 3.0 |
| raw, sliced, ½ cup . . . . . . | 19 | 1.2 | 4.3 | .1 | 0 | 14 | 2.5 |
| boiled, drained, sliced, | | | | | | | |
| ½ cup . . . . . . . . . . . . . | 24 | 1.5 | 5.5 | .1 | 0 | 17 | .9 |
| **Kumquat, fresh**: | | | | | | | |
| (*Frieda's*), 10 pcs., | | | | | | | |
| 6.7 oz. . . . . . . . . . . . | 135 | 4.0 | 30.0 | 2.0 | 0 | 19 | 12.0 |
| 1 medium, .7 oz. . . . . . . | 12 | .2 | 3.1 | <.1 | 0 | 1 | 1.3 |
| seeded, 1 oz. . . . . . . . . . | 18 | .3 | 4.7 | <.1 | 0 | 2 | 1.9 |
| **Kumquat, in jars,** | | | | | | | |
| extra heavy syrup | | | | | | | |
| (*Roland*), 2 pcs. . . . . . | 80 | 0 | 20.0 | 0 | 0 | 20 | 0 |
| **Kung pao sauce**: | | | | | | | |
| (*Annie Chun's*), 1 tbsp. . . | 30 | 1.0 | 4.0 | .5 | 0 | 350 | 0 |
| cooking (*Tiger Tiger* | | | | | | | |
| Shanghai), ½ cup . . . . | 223 | 4.0 | 36.0 | 7.0 | 0 | 950 | <1.0 |
| **Kuri squash**, see | | | | | | | |
| "Red kuri squash" | | | | | | | |
| **Kuzu root starch** | | | | | | | |
| (*Eden* Organic), 1 tbsp. | 30 | 0 | 8.0 | 0 | 0 | 0 | 0 |

# L

| Food and Measure | cal. | prot. (gms) | carbo. (gms) | fat (gms) | chol. (mgs) | sod. (mgs) | fiber (gms) |
|---|---|---|---|---|---|---|---|
| **Lamb**, choice grade, trimmed to ¼" fat, meat only, 4 oz., except as noted: | | | | | | | |
| cubed, leg/shoulder: | | | | | | | |
| braised or stewed .... | 253 | 38.2 | 0 | 10.0 | 122 | 79 | 0 |
| broiled ............ | 211 | 31.8 | 0 | 8.3 | 102 | 86 | 0 |
| foreshank, braised: | | | | | | | |
| lean w/fat ......... | 276 | 32.2 | 0 | 15.3 | 120 | 82 | 0 |
| lean only .......... | 212 | 35.2 | 0 | 6.8 | 118 | 84 | 0 |
| ground: | | | | | | | |
| raw .............. | 320 | 18.8 | 0 | 26.5 | 83 | 67 | 0 |
| broiled ........... | 321 | 28.1 | 0 | 22.3 | 110 | 92 | 0 |
| broiled, 1 cup ....... | 328 | 28.7 | 0 | 23.1 | 113 | 94 | 0 |
| leg, whole, roasted: | | | | | | | |
| lean w/fat ......... | 293 | 29.0 | 0 | 18.7 | 105 | 75 | 0 |
| lean w/fat, 1 slice, 3" diam. x ¼" ..... | 73 | 7.2 | 0 | 4.7 | 26 | 19 | 0 |
| lean only .......... | 217 | 32.1 | 0 | 8.8 | 101 | 77 | 0 |
| lean only, 3" slice .... | 54 | 8.0 | 0 | 2.2 | 25 | 19 | 0 |
| leg, shank, roasted: | | | | | | | |
| lean w/fat ......... | 255 | 29.9 | 0 | 14.1 | 102 | 74 | 0 |
| lean w/fat, 1 slice, 3" diam. x ¼" ..... | 64 | 7.5 | 0 | 3.5 | 26 | 18 | 0 |
| lean only .......... | 204 | 31.9 | 0 | 7.6 | 99 | 75 | 0 |
| lean only, 3" slice .... | 51 | 8.0 | 0 | 1.9 | 25 | 19 | 0 |
| leg, sirloin, roasted: | | | | | | | |
| lean w/fat ......... | 331 | 27.9 | 0 | 23.4 | 110 | 77 | 0 |
| lean w/fat, 1 slice, 3" diam. x ¼" ..... | 83 | 7.0 | 0 | 5.9 | 27 | 19 | 0 |
| lean only .......... | 231 | 32.1 | 0 | 10.4 | 104 | 81 | 0 |
| lean only, 3" slice .... | 58 | 8.0 | 0 | 2.6 | 26 | 20 | 0 |

| Food and Measure | cal. | prot. (gms) | carbo. (gms) | fat (gms) | chol. (mgs) | sod. (mgs) | fiber (gms) |
|---|---|---|---|---|---|---|---|
| loin chop, broiled: | | | | | | | |
| lean w/fat, 2¼ oz. | | | | | | | |
| (4.2 oz. raw | | | | | | | |
| w/bone) ......... | 201 | 16.1 | 0 | 14.7 | 64 | 49 | 0 |
| lean w/fat .......... | 358 | 28.5 | 0 | 26.2 | 113 | 87 | 0 |
| lean only, 1.6 oz. | | | | | | | |
| (4.2 oz. raw | | | | | | | |
| w/bone and fat) ... | 100 | 13.9 | 0 | 4.5 | 44 | 39 | 0 |
| lean only .......... | 245 | 34.0 | 0 | 11.0 | 108 | 95 | 0 |
| loin, roasted: | | | | | | | |
| lean w/fat ........ | 350 | 25.6 | 0 | 26.8 | 108 | 73 | 0 |
| lean only ........ | 229 | 30.2 | 0 | 11.1 | 99 | 75 | 0 |
| rib: | | | | | | | |
| broiled, lean w/fat .... | 409 | 25.1 | 0 | 33.6 | 112 | 86 | 0 |
| broiled, lean only .... | 266 | 31.5 | 0 | 14.7 | 103 | 96 | 0 |
| roasted, lean w/fat ... | 407 | 24.0 | 0 | 33.8 | 110 | 83 | 0 |
| roasted, lean only .... | 263 | 29.7 | 0 | 15.1 | 100 | 92 | 0 |
| shoulder, whole: | | | | | | | |
| braised, lean w/fat ... | 390 | 32.5 | 0 | 27.8 | 132 | 85 | 0 |
| braised, lean only .... | 321 | 37.2 | 0 | 10.0 | 133 | 90 | 0 |
| roasted, lean w/fat ... | 313 | 25.5 | 0 | 22.6 | 104 | 75 | 0 |
| roasted, lean only .... | 231 | 28.3 | 0 | 12.2 | 99 | 77 | 0 |
| **Lamb entree**, frozen, | | | | | | | |
| shepherd's pie (*Pacific* | | | | | | | |
| Organic), 1 cup ...... | 250 | 19.0 | 19.0 | 9.0 | 60 | 620 | 1.0 |
| **Lamb's quarters**, | | | | | | | |
| boiled, drained, | | | | | | | |
| chopped, ½ cup ..... | 29 | 2.9 | 4.5 | .6 | 0 | 26 | 1.9 |
| **Lard**, 1 tbsp. .......... | 120 | 0 | 0 | 13.0 | 10 | 0 | 0 |
| **Lasagna entree,** | | | | | | | |
| **canned**, 1 cup: | | | | | | | |
| (*Chef Boyardee*) ....... | 270 | 9.0 | 36.0 | 10.0 | 25 | 830 | 2.0 |
| (*Chef Boyardee* | | | | | | | |
| Whole Grain) ....... | 270 | 9.0 | 35.0 | 10.0 | 15 | 670 | 4.0 |
| **Lasagna entree, frozen**, | | | | | | | |
| 1 pkg., except as noted: | | | | | | | |
| (*Banquet* Family | | | | | | | |
| Size), 1 cup ........ | 220 | 11.0 | 27.0 | 8.0 | 20 | 770 | 4.0 |
| Alfredo: | | | | | | | |
| (*Michelina's* | | | | | | | |
| *Authentico*), 9 oz. ... | 350 | 12.0 | 40.0 | 15.0 | 40 | 720 | 2.0 |
| w/broccoli | | | | | | | |
| (*Michelina's Budget* | | | | | | | |
| *Gourmet*), 7.5 oz. ... | 290 | 10.0 | 35.0 | 11.0 | 30 | 550 | 2.0 |

| Food and Measure | cal. | prot. (gms) | carbo. (gms) | fat (gms) | chol. (mgs) | sod. (mgs) | fiber (gms) |
|---|---|---|---|---|---|---|---|
| **Lasagna entree, frozen** *(cont.)* | | | | | | | |
| cheese: | | | | | | | |
| (*Amy's*), 10.3 oz. .... | 380 | 20.0 | 44.0 | 14.0 | 45 | 680 | 4.0 |
| (*Cedarlane*), 10 oz. ... | 380 | 25.0 | 45.0 | 12.0 | 35 | 570 | 3.0 |
| (*Celentano*), ½ of | | | | | | | |
| 14-oz. pkg. ....... | 300 | 13.0 | 37.0 | 10.0 | 30 | 710 | 4.0 |
| (*Celentano* Light), | | | | | | | |
| 10 oz. ........... | 340 | 18.0 | 52.0 | 7.0 | 30 | 800 | 7.0 |
| cheese, 5: | | | | | | | |
| (*Lean Cuisine*), | | | | | | | |
| 11.5 oz. ......... | 360 | 21.0 | 51.0 | 8.0 | 20 | 600 | 4.0 |
| (*Michelina's Lean* | | | | | | | |
| *Gourmet*), 8 oz. .... | 290 | 13.0 | 50.0 | 5.0 | 10 | 560 | 8.0 |
| (*Stouffer's*), 10.75 oz. . | 370 | 21.0 | 39.0 | 14.0 | 35 | 960 | 4.0 |
| (*Stouffer's*), ½ of | | | | | | | |
| 18.25-oz. pkg. .... | 330 | 18.0 | 33.0 | 14.0 | 35 | 870 | 3.0 |
| (*Stouffer's* Family), | | | | | | | |
| ½ of 60-oz. pkg. ... | 270 | 12.0 | 36.0 | 9.0 | 20 | 710 | 3.0 |
| cheese, 4: | | | | | | | |
| (*Michelina's* | | | | | | | |
| *Authentico*), 8 oz. ... | 280 | 12.0 | 43.0 | 6.0 | 15 | 500 | 3.0 |
| layered (*Michelina's* | | | | | | | |
| *Authentico*), 8 oz. ... | 280 | 12.0 | 46.0 | 7.0 | 10 | 650 | 8.0 |
| chicken: | | | | | | | |
| (*Stouffer's*), ⅕ of | | | | | | | |
| 39-oz. pkg. ....... | 400 | 16.0 | 54.0 | 13.0 | 20 | 740 | 3.0 |
| Florentine (*Lean* | | | | | | | |
| *Cuisine*), 10 oz. ... | 280 | 20.0 | 36.0 | 6.0 | 30 | 650 | 3.0 |
| Florentine (*Smart* | | | | | | | |
| *Ones*), 10.5 oz. ...... | 290 | 15.0 | 44.0 | 6.0 | 20 | 580 | 5.0 |
| garlic, cheesy (*Stouffer's* | | | | | | | |
| *Easy Express* | | | | | | | |
| 35 oz.*), 7.78 oz. ..... | 330 | 18.0 | 36.0 | 13.0 | 40 | 860 | 3.0 |
| meat/meat sauce | | | | | | | |
| (*Banquet*), 8 oz. ..... | 250 | 12.0 | 34.0 | 7.0 | 10 | 510 | 4.0 |
| (*Boston Market*), | | | | | | | |
| 12.5 oz. ......... | 500 | 22.0 | 49.0 | 23.0 | 85 | 1290 | 4.0 |
| (*Buitoni*), ½ of | | | | | | | |
| 24-oz. pkg. ....... | 500 | 32.0 | 38.0 | 24.0 | 100 | 1090 | 5.0 |
| (*Lean Cuisine*), | | | | | | | |
| 10.5 oz. ......... | 320 | 17.0 | 45.0 | 8.0 | 30 | 630 | 4.0 |
| (*Marie Callender's* | | | | | | | |
| Meat), 1 cup ...... | 260 | 10.0 | 32.0 | 10.0 | 35 | 960 | 4.0 |

| Food and Measure | cal. | prot. (gms) | carbo. (gms) | fat (gms) | chol. (mgs) | sod. (mgs) | fiber (gms) |
|---|---|---|---|---|---|---|---|
| (*Marie Callender's* Meat Sauce), 1 cup | 260 | 16.0 | 26.0 | 10.0 | 35 | 960 | 5.0 |
| (*Michelina's Authentico*), 8.5 oz. | 290 | 12.0 | 38.0 | 9.0 | 20 | 870 | 3.0 |
| (*Michelina's Budget Gourmet*), 8 oz. . . . | 260 | 10.0 | 34.0 | 8.0 | 15 | 680 | 3.0 |
| (*Michelina's Lean Gourmet*), 8 oz. . . . | 310 | 15.0 | 49.0 | 6.0 | 20 | 890 | 8.0 |
| (*Smart Ones* Bake), 9 oz. . . . . . . . . . . | 270 | 14.0 | 43.0 | 4.0 | 15 | 540 | 3.0 |
| (*Smart Ones* Traditional), 10.5 oz. | 300 | 17.0 | 43.0 | 6.0 | 25 | 780 | 5.0 |
| (*Stouffer's* Bake), 11.5 oz. . . . . . . . . | 350 | 17.0 | 49.0 | 10.0 | 30 | 960 | 5.0 |
| (*Stouffer's* Family), ⅕ of 38-oz. pkg. . . . | 290 | 18.0 | 27.0 | 12.0 | 35 | 730 | 2.0 |
| (*Stouffer's* Italiano), ½ of 19-oz. pkg. . . . | 290 | 16.0 | 30.0 | 12.0 | 35 | 690 | 3.0 |
| (*Stouffer's* Italiano Family), ⅕ of 38-oz. pkg. . . . . . . . | 250 | 13.0 | 30.0 | 9.0 | 30 | 720 | 3.0 |
| mozzarella: | | | | | | | |
| (*Michelina's Authentico*), 8 oz. . . | 260 | 9.0 | 39.0 | 7.0 | 20 | 540 | 3.0 |
| (*Michelina's Budget Gourmet*), 7.5 oz. . . | 250 | 9.0 | 38.0 | 7.0 | 20 | 510 | 3.0 |
| sausage, Italian (*Stouffer's*), 10.88 oz. . | 410 | 18.0 | 41.0 | 19.0 | 50 | 930 | 4.0 |
| soy cheese (*Rising Moon Organics*), 10 oz. . . . . | 380 | 16.0 | 56.0 | 10.0 | 0 | 460 | 6.0 |
| spinach (*Amy's* Light & Lean), 8 oz. . . . . . . | 240 | 11.0 | 40.0 | 5.0 | 10 | 540 | 5.0 |
| vegetable: | | | | | | | |
| (*Amy's*), 9.5 oz. . . . . . | 310 | 16.0 | 35.0 | 12.0 | 20 | 680 | 5.0 |
| (*Amy's* Light Sodium), 9.5 oz. . . . . . . . . . | 290 | 15.0 | 41.0 | 8.0 | 15 | 340 | 4.0 |
| (*Stouffer's*), 10.5 oz. . . | 390 | 17.0 | 40.0 | 18.0 | 25 | 730 | 4.0 |
| (*Stouffer's* Family), 1/12 of 96-oz. pkg. . . | 320 | 16.0 | 35.0 | 13.0 | 25 | 1010 | 3.0 |
| garden (*Amy's*), 10.3 oz. . . . . . . . . . . | 290 | 11.0 | 41.0 | 9.0 | 20 | 720 | 5.0 |
| roasted (*Amy's*), 9.8 oz. . . . . . . . . . | 350 | 16.0 | 47.0 | 11.0 | 15 | 680 | 4.0 |
| tofu (*Amy's*), 9.5 oz. . . | 330 | 16.0 | 41.0 | 11.0 | 0 | 680 | 5.0 |

| Food and Measure | cal. | prot. (gms) | carbo. (gms) | fat (gms) | chol. (mgs) | sod. (mgs) | fiber (gms) |
|---|---|---|---|---|---|---|---|
| **Lasagna entree, frozen** *(cont.)* | | | | | | | |
| vegetarian: | | | | | | | |
| (*Boca*), 10.5 oz. ..... | 290 | 21.0 | 42.0 | 5.0 | 15 | 880 | 5.0 |
| (*MorningStar Farms*), | | | | | | | |
| 10 oz. ........... | 270 | 20.0 | 41.0 | 6.0 | 10 | 590 | 6.0 |
| **Lasagne entree, microwave**, | | | | | | | |
| meat sauce.: | | | | | | | |
| (*Chef Boyardee*), | | | | | | | |
| ½ bowl, 1 cup ....... | 250 | 9.0 | 33.0 | 9.0 | 25 | 830 | 3.0 |
| (*Chef Boyardee* Single), | | | | | | | |
| 7.5 oz. ........... | 220 | 8.0 | 30.0 | 7.0 | 15 | 670 | 3.0 |
| (*Hormel* Microcup), 7.5 oz. | 210 | 9.0 | 31.0 | 5.0 | 10 | 840 | 3.0 |
| (*Hormel Compleats*), | | | | | | | |
| 10 oz. ............. | 280 | 13.0 | 42.0 | 7.0 | 50 | 1100 | 3.0 |
| **Lasagne entree mix** | | | | | | | |
| (see also "Hamburger | | | | | | | |
| entree mix") (*Banquet* | | | | | | | |
| *Homestyle Bakes*), | | | | | | | |
| 1 serving .......... | 330 | 14.0 | 39.0 | 13.0 | 25 | 850 | 7.0 |
| **Leek**, w/lower leaf | | | | | | | |
| portion, fresh: | | | | | | | |
| raw: | | | | | | | |
| (*Frieda's*), 1 cup, 3.1 oz. | 55 | 1.0 | 12.0 | 0 | 0 | 18 | 2.0 |
| 9.9-oz. leek .......... | 76 | 1.9 | 17.6 | .4 | 0 | 25 | 2.2 |
| chopped, ½ cup ..... | 32 | .8 | 7.4 | .2 | 0 | 10 | .9 |
| boiled, drained: | | | | | | | |
| 4.4-oz. leek .......... | 38 | .2 | 9.5 | .3 | 0 | 12 | 1.2 |
| chopped, ½ cup ..... | 16 | .4 | 4.0 | .1 | 0 | 5 | .5 |
| **Leek, freeze-dried**, 1 tbsp. | 1 | <.1 | .2 | tr. | 0 | <1 | <1.0 |
| **Lemon**, fresh: | | | | | | | |
| (*Frieda's* Meyer), | | | | | | | |
| 1 medium .......... | 25 | 0 | 4.0 | 0 | 0 | 0 | 0 |
| 2⅛" lemon, 3.8 oz. ..... | 22 | 1.3 | 11.6 | .3 | 0 | 3 | n.a. |
| 1 wedge, ¼ medium .... | 5 | .3 | 2.9 | .1 | 0 | 1 | n.a. |
| peeled, 2⅛" lemon ..... | 17 | .6 | 5.4 | .2 | 0 | 1 | 1.6 |
| **Lemon, preserved**, in | | | | | | | |
| jars (*Roland*), .5 oz. .. | 5 | 0 | 1.0 | 0 | 0 | 200 | 0 |
| **Lemon curd** | | | | | | | |
| (*Dickenson's*), 1 tbsp. . | 60 | 0 | 11.0 | 1.0 | 15 | 10 | 0 |
| **Lemon drink** (see also | | | | | | | |
| "Lemonade"), | | | | | | | |
| 8 fl. oz.: | | | | | | | |
| (*Santa Cruz Organic*) .... | 120 | 0 | 29.0 | 0 | 0 | 10 | 0 |
| (*Tropicana* Light) ....... | 10 | 0 | 2.0 | 0 | 0 | 25 | 0 |

| Food and Measure | cal. | prot. (gms) | carbo. (gms) | fat (gms) | chol. (mgs) | sod. (mgs) | fiber (gms) |
|---|---|---|---|---|---|---|---|
| **Lemon drink blend**, ginger echinacea, 8 fl. oz.: | | | | | | | |
| (*Santa Cruz Organic*) . . . . | 100 | <1.0 | 25.0 | 0 | 0 | 10 | 0 |
| (S*imply Nutritious*) . . . . . | 100 | <1.0 | 25.0 | 0 | 0 | 10 | 0 |
| **Lemon juice**, fresh: | | | | | | | |
| ½ cup . . . . . . . . . . . . . . | 31 | .5 | 10.5 | 0 | 0 | 1 | .5 |
| 1 tbsp. . . . . . . . . . . . . . | 4 | .1 | 1.3 | 0 | 0 | <1 | .1 |
| **Lemon pepper**: | | | | | | | |
| (*Lawry's*), ¼ tsp. . . . . . . . | 0 | 0 | 0 | 0 | 0 | 80 | 0 |
| (*McCormick Perfect Pinch*), ¼ tsp. . . . . . . . | 0 | 0 | 0 | 0 | 0 | 210 | 0 |
| 1 tsp. . . . . . . . . . . . . . . | 7 | .2 | 1.5 | 0 | 0 | 425 | .3 |
| w/garlic and onion (*McCormick California*), ¼ tsp. . . . . | 0 | 0 | 0 | 0 | 0 | 30 | 0 |
| herb (*Grill Mates*), ¼ tsp. | 0 | 0 | 0 | 0 | 0 | 95 | 0 |
| **Lemonade,** 8 fl. oz., except as noted: | | | | | | | |
| (*Apple & Eve*) . . . . . . . . | 130 | 0 | 32.0 | 0 | 0 | 5 | 0 |
| (*AriZona*) . . . . . . . . . . . . | 110 | 0 | 27.0 | 0 | 0 | 10 | 0 |
| (*Florida's Natural*) . . . . . . | 110 | 0 | 28.0 | 0 | 0 | 20 | 0 |
| (*Lipton Brisk*) . . . . . . . . . | 100 | 0 | 27.0 | 0 | 0 | 65 | 0 |
| (*Minute Maid*), 12 fl. oz. . | 150 | 0 | 42.0 | 0 | 0 | 50 | 0 |
| (*Minute Maid* 12%) . . . . . | 110 | 0 | 31.0 | 0 | 0 | 15 | 0 |
| (*Minute Maid* 3%) . . . . . . | 100 | 0 | 28.0 | 0 | 0 | 35 | 0 |
| (*Minute Maid* Can) . . . . . | 100 | 0 | 28.0 | 0 | 0 | 35 | 0 |
| (*Nantucket Nectars*) . . . . | 110 | 0 | 28.0 | 0 | 0 | 20 | 0 |
| (*Newman's Own* Lightly Sweetened) . . . | 80 | 0 | 20.0 | 0 | 0 | 40 | 0 |
| (*Newman's Own* Virgin Old Fashioned Roadside/Organic) . . . | 110 | 0 | 27.0 | 0 | 0 | 40 | 0 |
| (*Odwalla*) . . . . . . . . . . . | 120 | 0 | 30.0 | 0 | 0 | 10 | 0 |
| (*Odwalla* Light) . . . . . . . . | 50 | 0 | 14.0 | 0 | 0 | 15 | 0 |
| (*R.W. Knudsen* 100% Juice Box) . . . . | 130 | 1.0 | 32.0 | 0 | 0 | 15 | 0 |
| (*Santa Cruz Organic*) . . . . | 100 | 0 | 24.0 | 0 | 0 | 0 | 0 |
| (*Simply Lemonade*) . . . . . | 120 | 0 | 30.0 | 0 | 0 | 15 | 0 |
| (*Snapple*) . . . . . . . . . . . | 90 | 0 | 24.0 | 0 | 0 | 45 | 0 |
| (*Turkey Hill*) . . . . . . . . . | 120 | 0 | 29.0 | 0 | 0 | 10 | 0 |
| pink: | | | | | | | |
| (*Minute Maid* 13%) . . | 110 | 0 | 29.0 | 0 | 0 | 15 | 0 |
| (*Minute Maid* 3%) . . . | 100 | 0 | 28.0 | 0 | 0 | 35 | 0 |

| Food and Measure | cal. | prot. (gms) | carbo. (gms) | fat (gms) | chol. (mgs) | sod. (mgs) | fiber (gms) |
|---|---|---|---|---|---|---|---|
| **Lemonade, pink** *(cont.)* | | | | | | | |
| (*Minute Maid* Coolers), | | | | | | | |
| 6.75 fl. oz. . . . . . . . | 90 | 0 | 25.0 | 0 | 0 | 15 | 0 |
| (*Newman's Own* | | | | | | | |
| Virgin) . . . . . . . . . | 110 | 0 | 27.0 | 0 | 0 | 40 | 0 |
| (*Snapple*) . . . . . . . . . | 100 | 0 | 25.0 | 0 | 0 | 45 | 0 |
| (*Turkey Hill*) . . . . . . . | 120 | 0 | 29.0 | 0 | 0 | 10 | 0 |
| (*Veryfine*), 11.5 fl. oz. . . | 190 | 0 | 48.0 | 0 | 0 | 25 | 0 |
| frozen*: | | | | | | | |
| (*Cascadian Farm* | | | | | | | |
| Organic) . . . . . . . . | 110 | 0 | 28.0 | 0 | 0 | 15 | 0 |
| pink or white | | | | | | | |
| (*Minute Maid*) . . . . | 110 | 0 | 29.0 | 0 | 0 | 0 | 0 |
| sparkling (*Santa Cruz* | | | | | | | |
| *Organic*) . . . . . . . . . . | 110 | 0 | 27.0 | 0 | 0 | 0 | 0 |
| tea, see "Tea, iced" | | | | | | | |
| **Lemonade fruit** | | | | | | | |
| **blend**, 8 fl. oz.: | | | | | | | |
| agave (*SoBe Lifewater*) . . | 40 | 0 | 16.0 | 0 | 0 | 20 | 0 |
| cranberry: | | | | | | | |
| (*Honest Ade* Organic) . | 48 | 0 | 12.0 | 0 | 0 | 5 | 0 |
| white (*Langers*) . . . . . | 120 | 0 | 30.0 | 0 | 0 | 15 | 0 |
| limeade: | | | | | | | |
| (*Minute Maid* | | | | | | | |
| Limonada) . . . . . . . | 120 | 0 | 33.0 | 0 | 0 | 15 | 0 |
| (*Minute Maid* | | | | | | | |
| Limonada Light) . . . | 15 | 0 | 4.0 | 0 | 0 | 15 | 0 |
| (*Turkey Hill* | | | | | | | |
| Limonade) . . . . . . . | 120 | 0 | 28.0 | 0 | 0 | 10 | 0 |
| frozen* (*Minute Maid* | | | | | | | |
| Limonada) . . . . . . . | 90 | 0 | 25.0 | 0 | 0 | 0 | 0 |
| mango: | | | | | | | |
| (*Bolthouse Farms*) . . . | 120 | <1.0 | 30.0 | 0 | 0 | 0 | <1.0 |
| (*Santa Cruz Organic*) . | 100 | 0 | 24.0 | 0 | 0 | 10 | 0 |
| pomegranate: | | | | | | | |
| (*Newman's Own*) . . . . | 110 | 0 | 28.0 | 0 | 0 | 15 | 0 |
| (*Turkey Hill*) . . . . . . . | 110 | 0 | 28.0 | 0 | 0 | 10 | 0 |
| raspberry: | | | | | | | |
| (*Florida's Natural*) . . . . | 110 | 0 | 28.0 | 0 | 0 | 20 | 0 |
| (*Langers*) . . . . . . . . . . | 120 | 0 | 29.0 | 0 | 0 | 0 | 0 |
| (*Minute Maid*) . . . . . . . | 120 | 0 | 32.0 | 0 | 0 | 15 | 0 |
| (*Santa Cruz Organic*) . | 100 | 0 | 24.0 | 0 | 0 | 0 | 0 |
| (*Simply Lemonade*) . . | 110 | 0 | 28.0 | 0 | 0 | 15 | 0 |
| frozen* (*Minute Maid*) | 110 | 0 | 29.0 | 0 | 0 | 15 | 0 |

| Food and Measure | cal. | prot. (gms) | carbo. (gms) | fat (gms) | chol. (mgs) | sod. (mgs) | fiber (gms) |
|---|---|---|---|---|---|---|---|
| strawberry (*Santa Cruz Organic*) ....... | 100 | 0 | 24.0 | 0 | 0 | 0 | 0 |
| strawberry kiwi (*Turkey Hill*) ........ | 120 | 0 | 29.0 | 0 | 0 | 10 | 0 |
| **Lemonade mix** (*Country* Time), 8 fl. oz.*: | | | | | | | |
| pink or white .......... | 60 | 0 | 16.0 | 0 | 0 | 25 | 0 |
| raspberry ............ | 80 | 0 | 19.0 | 0 | 0 | 0 | 0 |
| strawberry ............ | 80 | 0 | 20.0 | 0 | 0 | 0 | 0 |
| **Lemongrass**, fresh: | | | | | | | |
| (*Frieda's*), 1 tbsp. ...... | 5 | 0 | 1.0 | 0 | 0 | 0 | 0 |
| sliced, 1 cup .......... | 66 | .5 | 16.9 | .3 | 0 | 4 | n.a. |
| **Lemongrass**, in jars: | | | | | | | |
| minced (*Tiger Tiger Thai*), 1 tbsp. ....... | 10 | 0 | 2.0 | 0 | 0 | 10 | <1.0 |
| sliced (*Roland*), 1 tbsp. .. | 5 | 0 | 2.0 | 0 | 0 | 10 | 0 |
| **Lentil**, dry, ¼ cup, except as noted: | | | | | | | |
| (*Bob's Red Mill*) ....... | 150 | 11.0 | 27.0 | 0 | 0 | 15 | 7.0 |
| green: | | | | | | | |
| (*Arrowhead Mills* Organic) .......... | 150 | 10.0 | 27.0 | 1.0 | 0 | 5 | 7.0 |
| (*Bob's Red Mill* Petite French) .......... | 160 | 12.0 | 29.0 | 0 | 0 | 15 | 7.0 |
| (*Eden* Organic) ...... | 170 | 11.0 | 30.0 | 1.0 | 0 | 10 | 12.0 |
| (*Roland* French) ..... | 120 | 10.0 | 20.0 | 0 | 0 | 5 | 5.0 |
| or beluga (*Roland*) ... | 100 | 9.0 | 21.0 | 0 | 0 | 0 | 5.0 |
| red: | | | | | | | |
| (*Arrowhead Mills* Organic) .......... | 170 | 13.0 | 28.0 | 1.0 | 0 | 5 | 7.0 |
| (*Bob's Red Mill*) ..... | 150 | 11.0 | 27.0 | 0 | 0 | 15 | 7.0 |
| (*Roland*) ........... | 120 | 8.0 | 22.0 | 0 | 0 | 0 | 5.0 |
| cooked, ½ cup ........ | 115 | 8.9 | 19.9 | .4 | 0 | 2 | 7.8 |
| **Lentil, canned** (see also "Rice and lentils"), (*Eden* Organic), ½ cup | 90 | 8.0 | 13.0 | 0 | 0 | 210 | 4.0 |
| **Lentil, sprouted**, raw, ½ cup .......... | 40 | 3.4 | 8.4 | .2 | 0 | 4 | n.a. |
| **Lentil dish**, mix: | | | | | | | |
| (*Neera's* Dal and Seasoning), 1 cup* ... | 140 | 11.0 | 23.0 | 1.0 | 0 | 4 | 12.0 |
| (*Neera's* Urad and Channa Dal), 1 cup* .. | 104 | 8.0 | 18.0 | 1.0 | 0 | 4 | 9.0 |

| Food and Measure | cal. | prot. (gms) | carbo. (gms) | fat (gms) | chol. (mgs) | sod. (mgs) | fiber (gms) |
|---|---|---|---|---|---|---|---|
| **Lentil dish, mix** *(cont.)* | | | | | | | |
| (*Tasty Bite* Magic), | | | | | | | |
| ½ of 8.8-oz. pkg. .... | 240 | 12.0 | 33.0 | 6.0 | 0 | 440 | 9.0 |
| w/peas (*Tasty Bite* | | | | | | | |
| Zesty), ½ of 8-oz. pkg. | 200 | 10.0 | 38.0 | 3.5 | 0 | 400 | 7.0 |
| rice and, see "Rice | | | | | | | |
| dish mix" | | | | | | | |
| **Lentil entree, microwave** | | | | | | | |
| (*Tasty Bite*), | | | | | | | |
| ½ of 10-oz. pkg.: | | | | | | | |
| Bengal .............. | 160 | 6.0 | 16.0 | 8.0 | 0 | 440 | 8.0 |
| Jodhpur ............. | 110 | 6.0 | 16.0 | 2.5 | 0 | 460 | 4.0 |
| w/red beans, Madras .... | 120 | 6.0 | 14.0 | 5.0 | 3 | 450 | 5.0 |
| **Lettuce** (see also | | | | | | | |
| "Salad blend"): | | | | | | | |
| bibb or Boston: | | | | | | | |
| (*Earthbound Farm* | | | | | | | |
| Organic), 3 oz. .... | 10 | 1.0 | 2.0 | 0 | 0 | 0 | 1.0 |
| 1 head, 5" diam. ..... | 21 | 2.1 | 3.8 | .4 | 0 | 8 | 1.6 |
| 2 inner leaves ....... | 2 | .2 | .4 | <.1 | 0 | 1 | .5 |
| butter: | | | | | | | |
| (*Dole*), ½ head, 3 oz. . | 10 | 1.0 | 3.0 | 0 | 0 | 0 | 1.0 |
| (*Fresh Express Sweet* | | | | | | | |
| *Butter*), 3 oz. ..... | 10 | 1.0 | 2.0 | 0 | 0 | 0 | <1.0 |
| butterhead (*Frieda's* | | | | | | | |
| Limestone), 3 oz. .... | 10 | 1.0 | 2.0 | 0 | 0 | 10 | 1.0 |
| frisée (*Earthbound* | | | | | | | |
| *Farm* Organic) ....... | 10 | 1.0 | 4.0 | 0 | 0 | 35 | 1.0 |
| iceberg: | | | | | | | |
| (*Dole*), ⅛ medium ... | 10 | 1.0 | 3.0 | 0 | 0 | 10 | 1.0 |
| 1 head, 6" diam. ..... | 70 | 5.4 | 11.3 | 1.0 | 0 | 48 | 7.5 |
| 1 leaf, .7 oz. ........ | 3 | .2 | .4 | <.1 | 0 | 2 | .3 |
| shredded (*Fresh* | | | | | | | |
| *Express Shreds!*), | | | | | | | |
| 1½ cups, 3.1 oz. .. | 10 | 1.0 | 3.0 | 0 | 0 | 10 | 1.0 |
| shredded, 1 cup ..... | 7 | .6 | 1.2 | .1 | 0 | 3 | .8 |
| leaf/looseleaf, shredded: | | | | | | | |
| (*Dole*), 3 oz. ........ | 15 | 1.0 | 3.0 | 0 | 0 | 10 | 1.0 |
| ½ cup ............. | 5 | .4 | 1.0 | .1 | 0 | 3 | .5 |
| green (*Dole*), ¼ head, | | | | | | | |
| 3.2 oz. .......... | 15 | 1.0 | 3.0 | 0 | 0 | 25 | 1.0 |
| mâche (*Earthbound* | | | | | | | |
| *Farm* Organic), 3 oz. .. | 30 | 2.0 | 5.0 | 0 | 0 | 20 | 2.0 |

| Food and Measure | cal. | prot. (gms) | carbo. (gms) | fat (gms) | chol. (mgs) | sod. (mgs) | fiber (gms) |
|---|---|---|---|---|---|---|---|
| romaine or cos: | | | | | | | |
| (*Ready Pac* Caesar), | | | | | | | |
| 3 oz., 2½ cups .... | 15 | 1.0 | 3.0 | 0 | 0 | 10 | 1.0 |
| baby (*Dole*), 3 oz. .... | 25 | 2.0 | 4.0 | 0 | 0 | 0 | 2.0 |
| baby (*Earthbound* | | | | | | | |
| *Farm* Organic), 3 oz. | 15 | 1.0 | 2.0 | 0 | 0 | 50 | 1.0 |
| 1 inner leaf ......... | 1 | .2 | .2 | 0 | 0 | 1 | .2 |
| chopped (*Dole*), 3 oz. . | 15 | 1.0 | 3.0 | 0 | 0 | 5 | 1.0 |
| shredded, ½ cup .... | 4 | .5 | .7 | .1 | 0 | 2 | .5 |
| romaine hearts, 3 oz.: | | | | | | | |
| (*Dole*) ............. | 15 | 1.0 | 3.0 | 0 | 0 | 10 | 1.0 |
| (*Fresh Express*) ..... | 15 | 1.0 | 3.0 | 0 | 0 | 5 | 2.0 |
| (*Ready* Pac Bella) .... | 15 | 1.0 | 3.0 | 0 | 0 | 10 | 1.0 |
| **Lima beans:** | | | | | | | |
| immature, ½ cup: | | | | | | | |
| raw, trimmed ....... | 88 | 5.3 | 15.7 | .7 | 0 | 6 | 3.8 |
| boiled, drained ...... | 104 | 5.8 | 20.1 | .3 | 0 | 14 | 4.5 |
| mature, dry: | | | | | | | |
| baby (*Bob's Red Mill*), | | | | | | | |
| ¼ cup ........... | 150 | 9.0 | 28.0 | 0 | 0 | 5 | 9.0 |
| baby, boiled, ½ cup .. | 115 | 7.3 | 21.2 | .3 | 0 | 2 | 7.0 |
| large (*Bob's Red Mill*), | | | | | | | |
| ¼ cup ........... | 150 | 9.0 | 28.0 | 0 | 0 | 10 | 8.0 |
| large, boiled, ½ cup .. | 108 | 7.3 | 19.6 | .4 | 0 | 2 | 6.6 |
| **Lima beans, canned** | | | | | | | |
| (see also "Butter | | | | | | | |
| beans"), ½ cup: | | | | | | | |
| (*Luck's* Giant) ......... | 130 | 7.0 | 22.0 | 1.5 | 0 | 370 | 5.0 |
| green: | | | | | | | |
| (*Allens* Medium/*East* | | | | | | | |
| *Texas Fair*) ....... | 120 | 7.0 | 23.0 | 0 | 0 | 370 | 8.0 |
| (*Del Monte*) ........ | 80 | 4.0 | 15.0 | 0 | 0 | 390 | 4.0 |
| green, baby: | | | | | | | |
| (*Freshlike*) ......... | 140 | 9.0 | 26.0 | .5 | 0 | 270 | 7.0 |
| (*Veg-All*) ........... | 90 | 4.0 | 15.0 | 1.0 | 0 | 330 | 3.0 |
| w/bacon (*Trappey's*) .. | 120 | 6.0 | 22.0 | 1.0 | 0 | 330 | 6.0 |
| seasoned (*Glory*) .... | 100 | 6.0 | 18.0 | 0 | 0 | 570 | 6.0 |
| green and white | | | | | | | |
| (*Allens*) ............. | 110 | 6.0 | 20.0 | 1.0 | 0 | 280 | 9.0 |
| **Lima beans, frozen,** | | | | | | | |
| ½ cup, except as | | | | | | | |
| noted: | | | | | | | |
| baby: | | | | | | | |
| (*Birds Eye/C&W*) .... | 110 | 6.0 | 20.0 | 0 | 0 | 240 | 5.0 |

| Food and Measure | cal. | prot. (gms) | carbo. (gms) | fat (gms) | chol. (mgs) | sod. (mgs) | fiber (gms) |
|---|---|---|---|---|---|---|---|
| **Lima beans, frozen, baby** (cont.) | | | | | | | |
| (Green Giant Simply Steam) .......... | 80 | 4.0 | 15.0 | 0 | 0 | 170 | 3.0 |
| or petite | | | | | | | |
| (McKenzie's) ..... | 110 | 6.0 | 20.0 | 0 | 0 | 240 | 5.0 |
| baby, in butter sauce | | | | | | | |
| (Green Giant), ⅔ cup . | 100 | 5.0 | 18.0 | 1.5 | <5 | 420 | 5.0 |
| Fordhook (Birds Eye) ... | 100 | 6.0 | 18.0 | 0 | 0 | 5 | 4.0 |
| **Lime**, fresh: | | | | | | | |
| (Frieda's Key Lime), | | | | | | | |
| 2.4-oz. lime ........ | 20 | 1.0 | 7.0 | 0 | 0 | 0 | 2.0 |
| 2"-diam. lime .......... | 20 | .5 | 7.1 | .1 | 0 | 1 | 1.9 |
| peeled, seeded, 1 oz. .... | 9 | .2 | 3.0 | .1 | 0 | 1 | .8 |
| **Lime curd** | | | | | | | |
| (Dickenson's), 1 tbsp. . | 60 | 0 | 11.0 | 1.0 | 15 | 10 | 0 |
| **Lime drink**, see "Lemonade fruit blend" and "Limeade" | | | | | | | |
| **Lime juice**, fresh: | | | | | | | |
| ½ cup .............. | 33 | .5 | 11.1 | .1 | 0 | 1 | .5 |
| 1 tbsp. ............. | 4 | .1 | 1.4 | <.1 | 0 | tr. | .1 |
| **Lime juice, bottled**, | | | | | | | |
| sweetened, 1 tsp.: | | | | | | | |
| (Angostura) ......... | 5 | 0 | 2.0 | 0 | 0 | 0 | 0 |
| (Roland) ........... | 10 | 0 | 2.0 | 0 | 0 | 0 | 0 |
| unsweetened, 2 tbsp. ... | 6 | <.1 | 2.0 | <.1 | 0 | 5 | .1 |
| **Limeade**, 8 fl. oz.: | | | | | | | |
| (Honest Ade Organic) ... | 48 | 0 | 12.0 | 0 | 0 | 5 | 0 |
| (Newman's Own | | | | | | | |
| Virgin) ............ | 140 | 0 | 34.0 | 0 | 0 | 35 | 0 |
| (Odwalla Light) ........ | 50 | 0 | 14.0 | 0 | 0 | 15 | 0 |
| (Odwalla | | | | | | | |
| Summertime Lime) .. | 120 | 0 | 29.0 | 0 | 0 | 10 | 0 |
| (Santa Cruz Organic) .... | 100 | 0 | 26.0 | 0 | 0 | 0 | 0 |
| (Simply Limeade) ...... | 120 | 0 | 30.0 | 0 | 0 | 15 | 0 |
| cherry (Minute Maid) ... | 120 | 0 | 34.0 | 0 | 0 | 15 | 0 |
| sparkling (Santa Cruz | | | | | | | |
| Organic) ........... | 100 | 0 | 26.0 | 0 | 0 | 10 | 0 |
| **Ling**, meat only: | | | | | | | |
| raw, 4 oz. ............ | 99 | 21.5 | 0 | .7 | 45 | 153 | 0 |
| baked or broiled, 4 oz. .. | 126 | 27.6 | 0 | .9 | 58 | 196 | 0 |
| **Ling cod**, meat only: | | | | | | | |
| raw, 4 oz. ............ | 96 | 20.0 | 0 | 1.2 | 59 | 67 | 0 |
| baked or broiled, 4 oz. .. | 124 | 25.7 | 0 | 1.5 | 76 | 86 | 0 |

| Food and Measure | cal. | prot. (gms) | carbo. (gms) | fat (gms) | chol. (mgs) | sod. (mgs) | fiber (gms) |
|---|---|---|---|---|---|---|---|
| **Lingonberries**, in jars, in syrup (*Roland*), 2 tbsp. . . . . . . . . . . . | 70 | 0 | 16.0 | 0 | 0 | 5 | 1.0 |
| **Lingonberry-apple drink**, sparkling (*Kristen Regale*), 8 fl. oz. . . . . . | 100 | 0 | 24.0 | 0 | 0 | 10 | 0 |
| **Linguine**, see "Pasta" | | | | | | | |
| **Linguine entree**, frozen, carbonara (*Lean Cuisine*), 9.25 oz. . . . . | 300 | 14.0 | 43.0 | 8.0 | 15 | 590 | 2.0 |
| **Liquor**[1], 1 fl. oz.: | | | | | | | |
| 80 proof . . . . . . . . . . . . | 64 | 0 | 0 | 0 | 0 | tr. | 0 |
| 90 proof . . . . . . . . . . . . | 73 | 0 | 0 | 0 | 0 | tr. | 0 |
| 100 proof . . . . . . . . . . . | 82 | 0 | 0 | 0 | 0 | tr. | 0 |
| **Litchi**, see "Lychee" | | | | | | | |
| **Liver**: | | | | | | | |
| beef, pan-fried, 4 oz. . . . . | 246 | 30.3 | 8.9 | 9.1 | 547 | 120 | 0 |
| calves (veal), 4 oz.: | | | | | | | |
| braised . . . . . . . . . . . . | 218 | 32.2 | 4.3 | 7.1 | 579 | 88 | 0 |
| pan-fried . . . . . . . . . . . | 219 | 31.0 | 5.1 | 7.4 | 550 | 96 | 0 |
| chicken, raw (*Tyson*), 3 pcs., 4.1 oz. . . . . . . . | 110 | 19.0 | 0 | 4.5 | 470 | 80 | 0 |
| chicken, simmered: | | | | | | | |
| 4 oz. . . . . . . . . . . . . . | 189 | 27.7 | 1.0 | 7.4 | 638 | 86 | 0 |
| chopped, 1 cup . . . . . . | 219 | 34.1 | 1.2 | 7.6 | 883 | 71 | 0 |
| chicken, pan-fried, 4 oz. . . | 195 | 29.2 | 1.3 | 7.3 | 640 | 104 | 0 |
| duck, raw, 1 oz. . . . . . . . | 39 | 5.3 | 1.0 | 1.3 | 146 | n.a. | 0 |
| goose, raw, 1 oz. . . . . . . | 38 | 4.6 | 1.8 | 1.2 | 146 | 40 | 0 |
| lamb, braised, 4 oz. . . . . . | 249 | 34.7 | 2.9 | 10.0 | 568 | 64 | 0 |
| lamb, pan-fried, 4 oz. . . . . | 270 | 29.0 | 4.3 | 14.3 | 559 | 141 | 0 |
| pork, braised, 4 oz. . . . . . | 187 | 29.5 | 4.3 | 5.0 | 403 | 56 | 0 |
| turkey, simmered: | | | | | | | |
| 4 oz. . . . . . . . . . . . . . | 192 | 27.2 | 3.9 | 6.7 | 710 | 73 | 0 |
| chopped, 1 cup . . . . . . | 237 | 33.6 | 4.8 | 8.3 | 876 | 89 | 0 |
| **"Liver," vegetarian**, see "Vegetable dip" | | | | | | | |
| **Liverwurst** (see also "Braunschweiger"): | | | | | | | |
| (*Boar's Head Strassburger*), 2 oz. . . | 170 | 8.0 | 1.0 | 15.0 | 85 | 560 | 0 |

---

[1] Includes all pure distilled liquors: bourbon, brandy, gin, rum, Scotch, tequila, vodka, etc.

| Food and Measure | cal. | prot. (gms) | carbo. (gms) | fat (gms) | chol. (mgs) | sod. (mgs) | fiber (gms) |
|---|---|---|---|---|---|---|---|
| **Liverwurst** *(cont.)* | | | | | | | |
| smoked, 2 oz.: | | | | | | | |
| (*Boar's Head*) ........ | 170 | 8.0 | 1.0 | 15.0 | 45 | 620 | 0 |
| (*Thumann's*) ......... | 160 | 9.0 | 3.0 | 12.0 | 80 | 580 | 0 |
| **Liverwurst spread** | | | | | | | |
| (*Underwood*), ¼ cup . | 160 | 8.0 | 4.0 | 13.0 | 70 | 440 | 1.0 |
| **Lo bok**, see "Radish, Oriental" | | | | | | | |
| **Lobster**, northern, meat only: | | | | | | | |
| raw, 4 oz. ............ | 102 | 21.3 | .6 | 1.0 | 108 | n.a. | 0 |
| boiled or steamed: | | | | | | | |
| 4 oz. ............. | 111 | 23.2 | 1.5 | .7 | 82 | 431 | 0 |
| 1 cup, 5.1 oz. ....... | 142 | 29.7 | 1.9 | .9 | 104 | 551 | 0 |
| **"Lobster," imitation**, chunk style (*Louis Kemp Lobster Delights*), ½ cup, 3 oz. | 90 | 6.0 | 15.0 | 0 | 5 | 340 | 0 |
| **Lobster, spiny**, see "Spiny lobster" | | | | | | | |
| **Lobster sauce**, canned (*Progresso*), ½ cup .. | 100 | 3.0 | 6.0 | 7.0 | 5 | 430 | 2.0 |
| **Loganberries**, fresh, 1 cup ............. | 89 | 1.4 | 21.5 | .9 | 0 | 1 | n.a. |
| **Long bean**, see "Yard-long bean" | | | | | | | |
| *Long John Silver's:* | | | | | | | |
| fish/seafood: | | | | | | | |
| clams, breaded, 3 oz. . | 320 | 9.0 | 29.0 | 19.0 | 35 | 1190 | 2.0 |
| fish, battered, 1 pc. ... | 260 | 12.0 | 17.0 | 16.0 | 35 | 790 | 0 |
| lobster bites, buttered, 3.2 oz. ... | 230 | 13.0 | 24.0 | 9.0 | 60 | 520 | 2.0 |
| lobster crab cake, 1 .. | 170 | 6.0 | 16.0 | 9.0 | 30 | 390 | 1.0 |
| salmon, grilled, 2 .... | 150 | 24.0 | 2.0 | 5.0 | 50 | 440 | 0 |
| shrimp: | | | | | | | |
| battered, 3 ....... | 130 | 5.0 | 8.0 | 9.0 | 45 | 480 | 0 |
| popcorn, 3 oz. .... | 270 | 9.0 | 23.0 | 16.0 | 75 | 570 | 1.0 |
| scampi, 8 ........ | 200 | 17.0 | 3.0 | 13.0 | 135 | 650 | 0 |
| tilapia, grilled, 1 ..... | 110 | 22.0 | 1.0 | 2.5 | 55 | 250 | 0 |
| whitefish, breaded, 1 .. | 190 | 9.0 | 17.0 | 10.0 | 20 | 540 | 1.0 |
| *Chicken Plank*, 1 pc. .... | 140 | 8.0 | 9.0 | 8.0 | 20 | 480 | 0 |
| *Freshside Grille:* | | | | | | | |
| salmon ............ | 280 | 27.0 | 27.0 | 7.0 | 50 | 1010 | 3.0 |

| Food and Measure | cal. | prot. (gms) | carbo. (gms) | fat (gms) | chol. (mgs) | sod. (mgs) | fiber (gms) |
|---|---|---|---|---|---|---|---|
| shrimp scampi | 330 | 20.0 | 29.0 | 15.0 | 135 | 1230 | 3.0 |
| tilapia | 250 | 25.0 | 27.0 | 4.5 | 60 | 820 | 3.0 |
| sandwiches: | | | | | | | |
| chicken | 440 | 22.0 | 47.0 | 30.0 | 50 | 1350 | 4.0 |
| fish | 470 | 18.0 | 49.0 | 23.0 | 40 | 1180 | 3.0 |
| *Ultimate Fish* | | | | | | | |
| *Sandwich* | 530 | 21.0 | 50.0 | 27.0 | 55 | 1500 | 3.0 |
| condiments/sauces: | | | | | | | |
| BBQ | 40 | 0 | 10.0 | 0 | 0 | 230 | 0 |
| cocktail sauce | 25 | 0 | 6.0 | 0 | 0 | 250 | 0 |
| honey mustard | 100 | 0 | 12.0 | 6.0 | 0 | 170 | 0 |
| hot sauce | 0 | 0 | 0 | 0 | 0 | 140 | 0 |
| ketchup | 10 | 0 | 2.0 | 0 | 0 | 100 | 0 |
| malt vinegar | 0 | 0 | 0 | 0 | 0 | 35 | 0 |
| marinara | 15 | 1.0 | 4.0 | 0 | 0 | 125 | 1.0 |
| ranch | 160 | 0 | 2.0 | 17.0 | 15 | 240 | 0 |
| sweet & sour | 45 | 0 | 12.0 | 0 | 0 | 120 | 0 |
| tartar sauce | 100 | 0 | 4.0 | 9.0 | 15 | 250 | 0 |
| sides/starters: | | | | | | | |
| breadstick, 1 | 170 | 6.0 | 29.0 | 3.5 | 0 | 290 | 1.0 |
| broccoli cheese bites | 230 | 5.0 | 25.0 | 12.0 | 15 | 550 | 2.0 |
| broccoli cheese soup | 220 | 5.0 | 8.0 | 18.0 | 30 | 650 | 1.0 |
| coleslaw, 4 oz. | 200 | 1.0 | 15.0 | 15.0 | 20 | 340 | 3.0 |
| corn cobbette, 1 | 90 | 3.0 | 14.0 | 3.0 | 0 | 0 | 3.0 |
| w/butter oil | 150 | 3.0 | 14.0 | 10.0 | 0 | 30 | 3.0 |
| *Crumblies*, 1 oz. | 170 | 1.0 | 14.0 | 12.0 | 0 | 410 | 1.0 |
| fries, platter size | 230 | 3.0 | 34.0 | 10.0 | 0 | 350 | 3.0 |
| fries, basket size | 310 | 3.0 | 45.0 | 14.0 | 0 | 460 | 4.0 |
| hushpuppy, 1 | 60 | 1.0 | 9.0 | 2.5 | 0 | 200 | 1.0 |
| jalapeño cheddar | | | | | | | |
| bites, 5 | 240 | 6.0 | 23.0 | 14.0 | 15 | 730 | 2.0 |
| jalapeño peppers, 1 | 15 | 1.0 | 2.0 | 0 | 0 | 190 | 0 |
| mozzarella sticks, 3 | 150 | 5.0 | 13.0 | 9.0 | 10 | 350 | 1.0 |
| rice, 5 oz. | 180 | 4.0 | 37.0 | 1.0 | 0 | 470 | 2.0 |
| vegetable medley, | | | | | | | |
| 4 oz. | 50 | 1.0 | 8.0 | 2.0 | 0 | 360 | 3.0 |
| dessert pie, 1 pc.: | | | | | | | |
| chocolate cream | 280 | 3.0 | 28.0 | 17.0 | 10 | 230 | 1.0 |
| pineapple cream cheese | 300 | 3.0 | 35.0 | 16.0 | 10 | 210 | 0 |
| turtle | 290 | 3.0 | 34.0 | 16.0 | 10 | 210 | 0 |
| **Longan**, fresh: | | | | | | | |
| (*Frieda's*), 10 pcs. | 20 | 0 | 5.0 | 0 | 0 | 0 | 0 |
| seeded, 1 oz. | 17 | .4 | 4.3 | <.1 | 0 | <1 | .3 |

| Food and Measure | cal. | prot. (gms) | carbo. (gms) | fat (gms) | chol. (mgs) | sod. (mgs) | fiber (gms) |
|---|---|---|---|---|---|---|---|
| **Longan, canned**, in heavy syrup (*Roland*), 2 tbsp. | 25 | 0 | 6.0 | 0 | 0 | 0 | 0 |
| **Longan, dried**, 1 oz. | 81 | 1.4 | 21.0 | .1 | 0 | 14 | <1.0 |
| **Loquat:** | | | | | | | |
| (*Frieda's*), 5 oz. | 70 | 1.0 | 17.0 | 0 | 0 | 0 | 2.0 |
| 1 large, .7 oz. | 9 | <.1 | 2.4 | 0 | 0 | tr. | .3 |
| cubed, 1 cup | 70 | .6 | 18.1 | .3 | 0 | 1 | 2.5 |
| peeled, seeded, 1 oz. | 13 | .1 | 3.4 | .1 | 0 | <1 | .5 |
| **Loquat, canned**, in light syrup (*Roland*), 1.1 oz. | 20 | 0 | 5.0 | 0 | 0 | 0 | 0 |
| **Lotus root:** | | | | | | | |
| raw: | | | | | | | |
| (*Frieda's*), 1 cup, 3 oz. | 50 | 2.0 | 15.0 | 0 | 0 | 35 | 4.0 |
| 10 slices | 60 | 2.1 | 14.0 | .1 | 0 | 32 | 4.0 |
| trimmed, 1 oz. | 16 | .7 | 4.9 | <.1 | 0 | 11 | 1.4 |
| boiled, drained, ½ cup | 40 | 1.0 | 9.6 | <.1 | 0 | 27 | 1.9 |
| **Lotus root, dried** (*Eden* Organic), about 5 slices, .4 oz. | 35 | 1.0 | 8.0 | 0 | 0 | 25 | 2.0 |
| **Lotus seeds:** | | | | | | | |
| raw, 1 oz. | 25 | 1.2 | 4.9 | .2 | 0 | <1 | n.a. |
| dried, 1 oz. | 94 | 4.4 | 18.3 | .6 | 0 | 1 | n.a. |
| fried, 1 cup | 106 | 4.9 | 20.6 | .6 | 0 | 1 | n.a. |
| **Lox**, see "Salmon, smoked" | | | | | | | |
| **Lunch meat** (see also specific listings), loaf, 2 oz.: | | | | | | | |
| deluxe (*Black Bear*) | 140 | 7.0 | 3.0 | 11.0 | 30 | 510 | 0 |
| Dutch (*Boar's Head*) | 150 | 7.0 | 2.0 | 12.0 | 25 | 610 | 0 |
| kielbasa loaf (*Thumann's*) | 150 | 9.0 | <1.0 | 13.0 | 28 | 470 | 0 |
| minced (*Thumann's*) | 150 | 7.0 | 1.0 | 13.0 | 28 | 470 | 0 |
| olive loaf: | | | | | | | |
| (*Black Bear*) | 140 | 7.0 | 3.0 | 11.0 | 30 | 580 | 0 |
| (*Boar's Head*) | 130 | 6.0 | <1.0 | 12.0 | 20 | 630 | 0 |
| (*Thumann's*) | 130 | 8.0 | <1.0 | 12.0 | 18 | 580 | 0 |
| pepper loaf (*Black Bear*) | 140 | 7.0 | 3.0 | 11.0 | 30 | 520 | 0 |
| pickle and pepper: | | | | | | | |
| (*Black Bear* P&P) | 140 | 7.0 | 3.0 | 11.0 | 30 | 580 | 0 |

| Food and Measure | cal. | prot. (gms) | carbo. (gms) | fat (gms) | chol. (mgs) | sod. (mgs) | fiber (gms) |
|---|---|---|---|---|---|---|---|
| (*Boar's Head*) . . . . . . . | 150 | 6.0 | 2.0 | 13.0 | 30 | 500 | 0 |
| (*Thumann's*) . . . . . . . . | 130 | 8.0 | <1.0 | 12.0 | 18 | 470 | 0 |
| spiced ham: | | | | | | | |
| (*Boar's Head*) . . . . . . . | 120 | 7.0 | 1.0 | 10.0 | 30 | 570 | 0 |
| (*Di Lusso*) . . . . . . . . . | 140 | 8.0 | 1.0 | 11.0 | 35 | 680 | 0 |
| (*Hormel*) . . . . . . . . . . | 140 | 8.0 | 1.0 | 11.0 | 35 | 690 | 0 |
| **Lunch meat, canned** (*Spam*), 2 oz., except as noted: | | | | | | | |
| classic . . . . . . . . . . . . . | 180 | 7.0 | 1.0 | 16.0 | 40 | 790 | 0 |
| classic single, 3 oz. . . . . | 250 | 11.0 | 2.0 | 22.0 | 60 | 990 | 0 |
| less salt . . . . . . . . . . . . | 180 | 7.0 | 1.0 | 16.0 | 40 | 580 | 0 |
| lite . . . . . . . . . . . . . . . | 110 | 9.0 | 1.0 | 8.0 | 40 | 580 | 0 |
| lite single, 3 oz. . . . . . . . | 160 | 13.0 | 2.0 | 11.0 | 60 | 740 | 0 |
| w/bacon . . . . . . . . . . . . | 180 | 7.0 | 1.0 | 16.0 | 40 | 520 | 0 |
| w/cheese . . . . . . . . . . . | 170 | 8.0 | 1.0 | 15.0 | 40 | 720 | 0 |
| garlic . . . . . . . . . . . . . . | 180 | 7.0 | 1.0 | 16.0 | 40 | 390 | 0 |
| hot and spicy . . . . . . . . | 180 | 7.0 | 2.0 | 16.0 | 40 | 600 | 0 |
| smoked . . . . . . . . . . . . | 180 | 7.0 | 1.0 | 16.0 | 40 | 640 | 0 |
| turkey, oven-roasted . . . . | 80 | 9.0 | 1.0 | 5.0 | 35 | 520 | 0 |
| **Lunch "meat," vegetarian**, frozen (*Worthington Wham*), 2 oz., ⅜" slice . . . . . . . | 110 | 10.0 | 3.0 | 6.0 | 0 | 390 | 0 |
| **Lupin**, boiled, ½ cup . . . . | 98 | 12.9 | 8.2 | 2.4 | 0 | 3 | 2.3 |
| **Lychee**, fresh: (*Frieda's*), 6–8 pcs., 3.5 oz. . . . . . . . . . . . | 60 | 1.0 | 14.0 | 0 | 0 | 0 | 1.0 |
| 1 fruit, .3 oz. . . . . . . . . . | 6 | .1 | 1.6 | 0 | 0 | 0 | .1 |
| shelled: | | | | | | | |
| 1 cup . . . . . . . . . . . . | 125 | 1.6 | 31.4 | .8 | 0 | 2 | 2.5 |
| 1 oz. . . . . . . . . . . . . . | 19 | .2 | 4.7 | .1 | 0 | <1 | .4 |
| **Lychee, canned**, in heavy syrup (*Roland*), 2 tbsp., 1.1 oz. . . . . . . | 30 | 0 | 7.0 | 0 | 0 | 5 | 0 |
| **Lychee, dried**, 10 fruits, .7 oz. . . . . . . | 69 | 1.0 | 17.7 | .3 | 0 | 0 | 1.2 |
| **Lychee juice** (*Ceres Litchi*), 8 fl. oz. . . . . . . | 120 | 0 | 30.0 | 0 | 0 | 10 | 1.0 |

# M

| Food and Measure | cal. | prot. (gms) | carbo. (gms) | fat (gms) | chol. (mgs) | sod. (mgs) | fiber (gms) |
|---|---|---|---|---|---|---|---|
| **Macadamia nut**: | | | | | | | |
| (*Mauna Loa*): | | | | | | | |
| coffee glazed, ¼ cup .. | 180 | 1.0 | 12.0 | 15.0 | 5 | 75 | 1.0 |
| dry-roasted, 1 oz. .... | 230 | 2.0 | 4.0 | 24.0 | 0 | 105 | 2.0 |
| honey roast, 1.1 oz. .. | 220 | 2.0 | 10.0 | 21.0 | 0 | 100 | 2.0 |
| onion garlic, .5 oz. ... | 100 | 1.0 | 2.0 | 11.0 | 0 | 85 | 1.0 |
| (*Planters*), 1 oz. ....... | 200 | 2.0 | 4.0 | 21.0 | 0 | 55 | 3.0 |
| raw, whole/halves: | | | | | | | |
| 1 oz. ............. | 204 | 2.2 | 3.9 | 21.5 | 0 | 1 | 2.4 |
| ¼ cup ............ | 241 | 2.7 | 4.6 | 25.4 | 0 | 2 | 2.9 |
| chopped: | | | | | | | |
| (*Diamond*), ¼ cup ... | 220 | 2.0 | 4.0 | 23.0 | 0 | 0 | 3.0 |
| (*Planters*), 2 oz. ..... | 400 | 5.0 | 8.0 | 42.0 | 0 | 0 | 5.0 |
| dried, shelled, 1 oz. ..... | 199 | 2.4 | 3.9 | 20.9 | 0 | 1 | 2.6 |
| oil-roasted, 1 oz. ....... | 204 | 2.1 | 3.7 | 21.7 | 0 | 2 | n.a. |
| **Macaroni** (see also "Pasta"): | | | | | | | |
| uncooked: | | | | | | | |
| 2 oz. .............. | 210 | 7.3 | 42.4 | .9 | 0 | 4 | 1.4 |
| elbow, 1 cup ........ | 389 | 13.4 | 78.4 | 1.7 | 0 | 8 | 2.5 |
| enriched, 2 oz. ...... | 213 | 11.3 | 38.3 | 1.3 | 0 | 5 | 1.4 |
| whole wheat, 2 oz. ... | 198 | .3 | 42.8 | .8 | 0 | 5 | 4.7 |
| cooked, 1 cup: | | | | | | | |
| enriched, elbows .... | 197 | 6.7 | 39.7 | .9 | 0 | 1 | 1.8 |
| enriched, spirals ..... | 189 | 6.4 | 38.0 | .9 | 0 | 1 | 1.7 |
| small shells ........ | 162 | 5.5 | 32.6 | .8 | 0 | 1 | 1.8 |
| vegetable, enriched, spirals ......... | 172 | 6.1 | 35.7 | .2 | 0 | 8 | 5.8 |
| whole-wheat, elbows . | 174 | 7.5 | 37.2 | .8 | 0 | 4 | 3.9 |
| **Macaroni entree, canned** (*Chef Boyardee*), 1 cup: | | | | | | | |
| *Beefaroni* .............. | 240 | 9.0 | 30.0 | 9.0 | 15 | 720 | 3.0 |
| *Beefaroni*, Big ......... | 240 | 9.0 | 30.0 | 9.0 | 15 | 720 | 3.0 |

| Food and Measure | cal. | prot. (gms) | carbo. (gms) | fat (gms) | chol. (mgs) | sod. (mgs) | fiber (gms) |
|---|---|---|---|---|---|---|---|
| *Beefaroni*, Whole Grain .. | 240 | 9.0 | 31.0 | 9.0 | 20 | 750 | 3.0 |
| cheesy burger ......... | 200 | 9.0 | 30.0 | 5.0 | 15 | 820 | 3.0 |
| cheesy nacho ......... | 220 | 8.0 | 32.0 | 7.0 | 15 | 950 | 2.0 |
| chili mac ............ | 260 | 9.0 | 26.0 | 13.0 | 20 | 940 | 3.0 |
| mac & cheese ........ | 240 | 9.0 | 28.0 | 10.0 | 15 | 750 | 4.0 |
| **Macaroni entree, frozen/ chilled**, 1 pkg., 8 oz., except as noted: | | | | | | | |
| and beef: | | | | | | | |
| (*Banquet* Dinner) .... | 290 | 9.0 | 32.0 | 4.5 | 10 | 820 | 4.0 |
| (*Blake's* Organic) .... | 321 | 14.0 | 45.0 | 11.0 | 33 | 404 | 3.0 |
| (*Lean Cuisine*), 9.5 oz. | 260 | 16.0 | 42.0 | 3.0 | 30 | 500 | 4.0 |
| (*Michelina's* Authentico) ...... | 280 | 12.0 | 33.0 | 10.0 | 25 | 690 | 2.0 |
| (*Michelina's* Budget Gourmet) ........ | 280 | 12.0 | 33.0 | 10.0 | 25 | 690 | 2.0 |
| (*Stouffer's*), 12 oz. ... | 410 | 22.0 | 45.0 | 16.0 | 40 | 990 | 4.0 |
| w/beans (*Michelina's* Chili-Mac) ....... | 320 | 13.0 | 38.0 | 11.0 | 25 | 820 | 3.0 |
| cheesy (*Banquet*), 7 oz. ............ | 230 | 11.0 | 30.0 | 7.0 | 20 | 810 | 3.0 |
| cheddar, sharp (*Michelina's* Authentico), 9 oz. .... | 390 | 14.0 | 44.0 | 16.0 | 40 | 740 | 2.0 |
| cheddar and Romano (*Michelina's* Budget Gourmet) .......... | 260 | 10.0 | 40.0 | 7.0 | 15 | 550 | 2.0 |
| and cheese: | | | | | | | |
| (*Amy's*), 9 oz. ....... | 410 | 16.0 | 47.0 | 16.0 | 40 | 590 | 3.0 |
| (*Amy's* Light Sodium), 9 oz. ............ | 400 | 16.0 | 47.0 | 16.0 | 40 | 290 | 3.0 |
| (*Banquet* Family), 1 cup ............ | 190 | 7.0 | 32.0 | 3.5 | 5 | 710 | 2.0 |
| (*Blake's* Organic) .... | 370 | 7.0 | 45.0 | 18.0 | 50 | 480 | 4.0 |
| (*Bob Evans*), 1 cup ... | 330 | 14.0 | 33.0 | 16.0 | 35 | 1220 | 2.0 |
| (*Bob Evans* Single Serve), 6-oz. cont. . | 220 | 10.0 | 22.0 | 10.0 | 25 | 810 | 1.0 |
| (*Boston Market* Side), 7.75 oz. ......... | 320 | 14.0 | 45.0 | 9.0 | 20 | 880 | 4.0 |
| (*Cedarlane*), 9 oz. .... | 270 | 17.0 | 42.0 | 3.0 | 10 | 680 | 2.0 |
| (*Glutino*), 10.5 oz. ... | 440 | 14.0 | 64.0 | 15.0 | 25 | 600 | 3.0 |
| (*Hormel Country Crock*), 1 cup ..... | 330 | 14.0 | 38.0 | 14.0 | 30 | 930 | 2.0 |
| (*Lean Cuisine*), 10 oz. . | 290 | 15.0 | 41.0 | 7.0 | 20 | 630 | 1.0 |

| Food and Measure | cal. | prot. (gms) | carbo. (gms) | fat (gms) | chol. (mgs) | sod. (mgs) | fiber (gms) |
|---|---|---|---|---|---|---|---|
| **Macaroni entree, frozen/chilled, and cheese** *(cont.)* | | | | | | | |
| (*Michelina's Authentico*) ...... | 300 | 10.0 | 41.0 | 10.0 | 20 | 620 | 2.0 |
| (*Michelina's Authentico* Bake) .. | 320 | 10.0 | 43.0 | 11.0 | 20 | 670 | 2.0 |
| (*Michelina's Budget Gourmet* Homestyle), 7.5 oz. | 280 | 9.0 | 38.0 | 10.0 | 20 | 580 | 2.0 |
| (*Michelina's Lean Gourmet*), 9 oz. .... | 280 | 11.0 | 48.0 | 4.5 | 10 | 490 | 2.0 |
| (*Simply Macaroni & Cheese*), 1 cup .... | 280 | 12.0 | 33.0 | 13.0 | 25 | 910 | 1.0 |
| (*Smart Ones*), 10 oz. . | 270 | 11.0 | 52.0 | 2.0 | 5 | 790 | 2.0 |
| (*Stouffer's*), ½ of 12-oz. pkg. ....... | 340 | 15.0 | 33.0 | 16.0 | 25 | 820 | 3.0 |
| (*Stouffer's*), ½ of 20-oz. pkg. ....... | 340 | 14.0 | 36.0 | 16.0 | 30 | 820 | 3.0 |
| (*Stouffer's* Family), ¼ of 40-oz. pkg. ... | 350 | 15.0 | 34.0 | 17.0 | 30 | 920 | 2.0 |
| (*Stouffer's* Party), ⅒ of 76-oz. pkg. .. | 350 | 15.0 | 34.0 | 17.0 | 25 | 920 | 2.0 |
| (*Tabatchnick*), ½ of 15-oz. pkg. ....... | 250 | 9.0 | 34.0 | 8.0 | 20 | 770 | <1.0 |
| 3 cheese (*Moosewood* Organic), 10 oz. ... | 400 | 17.0 | 45.0 | 17.0 | 35 | 670 | 2.0 |
| 3 cheese (*Smart Ones*), 9 oz. ...... | 300 | 14.0 | 48.0 | 6.0 | 10 | 570 | 3.0 |
| asiago/cheddar (*Helen's Kitchen* Organic), 10 oz. ........... | 390 | 22.0 | 47.0 | 13.0 | 35 | 600 | 5.0 |
| w/broccoli (*Stouffer's*), 12 oz. ........... | 480 | 22.0 | 52.0 | 20.0 | 35 | 1000 | 5.0 |
| w/chicken (*Blake's* Organic) ......... | 360 | 18.0 | 34.0 | 17.0 | 80 | 320 | 3.0 |
| w/ham (*Michelina's Authentico*) ...... | 300 | 14.0 | 33.0 | 12.0 | 40 | 790 | 2.0 |
| rice pasta (*Amy's* Rice Mac & Cheese), 9 oz. ............. | 400 | 16.0 | 47.0 | 16.0 | 50 | 590 | 1.0 |
| cheeseburger (*Michelina's* Mac) .... | 350 | 16.0 | 38.0 | 13.0 | 40 | 680 | 2.0 |
| lobster and cheese (*Blue Horizon*), ¼ of 16-oz. pkg. ......... | 150 | 11.0 | 16.0 | 5.0 | 15 | 570 | 0 |

| Food and Measure | cal. | prot. (gms) | carbo. (gms) | fat (gms) | chol. (mgs) | sod. (mgs) | fiber (gms) |
|---|---|---|---|---|---|---|---|
| vegetarian: | | | | | | | |
| rice (*Amy's*) ....... | 520 | 8.0 | 72.0 | 22.0 | 0 | 740 | 3.0 |
| soy (*Amy's* Cheeze), | | | | | | | |
| 9 oz. ........... | 370 | 16.0 | 42.0 | 15.0 | 0 | 500 | 4.0 |
| **Macaroni entree, microwave** (see also "Macaroni entree, canned"): | | | | | | | |
| Alfredo (*Kraft Easy Mac* Micro), 1 cont. .. | 220 | 7.0 | 39.0 | 4.5 | 5 | 590 | 1.0 |
| and beef: | | | | | | | |
| (*Chef Boyardee* Beefaroni), ½ bowl., 1 cup .... | 230 | 8.0 | 31.0 | 8.0 | 10 | 950 | 4.0 |
| (*Chef Boyardee* Beefaroni Single), 7.5 oz. .... | 210 | 8.0 | 27.0 | 8.0 | 15 | 800 | 3.0 |
| and cheddar, ¾ cup*: | | | | | | | |
| (*Annie's* Real Aged) .. | 230 | 9.0 | 39.0 | 4.5 | 10 | 580 | 2.0 |
| white (*Annie's*) ...... | 230 | 9.0 | 39.0 | 4.0 | 10 | 570 | 2.0 |
| and cheese: | | | | | | | |
| (*Chef Boyardee*), ½ bowl, 1 cup .... | 240 | 9.0 | 28.0 | 10.0 | 15 | 750 | 4.0 |
| (*Chef Boyardee* Single), 7.5 oz. .......... | 190 | 7.0 | 23.0 | 8.0 | 15 | 660 | 3.0 |
| (*Kraft Easy Mac* Micro), 1 cont. .... | 220 | 6.0 | 39.0 | 4.0 | 5 | 700 | 1.0 |
| (*Kraft Easy Mac* Micro Big Pack), ¼ of 12.9-oz. pkg. . | 350 | 10.0 | 63.0 | 6.0 | 10 | 830 | 2.0 |
| (*Kraft Easy Mac* Micro Extreme Cheese), ⅙ of 12.9-oz. pkg. . | 230 | 7.0 | 42.0 | 4.0 | 5 | 520 | 1.0 |
| w/bacon (*Kraft Easy Mac* Micro), 1 cont. | 220 | 7.0 | 38.0 | 4.5 | 5 | 580 | 1.0 |
| triple cheese (*Kraft Easy Mac* Micro), 1 cont. .......... | 220 | 7.0 | 39.0 | 4.5 | 5 | 660 | 1.0 |
| taco, cheesy (*Kraft Easy Mac* Micro), 1 cont. .. | 220 | 6.0 | 40.0 | 3.5 | 5 | 600 | 1.0 |
| **Macaroni entree mix** (see also "Pasta dish mix"), dry mix, except as noted: | | | | | | | |
| Alfredo, w/cheese (*Kraft* Dinner), ⅓ of 7.25-oz. pkg. ....... | 250 | 9.0 | 50.0 | 2.5 | 5 | 650 | 2.0 |

| Food and Measure | cal. | prot. (gms) | carbo. (gms) | fat (gms) | chol. (mgs) | sod. (mgs) | fiber (gms) |
|---|---|---|---|---|---|---|---|
| **Macaroni entree mix** *(cont.)* | | | | | | | |
| and cheddar: | | | | | | | |
| *(Kraft* Crackers), | | | | | | | |
| 1.5-oz. pkg. ...... | 210 | 4.0 | 26.0 | 10.0 | 5 | 390 | 1.0 |
| *(Kraft* Crackers), | | | | | | | |
| ⅛ of 8-oz. pkg. .... | 150 | 3.0 | 18.0 | 7.0 | 5 | 280 | 1.0 |
| *(Kraft* Deluxe), ¼ of | | | | | | | |
| 14-oz. pkg. ....... | 320 | 12.0 | 45.0 | 10.0 | 15 | 930 | 1.0 |
| *(Kraft* Deluxe Family), | | | | | | | |
| ⅛ of 28-oz. pkg. ... | 260 | 9.0 | 48.0 | 3.5 | 15 | 580 | 1.0 |
| *(Pasta Roni),* 1 cup* .. | 200 | 7.0 | 37.0 | 2.5 | 0 | 510 | 1.0 |
| crunchy *(Kraft* Crackers), | | | | | | | |
| ½ of 2.25-oz. pkg. . | 150 | 3.0 | 18.0 | 7.0 | 5 | 280 | 1.0 |
| mild *(Kraft* Crackers), | | | | | | | |
| ⅛ of 8-oz. pkg. .... | 150 | 3.0 | 18.0 | 7.0 | 5 | 310 | 1.0 |
| mild, creamy *(Annie's* | | | | | | | |
| Deluxe), 1 cup* ... | 290 | 11.0 | 44.0 | 8.0 | 25 | 590 | 2.0 |
| sharp *(Kraft* Deluxe), | | | | | | | |
| ¼ of 14-oz. pkg. ... | 320 | 12.0 | 47.0 | 9.0 | 15 | 840 | 2.0 |
| wheat *(Kraft* Harvest), | | | | | | | |
| ⅓ of 6-oz. pkg. ..... | 200 | 8.0 | 37.0 | 2.5 | 5 | 570 | 2.0 |
| white, w/broccoli, | | | | | | | |
| rotini *(Kraft* Deluxe), | | | | | | | |
| ½ of 9.4-oz. pkg. .. | 390 | 16.0 | 48.0 | 15.0 | 25 | 1470 | 2.0 |
| white, 5-grain *(Annie's* | | | | | | | |
| Organic), 1 cup* .. | 270 | 11.0 | 47.0 | 4.0 | 10 | 580 | 3.0 |
| and cheese: | | | | | | | |
| *(Annie's* Classic), | | | | | | | |
| 1 cup* .......... | 280 | 11.0 | 48.0 | 4.0 | 10 | 540 | 2.0 |
| *(Annie's* Classic | | | | | | | |
| Family), 1 cup* ... | 270 | 11.0 | 48.0 | 4.0 | 10 | 530 | 2.0 |
| *(Annie's* Classic | | | | | | | |
| Organic), 1 cup* .. | 280 | 11.0 | 47.0 | 5.0 | 15 | 530 | 2.0 |
| *(Annie's* 25% Less | | | | | | | |
| Sodium), 1 cup* .. | 280 | 11.0 | 48.0 | 4.0 | 10 | 440 | 2.0 |
| *(Kraft* The Cheesiest), | | | | | | | |
| ⅓ of 7.25-oz. pkg. . | 260 | 9.0 | 48.0 | 3.5 | 15 | 580 | 1.0 |
| *(Kraft* Dinner | | | | | | | |
| Family Size), ⅙ of | | | | | | | |
| 14.5-oz. pkg. ..... | 260 | 9.0 | 48.0 | 3.5 | 15 | 580 | 1.0 |
| *(Kraft* Dinner | | | | | | | |
| Thick 'n Creamy), | | | | | | | |
| ⅓ of 7.25-oz. pkg. . | 260 | 9.0 | 48.0 | 3.5 | 15 | 580 | 1.0 |

| Food and Measure | cal. | prot. (gms) | carbo. (gms) | fat (gms) | chol. (mgs) | sod. (mgs) | fiber (gms) |
|---|---|---|---|---|---|---|---|
| (*Kraft* Organic Mix), ½ of 6-oz. pkg. | 240 | 10.0 | 49.0 | 2.5 | 5 | 630 | 2.0 |
| (*Kraft* Side Dish Half the Fat), ¼ of 14-oz. pkg. | 290 | 13.0 | 50.0 | 4.5 | 15 | 850 | 2.0 |
| 4 (*Annie's* Deluxe), 1 cup* | 310 | 12.0 | 44.0 | 9.0 | 25 | 650 | 2.0 |
| 3 (*Kraft* Premium Dinner), ⅓ of 7.25-oz. pkg. | 260 | 9.0 | 50.0 | 2.5 | 5 | 610 | 1.0 |
| 3 (*Kraft* Bistro Deluxe* Italiano), ⅓ of 10-oz. pkg. | 310 | 12.0 | 40.0 | 11.0 | 30 | 920 | 3.0 |
| portobello mushroom (*Kraft* Bistro Deluxe*), ⅓ of 10-oz. pkg. | 310 | 12.0 | 40.0 | 11.0 | 35 | 800 | 3.0 |
| spirals (*Kraft*), ½ of 5.5-oz. pkg. | 260 | 9.0 | 48.0 | 3.5 | 15 | 580 | 1.0 |
| Parmesan, sun-dried tomato (*Kraft* Bistro Deluxe*), ⅓ of 10-oz. pkg. | 300 | 12.0 | 40.0 | 11.0 | 30 | 870 | 3.0 |
| **Macaroni and cheese**, see "Macaroni entree" | | | | | | | |
| **Mace**, ground, 1 tsp. | 8 | .1 | .9 | .6 | 0 | 1 | .1 |
| **Mackerel**, meat only: | | | | | | | |
| raw, 4 oz.: | | | | | | | |
| Atlantic | 230 | 21.1 | 0 | 15.8 | 80 | 102 | 0 |
| king | 119 | 23.0 | 0 | 2.3 | 61 | 179 | 0 |
| Pacific/jack | 179 | 22.8 | 0 | 9.0 | 53 | 98 | 0 |
| Spanish | 158 | 21.9 | 0 | 7.2 | 86 | 67 | 0 |
| baked or broiled, 4 oz.: | | | | | | | |
| Atlantic | 297 | 27.0 | 0 | 20.2 | 85 | 94 | 0 |
| king | 152 | 29.5 | 0 | 2.9 | 77 | 230 | 0 |
| Pacific/jack | 228 | 29.2 | 0 | 11.5 | 68 | 125 | 0 |
| Spanish | 179 | 26.8 | 0 | 7.2 | 83 | 75 | 0 |
| **Mackerel, canned**, Jack, drained: | | | | | | | |
| in oil, fillets: | | | | | | | |
| (*Crown Prince* 4.25 oz.), 3.1 oz. | 130 | 23.0 | 0 | 4.0 | 45 | 450 | 0 |
| (*Roland*), 2 oz. | 80 | 14.0 | 0 | 3.0 | 35 | 330 | 0 |
| (*Vigo*), 2 pcs. | 150 | 12.0 | 0 | 11.0 | 25 | 290 | 0 |
| in water, ⅓ cup: | | | | | | | |
| (*Chicken of the Sea*) | 90 | 13.0 | 0 | 4.0 | 55 | 280 | 0 |

| Food and Measure | cal. | prot. (gms) | carbo. (gms) | fat (gms) | chol. (mgs) | sod. (mgs) | fiber (gms) |
|---|---|---|---|---|---|---|---|
| **Mackerel, canned, in water** *(cont.)* | | | | | | | |
| (*Crown Prince*) . . . . . . | 80 | 13.0 | 0 | 3.0 | 64 | 200 | 0 |
| (*Roland*) . . . . . . . . . . . | 90 | 13.0 | 0 | 4.0 | 45 | 240 | 0 |
| **Mackerel, salted**, 2 oz. . . . | 171 | 10.4 | 0 | 14.1 | 53 | 2492 | 0 |
| **Mahi mahi**, fresh, meat only: | | | | | | | |
| raw, 4 oz. . . . . . . . . . . . . | 97 | 21.0 | 0 | .8 | 83 | 99 | 0 |
| baked or broiled, 4 oz. . . | 124 | 26.0 | 0 | 1.0 | 107 | 128 | 0 |
| **Mahi mahi**, frozen, sticks, coconut (*Phillips*), 3 pcs., 3.4 oz., and ⅔ oz. sauce . . . . . | 290 | 14.0 | 31.0 | 13.0 | 65 | 580 | 1.0 |
| **Malanga**, fresh: | | | | | | | |
| (*Frieda's*), 3 oz. . . . . . . . . | 90 | 1.0 | 23.0 | 0 | 0 | 10 | 2.0 |
| sliced, ½ cup . . . . . . . . . . | 66 | 1.0 | 16.0 | .3 | 0 | 14 | 1.0 |
| **Malt drink mix** (*Ovaltine*), 4 tbsp. . . . . | 80 | 2.0 | 18.0 | 0 | 0 | 55 | 0 |
| **Malt syrup**, see "Barley malt syrup" | | | | | | | |
| **Malted milk powder** (*King Arthur*), 1 tbsp. . | 25 | <1.0 | 4.0 | 0 | 0 | 35 | <1.0 |
| **Mammy apple:** | | | | | | | |
| ½ of 25-oz. fruit . . . . . . . | 216 | 2.1 | 52.9 | 2.1 | 0 | 63 | 12.7 |
| peeled, seeded, 1 oz. . . . . | 14 | .1 | 3.5 | .1 | 0 | 4 | .9 |
| **Mandarin orange**, see "Tangerine" | | | | | | | |
| **Mango**, fresh: | | | | | | | |
| (*Dole*), ½ pc., 3.6 oz. . . . | 70 | <1.0 | 18.0 | 0 | 0 | 0 | 2.0 |
| 10.6-oz. fruit, 7.3 oz. trimmed | 135 | 1.1 | 35.2 | .6 | 0 | 4 | 3.7 |
| sliced, 1 cup . . . . . . . . . . | 107 | 8.4 | 28.1 | .5 | 0 | 2 | 3.0 |
| **Mango, can/jar:** | | | | | | | |
| in light syrup, ½ cup: | | | | | | | |
| (*Del Monte SunFresh*) | 70 | 0 | 19.0 | 0 | 0 | 15 | <1.0 |
| sliced (*Roland*) . . . . . . | 90 | 0 | 22.0 | 0 | 0 | 15 | 1.0 |
| in syrup, sliced (*Herdez*), 2 pcs. . . . . . | 170 | 0 | 30.0 | 0 | 0 | 10 | 1.0 |
| **Mango, dried**, 1.4 oz.: | | | | | | | |
| (*Mariani* Philippine) . . . . . | 130 | 1.0 | 32.0 | 0 | 0 | 90 | 2.0 |
| (*Sunsweet* Philippine) . . . | 130 | 1.0 | 32.0 | 0 | 0 | 85 | 1.0 |
| **Mango, frozen**, chunks: | | | | | | | |
| (*Birds Eye*), ⅓ of 16-oz. pkg. . . . . . . . . . | 90 | 1.0 | 24.0 | 0 | 0 | 0 | 3.0 |
| (*Contessa*), 1 cup . . . . . . | 90 | 1.0 | 22.0 | 0 | 0 | 25 | 2.0 |

| Food and Measure | cal. | prot. (gms) | carbo. (gms) | fat (gms) | chol. (mgs) | sod. (mgs) | fiber (gms) |
|---|---|---|---|---|---|---|---|
| (*C&W*), ¾ cup . . . . . . . . | 90 | <1.0 | 24.0 | 0 | 0 | 0 | 3.0 |
| (*Dole*), ¾ cup . . . . . . . . | 90 | 0 | 24.0 | 0 | 0 | 0 | 3.0 |
| **Mango dip**, w/cream cheese, salsa (*Margaritaville*), 1 oz. . . | 60 | 1.0 | 7.0 | 4.0 | 10 | 560 | 1.0 |
| **Mango drink**, 8 fl. oz.: | | | | | | | |
| (*Apple & Eve Nectar*) . . . . | 140 | 0 | 33.0 | 0 | 0 | 25 | 0 |
| (*Bolthouse Farms Amazing Mango* Smoothie) . . . . | 150 | 1.0 | 38.0 | 0 | 0 | 15 | 1.0 |
| (*Langers* Mongo) . . . . . . | 120 | 0 | 30.0 | 0 | 0 | 0 | 0 |
| (*Langers* Nectar) . . . . . . . | 140 | 0 | 35.0 | 0 | 0 | 15 | 0 |
| (*Snapple* Madness) . . . . . | 100 | 0 | 26.0 | 0 | 0 | 10 | 0 |
| **Mango drink blend**, 8 fl. oz.: | | | | | | | |
| (*AriZona* Mucho) . . . . . . . | 120 | 0 | 27.0 | 0 | 0 | 10 | 0 |
| melon (*SoBe Nirvana*) . . . | 120 | 0 | 29.0 | 0 | 0 | 15 | 0 |
| orange (*Langers*) . . . . . . | 130 | 0 | 33.0 | 0 | 0 | 0 | 0 |
| passion fruit (*Welch's*) . . | 130 | 0 | 31.0 | 0 | 0 | 45 | 0 |
| peach (*V8 Splash*) . . . . . . | 80 | 0 | 20.0 | 0 | 0 | 40 | 0 |
| **Mango juice blend**, 8 fl. oz.: | | | | | | | |
| (*After the Fall*) . . . . . . . . | 150 | 1.0 | 37.0 | 0 | 0 | 15 | 0 |
| (*Ceres*) . . . . . . . . . . . . | 120 | 0 | 30.0 | 0 | 0 | 10 | 1.0 |
| (*Odwalla Mango Tango* Smoothie) . . . . . . . . . | 150 | 1.0 | 34.0 | 1.0 | 0 | 10 | 0 |
| (*R.W. Knudsen* Organic Nectar) . . . . . | 120 | 0 | 29.0 | 0 | 0 | 15 | 0 |
| peach (*R.W. Knudsen*) . . | 130 | <1.0 | 31.0 | 0 | 0 | 50 | 0 |
| strawberry (*Apple & Eve Organics*) . . . . . . . | 160 | 0 | 40.0 | 0 | 0 | 20 | 0 |
| **Mangosteen**, canned in syrup, ½ cup . . . . . | 70 | .4 | 6.7 | 5.7 | 0 | 7 | 1.8 |
| **Mangosteen juice blend** (*Bossa Nova*), 8 fl. oz.: | | | | | | | |
| w/dragonfruit . . . . . . . . | 85 | 0 | 22.0 | 0 | 0 | 10 | 0 |
| w/passion fruit . . . . . . . | 85 | 0 | 21.0 | 0 | 0 | 15 | 0 |
| **Manicotti entree, frozen**, 1 pkg., except as noted: | | | | | | | |
| cheese, w/sauce: | | | | | | | |
| (*Celentano*), 10 oz. . . . | 410 | 18.0 | 50.0 | 15.0 | 40 | 1030 | 6.0 |
| (*Celentano*), ½ of 14-oz. pkg. . . . . . . . | 300 | 14.0 | 38.0 | 10.0 | 35 | 710 | 4.0 |

| Food and Measure | cal. | prot. (gms) | carbo. (gms) | fat (gms) | chol. (mgs) | sod. (mgs) | fiber (gms) |
|---|---|---|---|---|---|---|---|
| **Manicotti entree, frozen, cheese, w/sauce** *(cont.)* | | | | | | | |
| (*Celentano* Light), 10 oz. ........... | 330 | 17.0 | 51.0 | 6.0 | 25 | 800 | 7.0 |
| (*Healthy Choice* Formaggio), 11.75 oz. ..... | 380 | 16.0 | 63.0 | 6.0 | 25 | 600 | 8.0 |
| (*Michelina's*), 8 oz. ... | 270 | 11.0 | 34.0 | 11.0 | 30 | 980 | 3.0 |
| (*Stouffer's Easy Express*), ⅓ of 29.5-oz. pkg. | 340 | 15.0 | 33.0 | 16.0 | 45 | 950 | 5.0 |
| Florentine (*Celentano* Light), 10 oz. ..... | 330 | 16.0 | 52.0 | 6.0 | 25 | 660 | 8.0 |
| soy ricotta (*Rising Moon Organics*), 10 oz. ........... | 370 | 16.0 | 54.0 | 10.0 | 0 | 470 | 6.0 |
| cheese, w/out sauce (*Celentano*), ½ of 14-oz. pkg. ......... | 360 | 19.0 | 45.0 | 11.0 | 55 | 810 | 2.0 |
| spinach and 3-cheese (*Cedarlane*), 9.5 oz. .. | 380 | 21.0 | 45.0 | 13.0 | 30 | 660 | 5.0 |
| **Manicotti entree, microwave**, cheese (*Hormel Compleats*), 10 oz. ... | 290 | 10.0 | 42.0 | 9.0 | 25 | 990 | 2.0 |
| **Manioc**, see "Yuca root" | | | | | | | |
| **Maple seasoning blend** (*Grill Mates* Smokehouse), ¼ tsp. . | 0 | 0 | <1.0 | 0 | 0 | 115 | 0 |
| **Maple syrup**, ¼ cup: | | | | | | | |
| (*Maple Grove Farms*) ... | 200 | 0 | 53.0 | 0 | 0 | 0 | 0 |
| (*Roland*) ............. | 200 | 0 | 53.0 | 0 | 0 | 5 | 0 |
| (*Smucker's*) .......... | 210 | 0 | 53.0 | 0 | 0 | 5 | 0 |
| **Margarine** (see also "Butter blend"), 1 tbsp.: | | | | | | | |
| soft tub/spread: | | | | | | | |
| (*Blue Bonnet*) ....... | 70 | 0 | 0 | 8.0 | 0 | 125 | 0 |
| (*Blue Bonnet* Light) .. | 40 | 0 | 0 | 4.5 | 0 | 90 | 0 |
| (*Fleischmann's*) ..... | 60 | 0 | 0 | 7.0 | 0 | 35 | 0 |
| (*I Can't Believe It's Not Butter!*) ....... | 70 | 0 | 0 | 8.0 | 0 | 90 | 0 |
| (*I Can't Believe It's Not Butter! Calcium*) | 50 | 0 | 0 | 5.0 | 0 | 90 | 0 |
| (*I Can't Believe It's Not Butter! Fat Free*) | 5 | 0 | 0 | 0 | 0 | 90 | 0 |
| (*I Can't Believe It's Not Butter! Light*) .. | 50 | 0 | 0 | 5.0 | 0 | 85 | 0 |

| Food and Measure | cal. | prot. (gms) | carbo. (gms) | fat (gms) | chol. (mgs) | sod. (mgs) | fiber (gms) |
|---|---|---|---|---|---|---|---|
| (*I Can't Believe It's Not Butter!* Mediterranean Blend) | 80 | 0 | 0 | 8.0 | 0 | 90 | 0 |
| (*Land O Lakes*) ...... | 100 | 0 | 0 | 11.0 | 0 | 125 | 0 |
| (*Land O Lakes Fresh Buttery Taste*) ..... | 70 | 0 | 0 | 8.0 | 0 | 80 | 0 |
| (*Parkay* Original) ..... | 70 | 0 | 0 | 7.0 | 0 | 80 | 0 |
| (*Shedd's Country Crock*) .......... | 70 | 0 | 0 | 7.0 | 0 | 100 | 0 |
| (*Shedd's Country Crock* Churn) ..... | 60 | 0 | 0 | 7.0 | 0 | 85 | 0 |
| (*Shedd's Country Crock* Light) ...... | 50 | 0 | 0 | 5.0 | 0 | 90 | 0 |
| (*Smart Balance* Organic Whipped) . | 80 | 0 | 0 | 9.0 | 0 | 100 | 0 |
| (*Smart Balance* Original) ......... | 80 | 0 | 0 | 9.0 | 0 | 90 | 0 |
| (*Smart Balance* HeartRight) ...... | 80 | 0 | 0 | 8.0 | 0 | 85 | 0 |
| (*Smart Balance* HeartRight* Light) .. | 45 | 0 | 0 | 5.0 | 0 | 80 | 0 |
| squeeze: | | | | | | | |
| (*I Can't Believe It's Not Butter!*) ...... | 60 | 0 | 0 | 7.0 | 0 | 80 | 0 |
| (*Shedd's Country Crock*) .......... | 60 | 0 | 0 | 7.0 | 0 | 85 | 0 |
| stick: | | | | | | | |
| (*Blue Bonnet* Light) .. | 50 | 0 | 0 | 5.0 | 0 | 80 | 0 |
| (*Fleischmann's*) ..... | 80 | 0 | 0 | 9.0 | 0 | 110 | 0 |
| (*I Can't Believe It's Not Butter!*) ...... | 100 | 0 | 0 | 11.0 | 0 | 95 | 0 |
| (*Land O Lakes*) ...... | 100 | 0 | 0 | 11.0 | 0 | 105 | 0 |
| (*Land O Lakes Fresh Buttery Taste*) ..... | 90 | 0 | 0 | 10.0 | 0 | 95 | 0 |
| (*Parkay* Light) ....... | 45 | 0 | 0 | 5.0 | 0 | 75 | 0 |
| (*Parkay* Original) ..... | 80 | 0 | 0 | 9.0 | 0 | 130 | 0 |
| (*Shedd's Country Crock* Spreadable) . | 80 | 0 | 0 | 8.0 | 0 | 90 | 0 |
| **Margarine, flavored** (*Shedd's Country Crock*), 1 tbsp.: | | | | | | | |
| cinnamon ............ | 60 | 0 | 2.0 | 6.0 | 0 | 45 | 0 |
| honey .............. | 50 | 0 | 0 | 5.0 | 0 | 95 | 0 |

| Food and Measure | cal. | prot. (gms) | carbo. (gms) | fat (gms) | chol. (mgs) | sod. (mgs) | fiber (gms) |
|---|---|---|---|---|---|---|---|
| **Margarita drink mixer**: | | | | | | | |
| (*Stirrings*), 3 fl. oz. . . . . . | 80 | 0 | 21.0 | 0 | 0 | 0 | 0 |
| lime (*Margaritaville*), | | | | | | | |
| 4 fl. oz. . . . . . . . . . . . . | 110 | 0 | 27.0 | 0 | 0 | 70 | 0 |
| mango (*Margaritaville*), | | | | | | | |
| 4 fl. oz. . . . . . . . . . . . . | 120 | 0 | 29.0 | 0 | 0 | 75 | 0 |
| frozen (*Bacardi*), 2 fl. oz. . | 90 | 0 | 25.0 | 0 | 0 | 0 | 0 |
| **Marinade** (see also | | | | | | | |
| "Barbecue sauce," | | | | | | | |
| "Stir-fry sauce," and | | | | | | | |
| specific listings), 1 tbsp., | | | | | | | |
| except as noted: | | | | | | | |
| (*House of Tsang* | | | | | | | |
| Mandarin Soy) . . . . . . | 25 | 0 | 6.0 | 0 | 0 | 680 | 0 |
| (*Marinade Bay* | | | | | | | |
| Santa Fe) . . . . . . . . . | 50 | 0 | 2.0 | 4.5 | 0 | 75 | 0 |
| (*Neera's Kashmiri*) . . . . . | 18 | 0 | 5.0 | 1.0 | 0 | 69 | 0 |
| all varieties (*Maull's*), | | | | | | | |
| 2 tbsp. . . . . . . . . . . . | 60 | 0 | 13.0 | 0 | 0 | 300 | 0 |
| balsamic-roasted | | | | | | | |
| onion (*Ken's*) . . . . . . . | 15 | 0 | 2.0 | 0 | 0 | 350 | 0 |
| cherry soy (*World | | | | | | | |
| Harbors Cheriyaki* | | | | | | | |
| Glaze), 2 tbsp. . . . . . . | 50 | 0 | 14.0 | 0 | 0 | 390 | 0 |
| chicken (*Lea & | | | | | | | |
| Perrins*) . . . . . . . . . . | 20 | 0 | 3.0 | 0 | 0 | 290 | 0 |
| chili and lime (*Lawry's | | | | | | | |
| Mexican*) . . . . . . . . . . | 25 | 1.0 | 3.0 | 0 | 0 | 380 | 0 |
| chipotle: | | | | | | | |
| (*Lawry's* Baja) . . . . . . . | 15 | 0 | 4.0 | 0 | 0 | 390 | 0 |
| Southwest (*Mrs. | | | | | | | |
| Dash*) . . . . . . . . . . | 25 | 0 | 2.0 | 1.5 | 0 | 0 | 0 |
| cilantro lime (*Marinade | | | | | | | |
| Bay*) . . . . . . . . . . . . . | 50 | 0 | 2.0 | 4.0 | 0 | 55 | 0 |
| fajita (*World Harbors | | | | | | | |
| Mexican*) . . . . . . . . . . | 45 | 0 | 10.0 | 0 | 0 | 290 | 0 |
| garlic, roasted, herbs | | | | | | | |
| (*Kikkoman*) . . . . . . . . . | 20 | 1.0 | 4.0 | 0 | 0 | 630 | 0 |
| garlic herb: | | | | | | | |
| (*Marinade Bay*) . . . . . . | 45 | 0 | 2.0 | 4.5 | 0 | 70 | 0 |
| (*Mrs. Dash* Zesty) . . . . | 30 | 0 | 3.0 | 2.0 | 0 | 0 | 0 |
| garlic lime: | | | | | | | |
| (*Lawry's* Havana) . . . . | 10 | 0 | 2.0 | 0 | 0 | 330 | 0 |
| (*Mrs. Dash*) . . . . . . . . | 30 | 0 | 4.0 | 1.5 | 0 | 0 | 0 |

| Food and Measure | cal. | prot. (gms) | carbo. (gms) | fat (gms) | chol. (mgs) | sod. (mgs) | fiber (gms) |
|---|---|---|---|---|---|---|---|
| Hawaiian (*Lawry's*) ..... | 25 | 0 | 5.0 | 0 | 0 | 250 | 0 |
| herb and garlic: | | | | | | | |
| (*Ken's*) ............. | 20 | 0 | 3.0 | 1.0 | 0 | 370 | 0 |
| (*Lawry's*) .......... | 10 | 0 | 2.0 | 0 | 0 | 420 | 0 |
| roasted (*Newman's Own*) .......... | 20 | 0 | 3.0 | 1.0 | 0 | 370 | 0 |
| honey: | | | | | | | |
| bourbon (*Marinade Bay*) ............ | 50 | 0 | 3.0 | 4.0 | 0 | 95 | 0 |
| Dijon (*Lawry's*) ...... | 20 | 0 | 4.0 | .5 | 0 | 440 | 0 |
| Dijon (*World Harbors*), 2 tbsp. .......... | 30 | 0 | 7.0 | 0 | 0 | 230 | 0 |
| garlic (*Ken's* No Salt) . | 35 | 0 | 3.0 | 2.5 | 0 | 0 | 0 |
| ginger soy (*Marinade Bay*) ... | 20 | 0 | 3.0 | 0 | 0 | 170 | 0 |
| mustard (*Kikkoman*) .. | 30 | 1.0 | 6.0 | 0 | 0 | 420 | 0 |
| soy (*Marinade Bay*) .. | 15 | 0 | 3.0 | 0 | 0 | 190 | 0 |
| horseradish (*Marinade Bay*), 2 tbsp. ..... | 110 | 0 | 5.0 | 10.0 | 10 | 200 | 0 |
| Italian (*World Harbors* Grill), 2 tbsp. ....... | 25 | 0 | 4.0 | 1.0 | 0 | 300 | 0 |
| jalapeño, lime ginger (*Marinade Bay* Thai) .. | 5 | 0 | 2.0 | 0 | 0 | 340 | 0 |
| jerk: | | | | | | | |
| (*Lawry's* Caribbean) .. | 25 | 0 | 5.0 | 0 | 0 | 430 | 0 |
| (*Marinade Bay* Jamaican) ....... | 20 | 0 | 3.0 | 0 | 0 | 220 | 0 |
| (*World Harbors* Jamaican), 2 tbsp. . | 70 | 0 | 18.0 | 0 | 0 | 200 | 0 |
| lemon herb: | | | | | | | |
| (*Marinade Bay*) ...... | 45 | 0 | 2.0 | 4.0 | 0 | 75 | 0 |
| peppercorn (*Mrs. Dash*) ........... | 25 | 0 | 2.0 | 2.0 | 0 | 0 | 0 |
| lemon pepper: | | | | | | | |
| (*Ken's* No Sodium) ... | 15 | 0 | 3.0 | 0 | 0 | 0 | 0 |
| (*Lawry's*) .......... | 10 | 0 | 2.0 | 0 | 0 | 390 | 0 |
| (*Marinade Bay*) ...... | 25 | 0 | 4.0 | 1.0 | 0 | 80 | 0 |
| (*Newman's Own*) .... | 15 | 0 | 3.0 | 0 | 0 | 300 | 0 |
| and garlic (*World Harbors*), 2 tbsp. .. | 35 | 0 | 8.0 | 0 | 0 | 140 | 0 |
| herbed (*Emeril's*) .... | 70 | 0 | 1.0 | 8.0 | 0 | 55 | 0 |
| lemon rosemary garlic (*Emeril's* Gaaahlic) ... | 70 | 0 | 1.0 | 8.0 | 0 | 120 | 0 |

| Food and Measure | cal. | prot. (gms) | carbo. (gms) | fat (gms) | chol. (mgs) | sod. (mgs) | fiber (gms) |
|---|---|---|---|---|---|---|---|
| **Marinade** (cont.) | | | | | | | |
| mango (*World Harbors Island*), 2 tbsp. ...... | 60 | 0 | 14.0 | 0 | 0 | 190 | 0 |
| mesquite: | | | | | | | |
| grille (*Mrs. Dash*) .... | 25 | 0 | 3.0 | 1.5 | 0 | 0 | 0 |
| lime (*Lawry's*) ....... | 5 | 0 | 1.0 | 0 | 0 | 350 | 0 |
| lime (*Newman's Own*) | 20 | 0 | 3.0 | 1.0 | 0 | 190 | 0 |
| mojo (*World Harbors Cuban*), 2 tbsp. ...... | 25 | 0 | 5.0 | 1.0 | 0 | 300 | 0 |
| orange herb poppy seed (*Emeril's*) .......... | 150 | 0 | 4.0 | 15.0 | 0 | 170 | 0 |
| orange soy (*Marinade Bay*) .............. | 30 | 0 | <1.0 | 3.0 | 0 | 210 | 0 |
| red pepper (*Lawry's Louisiana*) .......... | 10 | 0 | 2.0 | 0 | 0 | 390 | 0 |
| rosemary mint (*Marinade Bay*) ...... | 50 | 0 | 3.0 | 4.5 | 0 | 55 | 0 |
| sesame: | | | | | | | |
| (*Emeril's* Asian) ..... | 140 | <1.0 | 4.0 | 14.0 | 0 | 340 | 0 |
| (*Marinade Bay* Korean) | 25 | 0 | 4.0 | 1.0 | 0 | 350 | 0 |
| toasted (*Kikkoman's*) . | 40 | 1.0 | 8.0 | .5 | 0 | 590 | 0 |
| sesame ginger: | | | | | | | |
| (*Ken's* No Salt) ...... | 30 | 0 | 6.0 | 0 | 0 | 0 | 0 |
| (*Lawry's*) .......... | 30 | 0 | 7.0 | 0 | 0 | 580 | 0 |
| (*Newman's Own*) .... | 25 | 0 | 4.0 | 1.0 | 0 | 300 | 0 |
| steak: | | | | | | | |
| (*Marinade Bay* Theo's Steakhouse) | 30 | 0 | 3.0 | 2.0 | 0 | 170 | 0 |
| (*Simply Tsang* Japanese Steakhouse) | 40 | 0 | 6.0 | 1.5 | 0 | 770 | 0 |
| (*World Harbors* Steakhouse), 2 tbsp. | 35 | 0 | 7.0 | 0 | 0 | 135 | 0 |
| and chop (*Lawry's*) ... | 5 | 0 | 1.0 | 0 | 0 | 400 | 0 |
| sun-dried tomato, w/garlic, olive oil (*Lawry's* Tuscan) .... | 15 | 0 | 3.0 | 0 | 0 | 350 | 0 |
| sweet/sour, see "Sweet and sour sauce" | | | | | | | |
| tequila lime (*Marinade Bay*) .............. | 30 | 0 | 4.0 | 1.5 | 0 | 180 | 0 |
| teriyaki, see "Teriyaki sauce" | | | | | | | |
| Szechuan barbecue (*Lawry's*) .......... | 35 | 0 | 8.0 | 0 | 0 | 460 | 0 |

| Food and Measure | cal. | prot. (gms) | carbo. (gms) | fat (gms) | chol. (mgs) | sod. (mgs) | fiber (gms) |
|---|---|---|---|---|---|---|---|
| wasabi soy (*Marinade Bay*) ............. | 15 | <1.0 | 5.0 | 0 | 0 | 280 | 0 |
| **Marinade seasoning mix**, 1 tsp., except as noted: (*Adolph's Marinade in Minutes*), ¾ tsp. ..... | 5 | 0 | 1.0 | 0 | 0 | 370 | 0 |
| beef, tenderizing (*Lawry's*), ¾ tsp. .... | 0 | 0 | <1.0 | 0 | 0 | 550 | 0 |
| brown sugar bourbon (*Grill Mates*) ........ | 10 | 0 | 2.0 | 0 | 0 | 400 | 0 |
| chipotle (*Grill Mates*) ... | 10 | 0 | 2.0 | 0 | 0 | 520 | 0 |
| citrus (*Grill Mates Baja*) .............. | 10 | 0 | 1.0 | 0 | 0 | 310 | 0 |
| garlic, herb, and wine (*Grill Mates*) ........ | 5 | 0 | 1.0 | 0 | 0 | 430 | 0 |
| Hawaiian luau (*Grill Mates*) ............. | 10 | 0 | 2.0 | 0 | 0 | 290 | 0 |
| herb, zesty (*Grill Mates*) ............. | 10 | 0 | 1.0 | 0 | 0 | 260 | 0 |
| meat: | | | | | | | |
| (*Kikkoman*) ......... | 10 | 0 | 2.0 | 0 | 0 | 580 | 0 |
| (*McCormick*) ....... | 15 | 0 | 3.0 | 0 | 0 | 280 | 0 |
| tenderizing (*Adolph's Marinade in Minutes No Salt*), ¾ tsp. .... | 10 | 0 | 2.0 | 0 | 0 | 0 | 0 |
| mesquite (*Grill Mates*) .. | 10 | 0 | 2.0 | 0 | 0 | 500 | 0 |
| Mexican (*Grill Mates Fiesta*) ............. | 10 | 0 | 2.0 | 0 | 0 | 380 | 0 |
| mojito lime (*Grill Mates*), ¾ tsp. ...... | 10 | 0 | 2.0 | 0 | 0 | 350 | 0 |
| peppercorn and garlic (*Grill Mates*) ........ | 5 | 0 | 1.0 | 0 | 0 | 340 | 0 |
| seafood: | | | | | | | |
| citrus, Caribbean (*McCormick*) ..... | 10 | 0 | 1.0 | 0 | 0 | 310 | 0 |
| lemon pepper (*McCormick*) ..... | 10 | 0 | 2.0 | 0 | 0 | 330 | 0 |
| steak, ½ tsp.: | | | | | | | |
| (*Grill Mates* Montreal) | 0 | 0 | 0 | 0 | 0 | 350 | 0 |
| (*Grill Mates* Montreal 25% Less Sodium) | 5 | 0 | <1.0 | 0 | 0 | 260 | 0 |
| steak sauce tenderizing (*Adolph's Marinade in Minutes*), ¾ tsp. ... | 5 | 0 | 1.0 | 0 | 0 | 450 | 0 |

| Food and Measure | cal. | prot. (gms) | carbo. (gms) | fat (gms) | chol. (mgs) | sod. (mgs) | fiber (gms) |
|---|---|---|---|---|---|---|---|
| **Marinade seasoning mix** *(cont.)* | | | | | | | |
| tomato, garlic, basil | | | | | | | |
| (*Grill Mates*) . . . . . . . . | 5 | 0 | 1.0 | 0 | 0 | 330 | 0 |
| **Marionberry**, see | | | | | | | |
| "Blackberry, dried" | | | | | | | |
| **Marjoram**, dried, 1 tsp. . . . | 2 | .1 | .4 | <.1 | 0 | <1 | .1 |
| **Marmalade**, see "Jam | | | | | | | |
| and preserves" | | | | | | | |
| **Marrow squash**, raw, | | | | | | | |
| trimmed, 1 oz. . . . . . . | 4 | .2 | 1.0 | <.1 | 0 | n.a. | <1.0 |
| **Marshmallow topping**: | | | | | | | |
| (*Jet-Puffed* Creme), | | | | | | | |
| 1 tbsp. . . . . . . . . . . . . | 40 | 0 | 11.0 | 0 | 0 | 10 | 0 |
| (*Marshmallow Fluff*), | | | | | | | |
| 2 tbsp. . . . . . . . . . . . . | 40 | 0 | 10.0 | 0 | 0 | 5 | 0 |
| (*Smucker's*), 2 tbsp. . . . . | 110 | 0 | 28.0 | 0 | 0 | 5 | 0 |
| **Martini drink mixer**, | | | | | | | |
| (*Stirrings*), 3 fl. oz.: | | | | | | | |
| apple . . . . . . . . . . . . . . . | 90 | 0 | 22.0 | 0 | 0 | 0 | 0 |
| blood orange or | | | | | | | |
| pomegranate . . . . . . . | 70 | 0 | 18.0 | 0 | 0 | 0 | 0 |
| watermelon . . . . . . . . . . | 70 | 0 | 19.0 | 0 | 0 | 0 | 0 |
| **Matai**, see "Water | | | | | | | |
| chestnut" | | | | | | | |
| **Matzo**, see "Cracker" | | | | | | | |
| **Matzo ball mix** | | | | | | | |
| (*Manischewitz*), 2 tbsp. | 50 | 1.0 | 11.0 | 0 | 0 | 700 | 1.0 |
| **Matzo meal**, see "Cracker | | | | | | | |
| meal" | | | | | | | |
| **Mayonnaise**, 1 tbsp.: | | | | | | | |
| (*Cains* All Natural) . . . . . . | 100 | 0 | 0 | 11.0 | 5 | 75 | 0 |
| (*Cains* Light) . . . . . . . . . | 50 | 0 | 2.0 | 4.5 | 5 | 130 | 0 |
| (*Cains* Nonfat) . . . . . . . . | 10 | 0 | 2.0 | 0 | 0 | 140 | 0 |
| (*Cains Naturally* | | | | | | | |
| Delicious) . . . . . . . . . . | 90 | 0 | 0 | 0 | 10 | 75 | 0 |
| (*Blue Plate* Real) . . . . . . | 100 | 0 | 0 | 11.0 | 10 | 80 | 0 |
| (*Hellmann's/Best* | | | | | | | |
| *Foods* Canola) . . . . . . | 45 | 0 | <1.0 | 4.5 | 0 | 95 | 0 |
| (*Hellmann's/Best* | | | | | | | |
| *Foods* Light) . . . . . . . . | 35 | 0 | 1.0 | 3.5 | <5 | 130 | 0 |
| (*Hellmann's/Best* | | | | | | | |
| *Foods* Low Fat) . . . . . . | 15 | 0 | 2.0 | 1.0 | 0 | 130 | 0 |
| (*Hellmann's/Best* | | | | | | | |
| *Foods* Real) . . . . . . . . | 90 | 0 | 0 | 10.0 | 5 | 90 | 0 |

| Food and Measure | cal. | prot. (gms) | carbo. (gms) | fat (gms) | chol. (mgs) | sod. (mgs) | fiber (gms) |
|---|---|---|---|---|---|---|---|
| (*Kraft* Light) ......... | 45 | 0 | 2.0 | 4.0 | 5 | 95 | 0 |
| (*Kraft* Real) .......... | 90 | 0 | 0 | 10.0 | 5 | 70 | 0 |
| (*Nayonaise*) ........... | 35 | <1.0 | 1.0 | 3.5 | 0 | 115 | 0 |
| (*Nayonaise* Nonfat) ..... | 10 | <1.0 | 2.0 | 0 | 0 | 100 | 0 |
| chipotle (*Kraft*) ........ | 40 | 0 | 2.0 | 4.0 | 5 | 120 | 0 |
| Dijon (*Nayonaise*) ...... | 30 | <1.0 | 1.0 | 3.0 | 0 | 140 | 0 |
| dressing: | | | | | | | |
| (*Hellmann's/Best* | | | | | | | |
| *Foods* Olive Oil) ... | 50 | 0 | <1.0 | 5.0 | 5 | 120 | 0 |
| (*Kraft* Nonfat) ....... | 10 | 0 | 2.0 | 0 | 0 | 120 | 0 |
| (*Miracle Whip*) ...... | 40 | 0 | 2.0 | 3.5 | 5 | 105 | 0 |
| (*Miracle Whip* Light) .. | 20 | 0 | 2.0 | 1.5 | 5 | 130 | 0 |
| (*Miracle Whip* Nonfat) | 15 | 0 | 3.0 | 0 | 0 | 125 | 0 |
| garlic herb (*Kraft*) ...... | 40 | 0 | 2.0 | 3.5 | 5 | 100 | 0 |
| horseradish Dijon | | | | | | | |
| (*Kraft*) ............. | 40 | 0 | 2.0 | 3.5 | 5 | 105 | 0 |
| hot and spicy (*Kraft*) .... | 100 | 0 | 0 | 11.0 | 5 | 85 | 0 |
| lime (*Hellmann's/Best* | | | | | | | |
| *Foods* con Jugo de | | | | | | | |
| Limon) ............. | 90 | 0 | 0 | 10.0 | 15 | 85 | 0 |
| w/olive oil (*Kraft*) ...... | 45 | 0 | 2.0 | 4.0 | 5 | 95 | 0 |
| **Mayonnaise, chilled,** | | | | | | | |
| 1 tbsp.: | | | | | | | |
| (*Delouis fils*) ........... | 110 | 0 | 0 | 12.0 | 30 | 70 | 0 |
| garlic (*Delouis fils* | | | | | | | |
| Aioli) .............. | 102 | 0 | 0 | 11.2 | 27 | 97 | 0 |
| *McDonald's:* | | | | | | | |
| breakfast: | | | | | | | |
| bagel, egg/cheese: | | | | | | | |
| w/bacon ......... | 560 | 24.0 | 56.0 | 27.0 | 260 | 1300 | 3.0 |
| w/steak ......... | 660 | 33.0 | 56.0 | 33.0 | 300 | 1580 | 3.0 |
| *Big Breakfast* ....... | 740 | 28.0 | 51.0 | 48.0 | 555 | 1560 | 3.0 |
| w/hotcakes ....... | 1090 | 36.0 | 111.0 | 56.0 | 575 | 2150 | 6.0 |
| w/large biscuit .... | 800 | 28.0 | 56.0 | 52.0 | 555 | 1680 | 4.0 |
| biscuit, regular: | | | | | | | |
| bacon/egg/cheese . | 420 | 15.0 | 37.0 | 23.0 | 235 | 1160 | 2.0 |
| chicken .......... | 410 | 17.0 | 41.0 | 20.0 | 30 | 1180 | 2.0 |
| sausage ......... | 430 | 11.0 | 34.0 | 27.0 | 30 | 1080 | 2.0 |
| sausage/egg ...... | 510 | 18.0 | 36.0 | 33.0 | 250 | 1170 | 2.0 |
| biscuit, large: | | | | | | | |
| bacon/egg/cheese . | 480 | 15.0 | 43.0 | 27.0 | 235 | 1270 | 3.0 |
| chicken .......... | 470 | 17.0 | 46.0 | 24.0 | 30 | 1290 | 3.0 |
| sausage ......... | 480 | 11.0 | 39.0 | 31.0 | 30 | 1190 | 3.0 |
| sausage/egg ...... | 570 | 18.0 | 42.0 | 37.0 | 250 | 1280 | 3.0 |

| Food and Measure | cal. | prot. (gms) | carbo. (gms) | fat (gms) | chol. (mgs) | sod. (mgs) | fiber (gms) |
|---|---|---|---|---|---|---|---|
| **McDonald's** (cont.) | | | | | | | |
| burrito, sausage . . . . . | 300 | 12.0 | 26.0 | 16.0 | 115 | 830 | 1.0 |
| *McSkillet* . . . . . . . . | 610 | 27.0 | 44.0 | 36.0 | 410 | 1390 | 3.0 |
| w/steak . . . . . . . . . | 570 | 32.0 | 44.0 | 30.0 | 430 | 1470 | 3.0 |
| hash browns . . . . . . . . | 150 | 1.0 | 15.0 | 9.0 | 0 | 310 | 2.0 |
| hotcakes, plain . . . . . . | 350 | 8.0 | 60.0 | 9.0 | 20 | 590 | 3.0 |
| w/sausage . . . . . . . | 520 | 15.0 | 61.0 | 24.0 | 50 | 930 | 3.0 |
| hotcake syrup pkt. . . . . | 180 | 0 | 45.0 | 0 | 0 | 20 | 0 |
| margarine, 1 pat . . . . . | 40 | 0 | 0 | 4.5 | 0 | 55 | 0 |
| *McGriddles*: | | | | | | | |
| bacon/egg/cheese . | 420 | 15.0 | 48.0 | 18.0 | 240 | 1110 | 2.0 |
| sausage . . . . . . . . . | 420 | 11.0 | 44.0 | 22.0 | 35 | 1030 | 2.0 |
| sausage/egg/cheese | 560 | 20.0 | 48.0 | 32.0 | 265 | 1360 | 2.0 |
| *McMuffin*, egg . . . . . . | 300 | 18.0 | 30.0 | 12.0 | 260 | 820 | 2.0 |
| *McMuffin*, sausage . . . | 370 | 14.0 | 29.0 | 22.0 | 45 | 850 | 2.0 |
| w/egg . . . . . . . . . . . | 450 | 21.0 | 30.0 | 27.0 | 285 | 920 | 2.0 |
| muffin, English . . . . . . | 160 | 5.0 | 27.0 | 3.0 | 0 | 280 | 2.0 |
| oatmeal, fruit/maple . . | 260 | 5.0 | 48.0 | 4.5 | 5 | 115 | 5.0 |
| w/brown sugar . . . . | 290 | 5.0 | 57.0 | 4.5 | 10 | 160 | 5.0 |
| burgers/sandwiches: | | | | | | | |
| Angus burger: | | | | | | | |
| bacon/cheese . . . . . | 790 | 45.0 | 63.0 | 39.0 | 145 | 2070 | 4.0 |
| chipotle bacon . . . . | 800 | 45.0 | 66.0 | 39.0 | 145 | 2020 | 4.0 |
| deluxe . . . . . . . . . | 750 | 40.0 | 61.0 | 39.0 | 135 | 1700 | 4.0 |
| mushroom/Swiss . . | 770 | 44.0 | 59.0 | 40.0 | 135 | 1170 | 4.0 |
| *Big Mac* . . . . . . . . . . . | 540 | 25.0 | 45.0 | 29.0 | 75 | 1040 | 3.0 |
| *Big N' Tasty* . . . . . . . . | 460 | 24.0 | 37.0 | 24.0 | 70 | 720 | 3.0 |
| w/cheese . . . . . . . . | 510 | 27.0 | 38.0 | 28.0 | 85 | 960 | 3.0 |
| cheeseburger . . . . . . . | 300 | 15.0 | 33.0 | 12.0 | 40 | 750 | 2.0 |
| double . . . . . . . . . | 440 | 25.0 | 34.0 | 23.0 | 80 | 1150 | 2.0 |
| McDouble . . . . . . . . | 390 | 22.0 | 33.0 | 19.0 | 65 | 920 | 2.0 |
| chicken, crispy: | | | | | | | |
| classic . . . . . . . . . | 530 | 28.0 | 59.0 | 20.0 | 50 | 1150 | 3.0 |
| club . . . . . . . . . . | 630 | 35.0 | 60.0 | 28.0 | 75 | 1360 | 4.0 |
| ranch BLT . . . . . . . | 580 | 31.0 | 62.0 | 23.0 | 65 | 1400 | 3.0 |
| Southern style . . . . | 400 | 24.0 | 39.0 | 17.0 | 45 | 1030 | 1.0 |
| chicken, grilled: | | | | | | | |
| classic . . . . . . . . . | 420 | 32.0 | 51.0 | 10.0 | 70 | 1190 | 3.0 |
| club . . . . . . . . . . | 530 | 39.0 | 52.0 | 17.0 | 95 | 1410 | 4.0 |
| ranch BLT . . . . . . . | 470 | 36.0 | 54.0 | 12.0 | 80 | 1440 | 3.0 |
| *Filet-O-Fish* . . . . . . . . | 380 | 15.0 | 38.0 | 18.0 | 40 | 640 | 2.0 |
| hamburger . . . . . . . . | 250 | 12.0 | 31.0 | 9.0 | 25 | 520 | 2.0 |
| *McChicken* . . . . . . . . | 360 | 14.0 | 40.0 | 16.0 | 35 | 830 | 2.0 |

| Food and Measure | cal. | prot. (gms) | carbo. (gms) | fat (gms) | chol. (mgs) | sod. (mgs) | fiber (gms) |
|---|---|---|---|---|---|---|---|
| *McRib* | 500 | 22.0 | 44.0 | 26.0 | 70 | 980 | 3.0 |
| *Quarter Pounder* | | | | | | | |
| w/cheese | 510 | 29.0 | 40.0 | 26.0 | 90 | 1190 | 3.0 |
| w/cheese, double | 740 | 48.0 | 40.0 | 42.0 | 155 | 1380 | 3.0 |
| *Snack Wrap*, Angus: | | | | | | | |
| bacon cheese | 390 | 21.0 | 28.0 | 21.0 | 75 | 1080 | 1.0 |
| deluxe | 410 | 20.0 | 27.0 | 25.0 | 75 | 990 | 2.0 |
| mushroom/Swiss | 430 | 22.0 | 27.0 | 26.0 | 75 | 730 | 2.0 |
| *Snack Wrap*, crispy: | | | | | | | |
| chipotle barbecue | 330 | 14.0 | 35.0 | 15.0 | 30 | 810 | 1.0 |
| honey mustard | 330 | 14.0 | 34.0 | 16.0 | 30 | 780 | 1.0 |
| ranch | 340 | 14.0 | 33.0 | 17.0 | 30 | 810 | 1.0 |
| *Snack Wrap*, grilled: | | | | | | | |
| chipotle barbecue | 260 | 18.0 | 28.0 | 9.0 | 45 | 830 | 1.0 |
| honey mustard | 260 | 18.0 | 27.0 | 9.0 | 45 | 800 | 1.0 |
| ranch | 270 | 18.0 | 26.0 | 10.0 | 45 | 830 | 1.0 |
| *Snack Wrap*, Mac | 330 | 15.0 | 26.0 | 19.0 | 45 | 690 | 1.0 |
| *Chicken McNuggets*: | | | | | | | |
| 4 pcs. | 190 | 10.0 | 11.0 | 12.0 | 30 | 400 | 0 |
| 6 pcs. | 280 | 14.0 | 16.0 | 17.0 | 40 | 600 | 0 |
| 10 pcs. | 460 | 24.0 | 27.0 | 29.0 | 70 | 1000 | 0 |
| barbecue sauce | 50 | 0 | 12.0 | 0 | 0 | 260 | 0 |
| honey sauce | 50 | 0 | 12.0 | 0 | 0 | 0 | 0 |
| hot mustard sauce | 60 | 1.0 | 9.0 | 2.5 | 5 | 250 | 2.0 |
| sweet 'n sour sauce | 50 | 0 | 12.0 | 0 | 0 | 150 | 0 |
| *Chicken Selects*: | | | | | | | |
| 3 pcs. | 400 | 23.0 | 23.0 | 24.0 | 50 | 1010 | 0 |
| 5 pcs. | 660 | 38.0 | 39.0 | 40.0 | 85 | 1680 | 0 |
| Buffalo sauce, spicy | 60 | 0 | 1.0 | 6.0 | 0 | 800 | 1.0 |
| chipotle barbecue | 60 | 0 | 15.0 | 0 | 0 | 210 | 1.0 |
| honey mustard | 60 | 0 | 10.0 | 2.0 | 5 | 140 | 0 |
| ranch, creamy | 170 | 0 | 2.0 | 18.0 | 10 | 270 | 0 |
| fries, large | 500 | 6.0 | 63.0 | 25.0 | 0 | 350 | 6.0 |
| medium | 380 | 4.0 | 480 | 19.0 | 0 | 270 | 5.0 |
| small | 230 | 3.0 | 29.0 | 11.0 | 0 | 160 | 3.0 |
| ketchup pkt. | 15 | 0 | 3.0 | 0 | 0 | 110 | 0 |
| salad, no dressing: | | | | | | | |
| bacon ranch | 140 | 9.0 | 10.0 | 7.0 | 25 | 300 | 3.0 |
| w/crispy chicken | 370 | 29.0 | 20.0 | 20.0 | 75 | 970 | 3.0 |
| w/grilled chicken | 260 | 33.0 | 12.0 | 9.0 | 90 | 1010 | 3.0 |
| Caesar | 90 | 7.0 | 9.0 | 4.0 | 10 | 180 | 3.0 |
| w/crispy chicken | 330 | 26.0 | 20.0 | 17.0 | 60 | 840 | 3.0 |
| w/grilled chicken | 220 | 30.0 | 12.0 | 6.0 | 75 | 890 | 3.0 |

| Food and Measure | cal. | prot. (gms) | carbo. (gms) | fat (gms) | chol. (mgs) | sod. (mgs) | fiber (gms) |
|---|---|---|---|---|---|---|---|
| **McDonald's, salad** *(cont.)* | | | | | | | |
| Southwest ......... | 140 | 6.0 | 20.0 | 4.5 | 10 | 150 | 6.0 |
| w/crispy chicken .. | 430 | 26.0 | 38.0 | 20.0 | 55 | 920 | 6.0 |
| w/grilled chicken .. | 320 | 30.0 | 30.0 | 9.0 | 70 | 960 | 6.0 |
| side salad ......... | 20 | 1.0 | 4.0 | 0 | 0 | 10 | 1.0 |
| fruit/walnut pkg. ..... | 210 | 4.0 | 31.0 | 8.0 | 5 | 60 | 2.0 |
| croutons, butter garlic | 60 | 2.0 | 10.0 | 1.5 | 0 | 140 | 1.0 |
| salad dressing | | | | | | | |
| (*Newman's Own*): | | | | | | | |
| balsamic vinaigrette .. | 40 | 0 | 4.0 | 3.0 | 0 | 730 | 0 |
| Caesar, creamy ...... | 190 | 2.0 | 4.0 | 18.0 | 20 | 500 | 0 |
| ranch ............ | 170 | 1.0 | 9.0 | 15.0 | 20 | 530 | 0 |
| Southwest, creamy ... | 100 | 1.0 | 11.0 | 6.0 | 20 | 340 | 0 |
| shakes: | | | | | | | |
| *McCafé*, 16 fl. oz.: | | | | | | | |
| chocolate ........ | 720 | 15.0 | 119.0 | 20.0 | 60 | 300 | 1.0 |
| strawberry ....... | 710 | 14.0 | 116.0 | 20.0 | 65 | 210 | 0 |
| vanilla .......... | 680 | 14.0 | 111.0 | 20.0 | 60 | 220 | 0 |
| *McFlurry*, 12 fl. oz.: | | | | | | | |
| *M&M's* .......... | 710 | 15.0 | 105.0 | 25.0 | 60 | 220 | 4.0 |
| *Oreo* ............ | 580 | 13.0 | 89.0 | 19.0 | 50 | 320 | 3.0 |
| *Triple Thick*, 16 oz.: | | | | | | | |
| chocolate ........ | 580 | 13.0 | 102.0 | 14.0 | 50 | 250 | 1.0 |
| strawberry ....... | 560 | 13.0 | 97.0 | 13.0 | 50 | 170 | 0 |
| vanilla .......... | 550 | 13.0 | 96.0 | 13.0 | 50 | 190 | 0 |
| desserts/sundaes: | | | | | | | |
| apple pie, hot ....... | 250 | 2.0 | 32.0 | 13.0 | 0 | 170 | 4.0 |
| caramel dip ......... | 70 | 0 | 15.0 | .5 | 5 | 35 | 0 |
| cinnamon melts ..... | 460 | 6.0 | 66.0 | 19.0 | 15 | 370 | 3.0 |
| cone, vanilla ........ | 150 | 4.0 | 24.0 | 3.5 | 15 | 60 | 0 |
| cookies: | | | | | | | |
| chocolate chip .... | 160 | 2.0 | 21.0 | 8.0 | 10 | 90 | 1.0 |
| *McDonaldland* .... | 260 | 4.0 | 43.0 | 8.0 | 0 | 300 | 1.0 |
| oatmeal raisin .... | 150 | 2.0 | 22.0 | 6.0 | 10 | 135 | 1.0 |
| sugar ........... | 160 | 2.0 | 21.0 | 7.0 | 5 | 120 | 0 |
| fruit/yogurt parfait ... | 160 | 4.0 | 31.0 | 2.0 | 5 | 85 | 1.0 |
| sundaes: | | | | | | | |
| hot caramel ...... | 340 | 7.0 | 60.0 | 8.0 | 30 | 160 | 0 |
| hot fudge ........ | 330 | 8.0 | 54.0 | 10.0 | 25 | 180 | 2.0 |
| strawberry ....... | 280 | 6.0 | 49.0 | 6.0 | 25 | 95 | 1.0 |
| sundae peanuts ... | 45 | 2.0 | 2.0 | 3.5 | 0 | 0 | 1.0 |
| iced coffee, medium: | | | | | | | |
| regular ............ | 200 | 2.0 | 30.0 | 8.0 | 30 | 60 | 0 |
| hazelnut or vanilla .... | 190 | 2.0 | 29.0 | 8.0 | 30 | 60 | 0 |

| Food and Measure | cal. | prot. (gms) | carbo. (gms) | fat (gms) | chol. (mgs) | sod. (mgs) | fiber (gms) |
|---|---|---|---|---|---|---|---|
| *McCafé*, hot, w/whole milk, 16 fl. oz.: | | | | | | | |
| cappuccino ......... | 140 | 8.0 | 11.0 | 7.0 | 20 | 85 | 0 |
| caramel ......... | 240 | 6.0 | 41.0 | 6.0 | 20 | 150 | 0 |
| hazelnut or vanilla . | 240 | 6.0 | 42.0 | 6.0 | 20 | 85 | 0 |
| vanilla syrup ...... | 120 | 6.0 | 18.0 | 6.0 | 20 | 130 | 0 |
| latte ............. | 180 | 10.0 | 13.0 | 10.0 | 30 | 130 | 0 |
| caramel ......... | 280 | 8.0 | 43.0 | 8.0 | 25 | 170 | 0 |
| hazelnut ......... | 280 | 8.0 | 45.0 | 8.0 | 25 | 110 | 0 |
| vanilla .......... | 280 | 8.0 | 44.0 | 8.0 | 25 | 110 | 0 |
| vanilla syrup ...... | 160 | 8.0 | 21.0 | 8.0 | 25 | 150 | 0 |
| hot chocolate ....... | 380 | 10.0 | 53.0 | 15.0 | 30 | 170 | 0 |
| w/nonfat milk ..... | 310 | 11.0 | 55.0 | 6.0 | 10 | 190 | 0 |
| mocha ........... | 330 | 7.0 | 48.0 | 12.0 | 25 | 150 | 0 |
| caramel ......... | 290 | 8.0 | 39.0 | 12.0 | 25 | 180 | 0 |
| *McCafé*, iced, 16 fl. oz.: | | | | | | | |
| frappe, caramel ...... | 550 | 8.0 | 76.0 | 24.0 | 70 | 160 | 0 |
| frappe, mocha ...... | 560 | 8.0 | 78.0 | 24.0 | 65 | 160 | 0 |
| latte, whole milk ..... | 100 | 6.0 | 8.0 | 6.0 | 15 | 80 | 0 |
| caramel ......... | 180 | 4.0 | 31.0 | 4.5 | 15 | 120 | 0 |
| hazelnut ......... | 180 | 4.0 | 33.0 | 4.5 | 15 | 65 | 0 |
| vanilla .......... | 190 | 5.0 | 33.0 | 4.5 | 15 | 70 | 0 |
| vanilla syrup ...... | 90 | 5.0 | 14.0 | 5.0 | 15 | 105 | 0 |
| mocha, whole milk ... | 310 | 7.0 | 42.0 | 13.0 | 25 | 140 | 0 |
| caramel ......... | 300 | 8.0 | 36.0 | 14.0 | 30 | 160 | 0 |
| smoothie, strawberry banana .......... | 260 | 2.0 | 60.0 | 1.0 | 5 | 40 | 3.0 |
| smoothie, wild berry .. | 260 | 3.0 | 60.0 | 1.0 | 5 | 35 | 4.0 |
| **Meat loaf**, chilled, 5 oz., except as noted: | | | | | | | |
| and gravy: | | | | | | | |
| (*Bob Evans*) ........ | 240 | 14.0 | 10.0 | 15.0 | 65 | 750 | 1.0 |
| (*Hormel*) ........... | 190 | 16.0 | 11.0 | 9.0 | 40 | 920 | 0 |
| seasoned (*Tyson*) ...... | 320 | 14.0 | 16.0 | 23.0 | 60 | 600 | 0 |
| w/tomato sauce (*Hormel*) ........... | 260 | 22.0 | 13.0 | 13.0 | 60 | 870 | 1.0 |
| turkey, w/glaze (*Jennie-O* Pan Roasted), ⅛ of 28-oz. pkg. ..... | 200 | 20.0 | 6.0 | 10.0 | 85 | 650 | 0 |
| turkey, w/tomato sauce: | | | | | | | |
| (*Hormel*) ........... | 190 | 21.0 | 14.0 | 5.0 | 50 | 1000 | 0 |
| (*Jennie-O So Easy*) ... | 170 | 19.0 | 9.0 | 7.0 | 75 | 810 | 0 |
| rotisserie (*Jennie-O*), 3 oz. ............. | 140 | 15.0 | 5.0 | 7.0 | 65 | 620 | 0 |

| Food and Measure | cal. | prot. (gms) | carbo. (gms) | fat (gms) | chol. (mgs) | sod. (mgs) | fiber (gms) |
|---|---|---|---|---|---|---|---|
| **Meat loaf entree**, frozen, 1 pkg., except as noted: | | | | | | | |
| (*Banquet*), 9.5 oz. . . . . . . | 280 | 12.0 | 28.0 | 13.0 | 40 | 1000 | 4.0 |
| w/gravy (*Marie Callender's*), 14 oz. . . . | 450 | 29.0 | 41.0 | 18.0 | 75 | 1090 | 6.0 |
| w/potatoes, gravy: (*Boston Market*), 12 oz. . . . . . . . . . . | 570 | 22.0 | 43.0 | 35.0 | 85 | 1330 | 4.0 |
| (*Boston Market* Dinner), 16 oz. . . . . | 710 | 30.0 | 53.0 | 42.0 | 95 | 1590 | 5.0 |
| (*Healthy Choice* Complete), 12 oz. . . . | 360 | 16.0 | 55.0 | 8.0 | 35 | 550 | 8.0 |
| (*Michelina's*), 8 oz. . . . . | 190 | 11.0 | 21.0 | 6.0 | 35 | 860 | 2.0 |
| (*Michelina's Lean Gourmet*), 8 oz. . . . | 180 | 11.0 | 21.0 | 6.0 | 35 | 860 | 2.0 |
| (*Smart Ones*), 9.5 oz. . | 240 | 21.0 | 22.0 | 8.0 | 45 | 820 | 3.0 |
| (*Stouffer's*), 10 oz. . . . . | 340 | 22.0 | 0.0 | 19.0 | 80 | 780 | 2.0 |
| (*Stouffer's*), ½ of 16-oz. pkg. . . . . . . . | 600 | 35.0 | 45.0 | 31.0 | 90 | 1310 | 5.0 |
| (*Stouffer's*), ⅙ of 33-oz. pkg. . . . . . . . | 200 | 18.0 | 8.0 | 11.0 | 30 | 650 | 1.0 |
| whipped potato (*Lean Cuisine* Comfort), 9.4 oz. . . . . . . . . . | 250 | 20.0 | 25.0 | 8.0 | 45 | 590 | 3.0 |
| smothered, w/gravy, rice (*Zatarain's*), 12 oz. . . . | 410 | 16.0 | 59.0 | 12.0 | 50 | 1190 | 2.0 |
| **Meat loaf entree, microwave**, potato, gravy (*Hormel Compleats*), 10-oz. pkg. | 310 | 18.0 | 34.0 | 11.0 | 40 | 940 | 3.0 |
| **"Meat" loaf entree, vegetarian** (*Amy's* Veggie Loaf), 1 pkg.: | | | | | | | |
| whole meal, 10 oz. . . . . . | 290 | 9.0 | 47.0 | 8.0 | 0 | 690 | 10.0 |
| whole meal, light sodium, 10 oz. . . . . . . | 290 | 9.0 | 47.0 | 8.0 | 0 | 340 | 10.0 |
| **Meat loaf seasoning**: | | | | | | | |
| (*Adolph's Meal Makers*), 2 tsp. . . . . . . | 20 | 0 | 4.0 | 0 | 0 | 450 | 0 |
| (*Lawry's*), 1 tbsp. . . . . . . | 30 | <1.0 | 7.0 | 0 | 0 | 470 | <1.0 |
| (*McCormick*), 1 tsp. . . . . | 15 | 0 | 2.0 | 0 | 0 | 320 | 0 |
| (*McCormick Bag 'n Season*), 2 tsp. . . . . . . | 15 | 1.0 | 2.0 | 0 | 0 | 400 | 0 |

| Food and Measure | cal. | prot. (gms) | carbo. (gms) | fat (gms) | chol. (mgs) | sod. (mgs) | fiber (gms) |
|---|---|---|---|---|---|---|---|
| **Meat spread** (see also specific meats): | | | | | | | |
| (*Spam* Spread), 4 tbsp., 2 oz. . . . . . . . . | 140 | 8.0 | 1.0 | 12.0 | 40 | 570 | 0 |
| potted (*Armour*), ¼ cup . | 100 | 8.0 | 0 | 8.0 | 65 | 560 | 0 |
| **Meat tenderizer**: | | | | | | | |
| (*McCormick*), ¼ tsp. . . . . | 0 | 0 | 0 | 0 | 0 | 400 | 0 |
| seasoned, ¼ tsp.: | | | | | | | |
| (*Adolph's*) . . . . . . . . . . | 0 | 0 | 0 | 0 | 0 | 560 | 0 |
| (*McCormick*) . . . . . . . | 0 | 0 | 0 | 0 | 0 | 300 | 0 |
| **Meatball**, frozen/ chilled: | | | | | | | |
| (*Mama Lucia* Homestyle/Italian), 8 pcs., 3.2 oz. . . . . . . . | 210 | 13.0 | 7.0 | 14.0 | 45 | 550 | 1.0 |
| (*Rosina* Homestyle), 6 pcs., 3 oz. . . . . . . . . | 270 | 12.0 | 7.0 | 22.0 | 35 | 610 | 1.0 |
| beef, 3 oz.: | | | | | | | |
| (*Rosina* Organic), 6 pcs. . . . . . . . . . . . | 200 | 16.0 | 5.0 | 13.0 | 25 | 540 | 3.0 |
| Italian (*Rosina*), 6 pcs. | 240 | 14.0 | 5.0 | 19.0 | 40 | 640 | 1.0 |
| Italian (*Shady Brook Farms*), 3 pcs. . . . . | 260 | 15.0 | 5.0 | 20 | 55 | 510 | 1.0 |
| beef, w/tomato sauce (*Banquet* Family), 5 pcs. w/sauce, 5 oz. . | 200 | 12.0 | 9.0 | 13.0 | 40 | 750 | 3.0 |
| chicken/turkey: | | | | | | | |
| Buffalo (*Aidell's*), 3 oz. . . . . . . . . . . . | 180 | 14.0 | 3.0 | 13.0 | 80 | 690 | <1.0 |
| Italian, w/mozzarella (*Aidells* Zesty), 3 pcs., 2.25 oz. . . . | 140 | 12.0 | 2.0 | 10.0 | 60 | 490 | <1.0 |
| and gravy (*Hormel*), 5 oz. . . . . . . . . . . . . . | 240 | 12.0 | 9.0 | 17.0 | 50 | 660 | 0 |
| sausage: | | | | | | | |
| (*Mama Lucia's*), 8 pcs., 3.2 oz. . . . . | 220 | 14.0 | 3.0 | 17.0 | 50 | 690 | 1.0 |
| (*Rosina*), 6 pcs., 3 oz. | 270 | 11.0 | 5.0 | 22.0 | 45 | 690 | 0 |
| Swedish (*Rosina*), 6 pcs., 3 oz. . . . . . . . . | 250 | 14.0 | 6.0 | 19.0 | 45 | 620 | 1.0 |
| turkey, 3 oz.: | | | | | | | |
| (*Foster Farms* Chilled), 3 pcs. . . . . . . . . . . | 150 | 15.0 | 8.0 | 7.0 | 40 | 460 | 0 |

| Food and Measure | cal. | prot. (gms) | carbo. (gms) | fat (gms) | chol. (mgs) | sod. (mgs) | fiber (gms) |
|---|---|---|---|---|---|---|---|
| **Meatball, turkey** *(cont.)* | | | | | | | |
| (*Foster Farms* Homestyle), 3 pcs. | 160 | 18.0 | 3.0 | 9.0 | 30 | 280 | 0 |
| (*Jennie-O* Homestyle) | 180 | 16.0 | 2.0 | 12.0 | 75 | 370 | 0 |
| (*Mama Lucia's*), 8 pcs., 3.2 oz. | 200 | 15.0 | 8.0 | 12.0 | 45 | 740 | 1.0 |
| (*Perdue*), 4 pcs. | 180 | 15.0 | 5.0 | 10.0 | 45 | 520 | 0 |
| (*Rosina*), 6 pcs. | 170 | 12.0 | 5.0 | 11.0 | 70 | 600 | 1.0 |
| Italian (*Foster Farms*) | 160 | 16.0 | 5.0 | 8.0 | 40 | 380 | 0 |
| Italian (*Jennie-O*) | 170 | 16.0 | 1.0 | 11.0 | 90 | 380 | 0 |
| Italian (*Shady Brook Farms*), 3 pcs. | 190 | 17.0 | 6.0 | 10.0 | 65 | 600 | <1.0 |
| **"Meatball," vegetarian,** frozen: | | | | | | | |
| (*Nate's* Meatless Classic), 3 pcs., 1.5 oz. | 90 | 8.0 | 5.0 | 4.5 | 0 | 270 | 2.0 |
| (*Veggie Patch*), 3 pcs., 3 oz. | 120 | 16.0 | 7.0 | 4.5 | 0 | 480 | 4.0 |
| (*Yves* Classic), 4 pcs., 2.1 oz. | 80 | 13.0 | 8.0 | 2.0 | 0 | 440 | 2.0 |
| garlic and portobello (*Veggie Patch* Family Pack), 4 pcs., 3 oz. | 130 | 16.0 | 6.0 * | 4.5 | 0 | 460 | 3.0 |
| Italian (*Nate's* Zesty), 3 pcs., 1.5 oz. | 90 | 9.0 | 4.0 | 4.5 | 0 | 340 | 2.0 |
| mushroom (*Nate's* Savory), 3 pcs., 1.5 oz. | 100 | 8.0 | 6.0 | 4.5 | 0 | 230 | 2.0 |
| **Meatball entree, canned,** 1 cup: | | | | | | | |
| stew (*Dinty Moore*) | 250 | 13.0 | 19.0 | 15.0 | 40 | 1050 | 1.0 |
| vegetables, Italian, w/ (*Dinty Moore American classics*) | 190 | 9.0 | 25.0 | 6.0 | 20 | 660 | 3.0 |
| **Meatball entree, frozen,** Swedish, 1 pkg.: | | | | | | | |
| (*Banquet*), 10.25 oz. | 440 | 19.0 | 51.0 | 18.0 | 80 | 1020 | 5.0 |
| (*Boston Market* Dinner), 16 oz. | 760 | 36.0 | 57.0 | 43.0 | 170 | 1290 | 5.0 |
| (*Marie Callender's*), 13 oz. | 540 | 23.0 | 48.0 | 28.0 | 60 | 1310 | 6.0 |
| (*Michelina's*), 9 oz. | 380 | 13.0 | 41.0 | 17.0 | 35 | 1140 | 3.0 |
| (*Michelina's Lean Gourmet*), 8.5 oz. | 310 | 14.0 | 42.0 | 9.0 | 25 | 620 | 2.0 |
| (*Smart Ones*), 9.1 oz. | 270 | 20.0 | 35.0 | 5.0 | 30 | 730 | 3.0 |
| (*Stouffer's*), 11.5 oz. | 560 | 32.0 | 47.0 | 27.0 | 100 | 1250 | 3.0 |

| Food and Measure | cal. | prot. (gms) | carbo. (gms) | fat (gms) | chol. (mgs) | sod. (mgs) | fiber (gms) |
|---|---|---|---|---|---|---|---|
| w/pasta (*Lean Cuisine*), 9.125 oz. . . . | 290 | 19.0 | 35.0 | 8.0 | 35 | 670 | 3.0 |
| **Meatball entree, microwave**, 10-oz. cont.: | | | | | | | |
| stew, w/chipotle (*Doña Maria Platillos*) . . . . . . | 390 | 19.0 | 30.0 | 21.0 | 50 | 920 | 7.0 |
| Swedish, w/pasta (*Hormel Compleats*) . . | 350 | 15.0 | 32.0 | 18.0 | 70 | 980 | 1.0 |
| **Meatball seasoning**: | | | | | | | |
| Italian (*McCormick*), 2 tsp. | 20 | 1.0 | 3.0 | .5 | 0 | 320 | 0 |
| Swedish (*McCormick*), 2 tsp. seasoning and 1 tsp.sauce mix . . . . . | 40 | <1.0 | 6.0 | 1.0 | 0 | 490 | 0 |
| **Meatball sub**, frozen, toasted (*Stouffer's Corner Bistro* Italiano), 6.88-oz. pc. . . . . . . . . | 400 | 16.0 | 42.0 | 18.0 | 35 | 790 | 4.0 |
| **Melba sauce** (*Roland*), 2 tbsp. . . . . . . . . . . . | 100 | 0 | 24.0 | 0 | 0 | 10 | 0 |
| **Melogold** (*Frieda's*), ½ fruit, 5.9 oz. . . . . . . | 50 | 0 | 13.0 | 0 | 0 | 0 | 2.0 |
| **Melon**, see specific melon listings | | | | | | | |
| **Melon balls**, frozen, cantaloupe/ honeydew, ½ cup . . . . | 28 | .7 | 6.9 | .2 | 0 | 27 | .6 |
| **Melon berry juice** (*Snapple*), 11.5 fl. oz. . | 170 | 0 | 42.0 | 0 | 0 | 15 | 0 |
| **Melts**, flatbread, frozen, 1 pc.: | | | | | | | |
| cheese, 5, and spinach (*California Pizza Kitchen*) . . . . . . . . . . | 390 | 15.0 | 44.0 | 17.0 | 20 | 730 | 3.0 |
| chicken: | | | | | | | |
| Alfredo (*Stouffer's Corner Bistro*) . . . . | 420 | 20.0 | 41.0 | 19.0 | 45 | 710 | 4.0 |
| bacon club (*California Pizza Kitchen*) . . . . | 390 | 19.0 | 44.0 | 16.0 | 35 | 680 | 2.0 |
| bacon ranch (*DiGiorno*) . . . . . . . | 420 | 20.0 | 44.0 | 18.0 | 40 | 780 | 2.0 |
| barbecue (*California Pizza Kitchen*) . . . . | 360 | 20.0 | 45.0 | 12.0 | 40 | 910 | 2.0 |
| bruschetta (*Smart Ones*) . . . . . . . . . . | 310 | 17.0 | 42.0 | 8.0 | 20 | 570 | 4.0 |

| Food and Measure | cal. | prot. (gms) | carbo. (gms) | fat (gms) | chol. (mgs) | sod. (mgs) | fiber (gms) |
|---|---|---|---|---|---|---|---|
| **Melts, chicken** *(cont.)* | | | | | | | |
| club (*Michelina's* | | | | | | | |
| *Lean Gourmet*) .... | 280 | 12.0 | 43.0 | 8.0 | 15 | 780 | 2.0 |
| marinara w/mozzarella | | | | | | | |
| (*Smart Ones*) ..... | 290 | 18.0 | 41.0 | 6.0 | 20 | 640 | 3.0 |
| Parmesan (*DiGiorno*) . | 380 | 19.0 | 45.0 | 14.0 | 35 | 750 | 2.0 |
| Philly (*Lean Cuisine*) .. | 350 | 22.0 | 46.0 | 9.0 | 35 | 620 | 5.0 |
| quesadilla (*Stouffer's* | | | | | | | |
| *Corner Bistro*) .... | 370 | 18.0 | 41.0 | 15.0 | 40 | 640 | 4.0 |
| ranch club (*Lean Cuisine*) | 360 | 23.0 | 47.0 | 9.0 | 25 | 640 | 4.0 |
| sun-dried tomato | | | | | | | |
| basil (*Lean Cuisine*) | 360 | 23.0 | 49.0 | 8.0 | 30 | 610 | 5.0 |
| *sun-dried tomato | | | | | | | |
| Italian deli (*Michelina's* | | | | | | | |
| *Lean Gourmet*) ...... | 280 | 12.0 | 43.0 | 8.0 | 15 | 780 | 2.0 |
| meat, 3 (*Stouffer's* | | | | | | | |
| *Corner Bistro* Sicilian) | 520 | 21.0 | 58.0 | 23.0 | 45 | 1110 | 3.0 |
| meatball, Italian, 4 | | | | | | | |
| cheese (*DiGiorno*) .... | 400 | 18.0 | 46.0 | 17.0 | 30 | 780 | 3.0 |
| steak: | | | | | | | |
| fire-roasted | | | | | | | |
| vegetables (*DiGiorno*) | 380 | 19.0 | 44.0 | 14.0 | 25 | 740 | 2.0 |
| mushroom cheddar | | | | | | | |
| (*Stouffer's Corner* | | | | | | | |
| *Bistro*) ........... | 390 | 18.0 | 40.0 | 17.0 | 40 | 680 | 4.0 |
| ranch (*Smart Ones*) .. | 300 | 18.0 | 41.0 | 8.0 | 20 | 570 | 4.0 |
| steakhouse ranch (*Lean* | | | | | | | |
| *Cuisine*) ........... | 350 | 22.0 | 46.0 | 9.0 | 30 | 550 | 4.0 |
| *sun-dried tomato | | | | | | | |
| **Melts and soup**, frozen | | | | | | | |
| (*Stouffer's Corner* | | | | | | | |
| *Bistro*), 10-oz. pkg.: | | | | | | | |
| cheese, 3, and ham/ | | | | | | | |
| tomato bisque soup .. | 380 | 15.0 | 41.0 | 18.0 | 40 | 990 | 4.0 |
| chicken bacon ranch/ | | | | | | | |
| baked potato soup ... | 430 | 19.0 | 47.0 | 19.0 | 50 | 900 | 2.0 |
| steak and Swiss/ | | | | | | | |
| broccoli chedder soup | 400 | 17.0 | 41.0 | 10.0 | 45 | 880 | 2.0 |
| **Mexican beans**, see | | | | | | | |
| "Pinto beans" and | | | | | | | |
| specific listings | | | | | | | |
| **Mexican dip**, frozen, | | | | | | | |
| 5-layer (*Cedarlane* | | | | | | | |
| *Organic*), 2 tbsp. ...... | 60 | 3.0 | 4.0 | 3.0 | 10 | 100 | 1.0 |

| Food and Measure | cal. | prot. (gms) | carbo. (gms) | fat (gms) | chol. (mgs) | sod. (mgs) | fiber (gms) |
|---|---|---|---|---|---|---|---|
| **Mexican entree** (see also specific listings), frozen, 9.5-oz. pkg.: | | | | | | | |
| (*Amy's* Casserole Bowl) . | 470 | 11.0 | 70.0 | 16.0 | 20 | 780 | 7.0 |
| (*Amy's* Casserole Bowl Light Sodium) ...... | 370 | 12.0 | 48.0 | 16.0 | 20 | 390 | 7.0 |
| **Mexican sauce**, see "Mole sauce," "Salsa," and specific listings | | | | | | | |
| **Mexican seasoning** (*Chi-Chi's* Fiesta Restaurante), ⅛ pkg. . | 10 | 0 | 2.0 | 0 | 0 | 290 | 0 |
| **Mexican squash** (*Frieda's*), ½ cup, 3 oz. | 35 | 1.0 | 9.0 | 0 | 0 | 0 | 2.0 |
| **Milk**, 8 fl. oz.: | | | | | | | |
| buttermilk: | | | | | | | |
| (*Friendship*) ........ | 120 | 9.0 | 12.0 | 4.0 | 15 | 125 | 0 |
| cultured .......... | 99 | 8.1 | 11.7 | 2.2 | 9 | 257 | 0 |
| cultured, skim (*Hood*) . | 90 | 9.0 | 13.0 | 0 | <5 | 250 | 0 |
| whole, 3.3% fat ........ | 150 | 8.0 | 11.4 | 8.2 | 33 | 120 | 0 |
| reduced fat, 2% ........ | 121 | 8.1 | 11.7 | 4.7 | 18 | 122 | 0 |
| protein fortified ...... | 137 | 9.7 | 13.5 | 4.9 | 19 | 145 | 0 |
| lowfat, 1% ............. | 102 | 8.0 | 11.7 | 2.6 | 10 | 123 | 0 |
| protein fortified ...... | 119 | 9.7 | 13.6 | 2.9 | 10 | 143 | 0 |
| skim/fat free .......... | 86 | 8.4 | 11.9 | .4 | 4 | 126 | 0 |
| **Milk, canned**, 2 tbsp.: | | | | | | | |
| condensed, sweetened: | | | | | | | |
| (*Carnation*) ........ | 130 | 3.0 | 22.0 | 3.0 | 10 | 45 | 0 |
| (*Eagle Brand*) ....... | 130 | 3.0 | 22.0 | 3.0 | 10 | 35 | 0 |
| (*Eagle Brand* Low Fat) | 120 | 3.0 | 23.0 | 1.5 | 5 | 40 | 0 |
| (*Eagle Brand* Skim) ... | 110 | 4.0 | 25.0 | 0 | 0 | 55 | 0 |
| evaporated: | | | | | | | |
| (*Carnation*) ........ | 40 | 2.0 | 3.0 | 2.0 | 10 | 30 | 0 |
| (*Carnation* Lowfat) ... | 25 | 2.0 | 3.0 | .5 | 5 | 35 | 0 |
| (*Carnation* Skim) .... | 25 | 2.0 | 4.0 | 0 | 0 | 40 | 0 |
| (*Pet*) ............. | 40 | 2.0 | 3.0 | 2.0 | 5 | 25 | 0 |
| (*Pet* Skim) ......... | 25 | 2.0 | 3.0 | 0 | 0 | 35 | 0 |
| **Milk, chocolate**, see "Milk, flavored" | | | | | | | |
| **Milk, dry**: | | | | | | | |
| buttermilk, sweet cream, 1 tbsp. ...... | 25 | 2.2 | 3.2 | .4 | 4 | 34 | 0 |
| whole, 1 oz. ........... | 141 | 7.5 | 10.9 | 7.6 | 27 | 105 | 0 |
| whole, 1 cup .......... | 635 | 33.7 | 49.2 | 34.2 | 124 | 475 | 0 |

| Food and Measure | cal. | prot. (gms) | carbo. (gms) | fat (gms) | chol. (mgs) | sod. (mgs) | fiber (gms) |
|---|---|---|---|---|---|---|---|
| **Milk, dry** *(cont.)* | | | | | | | |
| nonfat: | | | | | | | |
| (*Carnation*), ⅓ cup ... | 80 | 8.0 | 12.0 | 0 | <5 | 125 | 0 |
| regular, 1 cup ....... | 435 | 43.4 | 62.4 | .9 | 24 | 642 | 0 |
| instant, 3.2-oz. pkt. ... | 244 | 23.9 | 35.5 | .5 | 12 | 373 | 0 |
| **Milk, flavored**, | | | | | | | |
| 8 fl. oz.: | | | | | | | |
| banana strawberry, low | | | | | | | |
| fat (*Nesquik*) ........ | 170 | 8.0 | 29.0 | 3.0 | 10 | 130 | 0 |
| chocolate (*Hood* Premium) | 230 | 9.0 | 31.0 | 9.0 | 35 | 170 | <1.0 |
| chocolate, low fat: | | | | | | | |
| (*Cool Moos*) ........ | 180 | 8.0 | 32.0 | 2.5 | 10 | 210 | 0 |
| (*Hood*) ........... | 170 | 9.0 | 28.0 | 3.0 | 15 | 170 | <1.0 |
| (*Hood Moostruck*) ... | 180 | 9.0 | 31.0 | 2.5 | 15 | 230 | <1.0 |
| (*Nesquik*) ......... | 170 | 8.0 | 29.0 | 2.5 | 10 | 160 | <1.0 |
| (*Nesquik* 100 Calorie) . | 100 | 8.0 | 13.0 | 2.0 | 10 | 140 | <1.0 |
| double (*Nesquik*) .... | 180 | 8.0 | 30.0 | 3.0 | 10 | 180 | 1.0 |
| chocolate, reduced fat: | | | | | | | |
| (*Land O Lakes* Swiss) | 190 | 8.0 | 26.0 | 5.0 | 20 | 220 | <1.0 |
| (*Nesquik*) ......... | 190 | 8.0 | 29.0 | 5.0 | 20 | 160 | <1.0 |
| (*Organic Valley*) ..... | 170 | 8.0 | 24.0 | 5.0 | 20 | 250 | <1.0 |
| double (*Nesquik*) .... | 190 | 8.0 | 30.0 | 5.0 | 15 | 180 | 1.0 |
| chocolate, skim: | | | | | | | |
| (*Hood Simply Smart*) . | 160 | 12.0 | 28.0 | 0 | <5 | 220 | <1.0 |
| (*Land O Lakes*) ...... | 160 | 8.0 | 31.0 | 0 | <5 | 220 | <1.0 |
| (*Nesquik*) ......... | 150 | 8.0 | 29.0 | 0 | <5 | 160 | <1.0 |
| coffee, low fat (*Hood*) ... | 170 | 8.0 | 28.0 | 2.5 | 15 | 125 | 0 |
| strawberry: | | | | | | | |
| (*Land O Lakes*) ...... | 190 | 7.0 | 22.0 | 8.0 | 30 | 125 | 0 |
| low fat (*Nesquik*) .... | 180 | 8.0 | 31.0 | 2.5 | 10 | 125 | 0 |
| reduced fat (*Nesquik*) . | 200 | 8.0 | 31.0 | 5.0 | 20 | 370 | 0 |
| vanilla: | | | | | | | |
| low fat (*Nesquik*) .... | 170 | 8.0 | 30.0 | 2.5 | 10 | 130 | 0 |
| reduced fat (*Nesquik*) . | 190 | 8.0 | 30.0 | 5.0 | 15 | 130 | 0 |
| **Milk, goat**, fresh, | | | | | | | |
| 8 fl. oz. ............ | 168 | 8.7 | 10.9 | 10.1 | 28 | 122 | 0 |
| **"Milk," nondairy**, see | | | | | | | |
| "Almond beverage," | | | | | | | |
| "Soy beverage," etc. | | | | | | | |
| **Milk, human**, 8 fl. oz. ... | 172 | 2.9 | 16.9 | 10.8 | 34 | 42 | 0 |
| **Milk, sheep**, 8 fl. oz. .... | 265 | 14.7 | 13.1 | 17.2 | 66 | 108 | 0 |
| **Milkfish**, meat only: | | | | | | | |
| raw, 4 oz. ........... | 168 | 23.3 | 0 | 7.6 | 59 | 82 | 0 |
| baked or broiled, 4 oz. .. | 215 | 29.8 | 0 | 9.8 | 76 | 104 | 0 |

| Food and Measure | cal. | prot. (gms) | carbo. (gms) | fat (gms) | chol. (mgs) | sod. (mgs) | fiber (gms) |
|---|---|---|---|---|---|---|---|
| **Millet**, grain: | | | | | | | |
| dry: | | | | | | | |
| (*Arrowhead Mills* Organic), ¼ cup ... | 150 | 4.0 | 33.0 | 1.5 | 0 | 0 | 1.0 |
| (*Bob's Red Mill*), 2 tbsp. | 90 | 3.0 | 18.0 | 1.0 | 0 | 0 | 4.0 |
| (*Eden* Organic), ¼ cup | 160 | 5.0 | 30.0 | 2.0 | 0 | 5 | 4.0 |
| cooked, 4 oz. ......... | 135 | 4.0 | 26.8 | 1.1 | 0 | 2 | 1.5 |
| **Millet flour**: | | | | | | | |
| (*Arrowhead Mills* Organic), ⅓ cup ..... | 130 | 4.0 | 26.0 | 1.5 | 0 | 0 | 3.0 |
| (*Bob's Red Mill*), ¼ cup . | 110 | 3.0 | 22.0 | 1.0 | 0 | 2 | 4.0 |
| **Mincemeat**, see "Pie filling" | | | | | | | |
| **Mint**, fresh: | | | | | | | |
| peppermint, 2 tbsp. ..... | 2 | .1 | .5 | 0 | 0 | .1 | <.1 |
| spearmint, 2 tbsp. ...... | 5 | .4 | .9 | .1 | 0 | 3 | .7 |
| **Mint, dried**, | | | | | | | |
| spearmint, 1 tbsp. ... | 5 | .3 | .8 | .1 | 0 | 6 | .5 |
| **Mint drink mixer** (*Angostura*), 2 fl. oz. ............ | 80 | 0 | 18.0 | 0 | 0 | 5 | 0 |
| **Mint sauce** (*Crosse & Blackwell*), 1 tsp. .... | 5 | 0 | 1.0 | 0 | 0 | 0 | 0 |
| **Mirin**, see "Wine, cooking" | | | | | | | |
| **Miso**, 1 tbsp., except as noted: | | | | | | | |
| (*Eden* Organic Hacho) ... | 40 | 3.0 | 4.0 | 1.5 | 0 | 680 | <1.0 |
| (*Eden* Organic Shiro) ... | 30 | 1.0 | 6.0 | .5 | 0 | 330 | <1.0 |
| ½ cup ............... | 284 | 16.3 | 38.6 | 8.4 | 0 | 5032 | 7.6 |
| brown rice (*Eden* Organic Genmai) ..... | 25 | 2.0 | 3.0 | .5 | 0 | 780 | 2.0 |
| soy and barley (*Eden* Organic Mugi) ....... | 25 | 2.0 | 4.0 | .5 | 0 | 640 | <1.0 |
| **Miso condiment**, see "Tekka" | | | | | | | |
| **Mochi** (*Eden*), 1.75 oz.: | | | | | | | |
| brown rice, sprouted or sweet ........... | 110 | 2.0 | 25.0 | 1.0 | 0 | 0 | 1.0 |
| brown rice/mugwort .... | 110 | 2.0 | 24.0 | 1.0 | 0 | 10 | 2.0 |
| **Mojito drink mixer**: | | | | | | | |
| (*Angostura*), 3 fl. oz. .... | 80 | 0 | 20.0 | 0 | 0 | 15 | 0 |
| (*Stirrings*), 2 fl. oz. ..... | 50 | 0 | 13.0 | 0 | 0 | 0 | 0 |
| frozen (*Bacardi*), 2 fl. oz. . | 110 | 0 | 30.0 | 0 | 0 | 0 | 0 |

| Food and Measure | cal. | prot. (gms) | carbo. (gms) | fat (gms) | chol. (mgs) | sod. (mgs) | fiber (gms) |
|---|---|---|---|---|---|---|---|
| **Molasses**, 1 tbsp.: | | | | | | | |
| (*Brer Rabbit*) .......... | 60 | 0 | 15.0 | 0 | 0 | 10 | 0 |
| (*Grandma's*) .......... | 50 | 0 | 12.0 | 0 | 0 | 0 | 0 |
| (*Plantation* Barbados) ... | 60 | 0 | 15.0 | 0 | 0 | 0 | 0 |
| blackstrap: | | | | | | | |
| (*Brer Rabbit*) ........ | 60 | 1.0 | 13.0 | 0 | 0 | 65 | 0 |
| (*Plantation*) ......... | 42 | 0 | 11.0 | 0 | 0 | 10 | 0 |
| (*Plantation* Organic) .. | 60 | 0 | 13.0 | 0 | 0 | 0 | 0 |
| blend (*Mrs. Renfro's* Country), ¼ cup ..... | 240 | 0 | 61.0 | 0 | 0 | 15 | 0 |
| **Mole sauce** (*Doña Maria*): | | | | | | | |
| original, 2 tbsp. ........ | 200 | 3.0 | 10.0 | 13.0 | 0 | 400 | 2.0 |
| pipian, 2 tbsp. ......... | 230 | 4.0 | 5.0 | 18.0 | 0 | 530 | 3.0 |
| ready to serve, ⅓ cup ... | 140 | 2.0 | 13.0 | 9.0 | 0 | 470 | 2.0 |
| verde, 2 tbsp. ......... | 220 | 5.0 | 5.0 | 16.0 | 0 | 600 | 2.0 |
| **Monkfish**, meat only: | | | | | | | |
| raw, 4 oz. ............. | 86 | 16.4 | 0 | 1.7 | 29 | 21 | 0 |
| baked or broiled, 4 oz. .. | 110 | 21.0 | 0 | 2.2 | 36 | 26 | 0 |
| **Moose**, meat only, roasted, 4 oz. ....... | 152 | 33.2 | 0 | 1.1 | 88 | 78 | 0 |
| **Mortadella**, 2 oz.: | | | | | | | |
| (*Black Bear*) .......... | 150 | 10.0 | 2.0 | 14.0 | 30 | 490 | 0 |
| (*Boar's Head*) ......... | 160 | 9.0 | 0 | 14.0 | 30 | 560 | 0 |
| (*Thumann's*) .......... | 170 | 8.0 | <1.0 | 14.0 | 35 | 660 | 0 |
| beef and pork ......... | 174 | 9.2 | 1.7 | 14.2 | 31 | 698 | 0 |
| w/pistachios: | | | | | | | |
| (*Boar's Head*) ....... | 170 | 10.0 | 2.0 | 14.0 | 30 | 560 | 0 |
| (*Thumann's*) ........ | 170 | 8.0 | <1.0 | 15.0 | 35 | 610 | 0 |
| **Mothbean**, boiled, 4 oz. . | 133 | 8.9 | 23.8 | .6 | 0 | 11 | n.a. |
| **Moussaka**, see "Eggplant entree" | | | | | | | |
| **Mousse, mix**: | | | | | | | |
| (*Dr. Oetker*), ¼ pkg.: | | | | | | | |
| chocolate, double .... | 130 | 3.0 | 21.0 | 4.0 | 0 | 45 | 1.0 |
| chocolate, milk ...... | 100 | 2.0 | 15.0 | 3.5 | 0 | 45 | 0 |
| chocolate, white ..... | 80 | 0 | 15.0 | 2.0 | 0 | 115 | 0 |
| chocolate raspberry .. | 130 | 2.0 | 21.0 | 4.0 | 0 | 45 | 1.0 |
| chocolate truffle, dark ............ | 100 | 2.0 | 15.0 | 3.5 | 0 | 85 | 1.0 |
| mocha chocolate .... | 70 | 0 | 13.0 | 2.5 | 0 | 80 | 0 |
| strawberry ......... | 80 | 0 | 13.0 | 3.0 | 0 | 140 | 0 |
| vanilla, French ...... | 90 | 0 | 15.0 | 3.0 | 0 | 130 | 0 |

| Food and Measure | cal. | prot. (gms) | carbo. (gms) | fat (gms) | chol. (mgs) | sod. (mgs) | fiber (gms) |
|---|---|---|---|---|---|---|---|
| (*Dr. Oetker* Light), ⅓ pkg.: | | | | | | | |
| chocolate, milk ...... | 40 | 0 | 4.0 | 2.5 | 0 | 130 | 0 |
| chocolate truffle, dark ............ | 45 | 1.0 | 4.0 | 2.5 | 0 | 125 | 0 |
| strawberry ......... | 35 | 0 | 3.0 | 2.0 | 0 | 70 | 0 |
| vanilla, French ...... | 35 | 0 | 3.0 | 2.0 | 0 | 85 | 0 |
| **Muffin**, 2.3-oz. pc., except as noted: | | | | | | | |
| apple cinnamon: | | | | | | | |
| (*Fiber One* 3 Pack) ... | 200 | 3.0 | 36.0 | 4.5 | 30 | 170 | 7.0 |
| (*Fiber One* 4 Pack) ... | 170 | 3.0 | 34.0 | 4.5 | 30 | 170 | 7.0 |
| banana chocolate chip: | | | | | | | |
| (*Fiber One* 3 Pack) ... | 200 | 3.0 | 37.0 | 4.0 | 30 | 180 | 7.0 |
| (*Fiber One* 4 Pack) ... | 180 | 3.0 | 36.0 | 4.5 | 30 | 190 | 7.0 |
| blueberry, wild/oats: | | | | | | | |
| (*Fiber One* 3 Pack) ... | 190 | 3.0 | 34.0 | 4.0 | 30 | 190 | 7.0 |
| (*Fiber One* 4 Pack) ... | 170 | 3.0 | 33.0 | 4.0 | 30 | 200 | 7.0 |
| corn, 2 oz. ............ | 174 | 3.6 | 29.0 | 4.8 | 15 | 297 | 1.9 |
| English, see "Muffin, English" | | | | | | | |
| fruits, mixed, nuts and honey (*Fiber One*) | 170 | 3.0 | 34.0 | 4.5 | 30 | 190 | 7.0 |
| oat bran, 2 oz. ........ | 154 | 4.0 | 27.5 | 4.2 | 0 | 224 | 2.6 |
| **Muffin, English**, 1 pc.: | | | | | | | |
| (*Fiber One* Original) ..... | 100 | 5.0 | 23.0 | 1.0 | 0 | 230 | 6.0 |
| (*Glutino* Gluten Free) .... | 190 | 4.0 | 38.0 | 2.5 | 0 | 410 | 1.0 |
| (*Nature's Own*) ........ | 130 | 5.0 | 26.0 | 1.0 | 0 | 240 | <1.0 |
| (*Pepperidge Farm*) ..... | 130 | 5.0 | 25.0 | 1.5 | 0 | 170 | 1.0 |
| (*Thomas'* Original) ..... | 120 | 4.0 | 25.0 | 1.0 | 0 | 200 | 1.0 |
| (*Thomas'* Original Whole Grain) ....... | 130 | 4.0 | 26.0 | 1.0 | 0 | 220 | 2.0 |
| (*Thomas'* Sandwich) .... | 190 | 6.0 | 37.0 | 1.5 | 0 | 310 | 1.0 |
| apple cinnamon (*Thomas'*) .......... | 140 | 4.0 | 28.0 | 1.0 | 0 | 210 | 1.0 |
| berry, mixed (*Thomas'*) .. | 160 | 5.0 | 32.0 | 1.0 | 0 | 240 | 1.0 |
| cinnamon raisin (*Thomas'*) .......... | 140 | 4.0 | 29.0 | 1.0 | 0 | 170 | 1.0 |
| cranberry (*Thomas'*) .... | 140 | 4.0 | 31.0 | 1.0 | 0 | 230 | 1.0 |
| honey wheat: | | | | | | | |
| (*Nature's Own*) ...... | 100 | 5.0 | 24.0 | 1.0 | 0 | 250 | 7.0 |
| (*Thomas'*) .......... | 130 | 5.0 | 26.0 | 1.5 | 0 | 230 | 1.0 |
| multigrain: | | | | | | | |
| (*Fiber One*) ......... | 100 | 5.0 | 24.0 | 1.0 | 0 | 160 | 8.0 |

| Food and Measure | cal. | prot. (gms) | carbo. (gms) | fat (gms) | chol. (mgs) | sod. (mgs) | fiber (gms) |
|---|---|---|---|---|---|---|---|
| **Muffin, English, multigrain** *(cont.)* | | | | | | | |
| (*Nature's Own*) ...... | 100 | 5.0 | 24.0 | 1.0 | 0 | 250 | 7.0 |
| (*Thomas'* Light) ..... | 100 | 5.0 | 26.0 | 1.0 | 0 | 180 | 8.0 |
| 12 (*Thomas'*) ....... | 140 | 6.0 | 25.0 | 1.5 | 0 | 200 | 2.0 |
| wheat (*Fiber One*) .... | 100 | 5.0 | 24.0 | 1.0 | 0 | 150 | 8.0 |
| raisin (*Sun•Maid*) ...... | 170 | 5.0 | 36.0 | .5 | 0 | 180 | 2.0 |
| whole grain (*Thomas'* Original) .......... | 130 | 4.0 | 26.0 | 1.0 | 0 | 220 | 2.0 |
| whole wheat: | | | | | | | |
| (*Fiber One*) ......... | 100 | 5.0 | 22.0 | 1.0 | 0 | 230 | 6.0 |
| (*Nature's Own*) ...... | 120 | 6.0 | 24.0 | 1.5 | 0 | 180 | 3.0 |
| (*Pepperidge Farm*) ... | 140 | 6.0 | 26.0 | 1.5 | 0 | 210 | 3.0 |
| (*Thomas'*) .......... | 120 | 6.0 | 23.0 | 1.0 | 0 | 220 | 3.0 |
| **Muffin mix** (see also "Bread mix, sweet"), ¼ cup mix, except as noted: | | | | | | | |
| apple cinnamon: | | | | | | | |
| (*Dr. Oetker* Organics), ¹⁄₁₂ pkg. ......... | 120 | 1.0 | 28.0 | 0 | 0 | 190 | 0 |
| (*Fiber One*), 1 pc.* ... | 160 | 4.0 | 29.0 | 10.0 | 70 | 250 | 5.0 |
| (*"Jiffy"*) ............. | 160 | 2.0 | 26.0 | 5.0 | <5 | 320 | 0 |
| (*Martha White*) ...... | 140 | 1.0 | 25.0 | 4.0 | 5 | 150 | 0 |
| (*Martha White* Whole Grain) ............ | 140 | 1.0 | 24.0 | 4.0 | 5 | 150 | 1.0 |
| (*Pillsbury* Pouch) .... | 160 | 1.0 | 28.0 | 4.5 | 5 | 170 | 0 |
| w/flax (*Hodgson Mill*) . | 130 | 4.0 | 27.0 | 1.0 | 0 | 340 | 3.0 |
| oatmeal granola top (*Duncan Hines*), 1 pc.* ........... | 220 | 4.0 | 34.0 | 8.0 | 35 | 240 | 3.0 |
| apple streusel (*Betty Crocker*), 1 pc.* ..... | 230 | 3.0 | 37.0 | 8.0 | 35 | 280 | <1.0 |
| banana (*"Jiffy"*) ........ | 150 | 2.0 | 25.0 | 4.5 | <5 | 310 | <1.0 |
| banana nut: | | | | | | | |
| (*Betty Crocker* Box), 1 pc.* ............ | 210 | 4.0 | 28.0 | 9.0 | 35 | 250 | <1.0 |
| (*Betty Crocker* Pouch), ⅙ pouch ......... | 120 | 2.0 | 22.0 | 3.0 | 0 | 240 | 0 |
| (*Martha White*) ...... | 150 | 2.0 | 25.0 | 5.0 | 5 | 220 | <1.0 |
| (*Martha White* Whole Grain) ........... | 150 | 2.0 | 25.0 | 5.0 | 5 | 220 | 1.0 |
| (*Pillsbury* Pouch) .... | 150 | 2.0 | 25.0 | 5.0 | 5 | 220 | 1.0 |
| berry, triple (*Betty Crocker*), ⅙ pouch ... | 120 | 2.0 | 23.0 | 2.5 | 0 | 230 | 0 |

| Food and Measure | cal. | prot. (gms) | carbo. (gms) | fat (gms) | chol. (mgs) | sod. (mgs) | fiber (gms) |
|---|---|---|---|---|---|---|---|
| blueberry: | | | | | | | |
| (*Betty Crocker*), | | | | | | | |
| ⅙ pouch .......... | 120 | 2.0 | 23.0 | 2.5 | 0 | 230 | 0 |
| (*Fiber One*), 1 pc.* ... | 160 | 3.0 | 29.0 | 6.0 | 35 | 250 | 5.0 |
| (*"Jiffy"*) .............. | 160 | 2.0 | 26.0 | 5.0 | <5 | 320 | 0 |
| (*Martha White*) ...... | 140 | 1.0 | 25.0 | 4.0 | 5 | 150 | 0 |
| (*Martha White* Low | | | | | | | |
| Fat) ............. | 130 | 1.0 | 27.0 | 1.5 | 0 | 135 | 1.0 |
| (*Martha White* Whole | | | | | | | |
| Grain) .......... | 140 | 1.0 | 24.0 | 4.0 | 5 | 150 | 1.0 |
| (*Pillsbury* Pouch) .... | 160 | 1.0 | 28.0 | 4.5 | 5 | 170 | 0 |
| streusel (*Duncan* | | | | | | | |
| *Hines*), 1 pc.* ..... | 210 | 3.0 | 32.0 | 8.0 | 35 | 230 | 3.0 |
| whole wheat (*Hodgson* | | | | | | | |
| *Mill*) ............. | 131 | 5.0 | 24.0 | 1.5 | 0 | 222 | 3.6 |
| wild (*Betty Crocker*), | | | | | | | |
| 1 pc.* ............. | 180 | 3.0 | 27.0 | 7.0 | 35 | 230 | <1.0 |
| wild (*Duncan Hines* | | | | | | | |
| Maine), 1 pc.* .... | 180 | 3.0 | 27.0 | 7.0 | 35 | 230 | 3.0 |
| blueberry cheesecake | | | | | | | |
| (*Martha White*) ...... | 150 | 2.0 | 22.0 | 6.0 | 10 | 180 | 0 |
| bran: | | | | | | | |
| (*Hodgson Mill*) ...... | 130 | 4.0 | 28.0 | 1.0 | 0 | 200 | 3.0 |
| w/dates (*"Jiffy"*) ..... | 130 | 2.0 | 24.0 | 4.0 | <5 | 280 | 2.0 |
| honey (*Martha White*) . | 140 | 2.0 | 26.0 | 3.5 | 5 | 210 | 3.0 |
| carrot (*Dr. Oetker* | | | | | | | |
| Organics), 1/12 pkg. ... | 120 | 1.0 | 28.0 | 0 | 0 | 190 | 0 |
| chocolate: | | | | | | | |
| (*"Jiffy"*) .............. | 170 | 2.0 | 27.0 | 6.0 | <5 | 280 | 1.0 |
| double (*Betty Crocker*), | | | | | | | |
| 1 pc.* ............. | 230 | 3.0 | 33.0 | 10.0 | 35 | 250 | 1.0 |
| chocolate chip: | | | | | | | |
| (*Betty Crocker* Box), | | | | | | | |
| 1 pc.* ............. | 210 | 3.0 | 30.0 | 9.0 | 35 | 210 | <1.0 |
| (*Betty Crocker* Pouch), | | | | | | | |
| ⅙ pouch .......... | 130 | 2.0 | 22.0 | 3.5 | 0 | 210 | 1.0 |
| (*Duncan Hines*), 1 pc.* | 190 | 3.0 | 32.0 | 7.0 | 35 | 290 | 3.0 |
| (*Martha White*) ...... | 150 | 2.0 | 25.0 | 4.5 | 5 | 160 | 1.0 |
| (*Pillsbury* Pouch), | | | | | | | |
| ⅓ cup ............. | 160 | 2.0 | 28.0 | 5.0 | 5 | 180 | 1.0 |
| chocolate (*Martha* | | | | | | | |
| *White*) .......... | 140 | 2.0 | 25.0 | 5.0 | 5 | 160 | 1.0 |
| chocolate chunk, triple | | | | | | | |
| (*Duncan Hines*), 1 pc.* | 240 | 4.0 | 35.0 | 11.0 | 35 | 290 | 3.0 |

| Food and Measure | cal. | prot. (gms) | carbo. (gms) | fat (gms) | chol. (mgs) | sod. (mgs) | fiber (gms) |
|---|---|---|---|---|---|---|---|
| **Muffin, English** *(cont.)* | | | | | | | |
| cinnamon streusel | | | | | | | |
| (*Betty Crocker*), 1 pc.* | 210 | 3.0 | 29.0 | 9.0 | 35 | 210 | 0 |
| cinnamon sugar | | | | | | | |
| (*Martha White*) . . . . . . | 140 | 1.0 | 25.0 | 4.0 | 5 | 150 | 0 |
| cinnamon swirl | | | | | | | |
| (*Duncan Hines*), 1 pc. . | 220 | 3.0 | 34.0 | 8.0 | 35 | 230 | 3.0 |
| corn: | | | | | | | |
| (*Glory*), 1.2-oz. pc.* . . | 160 | 2.0 | 24.0 | 4.5 | 35 | 480 | 2.0 |
| (*Hodgson Mill*) . . . . . . | 130 | 4.0 | 27.0 | 1.0 | 0 | 340 | 3.0 |
| (*"Jiffy"*) . . . . . . . . . . . . | 150 | 2.0 | 27.0 | 4.5 | <5 | 340 | <1.0 |
| yellow (*Martha* | | | | | | | |
| *White*) . . . . . . . . . . | 140 | 2.0 | 26.0 | 3.0 | 0 | 230 | 1.0 |
| cornmeal (*Dr. Oetker* | | | | | | | |
| Organics), 1/12 pkg. . . . | 140 | 2.0 | 32.0 | .5 | 0 | 270 | 1.0 |
| cranberry orange | | | | | | | |
| (*Martha White*) . . . . . . | 140 | 1.0 | 25.0 | 4.0 | 5 | 150 | 0 |
| lemon poppy seed: | | | | | | | |
| (*Betty Crocker*), | | | | | | | |
| 1/6 pouch . . . . . . . . . | 120 | 2.0 | 22.0 | 3.0 | 0 | 200 | 0 |
| (*Betty Crocker* | | | | | | | |
| *Sunkist* Box), 1 pc.* | 200 | 3.0 | 30.0 | 8.0 | 35 | 230 | 0 |
| (*Dr. Oetker* Organics), | | | | | | | |
| 1/12 pkg. . . . . . . . . . | 120 | 1.0 | 28.0 | 0 | 0 | 190 | 0 |
| (*Martha White*) . . . . . . | 150 | 2.0 | 27.0 | 4.0 | 5 | 160 | <1.0 |
| (*Pillsbury* Pouch) . . . . | 150 | 2.0 | 27.0 | 4.0 | 5 | 160 | <1.0 |
| oatmeal: | | | | | | | |
| (*Dr. Oetker* Organics), | | | | | | | |
| 1/12 pkg. . . . . . . . . . | 140 | 2.0 | 32.0 | .5 | 0 | 270 | 1.0 |
| (*"Jiffy"*) . . . . . . . . . . . . | 150 | 2.0 | 25.0 | 4.5 | <5 | 290 | <1.0 |
| raspberry (*"Jiffy"*) . . . . . . | 160 | 2.0 | 26.0 | 6.0 | <5 | 320 | 0 |
| strawberry (*Martha White*) | 140 | 1.0 | 25.0 | 4.0 | 5 | 150 | 0 |
| strawberry cheesecake | | | | | | | |
| (*Martha White*) . . . . . . | 150 | 2.0 | 22.0 | 6.0 | 10 | 180 | 0 |
| whole wheat (*Hodgson* | | | | | | | |
| *Mill*) . . . . . . . . . . . . . . | 130 | 4.0 | 27.0 | 1.0 | 0 | 235 | 3.0 |
| wildberry: | | | | | | | |
| (*Martha White*) . . . . . . | 140 | 1.0 | 25.0 | 4.0 | 5 | 150 | 0 |
| (*Pillsbury* Pouch) . . . . | 160 | 1.0 | 28.0 | 4.5 | 5 | 170 | 0 |
| **Muffin sandwich**, see | | | | | | | |
| "Breakfast sandwich" | | | | | | | |
| **Mulberries**, fresh: | | | | | | | |
| 10 berries, 1/2 oz. . . . . . . | 7 | .2 | 1.5 | .1 | 0 | 2 | .3 |
| 1/2 cup . . . . . . . . . . . . . | 31 | 1.0 | 6.9 | .3 | 0 | 7 | 1.2 |

| Food and Measure | cal. | prot. (gms) | carbo. (gms) | fat (gms) | chol. (mgs) | sod. (mgs) | fiber (gms) |
|---|---|---|---|---|---|---|---|
| **Mullet**, striped, meat only: | | | | | | | |
| raw, 4 oz. . . . . . . . . . . . . | 133 | 22.0 | 0 | 4.3 | 56 | 74 | 0 |
| baked or broiled, 4 oz. . . | 170 | 28.1 | 0 | 5.5 | 71 | 81 | 0 |
| **Multigrain chips**, see "Multigrain snack," "Tortilla chips, multigrain," and "Snack chips/crisps" | | | | | | | |
| **Multigrain dish**, microwave, pilaf (*Tasty Bite*), ½ of 8.8-oz. pkg. . . . . | 170 | 8.0 | 29.0 | 4.0 | 0 | 380 | 3.0 |
| **Multigrain dish mix** (*Seeds of Change Organic*), 1 cup*: | | | | | | | |
| herb, Velleron . . . . . . . . . | 190 | 6.0 | 36.0 | 2.5 | 0 | 640 | 3.0 |
| 7-grain pilaf, Persia . . . . . | 240 | 6.0 | 51.0 | 1.5 | 0 | 750 | 5.0 |
| **Multigrain flour**, whole grain (*Bob's Red Mill*), ¼ cup . . . . . | 140 | 5.0 | 26.0 | 2.0 | 0 | 5 | 2.0 |
| **Multigrain snack** (see also "Snack chips/crisps" and "Tortilla, multigrain"): | | | | | | | |
| (*Quaker Mini Delights*), .75-oz. bag: | | | | | | | |
| caramel drizzle . . . . . . | 90 | 1.0 | 15.0 | 3.5 | 0 | 75 | 1.0 |
| chocolatey drizzle . . . . | 90 | 1.0 | 14.0 | 3.5 | 0 | 65 | 1.0 |
| chocolatey mint . . . . . | 90 | 1.0 | 14.0 | 3.5 | 0 | 70 | 1.0 |
| cinnamon streusel . . . | 90 | 2.0 | 14.0 | 3.5 | 0 | 95 | 1.0 |
| (*Quaker True Delights Fiber Crisps*), 1 oz.: | | | | | | | |
| blackberry pomegranate | 100 | 2.0 | 23.0 | 1.5 | 0 | 135 | 5.0 |
| blueberry, wild . . . . . . | 110 | 2.0 | 23.0 | 1.5 | 0 | 135 | 3.0 |
| **Mung bean**, dry: | | | | | | | |
| (*Bob's Red Mill*), ½ cup . | 300 | 15.0 | 58.0 | .5 | 0 | 25 | 3.0 |
| boiled, ½ cup . . . . . . . . | 106 | 7.1 | 19.3 | .4 | 0 | 2 | 7.7 |
| **Mung bean sprouts**: | | | | | | | |
| raw, 1 cup . . . . . . . . . . . | 31 | 3.2 | 6.2 | .2 | 0 | 6 | 1.9 |
| boiled, drained, ½ cup . . | 13 | 1.3 | 2.6 | .1 | 0 | 6 | .5 |
| **Mung bean sprouts, canned**, drained, 1 cup . . . . . . . . . . . . | 15 | 1.8 | 2.7 | <.1 | 0 | 175 | 1.0 |

| Food and Measure | cal. | prot. (gms) | carbo. (gms) | fat (gms) | chol. (mgs) | sod. (mgs) | fiber (gms) |
|---|---|---|---|---|---|---|---|
| **Mungo bean**, boiled, ½ cup . . . . . . . . . . . . | 95 | 6.8 | 16.5 | .5 | 0 | 7 | 5.8 |
| **Mushroom** (see also specific listings), button or common: | | | | | | | |
| raw, ½ cup: | | | | | | | |
| (*Dole*), 1.2 oz. . . . . . . . | 9 | 1.0 | 1.0 | 0 | 0 | 0 | 0 |
| pieces or slices . . . . . . | 9 | 1.0 | 1.5 | .2 | 0 | 1 | .4 |
| boiled, drained, pieces, ½ cup . . . . . . . . . . . . | 21 | 1.7 | 4.0 | .4 | 0 | 2 | 1.7 |
| can/jar, all styles, ½ cup: | | | | | | | |
| (*Green Giant*) . . . . . . . | 25 | 2.0 | 4.0 | 0 | 0 | 440 | 1.0 |
| (*Ka•Me* Stir-Fry) . . . . . | 20 | 2.0 | 3.0 | 0 | 0 | 380 | 2.0 |
| (*Roland*) . . . . . . . . . . . | 25 | 1.0 | 4.0 | 0 | 0 | 370 | 2.0 |
| drained . . . . . . . . . . . . | 19 | 1.5 | 3.9 | .5 | 0 | 332 | 1.9 |
| w/liquid . . . . . . . . . . . . | 20 | 2.0 | 3.0 | 0 | 0 | 400 | <1.0 |
| **Mushroom, abalone**, canned (*Roland*), ½ cup . . . . . . . . . . . . | 20 | 2.0 | 3.0 | 0 | 0 | 360 | 2.0 |
| **Mushroom, breaded**, frozen, w/roasted garlic (*Alexia* Bites), 2 oz. . . . | 110 | 3.0 | 16.0 | 4.0 | 0 | 280 | 1.0 |
| **Mushroom, cepes**, see "Mushroom, porcini" | | | | | | | |
| **Mushroom, chanterelle**: | | | | | | | |
| canned (*Roland*), ½ cup . | 25 | 1.0 | 4.0 | .0 | 0 | 240 | 2.0 |
| dried: | | | | | | | |
| (*Frieda's*), 2 pcs., .14 oz. . . . . . . . . . . | 15 | 1.0 | 2.0 | 0 | 0 | 0 | 1.0 |
| (*Roland*), ¼ cup . . . . . | 25 | 2.0 | 5.0 | 0 | 0 | 0 | 2.0 |
| **Mushroom, cloud ear**: | | | | | | | |
| dried, .2-oz. pc. . . . . . . . | 13 | .4 | 3.3 | <.1 | 0 | 2 | 3.2 |
| dried, ½ cup . . . . . . . . . | 39 | 1.3 | 10.2 | .1 | 0 | 5 | 9.8 |
| **Mushroom, crimini**, brown, or Italian, raw, .5-oz. pc. . . . . . . . | 3 | .4 | .6 | 0 | 0 | 1 | <.1 |
| **Mushroom, enoki**, fresh: | | | | | | | |
| (*Frieda's*), ¼ pkg., .9 oz. . | 10 | 1.0 | 2.0 | 0 | 0 | 1 | 1.0 |
| trimmed, 1 oz. . . . . . . . . | 10 | .2 | 2.0 | .1 | 0 | 1 | .7 |
| 1 large, 4⅛" long . . . . . . | 2 | .1 | .4 | <.1 | 0 | <1 | <1.0 |
| **Mushroom, golden**, canned (*Roland*), ½ cup . . . . . . . . . . . . | 30 | 2.0 | 6.0 | 0 | 0 | 390 | 2.0 |

| Food and Measure | cal. | prot. (gms) | carbo. (gms) | fat (gms) | chol. (mgs) | sod. (mgs) | fiber (gms) |
|---|---|---|---|---|---|---|---|
| **Mushroom, maitake**, dried (*Eden*), .4 oz., about 10 pcs. . . . . . . . | 35 | 2.0 | 7.0 | 0 | 0 | 0 | 4.0 |
| **Mushroom, marinated**, can/jar: | | | | | | | |
| (*Vigo*), 3 pcs. . . . . . . . . . | 15 | 1.0 | 1.0 | .5 | 0 | 135 | 0 |
| pickled, escababeche: | | | | | | | |
| (*Herdez*), 2 tbsp. . . . . . | 10 | 0 | 1.0 | 0 | 0 | 310 | 0 |
| (*Sabores Aztecas*), 2.1 oz. . . . . . . . . . . | 45 | 0 | 1.0 | 5.0 | 0 | 312 | 1.0 |
| **Mushroom, morel**, dried: | | | | | | | |
| (*Frieda's*), 3 pcs. .14 oz. . | 15 | 1.0 | 2.0 | 0 | 0 | 0 | 0 |
| (*Roland*), ½ cup . . . . . . | 25 | 2.0 | 5.0 | 0 | 0 | 0 | 2.0 |
| **Mushroom, oyster**: | | | | | | | |
| fresh: | | | | | | | |
| 1 large, 5.2 oz. . . . . . . | 55 | 6.1 | 9.2 | .8 | 0 | 46 | 3.6 |
| 1 small, .5 oz. . . . . . . . | 6 | .6 | .9 | .1 | 0 | 5 | .4 |
| canned (*Roland*), ½ cup | 20 | 2.0 | 3.0 | 0 | 0 | 360 | 2.0 |
| dried (*Frieda's*), 3 pcs., .14 oz. . . . . . . . . . | 15 | 1.0 | 2.0 | 0 | 0 | 0 | 0 |
| **Mushroom, pickled**, see "Mushroom, marinated" | | | | | | | |
| **Mushroom, porcini**, dried: | | | | | | | |
| (*Frieda's*), 5 pcs., .14 oz. . | 15 | 1.0 | 2.0 | 0 | 0 | 0 | 1.0 |
| (*Roland*), ¼ cup . . . . . . | 30 | 3.0 | 4.0 | 0 | 0 | 0 | 2.0 |
| (*Roland* Cepes), ½ cup . . | 50 | 5.0 | 6.0 | 1.0 | 0 | 70 | 3.0 |
| **Mushroom, portobello**: | | | | | | | |
| fresh, 1 oz. . . . . . . . . . . | 7 | .7 | 1.4 | <.1 | 0 | 2 | .4 |
| dried (*Frieda's*), 7 pcs., .14 oz. . . . . . . . . . . | 0 | 1.0 | 1.0 | 0 | 0 | 0 | 0 |
| grilled, 1 oz. . . . . . . . . . | 10 | 1.1 | 1.4 | .2 | 0 | 3 | .7 |
| **Mushroom, shiitake**, fresh, cooked: | | | | | | | |
| (*Frieda's*), 4 pcs. . . . . . . | 40 | 1.0 | 10.0 | 0 | 0 | 3 | 2.0 |
| 4 medium, ½ cup pcs. . . | 40 | 1.1 | 10.4 | .2 | 0 | 3 | 1.5 |
| **Mushroom, shiitake, dried**: | | | | | | | |
| (*Frieda's*), ¼ cup, .14 oz. . . . . . . . . . . | 10 | 0 | 3.0 | 0 | 0 | 0 | 0 |
| 4 medium, .5 oz. . . . . . . | 44 | 1.4 | 11.3 | .2 | 0 | 2 | 1.7 |
| whole: | | | | | | | |
| (*Roland*), ½ cup . . . . . | 50 | 3.0 | 10.0 | 0 | 0 | 0 | 6.0 |
| (*Eden*), 3 pcs., .4 oz. . . | 35 | 2,0 | 7.0 | 0 | 0 | 0 | 5.0 |

| Food and Measure | cal. | prot. (gms) | carbo. (gms) | fat (gms) | chol. (mgs) | sod. (mgs) | fiber (gms) |
|---|---|---|---|---|---|---|---|
| **Mushroom, shiitake, dried** *(cont.)* | | | | | | | |
| sliced: | | | | | | | |
| (*Eden*), 6 pcs., .4 oz. .. | 35 | 2.0 | 7.0 | 0 | 0 | 0 | 5.0 |
| (*Roland*), ¼ cup ..... | 30 | 2.0 | 5.0 | 0 | 0 | 0 | 2.0 |
| **Mushroom, straw:** | | | | | | | |
| canned, ½ cup: | | | | | | | |
| whole (*Ka•Me*) ...... | 20 | 2.0 | 3.0 | 0 | 0 | 380 | 2.0 |
| whole/pieces (*Roland*) | 20 | 2.0 | 3.0 | 0 | 0 | 380 | 2.0 |
| drained ............ | 29 | 3.5 | 4.2 | .6 | 0 | 350 | 2.3 |
| dried (*Frieda's* Padi | | | | | | | |
| Straw), 6 pcs., .14 oz. | 15 | 1.0 | 2.0 | 0 | 0 | 0 | 0 |
| **Mushroom, wild mix:** | | | | | | | |
| canned (*Roland* Wild | | | | | | | |
| Forest), ½ cup ...... | 25 | 1.0 | 3.0 | 0 | 0 | 240 | 1.0 |
| dried (*Roland*), ¼ cup ... | 25 | 2.0 | 5.0 | 0 | 0 | 0 | 2.0 |
| **Mushroom, wood ear,** | | | | | | | |
| dried (*Frieda's*), | | | | | | | |
| 3 pcs., .14 oz. ....... | 15 | 0 | 2.0 | 0 | 0 | 0 | 0 |
| **Mushroom batter mix** | | | | | | | |
| (*Don's Chuck Wagon*), | | | | | | | |
| ¼ cup .............. | 95 | 3.0 | 21.0 | 0 | 0 | 706 | 1.0 |
| **Mushroom bites,** | | | | | | | |
| frozen, Portobello, | | | | | | | |
| w/mozzarella (*Veggie* | | | | | | | |
| *Patch*), 3 pcs., 2.6 oz. . | 160 | 7.0 | 17.0 | 8.0 | 10.0 | 330 | 4.0 |
| **Mushroom burger,** see | | | | | | | |
| "Burger patty, | | | | | | | |
| vegetarian" | | | | | | | |
| **Mushroom dish,** | | | | | | | |
| microwave, w/potatoes | | | | | | | |
| (*Tasty Bite Takatak*), | | | | | | | |
| ½ of 10-oz. pkg. ..... | 120 | 3.0 | 17.0 | 3.0 | 0 | 420 | 3.0 |
| **Mushroom gravy,** ¼ cup: | | | | | | | |
| (*Campbell's*) .......... | 20 | 0 | 3.0 | 1.0 | <5 | 280 | 0 |
| (*Heinz* Home Style | | | | | | | |
| Rich) .............. | 20 | <1.0 | 3.0 | .5 | 0 | 320 | 0 |
| **Mushroom gravy mix:** | | | | | | | |
| (*McCormick*), 1 tbsp. ... | 20 | 0 | 2.0 | 1.0 | 0 | 280 | 0 |
| herb, for steak | | | | | | | |
| (*McCormick*), 1⅓ tbsp. | 40 | 1.0 | 5.0 | 1.0 | <5 | 220 | 0 |
| **Mushroom-leek pocket,** | | | | | | | |
| frozen (*Aunt Trudy's* | | | | | | | |
| Organic), 5-oz. pc. ... | 190 | 5.0 | 32.0 | 6.0 | 0 | 380 | 3.0 |

| Food and Measure | cal. | prot. (gms) | carbo. (gms) | fat (gms) | chol. (mgs) | sod. (mgs) | fiber (gms) |
|---|---|---|---|---|---|---|---|
| **Muskrat**, meat only, roasted, 4 oz. . . . . . . | 265 | 34.1 | 0 | 13.3 | 88 | 78 | 0 |
| **Mussels**, blue, meat only: | | | | | | | |
| raw, 4 oz. . . . . . . . . . . . | 98 | 13.5 | 4.2 | 2.5 | 32 | 324 | 0 |
| raw, 1 cup . . . . . . . . . . . | 129 | 17.9 | 3.4 | 5.5 | 42 | 429 | 0 |
| boiled or steamed, 4 oz. . | 195 | 27.0 | 8.4 | 5.1 | 64 | 418 | 0 |
| **Mussels**, can/jar: | | | | | | | |
| à la nicoise (*Roland*), ⅓ cup . . . . . . . . | 60 | 9.0 | 4.0 | 0 | 45 | 295 | 0 |
| marinated (*Roland* Jar), ⅓ cup . . . . . . . . | 50 | 11.0 | 4.0 | 0 | 70 | 520 | 0 |
| marinated, in oil: | | | | | | | |
| (*Roland*), ½ cup . . . . . | 75 | 11.0 | 0 | 4.0 | 25 | 290 | 0 |
| (*Vigo* Escabeche), 2 oz. | 75 | 11.0 | 0 | 4.0 | 25 | 250 | 0 |
| smoked, in oil (*Roland*), 2 oz. . . . . . . | 90 | 9.0 | 3.0 | 5.0 | 50 | 250 | 0 |
| tomato sauce, spices (*Roland*), ¼ cup . . . . . | 50 | 6.0 | 4.0 | 1.0 | 30 | 535 | 0 |
| in water (*Roland*), ¼ cup . . . . . . . . . . . | 50 | 10.0 | 1.0 | 2.0 | 60 | 220 | 0 |
| **Mussels, frozen**, Greenshell (*Seamazz*), 3 oz. . | 100 | 14.0 | 5.0 | 2.5 | 50 | 230 | 0 |
| **Mustard**, 1 tsp.: | | | | | | | |
| (*Jack Daniel's* Old No. 7) . . . . . . . . . . . | 5 | 0 | 0 | 0 | 0 | 70 | 0 |
| brown: | | | | | | | |
| (*Eden* Organic) . . . . . . | 0 | 0 | <1.0 | 0 | 0 | 80 | 0 |
| spicy (*French's*) . . . . . | 5 | 0 | 1.0 | 0 | 0 | 80 | 0 |
| spicy (*Grey Poupon*) . . | 5 | 0 | 0 | 0 | 0 | 50 | 0 |
| spicy (*Grey Poupon* Hearty) . . . . . . . . . | 5 | 0 | 0 | 0 | 0 | 65 | 0 |
| spicy (*Gulden's*) . . . . . | 5 | 0 | 0 | 0 | 0 | 50 | 0 |
| Chinese, hot: | | | | | | | |
| hot (*Mee Tu*) . . . . . . . | 2 | 0 | 1.0 | 0 | 0 | 40 | 0 |
| hot (*Roland*) . . . . . . . | 2 | 0 | 1.0 | 0 | 0 | 40 | 0 |
| Kobe (*Roland*) . . . . . . | 10 | 0 | 1.0 | 0 | 0 | 75 | 0 |
| chipotle (*Di Lusso*) . . . . | 5 | 0 | 0 | 0 | 0 | 60 | 0 |
| coarse ground (*Grey Poupon* Harvest) . . . . | 10 | 0 | 0 | 0 | 0 | 120 | 0 |
| Creole (*Zatarain's*) . . . . . | 10 | 0 | <1.0 | .5 | 0 | 150 | 0 |
| deli style: | | | | | | | |
| (*Boar's Head*) . . . . . . . | 0 | 0 | 0 | 0 | 0 | 40 | 0 |

| Food and Measure | cal. | prot. (gms) | carbo. (gms) | fat (gms) | chol. (mgs) | sod. (mgs) | fiber (gms) |
|---|---|---|---|---|---|---|---|
| **Mustard, deli style** *(cont.)* | | | | | | | |
| (*Di Lusso*) . . . . . . . . . | 5 | 0 | 0 | 0 | 0 | 70 | 0 |
| (*Emeril's* New York) . . | 5 | 0 | 1.0 | 0 | 0 | 50 | 0 |
| (*Grey Poupon*) . . . . . . | 5 | 0 | 0 | 0 | 0 | 50 | 0 |
| Dijon: | | | | | | | |
| (*Annie's Naturals* | | | | | | | |
| Organic) . . . . . . . . | 0 | 0 | 0 | 0 | 0 | 120 | 0 |
| (*Di Lusso*) . . . . . . . . . | 5 | 0 | 0 | 0 | 0 | 100 | 0 |
| (*Emeril's*) . . . . . . . . . | 5 | 0 | 1.0 | 0 | 0 | 120 | 0 |
| (*Grey Poupon/Grey* | | | | | | | |
| *Poupon* Country) . . | 5 | 0 | 0 | 0 | 0 | 120 | 0 |
| (*Jack Daniel's* Stone | | | | | | | |
| Ground) . . . . . . . . | 5 | 0 | 0 | 0 | 0 | 150 | 0 |
| (*Maille* Original) . . . . . | 5 | 0 | 0 | .5 | 0 | 105 | 0 |
| (*Roland* European) . . . | 5 | 0 | 0 | .5 | 0 | 100 | 0 |
| extra hot (*Maille*) . . . . | 10 | 0 | 1.0 | .5 | 0 | 115 | 0 |
| extra strong, green | | | | | | | |
| peppercorn or w/ | | | | | | | |
| herbs (*Roland*) . . . . | 10 | 0 | 0 | .5 | 0 | 130 | 0 |
| grained, w/wine | | | | | | | |
| (*Roland*) . . . . . . . . . | 10 | 0 | 0 | .5 | 0 | 105 | 0 |
| Dusseldorf (*Thumann's*) . | 4 | 0 | 0 | 0 | 0 | 63 | 0 |
| hickory (*Jack Daniel's*) . . | 5 | 0 | 0 | 0 | 0 | 125 | 0 |
| spicy (*Jack Daniel's* | | | | | | | |
| Southwest) . . . . . . . . . | 0 | 0 | 0 | 0 | 0 | 80 | 0 |
| yellow: | | | | | | | |
| (*Annie's Naturals* | | | | | | | |
| Organic) . . . . . . . . . | 0 | 0 | 0 | 0 | 0 | 55 | 0 |
| (*Eden* Organic) . . . . . . | 0 | 0 | 0 | 0 | 0 | 80 | 0 |
| (*French's*) . . . . . . . . . | 0 | 0 | 1.0 | 0 | 0 | 55 | 0 |
| (*Gulden's*) . . . . . . . . . | 5 | 0 | 0 | 0 | 0 | 55 | 0 |
| **Mustard blends**, 1 tsp.: | | | | | | | |
| cranberry honey | | | | | | | |
| (*Di Lusso*) . . . . . . . . . | 100 | 0 | 2.0 | 0 | 0 | 50 | 0 |
| honey: | | | | | | | |
| (*Annie's Naturals* | | | | | | | |
| Organic) . . . . . . . . | 10 | 0 | 2.0 | 0 | 0 | 40 | 0 |
| (*Boar's Head*) . . . . . . . | 10 | 0 | 2.0 | 0 | 0 | 25 | 0 |
| (*Di Lusso*) . . . . . . . . . | 10 | 0 | 1.0 | 0 | 0 | 45 | 0 |
| (*Emeril's* Smooth) . . . | 10 | 0 | 1.0 | 0 | 0 | 25 | 0 |
| (*French's*) . . . . . . . . . | 10 | 0 | 1.0 | 0 | 0 | 30 | 0 |
| (*Grey Poupon*) . . . . . . | 10 | 0 | 2.0 | 0 | 0 | 5 | 0 |
| (*Gulden's* Zesty) . . . . . | 10 | 0 | 2.0 | 0 | 0 | 25 | 0 |

| Food and Measure | cal. | prot. (gms) | carbo. (gms) | fat (gms) | chol. (mgs) | sod. (mgs) | fiber (gms) |
|---|---|---|---|---|---|---|---|
| (Hellmann's/Best Foods) ......... | 10 | 0 | 2.0 | 0 | 0 | 25 | 0 |
| (Thumann's) ........ | 20 | 0 | 1.5 | 1.5 | 0 | 330 | 0 |
| Dijon (French's) ..... | 10 | 0 | 1.0 | 0 | 0 | 40 | 0 |
| Dijon (Jack Daniel's) .. | 10 | 0 | 2.0 | 0 | 0 | 70 | 0 |
| Dijon (Roland) ...... | 10 | 0 | 1.0 | 0 | 0 | 65 | 0 |
| savory (Grey Poupon) | 10 | 0 | 1.0 | 0 | 0 | 5 | 0 |
| horseradish: | | | | | | | |
| (Annie's Naturals Organic) ......... | 5 | 0 | 1.0 | 0 | 0 | 90 | 0 |
| (Emeril's Kicked Up) .. | 5 | 0 | 0 | 0 | 0 | 60 | 0 |
| (French's) .......... | 5 | 0 | 0 | 0 | 0 | 80 | 0 |
| (Hellmann's Deli) .... | 5 | 0 | <1.0 | 0 | 0 | 55 | 0 |
| (Jack Daniel's) ...... | 5 | 0 | 0 | 0 | 0 | 75 | 0 |
| (Thumann's) ........ | 4 | 0 | 0 | 0 | 0 | 63 | 0 |
| jalapeño (Di Lusso) ..... | 5 | 0 | 0 | 0 | 0 | 85 | 0 |
| mayonnaise (Dijonnaise) ........ | 5 | 0 | <1.0 | 0 | 0 | 70 | 0 |
| wasabi, Dijon (Thumann's) ........ | 18 | 0 | 2.0 | 1.0 | 25 | 55 | 0 |
| **Mustard cabbage**, see "Cabbage, mustard" | | | | | | | |
| **Mustard greens**, fresh: | | | | | | | |
| raw (Glory), 2 cups ..... | 20 | 2.0 | 4.0 | 0 | 0 | 20 | 3.0 |
| raw, chopped, 1 oz. or ½ cup ....... | 7 | .8 | 1.4 | .1 | 0 | 7 | .6 |
| boiled, drained, ½ cup .. | 11 | 1.6 | 1.5 | .2 | 0 | 11 | 1.4 |
| **Mustard greens, canned**, ½ cup: | | | | | | | |
| chopped: | | | | | | | |
| (Allens No Salt) ..... | 30 | 1.0 | 5.0 | .5 | 0 | 10 | 3.0 |
| (Bush's) ........... | 25 | 2.0 | 3.0 | 0 | 0 | 400 | 2.0 |
| seasoned: | | | | | | | |
| (Allens) ........... | 30 | 2.0 | 5.0 | 0 | 0 | 390 | 2.0 |
| (Allens/Sunshine Southern Style) ... | 45 | 4.0 | 6.0 | .5 | 0 | 830 | 1.0 |
| (Glory) ............ | 35 | 2.0 | 3.0 | 0 | 0 | 490 | 1.0 |
| **Mustard greens, frozen**, chopped: | | | | | | | |
| (Allens), 1 cup ........ | 25 | 2.0 | 3.0 | 0 | 0 | 10 | 2.0 |
| boiled, drained, 1 cup ... | 30 | 3.4 | 4.7 | .4 | 0 | 38 | 4.2 |
| **Mustard powder**, 1 tsp. . | 9 | .5 | .3 | .6 | 0 | <1 | <1.0 |
| **Mustard seeds**, 1 tsp. .... | 15 | .8 | 1.2 | 1.0 | 0 | <1 | <1.0 |

| Food and Measure | cal. | prot. (gms) | carbo. (gms) | fat (gms) | chol. (mgs) | sod. (mgs) | fiber (gms) |
|---|---|---|---|---|---|---|---|
| **Mustard spinach:** | | | | | | | |
| raw, chopped, 1 cup .... | 33 | 3.3 | 5.9 | .5 | 0 | 32 | 4.2 |
| boiled, drained, | | | | | | | |
| chopped, 1 cup ...... | 29 | 3.1 | 5.0 | .4 | 0 | 25 | 3.6 |
| **Mustard tallow**, 1 tbsp. . | 115 | 0 | 0 | 12.8 | 13 | 0 | 0 |

# N

| Food and Measure | cal. | prot. (gms) | carbo. (gms) | fat (gms) | chol. (mgs) | sod. (mgs) | fiber (gms) |
|---|---|---|---|---|---|---|---|
| **Nacho snack**, frozen (*Amy's*), ½ of 6-oz. pkg., 5–6 pcs. . . . . . . . | 220 | 9.0 | 25.0 | 9.0 | 25 | 420 | 2.0 |
| **Name yam** (*Frieda's*), ¾ cup, 3 oz. . . . . . . . . | 100 | 1.0 | 24.0 | 0 | 0 | 10 | 3.0 |
| **Nan**, see "Bread" | | | | | | | |
| **Natto**, ½ cup . . . . . . . . . . | 187 | 15.6 | 12.6 | 9.7 | 0 | 6 | 4.8 |
| **Navy beans**, dry: | | | | | | | |
| (*Eden* Organic), ¼ cup . . | 160 | 9.0 | 28.0 | .5 | 0 | 10 | 12.0 |
| boiled, ½ cup . . . . . . . . | 129 | 7.9 | 24.0 | .5 | 0 | 1 | 3.3 |
| **Navy beans, canned**: | | | | | | | |
| (*Allens*), ½ cup . . . . . . . . | 110 | 6.0 | 19.0 | 1.0 | 0 | 380 | 6.0 |
| (*Bush's*), ½ cup . . . . . . . | 80 | 6.0 | 17.0 | 0 | 0 | 470 | 7.0 |
| (*Eden* Organic), ½ cup . . | 110 | 7.0 | 20.0 | 0 | 0 | 15 | 7.0 |
| w/bacon, ½ cup: | | | | | | | |
| (*Trappey's*) . . . . . . . . . | 110 | 5.0 | 18.0 | 1.5 | 0 | 420 | 6.0 |
| jalapeño (*Trappey's*) . . | 110 | 5.0 | 17.0 | 1.5 | 0 | 420 | 7.0 |
| **Navy beans, sprouted**, ½ cup . . . . . . . . . . . . . | 35 | 3.2 | 6.8 | .4 | 0 | 14 | n.a. |
| **Nectarine**: | | | | | | | |
| (*Chiquita*), 1 cup, 5 oz. . . | 63 | 2.0 | 15.0 | 0 | 0 | 0 | 2.0 |
| (*Dole*), 4.9-oz. pc. . . . . . . | 60 | 1.0 | 15.0 | 0 | 0 | 0 | 2.0 |
| 1 medium, 2½" diam. . . . | 67 | 1.3 | 16.0 | .6 | 0 | <1 | 2.2 |
| sliced, ½ cup . . . . . . . . . | 34 | .7 | 8.1 | .3 | 0 | <1 | 1.1 |
| **Noni berry drink** (*Snapple*), 8 fl. oz. . . . | 15 | 0 | 2.0 | 0 | 0 | 5 | 0 |
| **Noodle, Asian**, 2 oz. dry, except as noted: | | | | | | | |
| cellophane: | | | | | | | |
| (*Roland* Bean Thread), 1.75-oz. nest . . . . . | 180 | 0 | 43.0 | 0 | 0 | 0 | 0 |
| or long rice . . . . . . . . | 200 | .1 | 48.8 | <.1 | 0 | 6 | <1.0 |
| Chinese (*Nasoya*), 1 cup . | 210 | 8.0 | 43.0 | .5 | 10 | 400 | 2.0 |

| Food and Measure | cal. | prot. (gms) | carbo. (gms) | fat (gms) | chol. (mgs) | sod. (mgs) | fiber (gms) |
|---|---|---|---|---|---|---|---|
| **Noodle, Asian** *(cont.)* | | | | | | | |
| chow mein: | | | | | | | |
|   (*Annie Chun's*) . . . . . . | 200 | 8.0 | 39.0 | 1.0 | 0 | 350 | 3.0 |
|   (*La Choy*), ½ cup . . . . | 130 | 3.0 | 19.0 | 5.0 | 0 | 230 | <1.0 |
|   dried, ½ cup . . . . . . . . | 119 | 1.9 | 13.0 | 6.9 | 0 | 99 | .9 |
| hokkien, stir-fry | | | | | | | |
|   (*Ka•Me*), 3.5 oz. . . . . . | 170 | 5.0 | 32.0 | 2.0 | 0 | 170 | 2.0 |
| Japanese (*Nasoya*), | | | | | | | |
|   1 cup . . . . . . . . . . . . | 210 | 8.0 | 43.0 | .5 | 0 | 410 | 2.0 |
| lo mein: | | | | | | | |
|   (*Roland* Organic) . . . . | 190 | 5.0 | 40.0 | 1.0 | 0 | 170 | 1.0 |
|   wide (*Ka•Me*) . . . . . . . | 190 | 7.0 | 41.0 | 0 | 0 | 210 | 1.0 |
| rice: | | | | | | | |
|   all styles (*A Taste of* | | | | | | | |
|    *Thai*) . . . . . . . . . . . . | 200 | 3.0 | 46.0 | 0 | 0 | 0 | 2.0 |
|   (*Annie Chun's* Maifun) | 210 | 2.0 | 50.0 | 0 | 0 | 75 | 0 |
|   (*Annie Chun's* Pad Thai) | 200 | 3.0 | 45.0 | 0 | 0 | 20 | 0 |
|   (*Roland* Hsinchu), 1 cup | 230 | 0 | 57.0 | 0 | 0 | 120 | 0 |
|   (*Roland* Pad Thai) . . . . | 200 | 3.0 | 46.0 | 0 | 0 | 200 | 2.0 |
|   brown (*Annie Chun's* | | | | | | | |
|    Maifun) . . . . . . . . . | 200 | 4.0 | 44.0 | 1.0 | 0 | 10 | 4.0 |
|   canned (*La Choy*), | | | | | | | |
|    ½ cup . . . . . . . . . . . | 130 | 2.0 | 21.0 | 4.0 | 0 | 350 | <1.0 |
|   Thai, stir-fry (*Ka•* | | | | | | | |
|    *Me*), 3.5 oz. . . . . . . | 160 | 6.0 | 30.0 | 2.0 | 0 | 160 | 2.0 |
| soba: | | | | | | | |
|   (*Annie Chun's*) . . . . . . | 200 | 8.0 | 39.0 | 1.0 | 0 | 390 | 3.0 |
|   (*Eden* Organic) . . . . . . | 200 | 8.0 | 38.0 | 1.5 | 0 | 120 | 2.0 |
|   buckwheat (*Eden* | | | | | | | |
|    100%) . . . . . . . . . . . | 200 | 6.0 | 43.0 | 0 | 0 | 5 | 3.0 |
|   buckwheat (*Eden* | | | | | | | |
|    40%) . . . . . . . . . . . | 190 | 8.0 | 37.0 | 1.0 | 0 | 490 | 3.0 |
|   buckwheat (*Roland* | | | | | | | |
|    Organic) . . . . . . . . . | 200 | 7.0 | 40.0 | 1.0 | 0 | 170 | 1.0 |
|   kamut (*Eden* Organic) . | 200 | 7.0 | 38.0 | 1.0 | 0 | 120 | 3.0 |
|   lotus root (*Eden*) . . . . | 190 | 9.0 | 37.0 | 1.0 | 0 | 470 | 4.0 |
|   mugwort (*Eden* . . . . . . | 190 | 8.0 | 37.0 | .5 | 0 | 550 | 2.0 |
|    Organic) . . . . . . . . . | 200 | 9.0 | 37.0 | 1.5 | 0 | 120 | 2.0 |
|   wild yam (*Eden* | | | | | | | |
|    Jinenjo) . . . . . . . . . | 190 | 9.0 | 37.0 | .5 | 0 | 510 | 2.0 |
| soba, cooked, 1 cup . . . . | 113 | 5.8 | 24.4 | .1 | 0 | 40 | n.a. |
| somen: | | | | | | | |
|   uncooked . . . . . . . . . . | 203 | 6.5 | 42.2 | .5 | 0 | 1049 | 2.4 |
|   cooked, 1 cup . . . . . . . | 230 | 7.0 | 48.5 | .3 | 0 | 284 | n.a. |

| Food and Measure | cal. | prot. (gms) | carbo. (gms) | fat (gms) | chol. (mgs) | sod. (mgs) | fiber (gms) |
|---|---|---|---|---|---|---|---|
| sweet and sour, canned | | | | | | | |
|   (*La Choy*), 1 cup ...... | 180 | 5.0 | 35.0 | 1.5 | 15 | 910 | 4.0 |
| udon: | | | | | | | |
|   (*Eden* Japanese) ..... | 190 | 8.0 | 37.0 | 1.5 | 0 | 660 | 3.0 |
|   (*Eden* Organic 100% | | | | | | | |
|     Whole Grain) ..... | 200 | 8.0 | 38.0 | 1.5 | 0 | 120 | 3.0 |
|   (*Roland* Organic) .... | 190 | 5.0 | 40.0 | 1.0 | 0 | 170 | 1.0 |
|   brown rice (*Eden*) .... | 190 | 8.0 | 38.0 | 1.0 | 0 | 510 | 2.0 |
|   kamut (*Eden* Organic) . | 200 | 10.0 | 37.0 | 1.5 | 0 | 120 | 3.0 |
|   wheat and rice (*Eden* | | | | | | | |
|     Organic) .......... | 200 | 8.0 | 38.0 | 2.0 | 0 | 120 | 3.0 |
| udon, cooked, 4 oz. ..... | 115 | 2.8 | 23.0 | .6 | 0 | 51 | n.a. |
| **Noodle, Chinese,** | | | | | | | |
| **Japanese, or Thai**, | | | | | | | |
| see "Noodle, Asian" | | | | | | | |
| **Noodle, egg:** | | | | | | | |
| dry, 2 oz.: | | | | | | | |
|   all varieties (*Amish* | | | | | | | |
|     *Kitchen*) ......... | 220 | 8.0 | 38.0 | 4.0 | 115 | 10 | 1.0 |
|   enriched .......... | 216 | 7.9 | 40.3 | 2.4 | 54 | 12 | 1.5 |
|   spelt, whole grain | | | | | | | |
|     (*VitaSpelt* Organic) . | 200 | 9.0 | 38.0 | 3.0 | 45 | 15 | 5.0 |
| cooked: | | | | | | | |
|   1 cup ............. | 212 | 7.6 | 39.7 | 2.4 | 53 | 11 | 1.8 |
|   spinach, 1 cup ...... | 211 | 8.1 | 38.8 | 2.5 | 52 | 20 | 3.7 |
| **Noodle, egg, frozen** | | | | | | | |
|   (*Reames*), ½ cup, | | | | | | | |
|   except as noted: | | | | | | | |
| plain ................ | 170 | 5.0 | 32.0 | 2.0 | 70 | 10 | 1.0 |
| plain, 12-oz. pkg. ...... | 170 | 5.0 | 32.0 | 2.0 | 65 | 10 | 1.0 |
| yolk free ............ | 180 | 5.0 | 31.0 | .5 | 0 | 10 | 1.0 |
| golden ribbon, 1⅓ cups . | 210 | 8.0 | 39.0 | 2.5 | 90 | 15 | 1.0 |
| dumplings ............ | 180 | 6.0 | 34.0 | 2.5 | 75 | 10 | 1.0 |
| precooked, 1 cup ...... | 240 | 10.0 | 45.0 | 2.5 | 75 | 25 | 2.0 |
| **Noodle, spelt** | | | | | | | |
|   (*VitaSpelt* Organic): | | | | | | | |
| whole grain, 2 oz. ...... | 190 | 9.0 | 39.0 | 1.0 | 0 | 15 | 4.0 |
| white, 2 oz. .......... | 190 | 9.0 | 39.0 | 1.0 | 0 | 15 | 2.0 |
| **Noodle entree, canned** | | | | | | | |
|   (*Dinty Moore American* | | | | | | | |
|   *Classics*), 1 cup: | | | | | | | |
| and beef ............ | 230 | 9.0 | 23.0 | 11.0 | 35 | 890 | 2.0 |
| and chicken .......... | 220 | 8.0 | 25.0 | 10.0 | 35 | 1020 | 1.0 |

| Food and Measure | cal. | prot. (gms) | carbo. (gms) | fat (gms) | chol. (mgs) | sod. (mgs) | fiber (gms) |
|---|---|---|---|---|---|---|---|
| **Noodle entree, frozen**, 1 pkg., except as noted: | | | | | | | |
| Asian, stir-fry (*Amy's*), 10 oz. . . . . . . . . . . . . | 300 | 9.0 | 50.0 | 7.0 | 0 | 630 | 5.0 |
| and beef (*Banquet*), 1 cup . . . . . . . . . . . . | 170 | 10.0 | 22.0 | 4.5 | 15 | 970 | 2.0 |
| w/chicken, Thai style (*Lean Cuisine Spa Cuisine*), 1 pkg. . . . . . | 310 | 20.0 | 41.0 | 7.0 | 30 | 590 | 5.0 |
| pad Thai, 10 oz.: | | | | | | | |
| w/chicken (*Ethnic Gourmet*) . . . . . . . . | 410 | 20.0 | 66.0 | 7.0 | 25 | 830 | 3.0 |
| w/chicken (*Healthy Choice Café Steamers*) . . . . . . . | 270 | 19.0 | 40.0 | 3.5 | 25 | 540 | 5.0 |
| w/shrimp (*Ethnic Gourmet*) . . . . . . . . | 410 | 17.0 | 70.0 | 7.0 | 55 | 850 | 3.0 |
| w/tofu (*Ethnic Gourmet*) | 420 | 13.0 | 73.0 | 8.0 | 0 | 720 | 3.0 |
| **Noodle entree, microwave**: | | | | | | | |
| and chicken (*Dinty Moore* Cup), 7.5 oz. . . | 190 | 8.0 | 20.0 | 9.0 | 35 | 1100 | 1.0 |
| chili, sweet Korean (*Annie Chun's* Bowl), ½ of 8.4-oz. cont. . . . . | 320 | 7.0 | 60.0 | 4.5 | 0 | 830 | 2.0 |
| coconut ginger (*A Taste of Thai*), ½ of 4-oz. pkg. . . . . . . | 226 | 2.0 | 38.0 | 5.0 | 0 | 271 | 1.0 |
| curry: | | | | | | | |
| red (*A Taste of Thai*), ½ of 5¾-oz. pkg. . . | 290 | 2.0 | 52.0 | 8.0 | 0 | 360 | 1.0 |
| yellow (*A Taste of Thai*), 1 cup* . . . . . | 250 | 0 | 48.0 | 6.0 | 0 | 350 | 1.0 |
| garlic scallion (*Annie Chun's* Bowl), ½ of 8.25-oz. cont. . . . . . . | 310 | 8.0 | 57.0 | 5.0 | 0 | 980 | 2.0 |
| honey soy ginger (*Ka•Me*), ½ of 11.6-oz. pkg. . . . . . . | 320 | 6.0 | 57.0 | 8.0 | 0 | 670 | 2.0 |
| kung pao (*Annie Chun's* Bowl), ½ of 9-oz. cont. . . . . . . . . | 240 | 7.0 | 40.0 | 5.0 | 0 | 630 | 1.0 |
| lo mein (*Ka•Me*), ½ of 11.6-oz. pkg. . . . . . . | 230 | 7.0 | 39.0 | 6.0 | 0 | 620 | 2.0 |

| Food and Measure | cal. | prot. (gms) | carbo. (gms) | fat (gms) | chol. (mgs) | sod. (mgs) | fiber (gms) |
|---|---|---|---|---|---|---|---|
| **pad Thai:** | | | | | | | |
| (*Annie Chun's* Bowl), ½ of 9-oz. cont. .... | 230 | 7.0 | 45.0 | 4.5 | 0 | 710 | 1.0 |
| (*Ka•Me*), ½ of 11.6-oz. pkg. ..... | 310 | 9.0 | 45.0 | 11.0 | 0 | 790 | 2.0 |
| (*A Taste of Thai*), ½ of 5¾-oz. pkg. .. | 260 | 4.0 | 52.0 | 4.0 | 0 | 290 | 1.0 |
| **peanut, Thai:** | | | | | | | |
| (*A Taste of Thai*), ½ of 5.25-oz. pkg. ..... | 340 | 5.0 | 53.0 | 10.0 | 0 | 320 | 2.0 |
| satay (*Ka•Me*), ½ of 11.6-oz. pkg. ..... | 320 | 8.0 | 41.0 | 14.0 | 0 | 670 | 2.0 |
| sesame (*Annie Chun's* Bowl), ½ of 9-oz. cont. ....... | 280 | 8.0 | 40.0 | 11.0 | 0 | 340 | 1.0 |
| **ramen noodles** (*Annie Chun's* Noodle Express), ½ of 7-oz. tray: | | | | | | | |
| chow mein ········ | 160 | 5.0 | 27.0 | 4.0 | 0 | 510 | 1.0 |
| curry, Thai ......... | 180 | 4.0 | 29.0 | 7.0 | 0 | 500 | 2.0 |
| peanut, Thai ........ | 200 | 6.0 | 29.0 | 7.0 | 0 | 300 | 1.0 |
| spicy Szechuan ...... | 170 | 4.0 | 29.0 | 3.0 | 0 | 470 | 1.0 |
| teriyaki ............. | 160 | 5.0 | 31.0 | 2.0 | 0 | 510 | 1.0 |
| **Szechuan:** | | | | | | | |
| (*Ka•Me*), ½ of 11.6-oz. pkg. ..... | 230 | 7.0 | 39.0 | 6.0 | 0 | 620 | 2.0 |
| (*A Taste of China*), ½ of 6-oz. pkg. .... | 216 | 2.0 | 40.0 | 6.0 | 0 | 338 | 1.0 |
| **teriyaki:** | | | | | | | |
| (*Annie Chun's* Bowl), ½ of 8.2-oz. cont. .. | 200 | 6.0 | 38.0 | 2.5 | 0 | 440 | 1.0 |
| (*Ka•Me*), ½ of 11.6-oz. pkg. ..... | 320 | 8.0 | 41.0 | 14.0 | 0 | 670 | 2.0 |
| **Noodle entree mix**: | | | | | | | |
| chicken, savory (*Kraft Noodle Classics*), ⅓ pkg. .... | 270 | 10.0 | 46.0 | 5.0 | 55 | 1270 | 2.0 |
| chow mein (*Annie Chun's* Organic Meal Starter), ⅓ pkg. ..... | 220 | 8.0 | 42.0 | 1.5 | 0 | 570 | 1.0 |
| **pad Thai:** | | | | | | | |
| (*Annie Chun's* Meal Starter), ⅓ pkg. ... | 230 | 3.0 | 53.0 | 1.0 | 0 | 780 | 0 |

| Food and Measure | cal. | prot. (gms) | carbo. (gms) | fat (gms) | chol. (mgs) | sod. (mgs) | fiber (gms) |
|---|---|---|---|---|---|---|---|
| **Noodle entree mix, pad Thai** (cont.) | | | | | | | |
| (A Taste of Thai for Two), ½ pkg. ..... | 380 | 4.0 | 85.0 | 1.5 | 0 | 340 | 3.0 |
| peanut, sesame (Annie Chun's Organic Meal Starter), ⅓ pkg. ..... | 250 | 9.0 | 41.0 | 5.0 | 0 | 360 | 2.0 |
| soy ginger (Annie Chun's Organic Meal Starter), ⅓ pkg. ..... | 220 | 8.0 | 41.0 | 1.5 | 0 | 600 | 1.0 |
| teriyaki (Annie Chun's Organic Meal Starter), ⅓ pkg. ........... | 220 | 8.0 | 43.0 | 1.5 | 0 | 590 | 1.0 |
| **Nopales/Nopalitos**, see "Cactus pads" | | | | | | | |
| **Nori**, see "Seaweed" | | | | | | | |
| **Nut butter**, see specific nut listings | | | | | | | |
| **Nutmeg**, ground, 1 tsp. ... | 12 | .1 | 1.1 | .8 | 0 | tr. | .1 |
| **Nuts, mixed**, 1 oz., except as noted: | | | | | | | |
| (Frito Lay Deluxe) ...... | 170 | 4.0 | 6.0 | 16.0 | 0 | 115 | 2.0 |
| (Planters) ............ | 170 | 6.0 | 5.0 | 15.0 | 0 | 110 | 2.0 |
| (Planters Deluxe Lightly Salted) ...... | 170 | 5.0 | 6.0 | 15.0 | 0 | 50 | 2.0 |
| (Planters Deluxe w/Sea Salt) ......... | 170 | 5.0 | 6.0 | 15.0 | 0 | 100 | 2.0 |
| (Planters Lightly Salted) ............ | 170 | 6.0 | 5.0 | 15.0 | 0 | 55 | 2.0 |
| (Planters NUT-rition): | | | | | | | |
| antioxidant ......... | 160 | 4.0 | 15.0 | 11.0 | 0 | 0 | 2.0 |
| digestive ........... | 140 | 3.0 | 15.0 | 8.0 | 0 | 60 | 5.0 |
| energy ............. | 190 | 5.0 | 12.0 | 15.0 | 0 | 120 | 3.0 |
| heart healthy ........ | 170 | 6.0 | 5.0 | 16.0 | 0 | 45 | 3.0 |
| lightly salted ........ | 170 | 6.0 | 5.0 | 15.0 | 0 | 50 | 3.0 |
| omega-3............ | 160 | 3.0 | 16.0 | 10.0 | 0 | 0 | 2.0 |
| (Planters Sea Salt) ..... | 170 | 6.0 | 5.0 | 15.0 | 0 | 110 | 2.0 |
| cashew mix: | | | | | | | |
| almonds, macadamias (Planters NUT-rition) ....... | 170 | 5.0 | 7.0 | 15.0 | 0 | 50 | 2.0 |
| almonds, pecans (Planters Select) .. | 170 | 5.0 | 7.0 | 15.0 | 0 | 95 | 2.0 |
| sesame (Planters Salt & Pepper Mix) .... | 160 | 6.0 | 6.0 | 14.0 | 0 | 135 | 2.0 |

| Food and Measure | cal. | prot. (gms) | carbo. (gms) | fat (gms) | chol. (mgs) | sod. (mgs) | fiber (gms) |
|---|---|---|---|---|---|---|---|
| sesame (*Planters* Sea Salt) .......... | 170 | 6.0 | 5.0 | 15.0 | 0 | 110 | 2.0 |
| glazed (*Beer Nuts*) ..... | 180 | 7.0 | 4.0 | 15.0 | 0 | 60 | 2.0 |
| honey mustard mix (*Planters*) ......... | 160 | 6.0 | 6.0 | 14.0 | 0 | 135 | 2.0 |
| honey-roasted (*Planters*) | 160 | 5.0 | 9.0 | 12.0 | 0 | 120 | 2.0 |
| macadamia mix, cashew, almonds (*Planters* Select) ..... | 180 | 4.0 | 6.0 | 16.0 | 0 | 95 | 2.0 |
| peanuts/cashews, honey roasted (*Planters*) .... | 150 | 6.0 | 9.0 | 12.0 | 0 | 115 | 2.0 |
| pecan mix (*Planters* Pecan Lovers) ....... | 180 | 4.0 | 6.0 | 17.0 | 0 | 70 | 2.0 |
| pistachio mix: (*Planters*) .......... | 160 | 5.0 | 9.0 | 13.0 | 0 | 150 | 1.0 |
| (*Planters* Pistachio Lovers) .......... | 160 | 6.0 | 7.0 | 13.0 | 0 | 80 | 3.0 |

# O

| Food and Measure | cal. | prot. (gms) | carbo. (gms) | fat (gms) | chol. (mgs) | sod. (mgs) | fiber (gms) |
|---|---|---|---|---|---|---|---|
| **Oat** (see also "Cereal"): | | | | | | | |
| whole-grain, 1 oz. ...... | 110 | 4.8 | 18.8 | 2.0 | 0 | 1 | 3.0 |
| rolled or oatmeal: | | | | | | | |
| dry, 1 oz. ........... | 109 | 4.5 | 19.0 | 1.8 | 0 | 1 | 2.9 |
| cooked, 1 cup .:..... | 145 | 6.1 | 25.3 | 2.3 | 0 | 2 | 4.0 |
| **Oat beverage** (*Pacific* Organic), 8 fl. oz.: | | | | | | | |
| original ............. | 130 | 4.0 | 24.0 | 2.5 | 0 | 110 | 2.0 |
| vanilla .............. | 130 | 4.0 | 25.0 | 2.5 | 0 | 110 | 2.0 |
| **Oat bran**, dry: | | | | | | | |
| (*Shiloh Farms* Organic), ⅓ cup ............. | 150 | 8.0 | 23.0 | 2.5 | 0 | 0 | 7.0 |
| 1 oz. ................ | 70 | 4.9 | 18.8 | 2.0 | 0 | 1 | 4.5 |
| **Oat flakes** (see also "Cereal") (*Eden* Organic), ½ cup ..... | 170 | 5.0 | 31.0 | 3.0 | 0 | 0 . | 5.0 |
| **Oat flour**: | | | | | | | |
| (*Arrowhead Mills* Organic), ⅓ cup ..... | 120 | 4.0 | 21.0 | 3.0 | 0 | 0 | 3.0 |
| (*Bob's Red Mill*), ⅓ cup . | 160 | 7.0 | 26.0 | 3.0 | 0 | 0 | 4.0 |
| bran (*Hodgson Mill* Organic), ¼ cup ..... | 125 | 4.0 | 22.0 | 2.0 | 0 | 0 | 3.0 |
| **Oat groats** (*Arrowhead Mills* Organic), ¼ cup | 160 | 7.0 | 28.0 | 3.0 | 0 | 0 | 4.0 |
| **Ocean perch,** Atlantic, meat only: | | | | | | | |
| raw, 4 oz. ........... | 107 | 21.1 | 0 | 1.9 | 48 | 85 | 0 |
| baked or broiled, 4 oz. .. | 137 | 27.1 | 0 | 2.4 | 61 | 109 | 0 |
| **Oco** (*Frieda's*), ½ cup, 3 oz. ................ | 70 | 2.0 | 15.0 | 0 | 0 | 5 | 1.0 |
| **Octopus,** meat only: | | | | | | | |
| raw, 4 oz. ........... | 93 | 16.9 | 2.5 | 1.2 | 54 | 261 | 0 |
| boiled or steamed, 4 oz. . | 186 | 33.8 | 5.0 | 2.4 | 109 | 522 | 0 |

| Food and Measure | cal. | prot. (gms) | carbo. (gms) | fat (gms) | chol. (mgs) | sod. (mgs) | fiber (gms) |
|---|---|---|---|---|---|---|---|
| **Octopus, canned:** | | | | | | | |
| in soy/olive oil | | | | | | | |
| (*Vigo*), 4-oz. can, | | | | | | | |
| drained . . . . . . . . . . . | 100 | 14.0 | 3.0 | 4.0 | 40 | 250 | 0 |
| smoked, sliced | | | | | | | |
| (*Roland*), ⅓ cup, 2 oz. | 160 | 8.0 | 1.0 | 14.0 | 25 | 660 | 0 |
| spiced, w/tomato sauce, | | | | | | | |
| vegetables (*Roland*), | | | | | | | |
| 2 oz. . . . . . . . . . . . . . | 116 | 9.0 | 2.0 | 8.0 | 40 | 340 | 0 |
| **Oheloberry**, ½ cup . . . . . | 20 | .3 | 4.8 | .2 | 0 | 1 | n.a. |
| **Oil**, 1 tbsp., except | | | | | | | |
| as noted: | | | | | | | |
| (*House of Tsang* | | | | | | | |
| *Mongolian Fire*), 1 tsp. | 45 | 0 | 0 | 5.0 | 0 | 0 | 0 |
| all varieties (*Eden*) . . . . . | 120 | 0 | 0 | 14.0 | 0 | 0 | 0 |
| almond, canola, cocoa | | | | | | | |
| butter, corn, cottonseed, | | | | | | | |
| hazelnut, oat, palm, | | | | | | | |
| or poppy seed . . . . . . . | 120 | 0 | 0 | 13.6 | 0 | 0 | 0 |
| avocado, grapeseed, nut, | | | | | | | |
| pumpkinseed, or rice | | | | | | | |
| (*Roland*) . . . . . . . . . . . | 130 | 0 | 0 | 14.0 | 0 | 0 | 0 |
| avocado or mustard . . . . | 124 | 0 | 0 | 14.0 | 0 | 0 | 0 |
| butter oil | 112 | <.1 | 0 | 12.7 | 33 | 0 | 0 |
| chili, chive, garlic, ginger, | | | | | | | |
| olive, truffle, or sesame | | | | | | | |
| (*Roland*) . . . . . . . . . . . | 120 | 0 | 0 | 14.0 | 0 | 0 | 0 |
| chili, hot, or sesame | | | | | | | |
| (*House of Tsang*), | | | | | | | |
| 1 tsp. . . . . . . . . . . . . | 45 | 0 | 0 | 5.0 | 0 | 0 | 0 |
| coconut . . . . . . . . . . . . | 117 | 0 | 0 | 13.6 | 0 | 0 | 0 |
| cod liver . . . . . . . . . . . | 123 | 0 | 0 | 13.6 | 78 | 0 | 0 |
| herring . . . . . . . . . . . . | 123 | 0 | 0 | 13.6 | 104 | 0 | 0 |
| menhaden . . . . . . . . . . | 123 | 0 | 0 | 16.3 | 85 | 0 | 0 |
| olive, peanut, | | | | | | | |
| safflower, sesame, soybean, | | | | | | | |
| sunflower, vegetable, | | | | | | | |
| or walnut . . . . . . . . . | 120 | 0 | 0 | 14.0 | 0 | 0 | 0 |
| salmon | 123 | 0 | 0 | 13.6 | 66 | 0 | 0 |
| sardine . . . . . . . . . . . . | 123 | 0 | 0 | 13.6 | 97 | 0 | 0 |
| wok (*House of Tsang*) . . . | 130 | 0 | 0 | 14.0 | 0 | 0 | 0 |
| **Okra**, fresh: | | | | | | | |
| raw: | | | | | | | |
| (*Frieda's* Red), 3.5 oz. . | 33 | 2.0 | 8.0 | .2 | 0 | 8 | 3.0 |

| Food and Measure | cal. | prot. (gms) | carbo. (gms) | fat (gms) | chol. (mgs) | sod. (mgs) | fiber (gms) |
|---|---|---|---|---|---|---|---|
| **Okra, raw** *(cont.)* | | | | | | | |
| (*Green Giant*), 3.5 oz. . | 30 | 2.0 | 7.0 | 0 | 0 | 10 | 3.0 |
| sliced, ½ cup ....... | 19 | 1.0 | 3.8 | .1 | 0 | 4 | 1.3 |
| boiled, drained: | | | | | | | |
| 8 pods, 3" x ⅝" ...... | 27 | 1.6 | 6.1 | .1 | 0 | 5 | 2.1 |
| sliced, ½ cup ....... | 25 | 1.5 | 5.8 | .1 | 0 | 4 | 2.0 |
| **Okra, canned**, ½ cup: | | | | | | | |
| cut (*Allens/Trappey's*) ... | 30 | 1.0 | 6.0 | 0 | 0 | 400 | 3.0 |
| Creole gumbo | | | | | | | |
| (*Trappey's*) ......... | 35 | 2.0 | 6.0 | 0 | 0 | 290 | 3.0 |
| w/tomatoes: | | | | | | | |
| (*Allens/Trappey's*) .... | 30 | 1.0 | 5.0 | 0 | 0 | 380 | 3.0 |
| (*Glory* Sensibly | | | | | | | |
| Seasoned) ....... | 30 | 1.0 | 6.0 | 0 | 0 | 170 | 2.0 |
| w/tomatoes and corn: | | | | | | | |
| (*Allens/Trappey's*) .... | 30 | 1.0 | 6.0 | 0 | 0 | 280 | 4.0 |
| (*Glory* Sensibly | | | | | | | |
| Seasoned) ....... | 35 | 1.0 | 8.0 | 0 | 0 | 150 | 2.0 |
| **Okra, frozen**: | | | | | | | |
| whole, 9 pods, 3 oz.: | | | | | | | |
| (*Allens*) ............ | 35 | 1.0 | 7.0 | 0 | 0 | 10 | 3.0 |
| (*McKenzie's*) ........ | 30 | 1.0 | 6.0 | 0 | 0 | 20 | 2.0 |
| cut, ¾ cup: | | | | | | | |
| (*Allens*) ............ | 35 | 1.0 | 7.0 | 0 | 0 | 10 | 3.0 |
| (*McKenzie's*) ........ | 30 | 1.0 | 6.0 | 0 | 0 | 20 | 2.0 |
| boiled, drained, | | | | | | | |
| sliced, ½ cup ....... | 34 | 1.9 | 7.5 | .3 | 0 | 3 | 2.6 |
| breaded, ¾ cup: | | | | | | | |
| (*Allens* 16 oz.) ...... | 100 | 3.0 | 23.0 | 0 | 0 | 150 | 2.0 |
| (*McKenzie's*) ........ | 80 | 2.0 | 19.0 | 0 | 0 | 660 | 2.0 |
| **Olive**, pickled: | | | | | | | |
| black, oil cured: | | | | | | | |
| (*Vigo*), 4 pcs. ....... | 80 | 0 | 7.0 | 6.0 | 0 | 420 | 1.0 |
| pitted (*Roland*), | | | | | | | |
| 8 pcs., .5 oz. ..... | 70 | 0 | 7.0 | 4.0 | 0 | 440 | 0 |
| black, ripe, pitted: | | | | | | | |
| whole (*Lindsay*), .5 oz. | 25 | 0 | 1.0 | 2.5 | 0 | 115 | 0 |
| whole, large (*Roland*), | | | | | | | |
| 4 pcs. ........... | 20 | 0 | 1.0 | 2.0 | 0 | 110 | 1.0 |
| whole, medium | | | | | | | |
| (*Roland*), 5 pcs. ... | 30 | 0 | 1.0 | 2.0 | 0 | 110 | 1.0 |
| sliced (*Lindsay*), | | | | | | | |
| 2 tbsp. .......... | 25 | 0 | 1.0 | 2.5 | 0 | 125 | 0 |

| Food and Measure | cal. | prot. (gms) | carbo. (gms) | fat (gms) | chol. (mgs) | sod. (mgs) | fiber (gms) |
|---|---|---|---|---|---|---|---|
| sliced (*Roland*), 1 tbsp. . . . . . . . . . | 20 | 0 | 1.0 | 2.0 | 0 | 110 | 1.0 |
| chopped (*Lindsay*), 1⅓ tbsp. . . . . . . . . | 25 | 1.0 | 0 | 2.5 | 0 | 115 | 0 |
| Greek, black, whole: | | | | | | | |
| (*Peloponnese* Kalamata), 5 pcs. . . | 45 | 0 | 1.0 | 4.5 | 0 | 210 | 0 |
| (*Roland* Kalamata), 3 pcs. . . . . . . . . | 40 | 0 | 2.0 | 4.0 | 0 | 230 | 0 |
| (*Roland* Mt. Pelion), 3 pcs. . . . . . . . . | 30 | 0 | 2.0 | 2.0 | 0 | 260 | 0 |
| (*Vigo*), 4 pcs. . . . . . . . | 40 | 0 | 1.0 | 4.0 | 0 | 260 | 0 |
| (*Vigo* Calamata), 4 pcs. . . . . . . . . . . | 35 | 0 | 2.0 | 3.0 | 0 | 270 | 0 |
| 10 medium . . . . . . . . | 65 | .4 | 1.7 | 6.9 | 0 | 631 | 0 |
| 10 extra large . . . . . . . | 89 | .6 | 2.3 | 9.5 | 0 | 868 | 0 |
| Greek, black, pitted: | | | | | | | |
| (*Di Lusso* Kalamata), 1 tbsp., .5 oz. . . . . . | 45 | 0 | 1.0 | 4.5 | 0 | 210 | 0 |
| (*Peloponnese*), .5 oz. . | 45 | 0 | 1.0 | 4.5 | 0 | 210 | 0 |
| (*Roland* Kalamata), 3 pcs. . . . . . . . . | 40 | 0 | 2.0 | 4.0 | 0 | 230 | 0 |
| (*Vigo* Calamata), 4 pcs. | 35 | 0 | 2.0 | 3.0 | 0 | 270 | 0 |
| 1 oz. . . . . . . . . . . . . . | 96 | .6 | 2.5 | 10.2 | 0 | 932 | 0 |
| halves (*Peloponnese*), .5 oz. . . . . . . . . . | 45 | 0 | 1.0 | 4.5 | 0 | 190 | 0 |
| halves (*Roland* Kalamata), 16 pcs. . | 40 | 0 | 1.0 | 4.0 | 0 | 190 | 0 |
| sliced (*Roland* Kalamata), 1 tbsp. . | 40 | 0 | 2.0 | 4.0 | 0 | 230 | 0 |
| sliced (*Vigo* Calamata), 1 tbsp. . . . . . . . . . | 35 | 0 | 2.0 | 3.0 | 0 | 270 | 0 |
| Greek, blonde (*Roland*), 2 pcs. . . . . . | 30 | 0 | 2.0 | 2.0 | 0 | 260 | 0 |
| Greek, green: | | | | | | | |
| (*Di Lusso* Ionian), .5 oz. . . . . . . . . . . | 25 | 0 | 1.0 | 2.0 | 0 | 280 | 0 |
| (*Peloponnese* Ionian), 3 pcs. . . . . . . . . | 25 | 0 | 1.0 | 2.5 | 0 | 250 | 0 |
| (*Roland* Mt. Pelion), 3 pcs. . . . . . . . . | 15 | 0 | 2.0 | 1.0 | 0 | 190 | 0 |
| Greek, mixed: | | | | | | | |
| (*Di Lusso*), .5 oz. . . . . | 35 | 0 | 1.0 | 3.5 | 0 | 250 | 0 |
| (*Peloponnese*), 4 pcs. . | 30 | 0 | 1.0 | 3.0 | 0 | 250 | 0 |

| Food and Measure | cal. | prot. (gms) | carbo. (gms) | fat (gms) | chol. (mgs) | sod. (mgs) | fiber (gms) |
|---|---|---|---|---|---|---|---|
| **Olive, Greek, mixed** *(cont.)* | | | | | | | |
| (*Roland*), 3 pcs. . . . . . | 20 | 0 | 0 | 2.0 | 0 | 180 | 1.0 |
| pitted (*Roland*), 2 pcs. | 40 | 0 | 1.0 | 4.0 | 0 | 180 | 1.0 |
| green, cocktail | | | | | | | |
| (*Zatarain's*), 7 pcs. . . . | 25 | 0 | 0 | 3.0 | 0 | 350 | 0 |
| green, w/pits: | | | | | | | |
| (*Roland* Queen | | | | | | | |
| Cannonball), 2 pcs. | 20 | 0 | 1.0 | 2.0 | 0 | 310 | 0 |
| 10 small . . . . . . . . . . | 33 | .4 | .4 | 3.6 | 0 | 686 | .7 |
| 10 large . . . . . . . . . . | 45 | .5 | .5 | 4.9 | 0 | 926 | 1.0 |
| 10 giant . . . . . . . . . . | 76 | .9 | .9 | 8.3 | 0 | 1572 | 1.7 |
| green, cracked: | | | | | | | |
| (*Peloponnese*), 4 pcs. . | 30 | 0 | 1.0 | 2.5 | 0 | 250 | 0 |
| (*Roland* Sicilian), | | | | | | | |
| 2 pcs. . . . . . . . . . . | 40 | 0 | 1.0 | 4.0 | 0 | 200 | 0 |
| spiced (*Roland*), 3 pcs. | 30 | 0 | 1.0 | 3.0 | 0 | 210 | 0 |
| green, pitted: | | | | | | | |
| (*Lindsay* Ripe | | | | | | | |
| Naturals), 5 pc., .5 oz. | 25 | 0 | 1.0 | 2.5 | 0 | 115 | 0 |
| (*Roland* Queen), 3 pcs. | 15 | 0 | 1.0 | 2.0 | 0 | 170 | 0 |
| (*Zatarain's*), 6 pcs. . . . | 25 | 0 | 0 | 2.5 | 0 | 280 | .5 |
| niçoise (*Roland*), .5 oz. . . | 45 | 0 | 3.0 | 4.0 | 0 | 125 | 1.0 |
| picholine (*Roland*), | | | | | | | |
| .5 oz. . . . . . . . . . . . . | 25 | 0 | 2.0 | 2.0 | 0 | 200 | 1.0 |
| Provencal, w/herbs/hot | | | | | | | |
| pepper (*Roland*), | | | | | | | |
| 3 pcs. . . . . . . . . . . . . | 25 | 0 | 2.0 | 2.0 | 0 | 160 | 1.0 |
| stuffed, green: | | | | | | | |
| almonds (*Roland*), | | | | | | | |
| 4 pcs. . . . . . . . . . . | 35 | 0 | 1.0 | 3.5 | 0 | 310 | 0 |
| almonds (*Roland* | | | | | | | |
| Queen), 2 pcs. . . . . | 35 | 0 | 1.0 | 4.0 | 0 | 310 | 0 |
| anchovies (*Roland*), | | | | | | | |
| 5 pcs. . . . . . . . . . . | 25 | 0 | 1.0 | 2.0 | 0 | 170 | 0 |
| capers (*Roland* | | | | | | | |
| Queen), 2 pcs. . . . . | 20 | 0 | 1.0 | 2.0 | 0 | 330 | 0 |
| cheese, in oil (*Roland*), | | | | | | | |
| ½ cup, 4.6 oz. . . . . | 520 | 3.0 | 7.0 | 54.0 | 0 | 640 | 3.0 |
| garlic (*Roland* | | | | | | | |
| Queen), 2 pcs. . . . . | 20 | 0 | 1.0 | 2.0 | 0 | 300 | 0 |
| jalapeño (*Roland*), | | | | | | | |
| 2 pcs. . . . . . . . . . . | 25 | 0 | 1.0 | 2.0 | 0 | 330 | 0 |
| jalapeño (*Vigo*), 2 pcs. | 25 | 0 | 0 | 2.0 | 0 | 95 | 0 |

| Food and Measure | cal. | prot. (gms) | carbo. (gms) | fat (gms) | chol. (mgs) | sod. (mgs) | fiber (gms) |
|---|---|---|---|---|---|---|---|
| piri piri (*Roland*), 2 pcs. | 20 | 0 | 1.0 | 1.5 | 0 | 310 | 0 |
| onion or triple-stuffed (*Roland*), 5 pcs. | 25 | 0 | 1.0 | 2.0 | 0 | 330 | 0 |
| stuffed, pimento: | | | | | | | |
| (*Lindsay* Manzanilla), 5 pcs., .5 oz. | 25 | 0 | <1.0 | 2.5 | 0 | 240 | 0 |
| (*Lindsay* Queen), .3-oz. pc. | 10 | 0 | <1.0 | 1.0 | 0 | 160 | 0 |
| (*Roland* Jar), 6 pcs. | 25 | 0 | 1.0 | 2.0 | 0 | 330 | 0 |
| (*Roland* Manzanilla), 5 pcs. | 25 | 0 | 0 | 2.0 | 0 | 230 | 0 |
| (*Roland* Queen), 2 pcs. | 25 | 0 | 1.0 | 2.0 | 0 | 330 | 0 |
| (*Vigo* Manzanilla), 5 pcs. or ¼ cup | 25 | 0 | 1.0 | 2.5 | 0 | 230 | 0 |
| (*Vigo* Queen), 2 pcs. | 20 | 0 | 1.0 | 1.5 | 0 | 290 | 0 |
| **Olive antipasto**, and vegetables (*Peloponnese*), ⅓ cup | 35 | 1.0 | 2.0 | 3.0 | 0 | 740 | 1.0 |
| **Olive loaf**, see "Lunch meat" | | | | | | | |
| **Olive oil**, see "Oil" | | | | | | | |
| **Olive paste or pâté**, see "Olive spread" | | | | | | | |
| **Olive salad**, mixed (*Roland* Muffuletta), 2 tbsp. | 10 | 0 | 0 | 1.0 | 0 | 320 | 0 |
| **Olive sauce** (*Italia In Tavola*), 2 tbsp. | 90 | 0 | 0 | 10.0 | 0 | 970 | 0 |
| **Olive spread**: | | | | | | | |
| (*Peloponnese* Kalamata), 1 tsp. | 15 | 0 | 0 | 1.5 | 0 | 160 | 0 |
| (*Roland* Greek Kalamata), 1 tbsp. | 60 | 0 | 3.0 | 6.0 | 0 | 450 | 1.0 |
| paste, 1 tbsp.: | | | | | | | |
| black (*Roland*) | 70 | 0 | 3.0 | 7.0 | 0 | 200 | 1.0 |
| green (*Roland*) | 70 | 0 | 3.0 | 7.0 | 0 | 205 | 1.0 |
| pâté, 2 tbsp.: | | | | | | | |
| black (*Alessi*) | 187 | 1.0 | 2.7 | 19.0 | 0 | 817 | 1.4 |
| green (*Alessi*) | 160 | 1.0 | 2.0 | 17.0 | 0 | 460 | 1.0 |
| tapenade: | | | | | | | |
| (*Progresso*), 1 tbsp. | 20 | 0 | 1.0 | 2.0 | 0 | 180 | 0 |
| w/vegetables (*Alessi*), 2 tbsp. | 140 | 0 | 1.0 | 15.0 | 0 | 500 | 0 |

| Food and Measure | cal. | prot. (gms) | carbo. (gms) | fat (gms) | chol. (mgs) | sod. (mgs) | fiber (gms) |
|---|---|---|---|---|---|---|---|
| **Onion**, fresh/stored: | | | | | | | |
| raw: | | | | | | | |
| (*Frieda's* Boiler/ | | | | | | | |
| Pearl), 3 oz. . . . . . . | 30 | 1.0 | 8.0 | 0 | 0 | 3 | 1.0 |
| (*Frieda's* Hawaiian | | | | | | | |
| Maui), 4 oz. . . . . . . | 35 | 1.0 | 8.0 | 0 | 0 | 9 | 1.0 |
| chopped (*Frieda's* | | | | | | | |
| Cipolline), ½ cup . . | 30 | 1.0 | 6.0 | 0 | 0 | 3 | 1.0 |
| chopped, ½ cup . . . . . | 30 | .9 | 6.9 | 0.1 | 0 | 2 | 1.4 |
| chopped, 1 tbsp. . . . . . | 4 | .1 | .9 | <.1 | 0 | tr. | .2 |
| boiled, drained: | | | | | | | |
| chopped, ½ cup . . . . . | 46 | 1.4 | 10.7 | .2 | 0 | 3 | 1.5 |
| chopped, 1 tbsp. . . . . . | 7 | .2 | 1.5 | <.1 | 0 | <1 | .2 |
| **Onion, can/jar**, whole: | | | | | | | |
| baby (*Roland*), ⅔ cup . . . | 25 | 1.0 | 5.0 | 0 | 0 | 300 | 2.0 |
| w/balsamic vinegar: | | | | | | | |
| (*Roland*), 2 tbsp. . . . . | 20 | 1.0 | 4.0 | 0 | 0 | 240 | 0 |
| (*Roland* Borretane), | | | | | | | |
| 1 oz. . . . . . . . . . . . | 20 | 0 | 5.0 | 0 | 0 | 55 | 0 |
| cocktail: | | | | | | | |
| (*Crosse & Blackwell*), | | | | | | | |
| 1 tbsp. . . . . . . . . . | 5 | 0 | 1.0 | 0 | 0 | 250 | 0 |
| (*Lindsay*), 6 pcs., 1.1 oz. | 5 | 0 | 1.0 | 0 | 0 | 420 | 0 |
| (*Roland*), 2 tbsp. . . . . | 0 | 0 | 1.0 | 0 | 0 | 55 | 0 |
| (*Vigo*), 1 pc. . . . . . . . . | 0 | 0 | 0 | 0 | 0 | 30 | 0 |
| **Onion, dried**: | | | | | | | |
| flakes, 1 tbsp. . . . . . . . . | 16 | .5 | 4.2 | <.1 | 0 | 1 | .5 |
| minced, 1 tsp. . . . . . . . . . | 7 | .2 | 1.9 | 0 | 0 | <1 | .2 |
| **Onion, french fried**, | | | | | | | |
| canned, 2 tbsp.: | | | | | | | |
| (*French's* Original) . . . . . . | 45 | 0 | 3.0 | 3.5 | 0 | 60 | 0 |
| cheddar (*French's*) . . . . . | 45 | 0 | 3.0 | 3.5 | 0 | 65 | 0 |
| **Onion, frozen** (see | | | | | | | |
| also "Onion rings"): | | | | | | | |
| whole: | | | | | | | |
| (*C&W* Petite), ⅔ cup . | 30 | 0 | 6.0 | 0 | 0 | 10 | <1.0 |
| boiled, drained, | | | | | | | |
| ½ cup . . . . . . . . . . . | 30 | .7 | 7.0 | 0 | 0 | 8 | 1.5 |
| pearl (*Birds Eye* | | | | | | | |
| White), ⅔ cup . . . . | 30 | 0 | 6.0 | 0 | 0 | 10 | 1.0 |
| pearl, in cream sauce | | | | | | | |
| (*Birds Eye*), ½ cup . | 60 | 2.0 | 8.0 | 2.0 | 10 | 280 | 1.0 |
| chopped: | | | | | | | |
| (*McKenzie's*), ⅔ cup . . | 30 | 0 | 6.0 | 0 | 0 | 10 | 1.0 |

| Food and Measure | cal. | prot. (gms) | carbo. (gms) | fat (gms) | chol. (mgs) | sod. (mgs) | fiber (gms) |
|---|---|---|---|---|---|---|---|
| *(Ore-Ida)*, 2.8 oz. | 20 | >1.0 | 5.0 | 0 | 0 | 10 | 2.0 |
| boiled, drained, 1 tbsp. | 4 | .1 | 1.0 | <.1 | 0 | 2 | .2 |
| **Onion, green**, fresh, trimmed: | | | | | | | |
| bulb, w/top, 2 oz. | 18 | 1.0 | 4.0 | 0 | 0 | 9 | 1.5 |
| chopped: | | | | | | | |
| ½ cup | 16 | .9 | 3.7 | .1 | 0 | 8 | 1.3 |
| 1 tbsp. | 2 | .1 | .4 | <.1 | 0 | 1 | .2 |
| **Onion, Welsh**, 1 oz. | 10 | .5 | 1.8 | .1 | 0 | 5 | <1.0 |
| **Onion dip**, 2 tbsp.: | | | | | | | |
| *(Heluva Good! Bodacious)* | 60 | 1.0 | 3.0 | 5.0 | 20 | 210 | 0 |
| French: | | | | | | | |
| *(Cabot)* | 50 | 1.0 | 1.0 | 5.0 | 15 | 200 | 0 |
| *(Frito-Lay)* | 60 | 1.0 | 4.0 | 5.0 | 15 | 230 | 0 |
| *(Heluva Good!)* | 60 | 1.0 | 2.0 | 5.0 | 20 | 170 | 0 |
| *(Heluva Good!* Nonfat) | 25 | 1.0 | 3.0 | 0 | 0 | 210 | 0 |
| *(Kraft)* | 60 | 1.0 | 3.0 | 4.5 | 0 | 220 | 0 |
| *(Lay's)* | 60 | 1.0 | 2.0 | 5.0 | <5 | 230 | 0 |
| *(Marzetti)* | 120 | 1.0 | 2.0 | 12.0 | 20 | 220 | 0 |
| *(Marzetti* Light) | 60 | 0 | 3.0 | 6.0 | 5 | 230 | 0 |
| *(Wise)* | 60 | <1.0 | 3.0 | 5.0 | 0 | 230 | 0 |
| roasted *(Marie's)* | 100 | 1.0 | 2.0 | 10.0 | 15 | 220 | 0 |
| green *(Kraft)* | 60 | 1.0 | 3.0 | 4.5 | 0 | 170 | 0 |
| **Onion dip mix**: | | | | | | | |
| French *(McCormick)*, ¾ tsp. | 5 | 0 | <1.0 | 0 | 0 | 140 | 0 |
| garden *(Lay's* Dip Creations), 2 tbsp.* | 70 | 1.0 | 2.0 | 6.0 | 10 | 160 | 0 |
| **Onion gravy mix** *(McCormick)*, 2 tsp. | 30 | 0 | 3.0 | 1.0 | 0 | 330 | 0 |
| **Onion powder**, 1 tsp. | 7 | .2 | 1.7 | 0 | 0 | 1 | .1 |
| **Onion relish**, sweet *(Vidalia Valley)*, 1 tbsp. | 10 | 0 | 2.0 | 0 | 0 | 5 | 0 |
| **Onion ring batter mix**, ¼ cup dry: | | | | | | | |
| *(Don's Chuck Wagon)* | 100 | 3.0 | 21.0 | 0 | 0 | 690 | 1.0 |
| *(Golden Dipt Fry Easy)* | 100 | 1.0 | 20.0 | 0 | 0 | 660 | 0 |
| *(Zatarain's)* | 100 | 2.0 | 22.0 | .5 | 0 | 700 | <1.0 |
| **Onion ring snack**, see "Corn chips/crisps" | | | | | | | |

| Food and Measure | cal. | prot. (gms) | carbo. (gms) | fat (gms) | chol. (mgs) | sod. (mgs) | fiber (gms) |
|---|---|---|---|---|---|---|---|
| **Onion rings**, breaded, frozen: | | | | | | | |
| (*Alexia*), 6 pcs., 3 oz. . . . | 240 | 4.0 | 27.0 | 13.0 | 0 | 150 | 2.0 |
| (*Ore-Ida* Gourmet), 2.7 oz. . . . . . . . . . . | 180 | 3.0 | 25.0 | 8.0 | 0 | 520 | 1.0 |
| (*Ore-Ida* Onion Ringers), 2.8 oz. . . . . . | 180 | 2.0 | 21.0 | 10.0 | 0 | 160 | 2.0 |
| heated, 10 rings . . . . . . . | 289 | 3.8 | 27.1 | 19.0 | 0 | 17 | 2.9 |
| **Onion salt** (*McCormick*), ¼ tsp. . | 0 | 0 | 0 | 0 | 0 | 450 | 0 |
| **Onion sauce**, 1 tbsp.: | | | | | | | |
| (*Boar's Head* Sweet Vidalia) . . . . . . . . . . . | 10 | 0 | 2.0 | 0 | 0 | 15 | 0 |
| (*Di Lusso* Sweet) . . . . . . | 30 | 0 | 8.0 | 0 | 0 | 75 | 0 |
| (*Sabrett* Pushcart) . . . . . . | 10 | 0 | 3.0 | 0 | 0 | 105 | 0 |
| **Opo squash** (*Frieda's*), ⅔ cup, 3 oz. . . . . . . . . | 10 | 1.0 | 3.0 | 0 | 0 | 0 | 0 |
| **Opossum**, meat only, roasted, 4 oz. . . . . . . . | 251 | 34.3 | 0 | 11.6 | 146 | 66 | 0 |
| **Orange**, fresh: | | | | | | | |
| (*Dole*), 5.4-oz. fruit . . . . . | 80 | 1.0 | 19.0 | 0 | 0 | 0 | 3.0 |
| (*Frieda's* Blood), 5.4-oz. fruit . . . . . . . . | 70 | 1.0 | 15.0 | .5 | 0 | 0 | 3.0 |
| (*Frieda's* Cara Cara), 5-oz. fruit . . . . . . . . | 70 | 1.0 | 16.0 | 0 | 0 | 0 | 3.0 |
| (*Frieda's* Seville), 3 oz. . . | 40 | 1.0 | 10.0 | 0 | 0 | 0 | 2.0 |
| all varieties: | | | | | | | |
| 3¹/₁₆" fruit, 6.5 oz. . . . . | 87 | 1.7 | 21.6 | .2 | 0 | 0 | 4.4 |
| sections, 1 cup . . . . . . | 85 | 1.7 | 21.2 | .2 | 0 | 0 | 4.3 |
| California navel: | | | | | | | |
| 2⅞" fruit, 5 oz. . . . . . . | 65 | 1.4 | 16.3 | .1 | 0 | 1 | 3.4 |
| sections, 1 cup . . . . . . | 76 | 1.7 | 19.2 | .2 | 0 | 2 | 4.0 |
| California Valencia: | | | | | | | |
| 2⅝" fruit, 4.25 oz. . . . . | 59 | 1.3 | 14.4 | .4 | 0 | 0 | 3.0 |
| sections, 1 cup . . . . . . | 88 | 1.9 | 21.4 | .5 | 0 | 0 | 4.5 |
| Florida: | | | | | | | |
| 2¹¹/₁₆" fruit, 5 oz. . . . . . | 65 | 1.0 | 16.3 | .3 | 0 | 1 | 3.4 |
| sections, 1 cup . . . . . . | 85 | 1.3 | 21.4 | .4 | 0 | 1 | 4.4 |
| **Orange, blood, drink mixer** (*Angostura*), 2 fl. oz. . . . . . . . . . . . | 70 | 0 | 18.0 | 0 | 0 | 5 | 0 |
| **Orange, can/jar**, mandarin, see "Tangerine" | | | | | | | |

| Food and Measure | cal. | prot. (gms) | carbo. (gms) | fat (gms) | chol. (mgs) | sod. (mgs) | fiber (gms) |
|---|---|---|---|---|---|---|---|
| **Orange crème topping** (*Smucker's Magic Shell*), 2 tbsp. ....... | 210 | 1.0 | 17.0 | 15.0 | 0 | 50 | 0 |
| **Orange drink**, 8 fl. oz., except as noted: | | | | | | | |
| (*Minute Maid* Light) .... | 50 | 0 | 13.0 | 0 | 0 | 15 | 0 |
| (*Santa Cruz Organic* Box) .............. | 100 | 1.0 | 25.0 | 0 | 0 | 10 | 0 |
| (*Tropicana Trop50*) ..... | 50 | <1.0 | 13.0 | 0 | 0 | 10 | 0 |
| orange flavor, frozen* (*Bright & Early*) ..... | 110 | 0 | 29.0 | 0 | 0 | 10 | 0 |
| orangeade: | | | | | | | |
| (*AriZona*) .......... | 120 | 0 | 27.0 | 0 | 0 | 20 | 0 |
| (*Minute Maid*), 12 fl. oz. ......... | 160 | 0 | 43.0 | 0 | 0 | 110 | 0 |
| (*Minute Maid* 10%) .. | 110 | 0 | 30.0 | 0 | 0 | 15 | 0 |
| (*Minute Maid* 3%) ... | 110 | 0 | 29.0 | 0 | 0 | 75 | 0 |
| (*Minute Maid* Light) .. | 10 | 0 | 2.0 | 0 | 0 | 110 | 0 |
| (*Snapple*) .......... | 100 | 0 | 26.0 | 0 | 0 | 5 | 0 |
| (*Tropicana*) ......... | 130 | 0 | 33.0 | 0 | 0 | 0 | 0 |
| (*Turkey Hill*) ........ | 110 | 0 | 26.0 | 0 | 0 | 10 | 0 |
| **Orange drink blend**, 8 fl. oz., except as noted: | | | | | | | |
| carrot: | | | | | | | |
| (*Apple & Eve*) ....... | 130 | 0 | 32.0 | 0 | 0 | 20 | 0 |
| (*SoBe Elixir*) ........ | 90 | 0 | 23.0 | 0 | 0 | 10 | 0 |
| cream (*SoBe Tsunami*) .. | 100 | 0 | 25.0 | 0 | 0 | 25 | 0 |
| mango: | | | | | | | |
| (*Apple & Eve*) ....... | 120 | 0 | 30.0 | 0 | 0 | 30 | 0 |
| (*Nantucket Nectars*) .. | 120 | 0 | 30.0 | 0 | 0 | 25 | 0 |
| (*Newman's Own* Tango) | 130 | 0 | 33.0 | 0 | 0 | 5 | 0 |
| w/mangosteen (*Honest Ade* Organic) | 48 | 0 | 12.0 | 0 | 0 | 5 | 0 |
| pineapple: | | | | | | | |
| (*Welch's*) .......... | 120 | 0 | 31.0 | 0 | 0 | 50 | 0 |
| apple (*Welch's*) ...... | 140 | 0 | 35.0 | 0 | 0 | 20 | 0 |
| mango (*Nantucket Nectars*) .......... | 120 | 1.0 | 30.0 | 0 | 0 | 30 | 0 |
| starfruit (*Snapple Antioxidant Water*) ... | 50 | 0 | 13.0 | 0 | 0 | 0 | 0 |
| strawberry (*Minute Maid* Coolers), 6.75 fl. oz. ......... | 100 | 0 | 26.0 | 0 | 0 | 15 | 0 |

| Food and Measure | cal. | prot. (gms) | carbo. (gms) | fat (gms) | chol. (mgs) | sod. (mgs) | fiber (gms) |
|---|---|---|---|---|---|---|---|
| **Orange drink blend** *(cont.)* | | | | | | | |
| strawberry banana | | | | | | | |
| (*Tropicana Twister* Burst) | 130 | 0 | 33.0 | 0 | 0 | 25 | 0 |
| tangerine: | | | | | | | |
| (*Minute Maid* Light) .. | 15 | 0 | 4.0 | 0 | 0 | 15 | 0 |
| (*SoBe Lifewater*) ..... | 40 | 0 | 16.0 | 0 | 0 | 20 | 0 |
| **Orange juice**, 8 fl. oz.: | | | | | | | |
| (*Apple & Eve*) ......... | 110 | 1.0 | 27.0 | 0 | 0 | 10 | 0 |
| (*Dole* Chilled) ........ | 120 | <1.0 | 27.0 | 0 | 0 | 10 | 0 |
| (*Dole* Single Serve) ..... | 110 | 2.0 | 27.0 | 0 | 0 | 0 | 0 |
| (*Florida's Natural*) ...... | 110 | 2.0 | 26.0 | 0 | 0 | 0 | 0 |
| (*Minute Maid* Original/ Calcium + D/Low Acid/ Country/Home Squeezed Style/ Pulp Free) .......... | 110 | 2.0 | 27.0 | 0 | 0 | 15 | 0 |
| (*Minute Maid Heart Wise*) ............. | 110 | 2.0 | 27.0 | 0 | 0 | 20 | 0 |
| (*Nantucket Nectars* Premium) .......... | 110 | 2.0 | 26.0 | 0 | 0 | 0 | 0 |
| (*Odwalla*) ............ | 110 | 1.0 | 25.0 | 0 | 0 | 15 | 0 |
| (*R.W. Knudsen*) ...... | 110 | 2.0 | 26.0 | 0 | 0 | 10 | 0 |
| (*R.W. Knudsen* Organic) . | 110 | 2.0 | 25.0 | 0 | 0 | 0 | 0 |
| (*Simply Orange*) ....... | 110 | 2.0 | 26.0 | 0 | 0 | 0 | 0 |
| (*Tropicana* 15.2 oz.) .... | 110 | 2.0 | 27.0 | 0 | 0 | 15 | 0 |
| (*Tropicana Pure Valencia*) ........... | 120 | 2.0 | 27.0 | 0 | 0 | 0 | 0 |
| (*Tropicana Pure Premium* Healthy Heart) | 120 | 2.0 | 26.0 | 0 | 0 | 0 | 0 |
| (*Veryfine*) ............ | 120 | 0 | 30.0 | 0 | 0 | 20 | 0 |
| canned ............. | 105 | 1.5 | 24.5 | .4 | 0 | 5 | .5 |
| chilled .............. | 110 | 2.0 | 25.1 | .7 | 0 | 3 | .5 |
| fresh ................ | 112 | 1.7 | 25.8 | .5 | 0 | 2 | .5 |
| frozen*: | | | | | | | |
| (*Cascadian Farm* Organic) ......... | 110 | 1.0 | 27.0 | 0 | 0 | 0 | 0 |
| (*Langers/Langers* Plus) ........... | 120 | 0 | 29.0 | 0 | 0 | 15 | 0 |
| (*Minute Maid* Low Acid) ........... | 110 | 2.0 | 27.0 | 0 | 0 | 15 | 0 |
| (*Minute Maid* Original/ Pulp Free) ....... | 110 | 0 | 27.0 | 0 | 0 | 0 | 0 |
| (*Minute Maid* Calcium + D) ..... | 120 | 0 | 27.0 | 0 | 0 | 0 | 0 |

| Food and Measure | cal. | prot. (gms) | carbo. (gms) | fat (gms) | chol. (mgs) | sod. (mgs) | fiber (gms) |
|---|---|---|---|---|---|---|---|
| **Orange juice blend**, 8 fl. oz., except as noted: | | | | | | | |
| carrot (*R.W. Knudsen Organic*) | 120 | 1.0 | 29.0 | 0 | 0 | 35 | 0 |
| mango: | | | | | | | |
| (*Florida's Natural*) | 110 | 1.0 | 27.0 | 0 | 0 | 0 | 0 |
| (*R.W. Knudsen*) | 120 | 1.0 | 30.0 | 0 | 0 | 5 | 0 |
| (*Santa Cruz Organic*) | 130 | 1.0 | 32.0 | 0 | 0 | 15 | 0 |
| (*Simply Orange*) | 120 | 2.0 | 28.0 | 0 | 0 | 0 | 0 |
| (*Snapple*), 11.5 fl. oz. | 170 | 0 | 41.0 | 0 | 0 | 15 | 0 |
| (*Tropicana Pure Valencia*) | 130 | 2.0 | 30.0 | 0 | 0 | 0 | 0 |
| peach mango: | | | | | | | |
| (*Dole*) | 120 | <1.0 | 29.0 | 0 | 0 | 25 | 0 |
| (*Tropicana Tropics*) | 120 | 1.0 | 29.0 | 0 | 0 | 10 | 0 |
| frozen (*Dole*), ¼ cup | 120 | <1.0 | 29.0 | 0 | 0 | 25 | 0 |
| pineapple: | | | | | | | |
| (*Florida's Natural*) | 130 | 1.0 | 31.0 | 0 | 0 | 0 | 0 |
| (*Santa Cruz Organic*) | 130 | 0 | 31.0 | 0 | 0 | 20 | 0 |
| (*Simply Orange*) | 110 | 2.0 | 27.0 | 0 | 0 | 0 | 0 |
| (*Tropicana Pure Premium*) | 130 | 2.0 | 31.0 | 0 | 0 | 0 | 0 |
| strawberry (*Florida's Natural*) | 110 | 2.0 | 26.0 | 0 | 0 | 0 | 0 |
| strawberry banana: | | | | | | | |
| (*Dole*) | 120 | 2.0 | 30.0 | 0 | 0 | 10 | 0 |
| (*Tropicana Pure Premium*) | 130 | 2.0 | 30.0 | 0 | 0 | 0 | 0 |
| (*Tropicana Tropics*) | 120 | 1.0 | 29.0 | 0 | 0 | 10 | 0 |
| frozen (*Dole*), ¼ cup | 120 | <1.0 | 30.0 | 0 | 0 | 10 | 0 |
| tangerine: | | | | | | | |
| (*Tropicana Pure Premium*) | 110 | 2.0 | 25.0 | 0 | 0 | 0 | 0 |
| frozen* (*Minute Maid*) | 110 | 0 | 27.0 | 0 | 0 | 0 | 0 |
| **Orange roughy**, see "Roughy, orange" | | | | | | | |
| **Oregano**, dried, 1 tsp. | 3 | .1 | .5 | 0 | 0 | 0 | .1 |
| **Oriental 5-spice** (*Tone's*), 1 tsp. | 9 | .3 | 1.9 | .3 | 0 | 2 | .5 |
| **Oroblanco** (*Frieda's*), 5.4-oz. fruit | 100 | 1.0 | 22.0 | 1.0 | 0 | 0 | 4.0 |

| Food and Measure | cal. | prot. (gms) | carbo. (gms) | fat (gms) | chol. (mgs) | sod. (mgs) | fiber (gms) |
|---|---|---|---|---|---|---|---|
| **Ostrich**, ground, | | | | | | | |
| pan-broiled, 4 oz. . . . . | 187 | 22.9 | 0 | 10.0 | 81 | 82 | 0 |
| **Oyster**, meat only, 4 oz., | | | | | | | |
| except as noted: | | | | | | | |
| Eastern, farmed: | | | | | | | |
| raw . . . . . . . . . . . . . . | 67 | 5.9 | 6.3 | 1.8 | 29 | 202 | 0 |
| baked or broiled . . . . . | 90 | 7.9 | 8.3 | 2.4 | 43 | 185 | 0 |
| Eastern, wild: | | | | | | | |
| raw, 1 lb. . . . . . . . . . . | 310 | 32.0 | 17.7 | 11.1 | 238 | 957 | 0 |
| raw, 6 medium, 3 oz. . | 57 | 5.9 | 3.3 | 2.1 | 44 | 177 | 0 |
| baked or broiled . . . . . | 82 | 9.4 | 5.4 | 2.2 | 56 | 277 | 0 |
| steamed or poached . . | 155 | 16.0 | 8.9 | 5.6 | 119 | 478 | 0 |
| Pacific: | | | | | | | |
| raw . . . . . . . . . . . . . . | 92 | 10.7 | 5.6 | 2.6 | 57 | 120 | 0 |
| raw, steamed, or | | | | | | | |
| poached, 1 medium | 41 | 4.7 | 2.5 | 1.2 | 25 | 53 | 0 |
| boiled or steamed . . . . | 185 | 21.4 | 11.2 | 5.2 | 113 | 240 | 0 |
| **Oyster, canned**: | | | | | | | |
| whole, 2 oz.: | | | | | | | |
| (*Bumble Bee*) . . . . . . . | 70 | 9.0 | 2.0 | 2.5 | 50 | 160 | 0 |
| (*Chicken of the Sea*) . . | 80 | 7.0 | 6.0 | 3.0 | 35 | 220 | 0 |
| (*Crown Prince*) . . . . . . | 70 | 7.0 | 4.0 | 3.0 | 35 | 150 | 0 |
| boiled (*Reese*) . . . . . . | 70 | 7.0 | 3.0 | 3.0 | 45 | 140 | 0 |
| Eastern, wild: | | | | | | | |
| w/liquid, 4 oz. . . . . . . . | 78 | 8.0 | 4.4 | 2.8 | 62 | 127 | 0 |
| w/liquid, 1 cup . . . . . . | 170 | 17.5 | 9.7 | 6.1 | 136 | 277 | 0 |
| in teriyaki sauce | | | | | | | |
| (*Reese*), 2 oz. . . . . . . . | 70 | 8.0 | 6.0 | 2.0 | 65 | 370 | |
| **Oyster, smoked**, | | | | | | | |
| canned, 1 can, | | | | | | | |
| except as noted: | | | | | | | |
| in oil, drained: | | | | | | | |
| (*Brunswick* 3 oz.) . . . . | 150 | 12.0 | 7.0 | 8.0 | 40 | 240 | 0 |
| (*Bumble Bee*), 2 oz. . . | 110 | 11.0 | 2.0 | 6.0 | 70 | 160 | 0 |
| (*Chicken of the Sea* | | | | | | | |
| 3.75 oz.) . . . . . . . . . | 170 | 10.0 | 8.0 | 8.0 | 45 | 280 | 0 |
| (*Crown Prince* 3 oz.) . . | 170 | 14.0 | 8.0 | 9.0 | 60 | 280 | <1.0 |
| (*Reese*), 2 oz. . . . . . . . | 120 | 10.0 | 6.0 | 7.0 | 35 | 210 | 0 |
| (*Roland*), ⅓ cup . . . . . | 100 | 8.0 | 4.0 | 5.0 | 10 | 160 | 0 |
| in water, drained | | | | | | | |
| (*Reese*), 2 oz. . . . . . . . | 60 | 9.0 | 3.0 | 1.5 | 50 | 260 | 0 |
| **Oyster plant**, see | | | | | | | |
| "Salsify" | | | | | | | |

| Food and Measure | cal. | prot. (gms) | carbo. (gms) | fat (gms) | chol. (mgs) | sod. (mgs) | fiber (gms) |
|---|---|---|---|---|---|---|---|
| **Oyster sauce**, Asian: | | | | | | | |
| (*Kikkoman*), 1 tbsp. . . . . | 25 | 0 | 5.0 | 0 | 0 | 860 | 0 |
| (*Roland*), 1 tbsp. . . . . . . . | 10 | 0 | 3.0 | 0 | 0 | 460 | 0 |
| (*Tiger Tiger*), 2 tsp. . . . . . | 20 | 0 | 5.0 | 0 | 0 | 670 | 0 |
| vegetarian (*Roland*), | | | | | | | |
|   1 tbsp. . . . . . . . . . . . | 15 | 0 | 4.0 | 0 | 0 | 620 | 0 |
| **Oyster stew**, see | | | | | | | |
|   "Soup, condensed" | | | | | | | |

# P

| Food and Measure | cal. | prot. (gms) | carbo. (gms) | fat (gms) | chol. (mgs) | sod. (mgs) | fiber (gms) |
|---|---|---|---|---|---|---|---|
| **Pad Thai**, see "Noodle entree" | | | | | | | |
| **Pad Thai sauce**, see "Thai sauce" | | | | | | | |
| **Pad Thai seasoning** (*Kikkoman*), 2 tsp. . . . | 20 | 0 | 4.0 | 0 | 0 | 380 | 0 |
| **Paella entree**, frozen (*Contessa On the Stove*), ⅓ pkg.: | | | | | | | |
| w/sauce, 7.3 oz. . . . . . | 220 | 19.0 | 29.0 | 3.0 | 55 | 890 | 3.0 |
| w/out sauce . . . . . . . . | 200 | 18.0 | 26.0 | 3.0 | 55 | 350 | 3.0 |
| **Palm, hearts of,** can/jar, ½ cup: | | | | | | | |
| (*Roland*) . . . . . . . . . . . . | 25 | 2.0 | 4.0 | 0 | 0 | 450 | 2.0 |
| (*Roland* Organic) . . . . . . | 35 | 3.0 | 5.0 | 0 | 0 | 400 | 1.0 |
| marinated (*Roland*) . . . . . | 100 | 1.0 | 6.0 | 8.0 | 0 | 410 | 1.0 |
| **Pancake, frozen**, 3 pcs., except as noted: | | | | | | | |
| (*Aunt Jemima* Homestyle) | 240 | 5.0 | 41.0 | 6.0 | 30 | 500 | 1.0 |
| (*Aunt Jemima* Mini), 10 pcs. . . . . . . . . . . | 280 | 7.0 | 46.0 | 8.0 | 50 | 620 | 1.0 |
| (*Cinnabon* Original) . . . . . | 270 | 5.0 | 45.0 | 8.0 | 15 | 480 | 1.0 |
| (*Pillsbury* Original) . . . . . | 240 | 4.0 | 47.0 | 4.0 | 10 | 400 | 1.0 |
| (*Van's*), 2 pcs. . . . . . . . . | 170 | 4.0 | 34.0 | 2.0 | 5 | 300 | 1.0 |
| blueberry: | | | | | | | |
| (*Aunt Jemima*) . . . . . . | 250 | 6.0 | 43.0 | 6.0 | 25 | 470 | 1.0 |
| (*Eggo*) . . . . . . . . . . . . | 260 | 6.0 | 42.0 | 8.0 | 15 | 500 | 1.0 |
| buttermilk: | | | | | | | |
| (*Aunt Jemima*) . . . . . . | 240 | 6.0 | 41.0 | 6.0 | 30 | 490 | 1.0 |
| (*Aunt Jemima* Low Fat) | 200 | 5.0 | 39.0 | 3.0 | 25 | 460 | 1.0 |
| (*Eggo*) . . . . . . . . . . . . | 280 | 6.0 | 44.0 | 9.0 | 15 | 580 | 1.0 |
| (*Pillsbury*) . . . . . . . . . . | 240 | 4.0 | 47.0 | 4.0 | 10 | 400 | 1.0 |
| mini (*Eggo*), 11 pcs. . . | 260 | 5.0 | 42.0 | 8.0 | 10 | 550 | 1.0 |

| Food and Measure | cal. | prot. (gms) | carbo. (gms) | fat (gms) | chol. (mgs) | sod. (mgs) | fiber (gms) |
|---|---|---|---|---|---|---|---|
| mini (*Pillsbury*), 11 pcs. | 240 | 4.0 | 45.0 | 4.0 | 10 | 390 | 1.0 |
| caramel (*Cinnabon*) | 270 | 5.0 | 46.0 | 7.0 | 15 | 480 | 1.0 |
| chocolate chip (*Eggo*) | 270 | 6.0 | 42.0 | 9.0 | 15 | 490 | 1.0 |
| confetti (*Aunt Jemima*) | 260 | 5.0 | 43.0 | 6.0 | 25 | 490 | 1.0 |
| whole grain (*Aunt Jemima*) | 240 | 5.0 | 42.0 | 6.0 | 20 | 460 | 3.0 |
| **Pancake, mix**, ⅓ cup, except as noted: | | | | | | | |
| (*Arrowhead Mills Organic Gluten Free*), ¼ cup | 150 | 2.0 | 36.0 | 0 | 0 | 290 | 0 |
| (*Aunt Jemima Original*) | 150 | 4.0 | 33.0 | .5 | 0 | 470 | 1.0 |
| (*Aunt Jemima Original Complete*), 2 cakes* | 160 | 5.0 | 32.0 | 1.5 | 5 | 470 | 1.0 |
| (*Betty Crocker Original Complete*), 3 cakes* | 200 | 5.0 | 40.0 | 2.5 | 0 | 490 | <1.0 |
| (*Bob's Red Mill Gluten Free*) | 140 | 2.0 | 32.0 | .5 | 0 | 540 | 2.0 |
| (*Bob's Red Mill High Fiber Organic*) | 130 | 6.0 | 26.0 | 1.0 | 0 | 320 | 5.0 |
| (*Bisquick Gluten Free*) | 140 | 2.0 | 31.0 | .5 | 0 | 340 | <1.0 |
| (*Bisquick Heart Smart*) | 140 | 3.0 | 27.0 | 2.5 | 0 | 430 | 1.0 |
| (*Bisquick Original*) | 160 | 3.0 | 26.0 | 4.5 | 0 | 410 | 1.0 |
| (*Dr. Oetker Organics*) | 170 | 5.0 | 38.0 | 0 | 0 | 300 | 1.0 |
| (*Fiber One Complete*), 3 cakes* | 190 | 6.0 | 36.0 | 3.5 | 20 | 440 | 5.0 |
| (*Hungry Jack Extra Light/Fluffy*) | 150 | 4.0 | 31.0 | 1.5 | 0 | 570 | <1.0 |
| (*Hungry Jack Extra Light/Fluffy Complete*), 3 cakes* | 150 | 4.0 | 30.0 | 2.0 | 0 | 600 | <1.0 |
| (*Hungry Jack Original*) | 150 | 4.0 | 31.0 | 1.5 | 0 | 640 | <1.0 |
| blueberry, wheat (*Hungry Jack Complete*), 3 cakes* | 160 | 4.0 | 32.0 | 2.5 | 0 | 460 | 2.0 |
| buckwheat: (*Arrowhead Mills Organic*) | 170 | 7.0 | 29.0 | 2.0 | 0 | 290 | 7.0 |
| (*Bob's Red Mill*) | 140 | 6.0 | 26.0 | 1.0 | 0 | 320 | 6.0 |
| (*Hodgson Mill*) | 140 | 5.0 | 28.0 | 1.0 | 0 | 290 | 3.0 |
| buttermilk: (*Arrowhead Mills Organic*), ¼ cup | 140 | 6.0 | 27.0 | 1.0 | 5 | 340 | 2.0 |

| Food and Measure | cal. | prot. (gms) | carbo. (gms) | fat (gms) | chol. (mgs) | sod. (mgs) | fiber (gms) |
|---|---|---|---|---|---|---|---|
| **Pancake, mix, buttermilk** *(cont.)* | | | | | | | |
| (*Aunt Jemima*) ...... | 110 | 4.0 | 23.0 | .5 | 0 | 480 | 1.0 |
| (*Aunt Jemima* Complete), 3 cakes* | 160 | 5.0 | 31.0 | 2.0 | 10 | 460 | 1.0 |
| (*Bob's Red Mill*) ..... | 140 | 6.0 | 27.0 | .5 | 0 | 340 | 4.0 |
| (*Betty Crocker* Complete Box), 3 cakes* .... | 200 | 5.0 | 40.0 | 2.5 | 0 | 500 | <1.0 |
| (*Betty Crocker* Complete Pouch), 3 cakes* ......... | 210 | 6.0 | 37.0 | 4.0 | 25 | 780 | 1.0 |
| (*Bisquick Shake 'n Pour*), 3 cakes* ... | 220 | 6.0 | 42.0 | 3.0 | 0 | 800 | 1.0 |
| (*Fiber One* Complete), 3 cakes* ......... | 190 | 6.0 | 36.0 | 3.5 | 25 | 450 | 5.0 |
| (*Hungry Jack*) ....... | 150 | 4.0 | 31.0 | 1.5 | 0 | 630 | <1.0 |
| (*Hungry Jack* Complete), 3 cakes* | 150 | 4.0 | 31.0 | 1.5 | <5 | 550 | <1.0 |
| (*"Jiffy"* Complete) .... | 170 | 3.0 | 30.0 | 4.5 | <5 | 380 | <1.0 |
| apple cinnamon (*Arrowhead Mills* Organic), ¼ cup ... | 130 | 5.0 | 27.0 | .5 | 5 | 340 | 2.0 |
| multigrain, w/flax, soy (*Hodgson Mill*) | 150 | 10.0 | 31.0 | 2.0 | 0 | 321 | 5.0 |
| whole wheat (*Hodgson Mill*) ............. | 130 | 4.0 | 28.0 | 1.0 | 0 | 321 | 4.0 |
| cornmeal (*Bob's Red Mill* Organic) ........ | 130 | 4.0 | 28.0 | 1.0 | 0 | 320 | 4.0 |
| w/flax (*Hodgson Mill* Gluten Free) ........ | 140 | 4.0 | 30.0 | 2.0 | 0 | 200 | 3.0 |
| kamut (*Arrowhead Mills* Organic), ¼ cup . | 140 | 6.0 | 24.0 | 2.0 | 0 | 200 | 4.0 |
| multigrain: | | | | | | | |
| (*Arrowhead Mills* Organic), ¼ cup ... | 130 | 5.0 | 27.0 | 1.0 | 5 | 260 | 3.0 |
| 7 (*Bob's Red Mill* Organic) .......... | 130 | 5.0 | 27.0 | 1.0 | 5 | 320 | 4.0 |
| 10 (*Bob's Red Mill*), ½ cup ............ | 180 | 8.0 | 35.0 | 1.0 | 5 | 630 | 4.0 |
| chocolate chip (*Arrowhead Mills* Organic), ¼ cup ... | 140 | 4.0 | 26.0 | 2.5 | 5 | 240 | 3.0 |
| oat bran (*Arrowhead Mills* Organic), ¼ cup | 120 | 7.0 | 21.0 | 2.0 | 0 | 75 | 6.0 |
| oatmeal (*Quaker*) ...... | 150 | 5.0 | 31.0 | 2.0 | 0 | 360 | 4.0 |

| Food and Measure | cal. | prot. (gms) | carbo. (gms) | fat (gms) | chol. (mgs) | sod. (mgs) | fiber (gms) |
|---|---|---|---|---|---|---|---|
| wheat blends (*Hungry Jack*) . . . . . . . . . . . . . | 150 | 4.0 | 31.0 | 1.5 | 0 | 460 | 2.0 |
| whole wheat (*Aunt Jemima*), ¼ cup . . . . . | 120 | 4.0 | 26.0 | .5 | 0 | 620 | 3.0 |
| wild rice (*Arrowhead Mills* Organic), ¼ cup . | 130 | 6.0 | 28.0 | 1.0 | 0 | 70 | 2.0 |
| **Pancake breakfast**, frozen, and sausage: | | | | | | | |
| (*Aunt Jemima*), 6.8 oz. . . | 410 | 15.0 | 57.0 | 14.0 | 80 | 1030 | 1.0 |
| on a stick, 2.5-oz. pc.: | | | | | | | |
| (*Jimmy D's* Griddle Sticks) . . . . . . . . . . | 160 | 7.0 | 21.0 | 6.0 | 25 | 410 | 0 |
| (*Jimmy Dean*) . . . . . . . | 220 | 6.0 | 21.0 | 13.0 | 20 | 350 | 0 |
| blueberry cakes (*Jimmy Dean*) . . . . | 230 | 6.0 | 21.0 | 13.0 | 20 | 340 | 0 |
| stuffed, 3 pcs., 2.5 oz.: | | | | | | | |
| minis (*Jimmy Dean*) . . | 260 | 5.0 | 19.0 | 18.0 | 30 | 510 | 0 |
| minis, blueberry (*Jimmy Dean*) . . . . | 260 | 5.0 | 19.0 | 18.0 | 30 | 470 | 0 |
| w/syrup (*Jimmy Dean* Bowl), 8.6 oz. . . . . . . . | 710 | 12.0 | 91.0 | 34.0 | 65 | 1000 | 2.0 |
| **Pancake syrup**, ¼ cup: | | | | | | | |
| (*Aunt Jemima*) . . . . . . . . | 210 | 0 | 52.0 | 0 | 0 | 120 | 0 |
| (*Aunt Jemima* Country Rich) . . . . . . . . . . . . | 210 | 0 | 53.0 | 0 | 0 | 120 | 0 |
| (*Aunt Jemima* Country Rich Lite) . . . . . . . . . | 100 | 0 | 26.0 | 0 | 0 | 180 | 1.0 |
| (*Aunt Jemima* Lite) . . . . . | 100 | 0 | 26.0 | 0 | 0 | 190 | 1.0 |
| (*Eggo*) . . . . . . . . . . . . . . | 240 | 0 | 60.0 | 0 | 0 | 35 | 0 |
| (*Eggo* Lite) . . . . . . . . . . . | 110 | 0 | 27.0 | 0 | 0 | 180 | 0 |
| (*Hungry Jack*) . . . . . . . . | 210 | 0 | 53.0 | 0 | 0 | 140 | 0 |
| (*Hungry Jack* Lite) . . . . . | 100 | 0 | 24.0 | 0 | 0 | 180 | 0 |
| (*Hungry Jack* No Sugar) . | 20 | 0 | 8.0 | 0 | 0 | 140 | 0 |
| (*Smucker's* No Sugar) . . . | 20 | 0 | 8.0 | 0 | 0 | 150 | 0 |
| butter flavor: | | | | | | | |
| (*Aunt Jemima* Lite) . . . | 100 | 0 | 26.0 | 0 | 0 | 210 | 1.0 |
| (*Aunt Jemima* Rich) . . | 210 | 0 | 53.0 | 0 | 0 | 210 | 0 |
| (*Eggo* Buttery) . . . . . . | 160 | 0 | 41.0 | 0 | 0 | 90 | 0 |
| (*Hungry Jack*) . . . . . . . | 210 | 0 | 52.0 | 0 | 0 | 200 | 0 |
| **Pancetta**, see "Bacon, Italian" | | | | | | | |
| **Pancreas**, braised: | | | | | | | |
| beef, 4 oz. . . . . . . . . . . . | 307 | 30.7 | 0 | 19.5 | 297 | 68 | 0 |
| lamb, 4 oz. . . . . . . . . . . | 265 | 25.9 | 0 | 17.1 | 454 | 59 | 0 |

| Food and Measure | cal. | prot. (gms) | carbo. (gms) | fat (gms) | chol. (mgs) | sod. (mgs) | fiber (gms) |
|---|---|---|---|---|---|---|---|
| **Pancreas** *(cont.)* | | | | | | | |
| pork, 4 oz. | 248 | 32.3 | 0 | 12.2 | 357 | 48 | 0 |
| veal (calves), 4 oz. | 290 | 33.0 | 0 | 16.6 | n.a. | 77 | 0 |
| ***Panda Express:*** | | | | | | | |
| appetizers: | | | | | | | |
| chicken egg roll | 200 | 8.0 | 16.0 | 12.0 | 20 | 390 | 2.0 |
| chicken potstickers. | 220 | 7.0 | 23.0 | 11.0 | 20 | 280 | 1.0 |
| cream cheese Rangoon | 190 | 5.0 | 24.0 | 8.0 | 35 | 180 | 2.0 |
| veggie spring roll | 160 | 4.0 | 22.0 | 7.0 | 0 | 540 | 4.0 |
| soup: | | | | | | | |
| egg flower | 90 | 3.0 | 15.0 | 2.0 | 60 | 810 | 1.0 |
| hot and sour | 90 | 4.0 | 12.0 | 3.5 | 65 | 970 | 1.0 |
| rice and noodles: | | | | | | | |
| chow mein, 8.3 oz. | 400 | 12.0 | 61.0 | 12.0 | 0 | 1060 | 8.0 |
| fried rice, 10 oz. | 570 | 16.0 | 85.0 | 18.0 | 130 | 900 | 8.0 |
| steamed rice, 8.7 oz. | 420 | 8.0 | 93.0 | 0 | 0 | 0 | 0 |
| veggies: | | | | | | | |
| eggplant and tofu | 310 | 7.0 | 19.0 | 24.0 | 0 | 680 | 3.0 |
| mixed, entree, 8.6 oz. | 70 | 4.0 | 13.0 | .5 | 0 | 530 | 5.0 |
| mixed, side, 4.3 oz. | 35 | 2.0 | 7.0 | 0 | 0 | 260 | 3.0 |
| chicken: | | | | | | | |
| black pepper | 250 | 19.0 | 12.0 | 14.0 | 120 | 980 | 2.0 |
| broccoli | 180 | 13.0 | 11.0 | 9.0 | 65 | 670 | 3.0 |
| kung pao | 300 | 19.0 | 13.0 | 19.0 | 110 | 880 | 2.0 |
| mandarin | 310 | 34.0 | 8.0 | 16.0 | 115 | 740 | 0 |
| mushroom | 220 | 17.0 | 9.0 | 13.0 | 100 | 780 | 2.0 |
| orange | 400 | 15.0 | 42.0 | 20.0 | 90 | 640 | 0 |
| pineapple | 240 | 15.0 | 19.0 | 12.0 | 95 | 690 | 2.0 |
| potato | 220 | 11.0 | 19.0 | 11.0 | 60 | 810 | 3.0 |
| string bean | 190 | 12.0 | 11.0 | 10.0 | 75 | 760 | 2.0 |
| sweet & sour | 390 | 15.0 | 45.0 | 17.0 | 40 | 350 | 1.0 |
| chicken breast: | | | | | | | |
| pineapple | 220 | 17.0 | 20.0 | 8.0 | 45 | 640 | 1.0 |
| string bean | 170 | 15.0 | 13.0 | 7.0 | 35 | 760 | 2.0 |
| SweetFire | 440 | 17.0 | 53.0 | 18.0 | 45 | 370 | 1.0 |
| Thai cashew | 240 | 18.0 | 14.0 | 12.0 | 40 | 640 | 2.0 |
| beef: | | | | | | | |
| Beijing | 690 | 26.0 | 56.0 | 41.0 | 65 | 930 | 4.0 |
| broccoli | 130 | 10.0 | 13.0 | 4.0 | 15 | 740 | 3.0 |
| *Kobari* | 210 | 15.0 | 20.0 | 7.0 | 25 | 840 | 2.0 |
| Mongolian | 200 | 16.0 | 18.0 | 7.0 | 25 | 1000 | 2.0 |
| pork: | | | | | | | |
| BBQ | 360 | 34.0 | 13.0 | 19.0 | 120 | 1310 | 1.0 |
| sweet & sour | 450 | 14.0 | 40.0 | 26.0 | 35 | 400 | 3.0 |

| Food and Measure | cal. | prot. (gms) | carbo. (gms) | fat (gms) | chol. (mgs) | sod. (mgs) | fiber (gms) |
|---|---|---|---|---|---|---|---|
| shrimp: | | | | | | | |
| crispy ............ | 260 | 9.0 | 26.0 | 13.0 | 60 | 810 | 1.0 |
| honey walnut ....... | 370 | 14.0 | 27.0 | 23.0 | 110 | 470 | 2.0 |
| kung pao ......... | 250 | 14.0 | 14.0 | 15.0 | 115 | 880 | 2.0 |
| tangy ............ | 190 | 13.0 | 19.0 | 7.0 | 130 | 820 | 2.0 |
| sauces: | | | | | | | |
| mandarin .......... | 160 | 0 | 40.0 | 0 | 0 | 340 | 0 |
| sweet & sour ....... | 80 | 0 | 20.0 | 0 | 0 | 160 | 0 |
| fortune cookie, 1 pc. .... | 32 | 1.0 | 7.0 | 0 | 0 | 8 | 0 |
| *Panera Bread Café:* | | | | | | | |
| breakfast, egg soufflé: | | | | | | | |
| four cheese ......... | 480 | 16.0 | 36.0 | 29.0 | 195 | 700 | 2.0 |
| ham and Swiss ...... | 490 | 19.0 | 35.0 | 30.0 | 175 | 760 | 2.0 |
| spinach/artichoke .... | 540 | 19.0 | 38.0 | 34.0 | 165 | 910 | 2.0 |
| spinach/bacon ...... | 570 | 23.0 | 36.0 | 37.0 | 170 | 930 | 2.0 |
| breakfast sandwich: | | | | | | | |
| asiago bagel, egg/ | | | | | | | |
| cheese .......... | 480 | 23.0 | 54.0 | 18.0 | 200 | 800 | 2.0 |
| w/bacon ......... | 610 | 33.0 | 55.0 | 27.0 | 225 | 1250 | 2.0 |
| w/sausage ....... | 640 | 31.0 | 56.0 | 31.0 | 240 | 1130 | 2.0 |
| bacon/egg/cheese .... | 510 | 28.0 | 44.0 | 24.0 | 215 | 1060 | 2.0 |
| egg/cheese ......... | 380 | 18.0 | 43.0 | 14.0 | 190 | 620 | 2.0 |
| French toast bagel, | | | | | | | |
| sausage/egg/cheese | 660 | 27.0 | 69.0 | 30.0 | 230 | 1190 | 2.0 |
| jalapeño/cheddar | | | | | | | |
| bagel, egg/cheese . | 460 | 22.0 | 57.0 | 15.0 | 195 | 990 | 3.0 |
| w/bacon ......... | 590 | 32.0 | 58.0 | 25.0 | 220 | 1430 | 3.0 |
| w/ham .......... | 490 | 27.0 | 58.0 | 16.0 | 205 | 1290 | 3.0 |
| w/sausage ....... | 620 | 31.0 | 59.0 | 28.0 | 235 | 1310 | 3.0 |
| sausage/egg/cheese .. | 540 | 26.0 | 44.0 | 28.0 | 230 | 980 | 2.0 |
| power sandwich ..... | 330 | 22.0 | 31.0 | 14.0 | 200 | 830 | 4.0 |
| soup, full portion: | | | | | | | |
| black bean ......... | 170 | 10.0 | 29.0 | 4.0 | 0 | 1590 | 5.0 |
| broccoli cheddar ..... | 290 | 12.0 | 24.0 | 16.0 | 30 | 1540 | 7.0 |
| chicken, cream of, | | | | | | | |
| and wild rice ..... | 310 | 10.0 | 29.0 | 17.0 | 60 | 1470 | 3.0 |
| chicken noodle ...... | 140 | 5.0 | 23.0 | 3.0 | 30 | 1450 | 0 |
| clam chowder ....... | 450 | 8.0 | 29.0 | 34.0 | 50 | 1190 | 3.0 |
| onion, French, | | | | | | | |
| w/croutons ....... | 250 | 10.0 | 30.0 | 11.0 | 25 | 2380 | 3.0 |
| mac & cheese, small . | 490 | 17.0 | 37.0 | 30.0 | 55 | 1020 | 1.0 |
| mac & cheese, large .. | 980 | 33.0 | 75.0 | 61.0 | 110 | 2030 | 3.0 |
| potato, baked ....... | 350 | 9.0 | 33.0 | 21.0 | 70 | 1180 | 3.0 |
| tomato, w/croutons .. | 370 | 4.0 | 39.0 | 23.0 | 15 | 740 | 5.0 |

| Food and Measure | cal. | prot. (gms) | carbo. (gms) | fat (gms) | chol. (mgs) | sod. (mgs) | fiber (gms) |
|---|---|---|---|---|---|---|---|
| **Panera Bread Café**, soup *(cont.)* | | | | | | | |
| steak chili, w/ | | | | | | | |
| cornbread . . . . . . . . | 580 | 29.0 | 58.0 | 26.0 | 100 | 1330 | 7.0 |
| vegetable, w/pesto . . . | 160 | 5.0 | 28.0 | 3.5 | 0 | 1240 | 6.0 |
| sandwich, whole: | | | | | | | |
| asiago roast beef . . . . | 690 | 48.0 | 64.0 | 27.0 | 115 | 1270 | 3.0 |
| *Bacon Turkey Bravo* . . | 830 | 53.0 | 88.0 | 29.0 | 95 | 3010 | 4.0 |
| chicken Caesar . . . . . . | 720 | 43.0 | 69.0 | 32.0 | 130 | 1270 | 4.0 |
| chicken salad, Napa | | | | | | | |
| almond . . . . . . . . . . | 690 | 29.0 | 90.0 | 26.0 | 60 | 1200 | 5.0 |
| chipotle chicken . . . . . | 840 | 53.0 | 73.0 | 38.0 | 140 | 2170 | 4.0 |
| ham and Swiss . . . . . . | 590 | 45.0 | 64.0 | 17.0 | 90 | 2250 | 5.0 |
| Italian combo . . . . . . . | 990 | 59.0 | 95.0 | 40.0 | 150 | 2840 | 5.0 |
| Mediterranean veggie . | 610 | 22.0 | 100.0 | 13.0 | 10 | 1450 | 10.0 |
| tuna salad . . . . . . . . . . | 470 | 19.0 | 65.0 | 16.0 | 25 | 980 | 5.0 |
| turkey, Sierra . . . . . . . | 970 | 41.0 | 82.0 | 51.0 | 85 | 2050 | 4.0 |
| turkey, smoked . . . . . . | 440 | 34.0 | 68.0 | 2.5 | 50 | 1860 | 3.0 |
| sandwich, hot panini: | | | | | | | |
| Cuban chicken . . . . . . | 870 | 47.0 | 88.0 | 37.0 | 95 | 1890 | 4.0 |
| *Frontago Chicken* . . . . | 860 | 46.0 | 80.0 | 39.0 | 100 | 2150 | 4.0 |
| tomato mozzarella . . . | 770 | 30.0 | 96.0 | 29.0 | 35 | 1290 | 6.0 |
| *Smokehouse Turkey* . . | 720 | 53.0 | 67.0 | 26.0 | 115 | 2540 | 4.0 |
| turkey artichoke . . . . . | 750 | 42.0 | 90.0 | 24.0 | 85 | 2420 | 7.0 |
| salad, full portion: | | | | | | | |
| Caesar . . . . . . . . . . . . | 390 | 12.0 | 25.0 | 27.0 | 50 | 610 | 3.0 |
| Caesar, chicken . . . . . . | 510 | 37.0 | 29.0 | 29.0 | 115 | 820 | 3.0 |
| chicken, Asian sesame | 400 | 31.0 | 31.0 | 20.0 | 60 | 810 | 3.0 |
| chicken, BBQ . . . . . . . | 500 | 31.0 | 50.0 | 22.0 | 75 | 770 | 6.0 |
| chicken, Fuji apple . . . | 520 | 32.0 | 36.0 | 31.0 | 80 | 830 | 5.0 |
| classic café . . . . . . . . . | 170 | 2.0 | 18.0 | 11.0 | 0 | 270 | 4.0 |
| cobb, chicken . . . . . . . | 500 | 38.0 | 11.0 | 36.0 | 140 | 1120 | 3.0 |
| Greek . . . . . . . . . . . . . | 380 | 8.0 | 14.0 | 34.0 | 20 | 1670 | 5.0 |
| Thai chopped chicken . | 390 | 34.0 | 36.0 | 15.0 | 60 | 1380 | 5.0 |
| sides: | | | | | | | |
| apple . . . . . . . . . . . . . | 80 | 0 | 21.0 | 0 | 0 | 0 | 4.0 |
| baguette . . . . . . . . . . . | 180 | 6.0 | 36.0 | 1.0 | 0 | 440 | 1.0 |
| baguette, whole grain . | 180 | 7.0 | 36.0 | 1.5 | 0 | 400 | 4.0 |
| chips, *Lay's* baked . . . | 130 | 2.0 | 26.0 | 2.0 | 0 | 200 | 2.0 |
| chips, *Panera's* . . . . . . | 160 | 2.0 | 19.0 | 8.0 | 0 | 130 | 2.0 |
| fruit cup, 5 oz. . . . . . . . . | 60 | 1.0 | 16.0 | 0 | 0 | 15 | 1.0 |
| drinks, frozen: | | | | | | | |
| caramel, grande . . . . . | 600 | 5.0 | 97.0 | 22.0 | 60 | 170 | 0 |
| mango, grande . . . . . . | 330 | 2.0 | 61.0 | 10.0 | 20 | 20 | 2.0 |
| mocha, grande . . . . . . | 570 | 7.0 | 92.0 | 21.0 | 50 | 140 | 2.0 |

| Food and Measure | cal. | prot. (gms) | carbo. (gms) | fat (gms) | chol. (mgs) | sod. (mgs) | fiber (gms) |
|---|---|---|---|---|---|---|---|
| smoothie, low fat: | | | | | | | |
| black cherry ...... | 290 | 6.0 | 63.0 | 1.5 | 5 | 90 | 2.0 |
| mango .......... | 230 | 6.0 | 51.0 | 1.5 | 5 | 90 | 2.0 |
| strawberry ginseng | 260 | 6.0 | 59.0 | 1.5 | 5 | 90 | 2.0 |
| wild berry ........ | 290 | 6.0 | 67.0 | 1.5 | 5 | 90 | 1.0 |
| drinks, hot/espresso: | | | | | | | |
| caffee latte ........ | 120 | 8.0 | 11.0 | 4.5 | 20 | 95 | 0 |
| caffee mocha ....... | 380 | 11.0 | 49.0 | 17.0 | 40 | 160 | 2.0 |
| cappuccino ......... | 120 | 8.0 | 11.0 | 4.5 | 20 | 95 | 0 |
| caramel latte ........ | 420 | 10.0 | 53.0 | 18.0 | 50 | 190 | 0 |
| chai tea latte ........ | 200 | 7.0 | 32.0 | 4.5 | 15 | 85 | 0 |
| hot chocolate ....... | 380 | 11.0 | 48.0 | 17.0 | 40 | 160 | 2.0 |
| **Pangasius**, striped, frozen, raw (*Seamazz Swai*), 4 oz. ......... | 100 | 20.0 | 0 | 3.0 | 35 | 200 | 0 |
| **Panini**, frozen, 6 oz., except as noted: | | | | | | | |
| breakfast (*Lean Cuisine*), 5 oz.: | | | | | | | |
| Denver style ........ | 280 | 14.0 | 38.0 | 8.0 | 15 | 500 | 5.0 |
| sausage/egg/cheese .. | 290 | 14.0 | 44.0 | 6.0 | 10 | 450 | 5.0 |
| cheese, 3, and ham (*Stouffer's Corner Bistro*) ............ | 420 | 22.0 | 42.0 | 18.0 | 60 | 940 | 4.0 |
| chicken: | | | | | | | |
| club (*Lean Cuisine*) ... | 360 | 24.0 | 46.0 | 9.0 | 40 | 740 | 4.0 |
| mesquite (*Stouffer's Corner Bistro*) .... | 370 | 19.0 | 41.0 | 14.0 | 60 | 670 | 4.0 |
| Southwest (*Lean Cuisine*) ......... | 320 | 20.0 | 41.0 | 8.0 | 50 | 570 | 4.0 |
| Southwest (*Stouffer's Corner Bistro*) .... | 400 | 16.0 | 42.0 | 18.0 | 35 | 790 | 4.0 |
| spinach, mushroom (*Lean Cuisine*) .... | 310 | 22.0 | 42.0 | 7.0 | 30 | 600 | 5.0 |
| Philly cheesesteak (*Lean Cuisine*) ...... | 320 | 21.0 | 42.0 | 9.0 | 30 | 540 | 4.0 |
| spinach/artichoke/ chicken (*Lean Cuisine*) | 310 | 18.0 | 40.0 | 9.0 | 30 | 660 | 4.0 |
| steak/cheddar/mushroom (*Lean Cuisine*) ...... | 340 | 20.0 | 43.0 | 9.0 | 30 | 640 | 4.0 |
| turkey, smoked, club (*Stouffer's Corner Bistro*) ............ | 380 | 24.0 | 37.0 | 15.0 | 55 | 670 | 4.0 |

| Food and Measure | cal. | prot. (gms) | carbo. (gms) | fat (gms) | chol. (mgs) | sod. (mgs) | fiber (gms) |
|---|---|---|---|---|---|---|---|
| **Panko coating mix** (*McCormick Crusting Blends*), 1⅓ tbsp.: | | | | | | | |
| garlic/lemon/rosemary .. | 45 | 3.0 | 7.0 | 0 | 0 | 400 | 2.0 |
| Italian herb/cheese ..... | 40 | 3.0 | 5.0 | 1.0 | 5 | 390 | 1.0 |
| onion/pepper/herb ..... | 45 | 4.0 | 7.0 | 0 | 0 | 390 | 2.0 |
| **Panko crumbs**, see "Bread crumbs" | | | | | | | |
| **Pappadum** (*Devya Organic*), 3.5-oz. pkg.: | | | | | | | |
| plain ............. | 321 | 16.7 | 61.9 | .8 | 0 | 1638 | 4.5 |
| cumin or garlic ........ | 280 | 7.0 | 55.0 | 3.7 | 0 | 1550 | 10.0 |
| spicy .............. | 320 | 16.7 | 60.4 | 1.3 | 0 | 1902 | 4.5 |
| **Papaya**, fresh: | | | | | | | |
| (*Dole*), ½ pc., 5 oz. ..... | 60 | <1.0 | 15.0 | 0 | 0 | 5 | 3.0 |
| (*Frieda's* Golden Sunrise/Mexican), 1 cup, 5 oz. ....... | 50 | 1.0 | 14.0 | 0 | 0 | 0 | 3.0 |
| 1 lb., 3½" x 5⅛" ........ | 117 | 1.9 | 29.8 | .4 | 0 | 8 | 5.5 |
| cubed, 1 cup ......... | 55 | .9 | 13.7 | .2 | 0 | 4 | 2.5 |
| mashed, 1 cup ........ | 90 | 1.4 | 22.6 | .3 | 0 | 7 | 4.1 |
| **Papaya, can/jar**, ½ cup: | | | | | | | |
| in extra light syrup (*Del Monte SunFresh*) | 70 | 1.0 | 17.0 | 0 | 0 | 5 | 1.0 |
| in light syrup (*Roland*) .. | 70 | 0 | 18.0 | 0 | 0 | 10 | 1.0 |
| **Papaya juice**, 8 fl. oz.: | | | | | | | |
| (*Ceres*). .............. | 120 | 0 | 31.0 | 0 | 0 | 15 | 0 |
| (*R.W. Knudsen* Nectar) .. | 130 | <1.0 | 31.0 | 0 | 0 | 35 | 0 |
| **Papaya nectar**, canned, 8 fl. oz. ............ | 143 | .4 | 36.3 | .4 | 0 | 12 | 1.5 |
| **Paprika**, 1 tsp. ........ | 6 | .3 | 1.2 | .3 | 0 | 1 | .6 |
| **Parsley**, fresh: | | | | | | | |
| 10 sprigs ............. | 4 | .3 | .6 | .1 | 0 | 6 | .3 |
| chopped, ½ cup ....... | 11 | .9 | 1.9 | .2 | 0 | 17 | 1.0 |
| **Parsley, dried**: | | | | | | | |
| 1 tsp. ............... | 1 | .1 | .2 | .1 | 0 | 1 | .2 |
| freeze-dried, 1 tbsp. .... | 1 | .1 | .2 | <.1 | 0 | 2 | .2 |
| **Parsley root**, 1 oz. ..... | 3 | .8 | .7 | .2 | 0 | 28 | .4 |
| **Parsnip**: | | | | | | | |
| raw, sliced: | | | | | | | |
| (*Frieda's*), 1 cup ..... | 100 | 2.0 | 24.0 | 0 | 0 | 10 | 7.0 |
| ½ cup ............. | 50 | .8 | 12.1 | .2 | 0 | 7 | 3.3 |

| Food and Measure | cal. | prot. (gms) | carbo. (gms) | fat (gms) | chol. (mgs) | sod. (mgs) | fiber (gms) |
|---|---|---|---|---|---|---|---|
| boiled, drained: | | | | | | | |
| 1 medium, 9" ....... | 130 | 2.1 | 31.3 | .5 | 0 | 17 | 6.4 |
| sliced, ½ cup ....... | 63 | 1.0 | 15.2 | .2 | 0 | 8 | 3.1 |
| **Passion fruit**, fresh: | | | | | | | |
| (*Frieda's*), 5 oz. ........ | 140 | 3.0 | 33.0 | 1.0 | 0 | 40 | 15.0 |
| purple, 1 medium ...... | 18 | .4 | 4.2 | .1 | 0 | 5 | 1.9 |
| purple, trimmed, ½ cup . | 115 | .3 | 27.5 | .8 | 0 | 33 | 12.2 |
| **Passion fruit drink blend**, citrus (*SoBe Lifewater*), 8 fl. oz. ... | 40 | 0 | 17.0 | 0 | 0 | 20 | 0 |
| **Passion fruit juice**, 8 fl. oz.: | | | | | | | |
| (*Ceres*) ............. | 130 | 0 | 32.0 | 0 | 0 | 15 | 0 |
| (*Santa Cruz Organic* Nectar) ............ | 150 | 1.0 | 40.0 | 0 | 0 | 15 | 0 |
| fresh, purple .......... | 126 | 1.0 | 33.6 | .1 | 0 | 15 | .5 |
| fresh, yellow .......... | 148 | 1.7 | 35.7 | .4 | 0 | 15 | .5 |
| **Passion fruit juice blend**, 8 fl. oz.: | | | | | | | |
| orange guava (*Bolthouse Farms*) ............ | 150 | 1.0 | 35.0 | 0 | 0 | 15 | 0 |
| tangerine (*V8 V-Fusion*) . | 110 | 0 | 27.0 | 0 | 0 | 115 | 0 |
| **Pasta** (see also "Macaroni" and "Noodles"), dry, 2 oz., except as noted: | | | | | | | |
| plain ................ | 211 | 7.3 | 42.6 | .9 | 0 | 4 | 1.4 |
| all styles: | | | | | | | |
| (*Alessi*) ............ | 210 | 6.0 | 44.0 | 1.0 | 0 | 0 | 2.0 |
| (*Barilla Piccolini*) .... | 200 | 7.0 | 42.0 | 1.0 | 0 | 0 | 2.0 |
| (*Barilla Plus*) ........ | 210 | 10.0 | 38.0 | 2.0 | 0 | 25 | 4.0 |
| (*Delverde*) .......... | 200 | 7.0 | 41.0 | .5 | 0 | 0 | 1.0 |
| (*De Boles* Artichoke) .. | 210 | 7.0 | 41.0 | 1.0 | 0 | 0 | 1.0 |
| (*VitaSpelt* White) .... | 210 | 9.0 | 42.0 | .5 | 0 | 0 | 2.0 |
| (*VitaSpelt* Whole Grain) ............ | 190 | 8.0 | 40.0 | 1.5 | 0 | 0 | 5.0 |
| all styles, except: | | | | | | | |
| angel hair w/flax (*DeBoles* Gluten Free Rice) ........ | 210 | 4.0 | 46.0 | .5 | 0 | 15 | <1.0 |
| angel hair w/flax (*DeBoles* Organic Whole Wheat) .... | 210 | 7.0 | 42.0 | 1.5 | 0 | 10 | 5.0 |

| Food and Measure | cal. | prot. (gms) | carbo. (gms) | fat (gms) | chol. (mgs) | sod. (mgs) | fiber (gms) |
|---|---|---|---|---|---|---|---|
| **Pasta, all styles, except** *(cont.)* | | | | | | | |
| egg fettuccine (*Ronzoni*) . . . . . . . . | 210 | 7.0 | 42.0 | 1.0 | 0 | 0 | 2.0 |
| lasagna and penne (*DeBoles* Organic Artichoke) . . . . . . . | 210 | 7.0 | 43.0 | 1.0 | 0 | 5 | 1.0 |
| lasagna and whole grain (*Barilla* Blue Box) . . . . . . . . . . | 200 | 7.0 | 42.0 | 1.0 | 0 | 0 | 2.0 |
| whole grain (*Barilla*) . . | 200 | 7.0 | 41.0 | 1.5 | 0 | 0 | 6.0 |
| alphabets, vegetable (*Eden* Organic) . . . . . . | 210 | 9.0 | 40.0 | 2.0 | 0 | 20 | 4.0 |
| angel hair w/flax (*DeBoles*): | | | | | | | |
| gluten free rice . . . . . . | 210 | 4.0 | 44.0 | 1.5 | 0 | 10 | 1.0 |
| organic whole wheat . . | 190 | 6.0 | 38.0 | 1.5 | 0 | 10 | 6.0 |
| capellini (*Vigo*) . . . . . . . . | 210 | 7.0 | 44.0 | 1.0 | 0 | 0 | 2.0 |
| corn, elbow or spaghetti (*DeBoles*) . . | 200 | 4.0 | 43.0 | 2.0 | 0 | 15 | 5.0 |
| ditalini, kamut (*Eden* Organic) . . . . . . | 210 | 10.0 | 38.0 | 1.5 | 0 | 0 | 6.0 |
| fettuccine: | | | | | | | |
| (*Vigo*) . . . . . . . . . . . . . | 210 | 7.0 | 42.0 | 1.0 | 0 | 0 | 2.0 |
| egg (*Ronzoni*) . . . . . . . | 210 | 8.0 | 40.0 | 2.5 | 70 | 15 | 2.0 |
| gemelli, spelt and buckwheat (*Eden* Organic) . . . . . . . . . . | 210 | 6.0 | 41.0 | 2.0 | 0 | 15 | 4.0 |
| kamut/quinoa (*Eden* *Twisted Pair* Organic) . | 210 | 8.0 | 40.0 | 2.0 | 0 | 0 | 5.0 |
| kuzu (Eden) . . . . . . . . . . | 200 | 0 | 48.0 | 0 | 0 | 0 | 2.0 |
| lasagna: | | | | | | | |
| (*Barilla*), 2 pcs. . . . . . . | 180 | 6.0 | 38.0 | 1.0 · | 0 | 0 | 2.0 |
| (*DeBoles* Gluten Free Rice), 2.5 oz. . . . . . | 260 | 5.0 | 54.0 | .5 | 0 | 15 | 1.0 |
| (*DeBoles* Organic Artichoke), 2.5 oz. . | 260 | 9.0 | 54.0 | 1.0 | 0 | 5 | 1.0 |
| oven ready (*Barilla*), 3 pcs. . . . . . . . . . . | 190 | 6.0 | 38.0 | 1.5 | 15 | 10 | 2.0 |
| precooked (*Vigo*), 3 pcs. . . . . . . . . . . | 200 | 8.0 | 40.0 | .5 | 0 | 0 | 2.0 |
| linguine (*Vigo*) . . . . . . . . | 210 | 7.0 | 44.0 | 1.0 | 0 | 0 | 2.0 |
| mung bean (*Eden* Harusame) . . . . . . . . . | 190 | 0 | 47.0 | 0 | 0 | 5 | 0 |

| Food and Measure | cal. | prot. (gms) | carbo. (gms) | fat (gms) | chol. (mgs) | sod. (mgs) | fiber (gms) |
|---|---|---|---|---|---|---|---|
| orzo: | | | | | | | |
|   (*RiceSelect* Original) .. | 210 | 7.0 | 42.0 | 1.0 | 0 | 0 | 2.0 |
|   Greek (*Roland*), | | | | | | | |
|     4 tbsp., 2.7 oz. .... | 250 | 6.0 | 54.0 | 0 | 0 | 0 | 7.0 |
|   tri-color (*RiceSelect*) . | 210 | 7.0 | 42.0 | 1.0 | 0 | 20 | 2.0 |
|   whole wheat | | | | | | | |
|     (*RiceSelect*) ...... | 195 | 7.0 | 39.0 | 1.0 | 0 | 0 | 9.0 |
| penne: | | | | | | | |
|   (*DeBoles* Gluten Free | | | | | | | |
|     Multi Grain) ...... | 200 | 5.0 | 46.0 | 1.5 | 0 | 0 | 3.0 |
|   (*DeBoles* Organic | | | | | | | |
|     Artichoke) ....... | 210 | 7.0 | 41.0 | 1.0 | 0 | 0 | 1.0 |
|   whole wheat | | | | | | | |
|     (*Hodgson Mill*) .... | 210 | 9.0 | 40.0 | 1.0 | 0 | 10 | 6.0 |
| penne or rigatoni | | | | | | | |
|   (*Vigo*) ............. | 210 | 7.0 | 44.0 | 1.0 | 0 | 0 | 2.0 |
| ribbons: | | | | | | | |
|   artichoke (*Eden* | | | | | | | |
|     Organic) ......... | 210 | 9.0 | 40.0 | 1.5 | 0 | 10 | 2.0 |
|   parsley garlic, | | | | | | | |
|     saffron, or vegetable | | | | | | | |
|     (*Eden* Organic) .... | 210 | 9.0 | 40.0 | 1.5 | 0 | 0 | 3.0 |
|   spelt (*Eden* Organic) .. | 210 | 7.0 | 41.0 | 2.0 | 0 | 10 | 5.0 |
|   spinach (*Eden* | | | | | | | |
|     Organic) ......... | 210 | 8.0 | 41.0 | 1.0 | 0 | 30 | 5.0 |
| rice (*Eden* Bifun) ....... | 200 | 5.0 | 44.0 | .5 | 0 | 5 | 0 |
| rice, brown, all styles: | | | | | | | |
|   (*Lundberg* Organic) .. | 190 | 4.0 | 40.0 | 3.0 | 0 | 0 | 4.0 |
|   w/flax (*Hodgson Mill*) . | 190 | 4.0 | 40.0 | 3.0 | 0 | 0 | 4.0 |
| rigatoni, kamut and | | | | | | | |
|   buckwheat (*Eden* | | | | | | | |
|     Organic) .......... | 200 | 9.0 | 39.0 | 1.5 | 0 | 10 | 5.0 |
| shells, vegetable: | | | | | | | |
|   (*Eden* Organic) ...... | 200 | 8.0 | 40.0 | 1.0 | 0 | 0 | 2.0 |
|   small (*Eden* Organic) . | 210 | 9.0 | 40.0 | 2.0 | 0 | 20 | 4.0 |
| spaghetti (*Eden* Organic): | | | | | | | |
|   100% whole grain ... | 210 | 10.0 | 40.0 | 1.5 | 0 | 0 | 6.0 |
|   kamut ............. | 210 | 10.0 | 38.0 | 1.5 | 0 | 0 | 6.0 |
|   parsley garlic ...... | 210 | 8.0 | 41.0 | 1.0 | 0 | 0 | 5.0 |
|   spelt ............. | 210 | 7.0 | 41.0 | 2.0 | 0 | 10 | 5.0 |
| spirals (*Eden* Organic): | | | | | | | |
|   flax rice ........... | 200 | 9.0 | 40.0 | 2.0 | 0 | 10 | 4.0 |
|   kamut ............. | 210 | 10.0 | 38.0 | 1.5 | 0 | 0 | 6.0 |
|   kamut vegetable ..... | 210 | 8.0 | 40.0 | 2.0 | 0 | 45 | 6.0 |

| Food and Measure | cal. | prot. (gms) | carbo. (gms) | fat (gms) | chol. (mgs) | sod. (mgs) | fiber (gms) |
|---|---|---|---|---|---|---|---|
| **Pasta, spirals** (cont.) | | | | | | | |
| rye | 200 | 6.0 | 44.0 | 0 | 0 | 10 | 8.0 |
| spinach | 210 | 8.0 | 41.0 | 1.0 | 0 | 30 | 5.0 |
| vegetable | 200 | 8.0 | 40.0 | 1.0 | 0 | 0 | 2.0 |
| ziti rigati, spelt (*Eden* Organic) | 210 | 7.0 | 41.0 | 2.0 | 0 | 10 | 5.0 |
| **Pasta, cooked** (see also "Macaroni"): | | | | | | | |
| corn, 1 cup | 176 | 3.7 | 39.1 | 1.0 | 0 | 1 | 3.4 |
| spaghetti, 1 cup: | | | | | | | |
| plain | 197 | 6.7 | 39.7 | .9 | 0 | 1 | 2.4 |
| protein fortified | 230 | 11.3 | 44.3 | .3 | 0 | 7 | 2.4 |
| spinach | 182 | 6.4 | 36.6 | .9 | 0 | 20 | n.a. |
| whole wheat | 174 | 7.5 | 37.2 | .6 | 0 | 4 | 6.3 |
| **Pasta, chilled**: | | | | | | | |
| (*Buitoni*), 1¼ cups: | | | | | | | |
| angel hair | 230 | 10.0 | 43.0 | 2.5 | 45 | 20 | 2.0 |
| fettuccine | 260 | 12.0 | 46.0 | 3.0 | 70 | 90 | 2.0 |
| linguine | 240 | 10.0 | 45.0 | 2.5 | 50 | 20 | 2.0 |
| linguine, whole wheat | 240 | 13.0 | 41.0 | 3.0 | 50 | 250 | 6.0 |
| all styles, dry: | | | | | | | |
| w/egg, 2 oz. | 163 | 6.4 | 31.0 | 1.3 | 41 | 15 | 2.0 |
| spinach, w/egg, 2 oz. | 164 | 6.4 | 31.6 | 1.2 | 41 | 15 | n.a. |
| all styles, cooked: | | | | | | | |
| w/egg, 4 oz. | 149 | 5.8 | 28.3 | 1.2 | 37 | 7 | n.a. |
| spinach, w/egg, 4 oz. | 147 | 5.7 | 28.4 | 1.1 | 37 | 7 | n.a. |
| **Pasta dish, frozen** (see also "Pasta entree, frozen" and specific pastas): | | | | | | | |
| broccoli, Alfredo sauce (*Green Giant*), 1 cup* | 220 | 9.0 | 38.0 | 4.0 | 5 | 710 | 3.0 |
| broccoli, carrots: | | | | | | | |
| cheese sauce (*Green Giant*), 1 cup* | 200 | 8.0 | 36.0 | 3.5 | 0 | 880 | 3.0 |
| sugar snaps, garlic sauce (*Green Giant*), 1 cup* | 210 | 7.0 | 37.0 | 4.0 | 0 | 700 | 3.0 |
| cheddar (*Freshlike Combos*), 2 cups | 200 | 6.0 | 24.0 | 9.0 | 10 | 500 | 2.0 |
| garlic herb (*Freshlike Combos*), 2 cups | 250 | 6.0 | 32.0 | 10.0 | 50 | 310 | 2.0 |

| Food and Measure | cal. | prot. (gms) | carbo. (gms) | fat (gms) | chol. (mgs) | sod. (mgs) | fiber (gms) |
|---|---|---|---|---|---|---|---|
| vegetables, cheese sauce (*Birds Eye*), ½ cup .... | 160 | 5.0 | 26.0 | 3.5 | 5 | 590 | 2.0 |
| **Pasta dish mix** (see also "Pasta salad mix" and specific pastas), 1 cup*, except as noted: | | | | | | | |
| Alfredo: | | | | | | | |
| (*Zatarain's* Dinner) ... | 140 | 5.0 | 22.0 | 3.5 | 5 | 760 | <1.0 |
| whole wheat (*Annie's D.W.*) ........... | 270 | 11.0 | 49.0 | 4.0 | 10 | 560 | 5.0 |
| butter and (*Pasta Roni*): | | | | | | | |
| herb, Italiano ....... | 300 | 9.0 | 41.0 | 11.0 | 5 | 780 | 2.0 |
| garlic ............. | 250 | 8.0 | 39.0 | 8.0 | 5 | 690 | 2.0 |
| cheddar: | | | | | | | |
| rice pasta (*Annie's* Deluxe) .......... | 320 | 8.0 | 63.0 | 4.0 | 10 | 680 | 2.0 |
| rice pasta (*Annie's* Gluten Free) ...... | 280 | 7.0 | 53.0 | 4.0 | 10 | 400 | 1.0 |
| white, and broccoli (*Pasta Roni*) ...... | 300 | 9.0 | 39.0 | 13.0 | 5 | 710 | 2.0 |
| cheddar and Parmesan (*Annie's* Organic Peace Pasta) ........ | 270 | 11.0 | 48.0 | 3.5 | 10 | 620 | 2.0 |
| chicken: | | | | | | | |
| (*Pasta Roni*) ........ | 300 | 9.0 | 40.0 | 12.0 | 5 | 960 | 2.0 |
| broccoli (*Pasta Roni*) . | 360 | 10.0 | 49.0 | 15.0 | 5 | 870 | 3.0 |
| garlic: | | | | | | | |
| Alfredo (*Pasta Roni*) .. | 350 | 11.0 | 48.0 | 13.0 | 10 | 1000 | 2.0 |
| creamy (*Pasta Roni*) .. | 330 | 9.0 | 40.0 | 16.0 | 5 | 810 | 2.0 |
| gumbo (*Zatarain's* Dinner) ............ | 120 | 4.0 | 23.0 | .5 | 0 | 690 | 2.0 |
| jambalaya (*Zatarain's* Dinner) ............ | 140 | 5.0 | 28.0 | 1.0 | 0 | 540 | 2.0 |
| mushrooms, cream sauce (*Pasta Roni Nature's Way*) ....... | 280 | 9.0 | 41.0 | 9.0 | 5 | 590 | 3.0 |
| olive oil, Italian herb (*Pasta Roni Nature's Way*) .............. | 250 | 8.0 | 38.0 | 8.0 | 5 | 700 | 2.0 |
| Parmesan: | | | | | | | |
| (*Pasta Roni*) ........ | 310 | 9.0 | 39.0 | 13.0 | 5 | 800 | 2.0 |
| creamy (*Pasta Roni Nature's Way*) ...... | 270 | 9.0 | 43.0 | 7.0 | 5 | 430 | 3.0 |

| Food and Measure | cal. | prot. (gms) | carbo. (gms) | fat (gms) | chol. (mgs) | sod. (mgs) | fiber (gms) |
|---|---|---|---|---|---|---|---|
| **Pasta dish mix** *(cont.)* | | | | | | | |
| scampi (*Zatarain's* Dinner Mix) ......... | 110 | 4.0 | 21.0 | .5 | 0 | 470 | 1.0 |
| sour cream/chives (*Pasta Roni*) ........ | 310 | 8.0 | 38.0 | 14.0 | 5 | 800 | 2.0 |
| Stroganoff (*Pasta Roni*) ............. | 350 | 12.0 | 48.0 | 13.0 | 10 | 910 | 2.0 |
| tomato Parmesan (*Pasta Roni*) ........ | 270 | 10.0 | 40.0 | 9.0 | 5 | 840 | 2.0 |
| **Pasta entree, canned** | | | | | | | |
| (see also specific pastas), 1 cup: | | | | | | | |
| (*SpaghettiOs/ SpaghettiOs* A to Zs) . | 170 | 6.0 | 35.0 | 1.0 | 5 | 600 | 3.0 |
| (*SpaghettiOs* Plus Calcium) ........... | 170 | 6.0 | 35.0 | 1.0 | 5 | 600 | 3.0 |
| w/franks (*SpaghettiOs*) .. | 220 | 9.0 | 32.0 | 6.0 | 20 | 600 | 4.0 |
| w/meatballs: | | | | | | | |
| all varieties (*SpaghettiOs*) ..... | 240 | 11.0 | 32.0 | 7.0 | 20 | 600 | 4.0 |
| soy "meatballs" (*Annie's P'Sghetti Loops* Organic) ... | 190 | 9.0 | 29.0 | 4.0 | 0 | 650 | 2.0 |
| tomato cheese sauce: | | | | | | | |
| (*Annie's All Stars/ BernieO's* Organic) . | 150 | 4.0 | 31.0 | 1.0 | 0 | 680 | <1.0 |
| (*Annie's Arthur Loops* Organic) ... | 150 | 5.0 | 32.0 | 1.0 | 0 | 670 | 1.0 |
| **Pasta entree, frozen** | | | | | | | |
| (see also "Pasta dish, frozen" and specific pastas), 1 pkg., 10 oz., except as noted: | | | | | | | |
| baked (*Zatarain's* French Quarter) ..... | 370 | 19.0 | 40.0 | 15.0 | 35 | 970 | 4.0 |
| and beans (*Moosewood* Organic Pasta e Fagioli) | 230 | 9.0 | 39.0 | 3.0 | 0 | 180 | 6.0 |
| broccoli, Parmesan (*Moosewood* Organic) | 380 | 14.0 | 52.0 | 13.0 | 30 | 380 | 4.0 |
| w/chicken, see "Chicken entree, frozen" | | | | | | | |
| marinara, roasted red pepper (*Healthy Choice*), 8.5 oz. ..... | 270 | 10.0 | 43.0 | 6.0 | 5 | 580 | 5.0 |

| Food and Measure | cal. | prot. (gms) | carbo. (gms) | fat (gms) | chol. (mgs) | sod. (mgs) | fiber (gms) |
|---|---|---|---|---|---|---|---|
| pesto primavera (*Kashi*) . | 290 | 11.0 | 37.0 | 11.0 | 5 | 750 | 7.0 |
| portobello marsala (*Healthy Choice*), 9 oz. | 270 | 12.0 | 38.0 | 7.0 | 15 | 550 | 5.0 |
| primavera (*Smart Ones*), 9 oz. | 250 | 11.0 | 41.0 | 4.0 | 5 | 610 | 4.0 |
| puttanesca (*Organic Bistro*), 11.1 oz. | 320 | 11.0 | 55.0 | 6.0 | 0 | 380 | 8.0 |
| w/ricotta and spinach (*Smart Ones*), 9 oz. | 280 | 14.0 | 43.0 | 6.0 | 15 | 630 | 6.0 |
| Romano w/bacon (*Lean Cuisine*) | 260 | 12.0 | 42.0 | 5.0 | 10 | 570 | 3.0 |
| Stroganoff (*Michelina's*), 8 oz. | 400 | 13.0 | 38.0 | 18.0 | 35 | 740 | 2.0 |
| stuffed (*Marie Callender's* Medley), 13 oz. | 430 | 21.0 | 54.0 | 14.0 | 50 | 1110 | 8.0 |
| vegetables, zesty garlic (*Birds Eye* Pasta Secrets), 2 cups | 240 | 7.0 | 31.0 | 10.0 | 5 | 310 | 2.0 |
| **Pasta entree, microwave** (*Bowl Appetit!*), 1 cont.: | | | | | | | |
| Alfredo | 350 | 11.0 | 55.0 | 9.0 | 10 | 870 | 2.0 |
| cheddar broccoli | 310 | 10.0 | 52.0 | 7.0 | 10 | 960 | 2.0 |
| chicken flavor | 250 | 7.0 | 44.0 | 5.0 | 5 | 790 | 2.0 |
| garlic Parmesan | 310 | 9.0 | 51.0 | 8.0 | <5 | 1010 | 1.0 |
| **Pasta flour**, see "Semolina flour" | | | | | | | |
| **Pasta salad mix**: | | | | | | | |
| (*Suddenly Salad* Classic), ¾ cup* | 250 | 6.0 | 39.0 | 8.0 | 0 | 840 | 1.0 |
| w/bacon (*Kraft Pasta Salad*), ¼ pkg. | 170 | 7.0 | 34.0 | 1.0 | 0 | 300 | 1.0 |
| Caesar: | | | | | | | |
| (*Kraft Pasta Salad*), ¼ pkg. | 190 | 7.0 | 36.0 | 2.0 | 5 | 480 | 2.0 |
| (*Suddenly Salad*), 1 cup* | 310 | 6.0 | 38.0 | 14.0 | 0 | 640 | 1.0 |
| Italian: | | | | | | | |
| (*Kraft Pasta Salad*), ¼ pkg. | 160 | 6.0 | 31.0 | 1.5 | 0 | 320 | 2.0 |
| creamy (*Suddenly Salad*), ¾ cup* | 350 | 7.0 | 36.0 | 20.0 | 15 | 540 | 2.0 |

| Food and Measure | cal. | prot. (gms) | carbo. (gms) | fat (gms) | chol. (mgs) | sod. (mgs) | fiber (gms) |
|---|---|---|---|---|---|---|---|
| **Pasta salad mix** (cont.) | | | | | | | |
| Parmesan, creamy (Suddenly Salad), ¾ cup* ............ | 370 | 6.0 | 34.0 | 23.0 | 20 | 460 | 1.0 |
| ranch: | | | | | | | |
| bacon (Suddenly Salad), ¾ cup* .... | 350 | 6.0 | 34.0 | 21.0 | 15 | 470 | 2.0 |
| chipotle (Suddenly Salad), ¾ cup* .... | 290 | 6.0 | 32.0 | 26.0 | 15 | 450 | 1.0 |
| tuna (Kraft Pasta Salad), ⅕ pkg. .... | 300 | 9.0 | 27.0 | 18.0 | 15 | 410 | 1.0 |
| **Pasta sauce** (see also specific sauce), tomato, ½ cup, except as noted: | | | | | | | |
| (Barilla Italian Baking) ... | 60 | 2.0 | 12.0 | 1.0 | 0 | 460 | 2.0 |
| (Eden Organic Spaghetti) .......... | 70 | 2.0 | 9.0 | 2.5 | 0 | 300 | 5.0 |
| (Eden Organic Spaghetti No Salt) ... | 70 | 2.0 | 9.0 | 2.5 | 0 | 10 | 5.0 |
| (Eden Organic Pizza/ Pasta) .............. | 65 | 2.0 | 9.0 | 2.5 | 0 | 300 | 5.0 |
| (Emeril's Kicked Up) .... | 70 | 1.0 | 9.0 | 3.0 | 0 | 400 | 2.0 |
| (Hunt's Spicy/Zesty) .... | 60 | 1.0 | 10.0 | 2.0 | 0 | 700 | 3.0 |
| (Hunt's Traditional) ..... | 50 | 2.0 | 10.0 | 1.0 | 0 | 580 | 2.0 |
| (Mom's Traditional Organic) ........... | 60 | 1.0 | 7.0 | 3.0 | 0 | 390 | 1.0 |
| (Newman's Own Bombolina) ........ | 90 | 2.0 | 13.0 | 4.5 | 0 | 620 | 3.0 |
| (Newman's Own Sockarooni) ........ | 70 | 2.0 | 12.0 | 2.0 | 0 | 520 | 3.0 |
| (Prego Chunky Garden Combination) ....... | 70 | 2.0 | 13.0 | 1.5 | 0 | 470 | 3.0 |
| (Prego Traditional) ..... | 70 | 2.0 | 13.0 | 1.5 | 0 | 480 | 3.0 |
| (Prego Traditional Heart Smart) ........ | 70 | 2.0 | 13.0 | 1.5 | 0 | 360 | 3.0 |
| (Prego Veggie Smart Chunky/Savory) ..... | 90 | 2.0 | 16.0 | 1.5 | 0 | 360 | 3.0 |
| (Prego Veggie Smart Smooth/Simple) ..... | 90 | 2.0 | 18.0 | 1.5 | 0 | 410 | 3.0 |
| arrabiata: | | | | | | | |
| (Bertolli) ............ | 60 | 1.0 | 11.0 | 1.5 | 0 | 450 | 2.0 |
| (Cucina Antica) ...... | 45 | 1.0 | 6.0 | 2.0 | 0 | 239 | 1.0 |
| (Don Bruno) ........ | 70 | 1.0 | 7.0 | 5.0 | 0 | 290 | 1.0 |

| Food and Measure | cal. | prot. (gms) | carbo. (gms) | fat (gms) | chol. (mgs) | sod. (mgs) | fiber (gms) |
|---|---|---|---|---|---|---|---|
| (*Seeds of Change* Organic di Roma) .. | 80 | 1.0 | 6.0 | 6.0 | 0 | 300 | 2.0 |
| spicy (*Mom's*) ....... | 70 | 1.0 | 7.0 | 3.0 | 0 | 400 | 1.0 |
| artichoke hearts and asiago (*Mom's*) ...... | 90 | 3.0 | 7.0 | 6.0 | 5 | 410 | 3.0 |
| arugula, baby (*Cucina Antica*) ............ | 38 | 1.0 | 4.0 | 2.0 | 0 | 230 | 1.0 |
| basil, sweet (*Classico* Traditional) ........ | 70 | 2.0 | 13.0 | 1.0 | 0 | 520 | 3.0 |
| basil, tomato and: | | | | | | | |
| (*Amy's* Organic) ..... | 110 | 2.0 | 11.0 | 6.0 | 0 | 580 | 3.0 |
| (*Amy's* Organic Light Sodium) .... | 90 | 2.0 | 11.0 | 4.5 | 0 | 290 | 2.0 |
| (*Barilla*) ............ | 60 | 2.0 | 12.0 | 1.0 | 0 | 460 | 2.0 |
| (*Bertolli*) ........... | 80 | 2.0 | 13.0 | 2.0 | 0 | 520 | 3.0 |
| (*Bertolli* Organic) .... | 90 | 2.0 | 11.0 | 7.5 | 0 | 510 | 2.0 |
| (*Classico*) .......... | 50 | 2.0 | 11.0 | 1.0 | 0 | 310 | 2.0 |
| (*Cucina Antica*) ...... | 35 | 1.0 | 4.0 | 2.0 | 0 | 246 | 1.0 |
| (*Del Monte*) ........ | 70 | 2.0 | 16.0 | 1.0 | 0 | 600 | 3.0 |
| (*Muir Glen* Organic) .. | 60 | 2.0 | 12.0 | 1.0 | 0 | 370 | 2.0 |
| (*Newman's Own* Organic) ......... | 90 | 2.0 | 12.0 | 4.5 | 0 | 650 | <1.0 |
| (*Seeds of Change* Organic Genovese) . | 60 | 2.0 | 9.0 | 3.5 | 0 | 350 | 2.0 |
| garlic (*Prego*) ....... | 80 | 2.0 | 12.0 | 2.5 | 0 | 400 | 3.0 |
| spicy (*Classico*) ..... | 60 | 2.0 | 11.0 | 1.0 | 0 | 570 | 3.0 |
| beef Bolognese (*Muir Glen* Organic) ....... | 70 | 3.0 | 10.0 | 2.0 | 5 | 410 | 2.0 |
| w/cheese: | | | | | | | |
| 5 (*Bertolli*) ......... | 90 | 4.0 | 14.0 | 3.5 | <5 | 660 | <1.0 |
| 5 (*Newman's Own*) ... | 80 | 3.0 | 10.0 | 3.0 | 5 | 610 | 2.0 |
| 4 (*Classico*) ........ | 80 | 2.0 | 12.0 | 3.0 | 5 | 460 | 3.0 |
| 4 (*Del Monte*) ....... | 70 | 2.0 | 15.0 | 1.5 | 0 | 680 | 3.0 |
| 4 (*Hunt's*) .......... | 50 | 3.0 | 10.0 | 1.0 | 0 | 580 | 3.0 |
| 4 (*Muir Glen* Organic) . | 80 | 4.0 | 1.0 | 3.0 | 5 | 380 | 2.0 |
| 3 (*Barilla*) .......... | 80 | 3.0 | 11.0 | 2.0 | 0 | 490 | 2.0 |
| 3 (*Prego*) .......... | 80 | 3.0 | 14.0 | 1.5 | 5 | 430 | 3.0 |
| 3 (*Seeds of Change* Organic Romagna) . | 90 | 4.0 | 9.0 | 5.0 | 5 | 460 | 2.0 |
| and garlic, Italian (*Hunt's*) ......... | 50 | 3.0 | 9.0 | 1.0 | 0 | 600 | 2.0 |
| Fra Diavolo: | | | | | | | |
| (*Alessi*) ............ | 100 | 2.0 | 6.0 | 9.0 | 0 | 420 | 2.0 |
| (*Newman's Own*) .... | 70 | 0 | 10.0 | 3.0 | 0 | 510 | 2.0 |

| Food and Measure | cal. | prot. (gms) | carbo. (gms) | fat (gms) | chol. (mgs) | sod. (mgs) | fiber (gms) |
|---|---|---|---|---|---|---|---|
| **Pasta sauce** *(cont.)* | | | | | | | |
| garlic, roasted: | | | | | | | |
| (*Barilla*) . . . . . . . . . . . . | 60 | 2.0 | 12.0 | 1.0 | 0 | 460 | 2.0 |
| (*Classico*) . . . . . . . . . . | 50 | 2.0 | 9.0 | 1.0 | 0 | 350 | 2.0 |
| (*Emeril's* Gaaahlic) . . . | 70 | 2.0 | 9.0 | 3.0 | 0 | 480 | 2.0 |
| (*Muir Glen* Organic | | | | | | | |
| Garlic) . . . . . . . . . . | 60 | 2.0 | 12.0 | 1.0 | 0 | 380 | 2.0 |
| (*Newman's Own*) . . . . | 70 | 2.0 | 11.0 | 2.5 | 0 | 580 | 2.0 |
| and herb (*Prego*) . . . . | 90 | 2.0 | 13.0 | 3.0 | 0 | 460 | 3.0 |
| and onion (*Barilla*) . . . | 60 | 2.0 | 12.0 | 1.0 | 0 | 460 | 2.0 |
| Parmesan (*Prego*) . . . | 70 | 3.0 | 13.0 | .5 | 5 | 480 | 3.0 |
| and peppers | | | | | | | |
| (*Newman's Own*) . . | 70 | 2.0 | 11.0 | 2.5 | 0 | 460 | 2.0 |
| garlic, tomato and | | | | | | | |
| (*Seeds of Change* | | | | | | | |
| Organic Tuscan) . . . . . | 60 | 2.0 | 7.0 | 2.5 | 0 | 510 | 2.0 |
| garlic and: | | | | | | | |
| basil (*Mom's*) . . . . . . . | 70 | 2.0 | 7.0 | 3.0 | 0 | 380 | 2.0 |
| basil (*Rising Moon* | | | | | | | |
| *Organics*) . . . . . . . . | 35 | 2.0 | 8.0 | 0 | 0 | 190 | 2.0 |
| chanterelles (*Rising* | | | | | | | |
| *Moon Organics*) . . . | 40 | 2.0 | 9.0 | 0 | 0 | 250 | 2.0 |
| herb (*Del Monte*) . . . . | 60 | 2.0 | 11.0 | 1.5 | 0 | 490 | <1.0 |
| herb (*Hunt's*) . . . . . . . | 40 | 2.0 | 8.0 | 1.0 | 0 | 610 | 3.0 |
| Merlot (*Rising Moon* | | | | | | | |
| *Organics*) . . . . . . . . | 40 | 2.0 | 8.0 | 0 | 0 | 190 | 2.0 |
| onion (*Del Monte*) . . . | 80 | 2.0 | 16.0 | 1.0 | 0 | 490 | 2.0 |
| onion (*Hunt's*) . . . . . . | 50 | 2.0 | 10.0 | 1.0 | 0 | 540 | 3.0 |
| green pepper/ | | | | | | | |
| mushroom (*Del Monte*) | 80 | 2.0 | 16.0 | 1.0 | 0 | 490 | 3.0 |
| herb: | | | | | | | |
| (*Newman's Own* | | | | | | | |
| Organic) . . . . . . . . . | 90 | 2.0 | 13.0 | 4.0 | 0 | 660 | <1.0 |
| Italian (*Del Monte* | | | | | | | |
| Chunky) . . . . . . . . . | 60 | 2.0 | 12.0 | 1.0 | 0 | 520 | <1.0 |
| Italian (*Muir Glen* | | | | | | | |
| Organic) . . . . . . . . . | 60 | 2.0 | 11.0 | 1.0 | 0 | 350 | 2.0 |
| tomato and (*Muir* | | | | | | | |
| *Glen* Organic | | | | | | | |
| Chunky) . . . . . . . . . | 60 | 2.0 | 11.0 | 1.0 | 0 | 350 | 2.0 |
| marinara: | | | | | | | |
| (*Alessi* Smooth/ | | | | | | | |
| Chunky) . . . . . . . . . | 100 | 2.0 | 6.0 | 9.0 | 0 | 420 | 2.0 |
| (*Amy's* Organic) . . . . . | 80 | 1.0 | 10.0 | 4.5 | 0 | 590 | 3.0 |

| Food and Measure | cal. | prot. (gms) | carbo. (gms) | fat (gms) | chol. (mgs) | sod. (mgs) | fiber (gms) |
|---|---|---|---|---|---|---|---|
| (*Amy's* Organic Light Sodium) .... | 40 | 1.0 | 7.0 | 1.0 | 0 | 100 | 1.0 |
| (*Barilla*) ............ | 70 | 2.0 | 12.0 | 1.5 | 0 | 460 | 2.0 |
| (*Don Bruno*) ........ | 70 | 1.0 | 7.0 | 5.0 | 0 | 290 | 1.0 |
| (*Emeril's* Homestyle) . | 90 | 2.0 | 14.0 | 3.0 | 0 | 660 | 3.0 |
| (*Mom's*) ............ | 60 | 2.0 | 8.0 | 2.5 | 5 | 490 | 2.0 |
| (*Newman's Own*) .... | 70 | 2.0 | 12.0 | 2.0 | 0 | 510 | 3.0 |
| (*Newman's Own* Organic) ......... | 70 | 2.0 | 12.0 | 2.0 | 0 | 550 | <1.0 |
| (*Prego*) ............. | 80 | 2.0 | 10.0 | 3.0 | 0 | 480 | 3.0 |
| (*Seeds of Change* Organic di Venezia) | 60 | 1.0 | 6.0 | 3.5 | 0 | 380 | 2.0 |
| Burgundy (*Bertolli* Vineyard) ........ | 80 | 3.0 | 14.0 | 2.0 | 0 | 500 | 1.0 |
| Cabernet (*Classico*) .. | 70 | 2.0 | 11.0 | 2.0 | 0 | 330 | 2.0 |
| Cabernet (*Muir Glen* Organic) ......... | 60 | 2.0 | 11.0 | 1.0 | 0 | 360 | 2.0 |
| Cabernet (*Newman's Own*) ........... | 70 | 2.0 | 10.0 | 3.0 | 0 | 590 | 2.0 |
| garlic (*Cucina Antica*) . | 36 | 1.0 | 4.0 | 2.0 | 0 | 246 | 1.0 |
| mushroom (*Newman's Own*) ........... | 70 | 2.0 | 12.0 | 2.0 | 0 | 520 | 3.0 |
| w/plum tomatoes (*Classico*) ........ | 70 | 2.0 | 10.0 | 2.0 | 0 | 460 | 1.0 |
| roasted red pepper (*Cucina Antica*) ... | 40 | 1.0 | 6.0 | 2.0 | 0 | 248 | 1.0 |
| spicy (*Barilla*) ....... | 60 | 2.0 | 11.0 | 1.5 | 0 | 460 | 2.0 |
| spinach (*Cucina Antica*) .......... | 36 | 1.0 | 4.0 | 2.0 | 0 | 246 | 1.0 |
| martini (*Mom's*) ....... | 120 | 3.0 | 6.0 | 8.0 | 20 | 250 | 1.0 |
| meat: | | | | | | | |
| (*Del Monte*) ........ | 60 | 3.0 | 14.0 | 1.0 | 2 | 720 | 3.0 |
| (*Hunt's*) ........... | 60 | 3.0 | 11.0 | 1.0 | 0 | 610 | 3.0 |
| flavored w/ (*Prego*) ... | 80 | 2.0 | 13.0 | 2.5 | 5 | 480 | 3.0 |
| meatball, mini (*Prego*) .. | 100 | 4.0 | 13.0 | 3.0 | 5 | 480 | 3.0 |
| mushroom: | | | | | | | |
| (*Del Monte*) ........ | 60 | 2.0 | 14.0 | .5 | 0 | 630 | 2.0 |
| (*Hunt's*) ........... | 45 | 2.0 | 10.0 | .5 | 0 | 590 | 3.0 |
| fresh (*Prego*) ....... | 70 | 2.0 | 13.0 | 1.5 | 0 | 380 | 3.0 |
| portobello (*Bertolli* Vineyard) ........ | 80 | 2.0 | 12.0 | 2.5 | 0 | 450 | 1.0 |
| portobello (*Muir Glen* Organic) ......... | 50 | 2.0 | 10.0 | 0 | 0 | 350 | 2.0 |

| Food and Measure | cal. | prot. (gms) | carbo. (gms) | fat (gms) | chol. (mgs) | sod. (mgs) | fiber (gms) |
|---|---|---|---|---|---|---|---|
| **Pasta sauce, mushroom** (cont.) | | | | | | | |
| portobello, baby (*Prego* Chunky Garden Supreme) .. | 90 | 2.0 | 13.0 | 3.0 | 0 | 460 | 3.0 |
| triple (*Classico*) ..... | 70 | 3.0 | 13.0 | 1.0 | 0 | 380 | 3.0 |
| mushroom and: | | | | | | | |
| garlic (*Barilla*) ....... | 70 | 3.0 | 12.0 | 2.0 | 0 | 450 | 2.0 |
| green pepper (*Prego* Chunky Garden) ... | 90 | 2.0 | 13.0 | 3.0 | 0 | 470 | 3.0 |
| ripe olives (*Classico*) . | 60 | 2.0 | 10.0 | 2.0 | 0 | 360 | 2.0 |
| olive, green and black (*Barilla*) ....... | 80 | 2.0 | 10.0 | 3.0 | 0 | 770 | 4.0 |
| olive and asiago (*Rising Moon Organics*) ..... | 45 | 2.0 | 8.0 | 1.5 | 0 | 260 | 2.0 |
| olive oil and garlic: | | | | | | | |
| (*Bertolli*) ........... | 80 | 3.0 | 14.0 | 3.0 | 0 | 470 | <1.0 |
| basil (*Bertolli* Organic) ......... | 80 | 2.0 | 10.0 | 3.5 | 0 | 510 | 2.0 |
| onion and garlic: | | | | | | | |
| (*Newman's Own*) .... | 60 | 2.0 | 12.0 | 1.5 | 0 | 530 | 2.0 |
| (*Prego* Chunky Garden) ......... | 90 | 2.0 | 13.0 | 3.0 | 0 | 470 | 3.0 |
| caramelized, roasted garlic (*Classico*) ... | 85 | 3.0 | 13.0 | 3.0 | 0 | 510 | 3.0 |
| Vidalia, roasted garlic (*Bertolli*) .... | 80 | 3.0 | 14.0 | 2.5 | 0 | 470 | <1.0 |
| pepper, red: | | | | | | | |
| roasted (*Emeril's*) .... | 60 | 1.0 | 7.0 | 3.0 | 0 | 390 | 2.0 |
| roasted, and garlic (*Prego*) | 70 | 2.0 | 13.0 | 1.5 | 0 | 410 | 3.0 |
| spicy (*Classico*) ..... | 60 | 1.0 | 8.0 | 3.0 | 0 | 300 | 2.0 |
| peppers, sweet, and garlic (*Barilla*) ....... | 60 | 2.0 | 10.0 | 1.5 | 0 | 460 | 2.0 |
| pesto, tomato, and: | | | | | | | |
| (*Newman's Own*) .... | 80 | 2.0 | 10.0 | 4.0 | 0 | 640 | 2.0 |
| spicy (*Classico*) ..... | 90 | 2.0 | 10.0 | 5.0 | 0 | 480 | 3.0 |
| port and asiago (*Rising Moon Organics*) ..... | 45 | 5.0 | 8.0 | 1.0 | 0 | 200 | 2.0 |
| puttanesca: | | | | | | | |
| (*Alessi*) ............ | 100 | 2.0 | 6.0 | 9.0 | 0 | 470 | 2.0 |
| (*Cucina Antica*) ...... | 54 | 1.0 | 6.0 | 3.0 | 0 | 248 | 1.0 |
| (*Mom's*) ........... | 90 | 2.0 | 8.0 | 6.0 | 5 | 550 | 2.0 |
| red pepper, roasted (*Mom's* Organic) ..... | 50 | 1.0 | 5.0 | 3.0 | 0 | 390 | 1.0 |

| Food and Measure | cal. | prot. (gms) | carbo. (gms) | fat (gms) | chol. (mgs) | sod. (mgs) | fiber (gms) |
|---|---|---|---|---|---|---|---|
| ricotta Parmesan | | | | | | | |
| (*Prego*) . . . . . . . . . . . | 90 | 3.0 | 13.0 | 2.5 | 5 | 360 | 3.0 |
| sausage, Italian: | | | | | | | |
| (*Bertolli*) . . . . . . . . . . | 90 | 3.0 | 14.0 | 3.0 | <5 | 550 | <1.0 |
| (*Hunt's*) . . . . . . . . . . | 60 | 2.0 | 10.0 | 1.5 | 0 | 610 | 3.0 |
| and garlic (*Prego*) . . . . | 90 | 3.0 | 13.0 | 3.0 | 5 | 480 | 3.0 |
| w/pepper and onion | | | | | | | |
| (*Classico*) . . . . . . . . | 80 | 3.0 | 10.0 | 3.0 | 5 | 430 | 2.0 |
| and peppers | | | | | | | |
| (*Newman's Own*) . . | 90 | 4.0 | 11.0 | 4.0 | 10 | 630 | 2.0 |
| w/peppers (*Muir* | | | | | | | |
| *Glen* Organic) . . . . . | 80 | 3.0 | 10.0 | 3.0 | 5 | 420 | 2.0 |
| spinach and: | | | | | | | |
| cheese (*Classico* | | | | | | | |
| Florentine) . . . . . . . | 80 | 2.0 | 9.0 | 4.0 | 5 | 460 | 3.0 |
| garlic (*Classico* | | | | | | | |
| Organic) . . . . . . . . | 70 | 2.0 | 11.0 | 2.0 | 0 | 330 | 2.0 |
| tomato, fire-roasted: | | | | | | | |
| (*Bertolli* Vineyard) . . . . | 80 | 2.0 | 12.0 | 2.5 | 0 | 440 | 1.0 |
| (*Muir Glen* Organic) . . | 70 | 2.0 | 12.0 | 2.0 | 0 | 390 | 2.0 |
| and garlic (*Classico*) . . | 50 | 2.0 | 8.0 | 1.0 | 0 | 400 | 2.0 |
| and garlic (*Newman's* | | | | | | | |
| Own) . . . . . . . . . . | 70 | 2.0 | 9.0 | 3.5 | 0 | 500 | 2.0 |
| tomato, herbs and spices | | | | | | | |
| (*Classico* Organic) . . . | 70 | 2.0 | 12.0 | 1.0 | 0 | 400 | 2.0 |
| tomato, sun-dried | | | | | | | |
| (*Classico*) . . . . . . . . . | 80 | 2.0 | 11.0 | 4.0 | 0 | 420 | 3.0 |
| vegetable, garden: | | | | | | | |
| (*Barilla*) . . . . . . . . . . | 70 | 2.0 | 11.0 | 1.5 | 0 | 460 | 2.0 |
| (*Muir Glen* Organic) . . | 60 | 2.0 | 10.0 | 1.0 | 0 | 350 | 2.0 |
| vodka: | | | | | | | |
| (*Bertolli*) . . . . . . . . . . | 150 | 3.0 | 11.0 | 9.0 | 25 | 700 | 2.0 |
| (*Classico*) . . . . . . . . . | 120 | 3.0 | 12.0 | 7.0 | 15 | 490 | 2.0 |
| (*Cucina Antica*) . . . . . | 66 | 1.0 | 4.0 | 5.0 | 18 | 232 | 1.0 |
| (*Don Bruno*) . . . . . . . | 130 | 3.0 | 8.0 | 10.0 | 20 | 440 | 2.0 |
| (*Emeril's*) . . . . . . . . . | 130 | 2.0 | 13.0 | 8.0 | 10 | 490 | 2.0 |
| (*Newman's Own*) . . . . | 110 | 5.0 | 11.0 | 5.0 | 5 | 440 | 2.0 |
| (*Seeds of Change* | | | | | | | |
| Organic) . . . . . . . . | 120 | 2.0 | 8.0 | 10.0 | 20 | 310 | 2.0 |
| **Pasta sauce, chilled** | | | | | | | |
| (see also "Alfredo | | | | | | | |
| sauce"), tomato | | | | | | | |
| (*Buitoni*), ½ cup: | | | | | | | |
| marinara . . . . . . . . . . . | 70 | 1.0 | 10.0 | 3.0 | 0 | 560 | 2.0 |

| Food and Measure | cal. | prot. (gms) | carbo. (gms) | fat (gms) | chol. (mgs) | sod. (mgs) | fiber (gms) |
|---|---|---|---|---|---|---|---|
| **Pasta sauce, chilled** *(cont.)* | | | | | | | |
| marinara, roasted garlic . | 60 | 2.0 | 10.0 | 1.5 | 0 | 530 | 2.0 |
| tomato herb Parmesan .. | 130 | 4.0 | 10.0 | 8.0 | 10 | 740 | 2.0 |
| vodka .............. | 100 | 2.0 | 7.0 | 7.0 | 20 | 610 | 1.0 |
| **Pasta sauce mix**, see "Spaghetti sauce mix" and specific listings | | | | | | | |
| **Pastrami**, beef, 2 oz.: | | | | | | | |
| (*Black Bear*) .......... | 90 | 11.0 | 2.0 | 4.0 | 30 | 630 | 0 |
| (*Black Bear* Brisket) .... | 80 | 10.0 | 2.0 | 4.0 | 30 | 610 | 0 |
| (*Boar's Head* Brisket) ... | 90 | 12.0 | 2.0 | 4.0 | 30 | 670 | 0 |
| (*Boar's Head* Red) ...... | 80 | 12.0 | 1.0 | 3.0 | 35 | 610 | 0 |
| (*Boar's Head* Round) .... | 80 | 12.0 | 1.0 | 3.5 | 30 | 580 | 0 |
| (*Boar's Head* Top Round Cap-Off) ..... | 70 | 13.0 | 1.0 | 2.5 | 30 | 600 | 0 |
| (*Di Lusso*) ............ | 100 | 10.0 | 1.0 | 6.0 | 35 | 680 | 0 |
| (*Hebrew National*) ...... | 80 | 11.0 | 1.0 | 3.0 | 30 | 520 | 0 |
| (*Thumann's*) .......... | 80 | 14.0 | 0 | 3.0 | 30 | 520 | 0 |
| (*Thumann's* First Cut) ... | 70 | 12.0 | 0 | 2.0 | 32 | 520 | 0 |
| **Pastry sheets** (see also also "Fillo dough"), frozen/chilled: | | | | | | | |
| dough (*Pillsbury Recipe Creations*), ⅙ pkg. ... | 120 | 2.0 | 16.0 | 6.0 | 0 | 300 | <1.0 |
| puff (*Pepperidge Farm*), ⅙ sheet .......... | 170 | 3.0 | 14.0 | 11.0 | 0 | 140 | <1.0 |
| **Pastry shells**, baked: | | | | | | | |
| canapé (*Roland*): | | | | | | | |
| coquillettes or diamond, 3.5 oz. .. | 480 | 8.0 | 59.0 | 24.0 | 0 | 1309 | 2.0 |
| rounds, 10 pcs., 1.2 oz. | 160 | 2.0 | 24.0 | 6.0 | 0 | 240 | 0 |
| seashells, 3.5 oz. .... | 460 | 9.0 | 60.0 | 22.0 | 30 | 1230 | 2.0 |
| dessert (*Roland* 4.4"), 3.5 oz. ........... | 510 | 7.0 | 63.0 | 25.0 | 55 | n.a. | 2.0 |
| puff pastry (*Pepperidge Farm*), 1 pc. ........ | 190 | 3.0 | 16.0 | 13.0 | 0 | 160 | <1.0 |
| **Pâté, liver**, can/jar: | | | | | | | |
| 2 oz. ................ | 179 | 8.0 | .6 | 15.7 | 143 | 390 | 0 |
| 1 tbsp. .............. | 41 | 1.9 | .2 | 3.6 | 33 | 91 | 0 |
| chicken liver: | | | | | | | |
| 2 oz. .............. | 113 | 7.5 | 3.7 | 7.3 | 219 | 216 | 0 |
| 1 tbsp. ........... | 26 | 1.8 | .9 | 1.7 | 51 | 51 | 0 |

| Food and Measure | cal. | prot. (gms) | carbo. (gms) | fat (gms) | chol. (mgs) | sod. (mgs) | fiber (gms) |
|---|---|---|---|---|---|---|---|
| foie gras w/truffles: | | | | | | | |
| (*Maison Roland* Bloc | | | | | | | |
| 14.8 oz.), 2 oz. . . . . | 220 | 5.0 | 0 | 22.0 | 630 | 240 | 0 |
| (*Maison Roland* Bloc | | | | | | | |
| 7.4/11 oz.), 2 oz. . . | 220 | 4.0 | 0 | 24.0 | 540 | 300 | 0 |
| goose liver, smoked: | | | | | | | |
| 2 oz. . . . . . . . . . . . . . | 259 | 6.4 | 2.6 | 24.6 | 84 | 390 | 0 |
| 1 tbsp. . . . . . . . . . . . | 60 | 1.5 | .6 | 5.7 | 20 | 91 | 0 |
| truffle flavor, 2 oz. . . . . . . | 183 | 6.3 | 3.5 | 16.0 | 59 | 452 | 0 |
| w/truffle juice | | | | | | | |
| (*Roland*), ¼ cup, 2 oz. | 250 | 6.0 | 5.0 | 23.0 | 65 | 260 | 1.0 |
| **Peach**, fresh: | | | | | | | |
| (*Chiquita*), 5.3-oz. pc. . . . | 59 | 1.0 | 15.0 | 0 | 0 | 0 | 2.0 |
| (*Dole*), 5.2-oz. pc. . . . . . . | 60 | 1.0 | 14.0 | 0 | 0 | 0 | 2.0 |
| (*Frieda's Donut/* | | | | | | | |
| Late Season), 5 oz. . . . | 60 | 1.0 | 16.0 | 0 | 0 | 0 | 3.0 |
| 2½" pc., 4 per lb. . . . . . . . | 37 | .6 | 9.7 | .1 | 0 | 0 | 1.7 |
| sliced, 1 cup . . . . . . . . . | 73 | 1.2 | 18.9 | .2 | 0 | 0 | 3.4 |
| **Peach, can/jar,** halves | | | | | | | |
| or slices, ½ cup, | | | | | | | |
| except as noted: | | | | | | | |
| (*Del Monte Carb* | | | | | | | |
| *Clever*) . . . . . . . . . . . | 30 | 1.0 | 7.0 | 0 | 0 | 0 | 10 | 1.0 |
| in juice: | | | | | | | |
| (*Del Monte* 100%) . . . | 60 | 0 | 15.0 | 0 | 0 | 10 | 1.0 |
| (*Del Monte* Bowl) . . . . | 70 | 0 | 17.0 | 0 | 0 | 20 | 2.0 |
| (*S&W* Natural Style) . . | 80 | 1.0 | 19.0 | 0 | 0 | 20 | 1.0 |
| chunks (*Del Monte* | | | | | | | |
| *Fruit Naturals*) . . . . | 70 | <1.0 | 17.0 | 0 | 0 | 10 | <1.0 |
| chunks (*Del Monte* | | | | | | | |
| *Fruit Naturals* | | | | | | | |
| No Sugar) . . . . . . . | 40 | 1.0 | 12.0 | 0 | 0 | 0 | 2.0 |
| chunks, pomegranate/ | | | | | | | |
| orange juice (*Del* | | | | | | | |
| *Monte Superfruit*), | | | | | | | |
| 6-oz. cup . . . . . . . . | 100 | 2.0 | 26.0 | 0 | 0 | 15 | 3.0 |
| diced (*Del Monte* | | | | | | | |
| 100%), 4-oz. can . . | 60 | 0 | 13.0 | 0 | 0 | 10 | <1.0 |
| in extra light syrup: | | | | | | | |
| (*Del Monte* Lite | | | | | | | |
| Cling) . . . . . . . . . . . | 60 | 0 | 15.0 | 0 | 0 | 10 | 1.0 |
| (*Del Monte* Lite | | | | | | | |
| Freestone) . . . . . . . | 60 | 0 | 14.0 | 0 | 0 | 10 | 1.0 |

| Food and Measure | cal. | prot. (gms) | carbo. (gms) | fat (gms) | chol. (mgs) | sod. (mgs) | fiber (gms) |
|---|---|---|---|---|---|---|---|
| **Peach, can/jar, in extra light syrup** *(cont.)* | | | | | | | |
| diced (*Del Monte* Lite), 4-oz. can .... | 50 | 0 | 13.0 | 0 | 0 | 10 | <1.0 |
| in light syrup: | | | | | | | |
| (*Del Monte Orchard Select*) .......... | 80 | <1.0 | 20.0 | 0 | 0 | 10 | <1.0 |
| (*S&W*) ............. | 70 | 0 | 17.0 | 0 | 0 | 10 | 1.0 |
| diced (*Del Monte*), 4-oz. cup ........ | 70 | <1.0 | 17.0 | 0 | 0 | 10 | <1.0 |
| diced (*Dole* Bowl), 4 oz. | 70 | 0 | 20.0 | 0 | 0 | 0 | 1.0 |
| sliced (*Dole*) ........ | 90 | 1.0 | 21.0 | 0 | 0 | 10 | 1.0 |
| raspberry flavor (*Del Monte*) .......... | 80 | <1.0 | 20.0 | 0 | 0 | 10 | <1.0 |
| spiced (*Del Monte* Harvest Spice) .... | 80 | <1.0 | 21.0 | 0 | 0 | 10 | <1.0 |
| strawberry-banana flavor (*Del Monte*), 4-oz. cup ........ | 70 | <1.0 | 17.0 | 0 | 0 | 10 | <1.0 |
| white (*Roland*) ...... | 70 | 1.0 | 16.0 | 0 | 0 | 5 | 1.0 |
| in light syrup, chunks: | | | | | | | |
| (*S&W Sun*) .......... | 80 | <1.0 | 20.0 | 0 | 0 | 20 | 1.0 |
| (*S&W Tropical*) ...... | 80 | <1.0 | 19.0 | 0 | 0 | 15 | 0 |
| cinnamon brown sugar (*S&W Sweet Memory*) ... | 80 | <1.0 | 19.0 | 0 | 0 | 15 | <1.0 |
| hybrid (*S&W Snow*) .. | 80 | <1.0 | 20.0 | 0 | 0 | 15 | 1.0 |
| in heavy syrup: | | | | | | | |
| (*Del Monte*) ........ | 100 | 0 | 24.0 | 0 | 0 | 10 | 1.0 |
| diced (*Del Monte*), 4-oz. can ........ | 80 | 0 | 20.0 | 0 | 0 | 10 | <1.0 |
| spiced, whole (*Del Monte*) .......... | 100 | 0 | 24.0 | 0 | 0 | 10 | <1.0 |
| in gelatin, 4.5-oz. cont.: | | | | | | | |
| peach (*Del Monte*) ... | 90 | 0 | 22.0 | 0 | 0 | 40 | 0 |
| raspberry (*Del Monte*) ........... | 90 | 0 | 23.0 | 0 | 0 | 40 | 0 |
| strawberry (*Dole*) .... | 90 | 1.0 | 23.0 | 0 | 0 | 25 | 1.0 |
| strawberry banana (*Del Monte* Lite) .... | 60 | 0 | 14.0 | 0 | 0 | 40 | 0 |
| and crème (Dole Parfait), 4.3-oz. cup .. | 120 | 1.0 | 23.0 | 2.0 | 0 | 10 | 1.0 |
| **Peach, dried**, sulfured: | | | | | | | |
| halves, ½ cup ......... | 191 | 2.9 | 49.1 | .6 | 0 | 6 | 6.6 |
| 10 halves, 4.6 oz. ...... | 311 | 4.7 | 79.7 | 1.0 | 0 | 9 | 10.7 |

| Food and Measure | cal. | prot. (gms) | carbo. (gms) | fat (gms) | chol. (mgs) | sod. (mgs) | fiber (gms) |
|---|---|---|---|---|---|---|---|
| **Peach, frozen**, sliced: | | | | | | | |
| (*Birds Eye*), ⅓ of 16-oz. pkg. .......... | 50 | 1.0 | 13.0 | 0 | 0 | 0 | 2.0 |
| (*Cascadian Farm* Organic), 1 cup ...... | 50 | <1.0 | 14.0 | 0 | 0 | 0 | 2.0 |
| (*C&W* Ultimate), ¾ cup .. | 50 | 1.0 | 13.0 | 0 | 0 | 0 | 2.0 |
| (*Dole*), ¾ cup ......... | 50 | 1.0 | 13.0 | 0 | 0 | 0 | 2.0 |
| sweetened, ½ cup ...... | 118 | .8 | 30.0 | .2 | 0 | 8 | 1.8 |
| **Peach drink**, sparkling (*Kristian Regale*), 8 fl. oz. ............. | 100 | 0 | 24.0 | 0 | 0 | 10 | 0 |
| **Peach drink blend**, 8 fl. oz.: | | | | | | | |
| (*Snapple* Summer) ..... | 110 | 0 | 28.0 | 0 | 0 | 5 | 0 |
| (*Welch's* Medley) ...... | 140 | 0 | 35.0 | 0 | 0 | 5 | 0 |
| mango: | | | | | | | |
| (*V8 V-Fusion* Light) .. | 50 | 0 | 13.0 | 0 | 0 | 40 | 0 |
| frozen* (*Chiquita* Smoothies) ...... | 120 | 1.0 | 28.0 | 0 | 0 | 40 | 0 |
| mangosteen (*Snapple*) .. | 90 | 0 | 21.0 | 0 | 0 | 15 | 0 |
| punch (*Tropicana* Orchard) ........... | 130 | 0 | 33.0 | 0 | 0 | 5 | 0 |
| **Peach glaze**: | | | | | | | |
| (*Litehouse*), 3 tbsp. ..... | 70 | 0 | 17.0 | 0 | 0 | 45 | 0 |
| (*Marie's*), 2 tbsp. ....... | 40 | 0 | 10.0 | 0 | 0 | 35 | 0 |
| (*Marzetti*), 3 tbsp. ...... | 60 | 0 | 15.0 | 0 | 0 | 65 | 0 |
| **Peach juice**, 8 fl. oz.: | | | | | | | |
| (*After the Fall* Georgia) .. | 130 | 1.0 | 31.0 | 0 | 0 | 15 | 0 |
| (*Ceres*) ............. | 120 | 0 | 30.0 | 0 | 0 | 5 | 0 |
| (*R.W. Knudsen* Nectar) .. | 130 | 1.0 | 31.0 | 0 | 0 | 15 | 0 |
| (*Santa Cruz Organic* Nectar) ............. | 120 | 0 | 31.0 | 0 | 0 | 10 | 0 |
| **Peach juice blend**: | | | | | | | |
| mango, 8 fl. oz.: | | | | | | | |
| (*Apple & Eve* Organics) ........ | 130 | 0 | 31.0 | 0 | 0 | 25 | 0 |
| (*V8 V-Fusion*) ....... | 120 | 1.0 | 28.0 | 0 | 0 | 70 | 0 |
| orange (*Nantucket Nectars*), 8 fl. oz. .... | 130 | 1.0 | 32.0 | 0 | 0 | 30 | 0 |
| papaya mango (*Tropicana Pure*), 8 fl. oz. ... | 120 | 1.0 | 28.0 | 0 | 0 | 15 | 0 |
| **Peach nectar**, canned, 8 fl. oz. ............. | 135 | .7 | 34.7 | <.1 | 0 | 17 | 1.5 |

| Food and Measure | cal. | prot. (gms) | carbo. (gms) | fat (gms) | chol. (mgs) | sod. (mgs) | fiber (gms) |
|---|---|---|---|---|---|---|---|
| **Peach-apricot sauce** | | | | | | | |
| (*Saucy Susan*), 2 tbsp. | 80 | 0 | 19.0 | 0 | 0 | 260 | 1.0 |
| **Peanut**, shelled, 1 oz., | | | | | | | |
| except as noted: | | | | | | | |
| (*Beer Nuts* Kettle | | | | | | | |
| Cooked) . . . . . . . . . . | 185 | 8.0 | 6.0 | 15.0 | 0 | 60 | 2.0 |
| (*Beer Nuts* Original) . . . . | 170 | 7.0 | 7.0 | 14.0 | 0 | 80 | 2.0 |
| (*Frito-Lay* Salted), | | | | | | | |
| 1 pkg. . . . . . . . . . . . . | 260 | 13.0 | 8.0 | 22.0 | 0 | 190 | 4.0 |
| (*Frito-Lay* Salted in | | | | | | | |
| Shell) . . . . . . . . . . . . . | 160 | 7.0 | 6.0 | 14.0 | 0 | 170 | 2.0 |
| (*Planters* Cocktail) . . . . . . | 170 | 7.0 | 5.0 | 14.0 | 0 | 115 | 2.0 |
| (*Planters* Cocktail | | | | | | | |
| Lightly Salted) . . . . . . . | 170 | 7.0 | 5.0 | 14.0 | 0 | 55 | 2.0 |
| (*Planters* Cocktail | | | | | | | |
| Unsalted) . . . . . . . . . | 170 | 7.0 | 5.0 | 14.0 | 0 | 0 | 2.0 |
| (*Planters* Roasted in | | | | | | | |
| Shell Salted) . . . . . . . . | 160 | 7.0 | 5.0 | 14.0 | 0 | 135 | 2.0 |
| (*Planters* Salted) . . . . . . . | 170 | 7.0 | 5.0 | 14.0 | 0 | 115 | 2.0 |
| (*Planters* Salted), | | | | | | | |
| 1.75-oz. pkg. . . . . . . . | 290 | 13.0 | 8.0 | 25.0 | 0 | 200 | 4.0 |
| (*Planters* Salted), | | | | | | | |
| 2-oz. pkg. . . . . . . . . . | 330 | 15.0 | 9.0 | 29.0 | 0 | 230 | 5.0 |
| bacon, smoky | | | | | | | |
| (*Planters* Cocktail) . . . | 160 | 7.0 | 5.0 | 14.0 | 0 | 160 | 2.0 |
| boiled, salted . . . . . . . . . . | 90 | 3.8 | 6.0 | 6.2 | 0 | 213 | 2.5 |
| Buffalo wing | | | | | | | |
| (*Planters* Cocktail) . . . | 160 | 7.0 | 5.0 | 14.0 | 0 | 220 | 2.0 |
| Cajun (*Beer Nuts* | | | | | | | |
| Devil Crunch Nuts) . . . | 140 | 4.0 | 16.0 | 6.0 | 0 | 140 | 1.0 |
| chipotle (*Planters* | | | | | | | |
| Wicked Hot) . . . . . . . . | 170 | 7.0 | 5.0 | 14.0 | 0 | 75 | 2.0 |
| dry-roasted: | | | | | | | |
| (*Frito-Lay*), 1.75 oz. . . | 280 | 12.0 | 17.0 | 18.0 | 0 | 300 | 5.0 |
| (*Planters*) . . . . . . . . . . | 160 | 7.0 | 5.0 | 14.0 | 0 | 190 | 2.0 |
| (*Planters*), 1-oz. pkg. . . | 170 | 7.0 | 5.0 | 14.0 | 0 | 190 | 2.0 |
| (*Planters* 24 oz.) . . . . . | 170 | 8.0 | 5.0 | 14.0 | 0 | 190 | 2.0 |
| (*Planters* Lightly | | | | | | | |
| Salted) . . . . . . . . . . | 160 | 7.0 | 5.0 | 14.0 | 0 | 95 | 2.0 |
| (*Planters* Lightly | | | | | | | |
| Salted 24 oz.) . . . . . | 170 | 8.0 | 5.0 | 14.0 | 0 | 95 | 2.0 |
| (*Planters* Unsalted) . . . | 170 | 8.0 | 5.0 | 14.0 | 0 | 0 | 2.0 |
| (*Planters* Unsalted 8 oz.) | 160 | 8.0 | 6.0 | 14.0 | 0 | 0 | 2.0 |
| ½ cup . . . . . . . . . . . . . | 428 | 17.3 | 15.7 | 36.3 | 0 | 4 | 5.8 |

| Food and Measure | cal. | prot. (gms) | carbo. (gms) | fat (gms) | chol. (mgs) | sod. (mgs) | fiber (gms) |
|---|---|---|---|---|---|---|---|
| honey-roasted: | | | | | | | |
| (*Frito-Lay*), 1.75 oz. .. | 250 | 11.0 | 11.0 | 20.0 | 0 | 130 | 3.0 |
| (*Planters*) .......... | 160 | 6.0 | 7.0 | 13.0 | 0 | 110 | 2.0 |
| (*Planters* 3 oz.) ...... | 160 | 6.0 | 8.0 | 13.0 | 0 | 95 | 2.0 |
| (*Planters* 12 oz.) ..... | 160 | 6.0 | 8.0 | 12.0 | 0 | 115 | 2.0 |
| (*Planters*), 1.75 oz. .... | 280 | 11.0 | 13.0 | 22.0 | 0 | 190 | 4.0 |
| (*Planters* Party Size 34.5 oz.) ..... | 160 | 6.0 | 7.0 | 13.0 | 0 | 110 | 2.0 |
| honey dry-roasted | | | | | | | |
| (*Planters*) .......... | 160 | 6.0 | 7.0 | 13.0 | 0 | 110 | 2.0 |
| hot: | | | | | | | |
| (*Frito-Lay*), 1 pkg. .... | 310 | 12.0 | 10.0 | 25.0 | 0 | 390 | 4.0 |
| (*Planters* Heat), 1.75-oz. pkg. ..... | 290 | 12.0 | 9.0 | 25.0 | 0 | 350 | 4.0 |
| oil-roasted, ½ cup ...... | 419 | 19.0 | 13.6 | 35.5 | 0 | 4 | 6.6 |
| Spanish (*Planters* Redskin) ........... | 170 | 7.0 | 4.0 | 15.0 | 0 | 115 | 3.0 |
| sweet and crunchy (*Planters*) .......... | 140 | 4.0 | 15.0 | 8.0 | 0 | 20 | 1.0 |
| wasabi: | | | | | | | |
| (*Planters* Cocktail White Hot) ....... | 160 | 7.0 | 5.0 | 14.0 | 0 | 170 | 2.0 |
| (*Roland Feng Shui*), ¼ cup ..... | 150 | 6.0 | 10.0 | 9.0 | 0 | 140 | 0 |
| **Peanut butter**, 2 tbsp., except as noted: | | | | | | | |
| chunky or creamy: | | | | | | | |
| (*Arrowhead Mills* Valencia Natural/ Organic) ......... | 190 | 8.0 | 6.0 | 17.0 | 0 | 0 | 2.0 |
| (*Kettle* Organic), 1 oz. . | 160 | 7.0 | 5.0 | 14.0 | 0 | 0 | 2.0 |
| (*MaraNatha* Natural/ Organic) ......... | 190 | 8.0 | 7.0 | 16.0 | 0 | 80 | 3.0 |
| (*MaraNatha* Natural/ Organic No Stir) ... | 190 | 7.0 | 8.0 | 16.0 | 0 | 70 | 2.0 |
| (*Peter Pan* Reduced Fat) ............. | 200 | 8.0 | 14.0 | 13.0 | 0 | 150 | 2.0 |
| (*Santa Cruz Organic* Roasted) ........ | 210 | 8.0 | 6.0 | 16.0 | 0 | 50 | 2.0 |
| chunky/crunchy: | | | | | | | |
| (*Jif* Extra) .......... | 190 | 7.0 | 7.0 | 16.0 | 0 | 130 | 2.0 |
| (*Jif* Natural Spread) .. | 190 | 7.0 | 8.0 | 16.0 | 0 | 65 | 2.0 |
| (*Jif* Reduced Fat) .... | 190 | 8.0 | 15.0 | 12.0 | 0 | 220 | 1.0 |
| (*Peter Pan*) ......... | 200 | 8.0 | 6.0 | 16.0 | 0 | 110 | 3.0 |

| Food and Measure | cal. | prot. (gms) | carbo. (gms) | fat (gms) | chol. (mgs) | sod. (mgs) | fiber (gms) |
|---|---|---|---|---|---|---|---|
| **Peanut butter, chunky/crunchy** *(cont.)* | | | | | | | |
| (*Skippy Super Chunk*) | 190 | 7.0 | 7.0 | 16.0 | 0 | 120 | 2.0 |
| (*Skippy* Natural) ..... | 180 | 7.0 | 6.0 | 17.0 | 0 | 125 | 2.0 |
| (*Skippy* Reduced Fat) . | 180 | 7.0 | 15.0 | 12.0 | 0 | 160 | 2.0 |
| (*Smucker's*) ........ | 200 | 7.0 | 6.0 | 16.0 | 0 | 90 | 2.0 |
| (*Smucker's* Organic) .. | 210 | 7.0 | 6.0 | 16.0 | 0 | 45 | 2.0 |
| creamy: | | | | | | | |
| (*Jif*) .............. | 190 | 7.0 | 7.0 | 16.0 | 0 | 150 | 2.0 |
| (*Jif* Natural Spread) .. | 190 | 7.0 | 8.0 | 16.0 | 0 | 80 | 2.0 |
| (*Jif* Omega-3) ....... | 190 | 7.0 | 8.0 | 16.0 | 0 | 160 | 2.0 |
| (*Jif* Reduced Fat) .... | 190 | 8.0 | 15.0 | 12.0 | 0 | 250 | 1.0 |
| (*MaraNatha* Natural Omega-3/Calcium) . | 180 | 7.0 | 7.0 | 15.0 | 0 | 65 | 3.0 |
| (*Peter Pan*) ......... | 210 | 8.0 | 6.0 | 17.0 | 0 | 140 | 2.0 |
| (*Reese's*) .......... | 190 | 8.0 | 7.0 | 16.0 | 0 | 140 | 3.0 |
| (*Simply Jif*) ......... | 190 | 8.0 | 6.0 | 16.0 | 0 | 65 | 2.0 |
| (*Skippy*) ........... | 190 | 7.0 | 7.0 | 16.0 | 0 | 150 | 2.0 |
| (*Skippy* Natural) ..... | 190 | 7.0 | 6.0 | 16.0 | 0 | 150 | 2.0 |
| (*Skippy* Reduced Fat) . | 180 | 7.0 | 15.0 | 12.0 | 0 | 170 | 2.0 |
| (*Smucker's*) ........ | 200 | 7.0 | 6.0 | 16.0 | 0 | 105 | 2.0 |
| (*Smucker's* No Salt) .. | 210 | 7.0 | 6.0 | 16.0 | 0 | 0 | 2.0 |
| (*Smucker's* Organic) .. | 210 | 7.0 | 6.0 | 16.0 | 0 | 50 | 2.0 |
| (*Smucker's* Reduced Fat) .............. | 190 | 8.0 | 12.0 | 12.0 | 0 | 115 | 2.0 |
| whipped (*Peter Pan*) .. | 150 | 6.0 | 5.0 | 12.0 | 0 | 105 | 2.0 |
| w/honey: | | | | | | | |
| (*Arrowhead Mills*) .... | 190 | 7.0 | 7.0 | 16.0 | 0 | 100 | 2.0 |
| (*Jif*) .............. | 180 | 6.0 | 10.0 | 14.0 | 0 | 120 | 2.0 |
| (*Skippy* Natural) ..... | 200 | 6.0 | 9.0 | 16.0 | 0 | 140 | 2.0 |
| (*Smucker's*) ........ | 200 | 7.0 | 9.0 | 16.0 | 0 | 30 | 2.0 |
| chunky (*Peter Pan*) ... | 200 | 7.0 | 11.0 | 15.0 | 0 | 115 | 2.0 |
| creamy (*Peter Pan*) ... | 200 | 8.0 | 10.0 | 15.0 | 0 | 125 | 2.0 |
| honey nut, roasted: | | | | | | | |
| chunky (*Skippy*) ..... | 190 | 7.0 | 6.0 | 16.0 | 0 | 105 | 2.0 |
| creamy (*Skippy*) ..... | 190 | 7.0 | 7.0 | 16.0 | 0 | 125 | 2.0 |
| **Peanut butter baking chips**, 1 tbsp., .5 oz.: | | | | | | | |
| (*Reese's* Chips) ........ | 80 | 3.0 | 8.0 | 4.5 | 0 | 30 | 1.0 |
| w/chocolate: | | | | | | | |
| (*Reese's* Pieces) ..... | 70 | 1.0 | 10.0 | 3.0 | 0 | 35 | 0 |
| (*Nestlé Toll House*) ... | 70 | 1.0 | 9.0 | 4.5 | 0 | 25 | 0 |
| (*Nestlé Toll House* Swirled) ......... | 75 | 0 | 8.0 | 4.5 | 0 | 20 | 0 |

| Food and Measure | cal. | prot. (gms) | carbo. (gms) | fat (gms) | chol. (mgs) | sod. (mgs) | fiber (gms) |
|---|---|---|---|---|---|---|---|
| **Peanut butter and jelly**, grape or strawberry (*Smucker's Goober*), 3 tbsp. ..... | 240 | 7.0 | 24.0 | 13.0 | 0 | 140 | 2.0 |
| **Peanut butter sandwich**, frozen (*Smucker's Uncrustables*), 1 pc.: | | | | | | | |
| and grape jelly or strawberry jam ...... | 210 | 6.0 | 25.0 | 9.0 | 0 | 240 | 2.0 |
| and grape jelly or strawberry jam on whole wheat ........ | 210 | 7.0 | 26.0 | 9.0 | 0 | 230 | 3.0 |
| and honey on wheat .... | 210 | 7.0 | 26.0 | 9.0 | 0 | 230 | 3.0 |
| **Peanut butter sprinkles** (*Reese's*), 2 tbsp. .... | 90 | 1.0 | 12.0 | 4.0 | 0 | 55 | 1.0 |
| **Peanut butter topping** (*Reese's* Shell), 2 tbsp. ............ | 210 | 1.0 | 17.0 | 17.0 | 0 | 70 | 1.0 |
| **Peanut flour**, 1 cup: | | | | | | | |
| defatted .............. | 196 | 31.3 | 20.8 | .3 | 0 | 9 | 9.5 |
| low fat ............... | 257 | 20.3 | 18.8 | 13.1 | 0 | 0 | 9.5 |
| **Peanut sauce**, 1 tbsp., except as noted: | | | | | | | |
| (*Annie Chun's* Thai) ..... | 60 | 2.0 | 5.0 | 3.5 | 0 | 135 | 0 |
| (*Heaven and Earth*) ..... | 100 | 10.0 | 5.0 | 16.0 | 0 | 90 | 0 |
| (*Kikkoman*), 2 tbsp. .... | 80 | 2.0 | 10.0 | 3.5 | 0 | 650 | <1.0 |
| (*Marinade Bay*) ........ | 30 | 1.0 | 2.0 | 2.0 | 0 | 130 | 0 |
| (*San-J* Thai), 2 tbsp. .... | 80 | 3.0 | 10.0 | 3.5 | 0 | 690 | <1.0 |
| satay, 2 tbsp.: | | | | | | | |
| (*Roland*) ............ | 80 | 2.0 | 12.0 | 3.0 | 0 | 680 | 2.0 |
| (*A Taste of Thai*) ..... | 80 | 1.0 | 9.0 | 4.5 | 0 | 180 | 1.0 |
| **Peanut sauce mix** (*A Taste of Thai*), ¼ pkt. ............. | 60 | 1.0 | 8.0 | 2.5 | 0 | 140 | 1.0 |
| **Peanut seasoning** (*A Taste of Thai* Bake), ¼ pkt. ....... | 50 | 1.0 | 8.0 | 2.0 | 0 | 140 | 1.0 |
| **Peanut spread**, see "Peanut butter" | | | | | | | |
| **Pear**, fresh, w/peel: | | | | | | | |
| (*Chiquita*), 6.3-oz. pc. ... | 103 | 1.0 | 28.0 | 0 | 0 | 2 | 6.0 |
| (*Dole*), 5.9-oz. pc. ...... | 100 | <1.0 | 26.0 | 1.0 | 0 | 0 | 5.0 |
| 1 large, 2 per lb. ....... | 123 | .8 | 31.6 | .8 | 0 | 0 | 5.0 |

| Food and Measure | cal. | prot. (gms) | carbo. (gms) | fat (gms) | chol. (mgs) | sod. (mgs) | fiber (gms) |
|---|---|---|---|---|---|---|---|
| **Pear** *(cont.)* | | | | | | | |
| Bartlett, 1 medium, | | | | | | | |
| 2½ per lb. . . . . . . . . . | 98 | .7 | 25.1 | .7 | 0 | 1 | 4.0 |
| sliced, ½ cup . . . . . . . . . | 49 | .3 | 12.5 | .3 | 0 | 1 | 2.0 |
| **Pear, Asian**: | | | | | | | |
| (*Frieda's*), 4.3-oz. pc. . . . | 50 | 1.0 | 13.0 | 0 | 0 | 0 | 4.0 |
| 1 medium, 2¼" | | | | | | | |
| x 2½" diam. . . . . . . . . | 51 | .6 | 13.0 | .3 | 0 | 0 | 4.4 |
| **Pear, can/jar**, ½ cup | | | | | | | |
| halves or slices, | | | | | | | |
| except as noted: | | | | | | | |
| (*Del Monte Carb* | | | | | | | |
| *Clever*) . . . . . . . . . . . | 40 | 0 | 10.0 | 0 | 0 | 10 | 1.0 |
| in juice: | | | | | | | |
| (*Del Monte* 100%) . . . | 60 | 0 | 15.0 | 0 | 0 | 10 | 1.0 |
| (*S&W* Natural) . . . . . . | 80 | 0 | 21.0 | 0 | 0 | 10 | 2.0 |
| chunks, acai/ | | | | | | | |
| blackberry juice (*Del* | | | | | | | |
| *Monte Superfruit*), | | | | | | | |
| 6-oz. cup . . . . . . . . | 120 | 2.0 | 31.0 | 0 | 0 | 15 | 3.0 |
| w/liquid . . . . . . . . . . | 62 | .4 | 16.0 | .1 | 0 | 5 | 2.0 |
| in extra light syrup: | | | | | | | |
| (*Del Monte* Lite) . . . . . | 60 | 0 | 15.0 | 0 | 0 | 10 | 1.0 |
| diced (*Del Monte* | | | | | | | |
| Lite), 4-oz. can . . . . | 50 | 0 | 13.0 | 0 | 0 | 10 | <1.0 |
| in light syrup: | | | | | | | |
| (*S&W*) . . . . . . . . . . . | 80 | 0 | 19.0 | 0 | 0 | 10 | 2.0 |
| baby, whole (*Roland*) . | 80 | 0 | 21.0 | 0 | 0 | 10 | 1.0 |
| Bartlett (*Del Monte* | | | | | | | |
| *Orchard Select*) . . . | 80 | <1.0 | 20.0 | 0 | 0 | 10 | 2.0 |
| w/liquid . . . . . . . . . . . | 72 | .2 | 19.0 | <.1 | 0 | 6 | 2.0 |
| chunks (*S&W* Sun) . . . | 80 | <1.0 | 20.0 | 0 | 0 | 10 | <1.0 |
| cinnamon (*Del Monte*) | 80 | 0 | 21.0 | 0 | 0 | 10 | 1.0 |
| diced (*Dole* Bowl), 4 oz. | 80 | <1.0 | 19.0 | 0 | 0 | 5 | <1.0 |
| in heavy syrup: | | | | | | | |
| (*Del Monte*) . . . . . . . . | 100 | 0 | 24.0 | 0 | 0 | 10 | 1.0 |
| w/liquid . . . . . . . . . . . | 98 | .3 | 25.5 | .2 | 0 | 7 | 2.1 |
| diced (*Del Monte*), | | | | | | | |
| 4-oz. can . . . . . . . . | 80 | 0 | 20.0 | 0 | 0 | 10 | <1.0 |
| in gelatin, cherry | | | | | | | |
| pomegranate (*Jell-O*), | | | | | | | |
| 3.25-oz. cont. . . . . . . . | 30 | 2.0 | 5.0 | 0 | 0 | 50 | 0 |
| **Pear, dried**: | | | | | | | |
| 2 oz. . . . . . . . . . . . . . | 149 | 1.1 | 39.5 | .4 | 0 | 4 | 4.3 |

| Food and Measure | cal. | prot. (gms) | carbo. (gms) | fat (gms) | chol. (mgs) | sod. (mgs) | fiber (gms) |
|---|---|---|---|---|---|---|---|
| sulfured: | | | | | | | |
| halves, ½ cup ....... | 236 | 1.7 | 62.7 | .6 | 0 | 5 | 6.8 |
| stewed, ½ cup ...... | 162 | 1.2 | 43.1 | .4 | 0 | 4 | 8.2 |
| **Pear drink**, sparkling | | | | | | | |
| (*Kristian Regale*), | | | | | | | |
| 8 fl. oz. ............ | 100 | 0 | 25.0 | 0 | 0 | 10 | 0 |
| **Pear juice**, 8 fl. oz.: | | | | | | | |
| (*Bolthouse Farms* | | | | | | | |
| Merlot) ............ | 140 | 0 | 35.0 | 0 | 0 | 25 | 3.0 |
| (*Ceres*) ............. | 120 | 0 | 31.0 | 0 | 0 | 10 | 2.0 |
| (*R.W. Knudsen* | | | | | | | |
| Organic) .......... | 150 | <1.0 | 38.0 | 0 | 0 | 10 | 0 |
| (*R.W. Knudsen* | | | | | | | |
| Organic Box) ........ | 120 | 0 | 30.0 | 0 | 0 | 15 | <1.0 |
| (*Santa Cruz Organic* | | | | | | | |
| Nectar) ............ | 120 | 0 | 30.0 | 0 | 0 | 30 | 0 |
| sparkling (*R.W.* | | | | | | | |
| *Knudsen* Organic) .... | 120 | 0 | 29.0 | 0 | 0 | 15 | 0 |
| **Pear nectar**, canned, | | | | | | | |
| 8 fl. oz. ............ | 150 | .3 | 39.4 | <.1 | 0 | 10 | 1.5 |
| **Peas, black-eyed**, see | | | | | | | |
| "Black-eyed peas" | | | | | | | |
| **Peas, butter**, frozen | | | | | | | |
| (*Allens*), ⅔ cup ...... | 130 | 7.0 | 24.0 | 0 | 0 | 5 | 6.0 |
| **Peas, cream**, canned, | | | | | | | |
| (*East Texas Fair*), | | | | | | | |
| ½ cup ............. | 100 | 6.0 | 17.0 | 1.0 | 0 | 460 | 5.0 |
| **Peas, crowder**: | | | | | | | |
| canned, ½ cup: | | | | | | | |
| (*Allens/East Texas* | | | | | | | |
| *Fair*) ............ | 110 | 6.0 | 19.0 | 1.0 | 0 | 460 | 8.0 |
| (*Bush's*) ........... | 110 | 7.0 | 18.0 | 1.0 | 0 | 500 | 5.0 |
| frozen (*Allens*), ⅔ cup ... | 130 | n.a. | 23.0 | .5 | 0 | 10 | 5.0 |
| **Peas, edible-podded**: | | | | | | | |
| raw: | | | | | | | |
| (*Frieda's* Sugar | | | | | | | |
| Snap), 1 cup ..... | 25 | 2.0 | 5.0 | 0 | 0 | 3 | 2.0 |
| (*Green Giant* Fresh | | | | | | | |
| Snow Peas/Sugar | | | | | | | |
| Snap), 3 oz. ...... | 35 | 2.0 | 6.0 | 0 | 0 | 0 | 2.0 |
| w/sauce (*Frieda's* | | | | | | | |
| Snow), ½ cup .... | 40 | 2.0 | 8.0 | 0 | 0 | 180 | 2.0 |
| boiled, drained, ½ cup .. | 34 | 2.6 | 5.6 | .2 | 0 | 3 | 2.2 |

| Food and Measure | cal. | prot. (gms) | carbo. (gms) | fat (gms) | chol. (mgs) | sod. (mgs) | fiber (gms) |
|---|---|---|---|---|---|---|---|
| **Peas, edible-podded, frozen**, sugar snap: | | | | | | | |
| (*Birds Eye/Birds Eye Steamfresh/C&W*), ⅔ cup . . . . . . . . . . . . | 40 | 2.0 | 7.0 | 0 | 0 | 0 | 2.0 |
| (*Cascadian Farm Organic*), ¾ cup . . . . . | 35 | 2.0 | 6.0 | 0 | 0 | 140 | 2.0 |
| (*Green Giant Simply Steam*), ⅔ cup . . . . . . | 45 | 2.0 | 10.0 | 0 | 0 | 95 | 2.0 |
| boiled, drained, ½ cup . . | 42 | 2.8 | 7.2 | .3 | 0 | 4 | 2.5 |
| **Peas, edible-podded, combinations**, frozen, sugar snap, 1 cup: | | | | | | | |
| baby carrots, cauliflower, broccoli (*C&W Sugar Snap*) . . . | 30 | 1.0 | 5.0 | 0 | 0 | 25 | 2.0 |
| stir-fry (*Birds Eye*) . . . . . . | 40 | 2.0 | 7.0 | 0 | 0 | 25 | 2.0 |
| **Peas, field, canned** (see also "Peas, crowder" and "Peas, purple hull"), ½ cup: | | | | | | | |
| w/bacon (*Trappey's*) . . . . | 90 | 6.0 | 15.0 | 1.0 | 0 | 380 | 5.0 |
| w/jalapeño (*East Texas Fair* Pepper Peas) . . . . | 120 | 6.0 | 22.0 | 1.0 | 0 | 580 | 6.0 |
| w/pork (*East Texas Fair* Peas & Pork) . . . . | 110 | 6.0 | 19.0 | 1.5 | 0 | 540 | 5.0 |
| w/snaps: | | | | | | | |
| (*Allens/East Texas Fair/Sunshine*) . . . | 120 | 6.0 | 21.0 | 1.0 | 0 | 300 | 6.0 |
| (*Bush's*) . . . . . . . . . . | 80 | 5.0 | 16.0 | 0 | 0 | 430 | 2.0 |
| bacon (*Trappey's*) . . . . | 110 | 6.0 | 19.0 | 1.0 | 0 | 380 | 4.0 |
| seasoned (*Allens*) . . . . | 100 | 6.0 | 18.0 | .5 | 0 | 360 | 3.0 |
| seasoned (*Glory*) . . . . | 90 | 6.0 | 17.0 | .5 | 0 | 570 | 3.0 |
| **Peas, field, frozen**, w/snaps (*McKenzie's*), ⅔ cup . . . . . . . . . . . . . . . | 140 | 9.0 | 26.0 | .5 | 0 | 25 | 6.0 |
| **Peas, green**, fresh: | | | | | | | |
| raw: | | | | | | | |
| in pod, 1 lb. . . . . . . . . | 140 | 9.3 | 24.9 | .7 | 0 | 8 | 8.8 |
| shelled, ½ cup . . . . . . | 59 | 3.9 | 10.4 | .3 | 0 | 3 | 3.7 |
| boiled, drained, ½ cup . . | 67 | 4.3 | 12.5 | .2 | 0 | 2 | 4.4 |
| **Peas, green, can/jar**, ½ cup: | | | | | | | |
| (*Bush's* Petit Pois) . . . . . | 80 | 5.0 | 12.0 | 1.0 | 0 | 340 | 4.0 |

| Food and Measure | cal. | prot. (gms) | carbo. (gms) | fat (gms) | chol. (mgs) | sod. (mgs) | fiber (gms) |
|---|---|---|---|---|---|---|---|
| (*Del Monte*) . . . . . . . . . . | 60 | 3.0 | 13.0 | 0 | 0 | 390 | 4.0 |
| (*Del Monte* Very Young Small) . . . . . . . | 60 | 3.0 | 10.0 | 0 | 0 | 360 | 4.0 |
| (*Freshlike* Selects) . . . . . . | 90 | 5.0 | 16.0 | .5 | 0 | 410 | 5.0 |
| (*Freshlike* Tender Garden) . . . . . . . . . . | 110 | 6.0 | 19.0 | .5 | 0 | 370 | 6.0 |
| (*Freshlike* Tender Garden No Salt) . . . . . | 110 | 6.0 | 19.0 | .5 | 0 | 10 | 6.0 |
| (*Green Giant* Sweet) . . . . | 60 | 4.0 | 12.0 | 0 | 0 | 400 | 3.0 |
| (*Green Giant* Sweet Less Sodium) . . . . . . . | 60 | 4.0 | 11.0 | 0 | 0 | 200 | 3.0 |
| (*Le Sueur* Very Young) . . | 60 | 4.0 | 12.0 | 0 | 0 | 380 | 3.0 |
| (*Le Sueur* Very Young Less Sodium) . . . . . . . | 60 | 4.0 | 11.0 | 0 | 0 | 190 | 3.0 |
| (*Roland*) . . . . . . . . . . . . . | 120 | 7.0 | 21.0 | 0 | 0 | 450 | 6.0 |
| (*S&W* Petit Pois) . . . . . . . | 60 | 3.0 | 10.0 | 0 | 0 | 360 | 4.0 |
| (*Veg-All* Tender) . . . . . . . | 60 | 4.0 | 10.0 | .5 | 0 | 270 | 3.0 |
| drained . . . . . . . . . . . . . | 59 | 3.8 | 10.7 | .3 | 0 | 214 | 3.5 |
| seasoned, w/liquid . . . . . | 57 | 3.5 | 10.5 | .3 | 0 | 288 | 2.8 |
| **Peas, green, combinations, can/jar:** | | | | | | | |
| and carrots, ½ cup: | | | | | | | |
| (*Del Monte*) . . . . . . . . | 60 | 2.0 | 11.0 | 0 | 0 | 360 | 2.0 |
| (*Freshlike*) . . . . . . . . . | 60 | 4.0 | 11.0 | 0 | 0 | 350 | 3.0 |
| (*Roland*) . . . . . . . . . . | 90 | 4.0 | 17.0 | 0 | 0 | 250 | 4.0 |
| (*S&W*) . . . . . . . . . . . | 60 | 2.0 | 11.0 | 0 | 0 | 360 | 2.0 |
| (*Veg-All*) . . . . . . . . . . | 60 | 2.0 | 12.0 | 0 | 0 | 330 | 4.0 |
| w/liquid . . . . . . . . . . . | 48 | 2.8 | 10.8 | .3 | 0 | 332 | 2.6 |
| w/mushrooms, pearl onions (*Le Sueur*) . . . . | 60 | 3.0 | 11.0 | 0 | 0 | 380 | 2.0 |
| and onions, ½ cup: | | | | | | | |
| (*Freshlike* Selects) . . . | 60 | 3.0 | 11.0 | 0 | 0 | 440 | 3.0 |
| (*S&W*) . . . . . . . . . . . | 40 | 3.0 | 11.0 | 0 | 0 | 530 | 3.0 |
| w/liquid . . . . . . . . . . . | 31 | 2.0 | 5.1 | .2 | 0 | 265 | 1.4 |
| **Peas, green, combinations, frozen,** ⅔ cup, except as noted: | | | | | | | |
| and carrots: | | | | | | | |
| (*Cascadian Farm* Organic) . . . . . . . . | 50 | 2.0 | 10.0 | 0 | 0 | 75 | 3.0 |
| (*Veg-All* SteamSupreme) . . . | 60 | 3.0 | 11.0 | 0 | 0 | 25 | 4.0 |
| boiled, drained, ½ cup | 38 | 2.7 | 8.1 | .3 | 0 | 54 | 2.5 |

| Food and Measure | cal. | prot. (gms) | carbo. (gms) | fat (gms) | chol. (mgs) | sod. (mgs) | fiber (gms) |
|---|---|---|---|---|---|---|---|
| **Peas, green, combinations, frozen** *(cont.)* | | | | | | | |
| and corn, basil butter (*Green Giant Just for One*), 1 tray | 80 | 4.0 | 14.0 | 2.0 | <5 | 360 | 3.0 |
| and corn, carrots, sugar snaps (*C&W Early Harvest*) | 50 | 2.0 | 10.0 | 0 | 0 | 70 | 2.0 |
| and mushrooms, garlic seasoned (*Birds Eye Steamfresh*), ¾ cup | 80 | 4.0 | 12.0 | 2.0 | 0 | 340 | 3.0 |
| and pearl onions: | | | | | | | |
| (*Cascadian Farm Organic*), ¾ cup | 60 | 3.0 | 11.0 | 0 | 0 | 90 | 3.0 |
| (*C&W Petite*) | 60 | 4.0 | 11.0 | 0 | 0 | 160 | 3.0 |
| (*Green Giant Simply Steam*), ½ cup | 60 | 3.0 | 10.0 | 0 | 0 | 80 | 3.0 |
| baby (*Birds Eye*) | 60 | 4.0 | 12.0 | 0 | 0 | 0 | 3.0 |
| baby, and vegetables (*Birds Eye*), ¾ cup | 40 | 2.0 | 7.0 | 0 | 0 | 20 | 2.0 |
| in lightly seasoned sauce (*Birds Eye*) | 90 | 5.0 | 17.0 | 0 | 0 | 510 | 4.0 |
| boiled, drained, ½ cup | 41 | 2.3 | 7.8 | .2 | 0 | 33 | 2.0 |
| **Peas, green, dish**, microwave (*Tasty Bite*), ½ of 10-oz. pkg.: | | | | | | | |
| w/cheese, paneer | 150 | 3.0 | 7.0 | 10.0 | 13 | 350 | 6.0 |
| and greens, Agra | 140 | 4.0 | 9.0 | 10.0 | 3 | 410 | 4.0 |
| **Peas, green, dried**, rehydrated (*Frieda's*), ⅓ cup, 3 oz. | 130 | 9.0 | 22.0 | 0 | 0 | 290 | 9.0 |
| **Peas, green, frozen**, ⅔ cup, except as noted: | | | | | | | |
| (*Allens* Garden Peas) | 70 | 4.0 | 13.0 | 0 | 0 | 5 | 4.0 |
| (*Allens* Petite SteamSupreme) | 70 | 4.0 | 12.0 | 0 | 0 | 0 | 4.0 |
| (*Birds Eye* Baby) | 70 | 4.0 | 12.0 | 0 | 0 | 0 | 4.0 |
| (*Birds Eye/Freshlike* Garden/*Birds Eye Steamfresh* Sweet) | 70 | 5.0 | 12.0 | 0 | 0 | 0 | 4.0 |
| (*Birds Eye Steamfresh* Sweet Singles), 3.25-oz. bag | 70 | 5.0 | 13.0 | 0 | 0 | 0 | 4.0 |

| Food and Measure | cal. | prot. (gms) | carbo. (gms) | fat (gms) | chol. (mgs) | sod. (mgs) | fiber (gms) |
|---|---|---|---|---|---|---|---|
| (Cascadian Farm Organic Garden/Sweet) | 70 | 4.0 | 12.0 | 0 | 0 | 95 | 4.0 |
| (Cascadian Farm Organic Petite) ...... | 50 | 4.0 | 10.0 | .5 | 0 | 90 | 4.0 |
| (Cascadian Farm Purely Steam Organic Petite) ...... | 50 | 4.0 | 10.0 | 1.0 | 0 | 90 | 4.0 |
| (C&W/Freshlike Petite) ............. | 70 | 4.0 | 12.0 | 0 | 0 | 200 | 4.0 |
| (C&W Early Harvest Petite No Salt) ...... | 70 | 4.0 | 12.0 | 0 | 0 | 0 | 4.0 |
| (Green Giant Simply Steam Baby Sweet) .. | 60 | 4.0 | 13.0 | .5 | 0 | 190 | 4.0 |
| (Green Giant Valley Fresh Steamers) ..... | 60 | 4.0 | 12.0 | 0 | 0 | 0 | 4.0 |
| butter sauce, ¾ cup: (Allens SteamSupreme) ... | 100 | 4.0 | 14.0 | 2.5 | 5 | 130 | 4.0 |
| Green Giant Simply Steam) .......... | 80 | 5.0 | 14.0 | 1.5 | <5 | 340 | 4.0 |
| **Peas, pigeon,** see "Pigeon peas" | | | | | | | |
| **Peas, purple hull**: canned, ½ cup: (Allen/East Texas Fair) ............. | 120 | 7.0 | 21.0 | 1.0 | 0 | 350 | 6.0 |
| (Bush's) ........... | 90 | 6.0 | 19.0 | 0 | 0 | 460 | 5.0 |
| frozen: (Allens), ⅔ cup ...... | 150 | 10.0 | 26.0 | .5 | 0 | 0 | 6.0 |
| (McKenzie's), ½ cup .. | 120 | 8.0 | 22.0 | .5 | 0 | 21 | 5.0 |
| **Peas, split,** see "Split peas" | | | | | | | |
| **Peas, sprouted**: raw, ½ cup .......... | 77 | 5.3 | 17.0 | .4 | 0 | 12 | n.a. |
| boiled, drained, 4 oz. .... | 134 | 8.0 | 24.8 | .6 | 0 | 3 | 3.7 |
| **Peas, sugar snap or snow,** see "Peas, edible-podded" | | | | | | | |
| **Peas, sweet,** see "Peas, green" | | | | | | | |
| **Peas, wasabi** (Roland Feng Shui), ¼ cup ... | 120 | 6.0 | 21.0 | 1.0 | 0 | 155 | 3.0 |
| **Peas, white acre,** canned (East Texas Fair), ½ cup | 100 | 6.0 | 17.0 | 1.0 | 0 | 460 | 5.0 |

| Food and Measure | cal. | prot. (gms) | carbo. (gms) | fat (gms) | chol. (mgs) | sod. (mgs) | fiber (gms) |
|---|---|---|---|---|---|---|---|
| **Peas and carrots or** **onions**, see "Peas, green, combinations" | | | | | | | |
| **Pecan**, shelled: | | | | | | | |
| (*Beer Nuts*), 1 oz. . . . . . . | 200 | 3.0 | 4.0 | 19.0 | 0 | 65 | 1.0 |
| all style (*Diamond*), | | | | | | | |
| ¼ cup, 1.1 oz. . . . . . . . | 210 | 3.0 | 4.0 | 22.0 | 0 | 0 | 3.0 |
| halves: | | | | | | | |
| (*Planters*), 1 oz. . . . . . | 200 | 3.0 | 4.0 | 20.0 | 0 | 0 | 3.0 |
| (*Planters*), 2-oz. pkg. . | 390 | 5.0 | 8.0 | 41.0 | 0 | 5 | 5.0 |
| 1 cup . . . . . . . . . . . . . | 721 | 8.4 | 19.7 | 73.1 | 0 | 1 | 8.2 |
| chips (*Planters*), | | | | | | | |
| 2-oz. pkg. . . . . . . . . . | 390 | 5.0 | 8.0 | 41.0 | 0 | 0 | 5.0 |
| chopped, 1 cup . . . . . . . | 794 | 9.2 | 21.7 | 80.5 | 0 | 1 | 9.0 |
| dry-roasted: | | | | | | | |
| unsalted, 1 oz. . . . . . . | 201 | 2.7 | 3.8 | 21.1 | 0 | <1 | 2.7 |
| unsalted, 1 cup : . . . . . | 781 | 10.5 | 14.9 | 81.7 | 0 | 11 | 10.5 |
| oil-roasted: | | | | | | | |
| unsalted, 1 oz. . . . . . . | 203 | 2.7 | 3.7 | 21.3 | 0 | <1 | 2.7 |
| unsalted, 1 cup . . . . . . | 787 | 10.5 | 14.3 | 82.8 | 0 | 11 | 10.5 |
| pieces (*Planters*), 2-oz. pkg. | 390 | 5.0 | 8.0 | 41.0 | 0 | 0 | 5.0 |
| praline (*Frito-Lay*), | | | | | | | |
| 1 pkg. . . . . . . . . . . . . | 350 | 4.0 | 26.0 | 26.0 | 0 | 230 | 4.0 |
| **Pecan flour**, 1 oz. . . . . . | 93 | 9.1 | 14.4 | .4 | 0 | tr. | n.a. |
| **Pecan topping**, in syrup | | | | | | | |
| (*Smucker's*), 1 tbsp. . . | 160 | 1.0 | 19.0 | 9.0 | 0 | 0 | <1.0 |
| **Pectin**, see "Fruit pectin" | | | | | | | |
| **Penne**, see "Pasta" | | | | | | | |
| **Penne entree**, frozen, 1 pkg., except as noted: | | | | | | | |
| Alfredo (*Glutino* Gluten Free), 10.5 oz. . | 400 | 14.0 | 65.0 | 9.0 | 35 | 870 | 4.0 |
| w/chicken, see "Chicken entree" | | | | | | | |
| marinara (*Blue Horizon*), | | | | | | | |
| ¼ of 32-oz. pkg. . . . . . | 270 | 17.0 | 38.0 | 6.0 | 20 | 280 | 3.0 |
| portobello/spinach/ Parmesan (*Healthy* *Choice*), 9.4 oz. . . . . . | 270 | 11.0 | 40.0 | 7.0 | 10 | 600 | 5.0 |
| primavera (*Michelina's Lean* *Gourmet*), 8 oz. . . . . . | 280 | 11.0 | 43.0 | 6.0 | 15 | 470 | 3.0 |

| Food and Measure | cal. | prot. (gms) | carbo. (gms) | fat (gms) | chol. (mgs) | sod. (mgs) | fiber (gms) |
|---|---|---|---|---|---|---|---|
| puttanesca (*Moosewood Organic*), 10 oz. ..... | 300 | 8.0 | 45.0 | 10.0 | 0 | 300 | 2.0 |
| tomato basil (*Healthy Choice*), 10 oz. ...... | 280 | 13.0 | 39.0 | 6.0 | 15 | 600 | 7.0 |
| w/vegetables, Alfredo sauce (*Birds Eye Steamfresh* Lightly Sauced), 1⅓ cups ... | 260 | 9.0 | 37.0 | 8.0 | 20 | 420 | 2.0 |
| **Penne entree, microwave** (*Healthy Choice Fresh Mixers*), 6.9 oz.: | | | | | | | |
| Alfredo, roasted red pepper ........... | 290 | 10.0 | 51.0 | 5.0 | 10 | 500 | 6.0 |
| tomato basil, creamy .... | 290 | 10.0 | 50.0 | 5.0 | 5 | 490 | 6.0 |
| **Penne entree mix**, Alfredo cheese sauce (*Annie's*), 1 cup* .... | 290 | 12.0 | 39.0 | 10.5 | 30 | 490 | 2.0 |
| **Pepeao**, raw, sliced, 1 cup ............. | 25 | .5 | 6.7 | 0 | 0 | 9 | n.a. |
| **Pepeao, dried**, 1 cup ... | 72 | 1.2 | 19.5 | .1 | 0 | 17 | n.a. |
| **Pepitas**, see "Pumpkin seeds" | | | | | | | |
| **Pepper**, seasoning: | | | | | | | |
| (*Maull's* Four), ¾ tbsp. ... | 5 | 0 | 1.0 | 0 | 0 | 240 | 0 |
| black, 1 tsp.: | | | | | | | |
| ground ............ | 6 | .3 | 1.7 | .1 | 0 | 1 | .7 |
| whole ............ | 8 | .3 | 1.9 | 0 | 0 | 1 | .8 |
| chili, 1 tsp. ......... | 9 | .3 | 1.2 | .3 | 0 | <1 | .7 |
| red or cayenne, 1 tsp. ... | 6 | .2 | 1.0 | .3 | 0 | 1 | .7 |
| white, 1 tsp. ........ | 7 | .3 | 1.7 | .1 | 0 | 0 | .2 |
| **Pepper, ancho**, dried, .6-oz. pc. .......... | 48 | 2.0 | 8.7 | 1.4 | 0 | 7 | 3..7 |
| **Pepper, banana**, fresh, 1.2-oz. pc. .... | 9 | .6 | 1.8 | .2 | 0 | 4 | 1.1 |
| **Pepper, banana, in jars**, sliced (*Roland*), 14 slices, 1 oz. ...... | 0 | 0 | 0 | 0 | 0 | 580 | 0 |
| **Pepper, bell**, see "Pepper, sweet" | | | | | | | |
| **Pepper, cherry, in jars:** | | | | | | | |
| (*Roland*), 1 whole or 7 slices, 1 oz. ....... | 5 | 0 | 1.0 | 0 | 0 | 370 | 0 |
| (*Vigo*), 4 pcs. ......... | 10 | 0 | 2.0 | 0 | 0 | 480 | 0 |
| crushed (*Roland*), 1 tbsp. | 0 | 0 | 0 | 0 | 0 | 85 | 0 |

| Food and Measure | cal. | prot. (gms) | carbo. (gms) | fat (gms) | chol. (mgs) | sod. (mgs) | fiber (gms) |
|---|---|---|---|---|---|---|---|
| **Pepper, cherry** *(cont.)* | | | | | | | |
| hot or sweet (*B&G*), | | | | | | | |
| 1-oz. pc. . . . . . . . . . . | 10 | 0 | 2.0 | 0 | 0 | 310 | 0 |
| sliced, in oil (*B&G*), | | | | | | | |
| 7 pcs., 1 oz. . . . . . . . | 28 | 0 | 0 | 2.8 | 0 | 310 | 0 |
| **Pepper, chili**, fresh, | | | | | | | |
| green and red: | | | | | | | |
| (*Frieda's* Anaheim), | | | | | | | |
| chopped, ½ cup . . . . . | 30 | 2.0 | 7.0 | 0 | 0 | 5 | 1.0 |
| (*Frieda's* Habanero), | | | | | | | |
| 1.6-oz. pc. . . . . . . . . | 20 | 1.0 | 4.0 | 0 | 0 | 0 | 1.0 |
| 1 medium, 1.6 oz. . . . . . | 18 | .9 | 4.3 | .1 | 0 | 3 | .7 |
| chopped, ½ cup . . . . . . | 30 | 1.5 | 7.1 | .2 | 0 | 5 | 1.1 |
| **Pepper, chili, can/jar** | | | | | | | |
| (see also specific | | | | | | | |
| listings): | | | | | | | |
| whole (*Frieda's* | | | | | | | |
| Habanero), 4 pcs., 1 oz. | 10 | 0 | 2.0 | 0 | 0 | 270 | 1.0 |
| whole, green, 1 pc.: | | | | | | | |
| (*Chi-Chi's*) . . . . . . . . | 10 | 0 | 2.0 | 0 | 0 | 100 | 0 |
| (*Las Palmas*) . . . . . . . | 10 | 0 | 2.0 | 0 | 0 | 230 | 1.0 |
| (*Old El Paso*) . . . . . . . | 15 | 0 | 3.0 | 0 | 0 | 140 | 0 |
| fire-roasted (*La* | | | | | | | |
| *Victoria*) . . . . . . . . . | 5 | 0 | 1.0 | 0 | 0 | 190 | <1.0 |
| fire-roasted (*Ortega*) . . | 10 | <1.0 | 2.0 | 0 | 0 | 140 | <1.0 |
| large, 2.6 oz. . . . . . . . | 15 | .7 | 3.7 | <.1 | 0 | 856 | 1.0 |
| whole, green, ½ cup . . . . | 15 | .5 | 3.2 | .1 | 0 | 276 | 1.2 |
| chopped: | | | | | | | |
| (*Old El Paso*), 2 tbsp. | 10 | 0 | 2.0 | 0 | 0 | 120 | 0 |
| w/liquid, ½ cup . . . . . . | 17 | .6 | 4.2 | .1 | 0 | n.a. | 1.3 |
| diced, green, 2 tbsp.: | | | | | | | |
| (*Chi-Chi's*) . . . . . . . . | 10 | 0 | 2.0 | 0 | 0 | 85 | 0 |
| (*Las Palmas*) . . . . . . . | 5 | 0 | 1.0 | 0 | 0 | 110 | 1.0 |
| (*Ortega* 4 oz.) . . . . . . . | 5 | <1.0 | 1.0 | 0 | 0 | 70 | 0 |
| (*Ortega* 26 oz.) . . . . . . | 10 | <1.0 | 2.0 | 0 | 0 | 70 | 0 |
| fire-roasted (*La* | | | | | | | |
| *Victoria*) . . . . . . . . . | 10 | 1.0 | 2.0 | 0 | 0 | 120 | 0 |
| strips, green (*Las* | | | | | | | |
| *Palmas*), 1.3-oz. pc. . . | 10 | 0 | 2.0 | 0 | 0 | 240 | 1.0 |
| **Pepper, chili, dried**: | | | | | | | |
| (*Frieda's* Ancho | | | | | | | |
| Mulato), .25-oz. pc. . . | 25 | 1.0 | 4.0 | 1.0 | 0 | 6 | 2.0 |
| (*Frieda's* Bird/de Arbol/ | | | | | | | |
| Habanero), 1 tsp. . . . . | 15 | 0 | 1.0 | 0 | 0 | 1 | 0 |

| Food and Measure | cal. | prot. (gms) | carbo. (gms) | fat (gms) | chol. (mgs) | sod. (mgs) | fiber (gms) |
|---|---|---|---|---|---|---|---|
| (*Frieda's* California), 2 tbsp. . . . . . . . . . . . | 15 | 0 | 2.0 | 0 | 0 | 15 | 0 |
| (*Frieda's* Chipotle), .2-oz. pc. . . . . . . . . . | 20 | 1.0 | 4.0 | 0 | 0 | 22 | 0 |
| (*Frieda's* Guajillo), 2 tbsp. . . . . . . . . . | 15 | 0 | 3.0 | 0 | 0 | 4 | 1.0 |
| (*Frieda's* Japones), .5 oz. | 50 | 4.0 | 7.0 | 0 | 0 | 5 | 2.0 |
| (*Frieda's* Pasilla Negro), .25-oz. pc. . . . . . . . . | 25 | 1.0 | 4.0 | 1.0 | 0 | 5 | 2.0 |
| sun-dried, hot, 2 pcs. . . . | 3 | .1 | .8 | .1 | 0 | 1 | .3 |
| **Pepper, chipotle**, can/jar: | | | | | | | |
| (*Herdez*), 3 pcs, 1 oz. . . . | 30 | 0 | 3.0 | 1.0 | 0 | 360 | 0 |
| in adobo sauce (*Roland*), 2 tbsp. . . . . | 15 | 0 | 3.0 | 0 | 0 | 410 | 1.0 |
| **Pepper, green or red**, sweet, see "Pepper, sweet" | | | | | | | |
| **Pepper, hot**, in jars: | | | | | | | |
| (*B&G* Sandwich Toppers/Rings), 7 pcs., 1 oz. . . . . . . . . | 0 | 0 | 1.0 | 0 | 0 | 310 | 0 |
| roasted, chopped (*B&G*), 1 tsp., .5 oz. . . . . . . . . | 5 | 0 | 1.0 | 0 | 0 | 120 | 0 |
| **Pepper, Hungarian**, fresh, .94-oz. pc. . . . . | 8 | .2 | 1.8 | .1 | 0. | <1 | n.a. |
| **Pepper, jalapeño**, fresh, .5-oz. pc. . . . . . | 4 | .2 | .8 | .1 | 0 | <1 | .4 |
| **Pepper, jalapeño, can/jar**: whole, 2 pcs., except as noted: | | | | | | | |
| (*Chi-Chi's*) . . . . . . . . . | 10 | 0 | 2.0 | 0 | 0 | 190 | 0 |
| (*Herdez*), 3 pcs., 1.3 oz. | 15 | 0 | 1.0 | 0 | 0 | 620 | 1.0 |
| (*Las Palmas*) . . . . . . . | 15 | <1.0 | 2.0 | 0 | 0 | 190 | 0 |
| (*Mrs. Renfro's*), 1 pc. . | 5 | 0 | 0 | 0 | 0 | 410 | 0 |
| fire-roasted (*Ortega*) . . | 10 | <1.0 | 2.0 | 0 | 0 | 20 | 0 |
| chopped: | | | | | | | |
| (*B&G*), 2 tbsp. . . . . . . | 5 | 0 | 1.0 | 0 | 0 | 120 | 0 |
| hot (*Polaner*), 2 tbsp. . | 0 | 0 | 1.0 | 0 | 0 | 120 | 0 |
| w/liquid, ¼ cup . . . . . . | 7 | .2 | 1.2 | .2 | 0 | 434 | .8 |
| diced, 2 tbsp.: | | | | | | | |
| (*Ortega*) . . . . . . . . . . | 10 | <1.0 | 2.0 | 0 | 0 | 25 | 0 |
| fire-roasted, hot (*La Victoria*) . . . . . . . . . | 0 | 0 | <1.0 | 0 | 0 | 150 | 0 |

| Food and Measure | cal. | prot. (gms) | carbo. (gms) | fat (gms) | chol. (mgs) | sod. (mgs) | fiber (gms) |
|---|---|---|---|---|---|---|---|
| **Pepper, jalapeño, can/jar** *(cont.)* | | | | | | | |
| sliced: | | | | | | | |
| (*B&G*), 7 pcs., 1 oz. . . | 0 | 0 | <1.0 | 0 | 0 | 190 | 0 |
| (*Chi-Chi's* Wheels), | | | | | | | |
| ¼ cup . . . . . . . . . . . | 10 | 0 | 2.0 | 0 | 0 | 190 | 0 |
| (*Herdez*), ¼ cup . . . . . | 10 | 0 | 1.0 | 0 | 0 | 630 | 0 |
| (*Las Palmas*), 3 tbsp. . | 10 | <1.0 | 2.0 | 0 | 0 | 210 | 0 |
| (*Mission* Nacho), 1 oz. . | 5 | 0 | 1.0 | 0 | 0 | 270 | 0 |
| (*Mrs. Renfro's* Nacho), | | | | | | | |
| 12 pcs., 1 oz. . . . . . | 5 | 0 | 0 | 0 | 0 | 410 | 0 |
| (*Old El Paso*), 2 tbsp. . | 10 | 0 | 2.0 | 0 | 0 | 200 | 0 |
| (*Ortega*), 1 oz. . . . . . . | 5 | <1.0 | <1.0 | 0 | 0 | 300 | <1.0 |
| (*Pace* Nacho), 1 oz. . . | 5 | 0 | 1.0 | 0 | 0 | 300 | <1.0 |
| (*Roland*), ¼ cup . . . . . | 5 | 0 | 1.0 | 0 | 0 | 640 | 1.0 |
| (*Vigo*), 14 pcs. . . . . . . | 5 | 0 | 1.0 | 0 | 0 | 330 | 0 |
| fire-roasted (*La* | | | | | | | |
| *Victoria* Nacho), 1.1 oz. | 5 | 0 | <1.0 | 0 | 0 | 350 | 0 |
| w/liquid, ¼ cup . . . . . . | 9 | .3 | 1.6 | .3 | 0 | 568 | .9 |
| **Pepper, pasilla**, dried, | | | | | | | |
| 2 pcs., .5 oz. . . . . . . . . | 48 | 1.7 | 7.2 | 2.2 | 0 | 12 | 3.8 |
| **Pepper, piquillo**, can: | | | | | | | |
| (*Roland*), ½ cup . . . . . . | 60 | 2.0 | 11.0 | 0 | 0 | 25 | 2.0 |
| (*Roland* Organic), ½ cup . | 45 | 1.0 | 10.0 | 0 | 0 | 150 | 3.0 |
| stuffed w/cod (*El* | | | | | | | |
| *Navarrico* Bacalao), | | | | | | | |
| 7.8 oz., 4–5 pcs. . . . . . | 270 | 8.0 | 22.0 | 16.0 | 15 | 750 | 2.0 |
| **Pepper, poblano**, see | | | | | | | |
| "Pepper, chili" | | | | | | | |
| **Pepper, roasted**, see | | | | | | | |
| "Pepper, sweet, can/jar" | | | | | | | |
| **Pepper, serrano**, fresh: | | | | | | | |
| whole, .2-oz. pc. . . . . . . | 2 | .1 | .4 | <.1 | 0 | 2 | .2 |
| chopped, ½ cup . . . . . . . | 17 | .9 | 3.5 | .5 | 0 | 5 | 1.9 |
| **Pepper, serrano, in** | | | | | | | |
| **jars**, whole (*Herdez*), | | | | | | | |
| 4 pcs, 1.25 oz. . . . . . . | 15 | 0 | 1.0 | 0 | 0 | 570 | 1.0 |
| **Pepper, stuffed** | | | | | | | |
| (*Roland*), w/cheese: | | | | | | | |
| green, ½ cup . . . . . . . . . | 440 | 4.0 | 13.0 | 42.0 | 10 | 1320 | 6.0 |
| red, ½ cup . . . . . . . . . . . | 470 | 3.0 | 9.0 | 47.0 | 20 | 710 | 3.0 |
| **Pepper, stuffed, frozen:** | | | | | | | |
| green, w/meat, sauce: | | | | | | | |
| (*Stouffer's*), 10-oz. pkg. | 210 | 10.0 | 23.0 | 9.0 | 15 | 990 | 3.0 |

| Food and Measure | cal. | prot. (gms) | carbo. (gms) | fat (gms) | chol. (mgs) | sod. (mgs) | fiber (gms) |
|---|---|---|---|---|---|---|---|
| (*Stouffer's*), ½ of | | | | | | | |
| 15.5-oz. pkg. ..... | 150 | 8.0 | 17.0 | 6.0 | 15 | 750 | 2.0 |
| (*Stouffer's* Family), | | | | | | | |
| ¼ of 32-oz. pkg. ... | 190 | 9.0 | 20.0 | 8.0 | 20 | 730 | 2.0 |
| casserole (*Michelina's*), | | | | | | | |
| 8-oz. pkg. ........ | 270 | 10.0 | 31.0 | 10.0 | 30 | 920 | 1.0 |
| poblano, roasted | | | | | | | |
| (*Cedarlane* Chile | | | | | | | |
| Relleno), 10-oz. pkg. . | 400 | 23.0 | 37.0 | 20.0 | 55 | 770 | 5.0 |
| **Pepper, sweet**, fresh: | | | | | | | |
| green and/or red: | | | | | | | |
| raw, 1 medium, | | | | | | | |
| 3¾" x 3" or | | | | | | | |
| ½ cup chopped ... | 20 | .7 | 4.8 | .1 | 0 | 1 | 1.3 |
| raw, sliced, 1 cup .... | 25 | .8 | 5.9 | .2 | 0 | 2 | 1.7 |
| boiled, drained, | | | | | | | |
| 1 medium ........ | 20 | .7 | 4.9 | .1 | 0 | 1 | .9 |
| boiled, drained, | | | | | | | |
| chopped, 1 tbsp. .. | 3 | .1 | .8 | <.1 | 0 | <1 | .1 |
| boiled, drained, | | | | | | | |
| strips, ½ cup ..... | 19 | .6 | 4.6 | .1 | 0 | 1 | .8 |
| yellow, raw: | | | | | | | |
| 1 large, 5" x 3" ....... | 50 | 1.9 | 11.8 | .4 | 0 | 4 | 1.7 |
| 10 strips, 1.8 oz. ..... | 14 | .5 | 3.3 | .1 | 0 | 1 | .5 |
| **Pepper, sweet, can/jar** | | | | | | | |
| (see also "Pimiento"): | | | | | | | |
| fried (*B&G*), 1 oz. ...... | 25 | 0 | 2.0 | 1.5 | 0 | 160 | 1.0 |
| red: | | | | | | | |
| (*Peloponnese* Florina), | | | | | | | |
| 3.5 oz. .......... | 35 | .8 | 7.4 | .4 | 0 | 500 | 1.7 |
| fire-roasted (*Alessi*), | | | | | | | |
| 1 oz. ............ | 10 | 0 | 1.0 | 0 | 0 | 83 | 0 |
| marinated (*Roland*), | | | | | | | |
| 8 pcs., 1 oz. ...... | 10 | 0 | 2.0 | 0 | 0 | 100 | 0 |
| piquant (*Roland* | | | | | | | |
| Sweeties), 2 pcs., | | | | | | | |
| 1.1 oz. .......... | 30 | 0 | 7.0 | 0 | 0 | 0 | 0 |
| roasted (*Frieda's*), | | | | | | | |
| 1-oz. pc. ......... | 35 | 1.0 | 5.0 | 0 | 0 | 280 | 0 |
| roasted (*Roland*), ½ cup | 30 | 1.0 | 5.0 | 0 | 0 | 310 | 1.0 |
| roasted (*Vigo*), 1 oz. .. | 10 | 0 | 1.0 | 0 | 0 | 50 | 0 |
| roasted, w/garlic | | | | | | | |
| (*Roland*), 1 oz. ..... | 10 | 0 | 2.0 | 0 | 0 | 100 | 0 |

| Food and Measure | cal. | prot. (gms) | carbo. (gms) | fat (gms) | chol. (mgs) | sod. (mgs) | fiber (gms) |
|---|---|---|---|---|---|---|---|
| **Pepper, sweet, can/jar, red** *(cont.)* | | | | | | | |
| roasted, w/garlic, dill, oil (*Roland*), 1 oz. | 40 | 2.0 | 2.0 | 0 | 0 | 115 | 0 |
| roasted, strips (*Di Lusso*), 1 oz. | 10 | 0 | 1.0 | .5 | 0 | 250 | 0 |
| strips (*B&G*), 1 oz. | 20 | 0 | 5.0 | 0 | 0 | 75 | 0 |
| in water, drained, ½ cup | 13 | .6 | 2.7 | .2 | 0 | 958 | .8 |
| red and yellow: | | | | | | | |
| fire-roasted (*Alessi*), 1 oz. | 10 | 0 | 1.0 | 0 | 0 | 83 | 0 |
| fire-roasted (*Roland* Can), ½ cup | 30 | 1.0 | 5.0 | 0 | 0 | 310 | 1.0 |
| fire-roasted (*Roland* Jar), ½ cup | 40 | 2.0 | 2.0 | 0 | 0 | 115 | 0 |
| grilled (*Roland*), ½ cup | 35 | 1.0 | 4.0 | 2.0 | 0 | 500 | 3.0 |
| roasted (*B&G*), 1 oz.: | | | | | | | |
| w/balsamic vinegar | 10 | 0 | 2.0 | 0 | 0 | 70 | 0 |
| w/oregano/garlic | 15 | 0 | 1.0 | 1.5 | 0 | 75 | 0 |
| salad, w/oregano/ garlic (*B&G*), 1 oz. | 20 | 0 | 5.0 | 0 | 0 | 75 | 0 |
| **Pepper, sweet, freeze-dried**, ¼ cup | 5 | .3 | 1.1 | <.1 | 0 | 3 | .3 |
| **Pepper, sweet, frozen:** | | | | | | | |
| stir-fry, w/onion (*Birds Eye*), 1 cup | 25 | 1.0 | 5.0 | 0 | 0 | 10 | 1.0 |
| strips (*C&W*), ¾ cup | 25 | 1.0 | 4.0 | 0 | 0 | 10 | 1.0 |
| chopped: | | | | | | | |
| green (*McKenzie's*), ¾ cup | 25 | 1.0 | 4.0 | 0 | 0 | 5 | <1.0 |
| 1 oz. | 6 | .3 | 1.2 | .1 | 0 | 1 | .5 |
| **Pepper dip** (*Sabra* Moroccan Matbucha), 2 tbsp. | 20 | 1.0 | 3.0 | .5 | 0 | 180 | 0 |
| **Pepper relish**, sweet or hot (*Howard's*), 1 tbsp. | 20 | 0 | 5.0 | 0 | 0 | 55 | 0 |
| **Pepper sauce** (see also "Hot sauce"), black: | | | | | | | |
| (*Roland*), 2 tbsp. | 130 | 1.0 | 29.0 | 2.0 | 0 | 350 | 0 |
| (*Ka•Me*), 1 tbsp. | 20 | 0 | 4.0 | .5 | 0 | 200 | 0 |
| cayenne (*Frank's RedHot Thick*), 1 tbsp. | 20 | 0 | 4.0 | 0 | 0 | 290 | 0 |
| **Pepper spread:** | | | | | | | |
| jalapeño (*Roland*), 2 tbsp. | 40 | 0 | 1.0 | 4.0 | 0 | 460 | 0 |

| Food and Measure | cal. | prot. (gms) | carbo. (gms) | fat (gms) | chol. (mgs) | sod. (mgs) | fiber (gms) |
|---|---|---|---|---|---|---|---|
| red pepper: | | | | | | | |
| (*Peloponnese*), 1 tbsp. | 15 | 0 | 0 | 1.5 | 0 | 90 | 0 |
| (*Roland*), 2 tbsp. .... | 30 | 0 | 5.0 | 1.0 | 0 | 100 | 0 |
| **Pepper steak**, see | | | | | | | |
|   "Beef entree, frozen" | | | | | | | |
| **Peppercorn gravy mix**, | | | | | | | |
|   cracked, for steak | | | | | | | |
|   (*McCormick*), 1 tbsp. . | 35 | <1.0 | 5.0 | .5 | 0 | 380 | 0 |
| **Peppercorns, green** | | | | | | | |
|   (*Roland*): | | | | | | | |
| in brine, 1 tbsp. ........ | 10 | 0 | 2.0 | 0 | 0 | 55 | 1.0 |
| in vinegar, 1 tsp. ....... | 5 | 0 | 1.0 | 0 | 0 | 115 | 0 |
| **Pepperoncini**, in jars: | | | | | | | |
| (*Roland*), 1 pc. ........ | 10 | 0 | 2.0 | 0 | 0 | 330 | 1.0 |
| (*Roland* Golden), 3 pcs. .. | 0 | 0 | 1.0 | 0 | 0 | 460 | 0 |
| (*Vigo* Greek), 1 pc. ..... | 10 | 0 | 2.0 | 0 | 0 | 330 | 1.0 |
| **Pepperoni**, 1 oz., | | | | | | | |
|   except as noted: | | | | | | | |
| (*Applegate Farms*) ...... | 60 | 5.0 | 0 | 5.0 | 20 | 320 | 0 |
| (*Applegate Farms* | | | | | | | |
|   Sliced), 2 oz. ........ | 230 | 13.0 | 1.0 | 19.0 | 60 | 980 | 0 |
| (*Di Lusso*) ............. | 140 | 5.0 | 0 | 13.0 | 35 | 470 | 0 |
| (*Hormel*) ............. | 140 | 5.0 | 0 | 13.0 | 35 | 470 | 0 |
| (*Hormel* Twin) ......... | 140 | 5.0 | 0 | 13.0 | 30 | 500 | 0 |
| (*Thumann's* Stick), 2 oz. .. | 130 | 5.0 | 1.0 | 11.0 | 30 | 540 | 0 |
| all varieties, except | | | | | | | |
|   thick sliced and | | | | | | | |
|   twin (*Hormel* | | | | | | | |
|   Pillow Pack*) ........ | 140 | 5.0 | 0 | 13.0 | 35 | 490 | 0 |
| sandwich: | | | | | | | |
| (*Boar's Head*) ....... | 130 | 6.0 | 1.0 | 11.0 | 25 | 480 | 0 |
| (*Fiorucci*) ........... | 130 | 5.0 | 1.0 | 12.0 | 25 | 500 | 0 |
| (*Thumann's*) ........ | 150 | 5.0 | 0 | 14.0 | 55 | 420 | 0 |
| thick sliced (*Hormel* | | | | | | | |
|   Pillow Pack*) ........ | 140 | 5.0 | 0 | 13.0 | 35 | 470 | 0 |
| turkey, see "Turkey | | | | | | | |
|   pepperoni" | | | | | | | |
| uncured (*Hormel* | | | | | | | |
|   Natural Choice), 1.1 oz. | 150 | 5.0 | 0 | 14.0 | 35 | 510 | 0 |
| **"Pepperoni," vegetarian**: | | | | | | | |
| (*Tofurky*), 8 slices, 1 oz. . | 60 | 7.0 | 6.0 | .5 | 0 | 170 | 4.0 |
| (*Yves*), 6 slices, 1.7 oz. .. | 80 | 14.0 | 4.0 | 1.0 | 0 | 390 | 0 |
| **Perch**, meat only: | | | | | | | |
| raw, 4 oz. ............. | 103 | 22.0 | 0 | 1.1 | 102 | 70 | 0 |

| Food and Measure | cal. | prot. (gms) | carbo. (gms) | fat (gms) | chol. (mgs) | sod. (mgs) | fiber (gms) |
|---|---|---|---|---|---|---|---|
| **Perch** *(cont.)* | | | | | | | |
| baked or broiled, 4 oz. . . | 133 | 28.2 | 0 | 1.3 | 130 | 90 | 0 |
| ocean, see "Ocean perch" | | | | | | | |
| **Persimmon**, fresh: | | | | | | | |
| (*Frieda's* Fuyu/ Hachiya), 5 oz. . . . . . . | 100 | 1.0 | 26.0 | 0 | 0 | 0 | 5.0 |
| Japanese, 1 medium . . . . | 118 | 1.0 | 31.2 | .3 | 0 | 3 | 6.0 |
| native, 1 medium, 1.1 oz. | 32 | .2 | 8.4 | .1 | 0 | <1 | n.a. |
| **Persimmon, dried**: | | | | | | | |
| (*Frieda's* Fuyu), ⅓ cup, 1.4 oz. . . . . . . . | 140 | 1.0 | 35.0 | 0 | 0 | 10 | 3.0 |
| Japanese, 1 oz. . . . . . . . | 78 | .4 | 20.8 | .2 | 0 | 1 | 4.1 |
| **Pesto**, in jars: | | | | | | | |
| artichoke roasted garlic (*Campagna*), 1 tbsp. . . | 40 | 1.0 | 1.0 | 3.5 | 0 | 40 | <1.0 |
| basil: | | | | | | | |
| (*Alessi*), 2 tbsp. . . . . . | 175 | 2.0 | 4.0 | 18.0 | 0 | 490 | 0 |
| (*Campagna*), 1 tbsp. . . | 70 | 2.0 | 1.0 | 6.0 | 5 | 120 | 0 |
| (*Classico*), ¼ cup . . . . | 230 | 3.0 | 6.0 | 21.0 | 0 | 720 | 1.0 |
| (*Roland*), 1 tbsp. . . . . | 100 | 1.0 | 3.0 | 9.0 | 0 | 125 | 0 |
| cilantro pumpkin seed (*Campagna*), 1 tbsp. . . | 45 | 2.0 | 1.0 | 4.0 | 0 | 45 | 0 |
| olive and, 1 tbsp.: | | | | | | | |
| black fig (*Campagna*) . | 35 | 0 | 3.0 | 2.5 | 0 | 105 | 0 |
| sun-dried tomato (*Campagna*) . . . . . . | 45 | 0 | 2.0 | 4.0 | 0 | 65 | 0 |
| roasted red pepper (*Campagna*), 1 tbsp. . . | 45 | 1.0 | 1.0 | 4.0 | 0 | 80 | 0 |
| tomato, sun-dried: | | | | | | | |
| (*Alessi*), 2 tbsp. . . . . . | 175 | 2.0 | 4.0 | 18.0 | 0 | 490 | 0 |
| (*Classico*), ¼ cup . . . . | 90 | 3.0 | 8.0 | 5.0 | 0 | 630 | 1.0 |
| (*Roland*), ¼ cup . . . . . | 180 | 1.0 | 5.0 | 17.0 | 0 | 610 | 2.0 |
| **Pesto sauce, chilled** (*Buitoni*), ¼ cup: | | | | | | | |
| basil . . . . . . . . . . . . . . . | 300 | 7.0 | 6.0 | 28.0 | 20 | 540 | 2.0 |
| basil, reduced fat . . . . . . . | 240 | 7.0 | 9.0 | 19.0 | 15 | 540 | 2.0 |
| **Pesto sauce mix** (*McCormick*), 2 tsp. . . | 10 | <1.0 | <1.0 | 0 | 0 | 480 | 0 |
| **Pesto spread** (*Progresso*), 2 tbsp.: | | | | | | | |
| arrabiata . . . . . . . . . . . . | 130 | 3.0 | 7.0 | 11.0 | 5 | 140 | 2.0 |
| basil, original, lemon or roasted garlic . . . . . | 130 | 2.0 | 3.0 | 13.0 | 0 | 75 | 0 |

| Food and Measure | cal. | prot. (gms) | carbo. (gms) | fat (gms) | chol. (mgs) | sod. (mgs) | fiber (gms) |
|---|---|---|---|---|---|---|---|
| lemon artichoke ....... | 120 | 1.0 | 3.0 | 12.0 | 0 | 150 | <1.0 |
| roasted red pepper ..... | 120 | 1.0 | 1.0 | 13.0 | 0 | 150 | 0 |
| **Pheasant**, 4 oz., except as noted: | | | | | | | |
| raw, meat w/skin ....... | 205 | 25.7 | 0 | 10.5 | 81 | 45 | 0 |
| raw, meat only ........ | 151 | 26.7 | 0 | 4.1 | 75 | 42 | 0 |
| raw, breast, 6.4 oz. ..... | 243 | 44.4 | 0 | 5.9 | 106 | 60 | 0 |
| raw, leg, 3.8 oz. ........ | 143 | 23.8 | 0 | 4.6 | 112 | 48 | 0 |
| cooked, meat w/skin .... | 280 | 36.7 | 0 | 13.7 | 101 | 49 | 0 |
| **Picante sauce** (see also "Salsa"), 2 tbsp.: | | | | | | | |
| (*Chi-Chi's*) ............ | 10 | 0 | 2.0 | 0 | 0 | 150 | 0 |
| (*Pace*) ............... | 10 | 0 | 3.0 | 0 | 0 | 250 | 1.0 |
| hot (*Ortega*) .......... | 10 | 0 | 2.0 | 0 | 0 | 210 | 0 |
| medium (*Ortega*) ....... | 10 | 0 | 2.0 | 0 | 0 | 130 | 0 |
| mild (*Ortega*) .......... | 10 | 0 | 2.0 | 0 | 0 | 220 | 0 |
| **Pickle**, cucumber, 1 oz., except as noted: | | | | | | | |
| bread and butter: | | | | | | | |
| (*B&G*) ............. | 25 | 0 | 6.0 | 0 | 0 | 190 | 0 |
| chips (*Claussen*) ..... | 20 | 0 | 4.0 | 0 | 0 | 180 | 0 |
| sandwich slices (*Claussen*), 1.2 oz. . | 25 | 0 | 5.0 | 0 | 0 | 210 | 0 |
| cornichon, gherkins: | | | | | | | |
| (*Roland*) ........... | 5 | 0 | 1.0 | 0 | 0 | 360 | 1.0 |
| (*Trois Petits Cochons*) | 0 | 0 | 0 | 0 | 0 | 300 | 0 |
| deli style: | | | | | | | |
| (*B&G* New York Toppers) ......... | 0 | 0 | 1.0 | 0 | 0 | 190 | 0 |
| (*B&G* New York/ Zesty Spears) ..... | 0 | 0 | 1.0 | 0 | 0 | 170 | 0 |
| dill: | | | | | | | |
| chips (*Roland*), 8 pcs., 1 oz. ...... | 10 | 0 | 2.0 | 0 | 0 | 340 | 0 |
| chips (*Del Monte*) .... | 0 | 0 | 0 | 0 | 0 | 370 | 0 |
| hamburger (*B&G* Toppers) ......... | 0 | 0 | <1.0 | 0 | 0 | 200 | 0 |
| sandwich toppers (*Roland*), 1 slice ... | 10 | 0 | 2.0 | 0 | 0 | 340 | 0 |
| whole (*Roland*), 2 pcs., 1.1 oz. .... | 5 | 0 | 1.0 | 0 | 0 | 290 | 0 |
| whole or halves (*Del Monte*) .......... | 5 | 0 | 1.0 | 0 | 0 | 370 | 1.0 |

| Food and Measure | cal. | prot. (gms) | carbo. (gms) | fat (gms) | chol. (mgs) | sod. (mgs) | fiber (gms) |
|---|---|---|---|---|---|---|---|
| **Pickle, dill** *(cont.)* | | | | | | | |
| whole or hamburger | | | | | | | |
| chips (*B&G*) ...... | 0 | 0 | 0 | 0 | 0 | 320 | 0 |
| dill, kosher: | | | | | | | |
| all varieties (*B&G*) ... | 0 | 0 | 0 | 0 | 0 | 200 | 0 |
| burger slices | | | | | | | |
| (*Claussen*), .8 oz. .. | 5 | 0 | 1.0 | 0 | 0 | 300 | 0 |
| halves (*Claussen*) .... | 5 | 0 | 1.0 | 0 | 0 | 270 | 0 |
| halves (*Claussen* | | | | | | | |
| Deli) ........... | 5 | 0 | 1.0 | 0 | 0 | 450 | 0 |
| mini (*Claussen*), .8 oz. | 5 | 0 | 1.0 | 0 | 0 | 290 | 0 |
| sandwich slice | | | | | | | |
| (*Claussen*), 1.2 oz. . | 5 | 0 | 1.0 | 0 | 0 | 420 | 0 |
| spears (*Claussen* | | | | | | | |
| Deli), 1.2 oz. ...... | 5 | 0 | 1.0 | 0 | 0 | 310 | 0 |
| tiny (*Del Monte*) ..... | 5 | 0 | 1.0 | 0 | 0 | 240 | <1.0 |
| dill, Polish (*B&G* | | | | | | | |
| Toppers) ........... | 0 | 0 | <1.0 | 0 | 0 | 160 | 0 |
| garlic, hearty, whole | | | | | | | |
| (*Claussen* Deli) ...... | 5 | 0 | 1.0 | 0 | 0 | 270 | 0 |
| sour (*B&G*) ........... | 0 | 0 | 0 | 0 | 0 | 270 | 0 |
| sour, half (*Claussen* | | | | | | | |
| New York Deli) ...... | 5 | 0 | 1.0 | 0 | 0 | 270 | 0 |
| sweet: | | | | | | | |
| (*B&G* Tiny Treats) .... | 40 | 0 | 10.0 | 0 | 0 | 160 | 0 |
| all styles (*Del* | | | | | | | |
| *Monte*) ........... | 40 | 0 | 10.0 | 0 | 0 | 210 | <1.0 |
| all styles, except | | | | | | | |
| Tiny Treats | | | | | | | |
| (*B&G*) ........... | 35 | 0 | 9.0 | 0 | 0 | 115 | 0 |
| **Pickle relish** (see also | | | | | | | |
| specific listings), | | | | | | | |
| cucumber, 1 tbsp.: | | | | | | | |
| (*B&G* Emerald) ........ | 15 | 0 | 4.0 | 0 | 0 | 120 | 0 |
| (*Crosse & Blackwell* | | | | | | | |
| *Branston*) ........... | 25 | 0 | 7.0 | 0 | 0 | 160 | 0 |
| dill (*B&G*) ............. | 0 | 0 | 0 | 0 | 0 | 270 | 0 |
| hamburger: | | | | | | | |
| (*B&G*) ............. | 15 | 0 | 4.0 | 0 | 0 | 150 | 0 |
| (*Del Monte*) ........ | 20 | 0 | 5.0 | 0 | 0 | 125 | <1.0 |
| hot dog: | | | | | | | |
| (*B&G*) ............. | 20 | 0 | 5.0 | 0 | 0 | 75 | 0 |
| (*Del Monte*) ........ | 15 | 0 | 4.0 | 0 | 0 | 140 | <1.0 |
| India (*B&G*) ........... | 15 | 0 | 4.0 | 0 | 0 | 140 | 0 |

| Food and Measure | cal. | prot. (gms) | carbo. (gms) | fat (gms) | chol. (mgs) | sod. (mgs) | fiber (gms) |
|---|---|---|---|---|---|---|---|
| sweet: | | | | | | | |
| (*B&G*) | 15 | 0 | 4.0 | 0 | 0 | 120 | 0 |
| (*Cascadian Farm* Organic) | 15 | 0 | 4.0 | 0 | 0 | 65 | 0 |
| (*Claussen*) | 10 | 0 | 3.0 | 0 | 0 | 85 | 0 |
| (*Del Monte*) | 20 | 0 | 5.0 | 0 | 0 | 125 | 0 |
| **Pickling spice**, 1 tsp. | 10 | .3 | 1.2 | .6 | 0 | 1 | .3 |
| **Pie** (*Entenmann's*): | | | | | | | |
| apple, ⅙ pie | 350 | 3.0 | 55.0 | 14.0 | 0 | 410 | 2.0 |
| apple, single, snack 3.5-oz. pc. | 430 | 0 | 50.0 | 24.0 | 0 | 320 | <1.0 |
| cherry, single, snack, 3.5-oz. pc. | 420 | 3.0 | 50.0 | 24.0 | 0 | 320 | <1.0 |
| coconut custard, ⅕ pie | 370 | 7.0 | 38.0 | 21.0 | 120 | 330 | 2.0 |
| lemon, single, snack 3.5-oz. pc. | 450 | 2.0 | 50.0 | 26.0 | 0 | 310 | 0 |
| pumpkin, ⅕ pie | 300 | 4.0 | 42.0 | 13.0 | 35 | 340 | 2.0 |
| sweet potato, ⅙ pie | 320 | 5.0 | 42.0 | 14.0 | 75 | 300 | 1.0 |
| **Pie, frozen** (see also "Cobbler"), ⅛ pie, except as noted: | | | | | | | |
| apple: | | | | | | | |
| (*Amy's*), ½ of 8-oz. pie | 230 | 2.0 | 37.0 | 8.0 | 25 | 135 | 2.0 |
| (*Banquet*), 7-oz. pie | 370 | 3.0 | 59.0 | 14.0 | 10 | 730 | 2.0 |
| (*Michelina* Snackers), 2.25-oz. pc. | 170 | 3.0 | 35.0 | 5.0 | 10 | 150 | 1.0 |
| (*Mrs. Smith's*), ⅙ pie | 320 | 3.0 | 47.0 | 14.0 | 0 | 300 | 2.0 |
| (*Mrs. Smith's* PreBaked) | 340 | 3.0 | 46.0 | 16.0 | 0 | 440 | 2.0 |
| deep dish (*Mrs. Smith's*), ⅒ pie | 290 | 3.0 | 41.0 | 13.0 | 0 | 330 | 2.0 |
| raisin spice (*Mrs. Smith's* PreBaked) | 370 | 3.0 | 55.0 | 16.0 | 0 | 440 | 2.0 |
| apple crumb: | | | | | | | |
| cinnamon, deep dish (*Mrs. Smith's*) | 380 | 3.0 | 53.0 | 15.0 | 0 | 270 | 2.0 |
| Dutch (*Mrs. Smith's*), ⅙ pie | 340 | 3.0 | 52.0 | 14.0 | 0 | 240 | 2.0 |
| Dutch (*Mrs. Smith's* PreBaked) | 390 | 4.0 | 53.0 | 18.0 | 0 | 400 | 2.0 |
| blueberry: | | | | | | | |
| (*Mrs. Smith*), ⅙ pie | 310 | 3.0 | 45.0 | 14.0 | 0 | 420 | 2.0 |

| Food and Measure | cal. | prot. (gms) | carbo. (gms) | fat (gms) | chol. (mgs) | sod. (mgs) | fiber (gms) |
|---|---|---|---|---|---|---|---|
| **Pie, frozen, blueberry** *(cont.)* | | | | | | | |
| (*Mrs. Smith's* PreBaked) . . . . . . . | 330 | 3.0 | 45.0 | 16.0 | 0 | 430 | 2.0 |
| cherry: | | | | | | | |
| (*Mrs. Smith*), ⅙ pie . . | 300 | 3.0 | 40.0 | 14.0 | 0 | 300 | 2.0 |
| (*Mrs. Smith's* PreBaked) . . . . . . . | 350 | 3.0 | 48.0 | 16.0 | 0 | 360 | 1.0 |
| crumb, deep dish (*Mrs. Smith*), ¹⁄₁₀ pie | 300 | 3.0 | 45.0 | 12.0 | 0 | 280 | 1.0 |
| cherry berry (*Banquet*), 7-oz. pie . . . . . . . . . . . | 370 | 3.0 | 56.0 | 15.0 | 10 | 650 | 2.0 |
| chocolate crème: | | | | | | | |
| (*Mrs. Smith's*) . . . . . . . | 390 | 2.0 | 40.0 | 24.0 | 15 | 190 | 1.0 |
| mint (*Sara Lee Signature Selections*) | 420 | 3.0 | 44.0 | 27.0 | 5.0 | 300 | 2.0 |
| coconut crème (*Mrs. Smith's*) . . . . . . . . . . | 370 | 2.0 | 37.0 | 23.0 | 15 | 260 | 1.0 |
| coconut custard: | | | | | | | |
| (*Mrs. Smith*), ⅙ pie . . | 310 | 6.0 | 33.0 | 17.0 | 65 | 340 | 2.0 |
| (*Mrs. Smith's* PreBaked) . . . . . . . | 360 | 8.0 | 43.0 | 17.0 | 90 | 380 | 2.0 |
| cookies and crème (*Edwards* Single), 1 pc. | 290 | 3.0 | 34.0 | 16.0 | 5 | 140 | <1.0 |
| crème w/*Butterfinger* (*Edwards* Single), 1 pc. | 370 | 4.0 | 43.0 | 21.0 | 5 | 240 | <1.0 |
| lemon meringue (*Mrs. Smith's*) . . . . . . . | 310 | 2.0 | 46.0 | 12.0 | 40 | 170 | 1.0 |
| lime, Key: | | | | | | | |
| (*Edwards*) . . . . . . . . . . | 450 | 6.0 | 57.0 | 22.0 | 50 | 310 | <1.0 |
| (*Edwards* Single), 1 pc. | 330 | 4.0 | 42.0 | 16.0 | 35 | 240 | <1.0 |
| (*Sara Lee Signature Selections*) . . . . . . . | 380 | 4.0 | 50.0 | 18.0 | 0 | 230 | <1.0 |
| (*Smart Ones*), 2.8 oz. . . | 190 | 4.0 | 33.0 | 5.0 | 10 | 85 | 1.0 |
| mince (*Mrs. Smith's*), ⅙ pie . . . . . . . . . . . . . | 360 | 3.0 | 51.0 | 17.0 | 0 | 380 | 2.0 |
| peach: | | | | | | | |
| (*Banquet*), 7-oz. pie . . | 360 | 3.0 | 52.0 | 15.0 | 10 | 640 | 2.0 |
| (*Mrs. Smith*), ⅙ pie . . | 310 | 3.0 | 42.0 | 14.0 | 0 | 380 | 2.0 |
| (*Mrs. Smith's* PreBaked) . . . . . . . | 330 | 3.0 | 43.0 | 16.0 | 0 | 429 | 1.0 |
| deep dish (*Mrs. Smith's*), ¹⁄₁₀ pie . . . | 290 | 2.0 | 40.0 | 13.0 | 0 | 370 | 1.0 |
| pumpkin: | | | | | | | |
| (*Mrs. Smith's*), ⅙ pie . | 280 | 4.0 | 36.0 | 14.0 | 45 | 310 | 1.0 |

| Food and Measure | cal. | prot. (gms) | carbo. (gms) | fat (gms) | chol. (mgs) | sod. (mgs) | fiber (gms) |
|---|---|---|---|---|---|---|---|
| (*Mrs. Smith's* PreBaked) | 320 | 5.0 | 49.0 | 12.0 | 45 | 380 | 2.0 |
| (*Mrs. Smith's* Large), 1/10 pie | 290 | 4.0 | 42.0 | 13.0 | 40 | 320 | 1.0 |
| turtle (*Edwards*) | 390 | 4.0 | 46.0 | 22.0 | 10 | 270 | 1.0 |
| **Pie, mix** (*Jell-O* No Bake), dry: | | | | | | | |
| chocolate silk, 1/6 pkg. | 190 | 2.0 | 33.0 | 5.0 | 0 | 430 | 2.0 |
| *Oreo*, 1/6 pkg. | 280 | 2.0 | 48.0 | 8.0 | 0 | 440 | 2.0 |
| peanut butter cup, 1/8 pkg. | 290 | 4.0 | 39.0 | 15.0 | 0 | 330 | 2.0 |
| pumpkin pie style, 1/8 pkg. | 130 | 1.0 | 29.0 | 1.5 | 0 | 340 | 1.0 |
| **Pie crust** (see also "Pastry shell"), 1/8 of 9" crust, except as noted: | | | | | | | |
| (*Pet•Ritz*) | 80 | 1.0 | 9.0 | 4.0 | <5 | 70 | 0 |
| (*Pillsbury* Rolled) | 100 | <1.0 | 12.0 | 6.0 | <5 | 130 | 0 |
| chocolate: | | | | | | | |
| (*Arrowhead Mills* Organic) | 110 | 1.0 | 14.0 | 6.0 | 0 | 95 | <1.0 |
| (*Ready Crust*) | 100 | 1.0 | 14.0 | 4.5 | 0 | 110 | <1.0 |
| cookie, 1/6 crust: | | | | | | | |
| (*Nilla*) | 140 | 1.0 | 18.0 | 8.0 | 5 | 85 | 0 |
| (*Oreo*) | 130 | 1.0 | 19.0 | 7.0 | 0 | 170 | 1.0 |
| deep dish: | | | | | | | |
| (*Mrs. Smith's/Oronoque Orchards*) | 130 | 2.0 | 15.0 | 7.0 | 0 | 135 | <1.0 |
| (*Pet•Ritz*) | 90 | 1.0 | 11.0 | 5.0 | <5 | 85 | 0 |
| vegetable (*Pet•Ritz*) | 90 | 1.0 | 11.0 | 5.0 | 0 | 85 | 0 |
| graham cracker: | | | | | | | |
| (*Arrowhead Mills* Organic) | 110 | 1.0 | 14.0 | 5.0 | 0 | 65 | <1.0 |
| (*Honey Maid*), 1/6 crust | 150 | 1.0 | 18.0 | 8.0 | 0 | 115 | 0 |
| (*Ready Crust*) | 110 | 1.0 | 14.0 | 5.0 | 0 | 115 | <1.0 |
| (*Ready Crust* 10"), 1/10 crust | 130 | 1.0 | 18.0 | 6.0 | 0 | 140 | <1.0 |
| (*Ready Crust* Reduced Fat) | 100 | 1.0 | 15.0 | 3.5 | 0 | 100 | <1.0 |
| mini (*Ready Crust*), .8-oz. crust | 110 | 1.0 | 15.0 | 5.0 | 0 | 125 | <1.0 |

| Food and Measure | cal. | prot. (gms) | carbo. (gms) | fat (gms) | chol. (mgs) | sod. (mgs) | fiber (gms) |
|---|---|---|---|---|---|---|---|
| **Pie crust** *(cont.)* | | | | | | | |
| shortbread (*Ready Crust*) ............ | 110 | 1.0 | 14.0 | 5.0 | 0 | 110 | 0 |
| **Pie crust mix:** | | | | | | | |
| (*Betty Crocker*), ⅛ of 9" crust* ....... | 110 | 1.0 | 9.0 | 7.0 | 0 | 135 | 0 |
| (*Glutino* Gluten Free), ¹⁄₁₂ pkg., 4 tbsp. ..... | 130 | 2.0 | 29.0 | 0 | 0 | 150 | <1.0 |
| (*"Jiffy"*), ⅙ pkg. ....... | 80 | <1.0 | 8.0 | 5.0 | <5 | 120 | 0 |
| **Pie filling**, ⅓ cup, except as noted: | | | | | | | |
| apple: | | | | | | | |
|   (*Lucky Leaf* Lite) ..... | 30 | 0 | 7.0 | 0 | 0 | 10 | 0 |
|   (*Lucky Leaf/ Musselman's*) ..... | 90 | 0 | 22.0 | 0 | 0 | 40 | 2.0 |
| apricot (*Lucky Leaf*) .... | 90 | 0 | 22.0 | 0 | 0 | 55 | 0 |
| banana crème (*Lucky Leaf/Musselman's*) ... | 110 | 0 | 28.0 | 0 | 0 | 75 | 0 |
| blackberry (*Lucky Leaf*) .............. | 90 | 0 | 23.0 | 0 | 0 | 65 | 3.0 |
| blueberry: | | | | | | | |
|   (*Lucky Leaf*) ........ | 100 | 0 | 24.0 | 0 | 0 | 45 | 1.0 |
|   (*Musselman's*) ...... | 90 | 0 | 22.0 | 0 | 0 | 50 | 1.0 |
| cherry: | | | | | | | |
|   (*Lucky Leaf* Lite) ..... | 35 | 0 | 8.0 | 0 | 0 | 15 | 0 |
|   (*Lucky Leaf/ Musselman's*) ..... | 100 | 0 | 24.0 | 0 | 0 | 40 | 0 |
|   dark (*Lucky Leaf*) .... | 140 | 0 | 35.0 | 0 | 0 | 15 | 0 |
| chocolate crème (*Lucky Leaf/Musselman's*) ... | 100 | 0 | 25.0 | 0 | 0 | 95 | 0 |
| coconut crème: | | | | | | | |
|   (*Lucky Leaf*) ........ | 110 | 1.0 | 25.0 | 1.5 | 0 | 140 | 3.0 |
|   (*Musselman's*) ...... | 110 | 0 | 25.0 | 1.0 | 0 | 90 | 0 |
| lemon: | | | | | | | |
|   (*Lucky Leaf*) ........ | 120 | 0 | 29.0 | 1.0 | 15 | 220 | 0 |
|   (*Musselman's*) ..... | 120 | 0 | 30.0 | 0 | 0 | 220 | 0 |
|   crème (*Lucky Leaf*) ... | 130 | 0 | 31.0 | 1.0 | 10 | 220 | 0 |
|   crème (*Musselman's*) . | 100 | 0 | 25.0 | 0 | 0 | 160 | 0 |
| lime, Key (*Lucky Leaf/Musselman's*) ... | 130 | 0 | 31.0 | 0 | 0 | 210 | 0 |
| mince/mincemeat: | | | | | | | |
|   (*Crosse & Blackwell*), ¼ cup ........... | 180 | <1.0 | 43.0 | 0 | 0 | 220 | 0 |
|   w/apples (*None Such*) | 190 | 0 | 45.0 | .5 | 0 | 230 | 0 |

| Food and Measure | cal. | prot. (gms) | carbo. (gms) | fat (gms) | chol. (mgs) | sod. (mgs) | fiber (gms) |
|---|---|---|---|---|---|---|---|
| w/brandy and rum (*Crosse & Blackwell*), ¼ cup .. | 180 | <1.0 | 43.0 | 0 | 0 | 230 | 0 |
| w/brandy and rum (*None Such*) ...... | 200 | 0 | 47.0 | 1.0 | 0 | 250 | 0 |
| condensed (*None Such*), 4 tsp. ..... | 150 | 0 | 36.0 | .5 | 0 | 230 | 1.0 |
| peach (*Lucky Leaf*) ..... | 90 | 0 | 22.0 | 0 | 0 | 40 | 0 |
| pineapple (*Lucky Leaf*) .. | 100 | 0 | 23.0 | 0 | 0 | 35 | 1.0 |
| pumpkin: | | | | | | | |
| (*Arrowhead Mills Pour'n Bake*) ..... | 110 | 2.0 | 18.0 | 3.5 | 10 | 140 | <1.0 |
| (*Libby's* Pie Mix) ..... | 90 | 1.0 | 20.0 | .5 | 0 | 120 | 3.0 |
| raisin (*Lucky Leaf*) ..... | 90 | 0 | 22.0 | 0 | 0 | 75 | 1.0 |
| raspberry, red (*Lucky Leaf*) ............... | 80 | 0 | 19.0 | 0 | 0 | 35 | 2.0 |
| strawberry (*Lucky Leaf/Musselman's*) ... | 80 | 0 | 20.0 | 0 | 0 | 50 | 1.0 |
| **Pie filling mix**, see "Pudding and pie filling mix" | | | | | | | |
| **Pierogi**, frozen, 3 pcs., except as noted: | | | | | | | |
| potato cheddar: | | | | | | | |
| (*Mrs. T.'s*) .......... | 170 | 5.0 | 33.0 | 2.5 | 5 | 510 | 1.0 |
| (*Mrs. T.'s* 2 lb.) ...... | 180 | 6.0 | 34.0 | 2.5 | 10 | 540 | 1.0 |
| and bacon, mini (*Mrs. T.'s*), 7 pcs. .. | 150 | 5.0 | 26.0 | 3.0 | 5 | 470 | 1.0 |
| broccoli (*Mrs. T.'s*) ... | 190 | 5.0 | 32.0 | 4.5 | 5 | 520 | 2.0 |
| jalapeño (*Mrs. T.'s*) | 170 | 5.0 | 32.0 | 2.5 | 5 | 510 | 1.0 |
| mini (*Mrs. T.'s*), 7 pcs. | 140 | 4.0 | 27.0 | 2.0 | 5 | 390 | 1.0 |
| potato cheese: | | | | | | | |
| (*Golden*) ........... | 240 | 9.0 | 39.0 | 5.0 | 0 | 250 | <1.0 |
| American (*Mrs. T.'s*) .. | 200 | 7.0 | 30.0 | 6.0 | 15 | 550 | 1.0 |
| 4 (*Mrs. T.'s*) ........ | 220 | 6.0 | 34.0 | 7.0 | 5 | 540 | 1.0 |
| 4, mini (*Mrs. T.'s*), 7 pcs. ........... | 170 | 5.0 | 27.0 | 5.0 | 5 | 410 | 1.0 |
| potato onion: | | | | | | | |
| (*Golden*) ........... | 180 | 4.0 | 35.0 | 3.0 | 0 | 200 | <1.0 |
| (*Mrs. T.'s*) .......... | 160 | 5.0 | 32.0 | 2.0 | 5 | 390 | 1.0 |
| (*Mrs. T.'s* 2 lb.) ...... | 170 | 5.0 | 34.0 | 2.0 | 5 | 420 | 1.0 |
| potato sauerkraut: | | | | | | | |
| (*Golden*) ........... | 210 | 6.0 | 38.0 | 4.0 | 0 | 270 | 1.0 |
| (*Mrs. T.'s*) .......... | 190 | 5.0 | 32.0 | 5.0 | 10 | 480 | 1.0 |

| Food and Measure | cal. | prot. (gms) | carbo. (gms) | fat (gms) | chol. (mgs) | sod. (mgs) | fiber (gms) |
|---|---|---|---|---|---|---|---|
| **Pierogi** *(cont.)* | | | | | | | |
| potato sour cream/ | | | | | | | |
| chive *(Mrs. T.'s)* ..... | 190 | 5.0 | 32.0 | 5.0 | 10 | 480 | 1.0 |
| potato spinach/feta | | | | | | | |
| *(Mrs. T.)* ........... | 180 | 6.0 | 31.0 | 3.5 | 5 | 480 | 1.0 |
| **Pig's feet** (see also | | | | | | | |
| "Pork, pickled"): | | | | | | | |
| simmered, 4 oz. ....... | 220 | 21.8 | 0 | 14.1 | 113 | 34 | 0 |
| pickled, 2 oz.: | | | | | | | |
| *(Hormel)* ........... | 80 | 7.0 | 0 | 6.0 | 45 | 590 | 0 |
| jalapeño *(Hormel)* .... | 80 | 7.0 | 0 | 6.0 | 45 | 580 | 0 |
| **Pigeon peas**, fresh: | | | | | | | |
| raw, ½ cup ........... | 105 | 5.5 | 18.4 | 1.3 | 0 | 4 | 3.2 |
| boiled, drained, ½ cup .. | 86 | 4.6 | 15.0 | 1.1 | 0 | 3 | 2.5 |
| **Pigeon peas, canned**, | | | | | | | |
| green *(Roland)*, ½ cup | 80 | 4.0 | 15.0 | 0 | 0 | 610 | 4.0 |
| **Pigeon peas, dried**, | | | | | | | |
| boiled, ½ cup ....... | 102 | 5.7 | 19.5 | .3 | 0 | 5 | 3.9 |
| **Pignolia nuts**, see | | | | | | | |
| "Pine nuts" | | | | | | | |
| **Pike**, meat only: | | | | | | | |
| northern, 4 oz.: | | | | | | | |
| raw .............. | 100 | 21.8 | 0 | .8 | 44 | 44 | 0 |
| baked or broiled ..... | 128 | 28.0 | 0 | 1.0 | 57 | 56 | 0 |
| walleye, 4 oz.: | | | | | | | |
| raw .............. | 105 | 21.7 | 0 | 1.4 | 98 | 58 | 0 |
| baked or broiled ..... | 135 | 27.8 | 0 | 1.8 | 125 | 74 | 0 |
| **Pili nuts**, shelled, | | | | | | | |
| dried, 1 oz. ......... | 204 | 3.1 | 1.1 | 22.6 | 0 | 4 | <1.0 |
| **Pimiento**, can/jar, | | | | | | | |
| whole or diced | | | | | | | |
| *(Roland)*, ½ cup ..... | 30 | 1.0 | 5.0 | 0 | 0 | 310 | 1.0 |
| **Piña colada**, see | | | | | | | |
| "Pineapple drink/ | | | | | | | |
| juice blend" | | | | | | | |
| **Piña colada drink** | | | | | | | |
| **mixer**: | | | | | | | |
| *(Roland/Costamar)*, | | | | | | | |
| 3 fl. oz. ............ | 120 | 1.0 | 17.0 | 6.0 | 0 | 30 | 0 |
| *(Stirrings)*, 3 fl. oz. ..... | 160 | 0 | 37.0 | 2.0 | 10 | 15 | 0 |
| *(Vigo)*, 3 fl. oz. ........ | 120 | 1.0 | 17.0 | 6.0 | 0 | 30 | 0 |
| frozen *(Bacardi)*, | | | | | | | |
| 2 fl. oz. ............ | 170 | 0 | 36.0 | 4.0 | 0 | 20 | 0 |

| Food and Measure | cal. | prot. (gms) | carbo. (gms) | fat (gms) | chol. (mgs) | sod. (mgs) | fiber (gms) |
|---|---|---|---|---|---|---|---|
| **Pine nuts**, dried, shelled: | | | | | | | |
| (*Diamond*), ¼ cup | 200 | 4.0 | 4.0 | 20.0 | 0 | 0 | 1.0 |
| (*Frieda's*), ¼ cup, 1.1 oz. | 230 | 50 | 4.0 | 23.0 | 0 | 1 | 1.0 |
| (*Planters*), 2-oz. pkg. | 320 | 13.0 | 8.0 | 28.0 | 0 | 0 | 3.0 |
| pignolia: | | | | | | | |
| (*Alessi*), 4 tbsp. | 210 | 5.0 | 0 | 20.0 | 0 | 0 | 1.0 |
| 1 oz. | 160 | 6.8 | 4.0 | 14.2 | 0 | 1 | 1.3 |
| 1 tbsp. | 49 | 2.1 | 1.2 | 4.4 | 0 | <1 | .4 |
| pinyon: | | | | | | | |
| 1 oz. | 178 | 3.3 | 5.5 | 17.3 | 0 | 20 | 3.0 |
| 10 kernels | 6 | .1 | .2 | .6 | 0 | 1 | .1 |
| **Pineapple**, fresh: | | | | | | | |
| (*Chiquita*), 1 cup, 5.8 oz. | 82 | 1.0 | 22.0 | 0 | 0 | 2 | 2.0 |
| (*Dole*), 2 slices, 3" diam. x ¾" | 60 | <1.0 | 15.0 | 0 | 0 | 0 | 2.0 |
| (*Frieda's* Zulu Queen Baby), 1 cup, 5 oz. | 70 | 1.0 | 17.0 | .5 | 0 | 0 | 2.0 |
| plain or w/coconut (*Chiquita Fruit Bites*), 1 pc. or pkg. | 40 | 1.0 | 9.0 | 0 | 0 | 15 | <1.0 |
| whole, 1 lb. | 231 | 1.8 | 58.5 | 2.0 | 0 | 5 | 5.7 |
| diced, ½ cup | 38 | .3 | 9.6 | .3 | 0 | <1 | .9 |
| **Pineapple**, can/jar, ½ cup, except as noted: | | | | | | | |
| in juice: | | | | | | | |
| all styles (*Roland*) | 70 | 1.0 | 17.0 | 0 | 0 | 10 | 1.0 |
| chunks (*Del Monte*) | 70 | 0 | 17.0 | 0 | 0 | 10 | 1.0 |
| chunks (*Del Monte Fruit Naturals*) | 70 | <1.0 | 18.0 | 0 | 0 | 5 | <1.0 |
| chunks (*Del Monte SunFresh*) | 70 | 0 | 18.0 | 0 | 0 | 10 | <1.0 |
| chunks (*Dole*) | 60 | 0 | 16.0 | 0 | 0 | 10 | 1.0 |
| crushed (*Dole*) | 70 | 1.0 | 18.0 | 0 | 0 | 0 | 1.0 |
| sliced (*Del Monte*), 2 pcs. | 60 | 0 | 16.0 | 0 | 0 | 10 | 1.0 |
| sliced (*Dole*), 4 oz. | 60 | 0 | 15.0 | 0 | 0 | 10 | 1.0 |
| tidbits (*Del Monte*) | 70 | 0 | 17.0 | 0 | 0 | 10 | 1.0 |
| tidbits (*Del Monte Bowl*), 4 oz. | 70 | <1.0 | 18.0 | 0 | 0 | 5 | <1.0 |

| Food and Measure | cal. | prot. (gms) | carbo. (gms) | fat (gms) | chol. (mgs) | sod. (mgs) | fiber (gms) |
|---|---|---|---|---|---|---|---|
| **Pineapple, can/jar, in juice** *(cont.)* | | | | | | | |
| tidbits (*Del Monte* Pull-Top), 4 oz. . . . . | 50 | <1.0 | 15.0 | 0 | 0 | 10 | <1.0 |
| tidbits (*Dole*) . . . . . . . . | 60 | 0 | 15.0 | 0 | 0 | 10 | 1.0 |
| tidbits (*Dole* Fruit Bowl), 4 oz. . . . . . . | 60 | 1.0 | 16.0 | 0 | 0 | 10 | 1.0 |
| wedges (*Del Monte*) . . | 70 | 0 | 17.0 | 0 | 0 | 10 | 1.0 |
| in light syrup: | | | | | | | |
| chunks (*Dole*) . . . . . . . | 80 | 0 | 21.0 | 0 | 0 | 0 | 1.0 |
| sliced (*Roland*) . . . . . . | 100 | 1.0 | 25.0 | 0 | 0 | 10 | 1.0 |
| in heavy syrup: | | | | | | | |
| chunks (*Dole*) . . . . . . . | 90 | 1.0 | 24.0 | 0 | 0 | 10 | 1.0 |
| chunks or crushed (*Del Monte*) . . . . . . | 90 | 0 | 24.0 | 0 | 0 | 10 | 1.0 |
| crushed (*Dole*) . . . . . . | 90 | 0 | 24.0 | 0 | 0 | 10 | 1.0 |
| sliced (*Del Monte*), 2 pcs. . . . . . . . . . . | 90 | 0 | 23.0 | 0 | 0 | 10 | 1.0 |
| sliced (*Dole*), 2 pcs. . . | 90 | 0 | 24.0 | 0 | 0 | 10 | 1.0 |
| in gelatin, 1 cont.: | | | | | | | |
| lime (*Dole*), 4.3 oz. . . . | 90 | 0 | 23.0 | 0 | 0 | 50 | 1.0 |
| strawberry (*Dole* No Sugar), 4.3 oz. . . . . | 60 | 0 | 14.0 | 0 | 0 | 40 | 1.0 |
| tropical fusion (*Jell-O* No Sugar), 3.25 oz. . . . . . . . . | 35 | 2.0 | 7.0 | 0 | 0 | 35 | 0 |
| and crème (*Dole* Parfait), 2.3-oz. cup . . | 120 | 1.0 | 23.0 | 2.0 | 0 | 10 | 0 |
| **Pineapple, dried**, ⅓ cup, 1.4 oz.: | | | | | | | |
| (*Mariani* Tropical) . . . . . . | 130 | 0 | 34.0 | 0 | 0 | 100 | 1.0 |
| (*Sunsweet*) . . . . . . . . . . . | 130 | 0 | 33.0 | 0 | 0 | 95 | 2.0 |
| w/mango (*Mariani*) . . . . . | 130 | 0 | 33.0 | 0 | 0 | 110 | 2.0 |
| **Pineapple, frozen**, chunks (*Dole*), ¾ cup . | 100 | 0 | 25.0 | 0 | 0 | 0 | 2.0 |
| **Pineapple drink blend**, 8 fl. oz.: | | | | | | | |
| coconut: | | | | | | | |
| (*Santa Cruz Organic*) . | 130 | 1.0 | 30.0 | .5 | 0 | 20 | 0 |
| (*SoBe Liz Bizz* Piña Colada) . . . . . . . . . . | 130 | 0 | 32.0 | 0 | 0 | 50 | 0 |
| mango (*Trop50*) . . . . . . . | 50 | <1.0 | 14.0 | 0 | 0 | 10 | 0 |
| orange: | | | | | | | |
| (*Tropicana*) . . . . . . . . . | 130 | <1.0 | 32.0 | 0 | 0 | 25 | 0 |
| (*Veryfine*), 11.5 fl. oz. . | 180 | 0 | 45.0 | 0 | 0 | 30 | 0 |

| Food and Measure | cal. | prot. (gms) | carbo. (gms) | fat (gms) | chol. (mgs) | sod. (mgs) | fiber (gms) |
|---|---|---|---|---|---|---|---|
| orange guava: | | | | | | | |
| (*Langers*) .......... | 130 | 0 | 30.0 | 0 | 0 | 0 | 0 |
| (*Nantucket Nectars*) .. | 120 | 0 | 29.0 | 0 | 0 | 25 | 0 |
| **Pineapple guava**, see "Feijoa" | | | | | | | |
| **Pineapple juice**, 8 fl. oz.: | | | | | | | |
| (*Ceres*) .............. | 120 | 0 | 29.0 | 0 | 0 | 5 | 2.0 |
| (*Dole* Can), 6 fl. oz. ..... | 90 | 1.0 | 22.0 | 0 | 0 | 10 | 0 |
| (*Dole* Chilled) ........ | 130 | <1.0 | 30.0 | 0 | 0 | 10 | 0 |
| (*Langers*) ............ | 130 | 0 | 33.0 | 0 | 0 | 15 | 0 |
| (*R.W. Knudsen* Nectar) .. | 140 | 1.0 | 35.0 | 0 | 0 | 20 | 0 |
| (*R.W. Knudsen* Organic) .......... | 120 | 0 | 28.0 | 0 | 0 | 15 | 0 |
| frozen: | | | | | | | |
| (*Dole*), ¼ cup ....... | 130 | 1.0 | 30.0 | 0 | 0 | 20 | 0 |
| diluted ............ | 130 | 1.0 | 31.9 | <.1 | 0 | 3 | .5 |
| **Pineapple juice blend**, 8 fl. oz., except as noted: | | | | | | | |
| coconut: | | | | | | | |
| (*Dole* Piña Colada) ... | 120 | 1.0 | 29.0 | 0 | 0 | 10 | 0 |
| (*Langers*) .......... | 140 | 0 | 28.0 | 3.0 | 0 | 55 | 1.0 |
| (*R.W. Knudsen*) ..... | 170 | 1.0 | 39.0 | 1.0 | 0 | 25 | <1.0 |
| peach mango (*Dole*) .... | 130 | <1.0 | 31.00 | 0 | 0 | 10 | 0 |
| orange: | | | | | | | |
| (*Dole* Can), 6 fl. oz. ... | 100 | 1.0 | 24.0 | 0 | 0 | 15 | 0 |
| (*Dole* Chilled) ...... | 120 | <1.0 | 31.0 | 0 | 0 | 10 | 0 |
| (*Minute Maid*) ....... | 120 | 1.0 | 29.0 | 0 | 0 | 15 | 0 |
| (*Tropicana*), 10 fl. oz. . | 150 | <1.0 | 38.0 | 0 | 0 | 10 | 0 |
| (*Tropicana Tropics*) ... | 120 | 1.0 | 30.0 | 0 | 0 | 10 | 0 |
| frozen (*Dole*), ¼ cup .. | 120 | <1.0 | 29.0 | 0 | 0 | 10 | 0 |
| orange banana: | | | | | | | |
| (*Dole* Can), 6 fl. oz. ... | 100 | 0 | 25.0 | 0 | 0 | 15 | 0 |
| (*Dole* Chilled) ...... | 120 | <1.0 | 30.0 | 0 | 0 | 10 | 0 |
| (*Nantucket Nectars*) .. | 140 | 1.0 | 34.0 | 0 | 0 | 30 | 0 |
| frozen (*Dole*), ¼ cup .. | 120 | <1.0 | 30.0 | 0 | 0 | 10 | 0 |
| orange strawberry: | | | | | | | |
| (*Dole*) .............. | 120 | <1.0 | 29.0 | 0 | 0 | 10 | 0 |
| frozen (*Dole*), ¼ cup .. | 130 | 1.0 | 32.0 | 0 | 0 | 20 | 0 |
| **Pineapple mango crisp** (*Dole*), 4 oz. ........ | 150 | 2.0 | 29.0 | 3.5 | 0 | 20 | 2.0 |
| **Pineapple topping** (*Smucker's*), 2 tbsp. .. | 110 | 0 | 27.0 | 0 | 0 | 0 | 0 |

| Food and Measure | cal. | prot. (gms) | carbo. (gms) | fat (gms) | chol. (mgs) | sod. (mgs) | fiber (gms) |
|---|---|---|---|---|---|---|---|
| **Pink bean**, dried, | | | | | | | |
| boiled, ½ cup ........ | 125 | 7.6 | 23.5 | .4 | 0 | 2 | 4.5 |
| **Pink bean dish**, | | | | | | | |
| canned, w/chili, onion, | | | | | | | |
| cumin (*S&W* | | | | | | | |
| Pinquitos), ½ cup .... | 110 | 6.0 | 20.0 | .5 | 0 | 490 | 6.0 |
| *Pinkberry,* frozen | | | | | | | |
| yogurt, ½ cup: | | | | | | | |
| original ............. | 100 | 3.0 | 21.0 | 0 | 5 | 50 | 0 |
| chocolate ............ | 120 | 5.0 | 23.0 | 1.5 | <5 | 110 | 2.0 |
| coconut .............. | 140 | 4.0 | 30.0 | 5.0 | <5 | 50 | 0 |
| green tea ............ | 110 | 4.0 | 25.0 | 0 | 5 | 45 | 1.0 |
| mango ............... | 100 | 3.0 | 23.0 | 0 | 5 | 45 | 0 |
| passion fruit .......... | 110 | 3.0 | 24.0 | 0 | 5 | 45 | 0 |
| pomegranate .......... | 120 | 3.0 | 26.0 | 0 | 0 | 40 | 0 |
| **Pinto bean**: | | | | | | | |
| dry, ¼ cup: | | | | | | | |
| (*Arrowhead Mills* | | | | | | | |
| Organic) ......... | 150 | 9.0 | 27.0 | 0 | 0 | 0 | 10.0 |
| (*Bob's Red Mill*) ..... | 150 | 9.0 | 27.0 | .5 | 0 | 5 | 7.0 |
| (*Eden* Organic) ...... | 140 | 8.0 | 26.0 | .5 | 0 | 5 | 11.0 |
| boiled, ½ cup ........ | 117 | 7.0 | 21.8 | .4 | 0 | 1 | 7.3 |
| **Pinto bean, canned** | | | | | | | |
| (see also "Chili | | | | | | | |
| Beans" and "Refried | | | | | | | |
| beans"), ½ cup: | | | | | | | |
| (*Allens*) .............. | 110 | 5.0 | 20.0 | 1.0 | 0 | 290 | 7.0 |
| (*Bush's* Frijoles) ....... | 80 | 6.0 | 18.0 | 0 | 0 | 450 | 7.0 |
| (*Bush's* Frijoles | | | | | | | |
| Reduced Sodium) .... | 80 | 6.0 | 18.0 | 0 | 0 | 220 | 7.0 |
| (*Eden* Organic) ........ | 110 | 6.0 | 18.0 | 1.0 | 0 | 15 | 6.0 |
| (*Ranch* Style Premium) .. | 100 | 6.0 | 20.0 | 0 | 0 | 370 | 6.0 |
| (*Rosarita*) ............. | 100 | 6.0 | 20.0 | 0 | 0 | 580 | 6.0 |
| (*S&W*) .............. | 120 | 6.0 | 22.0 | 1.0 | 0 | 530 | 7.0 |
| w/bacon: | | | | | | | |
| (*Trappey's*) ......... | 120 | 6.0 | 20.0 | 1.0 | 0 | 270 | 7.0 |
| jalapeño (*Trappey's* | | | | | | | |
| Jalapinto) ........ | 120 | 6.0 | 22.0 | 1.0 | 0 | 540 | 8.0 |
| seasoned (*Bush's*) ... | 120 | 6.0 | 17.0 | 2.5 | 5 | 530 | 6.0 |
| w/jalapeños (*Ranch* | | | | | | | |
| Style) .............. | 110 | 6.0 | 20.0 | .5 | 0 | 650 | 7.0 |
| w/pork (*Bush's*) ........ | 120 | 6.0 | 17.0 | 2.5 | 5 | 530 | 6.0 |
| seasoned: | | | | | | | |
| (*Allens*) ............. | 220 | 13.0 | 40.0 | 1.0 | 0 | 540 | 9.0 |

| Food and Measure | cal. | prot. (gms) | carbo. (gms) | fat (gms) | chol. (mgs) | sod. (mgs) | fiber (gms) |
|---|---|---|---|---|---|---|---|
| (*Bush's* Frijoles) | 100 | 6.0 | 17.0 | 0 | 0 | 470 | 5.0 |
| (*Glory*) | 100 | 6.0 | 18.0 | 0 | 0 | 570 | 6.0 |
| (*Glory* Sensibly) | 100 | 6.0 | 18.0 | 0 | 0 | 250 | 6.0 |
| w/Vidalia onion | | | | | | | |
| (*Allens*) | 110 | 7.0 | 20.0 | 0 | 0 | 370 | 6.0 |
| spicy (*Eden* Organic) | 120 | 6.0 | 24.0 | 1.0 | 0 | 200 | 7.0 |
| w/tomato, corn, chili | | | | | | | |
| (*Del Monte Savory* | | | | | | | |
| *Sides* Rio Grande) | 70 | 2.0 | 14.0 | 0 | 0 | 470 | 2.0 |
| **Pinto bean, frozen,** | | | | | | | |
| boiled, drained, | | | | | | | |
| ⅓ of 10-oz. pkg. | 152 | 8.8 | 29.0 | .5 | 0 | 78 | 8.1 |
| **Pinto bean seasoning** | | | | | | | |
| (*Zatarain's*), 1 tsp. | 20 | <1.0 | 4.0 | 0 | 0 | 460 | 0 |
| **Pistachios,** shelled, | | | | | | | |
| except as noted: | | | | | | | |
| (*Frito-Lay* Salted), | | | | | | | |
| 1 pkg. | 150 | 4.0 | 7.0 | 13.0 | 0 | 180 | 3.0 |
| (*Seffon Farms*), ½ cup | | | | | | | |
| in shell or ¼ cup | | | | | | | |
| shelled, 1.1 oz. | 170 | 6.0 | 9.0 | 13.0 | 0 | 160 | 3.0 |
| dried, 1 oz. | 164 | 5.8 | 7.1 | 13.7 | 0 | 2 | 3.1 |
| dry-roasted: | | | | | | | |
| (*Eden* Organic), | | | | | | | |
| 3 tbsp., .9 oz. | 160 | 7.0 | 7.0 | 12.0 | 0 | 60 | 3.0 |
| (*Planters*), 1 oz. | 170 | 5.0 | 8.0 | 14.0 | 0 | 150 | 3.0 |
| unsalted, 1 oz. | 162 | 6.1 | 7.8 | 13.0 | 0 | 2 | 2.9 |
| unsalted, ¼ cup | 183 | 6.8 | 8.9 | 14.7 | 0 | 3 | 3.3 |
| **Pita,** see "Bread" | | | | | | | |
| **Pita chips,** 1 oz.: | | | | | | | |
| (*Garden of Eatin'* | | | | | | | |
| Greek Isle Whole | | | | | | | |
| Grain) | 120 | 3.0 | 20.0 | 3.0 | 0 | 190 | 2.0 |
| (*Stacy's* Multigrain) | 140 | 3.0 | 19.0 | 5.0 | 0 | 270 | 2.0 |
| (*Stacy's* Simply | | | | | | | |
| Naked/ Italian) | 130 | 3.0 | 19.0 | 5.0 | 0 | 270 | 1.0 |
| chili pepper (*New York* | | | | | | | |
| *Style* Red Hot) | 140 | 2.0 | 19.0 | 6.0 | 0 | 350 | 1.0 |
| cinnamon sugar | | | | | | | |
| (*Stacy's*) | 140 | 3.0 | 20.0 | 5.0 | 0 | 115 | 1.0 |
| garlic, roasted, and | | | | | | | |
| herb (*Athenos*) | 120 | 3.0 | 19.0 | 4.0 | 0 | 290 | 0 |
| herb (*Stacy's* Tuscan) | 130 | 3.0 | 19.0 | 5.0 | 0 | 270 | 1.0 |

| Food and Measure | cal. | prot. (gms) | carbo. (gms) | fat (gms) | chol. (mgs) | sod. (mgs) | fiber (gms) |
|---|---|---|---|---|---|---|---|
| **Pita chips** *(cont.)* | | | | | | | |
| Parmesan garlic herb: | | | | | | | |
| (*New York Style*) . . . . . | 140 | 3.0 | 19.0 | 6.0 | 0 | 320 | 1.0 |
| (*Stacy's*) . . . . . . . . . . | 140 | 3.0 | 18.0 | 5.0 | 0 | 270 | 1.0 |
| ranch (*New York Style*) . . | 140 | 3.0 | 18.0 | 6.0 | 0 | 340 | 1.0 |
| sea salt: | | | | | | | |
| (*Garden of Eatin'* | | | | | | | |
| Whole Grain) . . . . . | 120 | 3.0 | 21.0 | 3.0 | 0 | 260 | 2.0 |
| (*New York Style*) . . . . . | 140 | 3.0 | 19.0 | 6.0 | 0 | 350 | 1.0 |
| veggie (*Stacy's*) . . . . . . . . | 130 | 3.0 | 18.0 | 5.0 | 0 | 270 | 1.0 |
| **Pitanga**: | | | | | | | |
| 1 medium, .3 oz. . . . . . . . | 2 | .1 | .5 | <.1 | 0 | <1 | <1.0 |
| ½ cup . . . . . . . . . . . . . . | 29 | .7 | 6.5 | .3 | 0 | 3 | <1.0 |
| **Pitaya**, see "Dragon fruit" | | | | | | | |
| **Pizza**, frozen, 1 pie, except as noted: | | | | | | | |
| bacon Alfredo (*Lean Cuisine*) . . . . . . . . . . . | 320 | 17.0 | 42.0 | 9.0 | 15 | 670 | 2.0 |
| bacon cheeseburger: | | | | | | | |
| (*Jack's*), ¼ pie . . . . . . | 290 | 15.0 | 29.0 | 13.0 | 30 | 750 | 2.0 |
| (*Jack's* Naturally Rising), ⅙ pie . . . . | 320 | 16.0 | 41.0 | 11.0 | 25 | 710 | 3.0 |
| bacon/sausage/pepperoni (*DiGiorno* Cheese Stuffed), ⅕ pie . . . . . . | 390 | 20.0 | 37.0 | 19.0 | 40 | 1060 | 2.0 |
| bruschetta (*Shiloh Farms*), ½ pie . . . . . . . | 170 | 10.0 | 20.0 | 8.0 | 16 | 431 | 1.0 |
| Canadian bacon: | | | | | | | |
| (*Jack's*), ⅓ pie . . . . . . | 330 | 18.0 | 38.0 | 13.0 | 40 | 760 | 3.0 |
| (*Tombstone*), ¼ pie . . | 320 | 17.0 | 37.0 | 12.0 | 35 | 720 | 4.0 |
| (*Totino's* Crisp Crust Party), ½ pie . . . . . | 320 | 13.0 | 35.0 | 15.0 | 10 | 810 | 1.0 |
| uncured, w/pineapple (*Pacific*), ⅓ pie . . . . | 250 | 14.0 | 32.0 | 8.0 | 20 | 600 | 1.0 |
| Caribbean (*Kashi* Carnival), ⅓ pie . . . . . | 280 | 14.0 | 39.0 | 8.0 | 10 | 590 | 5.0 |
| cheese: | | | | | | | |
| (*Amy's*), ⅓ pie . . . . . . | 290 | 12.0 | 33.0 | 12.0 | 15 | 590 | 2.0 |
| (*Amy's* Single) . . . . . . | 420 | 18.0 | 49.0 | 17.0 | 20 | 720 | 3.0 |
| (*DiGiorno* Ultimate Toppings), ⅕ pie . . | 320 | 16.0 | 34.0 | 13.0 | 35 | 820 | 2.0 |
| (*Dr. Oetker* Ristorante), ⅓ pie . | 290 | 12.0 | 26.0 | 13.0 | 25 | 580 | 1.0 |

| Food and Measure | cal. | prot. (gms) | carbo. (gms) | fat (gms) | chol. (mgs) | sod. (mgs) | fiber (gms) |
|---|---|---|---|---|---|---|---|
| (*Ellio's*), 2 pcs. ...... | 290 | 13.0 | 42.0 | 6.0 | 15 | 530 | 3.0 |
| (*Jack's*), ⅓ pie ...... | 320 | 15.0 | 38.0 | 13.0 | 30 | 610 | 3.0 |
| (*Jack's* Naturally Rising), ⅕ pie .... | 340 | 14.0 | 49.0 | 9.0 | 20 | 580 | 3.0 |
| (*Jack's* Super), ¼ pie . | 320 | 16.0 | 30.0 | 15.0 | 35 | 700 | 3.0 |
| (*Jeno's* Crisp 'n Tasty) | 450 | 14.0 | 51.0 | 21.0 | 0 | 930 | 2.0 |
| (*Michelina's*) ........ | 390 | 14.0 | 41.0 | 19.0 | 25 | 720 | 2.0 |
| (*Tombstone* Brick Oven), ⅓ pie ..... | 350 | 17.0 | 38.0 | 15.0 | 35 | 680 | 3.0 |
| (*Tombstone* Garlic Bread), ⅙ pie ..... | 350 | 15.0 | 40.0 | 14.0 | 25 | 540 | 3.0 |
| (*Tombstone* Harvest Wheat Thin), ⅓ pie . | 300 | 17.0 | 37.0 | 10.0 | 25 | 620 | 3.0 |
| (*Totino's* Crisp Crust Party), ½ pie ..... | 320 | 11.0 | 35.0 | 15.0 | 10 | 670 | 1.0 |
| extra (*Tombstone* 11.3 oz.), ½ pie ... | 360 | 17.0 | 42.0 | 14.0 | 30 | 680 | 4.0 |
| extra (*Tombstone* 20.5 oz.), ¼ pie ... | 350 | 18.0 | 37.0 | 15.0 | 40 | 660 | 4.0 |
| rice crust (*Amy's*), ⅓ pie .......... | 320 | 10.0 | 34.0 | 16.0 | 10 | 590 | 2.0 |
| cheese, 5: |  |  |  |  |  |  |  |
| (*DiGiorno* Cheese Stuffed), ⅕ pie .... | 390 | 20.0 | 39.0 | 17.0 | 45 | 1160 | 2.0 |
| (*Michelina's* Lean Gourmet) ........ | 290 | 15.0 | 42.0 | 7.0 | 10 | 840 | 2.0 |
| tomato (*California Pizza Kitchen* Self-Rising), ⅕ pie .... | 330 | 15.0 | 41.0 | 11.0 | 20 | 750 | 2.0 |
| cheese, 4: |  |  |  |  |  |  |  |
| (*Amy's*), ⅓ pie ...... | 290 | 12.0 | 31.0 | 14.0 | 20 | 590 | 2.0 |
| (*California Pizza Kitchen* Small) .... | 510 | 22.0 | 69.0 | 17.0 | 25 | 730 | 3.0 |
| (*California Pizza Kitchen* Thin), ⅓ pie .......... | 330 | 17.0 | 31.0 | 16.0 | 35 | 690 | 2.0 |
| (*DiGiorno* Deep Dish), ½ pkg. .......... | 290 | 12.0 | 26.0 | 16.0 | 20 | 440 | 2.0 |
| (*DiGiorno* For One) ... | 720 | 28.0 | 84.0 | 30.0 | 35 | 1190 | 6.0 |
| (*DiGiorno* Garlic Bread), ⅙ pie ..... | 350 | 16.0 | 41.0 | 14.0 | 20 | 590 | 3.0 |
| (*DiGiorno* Thin Crust), ⅕ pie ..... | 330 | 19.0 | 33.0 | 14.0 | 35 | 670 | 3.0 |

| Food and Measure | cal. | prot. (gms) | carbo. (gms) | fat (gms) | chol. (mgs) | sod. (mgs) | fiber (gms) |
|---|---|---|---|---|---|---|---|
| **Pizza, cheese, 4** *(cont.)* | | | | | | | |
| (*DiGiorno Rising Crust*), ⅙ pie . . . . . | 310 | 15.0 | 40.0 | 11.0 | 25 | 850 | 2.0 |
| (*Dr. Oetker Ristorante*), ⅓ pie . | 300 | 12.0 | 27.0 | 16.0 | 30 | 550 | 1.0 |
| (*Lean Cuisine*) . . . . . . | 360 | 20.0 | 51.0 | 6.0 | 5 | 650 | 3.0 |
| (*Newman's Own* Thin & Crispy), ⅓ pie . . . | 300 | 16.0 | 31.0 | 13.0 | 30 | 610 | 2.0 |
| (*Smart Ones*) . . . . . . . | 370 | 18.0 | 57.0 | 7.0 | 10 | 690 | 4.0 |
| cheese, 3: | | | | | | | |
| (*Glutino* Gluten Free) . | 300 | 14.0 | 37.0 | 12.0 | 25 | 690 | 2.0 |
| (*Tombstone* Thin Crust), ¼ pie . . . . . | 310 | 16.0 | 28.0 | 15.0 | 40 | 660 | 3.0 |
| (*Totino's* Crisp Crust Party), ½ pie . . . . . | 330 | 12.0 | 34.0 | 16.0 | 15 | 640 | 1.0 |
| cornmeal crust (*Amy's*), ⅓ pie . . . . | 340 | 10.0 | 41.0 | 15.0 | 10 | 580 | 2.0 |
| Italian (*DiGiorno* Flatbread), ⅓ pie . . | 330 | 17.0 | 28.0 | 17.0 | 40 | 720 | 3.0 |
| "cheese," nondairy: | | | | | | | |
| (*Amy's* Cheeze), ⅓ pie | 290 | 12.0 | 37.0 | 11.0 | 0 | 590 | 2.0 |
| rice crust (*Amy's* Cheeze Single) . . . . | 460 | 10.0 | 46.0 | 28.0 | 0 | 680 | 4.0 |
| cheese/pesto, whole wheat (*Amy's*), ⅓ pie . | 360 | 13.0 | 37.0 | 18.0 | 15 | 680 | 4.0 |
| cheeseburger (*California Pizza Kitchen Thin*), ⅓ pie . . . . . . . . | 330 | 14.0 | 33.0 | 16.0 | 25 | 520 | 3.0 |
| chicken: | | | | | | | |
| fajita (*Smart Ones*) . . . | 380 | 21.0 | 58.0 | 7.0 | 25 | 690 | 4.0 |
| garlic (*California Pizza Kitchen Thin*), ⅓ pie . . . . . . . . . . | 270 | 16.0 | 33.0 | 9.0 | 30 | 650 | 2.0 |
| garlic, roasted (*Lean Cuisine*) . . . . . . . . | 330 | 23.0 | 42.0 | 8.0 | 20 | 600 | 2.0 |
| garlic, roasted (*Newman's Own* Thin & Crispy), ⅓ pie . . . | 270 | 14.0 | 31.0 | 10.0 | 30 | 540 | 2.0 |
| herb garlic (*Pacific*), ⅓ pie . . . . . . . . . . | 270 | 16.0 | 30.0 | 9.0 | 25 | 520 | 1.0 |
| pepper/onions (*DiGiorno* 200 Calorie), ½ pie . . . . | 200 | 11.0 | 22.0 | 9.0 | 20 | 470 | 1.0 |

| Food and Measure | cal. | prot. (gms) | carbo. (gms) | fat (gms) | chol. (mgs) | sod. (mgs) | fiber (gms) |
|---|---|---|---|---|---|---|---|
| pesto (*California Pizza Kitchen Natural*), ⅓ pie .... | 320 | 14.0 | 36.0 | 13.0 | 25 | 570 | 4.0 |
| pesto (*California Pizza Kitchen Small*) | 420 | 21.0 | 44.0 | 18.0 | 30 | 490 | 4.0 |
| Tuscan (*DiGiorno* Flatbread), ⅓ pie .. | 280 | 14.0 | 25.0 | 14.0 | 35 | 680 | 2.0 |
| chicken, barbecue: | | | | | | | |
| (*California Pizza Kitchen Self-Rising*), ⅕ pie .... | 320 | 16.0 | 43.0 | 10.0 | 25 | 750 | 2.0 |
| (*California Pizza Kitchen Small*) .... | 500 | 25.0 | 73.0 | 13.0 | 35 | 710 | 4.0 |
| (*California Pizza Kitchen Thin*), ⅓ pie | 290 | 17.0 | 35.0 | 9.0 | 30 | 560 | 2.0 |
| (*Glutino Gluten Free*) . | 360 | 16.0 | 55.0 | 12.0 | 25 | 870 | 3.0 |
| (*Lean Cuisine*) ...... | 340 | 20.0 | 48.0 | 7.0 | 35 | 430 | 2.0 |
| (*Pacific*), ⅓ pie ...... | 270 | 16.0 | 30.0 | 9.0 | 25 | 520 | 1.0 |
| combination: | | | | | | | |
| (*Jeno's Crisp 'n Tasty*) | 480 | 15.0 | 50.0 | 25.0 | 15 | 1060 | 2.0 |
| (*Totino's* Crisp Crust Party), ½ pie ..... | 370 | 12.0 | 35.0 | 20.0 | 10 | 830 | 1.0 |
| deluxe: | | | | | | | |
| (*Lean Cuisine*) ...... | 340 | 17.0 | 49.0 | 8.0 | 20 | 510 | 4.0 |
| (*Tombstone* Brick Oven), ¼ pie ..... | 280 | 14.0 | 30.0 | 12.0 | 30 | 560 | 2.0 |
| hamburger: | | | | | | | |
| (*Jack's*), ¼ pie ...... | 280 | 14.0 | 29.0 | 12.0 | 30 | 580 | 2.0 |
| (*Tombstone*), ¼ pie .. | 350 | 18.0 | 37.0 | 15.0 | 35 | 720 | 4.0 |
| (*Totino's* Crisp Crust Party), ½ pie ..... | 370 | 13.0 | 35.0 | 20.0 | 15 | 780 | 1.0 |
| Margherita: | | | | | | | |
| (*Amy's*), ⅓ pie ...... | 280 | 11.0 | 32.0 | 12.0 | 10 | 550 | 2.0 |
| (*Amy's Single*) ...... | 400 | 16.0 | 47.0 | 17.0 | 15 | 720 | 3.0 |
| (*California Pizza Kitchen Small*) .... | 420 | 20.0 | 45.0 | 18.0 | 30 | 680 | 2.0 |
| (*California Pizza Kitchen Thin*), ⅓ pie .......... | 290 | 13.0 | 31.0 | 13.0 | 20 | 520 | 2.0 |
| (*Kashi Thin*), ⅓ pie ... | 260 | 14.0 | 29.0 | 9.0 | 20 | 630 | 4.0 |
| (*Lean Cuisine*) ...... | 300 | 16.0 | 43.0 | 7.0 | 15 | 580 | 2.0 |
| (*Michelina's*) ........ | 390 | 13.0 | 41.0 | 21.0 | 20 | 680 | 2.0 |
| (*Newman's Own* Thin & Crispy), ⅓ pie ... | 280 | 12.0 | 31.0 | 12.0 | 25 | 650 | 1.0 |

| Food and Measure | cal. | prot. (gms) | carbo. (gms) | fat (gms) | chol. (mgs) | sod. (mgs) | fiber (gms) |
|---|---|---|---|---|---|---|---|
| **Pizza, Margherita** *(cont.)* | | | | | | | |
| (*Rising Moon* | | | | | | | |
| *Organics*), ½ pie .. | 330 | 13.0 | 45.0 | 11.0 | 15 | 600 | 5.0 |
| meat, 4, ⅕ pie: | | | | | | | |
| (*DiGiorno* Thin | | | | | | | |
| Crust) ........... | 340 | 18.0 | 34.0 | 15.0 | 35 | 860 | 3.0 |
| (*DiGiorno* Ultimate | | | | | | | |
| Toppings) ........ | 380 | 19.0 | 34.0 | 19.0 | 50 | 1140 | 2.0 |
| (*Tombstone*) ........ | 310 | 15.0 | 30.0 | 14.0 | 35 | 690 | 3.0 |
| meat, 3: | | | | | | | |
| (*DiGiorno* Cheese | | | | | | | |
| Stuffed), ⅙ pie .... | 350 | 17.0 | 34.0 | 16.0 | 40 | 950 | 2.0 |
| (*DiGiorno* Rising | | | | | | | |
| Crust), ⅙ pie ..... | 350 | 16.0 | 41.0 | 15.0 | 30 | 1010 | 2.0 |
| (*Jack's* Naturally | | | | | | | |
| Rising), ⅙ pie .... | 330 | 14.0 | 41.0 | 12.0 | 25 | 640 | 3.0 |
| (*Lean Cuisine*) ...... | 390 | 22.0 | 55.0 | 9.0 | 25 | 610 | 3.0 |
| (*Tombstone* Cheese | | | | | | | |
| Stuffed), ⅙ pie .... | 320 | 15.0 | 34.0 | 14.0 | 30 | 750 | 4.0 |
| (*Totino's* Crisp Crust | | | | | | | |
| Party), ½ pie ..... | 350 | 12.0 | 35.0 | 18.0 | 10 | 830 | 1.0 |
| Mediterranean | | | | | | | |
| (*Kashi*), ⅓ pie ....... | 290 | 15.0 | 37.0 | 9.0 | 20 | 640 | 5.0 |
| Mexican style (*Jack's*), | | | | | | | |
| ¼ pie ............. | 290 | 13.0 | 29.0 | 14.0 | 30 | 720 | 3.0 |
| mushroom: | | | | | | | |
| (*Dr. Oetker* Ristorante | | | | | | | |
| Funghi), ⅓ pie .... | 290 | 9.0 | 28.0 | 13.0 | 15 | 690 | 3.0 |
| (*Lean Cuisine*) ...... | 300 | 16.0 | 47.0 | 5.0 | 5 | 540 | 4.0 |
| olive (*Amy's*), ⅓ pie .. | 260 | 10.0 | 33.0 | 10.0 | 10 | 560 | 2.0 |
| olive (*Amy's* Single) .. | 450 | 18.0 | 56.0 | 19.0 | 20 | 780 | 3.0 |
| trio, and spinach | | | | | | | |
| (*Kashi*), ⅓ pie .... | 250 | 14.0 | 28.0 | 9.0 | 25 | 660 | 4.0 |
| pepperoni: | | | | | | | |
| (*Banquet* Meal) ...... | 340 | 11.0 | 47.0 | 12.0 | 10 | 730 | 4.0 |
| (*California Pizza* | | | | | | | |
| *Kitchen* Thin), ⅓ pie | 340 | 16.0 | 33.0 | 16.0 | 35 | 760 | 1.0 |
| (*DiGiorno* 200 | | | | | | | |
| Calorie), ½ pie .... | 200 | 10.0 | 21.0 | 9.0 | 15 | 520 | 1.0 |
| (*DiGiorno* Cheese | | | | | | | |
| Stuffed), ⅕ pie .... | 380 | 19.0 | 40.0 | 16.0 | 40 | 1040 | 3.0 |
| (*DiGiorno* Deep Dish), | | | | | | | |
| ½ pie ............ | 300 | 12.0 | 26.0 | 17.0 | 25 | 470 | 2.0 |
| (*DiGiorno* For One) ... | 770 | 30.0 | 83.0 | 35.0 | 45 | 1430 | 6.0 |

| Food and Measure | cal. | prot. (gms) | carbo. (gms) | fat (gms) | chol. (mgs) | sod. (mgs) | fiber (gms) |
|---|---|---|---|---|---|---|---|
| (*DiGiorno* For One Thin Crust) ....... | 590 | 31.0 | 63.0 | 24.0 | 50 | 1170 | 3.0 |
| (*DiGiorno* Garlic Bread), ⅙ pie ..... | 380 | 17.0 | 40.0 | 17.0 | 25 | 690 | 3.0 |
| (*DiGiorno* Thin Crust), ⅕ pie ..... | 340 | 17.0 | 33.0 | 16.0 | 35 | 800 | 3.0 |
| (*DiGiorno* Ultimate Toppings), ⅕ pie .. | 370 | 17.0 | 34.0 | 19.0 | 40 | 1080 | 2.0 |
| (*DiGiorno Rising Crust*), ⅙ pie ..... | 330 | 14.0 | 40.0 | 13.0 | 30 | 940 | 2.0 |
| (*Ellio's*), 2 pcs. ....... | 310 | 13.0 | 40.0 | 10.0 | 20 | 620 | 3.0 |
| (*Glutino* Gluten Free) . | 360 | 15.0 | 39.0 | 16.0 | 30 | 850 | 2.0 |
| (*Jack's*), ⅓ pie ....... | 390 | 18.0 | 38.0 | 19.0 | 45 | 890 | 3.0 |
| (*Jack's* Naturally Rising), ⅙ pie ..... | 330 | 14.0 | 41.0 | 13.0 | 30 | 680 | 3.0 |
| (*Jack's* Original), ½ pie ........... | 370 | 16.0 | 36.0 | 18.0 | 45 | 830 | 3.0 |
| (*Jeno's Crisp 'n Tasty*) | 490 | 15.0 | 50.0 | 25.0 | 15 | 1090 | 2.0 |
| (*Lean Cuisine*) ...... | 350 | 20.0 | 50.0 | 8.0 | 20 | 630 | 3.0 |
| (*Michelina's*) ........ | 450 | 12.0 | 41.0 | 27.0 | 25 | 870 | 2.0 |
| (*Michelina's Lean Gourmet*) ........ | 300 | 14.0 | 41.0 | 9.0 | 20 | 970 | 2.0 |
| (*Smart Ones*) ....... | 390 | 20.0 | 58.0 | 8.0 | 20 | 730 | 4.0 |
| (*Tombstone* 12 oz.), ⅓ pie ........... | 280 | 13.0 | 28.0 | 14.0 | 30 | 620 | 3.0 |
| (*Tombstone* Brick Oven), ¼ pie ..... | 310 | 14.0 | 29.0 | 16.0 | 40 | 720 | 2.0 |
| (*Tombstone* Garlic Bread), ⅙ pie ..... | 370 | 15.0 | 40.0 | 17.0 | 30 | 670 | 3.0 |
| (*Tombstone* Thin Crust), ¼ pie ..... | 320 | 15.0 | 28.0 | 18.0 | 40 | 780 | 3.0 |
| (*Totino's* Crisp Crust Party), ½ pie ..... | 360 | 12.0 | 35.0 | 19.0 | 10 | 830 | 1.0 |
| (*Totino's* Crisp Crust Party Classic), ½ pie | 360 | 12.0 | 35.0 | 19.0 | 10 | 810 | 1.0 |
| (*Totino's* Crisp Crust Party Triple), ½ pie . | 370 | 12.0 | 35.0 | 20.0 | 15 | 860 | 1.0 |
| pepperoni, uncured: | | | | | | | |
| (*Newman's Own* Thin & Crispy), ⅓ pie ... | 320 | 15.0 | 31.0 | 16.0 | 35 | 800 | 1.0 |
| (*Pacific*), ⅓ pie ...... | 260 | 14.0 | 31.0 | 10.0 | 30 | 600 | 1.0 |
| pepperoni/cheese | | | | | | | |
| (*Jack's* Half & Half), ⅓ pie ............ | 440 | 20.0 | 38.0 | 23.0 | 60 | 1070 | 3.0 |

| Food and Measure | cal. | prot. (gms) | carbo. (gms) | fat (gms) | chol. (mgs) | sod. (mgs) | fiber (gms) |
|---|---|---|---|---|---|---|---|
| **Pizza** (cont.) | | | | | | | |
| pepperoni/mushroom | | | | | | | |
| (*Jack's*), ¼ pie ...... | 300 | 14.0 | 29.0 | 15.0 | 35 | 680 | 2.0 |
| pepperoni/peppers: | | | | | | | |
| (*DiGiorno* Flatbread), | | | | | | | |
| ⅓ pie ........... | 340 | 16.0 | 26.0 | 20.0 | 45 | 920 | 2.0 |
| onions (*Dr. Oetker* | | | | | | | |
| Ristorante), ⅓ pie . | 300 | 10.0 | 27.0 | 17.0 | 25 | 890 | 3.0 |
| pepperoni/sausage: | | | | | | | |
| (*Jack's*), ½ pie ...... | 370 | 16.0 | 36.0 | 18.0 | 45 | 810 | 3.0 |
| (*Tombstone* 12.5 oz.), | | | | | | | |
| ⅓ pie ........... | 290 | 14.0 | 29.0 | 14.0 | 30 | 650 | 3.0 |
| (*Tombstone* 21.4 oz.), | | | | | | | |
| ¼ pie ........... | 370 | 18.0 | 37.0 | 17.0 | 40 | 800 | 4.0 |
| peppers, roasted, w/ | | | | | | | |
| fontina (*California Pizza* | | | | | | | |
| *Kitchen* Natural), ⅓ pie | 260 | 10.0 | 36.0 | 10.0 | 15 | 580 | 2.0 |
| pesto: | | | | | | | |
| (*Amy's*), ⅓ pie ...... | 310 | 12.0 | 39.0 | 12.0 | 10 | 480 | 2.0 |
| (*Amy's* Single) ...... | 440 | 18.0 | 52.0 | 19.0 | 15 | 780 | 3.0 |
| (*Rising Moon* | | | | | | | |
| *Organics*), ½ pie .. | 380 | 17.0 | 43.0 | 16.0 | 30 | 500 | 6.0 |
| sausage: | | | | | | | |
| (*DiGiorno* For One) ... | 760 | 30.0 | 85.0 | 33.0 | 45 | 1300 | 5.0 |
| (*Jack's* Naturally | | | | | | | |
| Rising), ⅙ pie .... | 330 | 13.0 | 41.0 | 12.0 | 25 | 580 | 3.0 |
| (*Jeno's* Crisp 'n Tasty) | 480 | 15.0 | 50.0 | 25.0 | 10 | 1030 | 2.0 |
| (*Tombstone* Brick | | | | | | | |
| Oven), ¼ pie ..... | 290 | 14.0 | 29.0 | 13.0 | 30 | 590 | 2.0 |
| (*Tombstone* Double | | | | | | | |
| Top), ⅙ pie ....... | 310 | 17.0 | 27.0 | 16.0 | 40 | 700 | 3.0 |
| (*Tombstone* Original | | | | | | | |
| 22.1 oz.), ⅕ pie ... | 290 | 14.0 | 30.0 | 13.0 | 30 | 590 | 3.0 |
| (*Tombstone* Original | | | | | | | |
| 12.1 oz.), ⅓ pie ... | 270 | 13.0 | 29.0 | 12.0 | 25 | 540 | 3.0 |
| (*Tombstone* Thin | | | | | | | |
| Crust), ¼ pie ..... | 330 | 17.0 | 29.0 | 17.0 | 40 | 760 | 3.0 |
| (*Totino's* Crisp Crust | | | | | | | |
| Party), ½ pie ..... | 370 | 12.0 | 35.0 | 20.0 | 10 | 820 | 1.0 |
| sausage, Italian: | | | | | | | |
| (*DiGiorno* Deep | | | | | | | |
| Dish), ½ pie ...... | 300 | 11.0 | 26.0 | 18.0 | 25 | 450 | 2.0 |
| (*DiGiorno* Rising | | | | | | | |
| Crust), ⅙ pie ..... | 350 | 15.0 | 40.0 | 14.0 | 30 | 960 | 2.0 |

| Food and Measure | cal. | prot. (gms) | carbo. (gms) | fat (gms) | chol. (mgs) | sod. (mgs) | fiber (gms) |
|---|---|---|---|---|---|---|---|
| (*Newman's Own* Thin & Crispy), ⅓ pie | 300 | 14.0 | 31.0 | 13.0 | 30 | 680 | 1.0 |
| onions (*DiGiorno* Flatbread), ⅓ pie | 400 | 18.0 | 27.0 | 26.0 | 60 | 1140 | 2.0 |
| spicy (*Jack's*), ⅓ pie | 380 | 18.0 | 38.0 | 17.0 | 40 | 720 | 3.0 |
| sausage/mushroom: | | | | | | | |
| (*Jack's*), ¼ pie | 290 | 13.0 | 29.0 | 14.0 | 30 | 570 | 3.0 |
| (*Tombstone*), ⅕ pie | 290 | 15.0 | 30.0 | 13.0 | 30 | 590 | 3.0 |
| sausage/pepperoni: | | | | | | | |
| (*DiGiorno Rising Crust*), ⅙ pie | 350 | 15.0 | 40.0 | 15.0 | 30 | 990 | 2.0 |
| (*Ellio's*), 2 pcs. | 310 | 14.0 | 41.0 | 10.0 | 15 | 610 | 4.0 |
| (*Jack's*), ¼ pie | 300 | 14.0 | 29.0 | 15.0 | 35 | 670 | 2.0 |
| (*Jack's* Half & Half), ¼ pie | 290 | 13.0 | 29.0 | 14.0 | 35 | 590 | 3.0 |
| (*Jack's* Naturally Rising), ⅙ pie | 330 | 14.0 | 41.0 | 13.0 | 30 | 640 | 3.0 |
| (*Tombstone* Brick Oven), ¼ pie | 320 | 15.0 | 29.0 | 17.0 | 40 | 710 | 3.0 |
| (*Tombstone* Double Top), ⅙ pie | 330 | 17.0 | 26.0 | 18.0 | 45 | 780 | 3.0 |
| Sicilian: | | | | | | | |
| (*California Pizza Kitchen* Small) | 450 | 21.0 | 42.0 | 22.0 | 35 | 820 | 2.0 |
| (*California Pizza Kitchen* Self-Rising), ⅕ pie | 380 | 18.0 | 42.0 | 16.0 | 35 | 1070 | 2.0 |
| (*California Pizza Kitchen* Thin), ⅓ pie | 310 | 17.0 | 30.0 | 14.0 | 30 | 920 | 2.0 |
| (*Michelina's*) | 400 | 15.0 | 40.0 | 20.0 | 30 | 860 | 2.0 |
| spinach: | | | | | | | |
| (*Amy's*), ⅓ pie | 310 | 12.0 | 38.0 | 12.0 | 15 | 590 | 2.0 |
| (*Amy's* Single) | 440 | 19.0 | 54.0 | 18.0 | 20 | 780 | 3.0 |
| (*Amy's* Single Light Sodium) | 440 | 19.0 | 54.0 | 18.0 | 20 | 390 | 3.0 |
| (*Dr. Oetker* Ristorante Spinaci), ⅓ pie | 290 | 9.0 | 28.0 | 16.0 | 15 | 750 | 2.0 |
| artichoke (*California Pizza Kitchen* Thin), ⅓ pie | 350 | 13.0 | 34.0 | 19.0 | 30 | 770 | 2.0 |
| "cheese," soy (*Glutino* Gluten Free) | 480 | 8.0 | 66.0 | 20.0 | 0 | 1000 | 6.0 |

| Food and Measure | cal. | prot. (gms) | carbo. (gms) | fat (gms) | chol. (mgs) | sod. (mgs) | fiber (gms) |
|---|---|---|---|---|---|---|---|
| **Pizza, spinach** *(cont.)* | | | | | | | |
| feta (*Glutino* Gluten Free) ............. | 300 | 11.0 | 39.0 | 11.0 | 25 | 840 | 2.0 |
| mushroom (*Lean Cuisine* Deep Dish) . | 340 | 18.0 | 52.0 | 7.0 | 10 | 450 | 2.0 |
| mushroom garlic (*DiGiorno Rising Crust*), ⅙ pie ..... | 290 | 15.0 | 41.0 | 9.0 | 15 | 790 | 2.0 |
| rice crust (*Amy's*), ⅓ pie ............ | 350 | 8.0 | 34.0 | 20.0 | 0 | 580 | 4.0 |
| supreme: | | | | | | | |
| (*DiGiorno* Cheese Stuffed), ⅙ pie .... | 350 | 17.0 | 34.0 | 16.0 | 40 | 950 | 3.0 |
| (*DiGiorno* Flatbread), ⅓ pie ............ | 380 | 16.0 | 28.0 | 22.0 | 45 | 980 | 4.0 |
| (*DiGiorno* For One) ... | 790 | 31.0 | 85.0 | 36.0 | 50 | 1460 | 6.0 |
| (*DiGiorno* For One Thin Crust) ....... | 570 | 29.0 | 64.0 | 22.0 | 45 | 1060 | 3.0 |
| (*DiGiorno* Garlic Bread), ⅛ pie ..... | 300 | 13.0 | 31.0 | 14.0 | 20 | 540 | 3.0 |
| (*DiGiorno* Thin Crust), ⅕ pie ..... | 340 | 16.0 | 35.0 | 15.0 | 30 | 730 | 3.0 |
| (*DiGiorno* Ultimate Toppings), ⅕ pie .. | 360 | 16.0 | 35.0 | 18.0 | 45 | 1010 | 2.0 |
| (*DiGiorno* Rising Crust.), ⅙ pie ..... | 360 | 16.0 | 41.0 | 15.0 | 30 | 990 | 3.0 |
| (*Ellio's*), 2 pcs. ...... | 310 | 15.0 | 41.0 | 10.0 | 20 | 630 | 5.0 |
| (*Jack's*), ¼ pie ...... | 300 | 14.0 | 29.0 | 15.0 | 35 | 650 | 3.0 |
| (*Jeno's Crisp 'n Tasty*) ............ | 480 | 15.0 | 49.0 | 24.0 | 15 | 1050 | 2.0 |
| (*Newman's Own* Thin & Crispy), ⅓ pie ... | 320 | 14.0 | 33.0 | 15.0 | 30 | 750 | 2.0 |
| (*Pacific*), ⅓ pie ...... | 270 | 15.0 | 31.0 | 11.0 | 25 | 650 | 2.0 |
| (*Tombstone*), ⅕ pie .. | 300 | 14.0 | 31.0 | 14.0 | 30 | 640 | 3.0 |
| (*Tombstone* Brick Oven), ¼ pie ..... | 320 | 15.0 | 29.0 | 16.0 | 40 | 700 | 3.0 |
| (*Tombstone* Garlic Bread), ⅙ pie ..... | 360 | 14.0 | 41.0 | 15.0 | 25 | 610 | 3.0 |
| (*Totino's* Crisp Crust Party), ½ pie ..... | 360 | 12.0 | 35.0 | 19.0 | 10 | 820 | 2.0 |
| tomato/basil/ mozzarella (*California Pizza Kitchen Natural*), ⅓ pie ...... | 420 | 16.0 | 50.0 | 19.0 | 25 | 800 | 2.0 |

| Food and Measure | cal. | prot. (gms) | carbo. (gms) | fat (gms) | chol. (mgs) | sod. (mgs) | fiber (gms) |
|---|---|---|---|---|---|---|---|
| vegan (*Tofurky*), ⅓ pie: | | | | | | | |
| "cheese" | 240 | 6.0 | 39.0 | 7.0 | 0 | 380 | 3.0 |
| Italian "sausage" | 270 | 13.0 | 40.0 | 6.0 | 0 | 320 | 5.0 |
| "pepperoni" | 270 | 13.0 | 39.0 | 7.0 | 0 | 400 | 7.0 |
| vegetable/veggie: | | | | | | | |
| (*Dr. Oetker* Ristorante), ⅓ pie | 250 | 8.0 | 28.0 | 12.0 | 15 | 750 | 2.0 |
| (*Tombstone* Light), ⅕ pie | 230 | 13.0 | 31.0 | 6.0 | 10 | 510 | 4.0 |
| grilled (*Rising Moon Organics*), ½ pie | 360 | 14.0 | 41.0 | 15.0 | 20 | 480 | 7.0 |
| vegetable, roasted: | | | | | | | |
| (*Amy's*), ⅓ pie | 280 | 7.0 | 42.0 | 9.0 | 0 | 540 | 3.0 |
| (*Amy's* Single) | 410 | 11.0 | 62.0 | 14.0 | 0 | 780 | 5.0 |
| (*Kashi* Thin), ⅓ pie | 250 | 14.0 | 28.0 | 9.0 | 20 | 630 | 4.0 |
| (*Lean Cuisine* Deep Dish) | 320 | 16.0 | 52.0 | 5.0 | 5 | 480 | 3.0 |
| rice crust (*Amy's*) | 430 | 7.0 | 55.0 | 20.0 | 0 | 680 | 5.0 |
| white, ⅓ pie: | | | | | | | |
| (*California Pizza Kitchen* Thin) | 290 | 15.0 | 31.0 | 12.0 | 25 | 600 | 2.0 |
| (*Newman's Own* Thin & Crispy) | 260 | 11.0 | 31.0 | 10.0 | 20 | 630 | 1.0 |
| broccoli spinach (*Amy's*) | 290 | 10.0 | 31.0 | 14.0 | 25 | 570 | 2.0 |
| the works (*Jack's* Naturally Rising), ⅙ pie | 330 | 14.0 | 42.0 | 12.0 | 25 | 590 | 3.0 |
| **Pizza, bagel,** frozen: | | | | | | | |
| (*Bagel Bites*), 4 pcs., 3.1 oz.: | | | | | | | |
| cheese, 3 | 200 | 8.0 | 29.0 | 6.0 | 10 | 350 | 1.0 |
| cheese/pepperoni | 210 | 8.0 | 28.0 | 7.0 | 15 | 430 | 1.0 |
| cheese/sausage/ pepperoni | 200 | 8.0 | 28.0 | 6.0 | 10 | 380 | 2.0 |
| mozzarella | 190 | 8.0 | 29.0 | 4.5 | 10 | 390 | 1.0 |
| supreme | 180 | 7.0 | 27.0 | 5.0 | 10 | 380 | 2.0 |
| cheese (*Dr. Praeger's*), 2-oz. pc. | 110 | 6.0 | 18.0 | 2.5 | 5 | 180 | 3.0 |
| **Pizza, flatbread melt,** see "Melts" | | | | | | | |
| **Pizza, French bread,** frozen, 1 pc.: | | | | | | | |
| (*Lean Cuisine*): | | | | | | | |
| cheese | 340 | 17.0 | 53.0 | 7.0 | 15 | 680 | 5.0 |

| Food and Measure | cal. | prot. (gms) | carbo. (gms) | fat (gms) | chol. (mgs) | sod. (mgs) | fiber (gms) |
|---|---|---|---|---|---|---|---|
| **Pizza, French bread** *(cont.)* | | | | | | | |
| deluxe . . . . . . . . . . . . . | 340 | 16.0 | 51.0 | 8.0 | 20 | 670 | 4.0 |
| pepperoni . . . . . . . . . . | 310 | 16.0 | 46.0 | 7.0 | 15 | 690 | 4.0 |
| *(Stouffer's):* | | | | | | | |
| cheese, 2 pack . . . . . . | 360 | 14.0 | 43.0 | 15.0 | 20 | 530 | 4.0 |
| cheese, 9 pack . . . . . . | 380 | 15.0 | 43.0 | 16.0 | 30 | 660 | 3.0 |
| cheese, extra . . . . . . . | 400 | 16.0 | 44.0 | 18.0 | 25 | 630 | 4.0 |
| cheese, five . . . . . . . . . | 420 | 17.0 | 44.0 | 20.0 | 35 | 600 | 3.0 |
| deluxe, 2 pack . . . . . . . | 430 | 15.0 | 44.0 | 21.0 | 25 | 820 | 4.0 |
| deluxe, 9 pack . . . . . . . | 430 | 15.0 | 45.0 | 21.0 | 30 | 880 | 3.0 |
| meat, three . . . . . . . . . | 470 | 19.0 | 43.0 | 25.0 | 40 | 990 | 4.0 |
| pepperoni, 2 pack . . . . | 410 | 15.0 | 43.0 | 20.0 | 25 | 810 | 4.0 |
| pepperoni, 9 pack . . . . | 430 | 16.0 | 44.0 | 21.0 | 30 | 930 | 3.0 |
| pepperoni/mushroom . | 430 | 16.0 | 44.0 | 21.0 | 25 | 920 | 4.0 |
| sausage . . . . . . . . . . . | 420 | 15.0 | 43.0 | 21.0 | 25 | 730 | 4.0 |
| sausage/pepperoni . . . | 460 | 17.0 | 43.0 | 24.0 | 30 | 880 | 4.0 |
| vegetables, grilled . . . . | 340 | 13.0 | 44.0 | 12.0 | 15 | 570 | 4.0 |
| **Pizza, fruit** *(Eggo)*, 5.3-oz. pc.: | | | | | | | |
| mixed berry granola . . . . | 390 | 10.0 | 62.0 | 13.0 | 15 | 390 | 4.0 |
| strawberry granola . . . . . | 400 | 10.0 | 66.0 | 12.0 | 10 | 390 | 4.0 |
| **Pizza, stuffed/pocket** (see also "Pizza snack"), frozen, 1 pc., 4.5 oz., except as noted: | | | | | | | |
| cheese: | | | | | | | |
| *(Amy's* Pocket) . . . . . . | 310 | 14.0 | 42.0 | 10.0 | 15 | 450 | 4.0 |
| *(Amy's* Toaster Pops), 2 oz. . . . . . . | 160 | 5.0 | 21.0 | 6.0 | 5 | 220 | 1.0 |
| and tomato *(Aunt Trudy's)*, 5 oz. . . . . | 320 | 11.0 | 36.0 | 15.0 | 20 | 490 | 2.0 |
| spinach *(Amy's* Pocket) . . . . . . . . . . . | 280 | 13.0 | 37.0 | 9.0 | 15 | 460 | 3.0 |
| **Pizza appetizer,** see "Pizza snacks" | | | | | | | |
| **Pizza crust,** 2.8-oz. pc.: | | | | | | | |
| *(Kontos)* . . . . . . . . . . . . . | 230 | 6.0 | 37.0 | 5.0 | 0 | 370 | 4.0 |
| multigrain *(Kontos)* . . . . . | 220 | 8.0 | 36.0 | 7.0 | 0 | 340 | 7.0 |
| **Pizza crust, frozen/ chilled:** | | | | | | | |
| *(Glutino* Gluten Free), 3.3-oz. crust . . . . . . . . | 270 | 1.0 | 56.0 | 4.5 | 0 | 550 | 3.0 |

| Food and Measure | cal. | prot. (gms) | carbo. (gms) | fat (gms) | chol. (mgs) | sod. (mgs) | fiber (gms) |
|---|---|---|---|---|---|---|---|
| (*Pillsbury* Classic), | | | | | | | |
| 1/6 pkg. | 160 | 5.0 | 31.0 | 2.0 | 0 | 470 | 1.0 |
| thins (*Pillsbury*), | | | | | | | |
| 1/5 pkg. | 180 | 5.0 | 29.0 | 5.0 | 0 | 360 | 1.0 |
| **Pizza crust mix**: | | | | | | | |
| (*Arrowhead Mills* | | | | | | | |
| Organic), 1/6 pkg. | 150 | 7.0 | 30.0 | .5 | 0 | 115 | 1.0 |
| (*Betty Crocker*), | | | | | | | |
| 1/4 crust | 160 | 4.0 | 33.0 | 2.0 | 0 | 340 | 1.0 |
| (*Hodgson Mill* Gluten | | | | | | | |
| Free), 1/6 pkg. | 192 | 3.0 | 45.0 | 1.0 | 0 | 228 | 1.7 |
| (*"Jiffy"*), 1/5 pkg. | 140 | 3.0 | 26.0 | 2.5 | 0 | 280 | <1.0 |
| (*Martha White*), 1/4 pkg. | 160 | 6.0 | 33.0 | 1.0 | 0 | 250 | 1.0 |
| (*Martha White* Deep | | | | | | | |
| Pan), 1/5 pkg. | 140 | 5.0 | 29.0 | 1.0 | 0 | 320 | 1.0 |
| ***Pizza Hut,*** 1/8 pie, | | | | | | | |
| except as noted: | | | | | | | |
| appetizers: | | | | | | | |
| breadsticks, 1 pc. | 150 | 5.0 | 19.0 | 7.0 | 0 | 250 | 1.0 |
| cheese | 180 | 7.0 | 20.0 | 7.0 | 15 | 370 | 1.0 |
| marinara sauce | 60 | 2.0 | 12.0 | 0 | 0 | 440 | 2.0 |
| wings, hot, 2 | 100 | 10.0 | 1.0 | 6.0 | 55 | 430 | 0 |
| wings, mild, 2 | 110 | 10.0 | 1.0 | 7.0 | 55 | 430 | 0 |
| wings sauce, ranch | 220 | 0 | 2.0 | 23.0 | 10 | 420 | 0 |
| blue cheese | 230 | 1.0 | 2.0 | 24.0 | 20 | 420 | 0 |
| *Fit 'n Delicious*, 12" | | | | | | | |
| chicken/onion/pepper | 180 | 11.0 | 23.0 | 4.5 | 20 | 510 | 1.0 |
| chicken/mushroom | 170 | 11.0 | 22.0 | 4.5 | 20 | 720 | 1.0 |
| ham/mushroom | 160 | 8.0 | 23.0 | 4.5 | 15 | 550 | 1.0 |
| ham/pineapple | 160 | 7.0 | 24.0 | 4.5 | 15 | 550 | 1.0 |
| pepper/onion | 150 | 6.0 | 24.0 | 4.0 | 10 | 400 | 2.0 |
| tomato/mushroom | 150 | 6.0 | 23.0 | 4.0 | 10 | 610 | 2.0 |
| hand-tossed, 12": | | | | | | | |
| cheese only | 220 | 10.0 | 26.0 | 8.0 | 25 | 560 | 1.0 |
| Dan's original | 260 | 12.0 | 26.0 | 12.0 | 30 | 670 | 2.0 |
| ham/pineapple | 200 | 9.0 | 27.0 | 7.0 | 20 | 560 | 1.0 |
| Hawaiian luau | 240 | 10.0 | 27.0 | 10.0 | 25 | 650 | 1.0 |
| *Meat Lover's* | 300 | 14.0 | 25.0 | 16.0 | 40 | 870 | 1.0 |
| pepperoni | 230 | 10.0 | 25.0 | 10.0 | 25 | 620 | 1.0 |
| pepperoni/mushroom | 210 | 10.0 | 26.0 | 8.0 | 20 | 550 | 2.0 |
| sausage/onion | 240 | 10.0 | 27.0 | 11.0 | 25 | 590 | 2.0 |
| spicy Sicilian | 250 | 10.0 | 26.0 | 11.0 | 25 | 740 | 2.0 |
| supreme | 260 | 11.0 | 26.0 | 12.0 | 30 | 690 | 2.0 |

| Food and Measure | cal. | prot. (gms) | carbo. (gms) | fat (gms) | chol. (mgs) | sod. (mgs) | fiber (gms) |
|---|---|---|---|---|---|---|---|
| **Pizza, French bread, hand-tossed** (cont.) | | | | | | | |
| triple meat ......... | 260 | 12.0 | 25.0 | 12.0 | 30 | 740 | 1.0 |
| *Veggie Lover's* ...... | 200 | 9.0 | 27.0 | 7.0 | 15 | 540 | 2.0 |
| hand-tossed, 14": | | | | | | | |
| cheese only ......... | 320 | 15.0 | 38.0 | 12.0 | 35 | 820 | 2.0 |
| Dan's original ....... | 380 | 17.0 | 38.0 | 18.0 | 40 | 960 | 2.0 |
| ham/pineapple ...... | 300 | 13.0 | 39.0 | 10.0 | 25 | 820 | 2.0 |
| Hawaiian luau ....... | 340 | 15.0 | 40.0 | 14.0 | 35 | 940 | 2.0 |
| *Meat Lover's* ........ | 440 | 20.0 | 38.0 | 23.0 | 60 | 1270 | 2.0 |
| pepperoni .......... | 340 | 15.0 | 37.0 | 14.0 | 35 | 920 | 2.0 |
| pepperoni/mushroom . | 310 | 14.0 | 38.0 | 12.0 | 30 | 810 | 2.0 |
| sausage/onion ...... | 350 | 15.0 | 39.0 | 15.0 | 35 | 850 | 2.0 |
| supreme ........... | 380 | 17.0 | 38.0 | 18.0 | 45 | 1000 | 2.0 |
| triple meat ......... | 380 | 17.0 | 38.0 | 18.0 | 45 | 1080 | 2.0 |
| spicy Sicilian ........ | 360 | 15.0 | 38.0 | 16.0 | 35 | 1050 | 2.0 |
| *Veggie Lover's* ...... | 290 | 12.0 | 39.0 | 10.0 | 20 | 770 | 3.0 |
| pan pizza, 12": | | | | | | | |
| cheese only ......... | 240 | 11.0 | 27.0 | 11.0 | 25 | 530 | 1.0 |
| Dan's original ....... | 280 | 12.0 | 27.0 | 14.0 | 30 | 630 | 1.0 |
| ham/pineapple ...... | 230 | 10.0 | 28.0 | 9.0 | 20 | 520 | 1.0 |
| Hawaiian luau ....... | 260 | 11.0 | 28.0 | 12.0 | 25 | 610 | 1.0 |
| *Meat Lover's* ........ | 330 | 14.0 | 27.0 | 18.0 | 40 | 830 | 1.0 |
| pepperoni .......... | 250 | 11.0 | 26.0 | 12.0 | 25 | 590 | 1.0 |
| pepperoni/mushroom . | 240 | 10.0 | 27.0 | 10.0 | 20 | 520 | 1.0 |
| sausage/onion ...... | 270 | 11.0 | 28.0 | 13.0 | 25 | 560 | 1.0 |
| spicy Sicilian ........ | 270 | 11.0 | 27.0 | 13.0 | 25 | 700 | 2.0 |
| supreme ........... | 290 | 12.0 | 27.0 | 14.0 | 30 | 650 | 2.0 |
| triple meat ......... | 290 | 13.0 | 27.0 | 15.0 | 30 | 700 | 2.0 |
| *Veggie Lover's* ...... | 230 | 9.0 | 28.0 | 9.0 | 15 | 500 | 2.0 |
| pan pizza, 14": | | | | | | | |
| cheese only ......... | 360 | 15.0 | 37.0 | 17.0 | 35 | 740 | 2.0 |
| Dan's original ....... | 420 | 17.0 | 37.0 | 22.0 | 40 | 880 | 2.0 |
| ham/pineapple ...... | 340 | 14.0 | 39.0 | 15.0 | 25 | 740 | 2.0 |
| Hawaiian luau ....... | 380 | 15.0 | 39.0 | 18.0 | 35 | 860 | 2.0 |
| *Meat Lover's* ........ | 480 | 20.0 | 37.0 | 28.0 | 60 | 1180 | 2.0 |
| pepperoni .......... | 380 | 15.0 | 36.0 | 19.0 | 35 | 840 | 2.0 |
| pepperoni/mushroom . | 350 | 14.0 | 37.0 | 17.0 | 30 | 730 | 2.0 |
| sausage/onion ...... | 390 | 15.0 | 38.0 | 20.0 | 35 | 770 | 2.0 |
| spicy Sicilian ........ | 400 | 16.0 | 38.0 | 21.0 | 35 | 960 | 2.0 |
| supreme ........... | 420 | 17.0 | 38.0 | 23.0 | 45 | 920 | 2.0 |
| triple meat ......... | 420 | 18.0 | 37.0 | 23.0 | 45 | 1000 | 2.0 |
| *Veggie Lover's* ...... | 330 | 13.0 | 38.0 | 15.0 | 20 | 690 | 2.0 |
| personal pan pizza, whole 6" pie: | | | | | | | |

| Food and Measure | cal. | prot. (gms) | carbo. (gms) | fat (gms) | chol. (mgs) | sod. (mgs) | fiber (gms) |
|---|---|---|---|---|---|---|---|
| cheese only | 590 | 26.0 | 69.0 | 24.0 | 55 | 1290 | 3.0 |
| Dan's original | 720 | 31.0 | 69.0 | 36.0 | 75 | 1600 | 4.0 |
| ham/pineapple | 550 | 23.0 | 71.0 | 20.0 | 45 | 1260 | 3.0 |
| Hawaiian luau | 620 | 26.0 | 71.0 | 25.0 | 55 | 1440 | 3.0 |
| *Meat Lover's* | 830 | 36.0 | 68.0 | 46.0 | 100 | 2110 | 3.0 |
| pepperoni | 610 | 26.0 | 67.0 | 26.0 | 55 | 1410 | 3.0 |
| pepperoni/mushroom | 570 | 24.0 | 68.0 | 23.0 | 45 | 1250 | 4.0 |
| sausage/onion | 690 | 28.0 | 71.0 | 32.0 | 65 | 1440 | 4.0 |
| spicy Sicilian | 680 | 29.0 | 69.0 | 32.0 | 70 | 1730 | 4.0 |
| supreme | 720 | 30.0 | 69.0 | 36.0 | 80 | 1680 | 4.0 |
| triple meat | 730 | 32.0 | 68.0 | 36.0 | 80 | 1770 | 3.0 |
| *Veggie Lover's* | 550 | 22.0 | 70.0 | 20.0 | 35 | 1190 | 4.0 |
| personal *PANormous*, whole 9" pie: | | | | | | | |
| cheese only | 1100 | 48.0 | 124.0 | 45.0 | 105 | 2400 | 6.0 |
| Dan's original | 1270 | 55.0 | 124.0 | 62.0 | 125 | 2810 | 7.0 |
| ham/pineapple | 1020 | 43.0 | 128.0 | 37.0 | 80 | 2300 | 6.0 |
| Hawaiian luau | 1150 | 49.0 | 129.0 | 49.0 | 105 | 2670 | 6.0 |
| *Meat Lover's* | 1470 | 64.0 | 123.0 | 80.0 | 175 | 3670 | 6.0 |
| pepperoni | 1100 | 47.0 | 121.0 | 48.0 | 100 | 2540 | 6.0 |
| pepperoni/mushroom | 1050 | 45.0 | 123.0 | 42.0 | 85 | 2290 | 7.0 |
| sausage/onion | 1210 | 50.0 | 128.0 | 56.0 | 110 | 2550 | 7.0 |
| spicy Sicilian | 1220 | 51.0 | 126.0 | 57.0 | 115 | 3150 | 7.0 |
| supreme | 1270 | 54.0 | 125.0 | 62.0 | 130 | 2920 | 7.0 |
| triple meat | 1280 | 56.0 | 123.0 | 62.0 | 135 | 3070 | 6.0 |
| *Veggie Lover's* | 1010 | 42.0 | 127.0 | 38.0 | 70 | 2240 | 8.0 |
| *Pizza Mia*, 12": | | | | | | | |
| cheese only | 200 | 9.0 | 24.0 | 7.0 | 15 | 490 | 1.0 |
| pepperoni | 200 | 8.0 | 24.0 | 8.0 | 15 | 510 | 1.0 |
| *P'Zone*, ½ order: | | | | | | | |
| classic | 630 | 28.0 | 77.0 | 23.0 | 65 | 1460 | 3.0 |
| meaty | 710 | 32.0 | 76.0 | 31.0 | 85 | 1800 | 2.0 |
| marinara sauce | 60 | 2.0 | 12.0 | 0 | 0 | 440 | 2.0 |
| pepperoni | 630 | 29.0 | 76.0 | 24.0 | 70 | 1570 | 2.0 |
| stuffed crust, 14": | | | | | | | |
| cheese only | 350 | 16.0 | 39.0 | 14.0 | 40 | 910 | 2.0 |
| Dan's original | 420 | 19.0 | 39.0 | 21.0 | 50 | 1090 | 2.0 |
| ham/pineapple | 340 | 15.0 | 41.0 | 13.0 | 35 | 950 | 2.0 |
| Hawaiian luau | 380 | 17.0 | 41.0 | 16.0 | 45 | 1070 | 2.0 |
| *Meat Lover's* | 480 | 22.0 | 39.0 | 26.0 | 70 | 1390 | 2.0 |
| pepperoni | 380 | 17.0 | 38.0 | 17.0 | 45 | 1050 | 2.0 |
| pepperoni/mushroom | 350 | 16.0 | 39.0 | 15.0 | 40 | 940 | 2.0 |
| sausage/onion | 390 | 17.0 | 40.0 | 18.0 | 45 | 980 | 2.0 |
| spicy Sicilian | 400 | 17.0 | 40.0 | 19.0 | 50 | 1170 | 2.0 |

| Food and Measure | cal. | prot. (gms) | carbo. (gms) | fat (gms) | chol. (mgs) | sod. (mgs) | fiber (gms) |
|---|---|---|---|---|---|---|---|
| **Pizza Hut**, stuffed crust *(cont.)* | | | | | | | |
| supreme .......... | 420 | 18.0 | 40.0 | 21.0 | 55 | 1140 | 2.0 |
| triple meat ........ | 420 | 19.0 | 39.0 | 21.0 | 55 | 1210 | 2.0 |
| *Veggie Lover's* ...... | 330 | 14.0 | 40.0 | 13.0 | 35 | 900 | 3.0 |
| stuffed rollers, 1 pc. .... | 230 | 9.0 | 24.0 | 10.0 | 25 | 590 | 1.0 |
| marinara sauce ...... | 60 | 2.0 | 12.0 | 0 | 0 | 440 | 2.0 |
| ranch sauce ........ | 220 | 0 | 2.0 | 23.0 | 10 | 420 | 0 |
| *Thin 'n Crispy*, 12": | | | | | | | |
| cheese only ........ | 190 | 9.0 | 22.0 | 8.0 | 25 | 550 | 1.0 |
| Dan's original ....... | 240 | 11.0 | 22.0 | 12.0 | 30 | 650 | 1.0 |
| ham/pineapple ...... | 180 | 8.0 | 23.0 | 6.0 | 20 | 540 | 1.0 |
| Hawaiian luau ....... | 220 | 10.0 | 24.0 | 10.0 | 25 | 650 | 1.0 |
| *Meat Lover's* ........ | 280 | 13.0 | 22.0 | 16.0 | 40 | 860 | 1.0 |
| pepperoni .......... | 200 | 9.0 | 21.0 | 9.0 | 25 | 610 | 1.0 |
| pepperoni/mushroom . | 190 | 9.0 | 22.0 | 8.0 | 20 | 540 | 1.0 |
| sausage/onion ...... | 220 | 9.0 | 23.0 | 10.0 | 25 | 580 | 1.0 |
| spicy Sicilian ....... | 220 | 9.0 | 22.0 | 10.0 | 25 | 750 | 1.0 |
| supreme .......... | 240 | 10.0 | 23.0 | 12.0 | 30 | 670 | 1.0 |
| triple meat ........ | 240 | 11.0 | 22.0 | 12.0 | 30 | 720 | 1.0 |
| *Veggie Lover's* ...... | 180 | 8.0 | 23.0 | 6.0 | 15 | 530 | 1.0 |
| *Thin 'n Crispy*, 14": | | | | | | | |
| cheese only ........ | 260 | 12.0 | 29.0 | 11.0 | 35 | 740 | 1.0 |
| Dan's original ....... | 320 | 15.0 | 29.0 | 16.0 | 40 | 890 | 1.0 |
| ham/pineapple ...... | 240 | 11.0 | 31.0 | 9.0 | 25 | 750 | 1.0 |
| Hawaiian luau ....... | 300 | 13.0 | 31.0 | 14.0 | 35 | 900 | 1.0 |
| *Meat Lover's* ........ | 390 | 18.0 | 28.0 | 23.0 | 60 | 1210 | 1.0 |
| pepperoni .......... | 280 | 13.0 | 28.0 | 13.0 | 35 | 850 | 1.0 |
| pepperoni/mushroom . | 260 | 12.0 | 29.0 | 11.0 | 30 | 740 | 1.0 |
| sausage/onion ...... | 300 | 13.0 | 30.0 | 14.0 | 35 | 780 | 1.0 |
| spicy Sicilian ........ | 300 | 13.0 | 30.0 | 15.0 | 35 | 1020 | 2.0 |
| supreme .......... | 330 | 15.0 | 30.0 | 17.0 | 45 | 930 | 2.0 |
| triple meat ........ | 320 | 15.0 | 28.0 | 17.0 | 45 | 1000 | 1.0 |
| *Veggie Lover's* ...... | 240 | 10.0 | 30.0 | 9.0 | 20 | 710 | 2.0 |
| Tuscani pastas, ½ pan: | | | | | | | |
| bacon mac/cheese ... | 520 | 24.0 | 54.0 | 22.0 | 60 | 1170 | 4.0 |
| chicken Alfredo ....... | 630 | 27.0 | 56.0 | 33.0 | 70 | 1180 | 4.0 |
| lasagna ............ | 600 | 31.0 | 43.0 | 33.0 | 100 | 1600 | 5.0 |
| meaty marinara ...... | 520 | 26.0 | 50.0 | 24.0 | 80 | 1310 | 6.0 |
| wings, bone-out, 2: | | | | | | | |
| all American ........ | 150 | 10.0 | 11.0 | 8.0 | 20 | 490 | 1.0 |
| Buffalo, hot ......... | 190 | 10.0 | 19.0 | 8.0 | 20 | 1000 | 1.0 |
| medium ......... | 190 | 10.0 | 18.0 | 9.0 | 20 | 990 | 1.0 |
| mild ............ | 190 | 10.0 | 18.0 | 9.0 | 20 | 1020 | 1.0 |
| Cajun ............ | 200 | 10.0 | 21.0 | 8.0 | 20 | 790 | 1.0 |

| Food and Measure | cal. | prot. (gms) | carbo. (gms) | fat (gms) | chol. (mgs) | sod. (mgs) | fiber (gms) |
|---|---|---|---|---|---|---|---|
| garlic Parmesan | 260 | 11.0 | 11.0 | 19.0 | 20 | 710 | 1.0 |
| honey BBQ | 220 | 10.0 | 27.0 | 8.0 | 20 | 720 | 1.0 |
| spicy BBQ | 200 | 10.0 | 21.0 | 8.0 | 25 | 940 | 1.0 |
| spicy Asian | 210 | 10.0 | 24.0 | 8.0 | 20 | 690 | 1.0 |
| wings, crispy, 2: | | | | | | | |
| all American | 200 | 9.0 | 8.0 | 14.0 | 45 | 500 | 1.0 |
| Buffalo, hot | 230 | 9.0 | 16.0 | 15.0 | 45 | 1020 | 1.0 |
| medium | 230 | 9.0 | 16.0 | 15.0 | 45 | 1010 | 1.0 |
| mild | 230 | 9.0 | 16.0 | 15.0 | 45 | 1040 | 1.0 |
| Cajun | 240 | 10.0 | 19.0 | 14.0 | 45 | 810 | 2.0 |
| garlic Parmesan | 300 | 10.0 | 9.0 | 25.0 | 45 | 730 | 1.0 |
| honey BBQ | 260 | 10.0 | 24.0 | 14.0 | 45 | 740 | 1.0 |
| spicy BBQ | 240 | 9.0 | 19.0 | 14.0 | 50 | 950 | 1.0 |
| spicy Asian | 250 | 10.0 | 21.0 | 14.0 | 45 | 710 | 1.0 |
| wings, traditional, 2: | | | | | | | |
| all American | 80 | 7.0 | 0 | 5.0 | 40 | 290 | 0 |
| Buffalo, hot | 110 | 8.0 | 8.0 | 6.0 | 40 | 810 | 1.0 |
| medium | 110 | 8.0 | 8.0 | 6.0 | 40 | 800 | 1.0 |
| mild | 110 | 8.0 | 8.0 | 6.0 | 40 | 830 | 1.0 |
| Cajun | 120 | 8.0 | 11.0 | 5.0 | 40 | 600 | 1.0 |
| garlic Parmesan | 180 | 8.0 | 1.0 | 16.0 | 45 | 520 | 0 |
| honey BBQ | 140 | 8.0 | 16.0 | 5.0 | 40 | 530 | 0 |
| spicy Asian | 130 | 8.0 | 13.0 | 5.0 | 40 | 500 | 0 |
| spicy BBQ | 120 | 8.0 | 11.0 | 5.0 | 45 | 750 | 0 |
| dessert/sides: | | | | | | | |
| apple pies, 2 | 330 | 2.0 | 40.0 | 17.0 | 0 | 190 | 2.0 |
| cheese sticks, 4 | 380 | 13.0 | 29.0 | 24.0 | 40 | 1020 | 2.0 |
| wedge fries, ½ order | 320 | 4.0 | 35.0 | 18.0 | 0 | 530 | 3.0 |
| **Pizza mix** (*Chef Boyardee* Pizza Maker): | | | | | | | |
| cheese, ¼ pkg. | 260 | 10.0 | 45.0 | 4.5 | 10 | 760 | 2.0 |
| cheese, two, ⅛ pkg. | 250 | 9.0 | 45.0 | 4.0 | 5 | 730 | 2.0 |
| pepperoni, ¼ pkg. | 290 | 11.0 | 44.0 | 8.0 | 15 | 740 | 2.0 |
| pepperoni, two, ⅛ pkg. | 280 | 11.0 | 44.0 | 7.0 | 15 | 710 | 2.0 |
| **Pizza pocket**, see "Pizza, stuffed/pocket" | | | | | | | |
| **Pizza rolls**, see "Pizza snacks" | | | | | | | |
| **Pizza sauce**, ¼ cup: | | | | | | | |
| (*Contadina* Original/ Squeeze) | 30 | 1.0 | 6.0 | .5 | 0 | 340 | 1.0 |
| (*Muir Glen* Organic) | 40 | 1.0 | 6.0 | 1.0 | 0 | 230 | 2.0 |
| cheese, 4 (*Contadina*) | 30 | 1.0 | 6.0 | .5 | 0 | 390 | 1.0 |

| Food and Measure | cal. | prot. (gms) | carbo. (gms) | fat (gms) | chol. (mgs) | sod. (mgs) | fiber (gms) |
|---|---|---|---|---|---|---|---|
| **Pizza sauce** *(cont.)* | | | | | | | |
| pepperoni flavor | | | | | | | |
| (*Contadina*) . . . . . . . . | 35 | 1.0 | 5.0 | 1.0 | 0 | 390 | 1.0 |
| **Pizza snacks** (see also "Pizza, stuffed/ pocket"), frozen: | | | | | | | |
| (*Cedarlane* Mini Bistro), 3 pcs., 4 oz. . . . | 280 | 10.0 | 27.0 | 15.0 | 25 | 660 | 2.0 |
| bites, in pastry (*Health is Wealth Munchees*), 6 pcs., 3 oz. . . . . . . . . | 180 | 6.0 | 29.0 | 5.0 | 0 | 480 | 2.0 |
| cheese: | | | | | | | |
| (*Amy's*), 5–6 pcs., 3 oz. . . . . . . . . . . . | 210 | 9.0 | 25.0 | 9.0 | 20 | 440 | 2.0 |
| minis (*Smart Ones*), 4 pcs. . . . . . . . . . . . | 270 | 13.0 | 38.0 | 7.0 | 10 | 480 | 5.0 |
| meat, 4, rolls (*Michelina's*), 4.5-oz. pkg. . . . . . . . . | 350 | 13.0 | 35.0 | 17.0 | 25 | 630 | 2.0 |
| pepperoni/cheese: | | | | | | | |
| (*Michelina's Budget Gourmet*), 5-oz. pkg. . . . . . . . . | 380 | 12.0 | 39.0 | 19.0 | 20 | 770 | 3.0 |
| (*Michelina's Lean Gourmet* Snackers), 11 pcs., 3 oz. . . . . . | 200 | 8.0 | 24.0 | 8.0 | 10 | 290 | 2.0 |
| baked (*Michelina's Lean Gourmet* Snackers), 4 pcs., 3.1 oz. . . . . | 240 | 10.0 | 33.0 | 8.0 | 15 | 510 | 2.0 |
| rolls (*Michelina's*), 5.5-oz. pkg. . . . . . . | 420 | 13.0 | 42.0 | 21.0 | 25 | 850 | 2.0 |
| rolls, 6 pcs., 3 oz.: | | | | | | | |
| cheese (*Totino's*) . . . . | 180 | 7.0 | 26.0 | 5.0 | <5 | 460 | 1.0 |
| cheesy taco (*Totino's*) . | 200 | 7.0 | 24.0 | 8.0 | 15 | 470 | 1.0 |
| combo (*Michelina's*) . . | 220 | 7.0 | 24.0 | 10.0 | 10 | 420 | 1.0 |
| combo (*Totino's*) . . . . | 210 | 7.0 | 24.0 | 9.0 | 5 | 470 | 1.0 |
| meat, 3 (*Totino's*) . . . . | 200 | 8.0 | 24.0 | 8.0 | 10 | 450 | 1.0 |
| pepperoni (*Michelina's*) . . . . . | 230 | 8.0 | 24.0 | 11.0 | 10 | 460 | 1.0 |
| pepperoni (*Totino's*) . . | 210 | 7.0 | 24.0 | 10.0 | 10 | 480 | 1.0 |
| pepperoni, triple (*Totino's*) . . . . . . . . | 220 | 8.0 | 24.0 | 11.0 | 10 | 530 | 1.0 |
| sausage (*Totino's*) . . . | 200 | 7.0 | 24.0 | 9.0 | 5 | 430 | 1.0 |
| supreme (*Totino's*) . . . | 200 | 7.0 | 25.0 | 8.0 | 5 | 390 | 1.0 |

| Food and Measure | cal. | prot. (gms) | carbo. (gms) | fat (gms) | chol. (mgs) | sod. (mgs) | fiber (gms) |
|---|---|---|---|---|---|---|---|
| spinach (*Amy's*), 5–6 pcs., 3 oz. | 190 | 8.0 | 24.0 | 7.0 | 20 | 380 | 2.0 |
| vegetable (*Smart Ones*), 4 pcs. | 270 | 11.0 | 41.0 | 7.0 | 10 | 470 | 6.0 |
| **Plantain**, fresh: | | | | | | | |
| raw: | | | | | | | |
| (*Frieda's*), 6.3 oz. | 218 | 2.0 | 57.0 | 1.0 | 0 | 7 | 4.0 |
| 1 medium, 6.3 oz. | 218 | 2.3 | 57.1 | .6 | 0 | 7 | 4.1 |
| sliced, ½ cup | 91 | 1.0 | 23.6 | .3 | 0 | 3 | 1.7 |
| cooked: | | | | | | | |
| (*Dole*), ½ medium | 100 | <1.0 | 28.0 | 0 | 0 | 0 | 2.0 |
| sliced, ½ cup | 89 | .6 | 24.0 | .1 | 0 | 4 | 1.8 |
| **Plantain chips** (*El Isleño*), 1 oz. | 150 | <1.0 | 17.0 | 9.0 | 0 | 35 | 2.0 |
| **Plum**, fresh: | | | | | | | |
| (*Chiquita*), 2.3-oz. pc. | 30 | 0 | 8.0 | 0 | 0 | 0 | 1.0 |
| (*Dole*), 2 medium, 5.3 oz. | 70 | 1.0 | 17.0 | 0 | 0 | 0 | 2.0 |
| Japanese or hybrid, 2⅛" fruit | 36 | .5 | 8.6 | .4 | 0 | tr. | <1.0 |
| sliced, ½ cup | 46 | .7 | 10.7 | .5 | 0 | 1 | 1.2 |
| **Plum, can/jar**, purple: | | | | | | | |
| in juice: | | | | | | | |
| ½ cup | 73 | .7 | 19.1 | <.1 | 0 | 2 | 1.3 |
| 3 plums and 2 tbsp. liquid | 55 | .5 | 14.4 | <.1 | 0 | 1 | 1.0 |
| in light syrup: | | | | | | | |
| ½ cup | 79 | .5 | 20.5 | .1 | 0 | 25 | 1.3 |
| 3 plums and 2¾ tbsp. liquid | 83 | .5 | 21.7 | .1 | 0 | 26 | 1.3 |
| in heavy syrup, ½ cup | 115 | .5 | 30.0 | .1 | 0 | 25 | 1.3 |
| **Plum, dried** (prune): | | | | | | | |
| (*Earthbound Farm Organic*), 5 pcs., 1.5 oz. | 110 | 1.0 | 25.0 | 0 | 0 | 0 | 3.0 |
| (*Mariani* Plum Support), ¼ cup, 1.4 oz. | 110 | 1.0 | 25.0 | 0 | 0 | 5 | 3.0 |
| (*Sunsweet*), 1.4 oz. | 100 | 1.0 | 24.0 | 0 | 0 | 5 | 3.0 |
| pitted, 1.4 oz.: | | | | | | | |
| (*Mariani*), ¼ cup | 110 | 1.0 | 25.0 | 0 | 0 | 0 | 3.0 |
| (*Mariani* Bite Size), ¼ cup | 110 | 1.0 | 27.0 | 0 | 0 | 5 | 3.0 |
| (*Mariani* Plus), ¼ cup | 110 | 1.0 | 25.0 | 0 | 0 | 5 | 3.0 |
| (*Sun•Maid*), ¼ cup | 100 | 1.0 | 26.0 | 0 | 0 | 0 | 3.0 |

| Food and Measure | cal. | prot. (gms) | carbo. (gms) | fat (gms) | chol. (mgs) | sod. (mgs) | fiber (gms) |
|---|---|---|---|---|---|---|---|
| **Plum, dried, pitted** *(cont.)* | | | | | | | |
| bite size (*Sunsweet*), | | | | | | | |
| 7 pcs. . . . . . . . . . . | 100 | 1.0 | 24.0 | 0 | 0 | 5 | 3.0 |
| cherry, lemon, or | | | | | | | |
| orange essence | | | | | | | |
| (*Sunsweet*), 5 pcs. . | 100 | 1.0 | 24.0 | 0 | 0 | 5 | 3.0 |
| cooked, w/pits: | | | | | | | |
| (*Sunsweet* Ready to | | | | | | | |
| Serve), ⅔ cup . . . . | 150 | 2.0 | 37.0 | 0 | 0 | 15 | 3.0 |
| unsweetened, ½ cup . | 113 | 1.2 | 29.8 | .2 | 0 | 2 | 7.0 |
| puree, 1 oz. . . . . . . . . | 73 | .6 | 18.5 | .1 | 0 | 7 | .9 |
| **Plum, dried, canned**, | | | | | | | |
| in heavy syrup: | | | | | | | |
| pitted, 4 oz. . . . . . . . . | 119 | 1.0 | 31.5 | .2 | 0 | 3 | 4.3 |
| ½ cup . . . . . . . . . . . . . | 123 | 1.0 | 32.5 | .2 | 0 | 3 | 4.4 |
| 5 pcs., 2 tbsp. liquid . . . | 90 | .8 | 23.9 | .2 | 0 | 2 | 3.3 |
| **Plum, pickled**, see | | | | | | | |
| "Umeboshi plum" | | | | | | | |
| **Plum drink**, 8 fl. oz.: | | | | | | | |
| (*Sunsweet PlumSmart* | | | | | | | |
| Light) . . . . . . . . . . . . | 60 | 0 | 15.0 | 0 | 0 | 20 | 3.0 |
| red (*Nantucket Nectars*) . | 120 | 0 | 30.0 | 0 | 0 | 25 | 0 |
| **Plum juice** (see also | | | | | | | |
| "Prune juice") | | | | | | | |
| (*Sunsweet* | | | | | | | |
| *PlumSmart*), 8 fl. oz. . | 160 | 0 | 36.0 | 0 | 0 | 55 | 3.0 |
| **Plum pudding** | | | | | | | |
| (*Crosse & Blackwell*), | | | | | | | |
| ⅓ of 14-oz. pkg. . . . . . | 460 | 6.0 | 87.0 | 10.0 | 0 | 240 | 5.0 |
| **Plum sauce**: | | | | | | | |
| (*Ka•Me*), 2 tbsp. . . . . . . . | 60 | 0 | 15.0 | 0 | 0 | 330 | 0 |
| (*Kikkoman*), 2 tbsp. . . . . | 80 | 0 | 18.0 | .5 | 0 | 280 | 0 |
| (*Roland*), 1 tbsp. . . . . . . . | 45 | 0 | 11.0 | 0 | 0 | 420 | 0 |
| **Poi**, ½ cup . . . . . . . . . . . | 134 | .5 | 32.7 | .2 | 0 | 14 | .5 |
| **Pokeberry shoots**: | | | | | | | |
| raw, ½ cup . . . . . . . . . . | 18 | 2.1 | 3.0 | .3 | 0 | 18 | 1.4 |
| boiled, drained, ½ cup . . | 16 | 1.9 | 2.5 | .3 | 0 | 15 | 1.2 |
| **Polenta** (see also "Corn- | | | | | | | |
| meal") (*Roland*), 2 tbsp. | 80 | 2.0 | 18.0 | 0 | 0 | 0 | 2.0 |
| **Polenta, prepared**, | | | | | | | |
| 2 slices, ½": | | | | | | | |
| (*Frieda's* Organic | | | | | | | |
| Traditional) . . . . . . . . . | 70 | 2.0 | 15.0 | 0 | 0 | 310 | 1.0 |

| Food and Measure | cal. | prot. (gms) | carbo. (gms) | fat (gms) | chol. (mgs) | sod. (mgs) | fiber (gms) |
|---|---|---|---|---|---|---|---|
| (*San Gennaro* Traditional) ......... | 70 | 2.0 | 15.0 | 0 | 0 | 310 | 1.0 |
| basil garlic (*San Gennaro*) .......... | 74 | 2.0 | 15.0 | 0 | 0 | 310 | 1.0 |
| sun-dried tomato garlic (*San Gennaro*) ...... | 74 | 2.0 | 16.0 | 0 | 0 | 310 | 1.0 |
| **Polenta, prepared, frozen,** 3 cheese (*San Gennaro*), 4-oz. pc. ... | 110 | 4.0 | 17.0 | 2.5 | 5 | 410 | 0 |
| **Polish sausage** (see also "Kielbasa"): | | | | | | | |
| beef (*Hebrew National*), 3-oz. link ............ | 250 | 10.0 | 1.0 | 23.0 | 40 | 870 | 0 |
| smoked (*Hillshire Farm Lit'l Polska*), 5 links .. | 160 | 7.0 | 2.0 | 14.0 | 40 | 550 | 0 |
| **Pollock**, meat only: | | | | | | | |
| Atlantic, 4 oz.: | | | | | | | |
| raw ............... | 104 | 22.1 | 0 | 1.1 | 80 | 98 | 0 |
| baked or broiled ..... | 134 | 28.3 | 0 | 1.4 | 103 | 125 | 0 |
| walleye, 4 oz.: | | | | | | | |
| raw ............... | 91 | 19.5 | 0 | .9 | 81 | 112 | 0 |
| baked or broiled ..... | 128 | 26.7 | 0 | 1.3 | 109 | 132 | 0 |
| **Pollock entree**, frozen, stuffed (*Oven Poppers Qwickies*), 3-oz. pc. .. | 100 | 10.0 | 11.0 | 2.0 | 20 | 150 | 0 |
| **Pomegranate**: | | | | | | | |
| whole, 9.7-oz. fruit ..... | 104 | 1.5 | 26.4 | .5 | 0 | 5 | .9 |
| seeds (*Frieda's* Arils), ½ cup ............. | 70 | 2.0 | 16.0 | 1.0 | 0 | 3 | 4.0 |
| **Pomegranate drink** (*Langers* Cocktail), 8 fl. oz. ............ | 140 | 0 | 34.0 | 0 | 0 | 15 | 0 |
| **Pomegranate drink blend**, 8 fl. oz.: | | | | | | | |
| apple, sparkling (*Kristian Regale*) ..... | 95 | 0 | 24.0 | 0 | 0 | 10 | 0 |
| blueberry: | | | | | | | |
| (*Apple & Eve*) ....... | 120 | 0 | 30.0 | 0 | 0 | 15 | 0 |
| (*Honest Ade* Organic) . | 48 | 0 | 12.0 | 0 | 0 | 5 | 0 |
| (*Langers*) .......... | 140 | 0 | 34.0 | 0 | 0 | 15 | 0 |
| (*Tropicana Trop50*) ... | 50 | 0 | 14.0 | 0 | 0 | 10 | 0 |
| (*V8 V-Fusion* Light) .. | 50 | 0 | 13.0 | 0 | 0 | 90 | 0 |
| acai (*Northland*) ..... | 100 | 0 | 26.0 | 0 | 0 | 10 | 0 |

| Food and Measure | cal. | prot. (gms) | carbo. (gms) | fat (gms) | chol. (mgs) | sod. (mgs) | fiber (gms) |
|---|---|---|---|---|---|---|---|
| **Pomegranate drink blend** *(cont.)* | | | | | | | |
| cherry: | | | | | | | |
| (*Apple & Eve Organics*) | 120 | 0 | 29.0 | 0 | 0 | 5 | 0 |
| (*SoBe Lifewater*) ..... | 40 | 0 | 17.0 | 0 | 0 | 25 | 0 |
| cranberry (*Langers*) .... | 140 | 0 | 34.0 | 0 | 0 | 15 | 0 |
| lemonade (*Minute Maid* Enhanced) ..... | 110 | 0 | 31.0 | 0 | 0 | 20 | 0 |
| limeade (*Odwalla PomaGrand*) ........ | 120 | 0 | 30.0 | 0 | 0 | 10 | 0 |
| pear (*Nantucket Nectars*) ........... | 110 | 0 | 28.0 | 0 | 0 | 25 | 0 |
| raspberry (*Snapple*) .... | 110 | 0 | 27.0 | 0 | 0 | 5 | 0 |
| strawberry (*Odwalla*) ... | 50 | 0 | 14.0 | 0 | 0 | 10 | 0 |
| **Pomegranate juice**, 8 fl. oz.: | | | | | | | |
| (*Apple & Eve Organics*) .. | 130 | 0 | 33.0 | 0 | 0 | 25 | 0 |
| (*Bolthouse Farms*) ..... | 150 | 0 | 38.0 | 0 | 0 | 20 | 0 |
| (*Langers* All Pomegranate) ....... | 140 | 0 | 34.0 | 0 | 0 | 15 | 0 |
| (*Northland* Pure) ....... | 140 | 0 | 34.0 | 0 | 0 | 25 | 0 |
| (*Pom* 100%) .......... | 160 | 0 | 40.0 | 0 | 0 | 10 | 0 |
| (*R.W. Knudsen* Organic/ Organic Nectar) ..... | 120 | 0 | 30.0 | 0 | 0 | 15 | 0 |
| (*R.W. Knudsen Just Pomegranate*) ....... | 150 | <1.0 | 38.0 | 0 | 0 | 20 | 0 |
| (*Simply Nutritious Vita Pomegranate*) ... | 130 | 0 | 33.0 | 0 | 0 | 10 | 0 |
| sparkling (*Langers*) ..... | 150 | 0 | 37.0 | 0 | 0 | 15 | 0 |
| **Pomegranate juice blend**, 8 fl. oz.: | | | | | | | |
| (*Odwalla PomaGrand*) ... | 160 | 0 | 40.0 | 0 | 0 | 30 | 0 |
| berry (*Odwalla PomaGrand*) ........ | 140 | 0 | 35.0 | 0 | 0 | 20 | 0 |
| black currant (*Santa Cruz Organic*) ....... | 110 | 0 | 29.0 | 0 | 0 | 15 | 0 |
| blueberry: | | | | | | | |
| (*Minute Maid*) ....... | 120 | 0 | 31.0 | .5 | 0 | 20 | 0 |
| (*Northland*) ......... | 120 | 0 | 28.0 | 0 | 0 | 25 | 0 |
| (*Pom*) ............. | 160 | 0 | 39.0 | 0 | 0 | 20 | 0 |
| (*V8 V-Fusion*) ....... | 100 | 0 | 25.0 | 0 | 0 | 60 | 0 |
| cherry: | | | | | | | |
| (*Nantucket Nectars*) .. | 120 | 0 | 29.0 | 0 | 0 | 30 | 0 |
| (*Pom*) ............. | 150 | <1.0 | 38.0 | 0 | 0 | 20 | 0 |

| Food and Measure | cal. | prot. (gms) | carbo. (gms) | fat (gms) | chol. (mgs) | sod. (mgs) | fiber (gms) |
|---|---|---|---|---|---|---|---|
| (*Tropicana Pure*) ..... | 130 | 1.0 | 32.0 | 0 | 0 | 10 | 0 |
| cranberry (*Apple & Eve*) ........... | 140 | 0 | 34.0 | 0 | 0 | 25 | 0 |
| kiwi (*Pom*) ........... | 150 | 0 | 36.0 | 0 | 0 | 15 | 0 |
| mango (*Pom*) ......... | 140 | 0 | 36.0 | 0 | 0 | 10 | 0 |
| nectarine (*Pom*) ....... | 130 | 0 | 31.0 | 0 | 0 | 25 | 0 |
| **Pomegranate juice concentrate** (*R.W. Knudsen*), 8 fl. oz.* .. | 150 | 1.0 | 37.0 | 0 | 0 | 10 | 0 |
| **Pomegranate syrup**, see "Grenadine" | | | | | | | |
| **Pompano**, Florida, meat only: | | | | | | | |
| raw, 4 oz. ............ | 186 | 21.0 | 0 | 10.7 | 57 | 74 | 0 |
| baked or broiled, 4 oz. .. | 239 | 26.4 | 0 | 13.8 | 73 | 86 | 0 |
| **Ponzu sauce**, 1 tbsp.: | | | | | | | |
| (*Eden*) ............... | 5 | 0 | 1.0 | 0 | 0 | 340 | 0 |
| (*Kikkoman*) ........... | 10 | <1.0 | 2.0 | 0 | 0 | 400 | 0 |
| citrus (*Mitsukan*) ....... | 10 | 0 | 1.0 | 0 | 0 | 580 | 0 |
| lime (*Kikkoman*) ....... | 10 | 0 | 2.0 | 0 | 0 | 360 | 0 |
| **Popcorn**, unpopped, 2 tbsp., except as noted: | | | | | | | |
| (*Act II* HomePop Classic) ............. | 150 | 2.0 | 16.0 | 10.0 | 0 | 210 | 3.0 |
| (*Act II* Kettle Corn) ..... | 160 | 3.0 | 18.0 | 10.0 | 0 | 150 | 3.0 |
| (*Arrowhead Mills* Organic), ¼ cup ..... | 170 | 5.0 | 7.0 | 2.0 | 0 | 0 | 7.0 |
| (*Jolly Time Crispy 'n White*) ........... | 150 | 3.0 | 16.0 | 10.0 | 0 | 410 | 6.0 |
| (*Jolly Time Crispy 'n White Light*) ...... | 120 | 3.0 | 20.0 | 5.0 | 0 | 320 | 7.0 |
| (*Jolly Time Healthy Pop* Crispy White) ... | 100 | 4.0 | 23.0 | 2.0 | 0 | 260 | 8.0 |
| (*Jolly Time Healthy Pop* Kettle Corn) ..... | 90 | 3.0 | 23.0 | 2.0 | 0 | 280 | 8.0 |
| (*Jolly Time Healthy Pop* 94% Fat Free) ... | 90 | 3.0 | 23.0 | 2.0 | 0 | 280 | 8.0 |
| (*Jolly Time KettleMania*) ........ | 150 | 2.0 | 15.0 | 11.0 | 0 | 230 | 3.0 |
| (*Newman's Own* Natural), 1.1 oz. ..... | 130 | 2.0 | 18.0 | 5.0 | 0 | 200 | 3.0 |
| (*Newman's Own* 94% Fat Free), 1.1 oz. ...... | 110 | 3.0 | 20.0 | 1.5 | 0 | 250 | 4.0 |

| Food and Measure | cal. | prot. (gms) | carbo. (gms) | fat (gms) | chol. (mgs) | sod. (mgs) | fiber (gms) |
|---|---|---|---|---|---|---|---|
| **Popcorn** *(cont.)* | | | | | | | |
| (*Orville Redenbacher's* Natural Simply Salted) ............ | 170 | 2.0 | 17.0 | 11.0 | 0 | 400 | 3.0 |
| (*Orville Redenbacher's* Natural Simply Salted Less Fat) ..... | 120 | 3.0 | 19.0 | 5.0 | 0 | 300 | 4.0 |
| (*Orville Redenbacher's* SmartPop! Kettle Korn) ............. | 140 | 4.0 | 29.0 | 2.5 | 0 | 230 | 6.0 |
| (*Smart Balance Movie Style*) ............. | 170 | 3.0 | 16.0 | 11.0 | 0 | 420 | 3.0 |
| (*Smart Balance Smart 'n Healthy*), 3 tbsp. ... | 120 | 4.0 | 24.0 | 2.0 | 0 | 85 | 5.0 |
| butter flavor: | | | | | | | |
| (*Act II*) ............ | 160 | 3.0 | 18.0 | 9.0 | 0 | 310 | 3.0 |
| (*Act II*), 1 mini bag ... | 190 | 4.0 | 25.0 | 11.0 | 0 | 440 | 5.0 |
| (*Act II 94% Fat Free*), 3 tbsp. ...... | 130 | 4.0 | 28.0 | 2.5 | 0 | 220 | 5.0 |
| (*Act II* Butter Lover's) . | 160 | 2.0 | 19.0 | 9.0 | 0 | 400 | 3.0 |
| (*Act II* Light), mini bag | 130 | 3.0 | 23.0 | 5.0 | 0 | 490 | 4.0 |
| (*Act II* Movie Theater) . | 150 | 3.0 | 18.0 | 9.0 | 0 | 300 | 3.0 |
| (*Act II* Xtreme) ...... | 180 | 3.0 | 18.0 | 12.0 | <5 | 330 | 3.0 |
| (*Jiffy Pop*) ......... | 140 | 3.0 | 19.0 | 7.0 | 0 | 220 | 3.0 |
| (*Jolly Time* Homemade) | 150 | 3.0 | 22.0 | 5.0 | 0 | 230 | 5.0 |
| (*Jolly Time Better Butter*) .......... | 160 | 3.0 | 18.0 | 10.0 | 0 | 350 | 5.0 |
| (*Jolly Time Blast O Butter*) ........ | 150 | 3.0 | 19.0 | 12.0 | 0 | 340 | 9.0 |
| (*Jolly Time Blast O Butter* Light) ...... | 130 | 3.0 | 21.0 | 6.0 | 0 | 340 | 6.0 |
| (*Jolly Time Butter• Licious*) ......... | 150 | 2.0 | 16.0 | 10.0 | 0 | 390 | 5.0 |
| (*Jolly Time Butter• Licious* Light) ..... | 130 | 3.0 | 22.0 | 5.0 | 0 | 230 | 4.0 |
| (*Jolly Time Healthy Pop* 94% Fat Free) . | 90 | 3.0 | 23.0 | 2.0 | 0 | 210 | 9.0 |
| (*Jolly Time White & Buttery*) ....... | 150 | 3.0 | 17.0 | 10.0 | 0 | 300 | 4.0 |
| (*Newman's Own*), 1.1 oz. | 130 | 2.0 | 18.0 | 5.0 | 0 | 180 | 3.0 |
| (*Newman's Own* Butter Boom), 1.1 oz. | 130 | 2.0 | 18.0 | 5.0 | 0 | 290 | 3.0 |
| (*Newman's Own* Light), 1.1 oz. ...... | 120 | 3.0 | 19.0 | 4.0 | 0 | 170 | 4.0 |

| Food and Measure | cal. | prot. (gms) | carbo. (gms) | fat (gms) | chol. (mgs) | sod. (mgs) | fiber (gms) |
|---|---|---|---|---|---|---|---|
| (*Orville Redenbacher's*) | 170 | 2.0 | 17.0 | 12.0 | 0 | 260 | 3.0 |
| (*Orville Redenbacher's*), mini bag ......... | 210 | 3.0 | 21.0 | 14.0 | 0 | 320 | 4.0 |
| (*Orville Redenbacher's Kettle Korn*) ...... | 170 | 2.0 | 16.0 | 13.0 | <5 | 130 | 3.0 |
| (*Orville Redenbacher's Light*) ............ | 120 | 3.0 | 19.0 | 5.0 | 0 | 190 | 4.0 |
| (*Orville Redenbacher's Movie Theater*) .... | 170 | 2.0 | 16.0 | 12.0 | 0 | 250 | 3.0 |
| (*Orville Redenbacher's Movie Theater*), mini bag ......... | 210 | 3.0 | 20.0 | 15.0 | 0 | 300 | 4.0 |
| (*Orville Redenbacher's Movie Theater Pour Over*) ....... | 180 | 2.0 | 14.0 | 14.0 | 0 | 320 | 3.0 |
| (*Orville Redenbacher's Natural*) ......... | 170 | 2.0 | 17.0 | 12.0 | 0 | 290 | 3.0 |
| (*Orville Redenbacher's Natural Less Fat*) .. | 120 | 3.0 | 19.0 | 6.0 | 0 | 250 | 4.0 |
| (*Popweaver*) ........ | 130 | 2.0 | 17.0 | 6.0 | 0 | 240 | 3.0 |
| (*Popweaver* Extra) ... | 140 | 2.0 | 17.0 | 7.0 | 0 | 300 | 3.0 |
| (*Popweaver* Light) ... | 110 | 2.0 | 17.0 | 3.5 | 0 | 190 | 3.0 |
| (*Smart Balance* Light) . | 120 | 3.0 | 18.0 | 4.5 | 0 | 290 | 4.0 |
| buttery garlic (*Orville Redenbacher's*) ...... | 230 | 3.0 | 20.0 | 17.0 | 0 | 450 | 4.0 |
| caramel: | | | | | | | |
| (*Orville Redenbacher's*) | 170 | 1.0 | 24.0 | 8.0 | 0 | 350 | 1.0 |
| apple (*Jolly Time Healthy Pop*) ..... | 100 | 4.0 | 23.0 | 2.0 | 0 | 260 | 7.0 |
| cheddar: | | | | | | | |
| (*Orville Redenbacher's*) | 180 | 2.0 | 15.0 | 14.0 | 0 | 340 | 3.0 |
| (*Orville Redenbacher's Pour Over*) ....... | 160 | 2.0 | 12.0 | 13.0 | 0 | 280 | 2.0 |
| cheese (*Jolly Time The Big Cheez*) ......... | 160 | 2.0 | 17.0 | 11.0 | 0 | 340 | 6.0 |
| kernels, popping: | | | | | | | |
| yellow (*Eden* Organic) | 80 | 2.0 | 20.0 | 1.0 | 0 | 0 | 5.0 |
| yellow/white (*Orville Redenbacher's*), 6 cups* ......... | 120 | 4.0 | 29.0 | 1.5 | 0 | 0 | 6.0 |
| yellow/white (*Jolly Time*) ............ | 100 | 4.0 | 24.0 | 1.0 | 0 | 0 | 6.0 |
| white (*Newman's Own*), 1.1 oz. .......... | 130 | 2.0 | 18.0 | 5.0 | 0 | 200 | 3.0 |

| Food and Measure | cal. | prot. (gms) | carbo. (gms) | fat (gms) | chol. (mgs) | sod. (mgs) | fiber (gms) |
|---|---|---|---|---|---|---|---|
| **Popcorn** (cont.) | | | | | | | |
| nacho (*Orville Redenbacher's*) ...... | 180 | 2.0 | 15.0 | 13.0 | 0 | 400 | 3.0 |
| salsa (*Jolly Time Sassy Salsa*) ........ | 160 | 2.0 | 16.0 | 11.0 | 0 | 320 | 3.0 |
| salt and (*Orville Redenbacher's* Mini Bag): | | | | | | | |
| cracked pepper ...... | 200 | 3.0 | 22.0 | 13.0 | 0 | 620 | 4.0 |
| lime .............. | 220 | 3.0 | 21.0 | 15.0 | 0 | 370 | 4.0 |
| white/yellow (*Bob's Red Mill*) .......... | 90 | 3.0 | 18.0 | 1.0 | 0 | 0 | 3.0 |
| **Popcorn, popped**, 1 oz., except as noted: | | | | | | | |
| (*Bachman* Air) ......... | 160 | 2.0 | 14.0 | 10.0 | 0 | 225 | 6.0 |
| (*Bachman* Air Lite) ..... | 110 | 4.0 | 22.0 | 1.5 | 0 | 110 | 4.0 |
| (*Herr's*) .............. | 140 | 2.0 | 11.0 | 10.0 | 0 | 250 | 3.0 |
| (*Herr's* Light) .......... | 120 | 2.0 | 19.0 | 4.0 | 0 | 80 | 3.0 |
| butter/butter flavor: | | | | | | | |
| (*Snyder's*), ⅝ oz. .... | 100 | 1.0 | 6.0 | 8.0 | 0 | 150 | 1.0 |
| (*Wise*) .............. | 150 | 1.0 | 14.0 | 10.0 | 0 | 280 | 3.0 |
| (*Wise* Reduced Fat) .. | 140 | 3.0 | 22.0 | 5.0 | 0 | 160 | 3.0 |
| caramel: | | | | | | | |
| (*Crunch 'n Munch*), ⅔ cup ........... | 160 | 2.0 | 20.0 | 8.0 | 5 | 100 | 1.0 |
| (*Rothbury Farms*), ¾ cup, 1.1. oz. .... | 140 | 1.0 | 21.0 | 6.0 | 15 | 240 | 1.0 |
| caramel nut: | | | | | | | |
| (*Cracker Jack*) ...... | 120 | 2.0 | 23.0 | 2.0 | 0 | 70 | 1.0 |
| almond/cashew (*Rothbury Farms*), ½ cup ........... | 150 | 2.0 | 17.0 | 9.0 | 10 | 180 | 1.0 |
| cheddar (*Chester's*) ..... | 150 | 2.0 | 15.0 | 10.0 | 0 | 200 | 3.0 |
| cheddar, white: | | | | | | | |
| (*Bachman*) ......... | 150 | 3.0 | 15.0 | 9.0 | <5 | 320 | 3.0 |
| (*Cape Cod*) ......... | 160 | 4.0 | 12.0 | 11.0 | 0 | 250 | 2.0 |
| (*Herr's*) ........... | 140 | 2.0 | 16.0 | 9.0 | 0 | 310 | 3.0 |
| (*Smartfood*) ........ | 160 | 3.0 | 14.0 | 10.0 | <5 | 290 | 2.0 |
| (*Smartfood* Reduced Fat) ............. | 130 | 4.0 | 17.0 | 6.0 | <5 | 260 | 3.0 |
| (*Wise*) .............. | 150 | 3.0 | 13.0 | 10.0 | 5 | 310 | 2.0 |
| (*Wise* Reduced Fat) .. | 140 | 3.0 | 18.0 | 6.0 | <5 | 250 | 3.0 |
| cheese: | | | | | | | |
| (*Bachman*), 1.1 oz. ... | 160 | 3.0 | 17.0 | 9.0 | <5 | 220 | 4.0 |

| Food and Measure | cal. | prot. (gms) | carbo. (gms) | fat (gms) | chol. (mgs) | sod. (mgs) | fiber (gms) |
|---|---|---|---|---|---|---|---|
| (*Herr's* Regular/Hot) .. | 140 | 2.0 | 13.0 | 8.0 | 0 | 240 | 3.0 |
| hot (*Wise*) .......... | 150 | 2.0 | 14.0 | 10.0 | <5 | 260 | 2.0 |
| cranberry almond (*Smartfood* Clusters), 1 pkg. ............. | 120 | 1.0 | 24.0 | 2.0 | 0 | 75 | 5.0 |
| honey mustard (*Smartfood* Clusters), 1 pkg. ..... | 110 | 1.0 | 25.0 | 1.0 | 0 | 150 | 5.0 |
| toffee, butter (*Crunch 'n Munch*), ⅔ cup .... | 150 | 2.0 | 22.0 | 6.0 | <5 | 170 | 1.0 |
| **Popcorn cakes**, see "Rice cakes" | | | | | | | |
| **Popcorn seasoning** (*Kernel Season's*), ¼ tsp.: | | | | | | | |
| barbecue ............. | 3 | 0 | 1.0 | 0 | 0 | 5 | 0 |
| butter flavor .......... | 3 | 0 | 1.0 | 0 | 0 | 80 | 0 |
| Cajun ............... | 2 | 0 | 0 | 0 | 0 | 57 | 0 |
| cheddar/Parmesan garlic | 2 | 0 | 0 | 0 | 0 | 75 | 0 |
| ranch ............... | 2 | 0 | 0 | 0 | 0 | 65 | 0 |
| ***Popeye's,*** 1 serving: | | | | | | | |
| chicken, mild: | | | | | | | |
| breast, breaded ...... | 350 | 33.0 | 8.0 | 20.0 | 179 | 1130 | 0 |
| no skin/breading .. | 120 | 24.0 | 0 | 2.0 | 120 | 540 | 0 |
| leg, breaded ........ | 110 | 11.0 | 3.0 | 7.0 | 92 | 280 | 0 |
| no skin/breading .. | 50 | 9.0 | 0 | 2.0 | 85 | 190 | 0 |
| thigh, breaded ...... | 280 | 16.0 | 7.0 | 20.0 | 135 | 710 | 0 |
| no skin/breading .. | 80 | 11.0 | 0 | 4.0 | 98 | 230 | 0 |
| wing, breaded ....... | 150 | 9.0 | 5.0 | 10.0 | 59 | 690 | 0 |
| no skin/breading .. | 40 | 7.0 | 0 | 1.5 | 58 | 400 | <1.0 |
| strips, 2 pc. ........ | 130 | 25.0 | 3.0 | 2.5 | 50 | 620 | 0 |
| chicken, spicy: | | | | | | | |
| breast, breaded ...... | 360 | 31.0 | 8.0 | 22.0 | 170 | 760 | 1.0 |
| no skin/breading .. | 120 | 25.0 | <1.0 | 2.0 | 112 | 380 | <1.0 |
| leg, breaded ........ | 100 | 9.0 | 3.0 | 5.0 | 71 | 230 | 0 |
| no skin/breading .. | 50 | 9.0 | 0 | 1.5 | 60 | 135 | 0 |
| thigh, breaded ...... | 300 | 15.0 | 7.0 | 24.0 | 131 | 490 | 0 |
| no skin/breading .. | 80 | 12.0 | 2.0 | 3.0 | 98 | 170 | 0 |
| wing, breaded ....... | 140 | 8.0 | 5.0 | 9.0 | 79 | 290 | 0 |
| no skin/breading .. | 40 | 6.0 | 0 | 2.0 | 66 | 125 | <1.0 |
| strips, 2 pcs. ........ | 150 | 23.0 | 5.0 | 4.0 | 55 | 820 | 0 |
| Big Deals: | | | | | | | |
| loaded chicken wrap .. | 400 | 19.0 | 44.0 | 17.0 | 35 | 1100 | 4.0 |
| Delta mini .......... | 300 | 15.0 | 30.0 | 13.0 | 30 | 780 | 1.0 |
| chicken biscuit ...... | 350 | 13.0 | 30.0 | 20.0 | 35 | 930 | <1.0 |

| Food and Measure | cal. | prot. (gms) | carbo. (gms) | fat (gms) | chol. (mgs) | sod. (mgs) | fiber (gms) |
|---|---|---|---|---|---|---|---|
| **Popeye's** *(cont.)* | | | | | | | |
| Big Easys: | | | | | | | |
|   chicken bowl ........ | 570 | 35.0 | 44.0 | 29.0 | 100 | 1600 | 8.0 |
|   crispy sandwich ..... | 560 | 33.0 | 56.0 | 23.0 | 75 | 1690 | 3.0 |
| Cajun wings, 6 pcs. ..... | 595 | 34.0 | 19.0 | 43.0 | 260 | 1274 | 0 |
| chicken strips, naked ... | 220 | 30.0 | 2.0 | 10.0 | 80 | 720 | 0 |
| Louisiana legends: | | | | | | | |
|   chicken/sausage | | | | | | | |
|     jambalaya ........ | 220 | 10.0 | 20.0 | 11.0 | 32 | 760 | 1.0 |
|   chicken, smothered .. | 210 | 10.0 | 24.0 | 8.0 | 23 | 743 | 1.0 |
|   etouffee, chicken .... | 160 | 12.0 | 6.0 | 10.0 | 20 | 870 | 2.0 |
|   etouffee, crawfish .... | 180 | 7.0 | 25.0 | 5.0 | 48 | 640 | 2.0 |
| Louisiana travelers: | | | | | | | |
|   nuggets, 6 ......... | 220 | 15.0 | 13.0 | 12.0 | 40 | 500 | <1.0 |
|   tenders, mild, 3 ..... | 375 | 33.0 | 24.0 | 17.0 | 84 | 1620 | 0 |
|   tenders, spicy, 3 ..... | 405 | 33.0 | 30.0 | 17.0 | 84 | 2160 | 0 |
| sandwiches: | | | | | | | |
|   deluxe, mild/spicy .... | 630 | 35.0 | 53.0 | 31.0 | 71 | 1480 | 3.0 |
|     mild, no mayo .... | 480 | 33.0 | 54.0 | 15.0 | 55 | 1290 | 3.0 |
|   Po Boy ........... | 330 | 8.0 | 36.0 | 17.0 | 10 | 560 | 0 |
| shrimp, butterfly ....... | 310 | 13.0 | 22.0 | 19.0 | 90 | 800 | 2.0 |
| shrimp, popcorn ....... | 280 | 12.0 | 22.0 | 16.0 | 95 | 1110 | <1.0 |
| sides, regular: | | | | | | | |
|   biscuit ............. | 240 | 4.0 | 26.0 | 13.0 | 0 | 490 | 1.0 |
|   coleslaw ........... | 260 | <1.0 | 14.0 | 23.0 | 15 | 260 | 9.0 |
|   corn on cob ........ | 190 | 6.0 | 37.0 | 2.0 | 0 | 0 | 4.0 |
|   french fries ......... | 310 | 4.0 | 35.0 | 17.0 | 7 | 660 | 3.0 |
|   green beans ........ | 70 | 2.0 | 14.0 | 1.0 | 5 | 400 | 2.0 |
|   mashed potatoes .... | 100 | 1.0 | 17.0 | 3.0 | 0 | 380 | <1.0 |
|     and gravy ........ | 120 | 3.0 | 18.0 | 4.0 | 5 | 570 | 2.0 |
|   red beans, rice ...... | 320 | 10.0 | 31.0 | 19.0 | 20 | 710 | 17.0 |
|   rice, Cajun ......... | 170 | 8.0 | 22.0 | 6.0 | 60 | 530 | 2.0 |
| cinnamon apple | | | | | | | |
|   turnover ........... | 250 | 3.0 | 34.0 | 12.0 | 5 | 320 | 2.0 |
| **Poppy seeds**: | | | | | | | |
| (*Bob's Red Mill*), 3 tbsp. . | 160 | 5.0 | 7.0 | 13.0 | 0 | 5 | 3.0 |
| 1 tsp. ................. | 15 | .5 | .7 | 1.3 | 0 | 1 | .8 |
| **Porgy**, see "Scup" | | | | | | | |
| **Pork** meat only, | | | | | | | |
|   4 oz.: | | | | | | | |
| backribs, roasted, | | | | | | | |
|   lean w/fat ......... | 420 | 27.5 | 0 | 33.5 | 134 | 115 | 0 |
| ground, cooked ........ | 337 | 29.1 | 0 | 23.6 | 107 | 83 | 0 |

| Food and Measure | cal. | prot. (gms) | carbo. (gms) | fat (gms) | chol. (mgs) | sod. (mgs) | fiber (gms) |
|---|---|---|---|---|---|---|---|
| leg, see "Ham" | | | | | | | |
| loin, whole: | | | | | | | |
| braised, lean w/fat ... | 271 | 30.9 | 0 | 15.4 | 90 | 54 | 0 |
| braised, lean only .... | 231 | 32.4 | 0 | 10.3 | 90 | 57 | 0 |
| broiled, lean w/fat .... | 274 | 30.9 | 0 | 15.8 | 90 | 70 | 0 |
| broiled, lean only .... | 238 | 32.4 | 0 | 11.1 | 90 | 73 | 0 |
| roasted, lean w/fat ... | 281 | 30.7 | 0 | 16.6 | 93 | 67 | 0 |
| roasted, lean only .... | 237 | 32.5 | 0 | 10.9 | 92 | 66 | 0 |
| loin, blade: | | | | | | | |
| braised, lean w/fat ... | 366 | 24.8 | 0 | 28.8 | 96 | 62 | 0 |
| braised, lean only .... | 255 | 28.4 | 0 | 14.8 | 94 | 70 | 0 |
| broiled, lean w/fat .... | 363 | 25.5 | 0 | 28.2 | 98 | 79 | 0 |
| broiled, lean only .... | 265 | 28.8 | 0 | 15.8 | 95 | 91 | 0 |
| roasted, lean w/fat ... | 366 | 26.9 | 0 | 27.9 | 106 | 34 | 0 |
| roasted, lean only .... | 280 | 30.2 | 0 | 16.8 | 106 | 33 | 0 |
| loin, center: | | | | | | | |
| braised, lean w/fat ... | 280 | 31.7 | 0 | 16.0 | 98 | 67 | 0 |
| braised, lean only .... | 229 | 33.8 | 0 | 9.4 | 96 | 70 | 0 |
| broiled, lean w/fat .... | 272 | 32.6 | 0 | 14.8 | 93 | 66 | 0 |
| broiled, lean only. .... | 229 | 34.2 | 0 | 9.2 | 93 | 68 | 0 |
| pan-fried, lean w/fat .. | 314 | 33.9 | 0 | 18.8 | 104 | 91 | 0 |
| pan-fried, lean only ... | 263 | 36.5 | 0 | 11.9 | 104 | 97 | |
| roasted, lean w/fat ... | 265 | 29.8 | 0 | 15.3 | 91 | 71 | 0 |
| roasted, lean only .... | 226 | 31.2 | 0 | 10.2 | 90 | 75 | 0 |
| loin, center rib: | | | | | | | |
| braised, lean w/fat ... | 284 | 30.2 | 0 | 17.1 | 83 | 45 | 0 |
| braised, lean only .... | 234 | 32.1 | 0 | 10.7 | 81 | 47 | 0 |
| broiled, lean w/fat .... | 298 | 32.6 | 0 | 17.6 | 93 | 70 | 0 |
| broiled, lean only .... | 248 | 34.9 | 0 | 11.0 | 92 | 74 | 0 |
| roasted, lean w/fat ... | 289 | 31.1 | 0 | 17.3 | 83 | 52 | 0 |
| roasted, lean only .... | 253 | 32.6 | 0 | 12.6 | 81 | 53 | 0 |
| loin, top, bone-in: | | | | | | | |
| braised, lean w/fat ... | 264 | 31.5 | 0 | 14.4 | 85 | 48 | 0 |
| braised, lean only .... | 229 | 33.0 | 0 | 9.7 | 83 | 48 | 0 |
| broiled, lean w/fat .... | 260 | 34.0 | 0 | 12.7 | 92 | 71 | 0 |
| broiled, lean only .... | 230 | 35.3 | 0 | 8.8 | 91 | 74 | 0 |
| roasted, lean w/fat ... | 256 | 31.9 | 0 | 13.0 | 89 | 50 | 0 |
| roasted, lean only .... | 220 | 34.3 | 0 | 8.2 | 89 | 51 | 0 |
| loin, top, boneless: | | | | | | | |
| pan-fried, lean w/fat .. | 291 | 32.9 | 0 | 16.8 | 89 | 62 | 0 |
| pan-fried, lean only ... | 255 | 34.6 | 0 | 11.9 | 87 | 65 | 0 |
| ribs, country style: | | | | | | | |
| braised, lean w/fat ... | 336 | 27.1 | 0 | 24.4 | 99 | 67 | 0 |
| braised, lean only .... | 265 | 29.5 | 0 | 15.4 | 98 | 71 | 0 |

| Food and Measure | cal. | prot. (gms) | carbo. (gms) | fat (gms) | chol. (mgs) | sod. (mgs) | fiber (gms) |
|---|---|---|---|---|---|---|---|
| **Pork, ribs, country style** *(cont.)* | | | | | | | |
| roasted, lean w/fat ... | 372 | 26.5 | 0 | 28.7 | 104 | 59 | 0 |
| roasted, lean only .... | 280 | 30.2 | 0 | 16.8 | 106 | 33 | 0 |
| shoulder, whole: | | | | | | | |
| roasted, lean w/fat ... | 331 | 26.4 | 0 | 24.3 | 102 | 77 | 0 |
| roasted, lean only .... | 261 | 28.7 | 0 | 15.4 | 102 | 85 | 0 |
| shoulder, arm (picnic): | | | | | | | |
| braised, lean w/fat ... | 374 | 31.7 | 0 | 26.3 | 124 | 100 | 0 |
| braised, lean only .... | 281 | 36.6 | 0 | 13.8 | 129 | 116 | 0 |
| roasted, lean w/fat ... | 360 | 26.6 | 0 | 27.2 | 107 | 79 | 0 |
| roasted, lean only .... | 259 | 30.3 | 0 | 14.3 | 108 | 91 | 0 |
| shoulder, Boston blade: | | | | | | | |
| braised, lean w/fat ... | 362 | 32.5 | 0 | 24.7 | 128 | 79 | 0 |
| braised, lean only .... | 310 | 35.3 | 0 | 17.6 | 132 | 85 | 0 |
| broiled, lean w/fat .... | 294 | 29.0 | 0 | 18.8 | 108 | 78 | 0 |
| broiled, lean only .... | 257 | 30.3 | 0 | 14.2 | 107 | 84 | 0 |
| roasted, lean w/fat ... | 305 | 26.2 | 0 | 21.4 | 98 | 76 | 0 |
| roasted, lean only .... | 263 | 27.5 | 0 | 16.2 | 96 | 100 | 0 |
| sirloin, bone-in: | | | | | | | |
| braised, lean w/fat ... | 278 | 28.8 | 0 | 17.1 | 93 | 58 | 0 |
| braised, lean only .... | 223 | 30.6 | 0 | 10.2 | 92 | 60 | 0 |
| broiled, lean w/fat .... | 294 | 30.2 | 0 | 18.2 | 98 | 77 | 0 |
| broiled, lean only .... | 242 | 32.3 | 0 | 11.5 | 96 | 82 | 0 |
| roasted, lean w/fat ... | 296 | 30.9 | 0 | 28.2 | 99 | 68 | 0 |
| roasted, lean only .... | 245 | 32.7 | 0 | 11.7 | 98 | 71 | 0 |
| sirloin, boneless: | | | | | | | |
| braised, lean w/fat ... | 214 | 30.1 | 0 | 9.5 | 92 | 52 | 0 |
| braised, lean only .... | 198 | 30.6 | 0 | 7.5 | 92 | 52 | 0 |
| broiled, lean w/fat .... | 236 | 34.6 | 0 | 9.8 | 103 | 64 | 0 |
| broiled, lean only .... | 219 | 35.3 | 0 | 7.6 | 104 | 64 | 0 |
| roasted, lean w/fat ... | 235 | 32.3 | 0 | 10.7 | 98 | 64 | 0 |
| roasted, lean only .... | 225 | 32.7 | 0 | 9.4 | 98 | 64 | 0 |
| spareribs, lean w/fat, | | | | | | | |
| braised ............ | 450 | 33.0 | 0 | 34.4 | 137 | 106 | 0 |
| tenderloin: | | | | | | | |
| broiled, lean w/fat .... | 228 | 33.9 | 0 | 9.2 | 107 | 73 | 0 |
| roasted, lean w/fat ... | 196 | 31.5 | 0 | 6.9 | 90 | 62 | 0 |
| roasted, lean only .... | 186 | 31.9 | 0 | 5.5 | 90 | 64 | 0 |
| **Pork, cured:** | | | | | | | |
| arm (picnic), roasted: | | | | | | | |
| lean w/fat, 4 oz. ..... | 318 | 23.2 | 0 | 24.2 | 66 | 1216 | 0 |
| lean w/fat, chopped | | | | | | | |
| or diced, 1 cup .... | 392 | 28.6 | 0 | 29.9 | 81 | 1501 | 0 |

| Food and Measure | cal. | prot. (gms) | carbo. (gms) | fat (gms) | chol. (mgs) | sod. (mgs) | fiber (gms) |
|---|---|---|---|---|---|---|---|
| lean only, 4 oz. ...... | 193 | 28.3 | 0 | 8.0 | 54 | 1396 | 0 |
| lean only, chopped or diced, 1 cup .... | 238 | 34.9 | 0 | 9.9 | 67 | 1723 | 0 |
| blade roll, lean w/fat, roasted, 4 oz. ....... | 325 | 19.6 | .4 | 26.6 | 76 | 1103 | 0 |
| leg, see "Ham" | | | | | | | |
| **Pork, frozen/chilled, raw,** 4 oz., except as noted: | | | | | | | |
| chops (see also "loin," below), boneless: | | | | | | | |
| center cut (*Farmland Extra Tender*) ..... | 130 | 22.0 | 1.0 | 3.0 | 60 | 230 | 0 |
| Southwest peppercorn rub (*Farmland Extra Tender*) ..... | 130 | 22.0 | 1.0 | 3.0 | 60 | 260 | 0 |
| crown roast (*Always Tender*) ........... | 190 | 21.0 | 0 | 12.0 | 60 | 350 | 0 |
| cubes or strips, boneless (*Farmland Extra Tender*) ........... | 120 | 23.0 | 1.0 | 2.0 | 70 | 230 | 0 |
| fillet, bacon-wrapped (*Farmland Extra Tender*), 5 oz. ....... | 290 | 38.0 | 1.0 | 14.0 | 115 | 610 | 0 |
| ground (*Farmland All Natural*) .......... | 250 | 16.0 | 0 | 19.0 | 70 | 55 | 0 |
| loin, bone-in: | | | | | | | |
| (*Always Tender*), 3.5 oz. .......... | 190 | 18.0 | 0 | 12.0 | 54 | 295 | 0 |
| (*Farmland Extra Tender*) .......... | 130 | 21.0 | 1.0 | 4.5 | 60 | 280 | 0 |
| center cut (*Farmland All Natural*) ....... | 130 | 26.0 | 0 | 2.0 | 70 | 60 | 0 |
| loin, boneless, center: | | | | | | | |
| (*Always Tender*) ..... | 170 | 21.0 | 0 | 9.0 | 60 | 330 | 0 |
| (*Farmland Extra Tender* for Chops) . | 130 | 21.0 | 1.0 | 4.5 | 60 | 220 | 0 |
| chop (*Hormel Natural Choice* Savory) .... | 120 | 18.0 | 0 | 5.0 | 50 | 480 | 0 |
| roast (*Farmland Extra Tender*) .......... | 230 | 19.0 | 1.0 | 16.0 | 65 | 270 | 0 |
| loin fillet (*Always Tender* Tenderloin) ... | 120 | 22.0 | 0 | 3.5 | 60 | 330 | 0 |

| Food and Measure | cal. | prot. (gms) | carbo. (gms) | fat (gms) | chol. (mgs) | sod. (mgs) | fiber (gms) |
|---|---|---|---|---|---|---|---|
| **Pork, frozen/chilled, raw** *(cont.)* | | | | | | | |
| loin fillet, seasoned | | | | | | | |
| (see also "tenderloin," below): | | | | | | | |
| bourbon maple (*Always Tender*) ... | 130 | 20.0 | 2.0 | 5.0 | 60 | 650 | 0 |
| brown sugar maple (*Always Tender*) ... | 140 | 20.0 | 3.0 | 5.0 | 45 | 480 | 0 |
| chipotle barbecue rub (*Farmland Extra Tender*) ..... | 130 | 22.0 | 1.0 | 3.0 | 60 | 290 | 0 |
| citrus, center cut (*Always Tender*) ... | 140 | 21.0 | 3.0 | 5.0 | 45 | 360 | 0 |
| cracked peppercorn rub (*Farmland Extra Tender*) ..... | 140 | 22.0 | 2.0 | 3.0 | 60 | 200 | 0 |
| garlic butter herb (*Farmland Extra Tender*) .......... | 140 | 22.0 | 2.0 | 3.0 | 60 | 200 | 0 |
| homestyle rub (*Farmland Extra Tender*) .......... | 140 | 22.0 | 3.0 | 3.0 | 55 | 220 | 0 |
| honey mustard (*Always Tender*) ... | 140 | 20.0 | 4.0 | 5.0 | 45 | 510 | 0 |
| horseradish black pepper (*Always Tender*) .......... | 120 | 20.0 | 3.0 | 3.5 | 40 | 420 | 0 |
| lemon garlic rub (*Farmland Extra Tender*) .......... | 130 | 22.0 | 2.0 | 3.0 | 55 | 220 | 0 |
| lemon pepper rub (*Farmland Extra Tender*) .......... | 130 | 22.0 | 2.0 | 3.0 | 60 | 240 | 0 |
| mesquite or peppercorn rub (*Farmland Extra Tender*) ..... | 130 | 22.0 | 2.0 | 3.0 | 55 | 220 | 0 |
| Parmesan (*Always Tender*) .......... | 120 | 20.0 | 1.0 | 4.0 | 45 | 390 | 0 |
| Parmesan (*Always Tender Old Smokehouse*) . | 120 | 20.0 | 2.0 | 4.0 | 45 | 360 | 0 |
| Parmesan garlic rub (*Farmland Extra Tender*) .......... | 140 | 22.0 | 2.0 | 3.0 | 60 | 210 | 0 |

| Food and Measure | cal. | prot. (gms) | carbo. (gms) | fat (gms) | chol. (mgs) | sod. (mgs) | fiber (gms) |
|---|---|---|---|---|---|---|---|
| Southwest peppercorn rub (*Farmland Extra Tender*) ..... | 130 | 22.0 | 1.0 | 3.0 | 60 | 260 | 0 |
| sun-dried tomato, center cut (*Always Tender*) .......... | 120 | 19.0 | 2.0 | 4.0 | 45 | 440 | 0 |
| tarragon mustard (*Always Tender*) ... | 130 | 20.0 | 4.0 | 3.5 | 35 | 480 | 0 |
| teriyaki ginger sesame rub (*Farmland Extra Tender*) ..... | 140 | 22.0 | 2.0 | 3.0 | 60 | 200 | 0 |
| medallions, peppered bacon (*Hormel Natural* Choice), 6 oz. .. | 260 | 30.0 | 0 | 15.0 | 100 | 700 | 0 |
| picnic (*Always Tender*) .. | 240 | 19.0 | 0 | 18.0 | 70 | 350 | 0 |
| rib ends, boneless (*Always Tender*) ..... | 160 | 20.0 | 0 | 9.0 | 60 | 330 | 0 |
| ribs/spareribs: | | | | | | | |
| (*Farmland Extra Tender* St. Louis) .. | 290 | 17.0 | 1.0 | 24.0 | 70 | 290 | 0 |
| baby back (*Always Tender*) .......... | 250 | 18.0 | 0 | 20.0 | 80 | 330 | 0 |
| Frenched rack (*Farmland Extra Tender*) ..... | 170 | 19.0 | 1.0 | 9.0 | 60 | 210 | 0 |
| loin/loin back (*Farmland Extra Tender*) ..... | 290 | 17.0 | 1.0 | 24.0 | 80 | 340 | 0 |
| riblets (*Farmland Extra Tender*) ..... | 190 | 21.0 | 0 | 11.0 | 70 | 50 | 0 |
| spareribs (*Always Tender*) .......... | 280 | 17.0 | 0 | 23.0 | 80 | 330 | 0 |
| spareribs (*Farmland Extra Tender*) ..... | 290 | 17.0 | 0 | 24.0 | 80 | 230 | 0 |
| strips (*Farmland Extra Tender*) ..... | 290 | 17.0 | 1.0 | 24.0 | 70 | 210 | 0 |
| roast, fresh (*Always Tender*) ............ | 170 | 20.0 | 0 | 10.0 | 60 | 330 | 0 |
| shoulder roast (*Always Tender*): | | | | | | | |
| barbecue, boneless ... | 200 | 18.0 | 2.0 | 13.0 | 60 | 340 | 0 |
| onion garlic ......... | 170 | 18.0 | 1.0 | 10.0 | 60 | 550 | 0 |
| sirloin: | | | | | | | |
| roast, boneless (*Always Tender*) .......... | 120 | 22.0 | 0 | 3.0 | 60 | 330 | 0 |

| Food and Measure | cal. | prot. (gms) | carbo. (gms) | fat (gms) | chol. (mgs) | sod. (mgs) | fiber (gms) |
|---|---|---|---|---|---|---|---|
| **Pork, frozen/chilled, raw, sirloin** *(cont.)* | | | | | | | |
| for strips (*Farmland Extra Tender*) ..... | 130 | 20.0 | 1.0 | 5.0 | 60 | 280 | 0 |
| tip roast (*Farmland Extra Tender*) ..... | 110 | 21.0 | 1.0 | 3.0 | 60 | 220 | 0 |
| tenderloin, see "loin fillet," above: | | | | | | | |
| tenderloin, seasoned: | | | | | | | |
| (*Always Tender Original*) ......... | 120 | 19.0 | 1.0 | 4.0 | 50 | 400 | 0 |
| apple bourbon (*Always Tender*) ... | 140 | 19.0 | 5.0 | 4.0 | 50 | 500 | 0 |
| chipotle barbecue rub (*Farmland Extra Tender*) .......... | 130 | 23.0 | 1.0 | 3.0 | 60 | 260 | 0 |
| cracked peppercorn rub (*Farmland Extra Tender*) .......... | 130 | 24.0 | 2.0 | 3.0 | 60 | 200 | 0 |
| garlic (*Always Tender*) | 130 | 19.0 | 1.0 | 5.0 | 45 | 600 | 0 |
| herb and olive oil or lemon garlic (*Always Tender*) ... | 130 | 19.0 | 1.0 | 5.0 | 45 | 600 | 0 |
| lemon pepper rub (*Farmland Extra Tender*) .......... | 130 | 23.0 | 2.0 | 3.0 | 65 | 240 | 0 |
| peppercorn (*Always Tender*) .......... | 120 | 18.0 | 2.0 | 4.0 | 50 | 630 | 0 |
| Southwest peppercorn rub (*Farmland Extra Tender*) ..... | 130 | 23.0 | 1.0 | 3.0 | 60 | 260 | 0 |
| teriyaki (*Always Tender*) .......... | 130 | 19.0 | 5.0 | 4.0 | 50 | 500 | 0 |
| **Pork, frozen/chilled, cooked**, 5 oz., except as noted: | | | | | | | |
| w/barbecue sauce: | | | | | | | |
| shredded (*Lloyd's Original*), ¼ cup ... | 80 | 6.0 | 9.0 | 2.0 | 15 | 360 | 0 |
| shredded, honey hickory (*Lloyd's*), ¼ cup ... | 80 | 6.0 | 10.0 | 2.0 | 15 | 440 | 0 |
| sweet/tangy (*Tyson*) .. | 180 | 17.0 | 13.0 | 7.0 | 50 | 810 | 0 |
| chop, apple bourbon (*Hormel*) .......... | 190 | 20.0 | 15.0 | 6.0 | 50 | 800 | 0 |

| Food and Measure | cal. | prot. (gms) | carbo. (gms) | fat (gms) | chol. (mgs) | sod. (mgs) | fiber (gms) |
|---|---|---|---|---|---|---|---|
| chops or roast, w/gravy | | | | | | | |
| (*Bob Evans*) ........ | 290 | 32.0 | 6.0 | 15.0 | 110 | 490 | 0 |
| loin, honey mustard | | | | | | | |
| (*Hormel*) .......... | 180 | 20.0 | 13.0 | 5.0 | 50 | 800 | 0 |
| ribs (*Lloyd's*), 2 ribs, | | | | | | | |
| w/barbecue sauce: | | | | | | | |
| baby back, honey | | | | | | | |
| hickory sauce, | | | | | | | |
| 4.8 oz. .......... | 340 | 21.0 | 19.0 | 20.0 | 85 | 810 | 0 |
| baby back, original | | | | | | | |
| sauce, 4.8 oz. ..... | 290 | 14.0 | 20.0 | 17.0 | 70 | 850 | 1.0 |
| spareribs, St. Louis, | | | | | | | |
| original sauce, 5 oz. | 350 | 18.0 | 25.0 | 20.0 | 70 | 1020 | <1.0 |
| roast: | | | | | | | |
| (*Hormel*) .......... | 180 | 28.0 | 1.0 | 7.0 | 85 | 600 | 0 |
| balsamic rosemary | | | | | | | |
| (*Hormel*) ....... | 200 | 31.0 | 2.0 | 8.0 | 95 | 400 | 0 |
| in gravy (*Tyson*) ..... | 190 | 19.0 | 5.0 | 10.0 | 55 | 590 | 0 |
| shoulder butt | | | | | | | |
| (*Thumann's*), 3 oz. ... | 225 | 21.0 | 0 | 18.0 | 45 | 765 | 0 |
| sweet and sour (*Simply | | | | | | | |
| Simmered*) ......... | 150 | 14.0 | 21.0 | 1.5 | 5 | 840 | 5.0 |
| **Pork, ground**, see "Pork" and "Pork, frozen/chilled, raw" | | | | | | | |
| **Pork, pickled** (see also "Pig's feet"), hocks or tidbits (*Hormel*), | | | | | | | |
| 2 oz. ............. | 100 | 8.0 | 0 | 8.0 | 45 | 690 | 0 |
| **Pork backfat**, 1 oz. ..... | 230 | 2.6 | 0 | 25.3 | 16 | 3 | 0 |
| **Pork belly**, raw, 1 oz. ... | 147 | 2.7 | 0 | 15.0 | 20 | 9 | 0 |
| **Pork coating/seasoning mix** (see also "Chicken coating mix"): | | | | | | | |
| (*Oven Fry* Extra Crispy), | | | | | | | |
| ⅛ pkg. ............ | 60 | 2.0 | 11.0 | 1.5 | 0 | 340 | 0 |
| (*Shake 'n Bake* Original | | | | | | | |
| w/Bags), 1 tbsp. ..... | 40 | 1.0 | 8.0 | 0 | 0 | 240 | 0 |
| (*Zatarain's* Bake & | | | | | | | |
| Crisp), 2 tbsp. ....... | 50 | 1.0 | 10.0 | .5 | 0 | 520 | 0 |
| barbecue, pulled | | | | | | | |
| (*McCormick* Slow | | | | | | | |
| Cookers), 1 tsp. ..... | 15 | 0 | 2.0 | 0 | 0 | 450 | 0 |

| Food and Measure | cal. | prot. (gms) | carbo. (gms) | fat (gms) | chol. (mgs) | sod. (mgs) | fiber (gms) |
|---|---|---|---|---|---|---|---|
| **Pork coating/seasoning mix** *(cont.)* | | | | | | | |
| chops (*McCormick Bag 'n Season*), 2 tsp. | 15 | 0 | 3.0 | 0 | 0 | 530 | 0 |
| steak (*Maull's*), 2 tbsp. | 20 | 0 | 4.0 | 0 | 0 | 480 | 0 |
| tenderloin, herb roast (*McCormick Bag 'n Season*), 1 tsp. | 10 | 0 | 2.0 | 0 | 0 | 180 | 0 |
| **Pork entree, frozen** (see also "Pork, frozen/chilled, cooked"), 1 pkg.: | | | | | | | |
| country fried chop (*Marie Callender's*), 15 oz. | 470 | 23.0 | 49.0 | 20.0 | 60 | 1380 | 8.0 |
| and mashed potato (*Stouffer's*), 10 oz. | 370 | 13.0 | 31.0 | 21.0 | 25 | 1110 | 3.0 |
| patty (*Banquet* Savory), 8 oz. | 250 | 11.0 | 26.0 | 11.0 | 25 | 770 | 4.0 |
| ribs, boneless (*Banquet*), 10 oz. | 320 | 15.0 | 42.0 | 11.0 | 30 | 830 | 5.0 |
| roast, w/gravy, potatoes (*Boston Market* Dinner), 15 oz. | 430 | 29.0 | 37.0 | 19.0 | 75 | 1740 | 3.0 |
| tangerine sauce (*Contessa On the Stove*), 9.8 oz. | 390 | 12.0 | 62.0 | 11.0 | 20 | 600 | 3.0 |
| w/out sauce | 310 | 12.0 | 42.0 | 11.0 | 20 | 170 | 3.0 |
| **Pork entree, microwave**, stew, w/salsa verde (*Doña Maria Platillos*), 10-oz. bowl | 290 | 18.0 | 22.0 | 14.0 | 60 | 940 | 4.0 |
| **Pork fat**, roasted, 1 oz. | 167 | 2.2 | 0 | 17.5 | 24 | 177 | 0 |
| **Pork gravy**, canned, golden (*Campbell's*), ¼ cup | 45 | 1.0 | 3.0 | 3.0 | 5 | 310 | 0 |
| **Pork gravy mix** (*McCormick*), 1 tbsp. | 20 | 0 | 4.0 | 0 | 0 | 350 | 0 |
| **Pork lunch meat** (see also "Ham lunch meat"), 2 oz.: | | | | | | | |
| (*Boar's Head* Porketta) | 80 | 15.0 | 0 | 2.0 | 35 | 540 | 0 |
| honey barbecue (*Black Bear*) | 60 | 9.0 | 3.0 | 1.0 | 30 | 290 | 0 |
| roast (*Thumann's* Home Style Fresh Ham) | 150 | 10.0 | 0 | 14.0 | 30 | 75 | 0 |

| Food and Measure | cal. | prot. (gms) | carbo. (gms) | fat (gms) | chol. (mgs) | sod. (mgs) | fiber (gms) |
|---|---|---|---|---|---|---|---|
| seasoned (*Boar's Head* Fresh Ham) . . . . . . . . | 80 | 14.0 | 0 | 3.0 | 35 | 310 | 0 |
| **Pork rind snack**, .5 oz.: | | | | | | | |
| (*Baken-ets* Fried Skins) . . | 80 | 7.0 | 0 | 5.0 | 20 | 310 | 0 |
| (*Herr's* Original) . . . . . . . | 80 | 9.0 | 0 | 5.0 | 20 | 270 | 0 |
| (*Mission* Chicharrones) . . | 80 | 9.0 | 0 | 5.0 | 20 | 270 | 0 |
| barbecue (*Herr's*) . . . . . . | 80 | 8.0 | 0 | 5.0 | 20 | 400 | 0 |
| hot: | | | | | | | |
| (*Baken-ets* Hot 'n Spicy Skins) . . . . . . | 80 | 7.0 | <1.0 | 5.0 | 20 | 470 | <1.0 |
| (*Mission* Chicharrones Picante) . . . . . . . . . | 80 | 8.0 | 0 | 4.5 | 15 | 370 | 0 |
| **Pot pie**, see specific entree listings | | | | | | | |
| **Pot roast**, see "Beef" | | | | | | | |
| **Pot stickers entree**, frozen, Asian: | | | | | | | |
| (*Healthy Choice*), 10-oz. pkg. . . . . . . . . . | 380 | 8.0 | 75.0 | 4.5 | 5 | 600 | 6.0 |
| (*Lean Cuisine*), 9-oz. pkg. | 260 | 8.0 | 49.0 | 4.0 | 10 | 530 | 2.0 |
| chicken and vegetable (*Annie Chun's* Organic), 7 pcs., 5 oz. . . . . . . . | 220 | 14.0 | 32.0 | 3.5 | 25 | 620 | 2.0 |
| pork and vegetable (*Annie Chun's* Organic), 7 pcs., 5 oz. . . . . . . . | 260 | 12.0 | 32.0 | 10.0 | 30 | 600 | 2.0 |
| **Potato**: | | | | | | | |
| raw: | | | | | | | |
| (*Frieda's* Assorted Fingerling Bag), 4 pcs., 5.2 oz. . . . . | 100 | 4.0 | 25.0 | 0 | 0 | 0 | 3.0 |
| (*Frieda's* Baby/ Fingerling/Red/Purple/ Yukon Gold/Yellow Finnish), 3 oz. . . . . | 70 | 2.0 | 15.0 | 0 | 0 | 5 | 1.0 |
| (*Green Giant*), 5.2 oz. . | 100 | 3.0 | 24.0 | 0 | 0 | 10 | 3.0 |
| unpeeled: | | | | | | | |
| 1 large, 6.5 oz. . . . . | 145 | 3.8 | 33.1 | .2 | 0 | 11 | 2.9 |
| 1 long, 7.1 oz. . . . . | 160 | 4.2 | 36.3 | .2 | 0 | 12 | 3.2 |
| peeled, 2½" potato . . . | 88 | 2.3 | 20.1 | .1 | 0 | 7 | 1.8 |
| peeled, diced, ½ cup . | 59 | 1.6 | 13.5 | .1 | 0 | 5 | 1.2 |
| baked: | | | | | | | |
| in skin, 4¾" x 2⅓" . . . . | 220 | 4.7 | 51.0 | .2 | 0 | 16 | 4.8 |
| w/out skin, 2⅓" . . . . . . | 145 | 3.1 | 33.6 | .2 | 0 | 8 | 2.3 |

| Food and Measure | cal. | prot. (gms) | carbo. (gms) | fat (gms) | chol. (mgs) | sod. (mgs) | fiber (gms) |
|---|---|---|---|---|---|---|---|
| **Potato, baked** *(cont.)* | | | | | | | |
| w/out skin, ½ cup .... | 57 | 1.2 | 13.2 | .1 | 0 | 3 | .9 |
| skin only, 1 oz. ...... | 56 | 1.2 | 13.1 | 0 | 0 | 6 | 2.2 |
| boiled in skin, peeled: | | | | | | | |
| 2½" potato, 4.8 oz. ... | 118 | 2.5 | 27.4 | .1 | 0 | 6 | 2.4 |
| ½ cup ............. | 68 | 1.5 | 15.7 | .1 | 0 | 3 | 1.4 |
| boiled w/out skin: | | | | | | | |
| 2½" potato ......... | 116 | 2.3 | 27.0 | .1 | 0 | 7 | 2.4 |
| ½ cup ............. | 67 | 1.3 | 15.6 | .1 | 0 | 4 | 1.4 |
| microwaved in skin: | | | | | | | |
| w/skin, 4¾" x 2⅓" | | | | | | | |
| potato ........... | 212 | 4.9 | 48.7 | .2 | 0 | 16 | 4.7 |
| peeled, ½ cup ....... | 78 | 1.6 | 18.2 | .1 | 0 | 5 | 1.2 |
| skin only, 2 oz. ..... | 75 | 2.5 | 16.8 | .1 | 0 | 9 | 3.2 |
| mashed, w/whole milk: | | | | | | | |
| ½ cup ............. | 81 | 2.0 | 18.4 | .6 | 2 | 318 | 2.1 |
| w/butter, ½ cup ..... | 111 | 2.0 | 17.5 | 4.4 | 13 | 309 | 2.1 |
| w/margarine, ½ cup .. | 111 | 2.0 | 17.5 | 4.4 | 2 | 309 | 2.1 |
| **Potato, can/jar:** | | | | | | | |
| whole: | | | | | | | |
| (*Butterfield* New), | | | | | | | |
| 3.5 pcs. ......... | 90 | 2.0 | 20.00 | 0 | 330 | 2.0 | |
| (*Del Monte* New), | | | | | | | |
| 2 pcs. ........... | 60 | 1.0 | 13.0 | 0 | 0 | 360 | 2.0 |
| (*Roland* Belgian | | | | | | | |
| Miniature), ⅔ cup . | 90 | 3.0 | 20.0 | 0 | 0 | 370 | 2.0 |
| (*Sunshine*), 3 pcs. ... | 90 | 2.0 | 20.0 | 0 | 0 | 330 | 2.0 |
| (*S&W* Small), 2 pcs. .. | 60 | 1.0 | 13.0 | 0 | 0 | 360 | 2.0 |
| diced, new potato: | | | | | | | |
| (*Butterfield*), ⅔ cup .. | 100 | 2.0 | 22.0 | 0 | 0 | 350 | 3.0 |
| (*Del Monte*), ½ cup .. | 45 | 1.0 | 11.0 | 0 | 0 | 280 | <1.0 |
| sliced, new potato: | | | | | | | |
| (*Butterfield*), ½ cup .. | 100 | 2.0 | 22.0 | 0 | 0 | 390 | 4.0 |
| (*Del Monte*), ⅔ cup .. | 60 | 1.0 | 13.0 | 0 | 0 | 360 | 2.0 |
| **Potato, dried**, see "Potato dish, mix" | | | | | | | |
| **Potato, frozen/chilled** (see also "Potato dish, frozen"), 3 oz., except as noted: | | | | | | | |
| (*McCain Purely Potatoes*): | | | | | | | |
| baby, whole, skin-on .. | 100 | 2.0 | 16.0 | 0 | 0 | 25 | <1.0 |
| slices, russet ....... | 70 | 2.0 | 15.0 | 0 | 0 | 50 | 1.0 |

| Food and Measure | cal. | prot. (gms) | carbo. (gms) | fat (gms) | chol. (mgs) | sod. (mgs) | fiber (gms) |
|---|---|---|---|---|---|---|---|
| diced, w/onion (*Simply* *Potatoes*), ⅔ cup .... | 80 | 2.0 | 19.0 | 0 | 0 | 170 | 2.0 |
| fried/fries: | | | | | | | |
| (*McCain* 5-Minute) ... | 110 | 1.0 | 16.0 | 5.0 | 0 | 290 | 1.0 |
| (*McCain Classic Cut*) . | 100 | 1.0 | 15.0 | 3.5 | 0 | 290 | 1.0 |
| (*McCaim Cross Trax*) . | 160 | 2.0 | 21.0 | 8.0 | 0 | 470 | 2.0 |
| (*McCain Golden Crisp*) | 140 | 2.0 | 24.0 | 4.5 | 0 | 200 | 1.0 |
| (*Ore-Ida Country*) .... | 130 | 2.0 | 20.0 | 4.5 | 0 | 300 | 2.0 |
| (*Ore-Ida Crispers!*) ... | 220 | 2.0 | 23.0 | 13.0 | 0 | 390 | 2.0 |
| (*Ore-Ida Crispy* *Crunchies!*) ...... | 150 | 2.0 | 21.0 | 7.0 | 0 | 310 | 2.0 |
| (*Ore-Ida Fast Food* *Fries* Extra Crispy) . | 160 | 2.0 | 23.0 | 6.0 | 0 | 440 | 2.0 |
| (*Ore-Ida Golden Fries*) | 130 | 2.0 | 21.0 | 3.5 | 0 | 310 | 2.0 |
| (*Ore-Ida Golden Fries* Easy Extra Crispy) . | 180 | 2.0 | 25.0 | 8.0 | 0 | 450 | 2.0 |
| (*Ore-Ida Golden Twirls*) | 160 | 2.0 | 24.0 | 6.0 | 0 | 400 | 2.0 |
| (*Ore-Ida Zesty Twirls*) . | 160 | 2.0 | 22.0 | 6.0 | 0 | 350 | 2.0 |
| beer batter (*McCain*) .. | 140 | 2.0 | 21.0 | 5.0 | 0 | 310 | 2.0 |
| cottage (*Ore-Ida*) .... | 130 | 2.0 | 21.0 | 4.5 | 0 | 300 | 2.0 |
| julienne, Yukon gold (*Alexia* Organic) ... | 130 | 2.0 | 22.0 | 3.5 | 0 | 180 | 2.0 |
| olive oil, Parmesan/ roasted garlic (*Alexia Oven Reds*) . | 120 | 3.0 | 19.0 | 3.5 | 0 | 270 | 2.0 |
| olive oil/rosemary/ garlic (*Alexia Oven* *Fries*) .......... | 130 | 2.0 | 22.0 | 3.5 | 0 | 240 | 2.0 |
| olive oil/sea salt (*Alexia Oven Fries*) . | 90 | 2.0 | 16.0 | 2.0 | 0 | 230 | 2.0 |
| shoestring (*Cascadian Farm* Organic) .... | 140 | 2.0 | 21.0 | 5.0 | 0 | 15 | 2.0 |
| spirals, seasoned (*McCain*) ........ | 150 | 2.0 | 21.0 | 7.0 | 0 | 350 | 2.0 |
| steak (*McCain*) ...... | 100 | 1.0 | 16.0 | 3.0 | 0 | 280 | 1.0 |
| steak (*Ore-Ida*) ...... | 110 | 2.0 | 19.0 | 3.0 | 0 | 300 | 2.0 |
| steak (*Ore-Ida* Country) | 120 | 2.0 | 18.0 | 4.0 | 0 | 300 | 2.0 |
| straight cut (*Cascadian Farm* Organic) .... | 130 | 2.0 | 21.0 | 4.0 | 0 | 15 | 2.0 |
| waffle (*Ore-Ida*) ..... | 160 | 2.0 | 22.0 | 6.0 | 0 | 390 | 2.0 |
| waffle, seasoned salt (*Alexia*) ...... | 160 | 2.0 | 21.0 | 7.0 | 0 | 330 | 2.0 |
| wedges (*Cascadian Farm* Organic Oven Fries) | 100 | 2.0 | 17.0 | 2.5 | 0 | 10 | 2.0 |

## Potato, frozen/chilled, fried/fries *(cont.)*

| Food and Measure | cal. | prot. (gms) | carbo. (gms) | fat (gms) | chol. (mgs) | sod. (mgs) | fiber (gms) |
|---|---|---|---|---|---|---|---|
| wedges (*Ore-Ida Texas Crispers!*) ........ | 150 | 2.0 | 21.0 | 6.0 | 0 | 230 | 2.0 |
| wedges, seasoned (*McCain*) ........ | 120 | 2.0 | 17.0 | 5.0 | 0 | 390 | 2.0 |
| wedges, seasoned (*McCain Route 66*) . | 170 | 2.0 | 20.0 | 9.0 | 0 | 630 | 2.0 |
| fries, crinkle cut: | | | | | | | |
| (*Alexia Oven Crinkles Organic Classic*) ... | 120 | 2.0 | 19.0 | 4.0 | 0 | 170 | 3.0 |
| (*Cascadian Farm Organic*) ........ | 110 | 2.0 | 17.0 | 4.0 | 0 | 10 | 2.0 |
| (*McCain*) ........... | 110 | 1.0 | 20.0 | 5.0 | 0 | 290 | 1.0 |
| (*McCain Golden Crisp*) | 140 | 2.0 | 24.0 | 4.5 | 0 | 200 | 1.0 |
| (*Ore-Ida Golden Crinkles*) | 120 | 2.0 | 20.0 | 3.5 | 0 | 310 | 2.0 |
| (*Ore-Ida Golden Crinkles Easy Fries Extra Crispy*) ..... | 180 | 2.0 | 25.0 | 8.0 | 0 | 400 | 2.0 |
| (*Ore-Ida Golden Crinkles Extra Crispy*) | 170 | 2.0 | 24.0 | 7.0 | 0 | 410 | 2.0 |
| (*Ore-Ida Pixie Crinkles*) | 140 | 2.0 | 21.0 | 5.0 | 0 | 300 | 2.0 |
| onion/garlic (*Alexia Oven Crinkles Organic*) ........ | 110 | 2.0 | 18.0 | 3.5 | 0 | 190 | 3.0 |
| salt/pepper (*Alexia Oven Crinkles Organic*) ........ | 120 | 2.0 | 20.0 | 4.0 | 0 | 310 | 3.0 |
| seasoned (*McCain*) ... | 150 | 2.0 | 21.0 | 6.0 | 0 | 440 | 3.0 |
| seasoned (*Ore-Ida Extra Crispy*) ..... | 150 | 2.0 | 22.0 | 6.0 | 0 | 450 | 2.0 |
| hash browns: | | | | | | | |
| (*Alexia Organic*) ..... | 70 | 2.0 | 15.0 | 0 | 0 | 300 | 1.0 |
| (*Cascadian Farm Organic*) ........ | 60 | 2.0 | 14.0 | 0 | 0 | 10 | 1.0 |
| (*Ore-Ida Country*) .... | 70 | 2.0 | 16.0 | 0 | 0 | 2 | 2.0 |
| (*Ore-Ida Southern*) ... | 70 | 2.0 | 16.0 | 0 | 0 | 30 | 2.0 |
| (*Simply Potatoes Shredded*), ½ cup . | 70 | 1.0 | 16.0 | 0 | 0 | 55 | <2.0 |
| cheesy (*Ore-Ida Country Creations*) ....... | 150 | 3.0 | 14.0 | 6.0 | 10 | 490 | 2.0 |
| O'Brien (*Ore-Ida*) .... | 60 | 1.0 | 14.0 | 0 | 0 | 40 | 2.0 |
| w/peppers/onions (*Ore-Ida Country Creations*) ....... | 90 | 2.0 | 13.0 | 3.5 | 0 | 370 | 2.0 |

| Food and Measure | cal. | prot. (gms) | carbo. (gms) | fat (gms) | chol. (mgs) | sod. (mgs) | fiber (gms) |
|---|---|---|---|---|---|---|---|
| seasoned (*Ore-Ida* Country Creations) | 110 | 2.0 | 15.0 | 4.5 | 0 | 450 | 2.0 |
| Southwest (*Simply Potatoes*), ⅔ cup | 80 | 2.0 | 17.0 | 0 | 0 | 240 | 2.0 |
| hash browns, patties: | | | | | | | |
| (*Ore-Ida Golden Patties*) | 170 | 1.0 | 15.0 | 8.0 | 0 | 170 | 2.0 |
| shredded (*Ore-Ida*) | 70 | 2.0 | 16.0 | 0 | 0 | 35 | 2.0 |
| toaster (*Ore-Ida*), ½ of 7-oz. pkg. | 220 | 2.0 | 25.0 | 13.0 | 0 | 510 | 2.0 |
| mashed, ½ cup, except as noted: | | | | | | | |
| (*Bob Evans* Original) | 150 | 3.0 | 20.0 | 7.0 | 15 | 410 | 2.0 |
| (*Bob Evans* Single Serve), 6-oz. cont. | 210 | 4.0 | 28.0 | 9.0 | 20 | 570 | 3.0 |
| (*Hormel Country Crock* Homestyle), ⅔ cup | 160 | 2.0 | 18.0 | 9.0 | 15 | 510 | 1.0 |
| (*Simply Potatoes* Country Style) | 100 | 2.0 | 18.0 | 2.0 | 5 | 95 | 2.0 |
| (*Simply Potatoes* Country Style Diner's Choice/Family) | 100 | 2.0 | 16.0 | 3.5 | 10 | 190 | 2.0 |
| (*Simply Potatoes* Traditional) | 100 | 2.0 | 14.0 | 4.0 | 10 | 440 | 2.0 |
| (*Simply Potatoes* Traditional Diner's Choice/Family) | 120 | 2.0 | 15.0 | 6.0 | 20 | 420 | 2.0 |
| cheddar (*Bob Evans*) | 170 | 3.0 | 20.0 | 7.0 | 15 | 580 | 2.0 |
| garlic (*Bob Evans*) | 140 | 3.0 | 19.0 | 5.0 | 10 | 430 | 2.0 |
| garlic (*Hormel Country Crock*), ⅔ cup | 140 | 2.0 | 18.0 | 7.0 | 10 | 450 | 1.0 |
| garlic (*Simply Potatoes*) | 110 | 2.0 | 15.0 | 5.0 | 10 | 400 | 2.0 |
| garlic (*Simply Potatoes* Diner's Choice/ Family) | 120 | 2.0 | 15.0 | 6.0 | 20 | 430 | 2.0 |
| loaded (*Hormel Country Crock*), ⅔ cup | 190 | 4.0 | 18.0 | 11.0 | 20 | 440 | 1.0 |
| red, w/garlic, Parmesan (*Alexia*) | 170 | 4.0 | 23.0 | 6.0 | 15 | 370 | 2.0 |
| sour cream and chive (*Bob Evans*) | 150 | 3.0 | 20.0 | 6.0 | 10 | 420 | 2.0 |
| sour cream and chive (*Simply Potatoes*) | 110 | 3.0 | 16.0 | 4.5 | 10 | 330 | 2.0 |

| Food and Measure | cal. | prot. (gms) | carbo. (gms) | fat (gms) | chol. (mgs) | sod. (mgs) | fiber (gms) |
|---|---|---|---|---|---|---|---|
| **Potato, frozen/chilled, mashed** *(cont.)* | | | | | | | |
| sour cream and chive (*Simply Potatoes* Diner's Choice/ Family) . . . . . . . . . . | 120 | 2.0 | 15.0 | 5.5 | 20 | 420 | 2.0 |
| Southwest (*Bob Evans*) | 160 | 3.0 | 20.0 | 7.0 | 15 | 510 | 2.0 |
| Yukon gold, w/sea salt (*Alexia*) . . . . . . . . . | 150 | 3.0 | 21.0 | 5.0 | 15 | 330 | 1.0 |
| mashing (*Ore-Ida Steam n' Mash*): | | | | | | | |
| cut red, ½ pkg. . . . . . . | 70 | 2.0 | 15.0 | 0 | 0 | 270 | 1.0 |
| cut russet, ½ pkg. . . . | 80 | 2.0 | 17.0 | 0 | 0 | 260 | 2.0 |
| garlic, ½ pkg. . . . . . . . | 110 | 2.0 | 17.0 | 4.0 | 10 | 330 | 2.0 |
| w/onions, peppers (*Cascadian Farm Organic Country*) . . . . | 50 | 1.0 | 12.0 | 0 | 0 | 10 | 1.0 |
| puffs/nuggets: | | | | | | | |
| (*Cascadian Farm Spud Puppies Organic*) . . . . . . . . . | 160 | 2.0 | 23.0 | 7.0 | 0 | 400 | 2.0 |
| (*McCain Tasti Taters*) . | 150 | 2.0 | 19.0 | 7.0 | 0 | 370 | 2.0 |
| (*Ore-Ida Crispy Crowns*) | 170 | 2.0 | 21.0 | 10.0 | 0 | 490 | 2.0 |
| (*Ore-Ida Mini Tater Tots*) . . . . . . . . . . . . | 170 | 2.0 | 22.0 | 9.0 | 0 | 430 | 2.0 |
| (*Ore-Ida Tater Tots*) . . | 170 | 2.0 | 20.0 | 8.0 | 0 | 420 | 2.0 |
| (*Ore-Ida Tater Tots Extra Crispy*) . . . . . | 170 | 2.0 | 20.0 | 9.0 | 0 | 460 | 2.0 |
| onion (*Ore-Ida Tater Tots*) . . . . . . . . . . . | 170 | 2.0 | 23.0 | 8.0 | 0 | 350 | 2.0 |
| Yukon gold (*Alexia*) . . | 150 | 2.0 | 19.0 | 7.0 | 0 | 440 | 3.0 |
| roasted, seasoned: | | | | | | | |
| (*McCain Roasters All-American*) . . . . . | 130 | 2.0 | 21.0 | 3.5 | 0 | 420 | 3.0 |
| (*Ore-Ida Original*), 2.6 oz. . . . . . . . . . | 130 | 2.0 | 18.0 | 4.5 | 0 | 310 | 2.0 |
| chive butter (*Birds Eye Steamfresh Lightly Sauced*), 1 cup . . . . . . . . . . | 140 | 3.0 | 29.0 | 1.5 | 0 | 450 | 3.0 |
| garlic butter (*Birds Eye Steamfresh Lightly Sauced*), 1¼ cups . | 190 | 3.0 | 30.0 | 7.0 | 20 | 390 | 3.0 |
| garlic and onion (*McCain Roasters*) . | 120 | 2.0 | 21.0 | 3.0 | 0 | 520 | 2.0 |

| Food and Measure | cal. | prot. (gms) | carbo. (gms) | fat (gms) | chol. (mgs) | sod. (mgs) | fiber (gms) |
|---|---|---|---|---|---|---|---|
| garlic Parmesan (*Ore-Ida*) ........ | 140 | 2.0 | 21.0 | 5.0 | 0 | 370 | 2.0 |
| slices (*Simply Potatoes* Homestyle), ⅔ cup ... | 90 | 2.0 | 21.0 | 0 | 0 | 75 | 2.0 |
| wedges, red, ½ cup: (*Simply Potatoes*) .... | 50 | 2.0 | 10.0 | 0 | 0 | 250 | 2.0 |
| rosemary/garlic (*Simply Potatoes*) . | 50 | 2.0 | 11.0 | 0 | 0 | 250 | 2.0 |
| **Potato, mix**, see "Potato dish, mix" | | | | | | | |
| **Potato, sweet**, see "Sweet potato" | | | | | | | |
| **Potato chips/crisps** (see also "Potato soy crisps" and "Sweet potato chips"), 1 oz.: | | | | | | | |
| (*Bachman* Golden Crisp) ............. | 150 | 2.0 | 16.0 | 9.0 | 0 | 115 | 0 |
| (*Bachman Golden Ridges*) ............ | 160 | 2.0 | 15.0 | 10.0 | <5 | 140 | 0 |
| (*Cape Cod* Classic) .... | 150 | 2.0 | 17.0 | 8.0 | 0 | 110 | 1.0 |
| (*Cape Cod* 40% Reduced Fat) ....... | 130 | 2.0 | 18.0 | 6.0 | 0 | 110 | 1.0 |
| (*Cape Cod* Robust Russet) ............ | 150 | 2.0 | 16.0 | 8.0 | 0 | 150 | 1.0 |
| (*Herr's* Baked) ......... | 120 | 2.0 | 23.0 | 2.0 | 0 | 180 | 2.0 |
| (*Herr's* Kettle) ......... | 160 | 2.0 | 14.0 | 10.0 | 0 | 180 | 1.0 |
| (*Herr's* Kettle Reduced Fat) ....... | 135 | 2.0 | 18.0 | 6.0 | 0 | 180 | 1.0 |
| (*Herr's* Kettle Russet) ... | 140 | 2.0 | 16.0 | 8.0 | 0 | 180 | 1.0 |
| (*Herr's* Lightly Salted) ... | 140 | 2.0 | 16.0 | 8.0 | 0 | 90 | 1.0 |
| (*Herr's* No Salt) ........ | 140 | 2.0 | 16.0 | 8.0 | 0 | 10 | 1.0 |
| (*Herr's* Old Bay) ........ | 150 | 2.0 | 14.0 | 10.0 | 0 | 360 | 1.0 |
| (*Herr's* Original/ Ripples) ............ | 140 | 2.0 | 16.0 | 8.0 | 0 | 180 | 1.0 |
| (*Kettle* Baked Lightly Salted) ............. | 120 | 3.0 | 21.0 | 3.0 | 0 | 135 | 2.0 |
| (*Kettle* Organic Lightly Salted) ...... | 150 | 2.0 | 16.0 | 9.0 | 0 | 115 | 1.0 |
| (*Kettle* Unsalted) ....... | 150 | 2.0 | 16.0 | 9.0 | 0 | 5 | 2.0 |
| (*Kettle* Krinkle Cut Lightly Salted) ...... | 150 | 2.0 | 16.0 | 9.0 | 0 | 115 | 1.0 |
| (*Lay's* Classic/Wavy) ... | 150 | 2.0 | 15.0 | 10.0 | 0 | 180 | 1.0 |

| Food and Measure | cal. | prot. (gms) | carbo. (gms) | fat (gms) | chol. (mgs) | sod. (mgs) | fiber (gms) |
|---|---|---|---|---|---|---|---|
| **Potato chips/crisps** *(cont.)* | | | | | | | |
| (*Lay's* Kettle Original/ | | | | | | | |
| Crinkle) ............ | 150 | 2.0 | 18.0 | 8.0 | 0 | 110 | 1.0 |
| (*Lay's* Kettle | | | | | | | |
| Reduced Fat) ....... | 140 | 2.0 | 19.0 | 6.0 | 0 | 160 | 2.0 |
| (*Lay's* Lightly Salted) ... | 150 | 2.0 | 15.0 | 10.0 | 0 | 90 | 1.0 |
| (*Lay's* Original | | | | | | | |
| Baked!) ........... | 120 | 2.0 | 23.0 | 2.0 | 0 | 180 | 2.0 |
| (*Lay's* Original Light) .... | 75 | 2.0 | 17.0 | 0 | 0 | 200 | 1.0 |
| (*Lay's Stax* Original) .... | 150 | 2.0 | 16.0 | 9.0 | 0 | 160 | 1.0 |
| (*Maui Style*) .......... | 150 | 2.0 | 16.0 | 9.0 | 0 | 150 | 1.0 |
| (*Munchos* Crisps) ...... | 160 | 1.0 | 16.0 | 10.0 | 0 | 230 | 1.0 |
| (*Pringles* Original) ...... | 150 | 1.0 | 15.0 | 9.0 | 0 | 160 | 1.0 |
| (*Pringles* Original | | | | | | | |
| Light) ............ | 70 | 1.0 | 15.0 | 0 | 0 | 180 | 1.0 |
| (*Pringles* Original | | | | | | | |
| Reduced Fat) ....... | 130 | 1.0 | 17.0 | 7.0 | 0 | 135 | 1.0 |
| (*Ruffles* Baked!) ....... | 120 | 2.0 | 21.0 | 3.0 | 0 | 200 | 2.0 |
| (*Ruffles* Light) .......... | 70 | 2.0 | 17.0 | 0.0 | 0 | 190 | 1.0 |
| (*Ruffles* Original) ....... | 160 | 2.0 | 14.0 | 10.0 | 0 | 160 | 1.0 |
| (*Ruffles* Reduced Fat) .... | 140 | 2.0 | 18.0 | 7.0 | 0 | 180 | 1.0 |
| (*Snyder's* Ripple) ...... | 140 | 2.0 | 18.0 | 6.0 | 0 | 100 | 4.0 |
| (*Terra* Au Naturel) ...... | 150 | 2.0 | 15.0 | 9.0 | 0 | 0 | 2.0 |
| (*Terra* Kettles | | | | | | | |
| Arrabiata) .......... | 140 | 1.0 | 18.0 | 7.0 | 0 | 190 | 1.0 |
| (*Terra* Kettles | | | | | | | |
| Chesapeake Bay & Beer) | 140 | 1.0 | 18.0 | 7.0 | 0 | 140 | 1.0 |
| (*Terra* Kettles General | | | | | | | |
| Tso) .............. | 140 | 1.0 | 18.0 | 7.0 | 0 | 190 | 1.0 |
| (*Terra Blues*) .......... | 130 | 2.0 | 19.0 | 6.0 | 0 | 115 | 3.0 |
| (*Terra Potpourri*) ....... | 140 | 2.0 | 17.0 | 7.0 | 0 | 110 | 4.0 |
| (*Terra Red Bliss*) ....... | 140 | 1.0 | 18.0 | 7.0 | 0 | 110 | 2.0 |
| (*Terra Stix*) ........... | 150 | 1.0 | 16.0 | 9.0 | 0 | 110 | 3.0 |
| (*Terra Yukon Gold*) ..... | 130 | 2.0 | 19.0 | 5.0 | 0 | 80 | 0 |
| (*Wise* All Natural) ...... | 150 | 2.0 | 14.0 | 10.0 | 0 | 160 | 1.0 |
| (*Wise* Lightly Salted) .... | 150 | 2.0 | 14.0 | 10.0 | 0 | 80 | 1.0 |
| (*Wise* Unsalted) ....... | 150 | 2.0 | 14.0 | 10.0 | 0 | 0 | 1.0 |
| (*Wise* Wavy) .......... | 150 | 2.0 | 14.0 | 10.0 | 0 | 160 | 1.0 |
| (*Wise* New York Deli) ... | 150 | 2.0 | 15.0 | 9.0 | 0 | 170 | 1.0 |
| (*Wise* Ridgies) ........ | 150 | 2.0 | 14.0 | 10.0 | 0 | 160 | 1.0 |
| all varieties, except | | | | | | | |
| barbecue (*Genisoy* | | | | | | | |
| Bakes) ............ | 110 | 5.0 | 16.0 | 2.5 | 0 | 270 | 2.0 |
| au gratin (*Lay's* Wavy) .. | 150 | 2.0 | 14.0 | 10.0 | <5 | 200 | 1.0 |

| Food and Measure | cal. | prot. (gms) | carbo. (gms) | fat (gms) | chol. (mgs) | sod. (mgs) | fiber (gms) |
|---|---|---|---|---|---|---|---|
| baked potato: | | | | | | | |
|   fully loaded (*Kettle*) .. | 150 | 2.0 | 16.0 | 9.0 | 0 | 180 | 1.0 |
|   loaded (*Pringles*) .... | 150 | 1.0 | 15.0 | 9.0 | 0 | 150 | 1.0 |
| balsamic sweet onion | | | | | | | |
|   (*Lay's*) ............ | 160 | 2.0 | 16.0 | 10.0 | 0 | 160 | 1.0 |
| barbecue: | | | | | | | |
|   (*Bachman* Bar-B-Q) .. | 150 | 2.0 | 15.0 | 9.0 | <5 | 320 | 0 |
|   (*Genisoy* Bakes) ..... | 110 | 5.0 | 16.0 | 2.5 | 0 | 190 | 2.0 |
|   (*Herr's* Baked) ....... | 120 | 2.0 | 22.0 | 3.0 | 0 | 330 | 2.0 |
|   (*Herr's* BBQ) ....... | 150 | 2.0 | 14.0 | 10.0 | 0 | 240 | 1.0 |
|   (*Kettle* Backyard) .... | 150 | 2.0 | 15.0 | 9.0 | 0 | 400 | 2.0 |
|   (*Kettle Krinkle Cut*) ... | 150 | 2.0 | 15.0 | 9.0 | 0 | 170 | 2.0 |
|   (*Lay's*) ............ | 150 | 2.0 | 15.0 | 10.0 | 0 | 200 | 1.0 |
|   (*Lay's* Baked!) ....... | 120 | 2.0 | 23.0 | 3.0 | 0 | 210 | 2.0 |
|   (*Pringles*) .......... | 150 | 1.0 | 15.0 | 9.0 | 0 | 150 | 1.0 |
|   (*Pringles* Light) ...... | 70 | 1.0 | 15.0 | 0 | 0 | 150 | 1.0 |
|   (*Ruffles* Authentic) ... | 150 | 2.0 | 16.0 | 10.0 | 0 | 190 | 1.0 |
|   (*Snyder's*) .......... | 150 | 2.0 | 20.0 | 6.0 | 0 | 300 | 4.0 |
|   (*Wise* BBQ) ......... | 150 | 2.0 | 14.0 | 10.0 | 0 | 210 | 1.0 |
|   bold/spicy (*Alexia* | | | | | | | |
|     Waffle Fries) ...... | 140 | 1.0 | 18.0 | 7.0 | 0 | 200 | 1.0 |
|   chipotle (*Kettle* | | | | | | | |
|     Organic) ......... | 150 | 2.0 | 16.0 | 9.0 | 0 | 150 | 2.0 |
|   hickory (*Lay's* Wavy) . | 150 | 2.0 | 16.0 | 9.0 | 0 | 210 | 1.0 |
|   hickory (*Terra*) ....... | 150 | 2.0 | 15.0 | 9.0 | 0 | 5 | 1.0 |
|   hickory honey (*Kettle* | | | | | | | |
|     Baked) .......... | 120 | 3.0 | 21.0 | 3.0 | 0 | 160 | 2.0 |
|   honey (*Herr's* BBQ) ... | 150 | 2.0 | 14.0 | 10.0 | 0 | 280 | 1.0 |
|   honey (*Wise*) ....... | 150 | 1.0 | 15.0 | 10.0 | 0 | 190 | 1.0 |
|   hot/spicy (*Lay's*) ..... | 160 | 2.0 | 15.0 | 10.0 | 0 | 200 | 1.0 |
|   mesquite (*Herr's* | | | | | | | |
|     Kettle) .......... | 160 | 2.0 | 14.0 | 10.0 | 0 | 300 | 1.0 |
|   mesquite (*Lay's* | | | | | | | |
|     Kettle) .......... | 150 | 2.0 | 17.0 | 8.0 | 0 | 190 | 1.0 |
|   mesquite (*Lay's Stax*) . | 150 | 1.0 | 15.0 | 9.0 | 0 | 190 | 1.0 |
|   mesquite, sweet | | | | | | | |
|     (*Cape Cod*) ....... | 140 | 2.0 | 18.0 | 6.0 | 0 | 150 | 2.0 |
|   spice rubbed (*Lay's* | | | | | | | |
|     Kettle Crinkle) .... | 140 | 2.0 | 18.0 | 8.0 | 0 | 190 | 1.0 |
|   sweet (Pringles | | | | | | | |
|     Xtreme Sizzlin') ... | 150 | 1.0 | 15.0 | 9.0 | 0 | 135 | 1.0 |
|   tangy Carolina | | | | | | | |
|     (*Lay's*) .......... | 160 | 2.0 | 15.0 | 10.0 | 0 | 190 | 1.0 |

**Potato chips/crisps** *(cont.)*

| Food and Measure | cal. | prot. (gms) | carbo. (gms) | fat (gms) | chol. (mgs) | sod. (mgs) | fiber (gms) |
|---|---|---|---|---|---|---|---|
| Buffalo, bleu (*Kettle Krinkle Cut*) ........ | 150 | 2.0 | 16.0 | 9.0 | 0 | 170 | 1.0 |
| Buffalo, wing: | | | | | | | |
| (*Pringles* Xtreme) .... | 150 | 1.0 | 15.0 | 9.0 | 0 | 280 | 1.0 |
| (*Wise New York Deli* Kettle) ....... | 140 | 2.0 | 16.0 | 8.0 | 0 | 220 | 1.0 |
| hot (*Snyder's*) ....... | 140 | 2.0 | 20.0 | 6.0 | 0 | 290 | 4.0 |
| Cajun: | | | | | | | |
| (*Pringles* Xtreme Ragin') .......... | 150 | 1.0 | 15.0 | 9.0 | 0 | 140 | 1.0 |
| herb/spice (*Lay's*) .... | 160 | 2.0 | 15.0 | 10.0 | 0 | 180 | 1.0 |
| cheddar: | | | | | | | |
| (*Lay's Stax*) ......... | 150 | 1.0 | 15.0 | 10.0 | 0 | 190 | 1.0 |
| (*Pringles*) ........... | 150 | 1.0 | 15.0 | 9.0 | 0 | 150 | 1.0 |
| (*Pringles* Reduced Fat Savory) ....... | 130 | 1.0 | 17.0 | 7.0 | 0 | 150 | 1.0 |
| aged (*Alexia* Waffle Fries) ...... | 140 | 1.0 | 18.0 | 7.0 | 0 | 200 | 1.0 |
| barbecue (*Pringles* Family Favs) ...... | 150 | 2.0 | 15.0 | 9.0 | 0 | 180 | 1.0 |
| w/herbs (*Kettle* New York) ....... | 150 | 2.0 | 16.0 | 9.0 | 0 | 190 | 1.0 |
| sharp (*Lay's* Kettle) ... | 150 | 2.0 | 16.0 | 9.0 | 0 | 180 | 1.0 |
| white, aged (*Kettle* Baked) .......... | 120 | 3.0 | 20.0 | 3.0 | 0 | 170 | 2.0 |
| cheddar/horseradish (*Herr's* Kettle) ....... | 160 | 2.0 | 14.0 | 10.0 | 0 | 300 | 1.0 |
| cheddar/sour cream: | | | | | | | |
| (*Herr's*) ............ | 150 | 2.0 | 14.0 | 10.0 | 0 | 310 | 1.0 |
| (*Herr's* Baked) ....... | 120 | 2.0 | 22.0 | 3.0 | 0 | 330 | 2.0 |
| (*Kettle Krinkle Cut*) ... | 150 | 2.0 | 16.0 | 9.0 | 0 | 140 | 1.0 |
| (*Lay's*) ............ | 160 | 2.0 | 15.0 | 10.0 | <5 | 230 | <1.0 |
| (*Ruffles*) ........... | 160 | 2.0 | 14.0 | 11.0 | 0 | 230 | 1.0 |
| (*Ruffles* Baked!) ..... | 120 | 2.0 | 21.0 | 3.5 | 0 | 270 | 2.0 |
| (*Wise Ridgies*) ...... | 150 | 2.0 | 15.0 | 9.0 | 0 | 190 | 1.0 |
| cheese: | | | | | | | |
| 5 (*Cape Cod*) ....... | 150 | 2.0 | 17.0 | 8.0 | 0 | 210 | 1.0 |
| 3 (*Kettle* Tuscan) .... | 150 | 2.0 | 16.0 | 9.0 | 0 | 140 | 1.0 |
| cheese and chilies (*Lay's* Southwest) .... | 160 | 2.0 | 15.0 | 10.0 | 0 | 200 | 1.0 |
| chili limón (*Lay's*) ...... | 150 | 2.0 | 14.0 | 10.0 | 0 | 210 | 1.0 |
| chipotle (*Kettle Death Valley Chipotle*) ...... | 150 | 2.0 | 16.0 | 9.0 | 0 | 170 | 2.0 |

| Food and Measure | cal. | prot. (gms) | carbo. (gms) | fat (gms) | chol. (mgs) | sod. (mgs) | fiber (gms) |
|---|---|---|---|---|---|---|---|
| dill: | | | | | | | |
| (*Lay's* Pickle) . . . . . . . | 160 | 2.0 | 13.0 | 10.0 | 0 | 360 | 1.0 |
| (*Pringles* Xtreme) . . . . | 150 | 1.0 | 15.0 | 9.0 | 0 | 110 | 1.0 |
| (*Snyder's* Kosher) . . . . | 140 | 2.0 | 20.0 | 6.0 | 0 | 360 | 4.0 |
| garlic: | | | | | | | |
| mashed (*Terra* Crinkles Yukon Gold) . . . . . . . . . . | 130 | 2.0 | 19.0 | 6.0 | 0 | 170 | 2.0 |
| roasted, Parmesan (*Terra Red Bliss*) . . | 140 | 2.0 | 16.0 | 7.0 | 0 | 115 | 2.0 |
| herbs, fine (*Terra Red Bliss*) . . . . . . . . . . . . . | 140 | 2.0 | 18.0 | 7.0 | 0 | 70 | 3.0 |
| honey: | | | | | | | |
| Dijon (*Kettle*) . . . . . . . | 150 | 2.0 | 16.0 | 9.0 | 0 | 160 | 1.0 |
| mustard (*Pringles*) . . . | 150 | 1.0 | 15.0 | 9.0 | 0 | 140 | 1.0 |
| hot: | | | | | | | |
| (*Herr's* Red Hot) . . . . . | 150 | 2.0 | 14.0 | 10.0 | 0 | 300 | 1.0 |
| (*Lay's* Flamin' Hot) . . . | 160 | 2.0 | 15.0 | 10.0 | 0 | 200 | 1.0 |
| pepper (*Alexia* Waffle Fries) . . . . . . . . . . . | 140 | 1.0 | 18.0 | 7.0 | 0 | 200 | 1.0 |
| jalapeño: | | | | | | | |
| (*Herr's* Kettle) . . . . . . . | 160 | 2.0 | 14.0 | 10.0 | 0 | 300 | 1.0 |
| (*Kettle*) . . . . . . . . . . . . | 150 | 2.0 | 16.0 | 9.0 | 0 | 200 | 1.0 |
| (*Lay's* Kettle) . . . . . . . | 140 | 2.0 | 16.0 | 8.0 | 0 | 170 | 1.0 |
| (*Pringles*) . . . . . . . . . . | 150 | 1.0 | 15.0 | 9.0 | 0 | 180 | 1.0 |
| (*Snyder's*) . . . . . . . . . . | 150 | 2.0 | 20.0 | 6.0 | 0 | 330 | 4.0 |
| (*Wise New York Deli*) . | 140 | 2.0 | 16.0 | 8.0 | 0 | 210 | 1.0 |
| chili (*Terra* Crinkles Blue) . . . . . . . . . . | 140 | 2.0 | 20.0 | 6.0 | 0 | 150 | 3.0 |
| sweet/spicy (*Cape Cod*) . . . . . . . . . . . | 150 | 2.0 | 16.0 | 8.0 | 0 | 160 | 1.0 |
| jalapeño/cheddar (*Wise*) . . . . . . . . . . . . . | 150 | 2.0 | 14.0 | 10.0 | 0 | 220 | <1.0 |
| ketchup (*Herr's Heinz*) . . | 150 | 2.0 | 15.0 | 10.0 | 0 | 300 | 1.0 |
| lemon pepper (*Terra* Unsalted) . . . . . . . . . . | 150 | 2.0 | 15.0 | 10.0 | 0 | 5 | 1.0 |
| lime (*Lay's* Limón) . . . . . | 160 | 2.0 | 15.0 | 10.0 | 0 | 370 | 1.0 |
| Mexican layered (*Pringles* Cravers) . . . . | 150 | 1.0 | 13.0 | 11.0 | 0 | 210 | 1.0 |
| mozzarella/marinara (*Pringles* Cravers) . . . . | 150 | 1.0 | 15.0 | 9.0 | 0 | 190 | 1.0 |
| onion: | | | | | | | |
| (*Lay's* Kettle Maui) . . . | 150 | 2.0 | 17.0 | 9.0 | 0 | 140 | 1.0 |

| Food and Measure | cal. | prot. (gms) | carbo. (gms) | fat (gms) | chol. (mgs) | sod. (mgs) | fiber (gms) |
|---|---|---|---|---|---|---|---|
| **Potato chips/crisps, onion** *(cont.)* | | | | | | | |
| (*Maui Style*) ........ | 150 | 2.0 | 17.0 | 9.0 | 0 | 140 | 1.0 |
| blossom (*Pringles* | | | | | | | |
| Cravers) ......... | 150 | 1.0 | 14.0 | 11.0 | 0 | 230 | 1.0 |
| sweet (*Kettle*) ....... | 150 | 2.0 | 16.0 | 9.0 | 0 | 150 | 1.0 |
| onion and garlic: | | | | | | | |
| (*Terra Yukon Gold*) ... | 130 | 2.0 | 19.0 | 5.0 | 0 | 65 | 1.0 |
| (*Wise*) ............. | 150 | 2.0 | 14.0 | 10.0 | 0 | 200 | 1.0 |
| Parmesan and: | | | | | | | |
| roasted garlic | | | | | | | |
| (*Cape Cod*) ....... | 140 | 2.0 | 17.0 | 7.0 | 0 | 230 | 1.0 |
| Tuscan herb (*Lay's* | | | | | | | |
| Baked!) ......... | 120 | 2.0 | 21.0 | 3.0 | 0 | 210 | 2.0 |
| pepper relish (*Lay's*) .... | 160 | 2.0 | 16.0 | 10.0 | 0 | 160 | 1.0 |
| pesto/smoked mozzarella | | | | | | | |
| (*Terra Kettles*) ....... | 140 | 1.0 | 18.0 | 7.0 | 0 | 200 | 1.0 |
| pizza flavor (*Pringles*) ... | 150 | 1.0 | 15.0 | 9.0 | 0 | 180 | 1.0 |
| ranch: | | | | | | | |
| (*Alexia* Waffle Fries) .. | 140 | 1.0 | 18.0 | 7.0 | 0 | 200 | 1.0 |
| (*Lay's* Baked! | | | | | | | |
| Southwestern) .... | 120 | 2.0 | 21.0 | 3.0 | 0 | 160 | 2.0 |
| (*Lay's* Kettle Harvest) . | 150 | 2.0 | 16.0 | 8.0 | 0 | 200 | 1.0 |
| (*Lay's* Wavy) ........ | 150 | 2.0 | 16.0 | 10.0 | 0 | 200 | 1.0 |
| (*Lay's Stax*) ......... | 150 | 1.0 | 15.0 | 9.0 | 0 | 180 | 1.0 |
| (*Pringles*) ......... | 150 | 1.0 | 15.0 | 9.0 | 0 | 190 | 1.0 |
| bacon (*Pringles*) ..... | 150 | 1.0 | 15.0 | 9.0 | 0 | 160 | 1.0 |
| salt and pepper: | | | | | | | |
| (*Herr's*) ............. | 150 | 2.0 | 14.0 | 10.0 | 0 | 420 | 1.0 |
| (*Terra Yukon Gold*) ... | 130 | 2.0 | 19.0 | 5.0 | 0 | 120 | 1.0 |
| (*Wise New York Deli*) . | 140 | 2.0 | 16.0 | 8.0 | 0 | 210 | 1.0 |
| fresh ground (*Kettle* | | | | | | | |
| Baked) .......... | 120 | 2.0 | 21.0 | 3.0 | 0 | 120 | 2.0 |
| fresh ground (*Kettle* | | | | | | | |
| Organic) ......... | 150 | 2.0 | 16.0 | 9.0 | 0 | 200 | 2.0 |
| fresh ground (*Kettle* | | | | | | | |
| Krinkle Cut*) ...... | 150 | 2.0 | 16.0 | 9.0 | 0 | 190 | 2.0 |
| sea salt (*Terra* | | | | | | | |
| Kettles Krinkle Cut) | 150 | 1.0 | 15.0 | 10.0 | 0 | 140 | 1.0 |
| sea salt/cracked | | | | | | | |
| pepper (*Cape Cod*) . | 140 | 2.0 | 16.0 | 7.0 | 0 | 160 | 1.0 |
| sea salt/cracked | | | | | | | |
| pepper (*Lay's* | | | | | | | |
| Kettle) .......... | 150 | 2.0 | 16.0 | 9.0 | 0 | 160 | 1.0 |

| Food and Measure | cal. | prot. (gms) | carbo. (gms) | fat (gms) | chol. (mgs) | sod. (mgs) | fiber (gms) |
|---|---|---|---|---|---|---|---|
| salt and vinegar: | | | | | | | |
| (*Herr's*) . . . . . . . . . . . | 150 | 2.0 | 14.0 | 10.0 | 0 | 340 | 1.0 |
| (*Herr's* Kettle | | | | | | | |
| Boardwalk) . . . . . . . | 140 | 2.0 | 16.0 | 8.0 | 0 | 300 | 1.0 |
| (*Lay's*) . . . . . . . . . . | 150 | 2.0 | 15.0 | 10.0 | 0 | 380 | 1.0 |
| (*Lay's Stax*) . . . . . . . . | 150 | 1.0 | 14.0 | 9.0 | 0 | 230 | 1.0 |
| (*Pringles*) . . . . . . . . . | 150 | 1.0 | 15.0 | 9.0 | 0 | 220 | 1.0 |
| (*Snyder's*) . . . . . . . . . | 140 | 2.0 | 19.0 | 6.0 | 0 | 250 | 4.0 |
| (*Terra Yukon Gold*) . . . | 130 | 2.0 | 20.0 | 5.0 | 0 | 110 | 2.0 |
| (*Wise*) . . . . . . . . . . . . | 150 | 2.0 | 14.0 | 10.0 | 0 | 290 | 1.0 |
| (*Wise New York Deli*) . | 140 | 2.0 | 16.0 | 8.0 | 0 | 240 | 1.0 |
| sea salt (*Cape Cod*) . . . | 150 | 2.0 | 15.0 | 8.0 | 0 | 170 | 1.0 |
| sea salt (*Cape Cod* | | | | | | | |
| 40% Less Fat) . . . . | 130 | 2.0 | 18.0 | 6.0 | 0 | 220 | 2.0 |
| sea salt (*Kettle*) . . . . . . | 150 | 2.0 | 16.0 | 9.0 | 0 | 190 | 1.0 |
| sea salt (*Kettle* | | | | | | | |
| Baked) . . . . . . . . . | 120 | 2.0 | 21.0 | 3.0 | 0 | 170 | 2.0 |
| sea salt (*Lay's* | | | | | | | |
| Kettle) . . . . . . . . . | 150 | 2.0 | 16.0 | 8.0 | 0 | 250 | 1.0 |
| sea salt: | | | | | | | |
| (*Kettle*) . . . . . . . . . . . | 150 | 2.0 | 16.0 | 9.0 | 0 | 115 | 1.0 |
| (*Ruffles* Natural | | | | | | | |
| Reduced Fat) . . . . . | 140 | 2.0 | 17.0 | 7.0 | 0 | 160 | 1.0 |
| (*Terra* Kettles Crinkle | | | | | | | |
| Cut) . . . . . . . . . . . | 140 | 1.0 | 18.0 | 7.0 | 0 | 100 | 1.0 |
| sour cream/onion: | | | | | | | |
| (*Bachman*) . . . . . . . . . | 150 | 2.0 | 15.0 | 9.0 | <5 | 240 | 0 |
| (*Herr's*) . . . . . . . . . . . | 150 | 2.0 | 14.0 | 10.0 | 0 | 310 | 1.0 |
| (*Herr's* Baked) . . . . . . . | 120 | 2.0 | 22.0 | 3.0 | 0 | 330 | 2.0 |
| (*Herr's* Kettle) . . . . . . . | 140 | 2.0 | 16.0 | 8.0 | 0 | 310 | 1.0 |
| (*Lay's*) . . . . . . . . . . | 160 | 2.0 | 15.0 | 10.0 | 0 | 210 | 1.0 |
| (*Lay's* Baked!) . . . . . . . | 120 | 2.0 | 21.0 | 3.0 | 0 | 210 | 2.0 |
| (*Lay's Stax*) . . . . . . . . | 150 | 1.0 | 15.0 | 10.0 | 0 | 190 | 1.0 |
| (*Pringles*) . . . . . . . . . . | 150 | 1.0 | 15.0 | 9.0 | 0 | 150 | 1.0 |
| (*Pringles* Light) . . . . . . | 70 | 2.0 | 15.0 | 0 | 0 | 190 | 1.0 |
| (*Pringles* Reduced Fat) | 130 | 1.0 | 17.0 | 7.0 | 0 | 180 | 1.0 |
| (*Ruffles*) . . . . . . . . . . . | 160 | 2.0 | 14.0 | 11.0 | 0 | 190 | 1.0 |
| (*Snyder's*) . . . . . . . . . | 150 | 2.0 | 20.0 | 6.0 | 0 | 210 | 4.0 |
| (*Wise Ridgies*) . . . . . . | 150 | 2.0 | 14.0 | 10.0 | 0 | 220 | 1.0 |
| and chive (*Kettle*) . . . . | 150 | 2.0 | 16.0 | 9.0 | 0 | 100 | 1.0 |
| green onion (*Cape* | | | | | | | |
| *Cod*) . . . . . . . . . . . . | 140 | 2.0 | 16.0 | 8.0 | 0 | 220 | 1.0 |
| steak flavor (*Herr's* | | | | | | | |
| Kansas City Prime) . . . | 150 | 2.0 | 14.0 | 10.0 | 0 | 360 | 1.0 |

| Food and Measure | cal. | prot. (gms) | carbo. (gms) | fat (gms) | chol. (mgs) | sod. (mgs) | fiber (gms) |
|---|---|---|---|---|---|---|---|
| **Potato chips/crisps** *(cont.)* | | | | | | | |
| sun-dried tomato/ | | | | | | | |
| balsamic vinegar | | | | | | | |
| (*Terra Red Bliss*) . . . . . | 140 | 2.0 | 18.0 | 7.0 | 0 | 85 | 3.0 |
| Thai, spicy (*Kettle*) . . . . . | 150 | 2.0 | 16.0 | 9.0 | 0 | 150 | 1.0 |
| tomato/basil, garden | | | | | | | |
| (*Lay's*) . . . . . . . . . . . . | 160 | 2.0 | 16.0 | 10.0 | 0 | 170 | 1.0 |
| vinegar (*Bachman*) . . . . . | 150 | 1.0 | 15.0 | 10.0 | <5 | 240 | 0 |
| yogurt/green onion | | | | | | | |
| (*Kettle*) . . . . . . . . . . . . | 150 | 2.0 | 16.0 | 9.0 | 0 | 150 | 1.0 |
| **Potato dish, canned,** | | | | | | | |
| au gratin (*Del Monte* | | | | | | | |
| *Savory Sides*), ½ cup . | 80 | 2.0 | 13.0 | 2.5 | 0 | 470 | 1.0 |
| **Potato dish, frozen** | | | | | | | |
| (see also "Potato, | | | | | | | |
| frozen/chilled"): | | | | | | | |
| au gratin (*Boston* | | | | | | | |
| *Market*), 5.4 oz. . . . . . | 210 | 8.0 | 23.0 | 9.0 | 25 | 380 | 3.0 |
| baby blend, w/ | | | | | | | |
| vegetables (*Birds Eye* | | | | | | | |
| *Steamfresh*), ¾ cup . . | 40 | 1.0 | 8.0 | 0 | 0 | 20 | 1.0 |
| baked, twice, 1 pc.: | | | | | | | |
| butter (*Ore-Ida*) . . . . . | 170 | 5.0 | 27.0 | 5.0 | 0 | 330 | 2.0 |
| cheddar (*Ore-Ida*) . . . . | 190 | 5.0 | 28.0 | 6.0 | 10 | 460 | 3.0 |
| sour cream/chive | | | | | | | |
| (*Ore-Ida*) . . . . . . . . | 180 | 5.0 | 26.0 | 7.0 | 10 | 450 | 3.0 |
| cakes/pancakes, see | | | | | | | |
| "Potato pancake" | | | | | | | |
| cheddar: | | | | | | | |
| (*Lean Cuisine* | | | | | | | |
| Deluxe), 10.4 oz. . . | 260 | 14.0 | 36.0 | 7.0 | 20 | 600 | 4.0 |
| (*Stouffer's* Bake), | | | | | | | |
| ½ of 10-oz. pkg. . . . . | 270 | 9.0 | 21.0 | 17.0 | 20 | 500 | 2.0 |
| w/broccoli (*Lean* | | | | | | | |
| *Cuisine*), 10.4 oz. . . | 230 | 12.0 | 35.0 | 6.0 | 15 | 640 | 4.0 |
| mashed (*Boston* | | | | | | | |
| *Market*), 5 oz. . . . . . . . | 170 | 3.0 | 21.0 | 8.0 | 5 | 470 | 2.0 |
| mashed (*Larry's*), 5 oz.: | | | | | | | |
| bacon/cheddar . . . . . . | 200 | 5.0 | 23.0 | 10.0 | 10 | 650 | 1.0 |
| bacon/onion/tomato . . | 180 | 3.0 | 25.0 | 8.0 | 5 | 650 | 2.0 |
| broccoli/cheddar . . . . . | 180 | 3.0 | 22.0 | 8.0 | 5 | 390 | 2.0 |
| cheddar . . . . . . . . . . . | 190 | 4.0 | 25.0 | 8.0 | 5 | 460 | 2.0 |
| sour cream/chives . . . | 180 | 3.0 | 25.0 | 8.0 | 5 | 440 | 2.0 |

| Food and Measure | cal. | prot. (gms) | carbo. (gms) | fat (gms) | chol. (mgs) | sod. (mgs) | fiber (gms) |
|---|---|---|---|---|---|---|---|
| roasted, w/broccoli, cheese sauce: | | | | | | | |
| (*Birds Eye*), ⅔ cup ... | 100 | 2.0 | 15.0 | 3.5 | 0 | 470 | 1.0 |
| (*Green Giant* Bag), 1 cup .......... | 110 | 4.0 | 20.0 | 2.0 | 0 | 640 | 2.0 |
| cheddar (*Smart Ones*), 10-oz. pkg. ....... | 240 | 10.0 | 35.0 | 7.0 | 20 | 520 | 4.0 |
| roasted, w/garlic, herbs: | | | | | | | |
| (*Green Giant* Bag), ½ cup* .......... | 90 | 2.0 | 15.0 | 2.0 | 0 | 420 | 1.0 |
| (*Green Giant* Box), ½ of 9-oz. box .... | 200 | 3.0 | 33.0 | 7.0 | 0 | 420 | 2.0 |
| roasted, w/green beans, rosemary butter (*Green Giant Valley Fresh Steamers*), ¾ cup* ... | 80 | 2.0 | 16.0 | 1.0 | 0 | 330 | 2.0 |
| skins (*Health is Wealth*), 2 pcs., 2.7 oz. ....... | 110 | 5.0 | 8.0 | 7.0 | 15 | 440 | 1.0 |
| **Potato dish, microwave:** | | | | | | | |
| w/chickpeas, tomato (*Tasty Bite* Bombay), ½ of 10-oz. pkg. ..... | 100 | 5.0 | 13.0 | 4.0 | 0 | 410 | 3.0 |
| scalloped, and ham (*Dinty Moore* Micro Cup), 7.5 oz. ........ | 240 | 9.0 | 20.0 | 13.0 | 35 | 1020 | 2.0 |
| w/spinach (*Tasty Bite* Aloo Palak), ½ of 10-oz. pkg. ....... | 100 | 3.0 | 13.0 | 3.0 | 0 | 400 | 3.0 |
| **Potato dish, mix**, ½ cup*, except as noted: | | | | | | | |
| (*Betty Crocker Seasoned Skillet* Traditional) ......... | 180 | 2.0 | 22.0 | 9.0 | 0 | 490 | 2.0 |
| au gratin: | | | | | | | |
| (*Betty Crocker*) ...... | 150 | 2.0 | 23.0 | 5.0 | <5 | 640 | 1.0 |
| (*Betty Crocker* Deluxe Loaded) ... | 140 | 3.0 | 24.0 | 4.0 | 5 | 660 | 1.0 |
| (*Hungry Jack*) ....... | 100 | 2.0 | 21.0 | 1.0 | 0 | 570 | 2.0 |
| cheesy (*Velveeta*), ⅕ pkg. .......... | 180 | 5.0 | 26.0 | 6.0 | 10 | 780 | 2.0 |
| cheesy cheddar (*Betty Crocker* Deluxe) ... | 180 | 3.0 | 23.0 | 8.0 | 5 | 700 | 1.0 |
| baked (*Betty Crocker* Loaded), ⅔ cup* .... | 150 | 3.0 | 23.0 | 6.0 | <5 | 650 | 1.0 |

| Food and Measure | cal. | prot. (gms) | carbo. (gms) | fat (gms) | chol. (mgs) | sod. (mgs) | fiber (gms) |
|---|---|---|---|---|---|---|---|
| **Potato dish, mix** *(cont.)* | | | | | | | |
| cheddar and bacon: | | | | | | | |
| (*Betty Crocker*), ⅔ cup* | 150 | 2.0 | 23.0 | 5.0 | 0 | 690 | 1.0 |
| (*Hungry Jack*), 1 oz. | 100 | 2.0 | 21.0 | 1.5 | 0 | 480 | 1.0 |
| cheese: | | | | | | | |
| 4 (*Hungry Jack*) | 100 | 3.0 | 20.0 | 1.5 | 0 | 530 | 2.0 |
| 3 (*Betty Crocker*) | 120 | 2.0 | 23.0 | 3.0 | 0 | 630 | 1.0 |
| 3 (*Betty Crocker Deluxe*), ⅔ cup* | 150 | 3.0 | 25.0 | 9.0 | <5 | 770 | 1.0 |
| garlic, roasted: | | | | | | | |
| (*Betty Crocker*) | 120 | 2.0 | 21.0 | 3.5 | 0 | 520 | 1.0 |
| herb (*Betty Crocker Seasoned Skillets*), ⅔ cup* | 170 | 2.0 | 21.0 | 9.0 | 0 | 410 | 2.0 |
| hash browns: | | | | | | | |
| (*Betty Crocker Seasoned Skillets*) | 120 | 2.0 | 18.0 | 4.0 | 0 | 440 | 2.0 |
| (*Hungry Jack*), ⅓ cup | 60 | 1.0 | 14.0 | 0 | 0 | 280 | 1.0 |
| jalapeño cheddar (*Hungry Jack*) | 100 | 2.0 | 22.0 | 1.5 | 0 | 420 | 1.0 |
| julienne (*Betty Crocker*), ⅔ cup* | 140 | 2.0 | 21.0 | 5.0 | <5 | 670 | 1.0 |
| mashed: | | | | | | | |
| (*Betty Crocker Loaded*), ⅔ cup* | 160 | 3.0 | 18.0 | 8.0 | 25 | 530 | 1.0 |
| (*Betty Crocker Loaded Pouch*), ⅔ cup* | 80 | 2.0 | 17.0 | 1.0 | 5 | 480 | 3.0 |
| (*Betty Crocker Potato Buds*), ⅔ cup* | 140 | 3.0 | 20.0 | 6.0 | 0 | 440 | 1.0 |
| (*Hungry Jack Original*), ⅓ cup | 80 | 2.0 | 19.0 | 0 | 0 | 20 | 1.0 |
| (*Hungry Jack Easy Mash'd Homestyle*), ¼ cup | 90 | 2.0 | 19.0 | 1.0 | 0 | 420 | 1.0 |
| (*Hungry Jack Idaho Spuds*), ⅓ cup | 80 | 2.0 | 17.0 | 0 | 0 | 20 | 2.0 |
| (*Idahoan Original*), ⅓ cup | 80 | 2.0 | 18.0 | 0 | 0 | 15 | 2.0 |
| baked, hearty (*Hungry Jack Easy Mash'd*), ¼ cup | 90 | 2.0 | 19.0 | 1.0 | 0 | 350 | 2.0 |
| baked flavor, loaded (*Idahoan*) | 110 | 2.0 | 20.0 | 2.5 | 0 | 500 | 1.0 |

| Food and Measure | cal. | prot. (gms) | carbo. (gms) | fat (gms) | chol. (mgs) | sod. (mgs) | fiber (gms) |
|---|---|---|---|---|---|---|---|
| butter, creamy (*Betty Crocker*), ⅔ cup* | 140 | 3.0 | 18.0 | 7.0 | 20 | 440 | 1.0 |
| butter, creamy (*Betty Crocker* Pouch), ⅔ cup* | 80 | 2.0 | 17.0 | 1.0 | <5 | 460 | 3.0 |
| butter, creamy (*Hungry Jack Easy Mash'd*), ¼ cup | 90 | 2.0 | 19.0 | 1.0 | 0 | 420 | 1.0 |
| butter herb (*Betty Crocker*), ⅔ cup* | 140 | 3.0 | 18.0 | 7.0 | 0 | 460 | 1.0 |
| butter herb (*Idahoan*) | 110 | 2.0 | 20.0 | 3.0 | 0 | 520 | 1.0 |
| buttery (*Idahoan Homestyle*) | 110 | 2.0 | 20.0 | 3.0 | 0 | 450 | 1.0 |
| cheddar and sour cream (*Betty Crocker* Pouch), ⅔ cup* | 80 | 2.0 | 18.0 | 1.0 | 0 | 470 | 3.0 |
| cheese, 4 (*Betty Crocker*), ⅔ cup* | 140 | 3.0 | 18.0 | 6.0 | 15 | 490 | 1.0 |
| cheese, 4 (*Idahoan*) | 100 | 2.0 | 20.0 | 2.5 | 0 | 590 | 1.0 |
| cheese, white (*Idahoan Italian Romano*) | 110 | 2.0 | 20.0 | 2.5 | 0 | 560 | 1.0 |
| cheesy (*Hungry Jack Easy Mash'd Homestyle*), ¼ cup | 90 | 2.0 | 18.0 | 1.5 | 0 | 460 | 1.0 |
| cheesy (*Hungry Jack Easy Mash'd Supreme*), ¼ cup | 90 | 2.0 | 19.0 | 1.0 | 0 | 350 | 2.0 |
| cheesy (*Velveeta* Twin), ⅛ pkg. | 140 | 4.0 | 19.0 | 5.0 | 10 | 460 | 1.0 |
| garlic, roasted (*Betty Crocker*), ⅔ cup* | 140 | 3.0 | 18.0 | 6.0 | 15 | 450 | 1.0 |
| garlic, roasted (*Betty Crocker* Pouch), ⅔ cup* | 80 | 2.0 | 17.0 | 1.0 | <5 | 420 | 3.0 |
| garlic, roasted (*Hungry Jack Easy Mash'd*), ¼ cup | 90 | 2.0 | 19.0 | 1.0 | 0 | 310 | 2.0 |
| garlic, roasted (*Idahoan*) | 110 | 2.0 | 20.0 | 3.0 | 0 | 590 | 1.0 |
| garlic, roasted, Parmesan (*Idahoan*) | 110 | 3.0 | 21.0 | 2.0 | 0 | 560 | 2.0 |
| reds (*Betty Crocker* Pouch), ⅔ cup* | 80 | 2.0 | 17.0 | 1.5 | <5 | 480 | 3.0 |

| Food and Measure | cal. | prot. (gms) | carbo. (gms) | fat (gms) | chol. (mgs) | sod. (mgs) | fiber (gms) |
|---|---|---|---|---|---|---|---|
| **Potato dish, mix, mashed** *(cont.)* | | | | | | | |
| reds, baby (*Idahoan*) | 110 | 2.0 | 21.0 | 3.0 | 0 | 400 | 2.0 |
| redskin/Yukon gold (*Hungry Jack*), ⅓ cup | 80 | 2.0 | 18.0 | 0 | 0 | 10 | 2.0 |
| sour cream chive (*Betty Crocker*), ⅔ cup* | 160 | 3.0 | 18.0 | 6.0 | 20 | 450 | 1.0 |
| sour cream chive (*Hungry Jack Easy Mash'd*), ¼ cup | 90 | 1.0 | 20.0 | 1.0 | 0 | 410 | 1.0 |
| Southwest (*Idahoan*) | 110 | 2.0 | 20.0 | 3.0 | 0 | 500 | 2.0 |
| Yukon gold (*Betty Crocker*) | 140 | 3.0 | 20.0 | 5.0 | 5 | 440 | 1.0 |
| sea salt/cracked pepper (*Hungry Jack*) | 100 | 2.0 | 22.0 | 1.0 | 0 | 380 | 2.0 |
| scalloped: | | | | | | | |
| (*Betty Crocker*), ⅔ cup* | 130 | 3.0 | 23.0 | 3.0 | <5 | 640 | 1.0 |
| cheesy (*Betty Crocker*) | 140 | 2.0 | 22.0 | 5.0 | 0 | 690 | 2.0 |
| cheesy (*Hungry Jack*) | 100 | 2.0 | 21.0 | 1.0 | 0 | 580 | 2.0 |
| cheesy, bacon (*Velveeta*), ⅕ pkg. | 190 | 6.0 | 26.0 | 7.0 | 15 | 250 | 2.0 |
| creamy (*Hungry Jack*) | 100 | 2.0 | 21.0 | 1.0 | 0 | 400 | 2.0 |
| sour cream and chive: | | | | | | | |
| (*Betty Crocker*), ⅔ cup* | 130 | 3.0 | 23.0 | 3.5 | <5 | 740 | 1.0 |
| (*Hungry Jack*) | 110 | 2.0 | 20.0 | 2.5 | 0 | 450 | 2.0 |
| **Potato flour**: | | | | | | | |
| (*Bob's Red Mill*), ¼ cup | 120 | 3.0 | 27.0 | .5 | 0 | 10 | 2.0 |
| 1 cup | 571 | 11.0 | 132.9 | .5 | 0 | 88 | 9.4 |
| **Potato pancake** (see also "Sweet potato dish"), frozen/ chilled, 1 pc., except as noted: | | | | | | | |
| (*Dr. Praeger's*), 2.25 oz. | 100 | 2.0 | 13.0 | 4.0 | 15 | 190 | 3.0 |
| (*Golden*), 1.3 oz. | 70 | 2.0 | 10.0 | 3.0 | <5 | 190 | 1.0 |
| (*Old Fashioned Kitchen 4 Pack*), 2.5 oz. | 130 | 4.0 | 18.0 | 6.0 | 8 | 350 | 2.0 |
| (*Old Fashioned Kitchen 12 Pack*), 3 oz. | 160 | 5.0 | 22.0 | 7.0 | 10 | 420 | 2.0 |
| mini (*McCain Baby Cakes* Homestyle), 4 pcs., 2.6 oz. | 150 | 1.0 | 17.0 | 9.0 | 0 | 440 | 2.0 |

| Food and Measure | cal. | prot. (gms) | carbo. (gms) | fat (gms) | chol. (mgs) | sod. (mgs) | fiber (gms) |
|---|---|---|---|---|---|---|---|
| **Potato pancake mix:** | | | | | | | |
| (*Carmel*), 3 tbsp. | 80 | 2.0 | 18.0 | 1.0 | 0 | 500 | 2.0 |
| (*Hungry Jack*), 2 tbsp. | 70 | 2.0 | 15.0 | 0 | 0 | 370 | 1.0 |
| **Potato salad**, chilled: | | | | | | | |
| (*Thumann's*), 4 oz. | 230 | 2.0 | 19.0 | 17.0 | 5 | 350 | 2.0 |
| red (*Thumann's*), 4 oz. | 180 | 3.0 | 15.0 | 13.0 | 5 | 460 | 0 |
| **Potato seasoning mix:** | | | | | | | |
| cheese, 4 (*McCormick*), | | | | | | | |
| 1 tbsp. | 30 | 1.0 | 3.0 | 1.5 | <5 | 280 | 0 |
| herb, Italian (*McCormick* | | | | | | | |
| Steamers), 2 tsp. | 20 | 0 | 4.0 | 0 | 0 | 430 | 0 |
| roasted garlic/rosemary | | | | | | | |
| (*McCormick* Steamers), | | | | | | | |
| 2 tsp. | 20 | 0 | 4.0 | 0 | 0 | 420 | 0 |
| toasted onion/garlic | | | | | | | |
| (*McCormick*), 1 tbsp. | 20 | 0 | 4.0 | 0 | 5 | 570 | 0 |
| **Potato soy crisps** | | | | | | | |
| (*Genisoy*), 1 oz.: | | | | | | | |
| barbecue | 120 | 6.0 | 17.0 | 3.0 | 0 | 410 | 2.0 |
| Parmesan/roasted garlic | | | | | | | |
| or ranch | 120 | 6.0 | 16.0 | 3.0 | 0 | 440 | 2.0 |
| sea salt/black pepper | 120 | 6.0 | 16.0 | 3.0 | 0 | 220 | 2.0 |
| **Potato sticks**, see | | | | | | | |
| "Potato chips/crisps" | | | | | | | |
| **Potato sticks, canned,** | | | | | | | |
| shoestring: | | | | | | | |
| (*Butterfield*), ⅔ cup | 150 | 2.0 | 16.0 | 9.0 | 0 | 90 | 2.0 |
| (*Butterfield* Single | | | | | | | |
| Serve), 1 cup | 250 | 3.0 | 26.0 | 15.0 | 0 | 150 | 3.0 |
| (*Herr's* Stix), 1 oz. | 150 | 2.0 | 15.0 | 10.0 | 0 | 200 | 1.0 |
| **Poultry seasoning** | | | | | | | |
| (see also "Chicken | | | | | | | |
| seasoning"), 1 tsp. | 5 | .1 | 1.0 | .1 | 0 | tr. | .2 |
| **Pout, ocean**, meat only: | | | | | | | |
| raw, 4 oz. | 90 | 18.9 | 0 | 1.0 | 59 | 69 | 0 |
| baked or broiled, 4 oz. | 116 | 24.2 | 0 | 1.3 | 76 | 88 | 0 |
| **Pretzel**, 1 oz.: | | | | | | | |
| (*Bachman* The Puzzle | | | | | | | |
| Pretzel) | 120 | 3.0 | 23.0 | 1.0 | 0 | 265 | 1.0 |
| (*Bachman* The Puzzle | | | | | | | |
| Pretzel Gluten | | | | | | | |
| Free) | 120 | 1.0 | 22.0 | 3.0 | 0 | 250 | 4.0 |
| (*Bachman* Kidzels) | 120 | 2.0 | 23.0 | 1.5 | 0 | 95 | 1.0 |

| Food and Measure | cal. | prot. (gms) | carbo. (gms) | fat (gms) | chol. (mgs) | sod. (mgs) | fiber (gms) |
|---|---|---|---|---|---|---|---|
| **Pretzel** *(cont.)* | | | | | | | |
| *(Bachman Nutzels)* ..... | 110 | 3.0 | 23.0 | 1.0 | 0 | 100 | 1.0 |
| *(Bachman Pita Pretzel)* .. | 110 | 2.0 | 23.0 | .5 | 0 | 220 | 1.0 |
| *(Herr's* Circle H | | | | | | | |
| Mini) ............... | 170 | 3.0 | 32.0 | 3.0 | 0 | 675 | 2.0 |
| *(Snyder's* Butter Snaps) . | 120 | 3.0 | 25.0 | 1.0 | 0 | 270 | <1.0 |
| *(Snyder's* Snaps) ........ | 110 | 3.0 | 24.0 | 1.0 | 0 | 340 | <1.0 |
| cheddar: | | | | | | | |
| *(Rold Gold* Tiny | | | | | | | |
| Twists) .......... | 110 | 3.0 | 22.0 | 1.0 | 0 | 370 | 1.0 |
| *(Rold Gold* Pretzel | | | | | | | |
| Waves) .......... | 120 | 2.0 | 21.0 | 3.0 | 0 | 420 | 1.0 |
| cheese filled: | | | | | | | |
| cheddar *(Combos)* ... | 130 | 3.0 | 19.0 | 5.0 | 0 | 440 | 0 |
| nacho *(Combos)* ..... | 130 | 3.0 | 19.0 | 5.0 | 0 | 460 | 1.0 |
| pizzeria *(Combos)* .... | 130 | 2.0 | 19.0 | 5.0 | 0 | 450 | 1.0 |
| chocolate, see "Candy" | | | | | | | |
| crackers/crisps, see | | | | | | | |
| "Cracker" | | | | | | | |
| garlic bread *(Snyder's* | | | | | | | |
| Nibblers) ........... | 130 | 2.0 | 24.0 | 3.0 | 0 | 180 | <1.0 |
| hard, bite size | | | | | | | |
| *(Herr's)*, 1.1 oz. ...... | 100 | 3.0 | 23.0 | 0 | 0 | 450 | 2.0 |
| honey mustard: | | | | | | | |
| *(Rold Gold* Tiny | | | | | | | |
| Twists) .......... | 110 | 3.0 | 23.0 | 1.0 | 0 | 430 | 1.0 |
| onion *(Snyder's* | | | | | | | |
| Nibblers) ........ | 130 | 3.0 | 23.0 | 3.0 | 0 | 95 | <1.0 |
| mustard, deli-style | | | | | | | |
| *(Gardetto's* Mix), | | | | | | | |
| ½ cup, 1.1 oz. ....... | 120 | 3.0 | 22.0 | 2.5 | 0 | 230 | <1.0 |
| Parmesan garlic *(Rold* | | | | | | | |
| *Gold* Pretzel Waves) .. | 120 | 2.0 | 22.0 | 2.5 | 0 | 340 | 1.0 |
| peanut butter filled | | | | | | | |
| *(Herr's)*, 1.1 oz. ...... | 160 | 8.0 | 15.0 | 8.0 | 0 | 250 | 1.0 |
| pieces *(Snyder's)*: | | | | | | | |
| barbecue, Southern .. | 140 | 2.0 | 17.0 | 7.0 | 0 | 390 | 1.0 |
| Buffalo wing, hot .... | 140 | 2.0 | 17.0 | 7.0 | 0 | 380 | <1.0 |
| buttermilk ranch ..... | 140 | 2.0 | 19.0 | 6.0 | 0 | 230 | 1.0 |
| cheddar ........... | 130 | 2.0 | 18.0 | 6.0 | 0 | 260 | <1.0 |
| garlic bread ......... | 140 | 3.0 | 18.0 | 7.0 | 0 | 160 | 1.0 |
| honey mustard onion . | 140 | 2.0 | 18.0 | 7.0 | 0 | 240 | <1.0 |
| jalapeño ........... | 140 | 2.0 | 20.0 | 5.0 | 0 | 370 | <1.0 |

| Food and Measure | cal. | prot. (gms) | carbo. (gms) | fat (gms) | chol. (mgs) | sod. (mgs) | fiber (gms) |
|---|---|---|---|---|---|---|---|
| rods: | | | | | | | |
| (*Bachman* "Rolled") | 110 | 3.0 | 24.0 | .5 | 0 | 260 | 1.0 |
| (*Rold Gold* Classic) | 110 | 3.0 | 22.0 | 1.0 | 0 | 610 | 1.0 |
| (*Snyder's*) | 120 | 3.0 | 24.0 | 1.0 | 0 | 290 | 1.0 |
| sandwich (*Snyder's*): | | | | | | | |
| cheddar | 150 | 3.0 | 16.0 | 8.0 | <5 | 200 | <1.0 |
| jalapeño cheddar | 140 | 3.0 | 17.0 | 7.0 | <5 | 190 | 1.0 |
| peanut butter | 140 | 4.0 | 16.0 | 7.0 | 0 | 140 | <1.0 |
| sesame rings (*Glutino* Gluten Free), 1.1 oz. | 150 | 1.0 | 19.0 | 8.0 | 0 | 390 | 0 |
| sourdough: | | | | | | | |
| (*Herr's* Specials), 1.5 oz. | 170 | 4.0 | 31.0 | 0 | 0 | 675 | 2.0 |
| (*Snyder's* Nibblers) | 120 | 3.0 | 25.0 | 0 | 0 | 200 | <1.0 |
| hard (*Rold Gold*), 1 pc. | 90 | 2.0 | 19.0 | 1.0 | 0 | 500 | 2.0 |
| hard (*Snyder's*) | 100 | 3.0 | 22.0 | 0 | 0 | 240 | 1.0 |
| nuggets (*Bachman* Bites) | 110 | 3.0 | 22.0 | 1.0 | 0 | 240 | 1.0 |
| twists (*Bachman* Specials) | 110 | 3.0 | 22.0 | 1.5 | 0 | 250 | <1.0 |
| spelt: | | | | | | | |
| (*VitaSpelt* Organic) | 110 | 4.0 | 21.0 | 1.5 | 0 | 260 | <1.0 |
| sourdough (*VitaSpelt* Organic) | 110 | 3.0 | 23.0 | 1.5 | 0 | 260 | 1.0 |
| sticks: | | | | | | | |
| (*Bachman*) | 100 | 2.0 | 20.0 | 1.0 | 0 | 520 | 1.0 |
| (*Glutino* Gluten Free), 33 pcs., 1.1 oz. | 140 | 0 | 21.0 | 6.0 | 0 | 420 | 0 |
| (*Herr's* Stix) | 115 | 3.0 | 21.0 | 2.0 | 0 | 450 | 2.0 |
| (*Rold Gold* Classic) | 100 | 2.0 | 23.0 | 0 | 0 | 580 | 1.0 |
| (*Snyder's* Dipping Stix) | 120 | 3.0 | 24.0 | 1.0 | 0 | 240 | 1.0 |
| (*Snyder's* Gluten Free), 1.1 oz. | 110 | 0 | 25.0 | 1.5 | 0 | 260 | <1.0 |
| (*Snyder's* Olde Tyme) | 120 | 3.0 | 23.0 | 1.5 | 0 | 200 | <1.0 |
| (*Wise* Thins) | 110 | 2.0 | 23.0 | 1.0 | 0 | 410 | <1.0 |
| butter sesame (*Snyder's*) | 120 | 3.0 | 22.0 | 2.0 | 0 | 250 | 2.0 |
| 8 grain and seeds (*Snyder's* Organic) | 120 | 4.0 | 20.0 | 2.5 | 0 | 100 | 3.0 |
| honey wheat (*Snyder's*) | | 120 | 3.0 | 24.0 | 2.0 | 0 | 230 |
| 2.0honey whole wheat (*Snyder's* Organic) | 110 | 4.0 | 20.0 | 2.0 | 0 | 100 | 3.0 |
| multigrain (*Snyder's*), 1.1 oz. | 120 | 3.0 | 23.0 | 2.0 | 0 | 160 | 3.0 |

| Food and Measure | cal. | prot. (gms) | carbo. (gms) | fat (gms) | chol. (mgs) | sod. (mgs) | fiber (gms) |
|---|---|---|---|---|---|---|---|
| **Pretzel, sticks** *(cont.)* | | | | | | | |
| pumpernickel onion | | | | | | | |
| (*Snyder's*) . . . . . . . | 120 | 3.0 | 23.0 | 2.0 | 0 | 280 | 2.0 |
| whole grain (*Herr's*), | | | | | | | |
| 1.1 oz. . . . . . . . . . | 110 | 3.0 | 22.0 | 1.0 | 0 | 300 | 4.0 |
| whole wheat and oat | | | | | | | |
| (*Snyder's* Organic) . | 110 | 4.0 | 21.0 | 1.5 | 0 | 100 | 3.0 |
| twists: | | | | | | | |
| (*Bachman* Original/ | | | | | | | |
| Butter) . . . . . . . . . | 100 | 3.0 | 22.0 | 1.0 | 0 | 440 | 1.0 |
| (*Bachman Thin 'n Right*) | 120 | 3.0 | 23.0 | 1.0 | 0 | 125 | 1.0 |
| (*Glutino* Gluten Free), | | | | | | | |
| 24 pcs., 1.1 oz. . . . | 140 | 0 | 21.0 | 6.0 | 0 | 420 | 0 |
| (*Glutino* Gluten Free | | | | | | | |
| Unsalted), 1.1 oz. . . | 140 | 0 | 21.0 | 6.0 | 0 | 120 | 0 |
| (*Herr's* Extra Thin) . . . | 100 | 3.0 | 22.0 | 1.0 | 0 | 450 | 2.0 |
| (*Herr's* Extra Thin | | | | | | | |
| No Salt) . . . . . . . . | 100 | 3.0 | 24.0 | 0 | 0 | 100 | 2.0 |
| (*Rold Gold* Thins) . . . . | 110 | 2.0 | 23.0 | 1.0 | 0 | 560 | 1.0 |
| (*Rold Gold* Tiny) . . . . . | 110 | 2.0 | 23.0 | 1.0 | 0 | 450 | 1.0 |
| (*Rold Gold* Tiny Fat | | | | | | | |
| Free) . . . . . . . . . . | 100 | 3.0 | 23.0 | 0 | 0 | 420 | 1.0 |
| (*Snyder's* Homestyle) . | 120 | 3.0 | 25.0 | 1.0 | 0 | 230 | 1.0 |
| (*Snyder's* Olde Tyme) . | 120 | 3.0 | 24.0 | 1.0 | 0 | 120 | 1.0 |
| (*Snyder's* Thins) . . . . . | 110 | 3.0 | 23.0 | 0 | 0 | 330 | <1.0 |
| (*Wise* Thins) . . . . . . . | 110 | 2.0 | 23.0 | 1.0 | 0 | 360 | <1.0 |
| honey wheat, | | | | | | | |
| braided (*Rold Gold*) | 110 | 2.0 | 23.0 | 1.0 | 0 | 230 | 1.0 |
| twists, mini: | | | | | | | |
| (*Bachman* Baked) . . . . | 110 | 3.0 | 25.0 | 0 | 0 | 190 | <1.0 |
| (*Bachman* Low | | | | | | | |
| Sodium Petite) . . . . | 110 | 3.0 | 25.0 | 0 | 0 | 50 | <1.0 |
| (*Snyder's*) . . . . . . . . . | 110 | 3.0 | 25.0 | 0 | 0 | 250 | <1.0 |
| (*Snyder's* Unsalted) . . | 110 | 3.0 | 25.0 | 0 | 0 | 75 | <1.0 |
| wheat and honey | | | | | | | |
| (*Bachman* Pretzelsnack) | 110 | 3.0 | 23.0 | 1.0 | 0 | 190 | 1.0 |
| **Pretzel, soft**, frozen: | | | | | | | |
| (*SuperPretzel*), 2.25-oz. | | | | | | | |
| pc., w/out added salt . | 160 | 5.0 | 34.0 | 1.0 | 0 | 130 | 1.0 |
| (*SuperPretzel*), 2.5-oz. | | | | | | | |
| pc., w/out added salt . | 190 | 6.0 | 40.0 | 1.0 | 0 | 160 | 2.0 |
| (*SuperPretzel Soft* | | | | | | | |
| *Pretzel Bites*), 5 pcs., | | | | | | | |
| w/out added salt . . . . . | 150 | 3.0 | 32.0 | .5 | 0 | 115 | 1.0 |

| Food and Measure | cal. | prot. (gms) | carbo. (gms) | fat (gms) | chol. (mgs) | sod. (mgs) | fiber (gms) |
|---|---|---|---|---|---|---|---|
| filled (*SuperPretzel Pretzelfils*) 2 pcs.: | | | | | | | |
| mozzarella | 130 | 7.0 | 18.0 | 4.0 | 10 | 310 | 1.0 |
| pepperjack | 130 | 5.0 | 19.0 | 4.5 | 10 | 490 | 1.0 |
| pizza | 120 | 5.0 | 20.0 | 2.0 | 5 | 230 | 1.0 |
| filled, cheddar (*SuperPretzel Softstix*), 2 pcs. | 130 | 4.0 | 22.0 | 3.0 | 10 | 270 | 1.0 |
| **Prickly pear**: | | | | | | | |
| (*Frieda's* Cactus Pear), 3.6-oz. pc. | 40 | 1.0 | 10.0 | .5 | 0 | 5 | 4.0 |
| 4.8-oz. fruit, 3.6 oz. trimmed | 42 | .8 | 9.9 | .5 | 0 | 5 | 3.7 |
| 1 cup | 61 | 1.1 | 14.3 | .8 | 0 | 7 | 5.4 |
| **Prosciutto**, 1 oz., except as noted: | | | | | | | |
| (*Applegate Farms*) | 70 | 9.0 | 0 | 4.0 | 25 | 640 | 0 |
| (*Black Bear*) | 60 | 8.0 | 1.0 | 3.0 | 15 | 500 | 0 |
| (*Boar's Head* Riserva Stradolce) | 60 | 8.0 | 0 | 3.0 | 15 | 750 | 0 |
| (*Boar's Head* Proscuitto di Parma) | 60 | 8.0 | 0 | 3.5 | 25 | 660 | 0 |
| (*Di Lusso*), 2 oz. | 120 | 15.0 | 0 | 7.0 | 50 | 1100 | 0 |
| (*Thumann's*) | 60 | 10.0 | 0 | 2.5 | 25 | 770 | 0 |
| **Protein bar**, see "Granola/cereal bar" | | | | | | | |
| **Protein shake** (*Special K*), 10 fl. oz.: | | | | | | | |
| chocolate, milk | 190 | 10.0 | 29.0 | 5.0 | 10 | 220 | 5.0 |
| vanilla, French | 180 | 10.0 | 29.0 | 5.0 | 15 | 230 | 5.0 |
| **Prune**, see "Plum, dried" | | | | | | | |
| **Prune juice**, 8 fl. oz., except as noted: | | | | | | | |
| (*R.W. Knudsen* Organic) | 170 | 1.0 | 46.0 | 0 | 0 | 20 | 3.0 |
| (*Sunsweet*) | 180 | 2.0 | 43.0 | 0 | 0 | 30 | 3.0 |
| canned | 182 | 1.6 | 44.7 | .1 | 0 | 10 | 2.6 |
| **Pudding** (see also "Bread pudding" and "Rice pudding"), ready-to-eat, 3.5-oz. cont., except as noted: | | | | | | | |
| banana: | | | | | | | |
| (*Handi-Snacks*) | 90 | 1.0 | 20.0 | 1.0 | 0 | 160 | 0 |
| (*Hunt's Snack Pack*) | 110 | 1.0 | 19.0 | 3.5 | 0 | 150 | 0 |

| Food and Measure | cal. | prot. (gms) | carbo. (gms) | fat (gms) | chol. (mgs) | sod. (mgs) | fiber (gms) |
|---|---|---|---|---|---|---|---|
| **Pudding, banana** *(cont.)* | | | | | | | |
| cream (*Kozy Shack*), | | | | | | | |
| ½ cup ........... | 130 | 3.0 | 19.0 | 4.5 | 15 | 120 | 0 |
| cream (*Swiss Miss* | | | | | | | |
| *Pie Lovers*), 4 oz. .. | 130 | 2.0 | 23.0 | 3.5 | <5 | 170 | 0 |
| cream pie (*Hunt's* | | | | | | | |
| *Snack Pack*) ...... | 110 | 1.0 | 18.0 | 3.5 | 0 | 150 | 0 |
| berry, mixed (*Jell-O* | | | | | | | |
| *Smoothie*), 4 oz. ..... | 100 | 1.0 | 18.0 | 2.5 | 10 | 40 | 0 |
| blueberry muffin or | | | | | | | |
| cinnamon roll | | | | | | | |
| (*Hunt's Snack Pack*) .. | 110 | 1.0 | 20.0 | 3.5 | 0 | 125 | 0 |
| butterscotch: | | | | | | | |
| (*Handi-Snacks*) ...... | 90 | 1.0 | 21.0 | 1.0 | 0 | 160 | 0 |
| (*Hunt's Snack Pack*) .. | 110 | 1.0 | 21.0 | 3.0 | 0 | 150 | 0 |
| (*Swiss Miss*), 4 oz. ... | 130 | 2.0 | 24.0 | 3.0 | <5 | 170 | <1.0 |
| caramel (*Hunt's Snack* | | | | | | | |
| *Pack* No Sugar) ..... | 60 | 0 | 11.0 | 3.0 | 0 | 105 | 0 |
| caramel, creamy: | | | | | | | |
| (*Handi-Snacks* | | | | | | | |
| Reduced Calorie) .. | 45 | 1.0 | 9.0 | 1.0 | 0 | 170 | 0 |
| (*Jell-O* No Sugar), | | | | | | | |
| 3.75 oz. ......... | 60 | 1.0 | 13.0 | 1.0 | 0 | 200 | 0 |
| caramel cream: | | | | | | | |
| (*Hunt's Snack Pack*) .. | 120 | 1.0 | 21.0 | 3.0 | 0 | 160 | 0 |
| (*Jell-O* Mousse No | | | | | | | |
| Sugar), 2.3 oz. .... | 60 | 1.0 | 9.0 | 3.0 | 10 | 135 | 0 |
| cheesecake, strawberry | | | | | | | |
| (*Jell-O*) ............ | 130 | 2.0 | 25.0 | 2.0 | 5 | 125 | 0 |
| chocolate: | | | | | | | |
| (*Handi-Snacks*) ...... | 90 | 1.0 | 23.0 | 1.0 | 0 | 150 | 0 |
| (*Handi-Snacks* No Sugar) | 45 | 2.0 | 9.0 | 1.0 | 0 | 160 | 1.0 |
| (*Handi-Snacks* Nonfat) | 90 | 2.0 | 21.0 | 0 | 0 | 170 | 0 |
| (*Hunt's Snack Pack*) .. | 130 | 1.0 | 23.0 | 3.0 | 0 | 140 | <1.0 |
| (*Hunt's Snack Pack* | | | | | | | |
| Daredevil Triples) .. | 130 | 1.0 | 23.0 | 3.5 | 0 | 125 | <1.0 |
| (*Hunt's Snack Pack* | | | | | | | |
| Nonfat) .......... | 80 | 2.0 | 20.0 | 0 | 0 | 140 | <1.0 |
| (*Hunt's Snack Pack* | | | | | | | |
| No Sugar) ....... | 70 | <1.0 | 15.0 | 3.5 | 0 | 110 | 1.0 |
| (*Jell-O*), 4 oz. ....... | 120 | 2.0 | 25.0 | 1.5 | 0 | 190 | 1.0 |
| (*Jell-O* No Sugar), | | | | | | | |
| 3.75 oz. ......... | 60 | 2.0 | 13.0 | 1.5 | 0 | 180 | 1.0 |
| (*Jell-O* Nonfat), 4 oz. . | 100 | 2.0 | 23.0 | 0 | 0 | 180 | 1.0 |

| Food and Measure | cal. | prot. (gms) | carbo. (gms) | fat (gms) | chol. (mgs) | sod. (mgs) | fiber (gms) |
|---|---|---|---|---|---|---|---|
| (*Kozy Shack*), 4 oz. ... | 140 | 4.0 | 24.0 | 3.5 | 15 | 140 | 1.0 |
| (*Kozy Shack* Low Fat Milk), 4 oz. ....... | 110 | 4.0 | 20.0 | 1.0 | 5 | 110 | 4.0 |
| (*Kozy Shack* No Sugar), ½ cup .... | 60 | 3.0 | 10.0 | 1.0 | 5 | 130 | 4.0 |
| (*Swiss Miss* No Sugar) | 70 | <1.0 | 15.0 | 3.5 | 0 | 110 | 1.0 |
| chocolate topping (*Jell-O Sundae Toppers*), 3.75 oz. . | 110 | 2.0 | 23.0 | 1.5 | 0 | 170 | 1.0 |
| cream (*Swiss Miss* Pie Lovers), 4 oz. ... | 150 | 3.0 | 26.0 | 4.0 | <5 | 170 | <1.0 |
| dark (*Jell-O* Mousse No Sugar), 2.3 oz. . | 60 | 2.0 | 10.0 | 2.5 | 10 | 100 | 1.0 |
| double (*Jell-O* No Sugar), 3.75 oz. ... | 60 | 2.0 | 13.0 | 1.5 | 0 | 170 | 1.0 |
| milk (*Swiss Miss*) .... | 160 | 3.0 | 30.0 | 3.5 | <5 | 170 | 2.0 |
| triple (*Swiss Miss* Dream), 4 oz. ..... | 150 | 3.0 | 26.0 | 4.0 | <5 | 170 | <1.0 |
| chocolate caramel (*Hunt's Snack Pack*) .. | 130 | 1.0 | 23.0 | 3.5 | 0 | 150 | 0 |
| chocolate fudge: | | | | | | | |
| (*Hunt's Snack Pack*) .. | 120 | 2.0 | 22.0 | 3.5 | 0 | 130 | <1.0 |
| sundae (*Jell-O*), 4 oz. . | 140 | 2.0 | 25.0 | 3.5 | 0 | 170 | 0 |
| chocolate hazelnut (*Kozy Shack*), 4 oz. ... | 110 | 4.0 | 20.0 | 1.5 | 5 | 150 | 1.0 |
| chocolate mint (*Kozy Shack* No Sugar), 4 oz. | 70 | 4.0 | 10.0 | 1.0 | 5 | 140 | 3.0 |
| chocolate mud pie (*Hunt's Snack Pack*) .. | 130 | 2.0 | 24.0 | 3.5 | 0 | 130 | <1.0 |
| chocolate/vanilla (*Hunt's Snack Pack*) .. | 120 | 1.0 | 21.0 | 3.5 | 0 | 130 | 0 |
| chocolate/vanilla swirl: | | | | | | | |
| (*Jell-O*), 4 oz. ....... | 110 | 2.0 | 24.0 | 1.5 | 0 | 190 | 1.0 |
| (*Jell-O* No Sugar), 3.75 oz. ......... | 60 | 1.0 | 13.0 | 1.5 | 0 | 180 | 1.0 |
| (*Jell-O* Nonfat), 4 oz. | 100 | 2.0 | 23.0 | 0 | 0 | 190 | 1.0 |
| (*Swiss Miss*), 4 oz. .. | 150 | 3.0 | 26.0 | 4.0 | 10 | 170 | <1.0 |
| w/cookies (*Jell-O Oreo*), 4 oz. .............. | 120 | 2.0 | 25.0 | 1.5 | 0 | 190 | 1.0 |
| devil's food/chocolate (*Jell-O* Nonfat), 4 oz. . | 100 | 2.0 | 22.0 | 0 | 0 | 190 | 1.0 |
| flan, ½ cup: | | | | | | | |
| crème caramel (*Kozy Shack*) .......... | 150 | 4.0 | 27.0 | 3.5 | 35 | 85 | 0 |

| Food and Measure | cal. | prot. (gms) | carbo. (gms) | fat (gms) | chol. (mgs) | sod. (mgs) | fiber (gms) |
|---|---|---|---|---|---|---|---|
| **Pudding, flan** *(cont.)* | | | | | | | |
| dulce de leche (*Kozy Shack* Restaurant) . | 190 | 5.0 | 28.0 | 6.0 | 50 | 135 | 0 |
| ice cream sandwich (*Hunt's Snack Pack*) .. | 120 | 1.0 | 21.0 | 3.5 | 0 | 130 | <1.0 |
| lemon: | | | | | | | |
| (*Hunt's Snack Pack*) .. | 130 | 0 | 25.0 | 2.5 | 0 | 65 | 0 |
| meringue (*Hunt's Snack Pack*) ...... | 120 | 0 | 25.0 | 2.5 | 0 | 60 | 0 |
| strawberries/cream swirl (*Creme Savers*), 4 oz. ....... | 130 | 2.0 | 25.0 | 3.0 | 10 | 85 | 0 |
| strawberry, 4 oz.: | | | | | | | |
| (*Kozy Shack*) ....... | 130 | 3.0 | 21.0 | 3.0 | 15 | 130 | 0 |
| (*Kozy Shack* No Sugar) | 80 | 3.0 | 10.0 | 1.0 | 5 | 125 | 3.0 |
| strawberry banana (*Jell-O Smoothie*), 4 oz. | 100 | 1.0 | 18.0 | 2.5 | 10 | 40 | 0 |
| tapioca: | | | | | | | |
| (*Hunt's Snack Pack*) .. | 120 | 2.0 | 20.0 | 3.5 | 0 | 135 | 0 |
| (*Hunt's Snack Pack Nonfat*) .......... | 80 | 1.0 | 18.0 | 0 | 0 | 160 | 0 |
| (*Jell-O*), 4 oz. ....... | 110 | 1.0 | 25.0 | 1.5 | 0 | 200 | 0 |
| (*Jell-O Nonfat*), 4 oz. . | 100 | 1.0 | 23.0 | 0 | 0 | 200 | 0 |
| (*Kozy Shack*), 4 oz. ... | 130 | 3.0 | 23.0 | 3.0 | 10 | 130 | 0 |
| (*Kozy Shack* No Sugar), 4 oz. ..... | 70 | 4.0 | 11.0 | .5 | 5 | 135 | 4.0 |
| (*Swiss Miss*) ........ | 140 | 2.0 | 24.0 | 3.5 | <5 | 170 | 0 |
| honey lemon (*Kozy Shack*), 4 oz. ..... | 130 | 3.0 | 24.0 | 3.0 | 10 | 125 | 0 |
| vanilla: | | | | | | | |
| (*Handi-Snacks*) ...... | 90 | 1.0 | 20.0 | 1.0 | 0 | 160 | 0 |
| (*Handi-Snacks* No Sugar) .......... | 45 | 1.0 | 9.0 | 1.0 | 0 | 160 | 0 |
| (*Hunt's Snack Pack*) .. | 120 | <1.0 | 21.0 | 3.5 | 0 | 135 | 1.0 |
| (*Hunt's Snack Pack No Sugar*) ....... | 60 | 0 | 11.0 | 3.0 | 0 | 100 | 0 |
| (*Hunt's Snack Pack Nonfat*) .......... | 80 | 1.0 | 18.0 | 0 | 0 | 140 | 0 |
| (*Jell-O*), 4 oz. ....... | 110 | 1.0 | 23.0 | 1.5 | 0 | 190 | 0 |
| (*Jell-O No Sugar*), 3.75 oz. ......... | 60 | 1.0 | 13.0 | 1.0 | 0 | 180 | 0 |
| (*Kozy Shack* No Sugar), ½ cup ........... | 90 | 3.0 | 10.0 | 3.0 | 10 | 115 | 4.0 |
| (*Swiss Miss*), 4 oz. ... | 140 | 1.0 | 25.0 | 4.0 | 15 | 150 | 0 |

| Food and Measure | cal. | prot. (gms) | carbo. (gms) | fat (gms) | chol. (mgs) | sod. (mgs) | fiber (gms) |
|---|---|---|---|---|---|---|---|
| (*Swiss Miss* No Sugar) | 60 | 0 | 11.0 | 3.0 | 0 | 100 | 0 |
| caramel or chocolate topping (*Jell-O Sundae Toppers*), 3.75 oz. | 110 | 1.0 | 23.0 | 1.0 | 0 | 160 | 0 |
| caramel sundae (*Jell-O Nonfat*), 4 oz. | 100 | 1.0 | 23.0 | 0 | 0 | 230 | 0 |
| **Pudding bar**, chocolate (*Jell-O X-Treme Stick*), 2.25-oz. pc. | 80 | 1.0 | 16.0 | 2.0 | 0 | 100 | 1.0 |
| **Pudding and pie filling mix** (see also "Mousse mix"), dry, ¼ pkg. or 1 serving, except as noted: | | | | | | | |
| banana cream: | | | | | | | |
| (*Dr. Oetker* Organics) | 90 | 0 | 23.0 | 0 | 0 | 100 | 0 |
| (*Jell-O* Cook & Serve) | 80 | 0 | 20.0 | 0 | 0 | 180 | 0 |
| (*Jell-O* Instant) | 90 | 0 | 23.0 | 0 | 0 | 360 | 0 |
| (*Jell-O* No Sugar/Fat) | 25 | 0 | 6.0 | 0 | 0 | 310 | 0 |
| (*Royal* No Sugar) | 40 | 0 | 10.0 | 0 | 0 | 370 | 0 |
| butterscotch: | | | | | | | |
| (*Dr. Oetker* Organics) | 100 | 0 | 24.0 | 0 | 0 | 100 | 0 |
| (*Jell-O* Cook & Serve) | 100 | 0 | 24.0 | 0 | 0 | 130 | 0 |
| (*Jell-O* Instant) | 90 | 0 | 23.0 | 0 | 0 | 400 | 0 |
| (*Jell-O* Instant No Sugar/Fat) | 25 | 0 | 6.0 | 0 | 0 | 300 | 0 |
| (*Royal* No Sugar) | 40 | 0 | 10.0 | 0 | 0 | 410 | 0 |
| cheesecake: | | | | | | | |
| (*Jell-O* Instant) | 100 | 0 | 24.0 | 0 | 0 | 360 | 0 |
| (*Jell-O* Instant No Sugar/Fat) | 25 | 0 | 6.0 | 0 | 0 | 310 | 0 |
| chocolate: | | | | | | | |
| (*Dr. Oetker*) | 40 | 0 | 9.0 | 0 | 0 | 30 | 0 |
| (*Dr. Oetker* Organics) | 120 | 0 | 30.0 | 0 | 0 | 100 | 0 |
| (*Jell-O* Cook & Serve) | 90 | 1.0 | 22.0 | 0 | 0 | 110 | 1.0 |
| (*Jell-O* Cook & Serve No Sugar) | 30 | 1.0 | 7.0 | 0 | 0 | 110 | 1.0 |
| (*Jell-O* Instant) | 100 | 0 | 25.0 | 0 | 0 | 420 | 1.0 |
| (*Jell-O* Instant No Sugar/Fat) | 35 | 1.0 | 8.0 | 0 | 0 | 310 | 1.0 |
| (*Mori-Nu Mates*) | 110 | 0 | 22.0 | 2.0 | 0 | 5 | 1.0 |

| Food and Measure | cal. | prot. (gms) | carbo. (gms) | fat (gms) | chol. (mgs) | sod. (mgs) | fiber (gms) |
|---|---|---|---|---|---|---|---|
| **Pudding and pie filling mix, chocolate** *(cont.)* | | | | | | | |
| (*Royal* Cook & Serve) . | 80 | 1.0 | 20.0 | 0 | 0 | 80 | 0 |
| (*Royal* No Sugar) .... | 40 | 1.0 | 10.0 | 0 | 0 | 430 | <1.0 |
| white (*Jell-O* Instant) . | 90 | 0 | 23.0 | 0 | 0 | 350 | 0 |
| white (*Jell-O* Instant No Sugar/Fat) ..... | 25 | 0 | 6.0 | 0 | 0 | 300 | 0 |
| chocolate fudge: | | | | | | | |
| (*Jell-O* Cook & Serve) .......... | 90 | 1.0 | 22.0 | 0 | 0 | 115 | 1.0 |
| (*Jell-O* Instant) ...... | 100 | 1.0 | 25.0 | 0 | 0 | 380 | 1.0 |
| (*Jell-O* Instant No Sugar/Fat) ....... | 35 | 1.0 | 8.0 | 0 | 0 | 310 | 1.0 |
| coconut: | | | | | | | |
| (*Dr. Oetker* Organics) . | 100 | 0 | 22.0 | 2.0 | 0 | 100 | 0 |
| cream (*Jell-O* Cook & Serve) ......... | 90 | 0 | 18.0 | 2.5 | 0 | 150 | 1.0 |
| cream (*Jell-O* Instant) . | 100 | 0 | 21.0 | 2.5 | 0 | 270 | 1.0 |
| cookies and cream (*Jell-O Oreo* Instant) .. | 120 | 0 | 28.0 | 1.0 | 0 | 390 | 0 |
| cream (*Dr. Oetker*) ..... | 40 | 0 | 10.0 | 0 | 0 | 30 | 0 |
| crème brûlée: | | | | | | | |
| (*Dr. Oetker*) ......... | 110 | 1.0 | 23.0 | 1.5 | 10 | 90 | 0 |
| milk chocolate (*Dr. Oetker*) .......... | 110 | 1.0 | 24.0 | 1.5 | 35 | 110 | 0 |
| crème caramel (*Dr. Oetker*) ............ | 100 | 0 | 23.0 | 0 | 15 | 45 | 0 |
| devil's food (*Jell-O* Instant) ............ | 140 | 0 | 25.0 | 0 | 0 | 360 | 1.0 |
| flan: | | | | | | | |
| (*Roland*), ⅛ pkt. ..... | 60 | 0 | 17.0 | 0 | 0 | 90 | 0 |
| (*Royal*) ............ | 70 | 0 | 18.0 | 0 | 0 | 30 | 0 |
| lemon: | | | | | | | |
| (*Jell-O* Cook & Serve 2.9 oz.) ..... | 50 | 0 | 12.0 | 0 | 0 | 70 | 0 |
| (*Jell-O* Cook & Serve 4.3 oz.) ..... | 60 | 0 | 14.0 | 0 | 0 | 80 | 0 |
| (*Jell-O* Instant) ...... | 90 | 0 | 24.0 | 0 | 0 | 310 | 0 |
| (*Jell-O* Instant No Sugar/Fat) ....... | 25 | 0 | 6.0 | 0 | 0 | 300 | 0 |
| or key lime (*Dr. Oetker* Pie Filling) .. | 100 | 0 | 26.0 | 0 | 0 | 80 | 0 |
| pistachio: | | | | | | | |
| (*Jell-O* Instant) ...... | 100 | 0 | 23.0 | .5 | 0 | 360 | 0 |

| Food and Measure | cal. | prot. (gms) | carbo. (gms) | fat (gms) | chol. (mgs) | sod. (mgs) | fiber (gms) |
|---|---|---|---|---|---|---|---|
| (*Jell-O* Instant No Sugar/Fat) . . . . . . . | 25 | 0 | 6.0 | 0 | 0 | 310 | 0 |
| (*Royal* No Sugar) . . . . | 40 | 0 | 9.0 | 0 | 0 | 290 | 0 |
| pumpkin spice | | | | | | | |
| (*Jell-O* Instant) . . . . . . | 90 | 0 | 23.0 | 0 | 0 | 340 | 0 |
| raspberry (*Dr. Oetker*) . . . | 40 | 0 | 10.0 | 0 | 0 | 30 | 0 |
| tapioca (*Jell-O* Cook & Serve) . . . . . . . . . . . | 90 | 0 | 22.0 | 0 | 0 | 115 | 0 |
| vanilla: | | | | | | | |
| (*Dr. Oetker*) . . . . . . . . . | 40 | 0 | 10.0 | 0 | 0 | 45 | 0 |
| (*Dr. Oetker* Organics) . | 100 | 0 | 26.0 | 0 | 0 | 100 | 0 |
| (*Jell-O* Cook & Serve) . . . . . . . . . | 80 | 0 | 21.0 | 0 | 0 | 135 | 0 |
| (*Jell-O* Cook & Serve No Sugar) . . | 20 | 0 | 5.0 | 0 | 0 | 115 | 0 |
| (*Jell-O* Instant) . . . . . . | 90 | 0 | 23.0 | 0 | 0 | 350 | 0 |
| (*Jell-O* Instant No Sugar/Fat) . . . . . . . | 25 | 0 | 6.0 | 0 | 0 | 300 | 0 |
| (*Mori-Nu Mates*) . . . . . | 110 | 0 | 23.0 | 2.0 | 0 | 5 | 0 |
| (*Royal* Cook & Serve) . | 70 | 0 | 18.0 | 0 | 0 | 160 | 0 |
| (*Royal* No Sugar) . . . . | 40 | 0 | 10.0 | 0 | 0 | 350 | 0 |
| French (*Jell-O* Instant) . . . . . . . . . | 90 | 0 | 23.0 | 0 | 0 | 350 | 0 |
| **Puff pastry**, see "Pastry, puff" | | | | | | | |
| **Pummelo** (see also "Melogold"): | | | | | | | |
| (*Frieda's*), ¼ fruit . . . . . . | 90 | 1.0 | 20.0 | .5 | 0 | 0 | 4.0 |
| 1 fruit, 1 lb. 3 oz. w/out rind . . . . . . . . . . | 231 | 4.6 | 58.6 | .2 | 0 | 6 | 6.1 |
| sections, 1 cup . . . . . . . . | 72 | 1.4 | 18.3 | .1 | 0 | 2 | 1.9 |
| **Pumpkin**, fresh: | | | | | | | |
| mini (*Frieda's* Orange/ White), ¾ cup, 3 oz. . . | 20 | 1.0 | 6.0 | 0 | 0 | 0 | 2.0 |
| pulp, ½ cup: | | | | | | | |
| raw, 1" cubes . . . . . . . | 15 | .6 | 3.8 | .1 | 0 | 1 | 1.0 |
| boiled, drained, mashed | 24 | .9 | 6.0 | .1 | 0 | 2 | 1.0 |
| **Pumpkin, canned**, ½ cup: | | | | | | | |
| (*Libby's* 100% Pure) . . . . | 40 | 2.0 | 9.0 | .5 | 0 | 5 | 5.0 |
| w/ or w/out winter squash | 41 | 1.3 | 9.9 | .3 | 0 | 6 | 3.4 |
| **Pumpkin flower**: | | | | | | | |
| raw, ½ cup . . . . . . . . . . | 3 | .2 | .5 | <.1 | 0 | 1 | <1.0 |
| boiled, drained, ½ cup . . | 10 | .7 | 2.2 | .1 | 0 | 4 | .6 |

| Food and Measure | cal. | prot. (gms) | carbo. (gms) | fat (gms) | chol. (mgs) | sod. (mgs) | fiber (gms) |
|---|---|---|---|---|---|---|---|
| **Pumpkin leaf**: | | | | | | | |
| raw, ½ cup . . . . . . . . . . | 4 | .6 | .5 | .1 | 0 | 2 | <1.0 |
| boiled, drained, ½ cup  . . | 7 | 1.0 | 1.2 | .1 | 0 | 3 | .9 |
| **Pumpkin pie mix**, | | | | | | | |
| see "Pie filling" | | | | | | | |
| **Pumpkin pie spice**, | | | | | | | |
| 1 tsp. . . . . . . . . . . . . | 6 | .1 | 1.2 | .2 | 0 | 1 | .3 |
| **Pumpkin seeds**: | | | | | | | |
| in shell, roasted: | | | | | | | |
| 1 oz. or 85 seeds  . . . . | 127 | 5.3 | 15.3 | 5.5 | 0 | 5 | n.a. |
| 1 cup  . . . . . . . . . . . . | 285 | 11.9 | 34.4 | 12.4 | 0 | 12 | n.a. |
| salted, 1 oz.  . . . . . . . | 127 | 5.3 | 15.3 | 5.5 | 0 | 163 | n.a. |
| in shell, dry-roasted: | | | | | | | |
| (*Eden* Organic), | | | | | | | |
| ¼ cup . . . . . . . . . . | 200 | 10.0 | 5.0 | 16.0 | 0 | 100 | 5.0 |
| spicy, w/tamari (*Eden* | | | | | | | |
| Organic), ¼ cup  . . . | 200 | 10.0 | 5.0 | 16.0 | 0 | 75 | 5.0 |
| in shell, seasoned | | | | | | | |
| (*Spitz*), 1 oz. . . . . . . . . | 160 | 7.0 | 8.0 | 11.0 | 0 | 730 | 8.0 |
| shelled: | | | | | | | |
| raw (*Bob's Red Mill*), | | | | | | | |
| 3 tbsp. . . . . . . . . . | 170 | 9.0 | 3.0 | 15.0 | 0 | 0 | 2.0 |
| 1 oz., 142 kernels  . . . . | 154 | 7.0 | 5.1 | 13.0 | 0 | 5 | n.a. |
| shelled, roasted: | | | | | | | |
| (*Frieda's* Pepitas), | | | | | | | |
| 1 oz. . . . . . . . . . . . | 160 | 10.0 | 4.0 | 13.0 | 0 | 172 | 1.0 |
| (*Planters* Pepitas), | | | | | | | |
| 1.2 oz. . . . . . . . . . | 200 | 10.0 | 4.0 | 15.0 | 0 | 270 | 3.0 |
| 1 oz. . . . . . . . . . . . . | 148 | 9.4 | 3.8 | 12.0 | 0 | 5 | 1.8 |
| salted, 1 oz. . . . . . . . . | 148 | 9.4 | 3.8 | 12.0 | 0 | 163 | 1.8 |
| shelled, seasoned | | | | | | | |
| (*Spitz*), 1 oz. . . . . . . . . | 180 | 8.0 | 4.0 | 15.0 | 0 | 920 | 4.0 |
| **Pumpkin spice topping** | | | | | | | |
| (*Smucker's*), 2 tbsp. . . | 110 | 1.0 | 27.0 | .5 | 0 | 115 | 0 |
| **Purslane**, ½ cup: | | | | | | | |
| raw . . . . . . . . . . . . . . | 4 | .3 | .7 | <.1 | 0 | 10 | <1.0 |
| boiled, drained  . . . . . . . | 10 | .9 | 2.1 | .1 | 0 | 26 | <1.0 |

# Q

| Food and Measure | cal. | prot. (gms) | carbo. (gms) | fat (gms) | chol. (mgs) | sod. (mgs) | fiber (gms) |
|---|---|---|---|---|---|---|---|
| **Quail**: | | | | | | | |
| raw, meat w/skin, (4.3 oz. w/bone), 3.8 oz. | 210 | 21.4 | 0 | 13.1 | 83 | 58 | 0 |
| raw, meat only (4.3 oz. w/bone, skin), 3.2 oz. | 123 | 20.0 | 0 | 4.2 | 64 | 47 | 0 |
| raw, breast meat only: 1 breast, 2 oz. | 69 | 12.7 | 0 | 1.8 | 32 | 31 | 0 |
| cooked, meat w/skin, 1 oz. | 66 | 7.1 | 0 | 4.0 | 25 | 15 | 0 |
| **Quail egg**, see "Egg, quail" | | | | | | | |
| **Quesadilla**, frozen: | | | | | | | |
| breakfast: (*Smart Ones*), 1 pc. | 230 | 12.0 | 29.0 | 7.0 | 15 | 730 | 6.0 |
| egg/sausage/cheese (*El Monterey*), 4-oz. pc. | 230 | 8.0 | 25.0 | 12.0 | 30 | 640 | 0 |
| cheese, 3 (*Cedarlane*), 3-oz. pc. | 250 | 10.0 | 27.0 | 11.0 | 25 | 420 | 0 |
| chicken: (*Lean Cuisine*), 5 oz. | 280 | 18.0 | 35.0 | 7.0 | 20 | 710 | 3.0 |
| barbecue (*Lean Cuisine*), 5 oz. | 270 | 18.0 | 34.0 | 7.0 | 20 | 680 | 2.0 |
| chicken/cheese: (*El Monterey*), 4-oz. pc. | 220 | 10.0 | 29.0 | 9.0 | 20 | 560 | 1.0 |
| (*El Monterey* 4 Pc.), 3-oz. pc. | 190 | 9.0 | 22.0 | 7.0 | 15 | 460 | 1.0 |
| (*Smart Ones*), 8-oz. pkg. | 220 | 11.0 | 28.0 | 6.0 | 15 | 620 | 7.0 |

| Food and Measure | cal. | prot. (gms) | carbo. (gms) | fat (gms) | chol. (mgs) | sod. (mgs) | fiber (gms) |
|---|---|---|---|---|---|---|---|
| **Quesadilla, chicken/cheese** *(cont.)* | | | | | | | |
| fajita (*Tyson Quesa-Dippers*), | | | | | | | |
| 2 wedges . . . . . . . . | 190 | 10.0 | 17.0 | 9.0 | 20 | 540 | 1.0 |
| salsa, 2 tbsp. . . . . . | 10 | 0 | 2.0 | 0 | 0 | 300 | 0 |
| grilled, 3-cheese (*El Monterey*), | | | | | | | |
| 3.5-oz. pc. . . . . . . . | 230 | 13.0 | 20.0 | 11.0 | 35 | 510 | 1.0 |
| grilled, 3-cheese, mini (*José Olé*), 3 pcs., | | | | | | | |
| 4 oz. . . . . . . . . . . . | 270 | 13.0 | 31.0 | 9.0 | 25 | 920 | 1.0 |
| taco seasoned (*Tyson QuesaDippers*), | | | | | | | |
| 2 wedges . . . . . . . . | 200 | 9.0 | 16.0 | 11.0 | 30 | 470 | 0 |
| salsa, 2 tbsp. . . . . . | 10 | 0 | 2.0 | 0 | 0 | 300 | 0 |
| steak/cheese, 1 pc.: | | | | | | | |
| (*El Monterey*), 4 oz. . . | 220 | 12.0 | 27.0 | 9.0 | 20 | 560 | 1.0 |
| (*El Monterey* 4 Pc.*), | | | | | | | |
| 3 oz. . . . . . . . . . . . | 200 | 11.0 | 20.0 | 8.0 | 30 | 410 | 1.0 |
| grilled, 3-cheese, mini (*José Olé*), 4 oz. . . . | 260 | 13.0 | 32.0 | 9.0 | 25 | 880 | <1.0 |
| **Quesadilla seasoning** (*McCormick* Recipe Inspirations), ¾ tsp. . . . | 5 | 0 | <1.0 | 0 | 0 | 0 | 0 |
| **Quiche**, frozen, mini (*The Fillo Factory*), 2.1 oz.: | | | | | | | |
| cheese and onion . . . . . . | 190 | 6.0 | 11.0 | 14.0 | 70 | 230 | 0 |
| mushroom and pepper . . | 160 | 3.0 | 11.0 | 11.0 | 60 | 170 | 0 |
| spinach and cheese . . . . . | 170 | 4.0 | 11.0 | 12.0 | 65 | 190 | 1.0 |
| **Quince**: | | | | | | | |
| (*Frieda's*), 5 oz. . . . . . . . . | 80 | 1.0 | 21.0 | 0 | 0 | 5 | 3.0 |
| 1 medium, 5.3 oz. . . . . . . | 53 | .4 | 14.1 | .1 | 0 | 4 | 1.7 |
| peeled, seeded, 1 oz. . . . . | 16 | .1 | 4.3 | <.1 | 0 | 1 | .5 |
| **Quinoa**, dry, ¼ cup, except as noted: | | | | | | | |
| (*Arrowhead Mills*), ⅓ cup | 160 | 6.0 | 30.0 | 2.5 | 0 | 10 | 3.0 |
| (*Bob's Red Mill* Organic) . | 170 | 7.0 | 30.0 | 2.5 | 0 | 2 | 3.0 |
| (*Eden* Organic) . . . . . . . | 170 | 5.0 | 31.0 | 2.5 | 0 | 0 | 4.0 |
| all varieties (*Roland*) . . . . | 160 | 6.0 | 30.0 | 2.0 | 0 | 10 | 2.0 |
| red (*Eden* Organic) . . . . . | 170 | 6.0 | 32.0 | 2.0 | 0 | 5 | 5.0 |
| **Quinoa dish**, microwave w/brown rice (*Seeds of Change* Uyuni Organic), 1 cup . . . . . . | 240 | 6.0 | 47.0 | 3.5 | 0 | 400 | 3.0 |

| Food and Measure | cal. | prot. (gms) | carbo. (gms) | fat (gms) | chol. (mgs) | sod. (mgs) | fiber (gms) |
|---|---|---|---|---|---|---|---|
| **Quinoa dish mix**, w/ brown rice (*Seeds of Change* Organic): | | | | | | | |
| Amantani, 1 cup* | 190 | 5.0 | 39.0 | 1.5 | 0 | 550 | 3.0 |
| Cuzco, 1 cup* | 190 | 6.0 | 37.0 | 2.0 | 0 | 580 | 4.0 |
| **Quinoa flour** (*Bob's Red Mill* Organic), ¼ cup | 110 | 4.0 | 18.0 | 1.5 | 0 | 0 | 2.0 |

# R

| Food and Measure | cal. | prot. (gms) | carbo. (gms) | fat (gms) | chol. (mgs) | sod. (mgs) | fiber (gms) |
|---|---|---|---|---|---|---|---|
| **Rabbit**, domesticated, meat only: | | | | | | | |
| roasted, 4 oz. . . . . . . . . . | 223 | 33.0 | 0 | 9.1 | 93 | 53 | 0 |
| stewed, 4 oz. . . . . . . . . . . | 234 | 34.5 | 0 | 9.6 | 98 | 42 | 0 |
| stewed, diced, 1 cup . . . . | 288 | 42.5 | 0 | 11.8 | 120 | 52 | 0 |
| **Rabbit, wild**, meat only, stewed: | | | | | | | |
| 4 oz. . . . . . . . . . . . . . . . | 196 | 37.4 | 0 | 4.0 | 139 | 51 | 0 |
| diced, 1 cup . . . . . . . . . | 242 | 46.2 | 0 | 4.9 | 172 | 63 | 0 |
| **Raccoon**, meat only, roasted, 4 oz. . . . . . . . | 289 | 33.1 | 0 | 16.4 | 109 | 90 | 0 |
| **Radiatore pasta mix**, basil and herb (*Near East*), 2 oz. . . . . . . . . | 190 | 7.0 | 39.0 | 1.5 | 0 | 390 | 2.0 |
| **Radicchio**, fresh: | | | | | | | |
| (*Frieda's*), 2 cups . . . . . . | 20 | 1.0 | 4.0 | 0 | 0 | 20 | 1.0 |
| 3 oz. . . . . . . . . . . . . . . . | 20 | 1.2 | 3.8 | .2 | 0 | 19 | .8 |
| 1 medium leaf, .3 oz. . . . . | 2 | .1 | .4 | <.1 | 0 | 2 | 0 |
| shredded, 1 cup . . . . . . . | 9 | .6 | 1.8 | .1 | 0 | 8 | .4 |
| **Radish**: | | | | | | | |
| (*Green Giant*), 3 oz. . . . . . | 15 | 1.0 | 3.0 | 0 | 0 | 35 | 1.0 |
| 10 medium, ¾"–1" . . . . . . | 7 | .3 | 1.6 | .2 | 0 | 11 | .7 |
| sliced, ½ cup . . . . . . . . . | 12 | .4 | 2.1 | .3 | 0 | 14 | .9 |
| **Radish, black** (*Frieda's*), sliced, ½ cup . . . . . . . | 10 | 1.0 | 2.0 | 0 | 0 | 10 | 1.0 |
| **Radish, Oriental**: | | | | | | | |
| (*Frieda's* Daikon/Lo Bok/Moo), sliced, 1 cup . . . . . . . . . . . . . | 20 | 1.0 | 5.0 | 0 | 0 | 24 | 2.0 |
| 7" pc., 11.9 oz. . . . . . . . . | 61 | 2.0 | 12.8 | .3 | 0 | 71 | 5.4 |
| sliced, ½ cup . . . . . . . . . | 8 | .3 | 1.8 | <.1 | 0 | 9 | .7 |
| boiled, drained, sliced, ½ cup . . . . . . . | 12 | .5 | 2.5 | .2 | 0 | 10 | 1.2 |

| Food and Measure | cal. | prot. (gms) | carbo. (gms) | fat (gms) | chol. (mgs) | sod. (mgs) | fiber (gms) |
|---|---|---|---|---|---|---|---|
| **Radish, Oriental, daikon:** | | | | | | | |
| dried, ½ cup, .5 oz. | 157 | 4.6 | 36.8 | .8 | 0 | 161 | 4.8 |
| dried, shredded (*Eden* Organic), 2 tbsp. | 45 | 1.0 | 9.0 | 0 | 0 | 20 | 3.0 |
| pickled (*Eden* Organic), 2 slices, .5 oz. | 5 | 0 | 1.0 | 0 | 0 | 250 | 0 |
| **Radish, white-icicle:** | | | | | | | |
| 1 medium, .6 oz. | 2 | .2 | .5 | <.1 | 0 | 3 | .2 |
| sliced, ½ cup | 7 | .6 | 1.3 | .1 | 0 | 8 | .7 |
| **Raisin sauce**, in jars (*Reese*), ¼ cup | 150 | 0 | 36.0 | 0 | 0 | 55 | 0 |
| **Raisins**, ¼ cup, except as noted: | | | | | | | |
| (*Mariani* Cinnamon Raisin Bread), ⅓ cup | 120 | 1.0 | 31.0 | 0 | 0 | 35 | 1.0 |
| seeded, not packed | 107 | .9 | 28.5 | .2 | 0 | 11 | 2.5 |
| seedless: | | | | | | | |
| (*Dole*) | 120 | 1.0 | 32.0 | 0 | 0 | 0 | 1.0 |
| (*Earthbound Farm* Organic Thompson) | 120 | 1.0 | 32.0 | 0 | 0 | 0 | 2.0 |
| (*Mariani*) | 120 | 1.0 | 32.0 | 0 | 0 | 0 | 1.0 |
| (*Sun•Maid*), 1-oz. box | 90 | 1.0 | 22.0 | 0 | 0 | 5 | 2.0 |
| (*Sun•Maid* Baking) | 110 | 1.0 | 27.0 | 0 | 0 | 5 | 2.0 |
| (*Sun•Maid* Regular/ Jumbo/Golden) | 130 | 1.0 | 31.0 | 0 | 0 | 10 | 2.0 |
| golden (*Dole*) | 120 | 1.0 | 32.0 | 0 | 0 | 5 | 2.0 |
| golden, not packed | 110 | 1.3 | 28.9 | .2 | 0 | 5 | 1.5 |
| golden, w/cherries (*Sun•Maid*) | 130 | 1.0 | 31.0 | 0 | 0 | 5 | 2.0 |
| not packed | 109 | 1.2 | 28.7 | .2 | 0 | 5 | 1.5 |
| red (*Sunsweet* Jumbo) | 130 | 1.0 | 31.0 | 0 | 0 | 10 | 2.0 |
| vine-dried (*Frieda's* Raisins on the Vine), 4 oz. | 340 | 3.0 | 90.0 | .5 | 0 | 12 | 4.0 |
| coated, see "Candy" | | | | | | | |
| **Raita seasoning**, see "Yogurt seasoning" | | | | | | | |
| **Rambuten**, canned, in syrup, ½ cup | 62 | .5 | 15.7 | .2 | 0 | 17 | 1.4 |
| **Ranch dip**, 2 tbsp: | | | | | | | |
| (*Cabot*) | 50 | 1.0 | 1.0 | 5.0 | 15 | 140 | 0 |
| (*Kraft* Creamy) | 60 | 1.0 | 3.0 | 4.5 | 0 | 190 | 0 |
| (*Lay's* Smooth) | 60 | 1.0 | 2.0 | 5.0 | <5 | 210 | 0 |

| Food and Measure | cal. | prot. (gms) | carbo. (gms) | fat (gms) | chol. (mgs) | sod. (mgs) | fiber (gms) |
|---|---|---|---|---|---|---|---|
| **Ranch dip** *(cont.)* | | | | | | | |
| (*Marie's* Homestyle) .... | 80 | 1.0 | 2.0 | 7.0 | 15 | 200 | 0 |
| (*Marzetti*) ............ | 120 | 1.0 | 2.0 | 12.0 | 20 | 210 | 0 |
| (*Marzetti* Light) ........ | 60 | 0 | 2.0 | 6.0 | 5 | 240 | 0 |
| (*Marzetti* Nonfat) ....... | 30 | 1.0 | 6.0 | 0 | 0 | 330 | 0 |
| (*Marzetti* Organic) ...... | 130 | 1.0 | 3.0 | 13.0 | 15 | 290 | 0 |
| (*Wise*) .............. | 50 | <1.0 | 3.0 | 4.0 | 0 | 230 | 0 |
| buttermilk: | | | | | | | |
| (*Heluva Good!*) ...... | 60 | 1.0 | 2.0 | 5.0 | 20 | 180 | 0 |
| (*Marie's*) .......... | 100 | 1.0 | 2.0 | 9.0 | 15 | 230 | 0 |
| (*Marie's* Lite) ....... | 60 | 2.0 | 3.0 | 5.0 | 10 | 310 | 0 |
| Southwest: | | | | | | | |
| (*Marzetti*) .......... | 120 | 1.0 | 2.0 | 12.0 | 20 | 170 | 0 |
| (*Marzetti* Nonfat) .... | 30 | 1.0 | 6.0 | 0 | 0 | 270 | 0 |
| creamy (*Tostitos*) .... | 60 | 1.0 | 2.0 | 5.0 | <5 | 160 | <1.0 |
| **Ranch dip mix**: | | | | | | | |
| (*Lay's* Dip Creations), | | | | | | | |
| 2 tbsp.* ........... | 70 | 1.0 | 2.0 | 6.0 | 10 | 160 | 0 |
| (*McCormick*), ¾ tsp. .... | 5 | 0 | <1.0 | 0 | 0 | 270 | 0 |
| **Raspberry**, fresh: | | | | | | | |
| (*Dole* Red), 1 cup ...... | 60 | 1.0 | 15.0 | 1.0 | 0 | 0 | 8.0 |
| (*Green Giant*), 3.5 oz. ... | 50 | 1.0 | 12.0 | .5 | 0 | 0 | 7.0 |
| ½ cup ............... | 31 | .6 | 7.1 | .3 | 0 | <1 | 4.2 |
| **Raspberry, dried** | | | | | | | |
| (*Frieda's*), ⅓ cup, | | | | | | | |
| 1.4 oz. ........... | 145 | 1.0 | 36.0 | .5 | 0 | 0 | 6.0 |
| **Raspberry, frozen**: | | | | | | | |
| (*Birds Eye*), 1⅓ cup .... | 70 | 2.0 | 15.0 | 0 | 0 | 0 | 7.0 |
| (*Cascadian Farm* | | | | | | | |
| Organic), 1¼ cup .... | 70 | 1.0 | 16.0 | 0 | 0 | 15 | 3.0 |
| (*C&W* Ultimate), | | | | | | | |
| 1½ cup ............ | 70 | 2.0 | 15.0 | 0 | 0 | 0 | 7.0 |
| (*Dole*), 1 cup .......... | 50 | 1.0 | 17.0 | 0 | 0 | 0 | 8.0 |
| sweetened, ½ cup ...... | 129 | .9 | 32.7 | .2 | 0 | 1 | 5.5 |
| **Raspberry drink** | | | | | | | |
| **blend**, 8 fl. oz.: | | | | | | | |
| blue (*Tropicana* | | | | | | | |
| *Twister*) ........... | 110 | 0 | 26.0 | 0 | 0 | 25 | 0 |
| peach (*Snapple*) ....... | 110 | 0 | 28.0 | 0 | 0 | 5 | 0 |
| **Raspberry juice** | | | | | | | |
| **blend**, 8 fl. oz.: | | | | | | | |
| acai (*Tropicana Pure*) ... | 140 | 1.0 | 31.0 | 0 | 0 | 10 | 0 |
| frozen* (*Cascadian* | | | | | | | |
| *Farm* Organic) ....... | 130 | 0 | 31.0 | 0 | 0 | 10 | 0 |

| Food and Measure | cal. | prot. (gms) | carbo. (gms) | fat (gms) | chol. (mgs) | sod. (mgs) | fiber (gms) |
|---|---|---|---|---|---|---|---|
| pomegranate goji (*Northland*) ........ | 130 | 0 | 32.0 | 0 | 0 | 20 | 0 |
| **Raspberry syrup** (*Maple Grove Farms*), ¼ cup . | 210 | 0 | 53.0 | 0 | 0 | 0 | 0 |
| **Raspberry topping** (*Smucker's Plate-Scrapers*), 2 tbsp. .... | 100 | 0 | 25.0 | 0 | 0 | 5 | 0 |
| **Ratatouille**, see "Eggplant dip/appetizer" | | | | | | | |
| **Ravioli** | | | | | | | |
| frozen/chilled: | | | | | | | |
| agnolotti (*Buitoni Riserva*), 1 cup: | | | | | | | |
| quatto formagie ..... | 360 | 17.0 | 35.0 | 17.0 | 90 | 698 | 2.0 |
| wild mushroom ..... | 320 | 14.0 | 39.0 | 13.0 | 75 | 760 | 3.0 |
| basil/asiago/pine nuts (*Rising Moon Organics*), ½ cup .... | 260 | 9.0 | 46.0 | 4.0 | 20 | 300 | 1.0 |
| beef: | | | | | | | |
| (*Celentano*), 3 pcs., 3 oz. ............ | 180 | 8.0 | 24.0 | 6.0 | 35 | 260 | 2.0 |
| (*Italian Village*), 6 pcs., 3 oz. ...... | 200 | 8.0 | 31.0 | 5.0 | 30 | 220 | 2.0 |
| spicy, sausage (*Buitoni Riserva*), 1 cup .... | 300 | 15.0 | 40.0 | 9.0 | 75 | 703 | 3.0 |
| cheese: | | | | | | | |
| (*Celentano* 13 oz.), 4 pcs., 4.3 oz. .... | 240 | 10.0 | 37.0 | 6.0 | 35 | 260 | 1.0 |
| (*Celentano* 30 oz.), 4 pcs., 4.3 oz. .... | 220 | 11.0 | 34.0 | 4.5 | 30 | 280 | 2.0 |
| (*Celentano* 64 oz.), 4 pcs., 4.3 oz. .... | 230 | 10.0 | 36.0 | 4.0 | 25 | 270 | 2.0 |
| (*Celentano* Light), 4 pcs., 4.3 oz. .... | 200 | 10.0 | 34.0 | 2.5 | 20 | 270 | 2.0 |
| (*Italian Village*), 9 pcs., 4 oz. ...... | 210 | 9.0 | 37.0 | 3.0 | 20 | 190 | 2.0 |
| (*Italian Village* Round), 4 pcs., 4.2 oz. .......... | 190 | 9.0 | 33.0 | 3.0 | 20 | 230 | 2.0 |
| mini (*Celentano*), 12 pcs., 4 oz. ..... | 210 | 10.0 | 35.0 | 3.5 | 25 | 200 | 2.0 |
| mini (*Italian Village*), 13 pcs., 4.3 oz. ... | 200 | 9.0 | 35.0 | 3.0 | 20 | 210 | 2.0 |

| Food and Measure | cal. | prot. (gms) | carbo. (gms) | fat (gms) | chol. (mgs) | sod. (mgs) | fiber (gms) |
|---|---|---|---|---|---|---|---|
| **Ravioli, cheese** *(cont.)* | | | | | | | |
| mini (*Rising Moon Organics* Itsy-Bitsy), ½ cup . . . . . . . . . . | 290 | 10.0 | 53.0 | 3.5 | 20 | 350 | <1.0 |
| cheese, 4 (*Italian Village*), 4 pcs., 4.2 oz. | 190 | 9.0 | 33.0 | 3.0 | 20 | 230 | 2.0 |
| cheese, 4, 1¼ cups: | | | | | | | |
| (*Buitoni*) . . . . . . . . . . . | 330 | 14.0 | 45.0 | 10.0 | 60 | 550 | 3.0 |
| (*Buitoni* Light) . . . . . . | 260 | 13.0 | 41.0 | 4.5 | 45 | 460 | 2.0 |
| (*Buitoni* Whole Wheat) | 320 | 15.0 | 40.0 | 11.0 | 70 | 700 | 5.0 |
| cheese, 3, mini (*Buitoni* Ravioletti), 1 cup . . . . . . . . . . . . . | 270 | 12.0 | 43.0 | 5.0 | 30 | 340 | 2.0 |
| chicken, 4-cheese (*Buitoni* Riserva), 1 cup | 300 | 16.0 | 35.0 | 11.0 | 85 | 793 | 2.0 |
| feta-hazelnut/butternut squash (*Rising Moon Organics*), ½ cup . . . . | 270 | 9.0 | 50.0 | 3.5 | 15 | 340 | 2.0 |
| garlic and, ½ cup: | | | | | | | |
| herb (*Rising Moon Organics*) . . . . . . . | 250 | 8.0 | 52.0 | .5 | 0 | 550 | 3.0 |
| mozzarella (*Rising Moon Organics*) . . . | 260 | 10.0 | 44.0 | 4.5 | 35 | 420 | 3.0 |
| roasted veggies (*Rising Moon Organics*) . . . | 230 | 8.0 | 46.0 | .5 | 0 | 320 | 2.0 |
| garlic/gorgonzola/ spinach (*Rising Moon Organics*), ½ cup . . . . | 270 | 10.0 | 45.0 | 5.0 | 35 | 420 | 3.0 |
| mushroom, wild chanterelle (*Rising Moon Organics*), ½ cup . . . . | 250 | 9.0 | 47.0 | 3.0 | 20 | 300 | 1.0 |
| spinach (*Rising Moon Organics*), ½ cup . . . . | 220 | 8.0 | 46.0 | 1.0 | 0 | 410 | 3.0 |
| **Ravioli entree, canned,** 1 cup: | | | | | | | |
| beef: | | | | | | | |
| (*Campbell's Raviolio's*) | 270 | 11.0 | 38.0 | 3.5 | 20 | 1090 | 4.0 |
| (*Chef Boyardee*) . . . . . | 230 | 8.0 | 31.0 | 8.0 | 15 | 750 | 3.0 |
| (*Chef Boyardee* Big) . . | 250 | 11.0 | 39.0 | 6.0 | 15 | 750 | 5.0 |
| (*Chef Boyardee* 99% Fat Free) . . . . . . . . . | 170 | 7.0 | 33.0 | 1.5 | 10 | 880 | 2.0 |
| mini (*Chef Boyardee*) . | 230 | 8.0 | 32.0 | 8.0 | 10 | 700 | 4.0 |
| mini, and meatballs (*Chef Boyardee*) . . . | 280 | 10.0 | 33.0 | 12.0 | 25 | 700 | 4.0 |

| Food and Measure | cal. | prot. (gms) | carbo. (gms) | fat (gms) | chol. (mgs) | sod. (mgs) | fiber (gms) |
|---|---|---|---|---|---|---|---|
| cheesy (*Annie's* Organic) | 180 | 6.0 | 31.0 | 3.5 | 5 | 730 | 3.0 |
| pepperoni pizza (*Chef Boyardee*) .......... | 250 | 9.0 | 38.0 | 7.0 | 10 | 950 | 4.0 |
| sausage, Italian (*Chef Boyardee* Big) ....... | 240 | 9.0 | 40.0 | 4.5 | 15 | 990 | 4.0 |
| **Ravioli entree, frozen,** 1 pkg., except as noted: | | | | | | | |
| beef: | | | | | | | |
| braised, and sausage (*Buitoni*), ½ of 24-oz. pkg. ....... | 590 | 33.0 | 72.0 | 19.0 | 120 | 1200 | 5.0 |
| marinara, w/carrots (*Michelina's* Bellisio), 8 oz. .... | 220 | 9.0 | 28.0 | 7.0 | 15 | 720 | 3.0 |
| butternut squash: | | | | | | | |
| (*Lean Cuisine Spa Cuisine*), 9.8 oz. ... | 270 | 10.0 | 42.0 | 7.0 | 19 | 590 | 5.0 |
| (*Buitoni*), ½ of 24-oz. pkg. ....... | 490 | 14.0 | 72.0 | 16.0 | 55 | 690 | 5.0 |
| cheese: | | | | | | | |
| (*Amy's* Bowls), 9.5 oz. | 380 | 14.0 | 55.0 | 12.0 | 25 | 680 | 4.0 |
| (*Lean Cuisine*), 8.5 oz. | 220 | 11.0 | 33.0 | 5.0 | 35 | 620 | 3.0 |
| (*Michelina's*), 8 oz. ... | 370 | 15.0 | 40.0 | 17.0 | 45 | 880 | 2.0 |
| (*Stouffer's*), 12 oz. ... | 380 | 19.0 | 47.0 | 13.0 | 80 | 1000 | 5.0 |
| 4, and spinach (*Buitoni*), ½ of 26-oz. pkg. ....... | 550 | 24.0 | 55.0 | 21.0 | 100 | 1270 | 7.0 |
| w/meat sauce (*Stouffer's* Family), ⅙ of 52.8-oz. pkg. . | 310 | 14.0 | 36.0 | 12.0 | 40 | 1030 | 3.0 |
| chicken/mushroom (*Buitoni*), ½ of 22-oz. pkg. ......... | 530 | 29.0 | 59.0 | 20.0 | 110 | 1140 | 5.0 |
| Florentine, 8.5 oz.: | | | | | | | |
| (*Smart Ones*) ....... | 250 | 11.0 | 40.0 | 5.0 | 30 | 720 | 4.0 |
| marinara (*Healthy Choice*) .......... | 240 | 11.0 | 38.0 | 4.0 | 28 | 540 | 6.0 |
| lobster, Maine (*Buitoni*), ¼ of 34-oz. pkg. ..... | 430 | 14.0 | 106.0 | 20.0 | 105 | 890 | 2.0 |
| lobster cheese (*Healthy Choice*), 9 oz. ....... | 250 | 10.0 | 37.0 | 6.0 | 15 | 580 | 4.0 |

| Food and Measure | cal. | prot. (gms) | carbo. (gms) | fat (gms) | chol. (mgs) | sod. (mgs) | fiber (gms) |
|---|---|---|---|---|---|---|---|
| **Ravioli entree, frozen** *(cont.)* | | | | | | | |
| pumpkin squash (*Healthy Choice*), 9.2 oz. . . . . . . . . . . . | 300 | 9.0 | 52.0 | 6.0 | 10 | 600 | 6.0 |
| shrimp/lobster (*Buitoni*), ½ of 22-oz. pkg. . . . . . . . . | 500 | 21.0 | 68.0 | 16.0 | 125 | 1170 | 0 |
| spinach/mozzarella (*Buitoni*), 5.6 oz. . . . . . | 310 | 14.0 | 42.0 | 8.0 | 55 | 770 | 3.0 |
| vegetable, grilled, and goat cheese agnolotti (*Buitoni*), ½ of 24-oz. pkg. . . . . . . . . | 530 | 18.0 | 65.0 | 20.0 | 75 | 940 | 4.0 |
| **Ravioli entree, microwave**, 7.5-oz. cont., except as noted: | | | | | | | |
| beef: | | | | | | | |
| (*Chef Boyardee*), ½ bowl, 1 cup . . . . | 220 | 8.0 | 32.0 | 7.0 | 15 | 900 | 3.0 |
| (*Chef Boyardee* Single) | 190 | 7.0 | 29.0 | 5.0 | 10 | 920 | 2.0 |
| beef, mini: | | | | | | | |
| (*Chef Boyardee*), ½ bowl, 1 cup . . . . | 240 | 8.0 | 33.0 | 8.0 | 15 | 950 | 3.0 |
| (*Chef Boyardee* Single) | 180 | 6.0 | 30.0 | 4.5 | 10 | 590 | 2.0 |
| and meatballs (*Chef Boyardee* Single) . . | 240 | 9.0 | 30.0 | 9.0 | 15 | 750 | 3.0 |
| cheese (*Chef Boyardee* Single) . . . . . . . . . . . . | 200 | 8.0 | 31.0 | 4.5 | 10 | 790 | 2.0 |
| cheese/spinach (*Hormel Compleats*), 10 oz. . . . | 230 | 9.0 | 37.0 | 5.0 | 15 | 500 | 3.0 |
| **Red bean** (see also "Kidney beans"), canned, ½ cup: | | | | | | | |
| (*Allens*) . . . . . . . . . . . . . | 100 | 6.0 | 19.0 | .5 | 0 | 310 | 9.0 |
| (*Bush's*) . . . . . . . . . . . . . | 110 | 6.0 | 19.0 | .5 | 0 | 460 | 6.0 |
| (*Eden* Organic Small) . . . | 100 | 6.0 | 17.0 | .5 | 0 | 25 | 5.0 |
| seasoned: | | | | | | | |
| (*Glory* New Orleans) . . | 110 | 7.0 | 20.0 | .5 | 0 | 540 | 5.0 |
| (*Glory* Sensibly) . . . . . | 100 | 6.0 | 18.0 | 0 | 0 | 250 | 4.0 |
| (*S&W* Louisiana) . . . . | 110 | 6.0 | 20.0 | .5 | 0 | 340 | 5.0 |
| and rice (*Glory*) . . . . . | 90 | 5.0 | 18.0 | .5 | 0 | 680 | 3.0 |
| **Red bean, dried**, small (*Bob's Red Mill*), ¼ cup . . . . . . . . . . . . . | 160 | 10.0 | 28.0 | 0 | 0 | 5 | 7.0 |

| Food and Measure | cal. | prot. (gms) | carbo. (gms) | fat (gms) | chol. (mgs) | sod. (mgs) | fiber (gms) |
|---|---|---|---|---|---|---|---|
| **Red bean seasoning** | | | | | | | |
| (*Zatarain's*), 1 tsp. ... | 15 | 0 | 3.0 | 0 | 0 | 370 | <1.0 |
| **Red kuri squash** | | | | | | | |
| (*Frieda's*), 3 oz. ...... | 30 | 1.0 | 7.0 | 0 | 0 | 0 | 1.0 |
| **Red snapper**, see "Snapper" | | | | | | | |
| **Redfish**, see "Ocean perch" | | | | | | | |
| **Refried beans**, | | | | | | | |
| canned, ½ cup: | | | | | | | |
| (*Allens*) ............. | 150 | 7.0 | 24.0 | 2.5 | 0 | 360 | 11.0 |
| (*Allens* Nonfat) ....... | 120 | 7.0 | 23.0 | 0 | 0 | 500 | 8.0 |
| (*Amy's* Organic) ....... | 140 | 7.0 | 22.0 | 3.0 | 0 | 390 | 6.0 |
| (*Amy's* Organic Light | | | | | | | |
| Sodium) ........... | 140 | 7.0 | 22.0 | 3.0 | 0 | 190 | 6.0 |
| (*Bush's*) ............. | 150 | 9.0 | 24.0 | 3.0 | 0 | 490 | 7.0 |
| (*Bush's* Nonfat) ....... | 130 | 9.0 | 24.0 | 0 | 0 | 490 | 7.0 |
| (*Las Palmas*) ........ | 150 | 8.0 | 23.0 | 3.0 | 0 | 540 | 9.0 |
| (*Old El Paso*) ......... | 90 | 5.0 | 16.0 | .5 | 0 | 580 | 5.0 |
| (*Old El Paso* Nonfat) .... | 100 | 6.0 | 18.0 | 0 | 0 | 580 | 6.0 |
| (*Old El Paso* | | | | | | | |
| Vegetarian) ........ | 90 | 5.0 | 16.0 | .5 | 0 | 570 | 5.0 |
| (*Ortega*) ............. | 150 | 8.0 | 25.0 | 2.5 | 0 | 570 | 9.0 |
| (*Ortega* Nonfat) ....... | 130 | 8.0 | 25.0 | 0 | 0 | 570 | 9.0 |
| (*Rosarita*) ........... | 120 | 6.0 | 18.0 | 2.5 | 0 | 540 | 6.0 |
| (*Rosarita* Nonfat) ...... | 100 | 6.0 | 18.0 | 0 | 0 | 540 | 5.0 |
| (*Rosarita* Vegetarian) ... | 120 | 6.0 | 19.0 | 2.0 | 0 | 540 | 6.0 |
| (*Taco Bell* Nonfat) ..... | 100 | 6.0 | 18.0 | 0 | 0 | 540 | 4.0 |
| (*Taco Bell* Vegetarian) ... | 120 | 7.0 | 20.0 | 1.0 | 0 | 610 | 6.0 |
| (*Zapata*) ............. | 130 | 8.0 | 22.0 | 0 | 0 | 290 | 7.0 |
| black bean: | | | | | | | |
| (*Amy's* Organic) ..... | 140 | 8.0 | 21.0 | 3.0 | 0 | 440 | 6.0 |
| (*Amy's* Organic Light | | | | | | | |
| Sodium) ......... | 140 | 8.0 | 21.0 | 3.0 | 0 | 220 | 6.0 |
| (*Rosarita* Nonfat) .... | 110 | 7.0 | 19.0 | 0 | 0 | 560 | 6.0 |
| regular or spicy | | | | | | | |
| (*Eden* Organic) .... | 110 | 6.0 | 18.0 | 1.5 | 0 | 180 | 7.0 |
| black soy and black | | | | | | | |
| beans (*Eden* Organic) . | 90 | 8.0 | 13.0 | 3.0 | 0 | 170 | 6.0 |
| w/green chiles: | | | | | | | |
| (*Amy's* Organic) ..... | 130 | 7.0 | 20.0 | 3.0 | 0 | 440 | 6.0 |
| (*Old El Paso*) ....... | 90 | 5.0 | 16.0 | .5 | 0 | 580 | 5.0 |
| (*Rosarita* Nonfat) .... | 100 | 7.0 | 19.0 | 0 | 0 | 580 | 6.0 |

| Food and Measure | cal. | prot. (gms) | carbo. (gms) | fat (gms) | chol. (mgs) | sod. (mgs) | fiber (gms) |
|---|---|---|---|---|---|---|---|
| **Refried beans** *(cont.)* | | | | | | | |
| kidney bean (*Eden* Organic) ......... | 80 | 7.0 | 15.0 | 1.0 | 0 | 180 | 6.0 |
| pinto bean, regular or spicy (*Eden* Organic) . | 90 | 6.0 | 19.0 | 1.0 | 0 | 180 | 7.0 |
| w/salsa (*Rosarita* Nonfat) ............ | 100 | 6.0 | 19.0 | 0 | 0 | 600 | 6.0 |
| spicy (*Old El Paso*) ..... | 90 | 5.0 | 16.0 | 0 | 0 | 510 | 5.0 |
| **Relish**, see "Pickle relish" and specific listings | | | | | | | |
| **Remoulade sauce**: | | | | | | | |
| (*Crosse & Blackwell*), 2 tbsp. ............ | 60 | 0 | 9.0 | 3.0 | 5 | 440 | 0 |
| (*Zatarain's*), 2 tbsp. ..... | 45 | <1.0 | 4.0 | 3.0 | 0 | 510 | <1.0 |
| dressing (*Louisiana*), 1 tbsp. ............ | 80 | 0 | 2.0 | 7.0 | 0 | 100 | 0 |
| **Rhubarb**, fresh: | | | | | | | |
| 1 stalk ............... | 11 | .5 | 2.3 | .1 | 0 | 2 | .9 |
| diced: | | | | | | | |
| (*Frieda's*), 1 cup ..... | 25 | 1.0 | 6.0 | 0 | 0 | 5 | 2.0 |
| ½ cup ............. | 13 | .6 | 2.8 | .1 | 0 | 2 | 1.1 |
| **Rhubarb, frozen**, sweetened, cooked, ½ cup ............. | 139 | .5 | 37.4 | .1 | 0 | 2 | 2.4 |
| **Rice** (see also "Wild rice"), dry, ¼ cup, except as noted: | | | | | | | |
| Arborio: | | | | | | | |
| (*Fantastic*) ......... | 160 | 3.0 | 36.0 | 0 | 0 | 0 | <1.0 |
| (*Lundberg*) ......... | 160 | 5.0 | 35.0 | 1.0 | 0 | 0 | 1.0 |
| (*RiceSelect* Organic) .. | 150 | 3.0 | 37.0 | 0 | 0 | 0 | 0 |
| (*Roland* Superfino) ... | 170 | 4.0 | 38.0 | 0 | 0 | 0 | 2.0 |
| (*Vigo*), ⅓ cup ....... | 150 | 3.0 | 35.0 | 0 | 0 | 0 | 0 |
| basmati, brown: | | | | | | | |
| (*Arrowhead Mills* Organic) ......... | 140 | 3.0 | 31.0 | 1.5 | 0 | 0 | 2.0 |
| (*Lundberg* Organic/ Eco-Farmed) ..... | 150 | 4.0 | 33.0 | 1.5 | 0 | 0 | 2.0 |
| (*RiceSelect Texmati* Regular/Organic) .. | 170 | 4.0 | 35.0 | 1.0 | 0 | 0 | 0 |
| light (*RiceSelect Texmati* Organic) .. | 160 | 4.0 | 33.0 | 1.0 | 0 | 0 | 1.0 |

| Food and Measure | cal. | prot. (gms) | carbo. (gms) | fat (gms) | chol. (mgs) | sod. (mgs) | fiber (gms) |
|---|---|---|---|---|---|---|---|
| basmati, white: | | | | | | | |
| (*Arrowhead Mills* | | | | | | | |
|   Organic) ......... | 150 | 3.0 | 33.0 | .5 | 0 | 0 | <1.0 |
| (*Carolina/Mahatma*) .. | 160 | 3.0 | 36.0 | 0 | 0 | 0 | 0 |
| (*Fantastic*) ......... | 160 | 3.0 | 36.0 | 0 | 0 | 0 | <1.0 |
| (*Lundberg* Eco- | | | | | | | |
|   Farmed) ......... | 160 | 3.0 | 36.0 | .5 | 0 | 0 | 0 |
| (*Lundberg* Organic) .. | 160 | 3.0 | 34.0 | .5 | 0 | 0 | 1.0 |
| (*RiceSelect Kasmati/* | | | | | | | |
|   *Texmati*) ......... | 150 | 3.0 | 34.0 | .5 | 0 | 0 | 0 |
| (*Vigo*), ⅓ cup ....... | 160 | 4.0 | 36.0 | 0 | 0 | 10 | 0 |
| blends (see also "Grains, mixed"): | | | | | | | |
| (*Lundberg Countrywild*) | 150 | 3.0 | 35.0 | 1.5 | 0 | 0 | 3.0 |
| (*Lundberg Jubilee*) ... | 170 | 4.0 | 39.0 | 1.5 | 0 | 0 | 3.0 |
| (*Lundberg Wild* | | | | | | | |
|   *Blend*) .......... | 150 | 4.0 | 35.0 | 1.5 | 0 | 0 | 3.0 |
| brown: | | | | | | | |
| (*Carolina/Mahatma* | | | | | | | |
|   Whole Grain) ..... | 150 | 3.0 | 12.0 | 1.0 | 0 | 0 | 1.0 |
| (*Lundberg* Sweet | | | | | | | |
|   Organic) ......... | 150 | 3.0 | 35.0 | 1.0 | 0 | 0 | 2.0 |
| (*Lundberg Golden* | | | | | | | |
|   *Rose* Organic) .... | 160 | 3.0 | 34.0 | 1.0 | 0 | 0 | 1.0 |
| (*Lundberg Wehani* | | | | | | | |
|   Organic) ......... | 170 | 4.0 | 37.0 | 1.5 | 0 | 0 | 3.0 |
| (*River*) ............ | 150 | 3.0 | 32.0 | 1.0 | 0 | 0 | 1.0 |
| (*Success* Boil-in-Bag), | | | | | | | |
|   ½ cup .......... | 150 | 4.0 | 33.0 | 1.0 | 0 | 0 | 2.0 |
| (*Uncle Ben's* Natural | | | | | | | |
|   Whole Grain) ..... | 170 | 5.0 | 35.0 | 1.5 | 0 | 0 | 2.0 |
| (*Uncle Ben's Fast &* | | | | | | | |
|   *Natural* Instant) ... | 170 | 4.0 | 36.0 | 1.0 | 0 | 20 | 2.0 |
| parboiled (*Minute*), | | | | | | | |
|   ½ cup .......... | 150 | 3.0 | 34.0 | 1.5 | 0 | 10 | 2.0 |
| brown, long grain: | | | | | | | |
| (*Arrowhead Mills* | | | | | | | |
|   Organic) ......... | 160 | 6.0 | 32.0 | 1.0 | 0 | 0 | 1.0 |
| (*Lundberg* Eco- | | | | | | | |
|   Farmed) ......... | 150 | 3.0 | 35.0 | 2.0 | 0 | 0 | 3.0 |
| (*Lundberg* Organic) .. | 150 | 3.0 | 35.0 | 1.5 | 0 | 0 | 3.0 |
| brown, roasted, "couscous" (*Lundberg* | | | | | | | |
| Organic), 1.6 oz. ..... | 150 | 3.0 | 35.0 | 1.5 | 0 | 0 | 3.0 |

| Food and Measure | cal. | prot. (gms) | carbo. (gms) | fat (gms) | chol. (mgs) | sod. (mgs) | fiber (gms) |
|---|---|---|---|---|---|---|---|
| **Rice** *(cont.)* | | | | | | | |
| brown, short grain: | | | | | | | |
| (*Arrowhead Mills* | | | | | | | |
| Organic) ......... | 180 | 4.0 | 38.0 | 1.0 | 0 | 0 | 2.0 |
| (*Lundberg* Organic/ | | | | | | | |
| Eco-Farmed) ..... | 150 | 3.0 | 35.0 | 1.5 | 0 | 0 | 3.0 |
| carnaroli (*Roland* | | | | | | | |
| Superfino) ..... | 170 | 4.0 | 38.0 | 0 | 0 | 0 | 2.0 |
| glutinous or sweet ..... | 171 | 3.2 | 37.8 | .3 | 0 | 3 | 1.3 |
| gold, parboiled | | | | | | | |
| (*Carolina/Mahatma*) .. | 160 | 3.0 | 37.0 | 0 | 0 | 0 | 1.0 |
| Japonica, black: | | | | | | | |
| (*Lundberg Black* | | | | | | | |
| *Japonica*) ........ | 170 | 5.0 | 38.0 | 2.0 | 0 | 0 | 3.0 |
| (*Roland*) ........... | 220 | 5.0 | 46.0 | 2.0 | 0 | 0 | 3.0 |
| jasmine: | | | | | | | |
| (*Carolina/Mahatma*) .. | 160 | 3.0 | 36.0 | 0 | 0 | 0 | 0 |
| (*Fantastic*) ......... | 160 | 3.0 | 36.0 | 0 | 0 | 0 | <1.0 |
| (*RiceSelect Jasmati*) .. | 150 | 3.0 | 34.0 | 0 | 0 | 0 | 0 |
| (*RiceSelect Jasmati* | | | | | | | |
| Organic) ......... | 150 | 3.0 | 34.0 | 1.0 | 0 | 0 | 0 |
| (*Roland*) ........... | 160 | 3.0 | 36.0 | 0 | 0 | 0 | 0 |
| (*Success* Boil-in-Bag) . | 150 | 3.0 | 36.0 | 0 | 0 | 0 | 0 |
| (*A Taste of Thai*) ..... | 160 | 3.0 | 36.0 | 0 | 0 | 0 | 0 |
| (*Vigo*), ⅓ cup ....... | 160 | 0 | 36.0 | 0 | 0 | 0 | 1.0 |
| brown (*Lundberg* | | | | | | | |
| Organic) ......... | 150 | 4.0 | 33.0 | 1.5 | 0 | 0 | 2.0 |
| white (*Lundberg* Eco- | | | | | | | |
| Farmed) ......... | 160 | 3.0 | 36.0 | .5 | 0 | 0 | 0 |
| white (*Lundberg* | | | | | | | |
| Organic) ......... | 160 | 3.0 | 36.0 | .5 | 0 | 0 | 1.0 |
| red: | | | | | | | |
| (*Lundberg Christmas* | | | | | | | |
| *Rice*) ........... | 170 | 4.0 | 37.0 | 1.5 | 0 | 0 | 3.0 |
| long grain (*Roland*) .. | 200 | 5.0 | 42.0 | 2.0 | 0 | 0 | 4.0 |
| sushi: | | | | | | | |
| (*Lundberg* Organic) .. | 150 | 4.0 | 35.0 | 0 | 0 | 0 | 1.0 |
| (*RiceSelect*) ........ | 190 | 3.0 | 45.0 | 0 | 0 | 0 | 0 |
| (*Roland*) ........... | 170 | 3.0 | 36.0 | 2.0 | 0 | 5 | 1.0 |
| (*Roland* Calrose) ..... | 160 | 3.0 | 36.0 | 0 | 0 | 0 | 0 |
| white, long grain: | | | | | | | |
| (*Carolina/Mahatma*) .. | 150 | 3.0 | 35.0 | 0 | 0 | 0 | 0 |
| (*Lundberg* Organic) .. | 160 | 4.0 | 36.0 | 0 | 0 | 0 | 0 |

| Food and Measure | cal. | prot. (gms) | carbo. (gms) | fat (gms) | chol. (mgs) | sod. (mgs) | fiber (gms) |
|---|---|---|---|---|---|---|---|
| (*Uncle Ben's* Instant), ½ cup | 190 | 3.0 | 43.0 | .5 | 0 | 15 | 1.0 |
| (*Uncle Ben's* Whole Grain) | 170 | 4.0 | 38.0 | 1.0 | 0 | 5 | 4.0 |
| (*Uncle Ben's Original Converted*) | 170 | 4.0 | 37.0 | 0 | 0 | 0 | 0 |
| parboiled (*Minute Premium*), ½ cup | 190 | 5.0 | 41.0 | 0 | 0 | 5 | 0 |
| white, medium grain: | | | | | | | |
| (*Carolina*) | 160 | 3.0 | 35.0 | 0 | 0 | 0 | 1.0 |
| (*River*) | 160 | 3.0 | 37.0 | 0 | 0 | 0 | 1.0 |
| (*Water Maid*) | 160 | 3.0 | 36.0 | 0 | 0 | 0 | 1.0 |
| white, parboiled (*Minute*), ½ cup | 200 | 5.0 | 45.0 | 0 | 0 | 5 | 0 |
| **Rice, cooked** (see also "Rice dish" and "Sushi wrap"), plain: | | | | | | | |
| (*Minute* Ready to Serve!), 1 cont.: | | | | | | | |
| brown, whole grain | 230 | 5.0 | 40.0 | 3.5 | 0 | 175 | 2.0 |
| brown and wild | 230 | 5.0 | 42.0 | 4.5 | 0 | 135 | 5.0 |
| white | 200 | 4.0 | 40.0 | 3.0 | 0 | 150 | 2.0 |
| (*Minute* Steamers): | | | | | | | |
| brown, 1 cup | 155 | 3.0 | 28.0 | 1.0 | 0 | 10 | 2.0 |
| white, ¾ cup | 170 | 4.0 | 42.0 | 0 | 0 | 0 | 0 |
| (*Tasty Bite*), ½ of 8.8-oz. pkg.: | | | | | | | |
| basmati | 170 | 3.0 | 37.0 | 2.0 | 0 | 0 | <1.0 |
| brown | 170 | 3.0 | 29.0 | 1.5 | 0 | 0 | 2.0 |
| jasmine | 210 | 3.0 | 39.0 | 4.0 | 0 | 0 | <1.0 |
| long grain | 170 | 3.0 | 36.0 | 2.0 | 0 | 0 | <1.0 |
| (*Uncle Ben's Ready Rice*), 1 cup: | | | | | | | |
| basmati | 220 | 6.0 | 44.0 | 3.0 | 0 | 15 | 1.0 |
| brown, whole grain | 220 | 5.0 | 41.0 | 4.0 | 0 | 5 | 2.0 |
| jasmine | 250 | 5.0 | 52.0 | 2.5 | 0 | 10 | 1.0 |
| white, long grain | 200 | 4.0 | 40.0 | 2.5 | 0 | 10 | 1.0 |
| black pearl (*Annie Chun's* Rice Express), ½ of 6.4-oz. pkg. | 140 | 3.0 | 28.0 | 1.0 | 0 | 0 | <1.0 |
| brown: | | | | | | | |
| (*Uncle Ben's* Boil-in-Bag), ¼ cup | 170 | 4.0 | 36.0 | 1.5 | 0 | 0 | 2.0 |

| Food and Measure | cal. | prot. (gms) | carbo. (gms) | fat (gms) | chol. (mgs) | sod. (mgs) | fiber (gms) |
|---|---|---|---|---|---|---|---|
| **Rice, cooked, brown** *(cont.)* | | | | | | | |
| (*Lundberg Countrywild* Heat & Eat Organic), 7.4 oz. .. | 290 | 6.0 | 65.0 | 3.0 | 0 | 0 | 6.0 |
| long grain (*Lundberg* Heat & Eat Organic), 7.4 oz. ........... | 290 | 6.0 | 65.0 | 3.0 | 0 | 5 | 6.0 |
| short grain (*Lundberg* Heat & Eat Organic), 7.4 oz. .......... | 290 | 5.0 | 65.0 | 2.5 | 0 | 10 | 5.0 |
| sprouted (*Annie Chun's* Rice Express), ½ of 6.4-oz. pkg. .. | 135 | 3.0 | 39.0 | 1.0 | 0 | 0 | 1.5 |
| frozen (*Birds Eye Steamfresh*), ¾ cup: | | | | | | | |
| brown .............. | 140 | 3.0 | 28.0 | 1.0 | 0 | 0 | 2.0 |
| white long grain ..... | 160 | 3.0 | 36.0 | 0 | 0 | 0 | 0 |
| sticky rice (*Annie Chun's* Rice Express), ½ of 6.4-oz. pkg.: | | | | | | | |
| multigrain .......... | 130 | 3.0 | 28.0 | 1.0 | 0 | 0 | 2.0 |
| white ............. | 150 | 2.0 | 34.0 | 0 | 0 | 0 | 0 |
| white (*Uncle Ben's* Boil-in-Bag), ⅓ cup .. | 190 | 4.0 | 44.0 | .5 | 0 | 0 | 1.0 |
| **Rice, w/grains**, see "Grains, mixed" | | | | | | | |
| **Rice and beans, canned** (*Eden* Organic), ½ cup: | | | | | | | |
| Cajun, small red ....... | 110 | 3.0 | 23.0 | 1.0 | 0 | 115 | 3.0 |
| Caribbean, black ....... | 120 | 4.0 | 23.0 | 1.0 | 0 | 100 | 4.0 |
| garbanzo ............. | 110 | 3.0 | 23.0 | 1.0 | 0 | 135 | 2.0 |
| kidney beans .......... | 110 | 3.0 | 23.0 | 1.0 | 0 | 135 | 3.0 |
| pinto beans ........... | 120 | 4.0 | 24.0 | 1.0 | 0 | 140 | 3.0 |
| Mexican, black ........ | 110 | 5.0 | 22.0 | 1.0 | 0 | 270 | 3.0 |
| Moroccan, garbanzo .... | 110 | 4.0 | 22.0 | 1.0 | 0 | 230 | 3.0 |
| Spanish, pinto ......... | 120 | 4.0 | 22.0 | 1.0 | 0 | 260 | 3.0 |
| **Rice and beans, frozen or mix**, see "Rice dish/entree" | | | | | | | |
| **Rice beverage** (see also "Rice-soy beverage"), 8 fl. oz.: | | | | | | | |
| (*Pacific*) ............. | 130 | 1.0 | 27.0 | 2.0 | 0 | 60 | 0 |
| (*Rice Dream* Chilled) .... | 120 | 1.0 | 23.0 | 2.5 | 0 | 80 | 0 |

| Food and Measure | cal. | prot. (gms) | carbo. (gms) | fat (gms) | chol. (mgs) | sod. (mgs) | fiber (gms) |
|---|---|---|---|---|---|---|---|
| (*Rice Dream* Classic) ... | 120 | 1.0 | 24.0 | 2.5 | 0 | 100 | 0 |
| (*Rice Dream* Heartwise) . | 130 | 1.0 | 27.0 | 2.0 | 0 | 80 | 3.0 |
| (*Rice Dream* Organic) ... | 120 | 1.0 | 23.0 | 2.5 | 0 | 100 | 0 |
| carob (*Rice Dream*) ..... | 150 | 1.0 | 30.0 | 2.5 | 0 | 80 | <1.0 |
| chocolate (*Rice Dream*) . | 160 | 2.0 | 34.0 | 3.0 | 0 | 90 | <1.0 |
| chocolate chai (*Rice Dream*) ........... | 160 | 1.0 | 35.0 | 3.0 | 0 | 70 | 1.0 |
| cinnamon vanilla (*Rice Dream* Horchata) .... | 160 | 1.0 | 32.0 | 2.5 | 0 | 5 | 0 |
| vanilla: | | | | | | | |
| (*Rice Dream* Chilled) . | 130 | 1.0 | 26.0 | 2.5 | 0 | 80 | 0 |
| (*Rice Dream* Classic) . | 130 | 1.0 | 27.0 | 2.5 | 0 | 105 | 0 |
| (*Rice Dream* Enriched) | 130 | 1.0 | 26.0 | 2.5 | 0 | 105 | 0 |
| vanilla hazelnut (*Rice Dream* Supreme) .... | 140 | 1.0 | 29.0 | 2.5 | 0 | 65 | 0 |
| **Rice bran** (*Bob's Red Mill*), ¼ cup ........ | 50 | 2.0 | 8.0 | 3.0 | 0 | 0 | 4.0 |
| **Rice cakes**, brown rice, 1 pc., except as noted: | | | | | | | |
| (*Lundberg* Eco-Farmed No Salt), .65 oz. ..... | 70 | 1.0 | 14.0 | 0 | 0 | 0 | 1.0 |
| (*Lundberg* Eco-Farmed/ Organic), .65 oz. ..... | 70 | 1.0 | 15.0 | 0 | 0 | 55 | 1.0 |
| (*Lundberg* Organic No Salt), .65 oz. ..... | 70 | 1.0 | 16.0 | 0 | 0 | 0 | 1.0 |
| (*Mother's*), .3 oz. ....... | 35 | 1.0 | 7.0 | 0 | 0 | 0 | 0 |
| (*Mother's* Salted), .3 oz. . | 35 | 1.0 | 7.0 | 0 | 0 | 15 | 0 |
| (*Quaker* Lightly Salted), .3 oz. ............ | 35 | 1.0 | 7.0 | 0 | 0 | 15 | 0 |
| (*Quaker* No Salt), .3 oz. ... | 35 | 1.0 | 7.0 | 0 | 0 | 0 | 0 |
| apple cinnamon: | | | | | | | |
| (*Lundberg* Eco-Farmed), .75 oz. ... | 80 | 2.0 | 18.0 | .5 | 0 | 0 | 1.0 |
| (*Quaker*), .5 oz. ...... | 50 | 1.0 | 11.0 | 0 | 0 | 0 | 0 |
| mini (*Quaker Quakes*), 8 pcs., .5 oz. ..... | 60 | 1.0 | 13.0 | 0 | 0 | 50 | 0 |
| barbecue, mini (*Quaker Quakes*), 10 pcs., .5 oz. | 70 | 1.0 | 12.0 | 2.0 | 0 | 140 | 0 |
| butter (*Mother's*), .3 oz. . | 35 | 1.0 | 8.0 | 0 | 0 | 45 | 0 |
| caramel, buttery (*Lundberg* Eco-Farmed), .75 oz. ............ | 80 | 2.0 | 18.0 | .5 | 0 | 0 | 1.0 |

| Food and Measure | cal. | prot. (gms) | carbo. (gms) | fat (gms) | chol. (mgs) | sod. (mgs) | fiber (gms) |
|---|---|---|---|---|---|---|---|
| **Rice cakes** *(cont.)* | | | | | | | |
| caramel, corn: | | | | | | | |
| (*Lundberg* Organic), | | | | | | | |
| .75 oz. . . . . . . . . . . | 80 | 1.0 | 18.0 | .5 | 0 | 40 | 1.0 |
| (*Mother's*), .45 oz. . . . | 45 | 1.0 | 10.0 | 0 | 0 | 30 | 0 |
| (*Quaker*), .45 oz. . . . . . | 50 | 1.0 | 11.0 | 0 | 0 | 30 | 0 |
| mini (*Quaker Quakes True Delights*), | | | | | | | |
| 7 pcs., .5 oz. . . . . . | 60 | 1.0 | 13.0 | 0 | 0 | 150 | 1.0 |
| cheddar, mini (*Quaker Quakes True Delights*), | | | | | | | |
| 9 pcs., .5 oz. . . . . . | 70 | 1.0 | 11.0 | 2.5 | 0 | 230 | 0 |
| cheddar, white: | | | | | | | |
| (*Quaker*), .4 oz. . . . . . . | 45 | 1.0 | 8.0 | .5 | 0 | 105 | 0 |
| popcorn (*Mother's*), | | | | | | | |
| .35 oz. . . . . . . . . . | 40 | 1.0 | 8.0 | 0 | 0 | 90 | 0 |
| cheese, nacho, mini (*Quaker Quakes*), | | | | | | | |
| 9 pcs., .5 oz. . . . . . . . | 70 | 1.0 | 10.0 | 2.5 | 0 | 210 | 1.0 |
| chocolate: | | | | | | | |
| crunch (*Quaker*), .5 oz. | 60 | 1.0 | 11.0 | 1.0 | 0 | 30 | 0 |
| mini (*Quaker Quakes*), | | | | | | | |
| 7 pcs., .5 oz. . . . . . | 60 | 1.0 | 13.0 | 1.0 | 0 | 50 | 0 |
| cinnamon toast (*Lundberg* Organic), .75 oz. . . . . . | 80 | 1.0 | 18.0 | .5 | 0 | 0 | 1.0 |
| w/corn/popcorn: | | | | | | | |
| (*Lundberg* Organic), | | | | | | | |
| .7 oz. . . . . . . . . . . | 70 | 1.0 | 16.0 | 0 | 0 | 55 | 1.0 |
| butter popped (*Quaker*), .3 oz. . . . | 35 | 1.0 | 8.0 | 0 | 0 | 45 | 0 |
| mini (*Quaker Quakes Kettle*), 15 pcs., | | | | | | | |
| 1.1 oz. . . . . . . . . . | 110 | 2.0 | 26.0 | 1.0 | 0 | 290 | 1.0 |
| green tea, sweet, w/lemon (*Lundberg* Organic), .75 oz. . . . . . | 80 | 1.0 | 17.0 | 0 | 0 | 0 | 1.0 |
| honey nut (*Lundberg* Eco-Farmed), .75 oz. . | 80 | 2.0 | 18.0 | .5 | 0 | 5 | 1.0 |
| koku seaweed (*Lundberg* Organic), .75 oz. . . . . . | 80 | 2.0 | 16.0 | 0 | 0 | 90 | 1.0 |
| mochi sweet (*Lundberg* Organic), .7 oz. . . . . . . | 70 | 1.0 | 15.0 | 0 | 0 | 55 | 1.0 |
| ranch, mini (*Quaker Quakes*), | | | | | | | |
| 10 pcs., .56 oz. . . . . . . | 70 | 1.0 | 10.0 | 2.5 | 0 | 200 | 0 |

| Food and Measure | cal. | prot. (gms) | carbo. (gms) | fat (gms) | chol. (mgs) | sod. (mgs) | fiber (gms) |
|---|---|---|---|---|---|---|---|
| sea salt, cracked pepper (*Quaker Quakes True Delights*), 9 pcs., .5 oz. .............. | 70 | 1.0 | 11.0 | 2.0 | 0 | 125 | 1.0 |
| sesame, toasted (*Lundberg* Eco-Farmed), .7 oz. ...... | 70 | 2.0 | 15.0 | 0 | 0 | 65 | 1.0 |
| sour cream/onion, mini (*Quaker Quakes*), 10 pcs., .6 oz. ....... | 70 | 1.0 | 12.0 | 2.5 | 0 | 140 | 0 |
| tamari: |  |  |  |  |  |  |  |
| flax w/ (*Lundberg* Organic), .75 oz. .. | 80 | 2.0 | 17.0 | 1.0 | 0 | 55 | 1.0 |
| w/seaweed (*Lundberg* Organic), .65 oz. .. | 70 | 1.0 | 15.0 | 0 | 0 | 125 | 1.0 |
| sesame (*Lundberg* Organic/Eco-Farmed), .7 oz. .... | 70 | 2.0 | 16.0 | .5 | 0 | 120 | 2.0 |
| vanilla crème brûlée, mini (*Quaker Quakes*), 10 pcs., .5 oz. ....... | 60 | 0 | 13.0 | 0 | 0 | 100 | 0 |
| wild (*Lundberg* Organic), .65 oz. ............. | 70 | 1.0 | 15.0 | 0 | 0 | 55 | 1.0 |
| **Rice chips/crisps** (see also "Cracker"), 1 oz., except as noted: |  |  |  |  |  |  |  |
| barbecue (*Lundberg* Santa Fe) .......... | 140 | 2.0 | 18.0 | 7.0 | 0 | 110 | <1.0 |
| brown (*Eden* Organic Chips), 1.1 oz. ...... | 150 | 2.0 | 19.0 | 7.0 | 0 | 100 | 0 |
| honey Dijon (*Lundberg*) . | 140 | 1.0 | 18.0 | 7.0 | 0 | 260 | 1.0 |
| lime (*Lundberg* Fiesta) .. | 140 | 2.0 | 18.0 | 7.0 | 0 | 270 | 1.0 |
| marinara, spicy (*New York Style Risotto Chips*) ............ | 140 | 2.0 | 19.0 | 7.0 | 0 | 160 | 2.0 |
| Parmesan roasted garlic (*New York Style Risotto Chips*) .. | 140 | 2.0 | 19.0 | 7.0 | 0 | 120 | 2.0 |
| pico de gallo (*Lundberg*) ......... | 140 | 2.0 | 18.0 | 7.0 | 0 | 230 | <1.0 |
| puffs, 5-flavor arare (*Eden* Organic), 1.1 oz. ............. | 110 | 3.0 | 24.0 | 0 | 0 | 160 | 2.0 |

| Food and Measure | cal. | prot. (gms) | carbo. (gms) | fat (gms) | chol. (mgs) | sod. (mgs) | fiber (gms) |
|---|---|---|---|---|---|---|---|
| **Rice chips/crisps** *(cont.)* | | | | | | | |
| sea salt: | | | | | | | |
| (*Lundberg*) . . . . . . . . . | 140 | 2.0 | 18.0 | 7.0 | 0 | 110 | <1.0 |
| (*New York Style Risotto Chips*) . . . . | 140 | 2.0 | 19.0 | 7.0 | 0 | 110 | 2.0 |
| sesame, black, sea salt (*Blue Ginger*) . . . . | 110 | 2.0 | 21.0 | 3.0 | 0 | 240 | 3.0 |
| sesame seaweed (*Lundberg*) . . . . . . . . . | 140 | 2.0 | 18.0 | 7.0 | 0 | 90 | <1.0 |
| sour cream scallion (*Blue Ginger*) . . . . . . . | 110 | 2.0 | 20.0 | 3.5 | 0 | 240 | 3.0 |
| wasabi (*Lundberg*) . . . . . | 140 | 2.0 | 18.0 | 6.0 | 0 | 210 | 1.0 |
| **Rice and corn chips** (*Tortillaz*), 1 oz.: | | | | | | | |
| cheesy nacho . . . . . . . . | 130 | 2.0 | 19.0 | 5.0 | 0 | 220 | 1.0 |
| garden salsa . . . . . . . . . | 120 | 2.0 | 21.0 | 4.0 | 0 | 210 | 1.0 |
| guacamole, zesty . . . . . . | 120 | 2.0 | 20.0 | 4.0 | 0 | 210 | 1.0 |
| **Rice dish, canned**: | | | | | | | |
| fried, Oriental Asian (*La Choy*), 1 cup* . . . . | 280 | 30.0 | 36.0 | 1.5 | 35 | 1120 | 2.0 |
| Spanish (*Zapata*), ⅔ cup . . . . . . . . . . . . | 100 | 2.0 | 21.0 | 1.0 | 0 | 320 | 3.0 |
| **Rice dish, frozen** (see also "Rice entree, frozen"): | | | | | | | |
| broccoli and cheese (*Veg-All Steam-Supreme*), 1 cup* . . . . | 200 | 6.0 | 29.0 | 5.0 | 15 | 470 | 1.0 |
| brown rice, 1½ cups: | | | | | | | |
| broccoli and carrots (*Birds Eye Steamfresh*) . . . . . . | 150 | 4.0 | 31.0 | 1.0 | 0 | 25 | 3.0 |
| multigrain, w/spinach, tomato, onion (*Birds Eye Steamfresh*) . . . | 180 | 6.0 | 36.0 | 1.0 | 0 | 40 | 4.0 |
| and wild, w/corn, carrots, peas (*Birds Eye Steamfresh*) . . . | 190 | 5.0 | 39.0 | 1.5 | 0 | 20 | 4.0 |
| cheesy, and broccoli (*Green GiantValley Fresh Steamers*), 1 cup* | 150 | 5.0 | 28.0 | 2.5 | 0 | 670 | 2.0 |
| chicken flavor (*Birds Eye Steamfresh*), 1½ cups . . . . . . . . . . | 240 | 6.0 | 41.0 | 4.5 | 0 | 720 | 1.0 |

| Food and Measure | cal. | prot. (gms) | carbo. (gms) | fat (gms) | chol. (mgs) | sod. (mgs) | fiber (gms) |
|---|---|---|---|---|---|---|---|
| long grain white, mixed vegetables (*Birds Eye Steamfresh*), 1½ cups ......... | 190 | 5.0 | 42.0 | .5 | 0 | 15 | 2.0 |
| Southwestern: | | | | | | | |
| (*Birds Eye Steamfresh*), 1½ cups ......... | 230 | 4.0 | 43.0 | 5.0 | 0 | 1010 | 1.0 |
| (*Veg-All Steam-Supreme*), 1 cup* . | 170 | 5.0 | 33.0 | 1.5 | 5 | 200 | 3.0 |
| vegetable, w/chicken (*Veg-All SteamSupreme*), 1 cup* ............. | 150 | 4.0 | 30.0 | 0 | 0 | 230 | 2.0 |
| **Rice dish, microwave** (see also "Rice entree, microwave"), 1 cup*, except as noted: | | | | | | | |
| (*Old El Paso* Fiesta) ..... | 240 | 5.0 | 47.0 | 4.5 | 0 | 680 | 1.0 |
| (*Seeds of Change* Organic Dharamsala) . | 230 | 8.0 | 41.0 | 3.5 | 0 | 480 | 4.0 |
| beans, red, and (*Seeds of Change* Organic Caribbean) ........ | 250 | 6.0 | 50.0 | 3.0 | 0 | 360 | 5.0 |
| broccoli and cheese (*Minute* Steamers) ... | 200 | 6.0 | 37.0 | 3.5 | 5 | 720 | 1.0 |
| brown and wild (*Uncle Ben's Whole Grain Medley*) ........... | 220 | 6.0 | 42.0 | 3.5 | 0 | 730 | 3.0 |
| butter/garlic (*Uncle Ben's Ready Rice*) .... | 220 | 4.0 | 41.0 | 4.0 | 0 | 750 | 2.0 |
| Cajun (*Uncle Ben's Ready Rice*) ........ | 210 | 6.0 | 42.0 | 2.0 | 0 | 980 | 3.0 |
| cheese, 4 (*Uncle Ben's Ready Rice*) .... | 230 | 6.0 | 44.0 | 3.5 | 0 | 900 | 2.0 |
| chicken flavor: | | | | | | | |
| (*Minute* Ready to Serve!), 1 cont. ... | 230 | 6.0 | 41.0 | 5.0 | 0 | 1020 | 2.0 |
| (*Uncle Ben's Whole Grain Medley*) .... | 210 | 5.0 | 41.0 | 3.5 | 0 | 730 | 4.0 |
| roasted (*Uncle Ben's Ready Rice*) ...... | 220 | 5.0 | 41.0 | 3.5 | 0 | 1020 | 2.0 |
| roasted (*Uncle Ben's Ready Rice* Family Size) ............ | 230 | 5.0 | 44.0 | 4.0 | 0 | 960 | 1.0 |

| Food and Measure | cal. | prot. (gms) | carbo. (gms) | fat (gms) | chol. (mgs) | sod. (mgs) | fiber (gms) |
|---|---|---|---|---|---|---|---|
| **Rice dish, microwave** *(cont.)* | | | | | | | |
| fried (*Minute* Steamers) . | 280 | 5.0 | 50.0 | 6.0 | 5 | 770 | 2.0 |
| garlic, roasted (*Uncle Ben's Whole Grain Medley*) . . . . . . . . . . | 200 | 5.0 | 38.0 | 3.0 | 0 | 560 | 3.0 |
| ginger lentil (*Tasty Bite*), ½ of 8.8-oz. pkg. . . . . . . . | 190 | 5.0 | 35.0 | 3.5 | 0 | 380 | 3.0 |
| herb (*Tasty Bite* Tehari), ½ of 8.8-oz. pkg. . . . . | 210 | 4.0 | 40.0 | 3.5 | 0 | 360 | 1.0 |
| and lentils, Masala (*A Taste of India*), ½ of 6-oz. pkg. . . . . . . | 260 | 6.0 | 47.0 | 5.0 | 0 | 310 | 2.0 |
| long grain and wild (*Uncle Ben's Ready Rice*) . . . . . . . . . . . . | 220 | 5.0 | 43.0 | 3.0 | 0 | 900 | 2.0 |
| Mexican: | | | | | | | |
| (*Old El Paso*) . . . . . . . | 250 | 5.0 | 48.0 | 4.5 | 0 | 930 | 1.0 |
| fiesta (*Tasty Bite*), ½ of 8.8-oz. pkg. . . | 160 | 3.0 | 33.0 | 2.5 | 0 | 380 | 2.0 |
| pilaf: | | | | | | | |
| (*Minute* Ready to Serve!), 1 cont. . . . | 220 | 5.0 | 41.0 | 4.0 | 0 | 1350 | 2.0 |
| (*Uncle Ben's Ready Rice*) . . . . . . . . . . . | 220 | 6.0 | 42.0 | 3.5 | 0 | 970 | 2.0 |
| Santa Fe (*Uncle Ben's Whole Grain Medley*) . | 220 | 7.0 | 42.0 | 3.0 | 0 | 700 | 5.0 |
| Spanish: | | | | | | | |
| (*Minute* Ready to Serve!), 1 cont. . . . | 230 | 6.0 | 41.0 | 4.5 | 0 | 420 | 2.0 |
| (*Minute* Steamers) . . . | 280 | 5.0 | 51.0 | 6.0 | 0 | 990 | 2.0 |
| (*Uncle Ben's Ready Rice*) . . . . . . . . . . | 200 | 4.0 | 41.0 | 2.5 | 0 | 680 | 3.0 |
| spiced, w/raisins (*A Taste of India*), ½ of 6.5-oz. pkg. . . . . . . . | 330 | 5.0 | 51.0 | 12.0 | 0 | 320 | 2.0 |
| sweet and sour (*A Taste of China*), ½ pkg., 3 oz. . . . . . . . | 260 | 4.0 | 53.0 | 3.0 | 0 | 340 | 2.0 |
| tandoori pilaf (*Tasty Bite*), ½ of 8.8-oz. pkg. | 160 | 3.0 | 33.0 | 3.0 | 0 | 400 | <1.0 |
| teriyaki (*Uncle Ben's Ready Rice*) . . . . . . . . | 220 | 6.0 | 42.0 | 3.0 | 5 | 870 | 3.0 |

| Food and Measure | cal. | prot. (gms) | carbo. (gms) | fat (gms) | chol. (mgs) | sod. (mgs) | fiber (gms) |
|---|---|---|---|---|---|---|---|
| Thai lime pilaf (*Tasty Bite*), ½ of 8.8-oz. pkg. | 180 | 3.0 | 33.0 | 5.0 | 0 | 200 | <1.0 |
| vegetable: | | | | | | | |
| garden (*Uncle Ben's Ready Rice*) ...... | 200 | 4.0 | 41.0 | 2.5 | 0 | 830 | 1.0 |
| harvest (*Uncle Ben's Whole Grain Medley*) .......... | 220 | 5.0 | 44.0 | 3.0 | 0 | 780 | 5.0 |
| yellow (*Minute* Ready to Serve!), 1 cont. .... | 190 | 3.0 | 35.0 | 4.0 | 0 | 1030 | 1.0 |
| **Rice dish, mix** (see also "Rice entree mix" and "Grains, mixed, dish"), 1 cup*, except as noted: | | | | | | | |
| almond, toasted, pilaf (*Near East*), 2 oz. .... | 200 | 5.0 | 40.0 | 3.0 | 0 | 580 | 2.0 |
| and beans: | | | | | | | |
| (*Seeds of Change Organic Tuscan*) ... | 190 | 5.0 | 39.0 | 1.5 | 0 | 560 | 3.0 |
| (*Vigo* Santa Fe), ⅓ cup | 200 | 8.0 | 38.0 | 2.0 | 0 | 950 | 3.0 |
| black (*Carolina*), 2 oz. . | 200 | 7.0 | 39.0 | 1.5 | 0 | 930 | 5.0 |
| black (*Mahatma*), 2 oz. | 200 | 6.0 | 41.0 | 1.0 | 0 | 900 | 3.0 |
| black (*Ortega*), 2 oz. .. | 200 | 6.0 | 41.0 | 1.0 | 0 | 910 | 3.0 |
| black (*Seeds of Change Organic Cuban*) ... | 190 | 6.0 | 38.0 | 1.5 | 0 | 400 | 5.0 |
| black (*Vigo*), ⅓ cup .. | 190 | 7.0 | 39.0 | 1.0 | 2 | 950 | 5.0 |
| black (*Zatarain's*) .... | 220 | 8.0 | 47.0 | .5 | 0 | 1190 | 6.0 |
| black (*Zatarain's* Reduced Sodium) . | 220 | 8.0 | 47.0 | .5 | 0 | 860 | 6.0 |
| red (*Carolina/ Mahatma*), 2 oz. ... | 190 | 7.0 | 41.0 | .5 | 0 | 890 | 3.0 |
| red (*Rice-A-Roni*) .... | 290 | 8.0 | 52.0 | 7.0 | 0 | 1070 | 5.0 |
| red (*Vigo*), ⅓ cup .... | 190 | 7.0 | 39.0 | 1.0 | 2 | 950 | 5.0 |
| red (*Zatarain's*) ...... | 190 | 8.0 | 40.0 | 0 | 0 | 1190 | 5.0 |
| red (*Zatarain's* Reduced Sodium) . | 190 | 8.0 | 40.0 | 0 | 0 | 720 | 5.0 |
| red, spicy (*Zatarain's*) . | 200 | 7.0 | 40.0 | 0 | 0 | 890 | 5.0 |
| white (*Zatarain's*) .... | 220 | 8.0 | 47.0 | .5 | 0 | 1410 | 7.0 |
| beef/beef favor: | | | | | | | |
| (*Rice-A-Roni*) ....... | 310 | 7.0 | 51.0 | 9.0 | 0 | 1020 | 2.0 |
| (*Rice-A-Roni* Lower Sodium) ......... | 270 | 7.0 | 50.0 | 5.0 | 0 | 650 | 2.0 |
| (*Zatarain's*) ......... | 200 | 5.0 | 45.0 | 0 | 0 | 760 | 1.0 |

| Food and Measure | cal. | prot. (gms) | carbo. (gms) | fat (gms) | chol. (mgs) | sod. (mgs) | fiber (gms) |
|---|---|---|---|---|---|---|---|
| **Rice dish, mix** *(cont.)* | | | | | | | |
| biryani (*Neera's*) ....... | 132 | 3.0 | 29.0 | 1.0 | 0 | 4 | 1.0 |
| black-eyed peas | | | | | | | |
|   (*Zatarain's*) ......... | 220 | 9.0 | 46.0 | .5 | 0 | 1330 | 4.0 |
| broccoli au gratin: | | | | | | | |
|   (*Rice-A-Roni*) ....... | 350 | 8.0 | 46.0 | 16.0 | 5 | 910 | 2.0 |
|   (*Uncle Ben's* | | | | | | | |
|     *Country Inn*) ...... | 200 | 4.0 | 43.0 | 2.0 | 5 | 790 | 1.0 |
| broccoli and cheese: | | | | | | | |
|   (*Carolina*), 2 oz. ..... | 200 | 5.0 | 39.0 | 3.0 | 5 | 820 | 1.0 |
|   (*Mahatma*), 2 oz. .... | 230 | 6.0 | 43.0 | 3.5 | 5 | 930 | 1.0 |
|   (*Vigo* Risotto con | | | | | | | |
|     Broccoli), ⅓ pkg. .. | 190 | 6.0 | 39.0 | 1.5 | 8 | 900 | 1.0 |
|   cheddar (*Uncle Ben's* | | | | | | | |
|     Whole Grain White) | 200 | 5.0 | 41.0 | 2.0 | 0 | 600 | 4.0 |
| Caribbean (*Zatarain's*) ... | 160 | 3.0 | 34.0 | 1.5 | 0 | 820 | <1.0 |
| cheddar (*Rice-A-Roni*) .. | 370 | 8.0 | 50.0 | 16.0 | 10 | 990 | 2.0 |
| cheddar broccoli | | | | | | | |
|   (*Zatarain's*) ......... | 220 | 5.0 | 45.0 | 1.5 | <5 | 820 | <1.0 |
| cheese: | | | | | | | |
|   4, creamy (*Rice-A-* | | | | | | | |
|     *Roni*) ............ | 270 | 6.0 | 37.0 | 12.0 | 5 | 740 | 1.0 |
|   Italian, and herb | | | | | | | |
|     (*Rice-A-Roni* | | | | | | | |
|     *Nature's Way*) ..... | 340 | 7.0 | 52.0 | 12.0 | 5 | 740 | 1.0 |
| chicken, roasted, | | | | | | | |
|   garlic pilaf (*Near* | | | | | | | |
|   *East*), 2 oz. ......... | 190 | 5.0 | 43.0 | .5 | 0 | 520 | 1.0 |
| chicken flavor: | | | | | | | |
|   (*Carolina*), 2 oz. ..... | 190 | 5.0 | 42.0 | 0 | 0 | 970 | <1.0 |
|   (*Mahatma*), 2 oz. .... | 190 | 5.0 | 42.0 | .5 | 0 | 930 | 1.0 |
|   (*Rice-A-Roni*) ....... | 300 | 7.0 | 50.0 | 9.0 | 0 | 1060 | 3.0 |
|   (*Rice-A-Roni* Lower | | | | | | | |
|     Sodium) ......... | 270 | 7.0 | 51.0 | 5.0 | 0 | 670 | 2.0 |
|   (*Uncle Ben's* | | | | | | | |
|     *Country Inn*) ...... | 200 | 6.0 | 41.0 | 1.0 | 0 | 940 | 1.0 |
|   (*Zatarain's*) ......... | 210 | 5.0 | 44.0 | 1.0 | 5 | 900 | 1.0 |
|   (*Zatarain's* Dinner) ... | 150 | 3.0 | 32.0 | 0 | 0 | 890 | 1.0 |
|   broccoli (*Rice-A-Roni*) | 220 | 6.0 | 40.0 | 5.0 | 0 | 920 | 2.0 |
|   broccoli (*Uncle Ben's* | | | | | | | |
|     *Country Inn*) ...... | 190 | 5.0 | 42.0 | 1.0 | 0 | 910 | 1.0 |
|   creamy (*Uncle Ben's* | | | | | | | |
|     Whole Grain White) | 200 | 5.0 | 44.0 | 2.0 | 0 | 590 | 5.0 |
|   Creole (*Zatarain's*) ... | 130 | 3.0 | 28.0 | .5 | 0 | 770 | 1.0 |

| Food and Measure | cal. | prot. (gms) | carbo. (gms) | fat (gms) | chol. (mgs) | sod. (mgs) | fiber (gms) |
|---|---|---|---|---|---|---|---|
| fajita (*Rice-A-Roni*) ... | 260 | 5.0 | 41.0 | 9.0 | 0 | 1090 | 2.0 |
| garlic (*Rice-A-Roni*) .. | 250 | 6.0 | 41.0 | 8.0 | 0 | 750 | 2.0 |
| herb (*Rice-A-Roni Whole Grain*) ..... | 260 | 6.0 | 41.0 | 8.0 | 0 | 760 | 4.0 |
| mushroom (*Rice-A-Roni*) ........... | 350 | 8.0 | 51.0 | 13.0 | 5 | 1290 | 2.0 |
| Parmesan (*Rice-A-Roni*) ........... | 370 | 8.0 | 52.0 | 15.0 | 5 | 1240 | 3.0 |
| pilaf (*Near East*), 2 oz. | 190 | 5.0 | 43.0 | .5 | 0 | 720 | 1.0 |
| smothered (*Zatarain's*) | 130 | 3.0 | 28.0 | 0 | 0 | 760 | <1.0 |
| teriyaki (*Rice-A-Roni*) . | 250 | 6.0 | 40.0 | 8.0 | 0 | 750 | 2.0 |
| vegetable (*Uncle Ben's Country Inn*) ...... | 200 | 5.0 | 41.0 | 1.5 | 0 | 720 | 1.0 |
| wild rice (*Uncle Ben's Country Inn*) ...... | 200 | 5.0 | 42.0 | 1.0 | 0 | 800 | 1.0 |
| coconut ginger (*A Taste of Thai*), ¾ cup* ..... | 200 | 4.0 | 36.0 | 3.0 | 0 | 400 | 1.0 |
| "couscous," roasted brown rice (*Lundberg*), 1.6 oz., ¼ pkg.: | | | | | | | |
| curry, Mediterranean . | 150 | 3.0 | 34.0 | 1.5 | 0 | 460 | 3.0 |
| garlic/olive oil ....... | 150 | 3.0 | 34.0 | 1.5 | 0 | 370 | 2.0 |
| herb, savory ........ | 150 | 3.0 | 34.0 | 1.5 | 0 | 400 | 2.0 |
| curry: | | | | | | | |
| pilaf (*Near East*), 2 oz. | 190 | 4.0 | 44.0 | .5 | 0 | 610 | 2.0 |
| yellow (*A Taste of Thai*), ¾ cup* ..... | 180 | 4.0 | 37.0 | 1.5 | 0 | 610 | 1.0 |
| dirty rice: | | | | | | | |
| (*Neera's* Jamaican) ... | 175 | 3.0 | 28.0 | 6.0 | 0 | 5 | 2.0 |
| (*Zatarain's*) .......... | 130 | 3.0 | 29.0 | 0 | 0 | 620 | <1.0 |
| (*Zatarain's* Reduced Sodium) ......... | 130 | 3.0 | 29.0 | 0 | 0 | 450 | <1.0 |
| brown (*Zatarain's*) ... | 140 | 3.0 | 30.0 | 1.0 | 0 | 780 | 2.0 |
| w/cheese (*Zatarain's*) . | 170 | 4.0 | 32.0 | 3.0 | <5 | 1040 | <1.0 |
| fried rice: | | | | | | | |
| (*Rice-A-Roni*) ....... | 310 | 7.0 | 50.0 | 10.0 | 0 | 1350 | 2.0 |
| Oriental (*Uncle Ben's Country Inn*) ...... | 200 | 6.0 | 42.0 | 1.0 | 0 | 580 | 1.0 |
| garlic: | | | | | | | |
| basil coconut (*A Taste of Thai*), ¾ cup* ... | 180 | 4.0 | 34.0 | 2.5 | 0 | 360 | 1.0 |
| herb (*Zatarain's*) ..... | 150 | 4.0 | 33.0 | 0 | 0 | 980 | <1.0 |
| herb pilaf (*Near East*), 2 oz. ............ | 190 | 4.0 | 44.0 | .5 | 0 | 500 | 1.0 |

| Food and Measure | cal. | prot. (gms) | carbo. (gms) | fat (gms) | chol. (mgs) | sod. (mgs) | fiber (gms) |
|---|---|---|---|---|---|---|---|
| **Rice dish, mix, garlic** *(cont.)* | | | | | | | |
| Italian creamy | | | | | | | |
| (*Rice-A-Roni*) ..... | 260 | 4.0 | 41.0 | 10.0 | 0 | 900 | 2.0 |
| roasted, Italiano | | | | | | | |
| (*Rice-A-Roni* | | | | | | | |
| Whole Grain) ..... | 270 | 6.0 | 41.0 | 9.0 | 0 | 760 | 3.0 |
| gravy and (*Zatarain's*) ... | 200 | 5.0 | 45.0 | .5 | 0 | 1200 | <1.0 |
| herb and butter | | | | | | | |
| (*Rice-A-Roni*) ....... | 310 | 6.0 | 53.0 | 9.0 | 0 | 1050 | 1.0 |
| jambalaya: | | | | | | | |
| (*Vigo* Cajun), ⅓ cup .. | 200 | 5.0 | 41.0 | 1.5 | 0 | 660 | 2.0 |
| (*Zatarain's*) ......... | 130 | 3.0 | 29.0 | 0 | 0 | 500 | <1.0 |
| (*Zatarain's* Reduced | | | | | | | |
| Sodium) ......... | 130 | 3.0 | 29.0 | 0 | 0 | 360 | <1.0 |
| brown (*Zatarain's*) ... | 140 | 4.0 | 31.0 | 1.0 | 0 | 610 | 2.0 |
| w/cheese (*Zatarain's*) . | 170 | 4.0 | 32.0 | 3.5 | <5 | 700 | <1.0 |
| mild (*Zatarain's*) ..... | 130 | 3.0 | 30.0 | 0 | 0 | 460 | 1.0 |
| spicy (*Zatarain's*) .... | 130 | 3.0 | 30.0 | 0 | 0 | 500 | 1.0 |
| and lentil pilaf: | | | | | | | |
| (*Near East*), 2 oz. .... | 180 | 11.0 | 36.0 | 3.5 | 0 | 650 | 8.0 |
| (*Vigo*), ¼ pkg. ...... | 190 | 7.0 | 40.0 | .5 | 0 | 810 | 4.0 |
| long grain and wild: | | | | | | | |
| (*Carolina/Mahatma*), | | | | | | | |
| 2 oz. ............ | 200 | 5.0 | 43.0 | .5 | 0 | 550 | 2.0 |
| (*Rice-A-Roni*) ....... | 240 | 5.0 | 43.0 | 6.0 | 0 | 840 | 1.0 |
| (*Rice-A-Roni Nature's* | | | | | | | |
| *Way*) .......... | 250 | 5.0 | 43.0 | 7.0 | 0 | 760 | 1.0 |
| (*Uncle Ben's* Fast | | | | | | | |
| Cook) ........... | 190 | 5.0 | 41.0 | .5 | 0 | 680 | 1.0 |
| (*Uncle Ben's* Original) . | 200 | 6.0 | 44.0 | 0 | 0 | 670 | 1.0 |
| (*Vigo*), ¼ pkg. ...... | 190 | 5.0 | 42.0 | 0 | 3 | 800 | 0 |
| (*Zatarain's*) ......... | 230 | 6.0 | 49.0 | 1.0 | 0 | 1000 | 2.0 |
| butter/herb (*Uncle* | | | | | | | |
| *Ben's*) ........... | 190 | 5.0 | 40.0 | 1.0 | 0 | 810 | 1.0 |
| chicken, herb-roasted | | | | | | | |
| (*Uncle Ben's*) ..... | 190 | 5.0 | 39.0 | 1.0 | 0 | 640 | 3.0 |
| garlic, roasted/olive | | | | | | | |
| oil (*Uncle Ben's*) ... | 180 | 5.0 | 39.0 | 1.0 | 0 | 590 | 3.0 |
| garlic herb (*Near* | | | | | | | |
| *East*), 2 oz. ....... | 190 | 5.0 | 43.0 | .5 | 0 | 620 | 2.0 |
| pilaf (*Near East*), 2 oz. . | 190 | 5.0 | 43.0 | .5 | 0 | 720 | 1.0 |
| tomato, sun-dried, | | | | | | | |
| Florentine (*Uncle* | | | | | | | |
| *Ben's*) ........... | 180 | 6.0 | 39.0 | 1.0 | 0 | 580 | 3.0 |

| Food and Measure | cal. | prot. (gms) | carbo. (gms) | fat (gms) | chol. (mgs) | sod. (mgs) | fiber (gms) |
|---|---|---|---|---|---|---|---|
| vegetable, roasted, and chicken (*Near East*), 2 oz. ....... | 190 | 5.0 | 43.0 | .5 | 0 | 660 | 2.0 |
| vegetable pilaf (*Uncle Ben's*) .......... | 180 | 5.0 | 40.0 | 1.0 | 0 | 610 | 3.0 |
| Mexican: | | | | | | | |
| (*Rice-A-Roni*) ....... | 250 | 6.0 | 40.0 | 8.0 | 0 | 720 | 2.0 |
| (*Uncle Ben's Country Inn* Fiesta) ...... | 200 | 5.0 | 42.0 | 1.0 | 0 | 680 | 1.0 |
| (*Vigo*), ¼ pkg. ...... | 190 | 5.0 | 42.0 | 0 | 10 | 600 | 1.0 |
| cheesy (*Old El Paso*), ⅓ pkg.* ......... | 280 | 5.0 | 55.0 | 4.5 | 0 | 640 | 1.0 |
| mushroom: | | | | | | | |
| whole grain and wild (*Uncle Ben's*) ..... | 200 | 6.0 | 42.0 | 1.5 | 0 | 570 | 3.0 |
| wild, and herb pilaf (*Near East*), 2 oz. .. | 190 | 5.0 | 43.0 | .5 | 0 | 480 | 1.0 |
| Parmesan and Romano (*Rice-A-Roni Nature's Way*) .............. | 280 | 7.0 | 42.0 | 9.0 | 10 | 770 | 1.0 |
| pilaf (see also specific listings): | | | | | | | |
| (*Carolina/Mahatma* Classic), 2 oz. ..... | 190 | 5.0 | 43.0 | .5 | 0 | 790 | 1.0 |
| (*Near East*), 2 oz. .... | 190 | 4.0 | 43.0 | .5 | 0 | 780 | 1.0 |
| (*Near East* Whole Grain), 2 oz. ...... | 180 | 5.0 | 41.0 | 1.0 | 0 | 600 | 3.0 |
| (*Rice-A-Roni*) ....... | 310 | 7.0 | 52.0 | 9.0 | 0 | 1060 | 2.0 |
| (*Uncle Ben's Country Inn*) ...... | 200 | 5.0 | 43.0 | .5 | 0 | 640 | 1.0 |
| (*Vigo*), ¼ pkg. ...... | 190 | 6.0 | 41.0 | 0 | 0 | 560 | 0 |
| (*Zatarain's*) ......... | 200 | 5.0 | 45.0 | 0 | 0 | 880 | <1.0 |
| pilau (*Neera's Shahi*) .... | 286 | 6.0 | 48.0 | 8.0 | 0 | 6 | 2.0 |
| pork (*Zatarain's* Dinner) ............. | 140 | 3.0 | 32.0 | 0 | 0 | 880 | 1.0 |
| risotto (see also specific listings): | | | | | | | |
| Alfredo (*Lundberg Organic*), ½ cup* .. | 140 | 3.0 | 31.0 | 0 | 0 | 410 | 1.0 |
| asparagus/mushroom (*Roland*), ¼ cup ... | 150 | 3.0 | 34.0 | 0 | 0 | 360 | 2.0 |
| butternut squash (*Lundberg*), ½ cup* | 143 | 4.0 | 31.0 | 1.0 | 0 | 496 | 1.0 |

| Food and Measure | cal. | prot. (gms) | carbo. (gms) | fat (gms) | chol. (mgs) | sod. (mgs) | fiber (gms) |
|---|---|---|---|---|---|---|---|
| **Rice dish, mix, risotto** *(cont.)* | | | | | | | |
| Florentine (*Lundberg* Organic), ½ cup* | 140 | 3.0 | 31.0 | 0 | 0 | 410 | 1.0 |
| garlic herb (*RiceSelect Chef's Original*), ¼ cup | 170 | 4.0 | 38.0 | 0 | <5 | 570 | <1.0 |
| garlic primavera (*Lundberg*), ½ cup* | 140 | 4.0 | 29.0 | 1.0 | 0 | 520 | 1.0 |
| Italian herb (*Lundberg* Eco-Farmed), ½ cup* | 140 | 4.0 | 28.0 | 1.0 | 0 | 530 | 1.0 |
| Milanese (*Alessi*), ⅓ cup* | 190 | 4.0 | 42.0 | 0 | 0 | 710 | 1.0 |
| mushroom, wild (*Marrakesh Express*), 2 oz. | 190 | 5.0 | 42.0 | .5 | 0 | 720 | 1.0 |
| Parmesan (*Marrakesh Express*), 2 oz. | 200 | 5.0 | 42.0 | 1.0 | 0 | 760 | 1.0 |
| Parmesan (*RiceSelect Chef's Original*), ¼ cup | 170 | 5.0 | 34.0 | 1.5 | 5 | 350 | <1.0 |
| Parmesan, creamy (*Lundberg*), ½ cup* | 140 | 5.0 | 27.0 | 1.5 | 5 | 490 | 1.0 |
| porcini (*Alessi*), ⅓ cup* | 190 | 3.0 | 44.0 | 0 | 0 | 810 | 1.0 |
| porcini (*Lundberg* Organic), ½ cup* | 143 | 4.0 | 31.0 | 1.0 | 0 | 535 | 1.0 |
| porcini (*Roland*), ¼ cup | 150 | 3.0 | 34.0 | 0 | 0 | 350 | 1.0 |
| portobello (*RiceSelect Chef's Original*), ¼ cup | 160 | 4.0 | 35.0 | .5 | 0 | 610 | <1.0 |
| primavera (*Vigo*), ¼ pkg. | 190 | 5.0 | 42.0 | 0 | 2.5 | 780 | 0 |
| w/saffron (*Roland*), ¼ cup | 150 | 3.0 | 34.0 | 0 | 0 | 420 | 2.0 |
| sun-dried tomato (*Alessi*), ⅓ cup* | 190 | 4.0 | 42.0 | 0 | 0 | 600 | 1.0 |
| sun-dried tomato (*Roland*), ¼ cup | 150 | 3.0 | 33.0 | 1.0 | 0 | 95 | 1.0 |
| sun-dried tomato herb (*Marrakesh Express*), 2 oz. | 190 | 5.0 | 42.0 | 0 | 0 | 500 | 1.0 |
| Tuscan (*Lundberg* Organic), ½ cup* | 140 | 3.0 | 31.0 | 0 | 0 | 735 | 1.0 |

| Food and Measure | cal. | prot. (gms) | carbo. (gms) | fat (gms) | chol. (mgs) | sod. (mgs) | fiber (gms) |
|---|---|---|---|---|---|---|---|
| vegetable primavera (*Roland*), ¼ cup ... | 150 | 3.0 | 34.0 | 0 | 0 | 360 | 2.0 |
| saffron, see "yellow," below | | | | | | | |
| sesame ginger (*Near East*), 2.5 oz. ...... | 250 | 5.0 | 55.0 | 1.5 | 0 | 460 | 1.0 |
| Spanish: | | | | | | | |
| (*Carolina/Mahatma* Authentic), 2 oz. ... | 180 | 4.0 | 42.0 | 0 | 0 | 650 | 1.0 |
| (*Old El Paso*), ⅓ pkg.* | 270 | 5.0 | 54.0 | 4.5 | 0 | 900 | 2.0 |
| (*Ortega*), 2 oz. ...... | 190 | 4.0 | 43.0 | 0 | 0 | 690 | 1.0 |
| (*Rice-A-Roni*) ....... | 260 | 6.0 | 44.0 | 8.0 | 0 | 1250 | 3.0 |
| (*Rice-A-Roni* Whole Grain) .......... | 250 | 5.0 | 42.0 | 8.0 | 0 | 760 | 3.0 |
| (*Zatarain's*) ......... | 180 | 4.0 | 41.0 | 0 | 0 | 520 | <1.0 |
| pilaf (*Near East*), 2.5 oz. .......... | 240 | 5.0 | 55.0 | .5 | 0 | 910 | 2.0 |
| taco (*Uncle Ben's* Whole Grain White) ........ | 160 | 4.0 | 35.0 | 1.5 | 0 | 570 | 4.0 |
| tomato: | | | | | | | |
| sun-dried, basil (*Near East*), 2.5 oz. ..... | 240 | 6.0 | 54.0 | .5 | 0 | 900 | 2.0 |
| sweet (*Uncle Ben's* Whole Grain White) | 210 | 5.0 | 46.0 | 1.5 | 0 | 480 | 5.0 |
| vegetables: | | | | | | | |
| fire-roasted (*Zatarain's*) ....... | 170 | 4.0 | 38.0 | 0 | 0 | 800 | 1.0 |
| French market (*Zatarain's*) ....... | 160 | 4.0 | 34.0 | 0 | 0 | 880 | 1.0 |
| garden (*Rice-A-Roni*) . | 270 | 7.0 | 40.0 | 10.0 | 0 | 830 | 2.0 |
| garden (*Uncle Ben's* Whole Grain White) | 180 | 4.0 | 40.0 | 1.0 | 0 | 470 | 3.0 |
| white and wild, see "long grain and wild," above | | | | | | | |
| yellow: | | | | | | | |
| (*Ortega*), 2 oz. ...... | 190 | 4.0 | 43.0 | 0 | 0 | 990 | 1.0 |
| (*Vigo*), ⅓ cup ....... | 190 | 5.0 | 43.0 | 0 | 0 | 730 | .5 |
| (*Zatarain's*) ......... | 190 | 4.0 | 43.0 | 0 | 0 | 930 | <1.0 |
| saffron (*Carolina/ Mahatma*), 2 oz. ... | 200 | 4.0 | 43.0 | 1.0 | 0 | 750 | 1.0 |
| spicy (*Carolina*), 2 oz. . | 180 | 4.0 | 41.0 | .5 | 0 | 1150 | <1.0 |
| spicy (*Mahatma*), 2 oz. | 190 | 4.0 | 42.0 | .5 | 0 | 1010 | 1.0 |

| Food and Measure | cal. | prot. (gms) | carbo. (gms) | fat (gms) | chol. (mgs) | sod. (mgs) | fiber (gms) |
|---|---|---|---|---|---|---|---|
| **Rice entree, frozen**, 1 pkg., except as noted: | | | | | | | |
| (*Zatarain's* Big Easy Bowl), 10 oz. ....... | 430 | 22.0 | 56.0 | 12.0 | 45 | 870 | 5.0 |
| and beans, w/chicken (*Banquet*), 7 oz. ..... | 190 | 6.0 | 31.0 | 4.5 | 5 | 540 | 3.0 |
| and beans, Santa Fe: | | | | | | | |
| (*Lean Cuisine*), 10.375 oz. ....... | 290 | 11.0 | 50.0 | 5.0 | 15 | 590 | 4.0 |
| (*Michelina's Lean Gourmet*), 9 oz. ... | 320 | 10.0 | 52.0 | 8.0 | 20 | 670 | 3.0 |
| (*Smart Ones*), 10 oz. . | 310 | 10.0 | 51.0 | 7.0 | 15 | 660 | 4.0 |
| beans, red, w/sausage (*Zatarain's*), 12 oz. ... | 510 | 16.0 | 68.0 | 20.0 | 30 | 1200 | 5.0 |
| broccoli/cheese/chicken (*Blue Horizon*), ¼ of 28-oz. pkg. .......... | 210 | 14.0 | 27.0 | 4.5 | 30 | 660 | 1.0 |
| brown, and vegetables (*Amy's* Bowls): | | | | | | | |
| 10 oz. ............. | 260 | 9.0 | 36.0 | 9.0 | 0 | 550 | 5.0 |
| light sodium, 10 oz. .. | 260 | 9.0 | 36.0 | 9.0 | 0 | 270 | 5.0 |
| black-eyed peas, 9 oz. | 290 | 11.0 | 38.0 | 11.0 | 0 | 580 | 8.0 |
| teriyaki, 9.5 oz. ...... | 290 | 12.0 | 52.0 | 4.5 | 0 | 780 | 6.0 |
| cheesy, and broccoli (*Green Giant*), 10 oz. . | 270 | 7.0 | 51.0 | 5.0 | 5 | 960 | 2.0 |
| chicken and, see "Chicken entree, frozen" | | | | | | | |
| curry (*Helen's Kitchen Organic*), 10 oz.: | | | | | | | |
| Indian, w/tofu ....... | 260 | 10.0 | 39.0 | 7.0 | 0 | 450 | 5.0 |
| Thai, red ........... | 330 | 11.0 | 45.0 | 13.0 | 0 | 390 | 6.0 |
| Thai, yellow, w/tofu, vegetables ........ | 310 | 10.0 | 50.0 | 9.0 | 0 | 430 | 5.0 |
| dirty, w/beef and pork (*Zatarain's*), 10 oz. ... | 460 | 14.0 | 62.0 | 16.0 | 35 | 740 | 2.0 |
| fried rice: | | | | | | | |
| chicken (*Contessa On the Stove*), ⅓ pkg.: | | | | | | | |
| w/sauce, 8 oz. ..... | 250 | 15.0 | 40.0 | 3.5 | 45 | 810 | 3.0 |
| w/out sauce ...... | 220 | 14.0 | 33.0 | 3.5 | 45 | 230 | 3.0 |
| chicken (*Lean Cuisine*), 9 oz. ............. | 260 | 12.0 | 41.0 | 5.0 | 25 | 380 | 4.0 |

| Food and Measure | cal. | prot. (gms) | carbo. (gms) | fat (gms) | chol. (mgs) | sod. (mgs) | fiber (gms) |
|---|---|---|---|---|---|---|---|
| chicken (*Michelina's*), 8 oz. | 410 | 12.0 | 64.0 | 12.0 | 40 | 1090 | 2.0 |
| shrimp (*Michelina's*), 8 oz. | 400 | 11.0 | 65.0 | 11.0 | 55 | 980 | 2.0 |
| shrimp (*Stouffer's Easy Express* Skillets), ½ of 25-oz. pkg. | 280 | 14.0 | 50.0 | 3.0 | 70 | 1220 | 8.0 |
| jambalaya, see "Rice dish, mix/entree" | | | | | | | |
| w/peas, mushrooms (*Green Giant Medley*), 10 oz. | 250 | 7.0 | 48.0 | 4.0 | 0 | 1000 | 3.0 |
| pilaf, vegetable: | | | | | | | |
| (*Green Giant*), 10 oz. | 210 | 5.0 | 41.0 | 3.5 | 5 | 1170 | 3.0 |
| herbed butter sauce (*Birds Eye*), 1 cup | 150 | 4.0 | 25.0 | 4.0 | 5 | 560 | 1.0 |
| wild rice (*Michelina's Budget Gourmet*), 8 oz. | 320 | 7.0 | 59.0 | 6.0 | 10 | 630 | 2.0 |
| risotto: | | | | | | | |
| Parmigiano (*Michelina's Authentico*), 8 oz. | 420 | 16.0 | 49.0 | 18.0 | 45 | 770 | 1.0 |
| portobello Parmesan (*Healthy Choice Steam*), 9.5 oz. | 220 | 9.0 | 35.0 | 4.0 | 10 | 590 | 4.0 |
| vegetable, stir-fry: | | | | | | | |
| (*Michelina's Authentico*), 8 oz. | 450 | 7.0 | 60.0 | 20.0 | 10 | 700 | 2.0 |
| (*Michelina's Budget Gourmet*), 7.5 oz. | 390 | 7.0 | 56.0 | 15.0 | 5 | 530 | 2.0 |
| **Rice entree, microwave** (*Bowl Appétit!*), 1 cont.: | | | | | | | |
| cheddar broccoli | 290 | 7.0 | 52.0 | 6.0 | 10 | 950 | 2.0 |
| herb chicken flavor | 250 | 6.0 | 51.0 | 3.0 | 5 | 780 | 2.0 |
| teriyaki | 250 | 5.0 | 57.0 | 1.0 | 0 | 940 | 2.0 |
| **Rice entree mix** (see also "Rice dish, mix"), ⅙ pkg., except as noted: | | | | | | | |
| fried, Asian style (*Banquet Homestyle Bakes*), ¼ pkg. | 240 | 10.0 | 47.0 | 1.5 | 5 | 1160 | 3.0 |

| Food and Measure | cal. | prot. (gms) | carbo. (gms) | fat (gms) | chol. (mgs) | sod. (mgs) | fiber (gms) |
|---|---|---|---|---|---|---|---|
| **Rice entree mix** *(cont.)* | | | | | | | |
| and cuttlefish (*Vigo* Calamares) ......... | 300 | 9.0 | 46.0 | 8.0 | 150 | 890 | 0 |
| yellow rice and: | | | | | | | |
| chicken (*Vigo*) ...... | 230 | 8.0 | 44.0 | 2.5 | 15 | 620 | 1.0 |
| seafood (*Vigo* Paella) . | 330 | 10.0 | 47.0 | 11.0 | 110 | 660 | 0 |
| **Rice flakes** (see also "Cereal"), brown (*Eden* Organic), ½ cup ..... | 180 | 3.0 | 40.0 | 1.5 | 0 | 0 | 1.0 |
| **Rice flour**: | | | | | | | |
| brown: | | | | | | | |
| (*Arrowhead Mills* Organic), ⅓ cup ... | 130 | 3.0 | 27.0 | 1.0 | 0 | 0 | 2.0 |
| (*Bob's Red Mill* Regular/ Organic), ¼ cup ... | 140 | 3.0 | 31.0 | 1.0 | 0 | 5 | 2.0 |
| (*Hodgson Mill*), <¼ cup .......... | 110 | 2.0 | 23.0 | 1.0 | 0 | 0 | 1.0 |
| (*Lundberg* Organic/ Eco-Farmed), ¼ cup .......... | 110 | 2.0 | 22.0 | 1.5 | 0 | 0 | 2.0 |
| all-purpose baking (*Hodgson Mill* Gluten Free), ¼ cup | 110 | 1.0 | 24.0 | 0 | 0 | 0 | 1.0 |
| white: | | | | | | | |
| (*Arrowhead Mills* Organic), ⅓ cup ... | 120 | 2.0 | 28.0 | 0 | 0 | 0 | <1.0 |
| (*Bob's Red Mill* Regular/ Organic), ¼ cup ... | 150 | 2.0 | 32.0 | .5 | 0 | 0 | 1.0 |
| sweet (*Bob's Red Mill*), ¼ cup .......... | 180 | 3.0 | 40.0 | .5 | 0 | 0 | 1.0 |
| **Rice and lentils**, canned (*Eden* Organic): | | | | | | | |
| regular, ½ cup ......... | 120 | 4.0 | 23.0 | 1.0 | 0 | 120 | 2.0 |
| curried, ½ cup ......... | 130 | 4.0 | 21.0 | 1.0 | 0 | 200 | 1.0 |
| **Rice pasta**, see "Pasta" | | | | | | | |
| **Rice pudding**, ready-to-eat, 1 cont.: | | | | | | | |
| (*Handi-Snacks*), 3.5 oz. .. | 140 | 3.0 | 19.0 | 6.0 | 0 | 130 | 0 |
| (*Kozy Shack*) .......... | 130 | 4.0 | 22.0 | 3.0 | 15 | 120 | 0 |
| (*Kozy Shack* European) .. | 130 | 4.0 | 21.0 | 3.5 | 20 | 135 | 0 |
| (*Kozy Shack* No Sugar) .. | 70 | 4.0 | 11.0 | 1.0 | 10 | 120 | 3.0 |
| cinnamon raisin (*Kozy Shack*) ............. | 140 | 4.0 | 24.0 | 3.0 | 15 | 120 | 0 |

| Food and Measure | cal. | prot. (gms) | carbo. (gms) | fat (gms) | chol. (mgs) | sod. (mgs) | fiber (gms) |
|---|---|---|---|---|---|---|---|
| crème brûlée (*Jell-O* Sugar Free), 3.75 oz. . | 70 | 2.0 | 12.0 | 2.0 | 10 | 170 | 0 |
| **Rice pudding mix**: (*Jell-O* Americana), | | | | | | | |
| ¼ pkg. . . . . . . . . . . | 90 | 1.0 | 23.0 | 0 | 0 | 100 | 0 |
| (*Zatarain's*), ½ cup* . . . . | 120 | 1.0 | 26.0 | 1.0 | 10 | 130 | 1.0 |
| cinnamon raisin (*Uncle Ben's*), ⅓ pkg. . . . . . . | 160 | 2.0 | 37.0 | 1.0 | 0 | 180 | 0 |
| French vanilla (*Uncle Ben's*), ⅓ pkg. . . . . . . | 120 | 2.0 | 28.0 | 0 | 0 | 90 | 1.0 |
| **Rice seasoning mix**, fried (Kikkoman), | | | | | | | |
| 1⅓ tbsp. . . . . . . . . . . | 330 | 1.0 | 6.0 | 0 | 0 | 460 | 0 |
| **Rice-soy beverage** (*EdenBlend* Organic), | | | | | | | |
| 8 fl. oz. . . . . . . . . . . | 120 | 7.0 | 18.0 | 3.0 | 0 | 90 | <1.0 |
| **Rice syrup**, brown (*Lundberg Sweet Dreams* Organic/ Eco-Farmed), 2 tbsp. . | 150 | 0 | 36.0 | 0 | 0 | 70 | 0 |
| **Rigatoni entree**, frozen, 1 pkg., except as noted: | | | | | | | |
| w/broccoli, chicken: (*Michelina's Lean Gourmet*), 8 oz. . . . | 280 | 12.0 | 37.0 | 8.0 | 30 | 660 | 2.0 |
| (*Smart Ones*), 9 oz. . . | 280 | 19.0 | 39.0 | 5.0 | 25 | 810 | 3.0 |
| cheese, 5 (*Lean Cuisine*), 10 oz. . . . . . . | 350 | 15.0 | 51.0 | 9.0 | 15 | 650 | 4.0 |
| cheese stuffed: (*Italian Village*), | | | | | | | |
| ½ of 10.5-oz. pkg. . | 270 | 12.0 | 38.0 | 8.0 | 30 | 260 | 2.0 |
| (*Michelina's*), 8.5 oz. . | 270 | 11.0 | 39.0 | 7.0 | 40 | 580 | 3.0 |
| (*Michelina's Lean Gourmet*), 8 oz. . . . | 220 | 8.0 | 33.0 | 6.0 | 30 | 510 | 3.0 |
| 3 cheese (*Lean Cuisine* Cafe), 10 oz. . . . . . . | 230 | 13.0 | 32.0 | 6.0 | 20 | 370 | 4.0 |
| w/chicken: (*Stouffer's Easy Express*), ⅙ of | | | | | | | |
| 28-oz. pkg. . . . . . . . | 260 | 14.0 | 29.0 | 10.0 | 20 | 430 | 2.0 |
| in pesto sauce (*Stouffer's*), 8.38 oz. | 400 | 22.0 | 44.0 | 15.0 | 40 | 770 | 3.0 |

| Food and Measure | cal. | prot. (gms) | carbo. (gms) | fat (gms) | chol. (mgs) | sod. (mgs) | fiber (gms) |
|---|---|---|---|---|---|---|---|
| **Rigatoni entree** (cont.) | | | | | | | |
| w/fish (Marie Callender's Pasta al Dente Pesce), 10.5 oz. | 340 | 16.0 | 44.0 | 12.0 | 75 | 990 | 7.0 |
| marinara (Marie Callender's Pasta al Dente Classico), 10.5 oz. ... | 460 | 19.0 | 41.0 | 24.0 | 45 | 990 | 7.0 |
| meatball, cheesy (Stouffer's Easy Express Skillets), ½ of 24-oz. pkg. ...... | 470 | 21.0 | 48.0 | 21.0 | 55 | 1190 | 5.0 |
| w/meatballs (Lean Cuisine Dinnertime Cuisine), 15.4 oz. .... | 400 | 23.0 | 56.0 | 9.0 | 35 | 830 | 7.0 |
| w/vegetables (Birds Eye Steamfresh Lightly Sauced), 2 cups | 220 | 7.0 | 35.0 | 5.0 | 0 | 400 | 2.0 |
| w/vodka cream sauce (Smart Ones), 9 oz. .. | 290 | 13.0 | 48.0 | 6.0 | 10 | 440 | 5.0 |
| **Risotto**, see "Rice dish, mix/entree" | | | | | | | |
| **Rockfish**, meat only: | | | | | | | |
| raw, 4 oz. ............. | 107 | 21.3 | 0 | 1.8 | 39 | 68 | 0 |
| baked or broiled, 4 oz. .. | 137 | 27.3 | 0 | 2.3 | 50 | 87 | 0 |
| **Roe** (see also "Caviar"), mixed species: | | | | | | | |
| raw, 1 oz., 2 tbsp. ...... | 40 | 6.3 | .4 | 1.8 | 106 | 26 | 0 |
| baked or broiled, 1 oz. .. | 58 | 8.1 | .5 | 2.3 | 135 | 33 | 0 |
| **Roll** (see also "Bagel," "Bialy," and "Biscuit"), 1 roll, except as noted: | | | | | | | |
| brown and serve (Cobblestone Mill Pistolettes) ......... | 90 | 4.0 | 19.0 | 1.0 | 0 | 125 | 1.0 |
| dinner: | | | | | | | |
| (Arnold Select) ...... | 110 | 3.0 | 21.0 | 1.5 | 0 | 200 | <1.0 |
| honey wheat (Nature's Own) ........... | 50 | 2.0 | 10.0 | 0 | 0 | 80 | <1.0 |
| soft (Pepperidge Farm Country Style) .... | 90 | 3.0 | 17.0 | 1.5 | 0 | 150 | 1.0 |
| egg, 2 oz. ............. | 174 | 5.4 | 29.5 | 3.6 | 28 | 309 | 2.1 |
| French: | | | | | | | |
| (Arnold Select) ...... | 230 | 7.0 | 43.0 | 3.0 | 0 | 450 | 2.0 |

| Food and Measure | cal. | prot. (gms) | carbo. (gms) | fat (gms) | chol. (mgs) | sod. (mgs) | fiber (gms) |
|---|---|---|---|---|---|---|---|
| (*Pepperidge Farm* Hearth) .......... | 120 | 4.0 | 23.0 | 1.5 | 0 | 170 | 1.0 |
| hamburger: | | | | | | | |
| (*Fiber One*) ......... | 110 | 5.0 | 25.0 | 1.5 | 0 | 220 | 5.0 |
| (*Nature's Own Whitewheat*) ...... | 100 | 5.0 | 22.0 | 1.0 | 0 | 220 | 4.0 |
| (*Pepperidge Farm*) ... | 120 | 5.0 | 22.0 | 2.0 | 0 | 180 | 1.0 |
| (*Roman Meal*) ....... | 110 | 4.0 | 20.0 | 2.0 | 0 | 200 | 2.0 |
| (*Wonder*) .......... | 110 | 3.0 | 21.0 | 1.5 | 0 | 210 | <1.0 |
| wheat (*Wonder*) ..... | 110 | 4.0 | 21.0 | 1.5 | 0 | 220 | 2.0 |
| wheat, whole (*Pepperidge Farm* 100%) . | 120 | 6.0 | 18.0 | 2.0 | 0 | 190 | 2.0 |
| white (*Arnold Select*) . | 150 | 5.0 | 30.0 | 2.0 | 0 | 350 | 1.0 |
| white, whole grain (*Pepperidge Farm*) . | 100 | 6.0 | 18.0 | 1.0 | 0 | 190 | 2.0 |
| hamburger sliders: | | | | | | | |
| (*Pepperidge Farm*) ... | 100 | 4.0 | 18.0 | 2.0 | 0 | 160 | 1.0 |
| wheat (*Pepperidge Farm*) .......... | 100 | 5.0 | 17.0 | 2.0 | 0 | 150 | 1.0 |
| herb, Italian (*Pepperidge Farm* Hearth) ....... | 130 | 5.0 | 24.0 | 1.5 | 0 | 190 | 1.0 |
| hoagie: | | | | | | | |
| (*Cobblestone Mill Philly Style*) ...... | 180 | 7.0 | 36.0 | 2.5 | 0 | 340 | 2.0 |
| (*Pepperidge Farm*) ... | 210 | 7.0 | 35.0 | 6.0 | 0 | 350 | 2.0 |
| hot dog: | | | | | | | |
| (*Arnold Select Chicago*) ......... | 140 | 5.0 | 25.0 | 2.5 | 0 | 230 | 1.0 |
| (*Cobblestone Mill*) ... | 120 | 5.0 | 22.0 | 2.5 | 0 | 200 | 1.0 |
| (*Fiber One*) ......... | 110 | 4.0 | 25.0 | 1.5 | 0 | 230 | 5.0 |
| (*Nature's Own Whitewheat*) ...... | 90 | 5.0 | 20.0 | 1.0 | 0 | 200 | 4.0 |
| (*Pepperidge Farm*) ... | 140 | 5.0 | 26.0 | 2.5 | 0 | 190 | <1.0 |
| (*Wonder*) .......... | 110 | 3.0 | 21.0 | 1.5 | 0 | 210 | <1.0 |
| honey wheat (*Nature's Own*) .......... | 100 | 5.0 | 19.0 | 1.0 | 0 | 170 | <1.0 |
| potato (*Arnold Select*) .......... | 140 | 4.0 | 28.0 | 2.0 | 0 | 240 | 1.0 |
| wheat (*Arnold Select*) . | 140 | 5.0 | 25.0 | 2.0 | 0 | 270 | 2.0 |
| wheat (*Wonder*) ..... | 110 | 4.0 | 21.0 | 1.5 | 0 | 220 | 2.0 |
| wheat, whole (*Nature's Own*) .......... | 100 | 5.0 | 19.0 | 1.5 | 0 | 160 | 3.0 |
| white (*Arnold Select*) . | 130 | 4.0 | 26.0 | 2.0 | 0 | 310 | 1.0 |

| Food and Measure | cal. | prot. (gms) | carbo. (gms) | fat (gms) | chol. (mgs) | sod. (mgs) | fiber (gms) |
|---|---|---|---|---|---|---|---|
| **Roll** *(cont.)* | | | | | | | |
| white (*Arnold Select* New England) ..... | 120 | 4.0 | 23.0 | 2.0 | 0 | 230 | 1.0 |
| white, whole grain (*Pepperidge Farm*) . | 110 | 6.0 | 21.0 | 1.0 | 0 | 220 | 2.0 |
| Italian (*Arnold Select*), ½ pc. ....... | 190 | 6.0 | 36.0 | 2.5 | 0 | 380 | 1.0 |
| Kaiser, see "sandwich," below | | | | | | | |
| multigrain, 7 (*Pepperidge Farm* Hearth) ....... | 140 | 4.0 | 25.0 | 2.0 | 0 | 180 | 2.0 |
| onion (*Cobblestone Mill*) . | 170 | 6.0 | 31.0 | 2.5 | 0 | 290 | 1.0 |
| oat bran, 2 oz. ......... | 134 | 5.4 | 22.8 | 2.6 | 0 | 234 | 2.3 |
| po boy, long (*Cobblestone Mill*) ... | 240 | 9.0 | 48.0 | 3.0 | 0 | 450 | 2.0 |
| rye, 2 oz. ............. | 162 | 5.8 | 30.1 | 1.9 | 0 | 506 | 2.8 |
| sandwich (see also specific listings): | | | | | | | |
| butter (*Nature's Own*) . | 120 | 5.0 | 23.0 | 2.0 | 5 | 115 | 1.0 |
| honey wheat (*Nature's Own*) .......... | 130 | 6.0 | 26.0 | 1.5 | 0 | 230 | 1.0 |
| Kaiser (*Cobblestone Mill* Gourmet) ..... | 230 | 8.0 | 44.0 | 4.0 | 0 | 470 | 2.0 |
| multigrain (*Arnold Select* Kaiser) ..... | 150 | 8.0 | 28.0 | 2.0 | 0 | 280 | 3.0 |
| onion (*Arnold Select*) . | 210 | 6.0 | 39.0 | 3.5 | 0 | 380 | 2.0 |
| onion, poppy seeds (*Pepperidge Farm*) . | 150 | 6.0 | 28.0 | 2.5 | 0 | 230 | 1.0 |
| potato (*Arnold Select*) | 160 | 5.0 | 31.0 | 2.0 | 0 | 280 | 1.0 |
| seeded (*Cobblestone Mill*) ............ | 200 | 8.0 | 34.0 | 4.0 | 0 | 350 | 1.0 |
| sesame seed (*Pepperidge Farm*) . | 130 | 6.0 | 22.0 | 3.0 | 0 | 220 | 1.0 |
| wheat (*Arnold Select*) . | 150 | 6.0 | 29.0 | 2.5 | 0 | 310 | 2.0 |
| wheat, whole (*Arnold Whole Grains*) .... | 160 | 8.0 | 26.0 | 2.0 | 0 | 310 | 4.0 |
| wheat, whole (*Nature's Own*) .......... | 100 | 5.0 | 19.0 | 1.5 | 0 | 160 | 3.0 |
| whole grain (*Nature's Own* Sugar Free) .. | 110 | 6.0 | 23.0 | 1.5 | 0 | 240 | 4.0 |
| sandwich, thin: (*Arnold Select Sandwich This*): | | | | | | | |
| honey wheat ...... | 100 | 5.0 | 22.0 | 1.0 | 0 | 220 | 5.0 |

| Food and Measure | cal. | prot. (gms) | carbo. (gms) | fat (gms) | chol. (mgs) | sod. (mgs) | fiber (gms) |
|---|---|---|---|---|---|---|---|
| multigrain | 100 | 5.0 | 22.0 | 1.0 | 0 | 230 | 5.0 |
| rye | 100 | 4.0 | 23.0 | 1.0 | 0 | 210 | 5.0 |
| white, whole grain | 100 | 4.0 | 22.0 | 1.0 | 0 | 230 | 5.0 |
| whole wheat | 100 | 5.0 | 21.0 | 1.0 | 0 | 230 | 5.0 |
| (*Nature's Own* Rounds): | | | | | | | |
| multigrain | 100 | 5.0 | 21.0 | 1.0 | 0 | 190 | 5.0 |
| whole grain | 100 | 5.0 | 20.0 | 1.0 | 0 | 180 | 5.0 |
| whole wheat | 100 | 5.0 | 21.0 | 1.0 | 0 | 180 | 5.0 |
| (*Pepperidge Farm Deli Flats*): | | | | | | | |
| honey wheat, soft | 100 | 5.0 | 21.0 | 1.0 | 0 | 170 | 5.0 |
| multigrain, 7 | 100 | 6.0 | 19.0 | 1.0 | 0 | 170 | 5.0 |
| white, whole grain | 100 | 6.0 | 20.0 | 1.5 | 0 | 170 | 5.0 |
| whole wheat, soft | 100 | 6.0 | 19.0 | 1.5 | 0 | 170 | 5.0 |
| sourdough (*Pepperidge Farm* Hearth) | 130 | 5.0 | 24.0 | 1.5 | 0 | 180 | 2.0 |
| steak (*Arnold Select*) | 200 | 6.0 | 37.0 | 2.0 | 0 | 510 | 1.0 |
| sub (*Cobblestone Mill*): | | | | | | | |
| wheat | 220 | 8.0 | 44.0 | 2.5 | 0 | 460 | 4.0 |
| white | 170 | 6.0 | 34.0 | 1.5 | 0 | 360 | 2.0 |
| wheat: | | | | | | | |
| (*Nature's Own* Double Fiber) | 80 | 6.0 | 15.0 | 1.5 | 0 | 160 | 5.0 |
| (*Pepperidge Farm Farmhouse*) | 220 | 8.0 | 36.0 | 4.5 | 0 | 310 | 1.0 |
| white (*Pepperidge Farm Farmhouse*) | 210 | 8.0 | 35.0 | 4.5 | 0 | 390 | <1.0 |
| **Roll, frozen/chilled** (see also "Biscuit, frozen/chilled"), 1 pc., except as noted: | | | | | | | |
| (*Alexia* Biscuits) | 170 | 3.0 | 20.0 | 9.0 | 0 | 450 | <1.0 |
| ciabatta: | | | | | | | |
| cheese (*New York*), 1.65-oz. slice | 160 | 5.0 | 17.0 | 8.0 | 5 | 330 | 1.0 |
| rosemary, olive oil (*Alexia* Artisan) | 100 | 3.0 | 19.0 | 1.5 | 0 | 220 | 1.0 |
| crescent (*Pillsbury*): | | | | | | | |
| big & buttery/flaky | 170 | 3.0 | 20.0 | 9.0 | 0 | 380 | <1.0 |
| butter flake/rounds | 110 | 1.0 | 11.0 | 6.0 | 0 | 220 | 0 |
| garlic butter | 110 | 2.0 | 11.0 | 6.0 | 0 | 270 | 0 |
| original | 110 | 2.0 | 11.0 | 6.0 | 0 | 220 | 0 |
| reduced fat | 90 | 2.0 | 12.0 | 4.5 | 0 | 220 | 0 |

| Food and Measure | cal. | prot. (gms) | carbo. (gms) | fat (gms) | chol. (mgs) | sod. (mgs) | fiber (gms) |
|---|---|---|---|---|---|---|---|
| **Roll, frozen/chilled** *(cont.)* | | | | | | | |
| dinner: | | | | | | | |
| (*Pillsbury* Chilled) . . . . | 100 | 3.0 | 20.0 | 1.5 | 0 | 290 | <1.0 |
| (*Sister Schubert's* Pre- | | | | | | | |
| Baked Yeast) . . . . . | 140 | 3.0 | 23.0 | 4.0 | 10 | 230 | 1.0 |
| soft (*Sister Schubert's*) | 190 | 4.0 | 28.0 | 7.0 | 15 | 240 | 1.0 |
| wheat (*Sister Schu-* | | | | | | | |
| *bert's* Pre-Baked) . . | 140 | 4.0 | 22.0 | 4.0 | 10 | 230 | 2.0 |
| focaccia, 3 cheese | | | | | | | |
| (*Alexia* Artisan) . . . . . . | 110 | 4.0 | 19.0 | 2.0 | 0 | 230 | 1.0 |
| French (*Alexia* Artisan) . . | 100 | 4.0 | 20.0 | 0 | 0 | 230 | 1.0 |
| multigrain, soft | | | | | | | |
| (*Sister Schubert's*) . . . | 180 | 5.0 | 27.0 | 5.0 | 20 | 260 | 3.0 |
| Parker House, 2 pcs.: | | | | | | | |
| (*Sister Schubert's*) . . . | 150 | 3.0 | 21.0 | 6.0 | 15 | 240 | 1.0 |
| honey butter wheat | | | | | | | |
| (*Sister Schubert's*) . | 140 | 4.0 | 20.0 | 5.0 | 15 | 240 | 2.0 |
| sausage wrap (*Sister* | | | | | | | |
| *Schubert's*) . . . . . . . . . | 110 | 3.0 | 13.0 | 5.0 | 15 | 210 | 0 |
| whole grain w/flax | | | | | | | |
| (*Alexia* Artisan) . . . . . . | 90 | 4.0 | 17.0 | 1.0 | 0 | 190 | 2.0 |
| **Roll, sweet**, see "Bun, sweet" | | | | | | | |
| **Roll mix** (see also "Biscuit mix"), hot | | | | | | | |
| (*Pillsbury*), ¼ cup . . . . | 110 | 4.0 | 21.0 | 1.5 | 0 | 210 | <1.0 |
| **Roseapple**, 1 oz. . . . . . . . | 7 | .2 | 1.6 | .1 | 0 | <1 | <1.0 |
| **Roselle**, 1 oz., ½ cup . . . | 14 | .3 | 3.2 | .2 | 0 | 2 | <1.0 |
| **Rosemary**, fresh, 1 oz. . . | 37 | .9 | 5.9 | 1.7 | 0 | 7 | 4.0 |
| **Rosemary, dried**, 1 tsp. . | 4 | .1 | .8 | .2 | 0 | 1 | .2 |
| **Rotelle pasta dish**, frozen, w/vegetables, herb butter sauce | | | | | | | |
| (*Birds Eye*), 1 cup . . . . | 100 | 3.0 | 18.0 | 1.5 | 5 | 400 | 1.0 |
| **Rotelli pasta entree**, frozen, primavera (*Helen's Kitchen* Organic), 10-oz. pkg. . | 330 | 15.0 | 57.0 | 5.0 | 0 | 350 | 8.0 |
| **Rotini entree, frozen:** | | | | | | | |
| and broccoli, cheese sauce (*Birds Eye Steamfresh* Lightly Sauced), 2 cups . . . . . | 210 | 7.0 | 37.0 | 4.0 | 10 | 600 | 2.0 |

| Food and Measure | cal. | prot. (gms) | carbo. (gms) | fat (gms) | chol. (mgs) | sod. (mgs) | fiber (gms) |
|---|---|---|---|---|---|---|---|
| meatball (*Stouffer's Easy Express*), ¼ of 29-oz. pkg. ......... | 300 | 14.0 | 38.0 | 10.0 | 25 | 490 | 3.0 |
| w/vegetables: | | | | | | | |
| w/cheese, tofu (*Amy's Country Cheddar Bowl*), 9.5-oz. pkg. . | 430 | 16.0 | 45.0 | 21.0 | 20 | 690 | 4.0 |
| w/cheese, tofu (*Amy's Country Cheddar Bowl Light Sodium*), 9.5-oz. pkg. ...... | 430 | 16.0 | 45.0 | 21.0 | 20 | 345 | 4.0 |
| garlic butter sauce (*Birds Eye Steamfresh Lightly Sauced*), 2 cups .......... | 230 | 6.0 | 35.0 | 8.0 | 20 | 350 | 3.0 |
| **Rotini entree, microwave**, 1 cont.: | | | | | | | |
| cheese, 3 (*Bowl Appetit!*) | 340 | 10.0 | 59.0 | 7.0 | 10 | 1020 | 2.0 |
| marinara (*Healthy Choice Fresh Mixers*) . | 300 | 10.0 | 56.0 | 3.5 | 0 | 600 | 7.0 |
| **Rotini entree mix**: | | | | | | | |
| cheddar (*Annie's Deluxe*), 1 cup* ..... | 280 | 10.0 | 41.0 | 8.0 | 20 | 630 | 2.0 |
| cheese: | | | | | | | |
| (*Velveeta*), ½ of 9.4-oz. pkg. ...... | 400 | 15.0 | 49.0 | 16.0 | 25 | 1230 | 2.0 |
| 4 (*Annie's*), 1 cup* ... | 300 | 12.0 | 41.0 | 11.5 | 30 | 600 | 2.0 |
| **Roughy, orange**, meat only: | | | | | | | |
| raw, 4 oz. ............ | 78 | 16.7 | 0 | .8 | 23 | 72 | 0 |
| baked or broiled, 4 oz. .. | 101 | 21.4 | 0 | 1.0 | 29 | 92 | 0 |
| **Roux and gravy mix** (*Zatarain's* Instant), ½ tbsp. ............ | 15 | 0 | 3.0 | 0 | 0 | 210 | <1.0 |
| **Rowal**, ½ cup, 4 oz. .... | 127 | 2.6 | 27.2 | 2.0 | 0 | 5 | 7.1 |
| **Rubs**, dry: | | | | | | | |
| (*Maull's* Briskette), 1 tbsp. ............ | 5 | 0 | 1.0 | 0 | 0 | 510 | 0 |
| applewood (*Grill Mates*), 2 tsp. ....... | 15 | 0 | 3.0 | 0 | 0 | 350 | 0 |
| chicken: | | | | | | | |
| (*Emeril's*), ½ tsp. .... | 0 | 0 | 0 | 0 | 0 | 80 | 0 |
| (*Grill Mates*), 2 tsp. .... | 15 | 0 | 2.0 | 0 | 0 | 260 | 0 |

| Food and Measure | cal. | prot. (gms) | carbo. (gms) | fat (gms) | chol. (mgs) | sod. (mgs) | fiber (gms) |
|---|---|---|---|---|---|---|---|
| **Rubs** (cont.) | | | | | | | |
| jerk (Neera's | | | | | | | |
| Jamaican), 1 tsp. .... | 5 | 0 | 2.0 | 0 | 0 | 185 | 0 |
| pork (Grill Mates), | | | | | | | |
| 2 tsp. ............. | 15 | 0 | 2.0 | 0 | 0 | 220 | 0 |
| ribs (Emeril's), ½ tsp. ... | 0 | 0 | 0 | 0 | 0 | 160 | 0 |
| salmon, citrus spice | | | | | | | |
| (McCormick), 2 tsp. .. | 5 | 0 | 3.0 | 0 | 0 | 240 | 0 |
| seafood: | | | | | | | |
| (Old Bay), ¾ tsp. .... | 5 | 0 | 0 | 0 | 0 | 210 | 0 |
| herb w/lemon | | | | | | | |
| (McCormick), 2 tsp. | 15 | 0 | 3.0 | 0 | 0 | 300 | 0 |
| steak: | | | | | | | |
| (Emeril's), ½ tsp. .... | 0 | 0 | 0 | 0 | 0 | 220 | 0 |
| (Grill Mates), 2 tsp. .... | 15 | 0 | 3.0 | 0 | 0 | 440 | 0 |
| sweet and smoke (Grill | | | | | | | |
| Mates), 2 tsp. ....... | 15 | 0 | 3.0 | 0 | 0 | 500 | 0 |
| **Rum runner**, drink | | | | | | | |
| mixer, frozen | | | | | | | |
| (Bacardi), 2 fl. oz. .... | 120 | 0 | 32.0 | 0 | 0 | 5 | 0 |
| **Rutabaga**, fresh: | | | | | | | |
| 1 large, 1.7 lbs. ........ | 278 | 9.3 | 62.8 | 1.5 | 0 | 154 | 19.3 |
| raw, cubed: | | | | | | | |
| (Glory), 1 cup ....... | 50 | 2.0 | 11.0 | 0 | 0 | 30 | 4.0 |
| ½ cup ............. | 25 | .8 | 5.7 | .1 | 0 | 14 | 1.8 |
| boiled, drained: | | | | | | | |
| cubed, ½ cup ....... | 33 | 1.1 | 7.4 | .2 | 0 | 17 | 1.5 |
| mashed, ½ cup ...... | 47 | 1.6 | 10.5 | .3 | 0 | 25 | 2.2 |
| **Rutabaga**, canned | | | | | | | |
| (Sunshine), ½ cup ... | 30 | <1.0 | 7.0 | 0 | 0 | 220 | 1.0 |
| **Rutabaga, frozen**, | | | | | | | |
| diced (Allens), ⅔ cup . | 35 | 1.0 | 7.0 | 0 | 0 | 15 | 2.0 |
| **Rye**, whole-grain: | | | | | | | |
| (Bob's Red Mill | | | | | | | |
| Organic Berries), ¼ cup | 150 | 6.0 | 33.0 | 1.0 | 0 | 0 | 6.0 |
| 1 cup ............... | 567 | 25.0 | 117.9 | 4.2 | 0 | 10 | 24.7 |
| **Rye flakes** (Eden | | | | | | | |
| Organic), ½ cup ..... | 170 | 4.0 | 37.0 | 1.0 | 0 | 0 | 5.0 |
| **Rye flour**: | | | | | | | |
| (Arrowhead Mills | | | | | | | |
| Organic), ¼ cup ..... | 110 | 3.0 | 23.0 | .5 | 0 | 0 | 4.0 |
| (Hodgson Mill 2 lb./ | | | | | | | |
| Organic), <¼ cup .... | 110 | 3.0 | 22.0 | .5 | 0 | 0 | 5.0 |

| Food and Measure | cal. | prot. (gms) | carbo. (gms) | fat (gms) | chol. (mgs) | sod. (mgs) | fiber (gms) |
|---|---|---|---|---|---|---|---|
| dark, 1 cup ........... | 415 | 18.0 | 88.0 | 3.4 | 0 | 2 | 28.9 |
| light: | | | | | | | |
| (*Bob's Red Mill* | | | | | | | |
| Unbleached), ¼ cup | 100 | 2.0 | 21.0 | .5 | 0 | 0 | 1.0 |
| 1 cup ............. | 374 | 8.6 | 81.8 | 1.4 | 0 | 2 | 14.9 |
| medium, 1 cup ........ | 361 | 9.9 | 79.0 | 1.8 | 0 | 3 | 14.9 |
| **Rye malt**, see "Malt syrup" | | | | | | | |

# S

| Food and Measure | cal. | prot. (gms) | carbo. (gms) | fat (gms) | chol. (mgs) | sod. (mgs) | fiber (gms) |
|---|---|---|---|---|---|---|---|
| **Sablefish**, meat only: | | | | | | | |
| raw, 4 oz. | 222 | 15.2 | 0 | 17.4 | 56 | 64 | 0 |
| baked, broiled, or | | | | | | | |
| microwaved, 4 oz. | 284 | 19.5 | 0 | 22.2 | 71 | 82 | 0 |
| smoked: | | | | | | | |
| (*Acme/Blue Hill* | | | | | | | |
| *Bay* Alaskan | | | | | | | |
| Black Cod), 2 oz. | 150 | 8.0 | 0 | 13.0 | 35 | 370 | 0 |
| 4 oz. | 291 | 20.0 | 0 | 22.8 | 73 | 836 | 0 |
| **Safflower kernels**, | | | | | | | |
| dried, 1 oz. | 147 | 4.6 | 9.7 | 10.9 | 0 | <1 | 1.0 |
| **Safflower meal**, | | | | | | | |
| partially defatted, 1 oz. | 97 | 10.1 | 13.8 | .7 | 0 | n.a. | <3.0 |
| **Saffron**, 1 tsp. | 2 | .1 | .5 | <.1 | 0 | 1 | 0 |
| **Sage**, ground, 1 tsp. | 2 | .1 | .4 | .1 | 0 | <1 | 0 |
| **Sake**, see "Wine" | | | | | | | |
| **Salad blend**, fresh | | | | | | | |
| (see also "Lettuce" | | | | | | | |
| and "Salad blend | | | | | | | |
| kit"), 3 oz., except | | | | | | | |
| as noted: | | | | | | | |
| (*Dole* American/ | | | | | | | |
| Italian) | 15 | 1.0 | 3.0 | 0 | 0 | 10 | 1.0 |
| (*Dole* European) | 15 | 1.0 | 3.0 | 0 | 0 | 15 | 1.0 |
| (*Dole* Mediterranean) | 15 | 1.0 | 3.0 | 0 | 0 | 20 | 2.0 |
| (*Fresh Express* | | | | | | | |
| American) | 15 | 1.0 | 3.0 | 0 | 0 | 15 | 1.0 |
| (*Fresh Express* Fancy | | | | | | | |
| Greens) | 20 | 1.0 | 3.0 | 0 | 0 | 30 | 1.0 |
| (*Fresh Express* Italian) | 15 | 1.0 | 3.0 | 0 | 0 | 5 | 2.0 |
| (*Fresh Express* Green | | | | | | | |
| & Crisp/Triple | | | | | | | |
| Hearts) | 15 | 1.0 | 3.0 | 0 | 0 | 10 | 1.0 |

| Food and Measure | cal. | prot. (gms) | carbo. (gms) | fat (gms) | chol. (mgs) | sod. (mgs) | fiber (gms) |
|---|---|---|---|---|---|---|---|
| (*Fresh Express Sierra Crisp* Herb) ......... | 15 | 2.0 | 2.0 | 0 | 0 | 25 | 1.0 |
| (*Fresh Express Tender Ruby* Reds) ......... | 20 | 2.0 | 2.0 | 0 | 0 | 35 | 1.0 |
| (*Fresh Express Veggie Lover's*) ........... | 20 | 1.0 | 4.0 | 0 | 0 | 20 | 2.0 |
| (*Glory* Southern) ....... | 20 | 2.0 | 4.0 | 0 | 0 | 20 | 2.0 |
| (*Ready Pac* Costa Brava) ............ | 15 | 1.0 | 3.0 | 0 | 0 | 20 | 1.0 |
| (*Ready Pac* Italiano/ St. Tropez) ......... | 15 | 1.0 | 3.0 | 0 | 0 | 10 | 1.0 |
| (*Ready Pac* Parisian) .... | 20 | 1.0 | 4.0 | 0 | 0 | 30 | 1.0 |
| (*Ready Pac* Veggie Medley) ........... | 15 | 1.0 | 4.0 | 0 | 0 | 15 | 1.0 |
| (*Ready Pac All American*) .......... | 15 | 1.0 | 3.0 | 0 | 0 | 15 | 1.0 |
| (*Ready Pac Lafayette*) ... | 10 | 1.0 | 3.0 | 0 | 0 | 5 | <1.0 |
| (*Ready Pac Ready Fixin's* Salad Mix) .... | 25 | 1.0 | 5.0 | 0 | 0 | 20 | 2.0 |
| arugula blend: | | | | | | | |
| (*Fresh Express* Wild Rocket Zest) ...... | 20 | 2.0 | 3.0 | 0 | 0 | 30 | 1.0 |
| baby, w/spinach (*Dole*) ........... | 40 | 4.0 | 8.0 | 1.0 | 0 | 95 | 4.0 |
| baby blends: | | | | | | | |
| (*Dole* Baby Garden) .. | 25 | 2.0 | 3.0 | 0 | 0 | 45 | 2.0 |
| (*Earthbound Farm* Organic Lettuces) .. | 15 | 1.0 | 3.0 | 0 | 0 | 60 | 1.0 |
| (*Earthbound Farm* Organic Mixed) ... | 15 | 1.0 | 4.0 | 0 | 0 | 70 | 2.0 |
| (*Ready Pac* Portofino) | 15 | 2.0 | 2.0 | 0 | 0 | 75 | 1.0 |
| w/herbs (*Earthbound Farm* Organic) .... | 15 | 2.0 | 4.0 | 0 | 0 | 70 | 2.0 |
| zesty (*Ready Pac*) .... | 20 | 2.0 | 4.0 | 0 | 0 | 25 | 2.0 |
| baby, spring mix: | | | | | | | |
| (*Earthbound Farm* Organic) ......... | 15 | 1.0 | 3.0 | 0 | 0 | 65 | 1.0 |
| (*Fresh Express*) ..... | 20 | 2.0 | 3.0 | 0 | 0 | 50 | <1.0 |
| (*Ready Pac*) ........ | 20 | 2.0 | 4.0 | 0 | 0 | 25 | 2.0 |
| (*Ready Pac* Spinach) . | 20 | 2.0 | 4.0 | 0 | 0 | 45 | 2.0 |
| butter/red leaf (*Dole*) .... | 10 | 1.0 | 3.0 | 0 | 0 | 10 | 1.0 |
| w/carrots (*Fresh Express Double Carrots*) ..... | 20 | 1.0 | 4.0 | 0 | 0 | 15 | 1.0 |

| Food and Measure | cal. | prot. (gms) | carbo. (gms) | fat (gms) | chol. (mgs) | sod. (mgs) | fiber (gms) |
|---|---|---|---|---|---|---|---|
| **Salad blend** *(cont.)* | | | | | | | |
| cole slaw/slaw: | | | | | | | |
| (*Dole* Angel Hair) .... | 20 | 1.0 | 5.0 | 0 | 0 | 15 | 2.0 |
| (*Dole* Classic) ....... | 25 | 1.0 | 5.0 | 0 | 0 | 25 | 2.0 |
| (*Fresh Express* Angel Hair) ............ | 20 | 1.0 | 5.0 | 0 | 0 | 15 | 2.0 |
| (*Fresh Express* 3-Color) ......... | 20 | 1.0 | 5.0 | 0 | 0 | 20 | 2.0 |
| (*Fresh Express* Old Fashioned) ....... | 25 | 1.0 | 5.0 | 0 | 0 | 15 | 2.0 |
| (*Green Giant* Fresh Broccoli/Rainbow) . | 25 | 2.0 | 5.0 | 0 | 0 | 25 | 2.0 |
| (*Green Giant* Fresh Sunshine) ........ | 25 | 1.0 | 5.0 | 0 | 0 | 25 | 2.0 |
| field greens (*Dole*) ..... | 15 | 1.0 | 4.0 | 0 | 0 | 30 | 2.0 |
| frisée blend (*Earthbound Farm* Organic) ....... | 15 | 1.0 | 4.0 | 0 | 0 | 30 | 1.0 |
| heirloom (*Earthbound Farm* Organic) ....... | 15 | 1.0 | 2.0 | 0 | 0 | 10 | 1.0 |
| iceberg: | | | | | | | |
| (*Dole* Classic) ....... | 15 | 1.0 | 4.0 | 0 | 0 | 15 | 1.0 |
| (*Fresh Express* Garden) | 15 | 1.0 | 4.0 | 0 | 0 | 20 | 1.0 |
| lettuce: | | | | | | | |
| (*Fresh Express* 5-Lettuce Mix) .... | 15 | 1.0 | 2.0 | 0 | 0 | 20 | 1.0 |
| (*Fresh Express* Lettuce Trio) ....... | 15 | 1.0 | 3.0 | 0 | 0 | 10 | 1.0 |
| 7 (*Dole*) .......... | 20 | 1.0 | 4.0 | 0 | 0 | 10 | 1.0 |
| mâche blend (*Earthbound Farm* Organic) ....... | 25 | 2.0 | 5.0 | 0 | 0 | 25 | 2.0 |
| romaine blend: | | | | | | | |
| (*Dole* Classic) ....... | 15 | 1.0 | 4.0 | 0 | 0 | 10 | 1.0 |
| (*Dole* Leafy) ........ | 15 | 1.0 | 3.0 | 0 | 0 | 15 | 1.0 |
| (*Fresh Express* Leafy Green) .......... | 15 | 1.0 | 3.0 | 0 | 0 | 10 | 2.0 |
| (*Fresh Express* Premium Romaine) | 20 | 1.0 | 4.0 | 0 | 0 | 15 | 2.0 |
| baby (*Ready Pac*) .... | 20 | 2.0 | 3.0 | 0 | 0 | 90 | 2.0 |
| spinach blend: | | | | | | | |
| (*Fresh Express* 50/50 Mix) ........ | 20 | 2.0 | 2.0 | 0 | 0 | 60 | 1.0 |
| (*Ready Pac* Florentine) | 20 | 2.0 | 3.0 | 0 | 0 | 55 | 2.0 |
| tender reds (*Dole*) ... | 50 | 3.0 | 12.0 | 0 | 0 | 210 | 6.0 |

| Food and Measure | cal. | prot. (gms) | carbo. (gms) | fat (gms) | chol. (mgs) | sod. (mgs) | fiber (gms) |
|---|---|---|---|---|---|---|---|
| **Salad blend kit**, fresh, w/dressing, 3.5 oz.*, except as noted: | | | | | | | |
| (*Dole* Asian Island Crunch) . . . . . . . . . . | 130 | 3.0 | 14.0 | 7.0 | 5 | n.a. | 2.0 |
| (*Dole* Autumn Splendor) . | 150 | 4.0 | 13.0 | 11.0 | 0 | 260 | 1.0 |
| (*Dole* Perfect Harvest) . . . | 160 | 2.0 | 12.0 | 12.0 | 0 | 105 | 2.0 |
| (*Dole* Summer Salad) . . . | 120 | 4.0 | 8.0 | 8.0 | 5 | 230 | 1.0 |
| (*Dole* Winter Jubilee) . . . | 160 | 3.0 | 10.0 | 13.0 | 5 | n.a. | 2.0 |
| (*Fresh Express* Orchard Harvest) . . . . . . . . . . | 250 | 6.0 | 13.0 | 19.0 | 15 | 280 | 2.0 |
| (*Fresh Express* House Italian Kit) . . . . . . . . . | 70 | 1.0 | 5.0 | 5.0 | 0 | 350 | 1.0 |
| (*Fresh Express* House Ranch Kit) . . . . . . . . | 100 | 1.0 | 5.0 | 9.0 | 5 | 210 | 1.0 |
| (*Fresh Express* Pear Gorgonzola Kit) . . . . . | 130 | 3.0 | 17.0 | 6.0 | 0 | 270 | 2.0 |
| (*Fresh Express* Strawberry Fields Kit) . | 200 | 3.0 | 17.0 | 13.0 | 0 | 65 | 2.0 |
| (*Ready Pac* Parisian/ Grand Parisian) . . . . . . | 140 | 3.0 | 11.0 | 11.0 | 5 | 190 | 2.0 |
| Asian: | | | | | | | |
| (*Fresh Express* Asian Kit) . . . . . . . . . . . . | 120 | 2.0 | 17.0 | 5.0 | 0 | 360 | 2.0 |
| (*Ready Pac*) . . . . . . . . | 120 | 2.0 | 14.0 | 7.0 | 0 | 270 | 1.0 |
| (*Ready Pac* Grand) . . . | 130 | 3.0 | 19.0 | 6.0 | 0 | 260 | 2.0 |
| baby greens (*Earthbound Farm* Organic) . . . . . . . | 230 | 3.0 | 5.0 | 24.0 | 0 | 270 | 2.0 |
| blue cheese (*Ready Pac* American) . . . . . . | 110 | 2.0 | 8.0 | 8.0 | 10 | 250 | 1.0 |
| Caesar: | | | | | | | |
| (*Dole*) . . . . . . . . . . . . | 140 | 3.0 | 8.0 | 11.0 | 5 | 300 | 2.0 |
| (*Dole* Light) . . . . . . . . | 90 | 3.0 | 8.0 | 6.0 | 5 | 340 | 1.0 |
| (*Dole* Ultimate) . . . . . . | 180 | 5.0 | 9.0 | 14.0 | 9 | 430 | 1.0 |
| (*Earthbound Farm* Organic), 5.6 oz. . . | 230 | 4.0 | 7.0 | 20.0 | 10 | 420 | 2.0 |
| (*Fresh Express* Caesar Kit) . . . . . . . . . . . . | 120 | 2.0 | 7.0 | 11.0 | 10 | 380 | 2.0 |
| (*Fresh Express* Caesar Lite) . . . . . . . . . . . . | 90 | 2.0 | 7.0 | 7.0 | 10 | 380 | 2.0 |
| (*Fresh Express* Caesar Supreme) . . . . . . . . | 140 | 2.0 | 6.0 | 12.0 | 10 | 430 | 1.0 |
| (*Ready Pac* Classic) . . | 190 | 5.0 | 8.0 | 15.0 | 10 | 390 | 1.0 |
| (*Ready Pac* Santa Fe) . | 150 | 3.0 | 7.0 | 12.0 | 10 | 250 | 1.0 |

| Food and Measure | cal. | prot. (gms) | carbo. (gms) | fat (gms) | chol. (mgs) | sod. (mgs) | fiber (gms) |
|---|---|---|---|---|---|---|---|
| **Salad blend kit, Caesar** *(cont.)* | | | | | | | |
| (*Ready Pac Bistro* Santa Fe), 6.2 oz. ... | 190 | 10.0 | 15.0 | 10.0 | 30 | 530 | 2.0 |
| garlic (*Dole*) ........ | 160 | 3.0 | 7.0 | 13.0 | 10 | 290 | 1.0 |
| chef salad: | | | | | | | |
| (*Ready Pac* Bistro), 7.8 oz. .......... | 270 | 15.0 | 10.0 | 20.0 | 55 | 890 | 2.0 |
| chopped turkey (*Fresh Express*) ......... | 140 | 6.0 | 7.0 | 10.0 | 20 | 290 | 1.0 |
| chicken: | | | | | | | |
| (*Fresh Express* Café Caribbean) ....... | 160 | 6.0 | 17.0 | 8.0 | 10 | 290 | 2.0 |
| (*Fresh Express* Café Tuscan Pesto) .... | 140 | 7.0 | 8.0 | 9.0 | 15 | 340 | 1.0 |
| (*Fresh Express* Café Waldorf) ......... | 170 | 7.0 | 19.0 | 9.0 | 20 | 250 | 2.0 |
| (*Fresh Express Chicken Caesar Kit*) | 90 | 8.0 | 5.0 | 5.0 | 20 | 310 | 2.0 |
| (*Fresh Express Chicken Taco Kit*) .. | 110 | 6.0 | 7.0 | 7.0 | 20 | 330 | 2.0 |
| Caesar (*Ready Pac Bistro*), 6.2 oz. .... | 230 | 16.0 | 8.0 | 16.0 | 50 | 980 | 1.0 |
| cranberry walnut (*Ready Pac Bistro*), 5 oz. ............. | 210 | 10.0 | 20.0 | 11.0 | 20 | 560 | 2.0 |
| cobb salad (*Ready Pac Bistro*), 7.23 oz. ...... | 300 | 13.0 | 7.0 | 23.0 | 140 | 950 | 2.0 |
| cole slaw: | | | | | | | |
| (*Fresh Express*) ..... | 150 | 1.0 | 14.0 | 10.0 | 5 | 160 | 2.0 |
| (*Ready Pac*) ........ | 130 | 1.0 | 13.0 | 9.0 | 5 | 160 | 2.0 |
| Italian (*Dole* Hearty) .... | 180 | 6.0 | 10.0 | 13.0 | 10 | 550 | 1.0 |
| Parisian (*Ready Pac*) .... | 140 | 3.0 | 11.0 | 11.0 | 5 | 190 | 2.0 |
| Southwest (*Dole*) ...... | 150 | 3.0 | 10.0 | 11.0 | 10 | n.a. | 2.0 |
| spinach, baby: | | | | | | | |
| (*Ready Pac*) ........ | 140 | 4.0 | 24.0 | 3.0 | 0 | 270 | 2.0 |
| (*Earthbound Farm* Organic) ......... | 130 | 5.0 | 12.0 | 11.0 | 0 | 330 | 6.0 |
| spinach bacon (*Ready Pac Bistro*), 4.8 oz. ... | 110 | 12.0 | 19.0 | 12.0 | 130 | 750 | 3.0 |
| **Salad dressing**, 2 tbsp., except as noted: | | | | | | | |
| (*Annie's Naturals* Goddess) .......... | 120 | 1.0 | 2.0 | 12.0 | 0 | 340 | 0 |

| Food and Measure | cal. | prot. (gms) | carbo. (gms) | fat (gms) | chol. (mgs) | sod. (mgs) | fiber (gms) |
|---|---|---|---|---|---|---|---|
| (*Annie's Naturals* Goddess Organic) .... | 130 | 1.0 | 1.0 | 13.0 | 0 | 390 | 0 |
| (*Annie's Naturals* Woodstock) ........ | 110 | 2.0 | 1.0 | 11.0 | 0 | 260 | 0 |
| (*Brianna's* New American) .......... | 160 | 0 | 6.0 | 17.0 | 0 | 290 | 0 |
| (*Brianna's* Santa Fe Blend) ............ | 25 | 0 | 5.0 | 0 | 0 | 480 | 0 |
| (*Wish-Bone Western* Nonfat) .......... | 50 | 0 | 12.0 | 0 | 0 | 280 | 0 |
| (*Wish-Bone Western* Original) .......... | 160 | 0 | 11.0 | 12.0 | 0 | 230 | 0 |
| (*Wish-Bone Western* Light!) ............ | 70 | 0 | 13.0 | 2.0 | 0 | 270 | 0 |
| apple poppy seed (*Girard's*) ......... | 110 | 0 | 8.0 | 9.0 | 0 | 105 | 0 |
| artichoke Parmesan (*Annie's Naturals*) .... | 130 | 1.0 | 1.0 | 13.0 | <5 | 250 | 0 |
| asiago, creamy (*Annie's Naturals*) .... | 80 | 1.0 | 0 | 9.0 | 5 | 340 | 0 |
| asiago pepper crème (*Teresa's*) ......... | 130 | 0 | 2.0 | 13.0 | 10 | 220 | 0 |
| asiago peppercorn: | | | | | | | |
| (*Marzetti* 15 oz.) ..... | 160 | 1.0 | 1.0 | 16.0 | 15 | 220 | 0 |
| (*Marzetti* 16 oz.) ..... | 130 | 1.0 | 2.0 | 14.0 | 10 | 230 | 0 |
| Asian: | | | | | | | |
| (*Newman's Own* Organic Low Fat) .. | 35 | 0 | 5.0 | 2.0 | 0 | 440 | 0 |
| creamy (*Litehouse*) ... | 130 | 0 | 4.0 | 13.0 | 10 | 170 | 0 |
| w/bacon flavor (*Wish-Bone Western*) . | 140 | 0 | 10.0 | 11.0 | 0 | 240 | 0 |
| basil Parmesan (*Bernstein's*) ........ | 100 | 1.0 | 2.0 | 10.0 | 5 | 400 | 0 |
| balsamic: | | | | | | | |
| (*Newman's Own* Organic Light) .... | 45 | 0 | 3.0 | 4.0 | 0 | 450 | 0 |
| creamy (*Ken's*) ...... | 90 | 0 | 8.0 | 7.0 | 0 | 160 | 0 |
| herb (*Annie's Naturals* Lite) ............ | 50 | 0 | 2.0 | 5.0 | 0 | 230 | 0 |
| white (*Litehouse*) ... | 90 | 0 | 4.0 | 9.0 | 0 | 70 | 0 |
| balsamic vinaigrette: | | | | | | | |
| (*Annie's Naturals*) .... | 110 | 0 | 2.0 | 11.0 | 0 | 60 | 0 |
| (*Annie's Naturals* Organic) ......... | 100 | 0 | 3.0 | 10.0 | 0 | 75 | 0 |

| Food and Measure | cal. | prot. (gms) | carbo. (gms) | fat (gms) | chol. (mgs) | sod. (mgs) | fiber (gms) |
|---|---|---|---|---|---|---|---|
| **Salad dressing, balsamic vinaigrette** *(cont.)* | | | | | | | |
| (*Bolthouse Farms*) ... | 30 | 0 | 6.0 | 0 | 0 | 150 | 0 |
| (*Cains*) ........... | 100 | 0 | 6.0 | 9.0 | 0 | 230 | 0 |
| (*Cardini's*) ......... | 100 | 0 | 5.0 | 8.0 | 0 | 250 | 0 |
| (*Cardini's* Light) ..... | 50 | 0 | 5.0 | 3.0 | 0 | 210 | 0 |
| (*Girard's* White) ..... | 110 | 0 | 5.0 | 9.0 | 0 · | 240 | 0 |
| (*Good Seasons*) ..... | 90 | 0 | 4.0 | 8.0 | 0 | 320 | 0 |
| (*Ken's Healthy Options*) ......... | 45 | 0 | 3.0 | 3.5 | 0 | 240 | 0 |
| (*Kraft*) ........... | 90 | 0 | 4.0 | 8.0 | 0 | 310 | 0 |
| (*Litehouse*) ......... | 100 | 0 | 5.0 | 10.0 | 0 | 150 | 0 |
| (*Litehouse* Organic) .. | 110 | 0 | 4.0 | 10.0 | 0 | 150 | 0 |
| (*Marie's*) ........... | 50 | 0 | 3.0 | 4.5 | 0 | 210 | 0 |
| (*Marzetti*) .......... | 100 | 0 | 4.0 | 9.0 | 0 | 340 | 0 |
| (*Marzetti* Light 16 oz.) .......... | 45 | 0 | 5.0 | 3.0 | 0 | 350 | 0 |
| (*Marzetti* Light 12 oz.) .......... | 50 | 0 | 5.0 | 3.0 | 0 | 210 | 0 |
| (*Marzetti* Organic) ... | 90 | 0 | 3.0 | 9.0 | 0 | 360 | 0 |
| (*Marzetti* White) .... | 100 | 0 | 5.0 | 9.0 | 0 | 220 | 0 |
| (*Newman's Own*) .... | 90 | 0 | 3.0 | 9.0 | 0 | 350 | 0 |
| (*Newman's Own Lighten Up!*) ...... | 45 | 0 | 2.0 | 4.0 | 0 | 390 | 0 |
| (*Seeds of Change* Organic) ......... | 60 | 0 | 6.0 | 4.0 | 0 | 105 · | 0 |
| (*Wish-Bone*) ........ | 60 | 0 | 3.0 | 5.0 | 0 | 280 | 0 |
| and basil (*Ken's*) ..... | 110 | 0 | 2.0 | 12.0 | 0 | 290 | 0 |
| and basil (*Ken's* Lite) . | 60 | 0 | 3.0 | 5.0 | 0 | 410 | 0 |
| and basil (*Wish-Bone* Light) ........... | 60 | 0 | 3.0 | 5.0 | 0 | 290 | 0 |
| cheese, 3 (*Newman's Own*) ........... | 100 | 0 | 2.0 | 11.0 | 0 | 380 | 0 |
| creamy (*Girard's*) .... | 100 | 0 | 6.0 | 9.0 | 0 | 220 | 0 |
| creamy (*Girard's* Light) ........... | 45 | 0 | 4.0 | 3.0 | 0 | 250 | 0 |
| creamy, w/honey (*Ken's*) .......... | 90 | 0 | 8.0 | 6.0 | 0 | 160 | 0 |
| Italian (*Wish-Bone*) ... | 70 | 0 | 4.0 | 6.0 | 0 | 340 | 0 |
| white (*Cains*) ....... | 130 | 0 | 10.0 | 10.0 | 0 | 240 | 0 |
| berry balsamic (*Marzetti* Light) ...... | 45 | 0 | 4.0 | 3.0 | 0 | 250 | 0 |
| berry lavender vinaigrette (*Teresa's*) . | 130 | 0 | 7.0 | 11.0 | 0 | 190 | 0 |

| Food and Measure | cal. | prot. (gms) | carbo. (gms) | fat (gms) | chol. (mgs) | sod. (mgs) | fiber (gms) |
|---|---|---|---|---|---|---|---|
| blackberry poppy | | | | | | | |
| seed (*Teresa's*) ...... | 110 | 0 | 5.0 | 9.0 | 0 | 160 | 0 |
| blue/bleu cheese: | | | | | | | |
| (*Brianna's* True) ..... | 120 | 1.0 | 5.0 | 11.0 | 5 | 250 | 0 |
| (*Kraft Roka*) ........ | 120 | 0 | 1.0 | 13.0 | 5 | 380 | 0 |
| (*Litehouse* Big Bleu) .. | 160 | 1.0 | 1.0 | 17.0 | 15 | 230 | 0 |
| (*Litehouse* Chunky/ | | | | | | | |
| Original) ......... | 150 | 1.0 | 1.0 | 16.0 | 15 | 220 | 0 |
| (*Litehouse* Light) .... | 70 | 1.0 | 2.0 | 6.0 | 5 | 240 | 0 |
| (*Litehouse* Yogurt | | | | | | | |
| Kefir) ........... | 80 | 1.0 | 2.0 | 7.0 | 5 | 270 | 0 |
| (*Marie's* Super) ...... | 160 | 2.0 | 1.0 | 17.0 | 20 | 210 | 0 |
| (*Marie's* Yogurt) ..... | 70 | 1.0 | 1.0 | 7.0 | 10 | 190 | 0 |
| (*Marzetti* Bistro) ..... | 180 | 1.0 | 1.0 | 19.0 | 15 | 210 | 0 |
| (*Marzetti* French) .,... | 160 | 1.0 | 11.0 | 13.0 | 0 | 270 | 0 |
| (*Marzetti* Organic) ... | 130 | 1.0 | 1.0 | 14.0 | 10 | 300 | 0 |
| (*Marzetti* Ultimate) ... | 160 | 1.0 | 1.0 | 17.0 | 15 | 250 | 0 |
| (*Wish-Bone* Light) ... | 40 | <1.0 | 6.0 | 2.0 | 0 | 310 | 0 |
| w/bacon (*Litehouse*) .. | 150 | 1.0 | 1.0 | 16.0 | 15 | 240 | 0 |
| w/bacon (*Marie's*) .... | 160 | 1.0 | 1.0 | 18.0 | 15 | 160 | 0 |
| w/gorgonzola (*Ken's*) . | 140 | 0 | 1.0 | 14.0 | 0 | 260 | 0 |
| w/gorgonzola | | | | | | | |
| (*WishBone*) ...... | 150 | 1.0 | 1.0 | 15.0 | <5 | 310 | 0 |
| blue cheese, chunky: | | | | | | | |
| (*Bernstein's*) ......... | 120 | 1.0 | 2.0 | 13.0 | 5 | 180 | 0 |
| (*Bolthouse Farms* | | | | | | | |
| Yogurt) .......... | 70 | 2.0 | 2.0 | 6.5 | 15 | 150 | 0 |
| (*Ken's*) ............ | 150 | 0 | 1.0 | 16.0 | 0 | 320 | <1.0 |
| (*Ken's* Lite) ........ | 80 | 1.0 | 4.0 | 7.0 | 0 | 350 | 0 |
| (*Marie's*) ........... | 160 | 1.0 | 0 | 17.0 | 15 | 160 | 0 |
| (*Marie's* Lite) ....... | 70 | 1.0 | 1.0 | 7.0 | 5 | 290 | 0 |
| (*Marzetti*) .......... | 150 | 1.0 | 1.0 | 15.0 | 15 | 320 | 0 |
| (*Marzetti* Light) ..... | 80 | 1.0 | 4.0 | 7.0 | 15 | 340 | 1.0 |
| (*Wish-Bone*) ........ | 150 | 0 | 1.0 | 15.0 | <5 | 270 | 0 |
| (*Wish-Bone* Nonfat) .. | 30 | <1.0 | 7.0 | 0 | 0 | 280 | <1.0 |
| blue cheese vinaigrette: | | | | | | | |
| (*Girard's*) .......... | 100 | 1.0 | 3.0 | 10.0 | 5 | 500 | 0 |
| (*Litehouse*) ......... | 80 | 1.0 | 4.0 | 7.0 | 5 | 280 | 0 |
| (*Marie's*) ........... | 120 | 1.0 | 4.0 | 11.0 | 5 | 190 | 0 |
| chunky (*Bolthouse* | | | | | | | |
| *Farms* Olive Oil) ... | 60 | 1.0 | 4.0 | 5.0 | 5 | 150 | 0 |
| Italian (*Marzetti*) ..... | 100 | 1.0 | 2.0 | 10.0 | 5 | 300 | 0 |
| blueberry pomegranate | | | | | | | |
| vinaigrette (*Teresa's*) . | 130 | 0 | 8.0 | 11.0 | 0 | 125 | 0 |

| Food and Measure | cal. | prot. (gms) | carbo. (gms) | fat (gms) | chol. (mgs) | sod. (mgs) | fiber (gms) |
|---|---|---|---|---|---|---|---|
| **Salad dressing** (cont.) | | | | | | | |
| blush wine vinaigrette: | | | | | | | |
| (*Brianna's*) ......... | 120 | 0 | 14.0 | 7.0 | 0 | 420 | 0 |
| (*Cains* Light) ........ | 70 | 0 | 8.0 | 4.5 | 0 | 480 | 0 |
| (*Cains* Nonfat) ...... | 35 | 0 | 8.0 | 0 | 0 | 490 | 0 |
| buttermilk (*Annie's* | | | | | | | |
| *Naturals* Organic) .... | 60 | 1.0 | 1.0 | 6.0 | 10 | 230 | 0 |
| Caesar: | | | | | | | |
| (*Annie's Naturals* | | | | | | | |
| Organic) ......... | 110 | 1.0 | 1.0 | 11.0 | 5 | 210 | 0 |
| (*Cains* Light) ........ | 70 | 1.0 | 5.0 | 6.0 | 5 | 490 | 0 |
| (*Cains* Nonfat) ...... | 30 | 0 | 6.0 | 0 | 0 | 600 | 0 |
| (*Cardini's* Light) ..... | 80 | 1.0 | 5.0 | 7.0 | 30 | 250 | 0 |
| (*Cardini's* Nonfat) .... | 40 | 0 | 9.0 | 0 | 0 | 510 | 0 |
| (*Cardini's* Original) ... | 160 | 1.0 | 1.0 | 17.0 | 30 | 240 | 0 |
| (*Girard's*) .......... | 140 | 1.0 | 1.0 | 15.0 | 10 | 360 | 0 |
| (*Girard's* Light) ...... | 90 | 1.0 | 5.0 | 8.0 | 10 | 370 | 0 |
| (*Ken's*) ............ | 170 | 0 | 1.0 | 18.0 | 0 | 430 | 0 |
| (*Ken's* Lite) ......... | 70 | 1.0 | 3.0 | 6.0 | 0 | 620 | 0 |
| (*Ken's* Tableside) .... | 150 | 1.0 | 2.0 | 16.0 | 0 | 420 | 0 |
| (*Kraft* Classic) ....... | 130 | 2.0 | 2.0 | 12.0 | 15 | 380 | 0 |
| (*Kraft* Classic Free) ... | 50 | 1.0 | 11.0 | 0 | 0 | 350 | 0 |
| (*Kraft* Light) ........ | 60 | 1.0 | 3.0 | 4.5 | 10 | 320 | 0 |
| (*Litehouse* Caesar | | | | | | | |
| Caesar) ......... | 130 | 1.0 | 2.0 | 13.0 | 15 | 250 | 0 |
| (*Litehouse* Caesar | | | | | | | |
| Caesar Family) .... | 140 | 1.0 | 1.0 | 15.0 | 15 | 170 | 0 |
| (*Litehouse* Lite) ...... | 70 | 0 | 2.0 | 7.0 | 5 | 220 | 0 |
| (*Litehouse* Organic) .. | 120 | 0 | 2.0 | 12.0 | 0 | 260 | 0 |
| (*Litehouse* Yogurt | | | | | | | |
| Kefir) ........... | 80 | 1.0 | 2.0 | 8.0 | 5 | 230 | 0 |
| (*Marie's*) ........... | 170 | 1.0 | 1.0 | 19.0 | 15 | 150 | 0 |
| (*Marzetti* Organic) ... | 150 | 0 | 1.0 | 16.0 | 5 | 250 | 0 |
| (*Marzetti* Supreme) .. | 140 | 1.0 | 1.0 | 15.0 | 10 | 320 | 0 |
| (*Marzetti* Supreme | | | | | | | |
| Light) ........... | 70 | 1.0 | 2.0 | 7.0 | 10 | 340 | 0 |
| (*Newman's Own*) .... | 150 | 1.0 | 1.0 | 16.0 | 0 | 420 | 0 |
| (*Newman's Own* | | | | | | | |
| Lighten Up!) ...... | 70 | 1.0 | 3.0 | 6.0 | 5 | 420 | 0 |
| (*Pfeiffer*) ........... | 120 | 1.0 | 2.0 | 12.0 | 5 | 310 | 0 |
| asiago (*Brianna's*) .... | 150 | 1.0 | 2.0 | 15.0 | 5 | 310 | 0 |
| bacon (*Kraft*) ........ | 130 | 1.0 | 2.0 | 13.0 | 0 | 360 | 0 |
| cilantro pepita (*El* | | | | | | | |
| *Torito*) .......... | 140 | 1.0 | 1.0 | 14.0 | 10 | 260 | 0 |

| Food and Measure | cal. | prot. (gms) | carbo. (gms) | fat (gms) | chol. (mgs) | sod. (mgs) | fiber (gms) |
|---|---|---|---|---|---|---|---|
| garlic (*Litehouse*) .... | 150 | 0 | 1.0 | 16.0 | 5 | 85 | 0 |
| Italian (*Kraft*) ....... | 130 | 0 | 3.0 | 13.0 | 5 | 250 | 0 |
| Parmesan (*Bolthouse Farms* Yogurt Parmigiano) ...... | 80 | 1.0 | 3.0 | 6.5 | 10 | 200 | 0 |
| Parmesan (*Litehouse*) | 100 | 1.0 | 3.0 | 10.0 | 5 | 220 | 0 |
| Parmesan (*Marie's* Yogurt) .......... | 50 | 1.0 | 2.0 | 5.0 | 10 | 200 | 0 |
| vinaigrette (*Cardini's* Light) ........... | 60 | 1.0 | 2.0 | 50 | | 450 | 0 |
| vinaigrette (*Ken's Healthy Options*) .. | 50 | 1.0 | 2.0 | 4.0 | 0 | 240 | 0 |
| vinaigrette (*Marzetti* Light) .......... | 70 | 1.0 | 2.0 | 6.0 | 5 | 420 | 0 |
| vinaigrette w/ Parmesan (*Kraft*) .. | 70 | 1.0 | 3.0 | 5.0 | 5 | 430 | 0 |
| Caesar, creamy: | | | | | | | |
| (*Bernstein's*) ........ | 120 | 0 | 1.0 | 13.0 | 15 | 200 | 0 |
| (*Cains*) ............. | 170 | 0 | 1.0 | 19.0 | 5 | 170 | 0 |
| (*Ken's Lite*) ........ | 90 | 1.0 | 4.0 | 8.0 | 5 | 320 | <1.0 |
| (*Marie's*) .......... | 120 | 1.0 | 1.0 | 13.0 | 25 | 160 | 0 |
| (*Marzetti*) .......... | 120 | 1.0 | 2.0 | 12.0 | 15 | 370 | 0 |
| (*Newman's Own*) .... | 170 | 0 | 1.0 | 18.0 | 20 | 340 | 0 |
| (*Wish-Bone*) ........ | 180 | <1.0 | 1.0 | 18.0 | 10 | 290 | 0 |
| (*Wish-Bone* Light) ... | 45 | <1.0 | 7.0 | 2.0 | 10 | 310 | 0 |
| w/aged Parmesan (*Good Seasons*) ... | 100 | 1.0 | 3.0 | 9.0 | 5 | 240 | 0 |
| w/roasted garlic (*Ken's*) .......... | 160 | 1.0 | 1.0 | 17.0 | 10 | 240 | 0 |
| Champagne: | | | | | | | |
| (*Girard's*) .......... | 150 | 0 | 1.0 | 16.0 | 0 | 490 | 0 |
| (*Girard's* Light) ...... | 60 | 0 | 2.0 | 5.0 | 0 | 500 | 0 |
| caper vinaigrette (*Brianna's*) ....... | 160 | 0 | 5.0 | 15.0 | 0 | 105 | 0 |
| cheddar chipotle (*Brianna's*) ......... | 110 | 1.0 | 4.0 | 11.0 | 0 | 240 | 0 |
| cheese: | | | | | | | |
| (*Bernstein's* Fantastico) ....... | 100 | 1.0 | 2.0 | 10.0 | 5 | 400 | 0 |
| (*Bernstein's* Fantastico Light) .. | 25 | 1.0 | 3.0 | 1.5 | 5 | 370 | 0 |
| chicken salad, Chinese (*Girard's*) .......... | 120 | 0 | 6.0 | 11.0 | 0 | 350 | 0 |

| Food and Measure | cal. | prot. (gms) | carbo. (gms) | fat (gms) | chol. (mgs) | sod. (mgs) | fiber (gms) |
|---|---|---|---|---|---|---|---|
| **Salad dressing** *(cont.)* | | | | | | | |
| cilantro, creamy | | | | | | | |
| (*Litehouse*) ......... | 110 | 1.0 | 3.0 | 10.0 | 10 | 230 | 0 |
| cole slaw/slaw: | | | | | | | |
| (*Bolthouse Farms* | | | | | | | |
| Yogurt) .......... | 70 | 1.0 | 10.0 | 4.0 | 5 | 60 | 0 |
| (*Litehouse*) ......... | 100 | 0 | 8.0 | 8.0 | 5 | 120 | 0 |
| (*Litehouse* Lite) ..... | 70 | 0 | 9.0 | 3.0 | 5 | 240 | 0 |
| (*Marie's*) ........... | 140 | 0 | 7.0 | 13.0 | 10 | 170 | 0 |
| (*Marzetti* 15 oz.) ..... | 160 | 0 | 6.0 | 15.0 | 20 | 390 | 0 |
| (*Marzetti* 16 oz.) ..... | 160 | 0 | 6.0 | 14.0 | 20 | 380 | 0 |
| (*Marzetti* Light) ...... | 90 | 0 | 7.0 | 7.0 | 20 | 390 | 0 |
| (*Marzetti* Lite 8 oz.) .. | 90 | 0 | 7.0 | 7.0 | 20 | 380 | 0 |
| (*Marzetti* Lite 16 oz.) . | 100 | 0 | 10.0 | 7.0 | 20 | 380 | 0 |
| (*Marzetti* Low Fat) ... | 60 | 0 | 12.0 | 1.5 | 15 | 370 | 0 |
| (*Marzetti* Southern) . | 150 | 0 | 12.0 | 11.0 | 15 | 220 | 0 |
| pineapple (*Litehouse*) . | 100 | 0 | 8.0 | 8.0 | 5 | 110 | 0 |
| cranberry vinaigrette | | | | | | | |
| (*Litehouse* Harvest) .. | 25 | 0 | 6.0 | 0 | 0 | 110 | 0 |
| cranberry walnut | | | | | | | |
| (*Newman's Own* | | | | | | | |
| *Lighten Up!*) ........ | 70 | 1.0 | 8.0 | 4.0 | 0 | 230 | 0 |
| feta: | | | | | | | |
| (*Marie's* Yogurt) ..... | 80 | 1.0 | 2.0 | 8.0 | 15 | 190 | 0 |
| chunky (*Marie's*) ..... | 150 | 1.0 | 1.0 | 17.0 | 15 | 150 | 0 |
| vinaigrette, Greek | | | | | | | |
| (*Seeds of Change* | | | | | | | |
| Organic) ......... | 60 | 1.0 | 5.0 | 4.5 | 0 | 270 | 0 |
| French: | | | | | | | |
| (*Annie's Naturals* | | | | | | | |
| Organic) ......... | 90 | 0 | 3.0 | 9.0 | 0 | 170 | 0 |
| (*Brianna's* Zesty) ..... | 150 | 0 | 4.0 | 15.0 | 0 | 240 | 0 |
| (*Cains*) ............ | 120 | 0 | 6.0 | 11.0 | 0 | 170 | 0 |
| (*Girard's* Original) .... | 120 | 0 | 0 | 13.0 | 0 | 410 | 0 |
| (*Marzetti* California) .. | 140 | 0 | 9.0 | 11.0 | 0 | 230 | 0 |
| (*Marzetti* Country) ... | 160 | 0 | 7.0 | 14.0 | 5 | 180 | 0 |
| (*Pfeiffer*) ............ | 150 | 0 | 7.0 | 13.0 | 5 | 220 | 0 |
| (*Pfeiffer* California) ... | 140 | 0 | 9.0 | 11.0 | 0 | 230 | 0 |
| (*Wish-Bone* Deluxe) .. | 130 | 0 | 5.0 | 11.0 | 0 | 170 | 0 |
| (*Wish-Bone* Deluxe | | | | | | | |
| Light) ........... | 50 | 0 | 8.0 | 2.0 | 0 | 260 | <1.0 |
| w/bacon (*Ken's*) ..... | 140 | 0 | 9.0 | 11.0 | 0 | 220 | 0 |
| creamy (*Ken's*) ...... | 130 | 0 | 6.0 | 12.0 | 0 | 150 | 0 |
| creamy (*Kraft*) ....... | 150 | 1.0 | 5.0 | 14.0 | 0 | 260 | 0 |

| Food and Measure | cal. | prot. (gms) | carbo. (gms) | fat (gms) | chol. (mgs) | sod. (mgs) | fiber (gms) |
|---|---|---|---|---|---|---|---|
| herb garden (*Bernstein's*) ...... | 130 | 0 | 6.0 | 12.0 | 0 | 260 | 0 |
| honey (*Ken's* Country) | 150 | 0 | 10.0 | 12.0 | 0 | 220 | 0 |
| honey (*Ken's* Country Lite) ............. | 100 | 0 | 11.0 | 6.0 | 0 | 230 | 0 |
| honey (*Ken's Healthy Options*) ......... | 70 | 0 | 8.0 | 4.0 | 0 | 230 | 0 |
| honey (*Marzetti*) ..... | 170 | 0 | 11.0 | 14.0 | 15 | 240 | 0 |
| honey (*Marzetti* Light) ........... | 80 | 0 | 12.0 | 3.5 | 0 | 270 | 0 |
| style (*Kraft* Free) ..... | 45 | 0 | 11.0 | 0 | 0 | 290 | 0 |
| style, creamy (*Kraft* Light) ........... | 80 | 0 | 10.0 | 5.0 | 0 | 330 | 0 |
| sweet (*Kraft Catalina*) . | 130 | 0 | 7.0 | 11.0 | 0 | 380 | 0 |
| sweet (*Kraft Catalina* Free) ............. | 50 | 0 | 11.0 | 0 | 0 | 350 | 0 |
| sweet (*Litehouse*) .... | 90 | 0 | 4.0 | 8.0 | 0 | 280 | 0 |
| sweet honey (*Kraft Catalina*) ......... | 130 | 0 | 8.0 | 10.0 | 0 | 340 | 0 |
| sweet and spicy (*Wish-Bone*) ...... | 140 | 0 | 6.0 | 12.0 | 0 | 340 | 0 |
| sweet and spicy (*Wish-Bone* Light) . | 50 | 0 | 9.0 | 2.0 | 0 | 240 | 0 |
| tomato (*Seeds of Change* Organic) .. | 60 | 0 | 8.0 | 3.0 | 0 | 210 | 0 |
| tomato/onion (*Cains*) . | 120 | 0 | 7.0 | 11.0 | 0 | 330 | 0 |
| vinaigrette (*Brianna's*) . | 130 | 0 | 0 | 14.0 | 0 | 260 | 0 |
| garlic, green (*Annie's Naturals* Organic) .... | 90 | 0 | 2.0 | 9.0 | 0 | 180 | 0 |
| garlic, roasted: | | | | | | | |
| balsamic (*Bernstein's Light Fantastic*) ... | 45 | 0 | 3.0 | 3.5 | 0 | 320 | 0 |
| balsamic (*Newman's Own Lighten Up!*) .. | 50 | 0 | 3.0 | 4.0 | 0 | 420 | 0 |
| vinaigrette (*Annie's Naturals* Organic) .. | 110 | 0 | 3.0 | 11.0 | 0 | 220 | 0 |
| garlic vinaigrette (*Litehouse*) ......... | 110 | 0 | 5.0 | 10.0 | 0 | 180 | 0 |
| ginger: | | | | | | | |
| (*Marzetti* Asian) ..... | 120 | 0 | 4.0 | 12.0 | 0 | 260 | 0 |
| (*Teresa's* Asian) ..... | 120 | 0 | 5.0 | 12.0 | 0 | 250 | 0 |
| mandarin (*Brianna's*) . | 150 | 0 | 8.0 | 14.0 | 0 | 340 | 0 |
| mango vinaigrette (*Marzetti*) ........ | 120 | 0 | 8.0 | 9.0 | 0 | 310 | 0 |

| Food and Measure | cal. | prot. (gms) | carbo. (gms) | fat (gms) | chol. (mgs) | sod. (mgs) | fiber (gms) |
|---|---|---|---|---|---|---|---|
| **Salad dressing, ginger** *(cont.)* | | | | | | | |
| soy (*Litehouse*) ...... | 100 | 1.0 | 4.0 | 9.0 | 0 | 390 | 0 |
| vinaigrette (*Annie's Naturals* Gingerly Lite) ........... | 40 | 0 | 3.0 | 3.0 | 0 | 290 | 0 |
| gorgonzola: | | | | | | | |
| (*Marzetti* Ultimate) ... | 150 | 1.0 | 2.0 | 16.0 | 15 | 290 | 0 |
| pear (*Litehouse*) ...... | 60 | 0 | 7.0 | 3.0 | 5 | 250 | 0 |
| green goddess: | | | | | | | |
| (*Annie's Naturals* Organic) ......... | 130 | <1.0 | 2.0 | 13.0 | <5 | 380 | 0 |
| (*Seven Seas*) ....... | 130 | 0 | 2.0 | 13.0 | 0 | 260 | 0 |
| Greek: | | | | | | | |
| creamy (*Ken's*) ...... | 130 | 0 | 2.0 | 13.0 | 5 | 230 | 0 |
| w/imported olive oil (*Ken's*) ......... | 100 | 0 | 2.0 | 11.0 | 0 | 220 | 0 |
| Greek vinaigrette: | | | | | | | |
| (*Cardini's* Light) ..... | 50 | 0 | 2.0 | 4.5 | 0 | 270 | 0 |
| (*Girard's*) .......... | 100 | 0 | 2.0 | 11.0 | 0 | 300 | 0 |
| (*Kraft*) ............. | 110 | 0 | 2.0 | 12.0 | 0 | 330 | 0 |
| (*Marie's*) ........... | 110 | 1.0 | 1.0 | 12.0 | 0 | 180 | 0 |
| (*Newman's Own*) .... | 100 | 0 | 1.0 | 10.0 | 0 | 270 | 0 |
| honey balsamic (*Marzetti*) .......... | 120 | 0 | 4.0 | 11.0 | 0 | 240 | 0 |
| honey Dijon: | | | | | | | |
| (*Brianna's*) ......... | 150 | 0 | 8.0 | 14.0 | 0 | 170 | 0 |
| (*Good Seasons* Grey Poupon Light) .... | 60 | 0 | 6.0 | 3.5 | 0 | 280 | 0 |
| (*Ken's*) ............. | 130 | 0 | 7.0 | 11.0 | 10 | 180 | 0 |
| (*Ken's* Healthy Options) ......... | 70 | 0 | 7.0 | 4.0 | 10 | 250 | 0 |
| (*Kraft*) ............. | 100 | 0 | 6.0 | 9.0 | 0 | 250 | 0 |
| (*Kraft* Free) ......... | 50 | 0 | 12.0 | 0 | 0 | 330 | 1.0 |
| (*Marie's*) ........... | 130 | 0 | 5.0 | 12.0 | 10 | 200 | 0 |
| (*Marzetti* 15 oz.) ..... | 130 | 0 | 6.0 | 12.0 | 10 | 170 | 0 |
| (*Marzetti* 16 oz.) ..... | 140 | 0 | 6.0 | 12.0 | 10 | 160 | 0 |
| (*Marzetti* Light) ...... | 90 | 0 | 8.0 | 6.0 | 10 | 190 | 0 |
| (*Marzetti* Nonfat) .... | 50 | 0 | 12.0 | 0 | 0 | 290 | 0 |
| (*Pfeiffer*) ........... | 130 | 0 | 6.0 | 12.0 | 10 | 180 | 0 |
| (*Teresa's* Light) ...... | 50 | 0 | 13.0 | 0 | 0 | 300 | 0 |
| (*Wish-Bone* Light) ... | 50 | 0 | 8.0 | 2.0 | 0 | 260 | <1.0 |
| vinaigrette (*Kraft*) .... | 90 | 0 | 6.0 | 7.0 | 0 | 340 | 0 |
| vinaigrette (*Litehouse* Lite) ... | 70 | 0 | 7.0 | 5.0 | 0 | 150 | 0 |

| Food and Measure | cal. | prot. (gms) | carbo. (gms) | fat (gms) | chol. (mgs) | sod. (mgs) | fiber (gms) |
|---|---|---|---|---|---|---|---|
| honey mustard: | | | | | | | |
| (*Bolthouse Farms* | | | | | | | |
| Yogurt) .......... | 45 | 1.0 | 7.0 | 2.0 | 5 | 80 | 0 |
| (*Cardini's*) .......... | 140 | 0 | 5.0 | 13.0 | 0 | 220 | 0 |
| (*Ken's*) ............ | 130 | 0 | 7.0 | 11.0 | 15 | 210 | 0 |
| (*Litehouse*) ........ | 130 | 0 | 4.0 | 12.0 | 10 | 160 | 0 |
| (*Marie's*) .......... | 140 | 0 | 6.0 | 13.0 | 10 | 200 | 0 |
| (*Newman's Own* | | | | | | | |
| Lighten Up!) ...... | 70 | 0 | 7.0 | 4.0 | 0 | 290 | 0 |
| vinaigrette (*Annie's* | | | | | | | |
| *Naturals* Lite) ..... | 40 | 0 | 5.0 | 3.0 | 0 | 130 | 0 |
| huckleberry vinaigrette | | | | | | | |
| (*Litehouse*) ........ | 25 | 0 | 6.0 | 0 | 0 | 105 | 0 |
| Italian: | | | | | | | |
| (*Annie's Naturals* | | | | | | | |
| Tuscany) ........ | 80 | 0 | 5.0 | 7.0 | 0 | 240 | 0 |
| (*Bernstein's* Dressing | | | | | | | |
| & Marinade) ...... | 110 | 0 | 1.0 | 12.0 | 0 | 330 | 0 |
| (*Bernstein's* | | | | | | | |
| Restaurant Recipe) | 120 | 1.0 | 1.0 | 12.0 | 5 | 360 | 0 |
| (*Cains*) ............ | 80 | 0 | 3.0 | 8.0 | 0 | 470 | 0 |
| (*Cains* Bellissimo) .... | 150 | 0 | 1.0 | 16.0 | 0 | 200 | 0 |
| (*Cains* Light) ........ | 50 | 0 | 4.0 | 3.5 | 0 | 410 | 0 |
| (*Cains* Nonfat) ...... | 15 | 0 | 4.0 | 0 | 0 | 490 | 0 |
| (*Cardini's*) .......... | 100 | 0 | 7.0 | 8.0 | 0 | 310 | 0 |
| (*Girard's* Olde | | | | | | | |
| Venice) .......... | 130 | 0 | 2.0 | 13.0 | 0 | 510 | 0 |
| (*Ken's* Dressing & | | | | | | | |
| Marinade) ........ | 150 | 0 | 1.0 | 16.0 | 0 | 450 | 0 |
| (*Ken's* Dressing & | | | | | | | |
| Marinade Lite) .... | 50 | 0 | 2.0 | 5.0 | 0 | 440 | 0 |
| (*Ken's* Zesty) ........ | 90 | 0 | 5.0 | 8.0 | 0 | 530 | 0 |
| (*Kraft* Free) ........ | 20 | 0 | 4.0 | 0 | 0 | 380 | 0 |
| (*Kraft* Zesty Free) .... | 15 | 0 | 3.0 | 0 | 0 | 480 | 0 |
| (*Kraft* Tuscan House) . | 130 | 0 | 3.0 | 13.0 | 5 | 250 | 0 |
| (*Kraft* Zesty) ........ | 70 | 0 | 3.0 | 6.0 | 0 | 370 | 0 |
| (*Marzetti* House) ..... | 120 | 0 | 2.0 | 12.0 | 0 | 320 | 0 |
| (*Marzetti* Nonfat) .... | 15 | 0 | 4.0 | 0 | 0 | 290 | 0 |
| (*Marzetti* Sweet) ..... | 160 | 0 | 7.0 | 14.0 | 0 | 260 | 0 |
| (*Marzetti* Venice) .... | 120 | 0 | 2.0 | 12.0 | 0 | 390 | 0 |
| (*Newman's Own* | | | | | | | |
| Family Recipe) .... | 120 | 1.0 | 1.0 | 13.0 | 0 | 400 | 0 |
| (*Newman's Own* | | | | | | | |
| Tuscan Organic) ... | 100 | 0 | 2.0 | 11.0 | 0 | 380 | 0 |

| Food and Measure | cal. | prot. (gms) | carbo. (gms) | fat (gms) | chol. (mgs) | sod. (mgs) | fiber (gms) |
|---|---|---|---|---|---|---|---|
| **Salad dressing, Italian** *(cont.)* | | | | | | | |
| (*Newman's Own* Lighten Up!) ...... | 60 | 0 | 0 | 6.0 | 0 | 260 | 0 |
| (*Pfeiffer*) ........... | 100 | 0 | 3.0 | 10.0 | 0 | 590 | 0 |
| (*Pfeiffer* Light) ...... | 50 | 0 | 3.0 | 4.0 | 0 | 300 | 0 |
| (*Pfeiffer* Nonfat) ..... | 20 | 0 | 4.0 | 0 | 0 | 290 | 0 |
| (*Pfeiffer* Tuscan) ..... | 110 | 0 | 1.0 | 12.0 | 0 | 420 | 0 |
| (*Seven Seas Viva* Fat Free) ......... | 15 | 0 | 2.0 | 0 | 0 | 480 | 0 |
| (*Seven Seas Viva* Reduced Fat) ...... | 45 | 0 | 2.0 | 4.0 | 0 | 370 | 0 |
| (*Seven Seas Viva* Robust) ......... | 90 | 0 | 2.0 | 9.0 | 0 | 380 | 0 |
| (*Wish-Bone*) ........ | 80 | 0 | 4.0 | 7.0 | 0 | 340 | 0 |
| (*Wish-Bone* House) ... | 110 | 0 | 3.0 | 10.0 | 5 | 260 | 0 |
| (*Wish-Bone* Light) ... | 35 | 0 | 3.0 | 2.5 | 0 | 340 | 0 |
| (*Wish-Bone* Light Country) ......... | 30 | 0 | 3.0 | 1.5 | 0 | 300 | 0 |
| (*Wish-Bone* Nonfat) .. | 15 | 0 | 3.0 | 0 | 0 | 350 | 0 |
| (*Wish-Bone* Robusto) . | 80 | 0 | 4.0 | 7.0 | 0 | 340 | 0 |
| balsamic (*Bernstein's*) | 110 | 0 | 2.0 | 11.0 | 0 | 270 | 0 |
| w/basil and Romano (*Ken's* Northern Lite) ............. | 50 | 0 | 1.0 | 5.0 | 0 | 330 | 0 |
| w/blue cheese crumbles (*Marzetti*) ........ | 130 | 1.0 | 2.0 | 13.0 | 5 | 180 | 0 |
| cheese, 3 (*Ken's*) .... | 110 | 1.0 | 4.0 | 11.0 | 0 | 340 | 0 |
| cheese/garlic (*Bernstein's*) ...... | 110 | 1.0 | 2.0 | 11.0 | 0 | 340 | 0 |
| cheese/garlic (*Bernstein's* Nonfat) | 10 | 0 | 2.0 | 0 | 0 | 380 | 0 |
| cheese trio (*Cains*) ... | 170 | 1.0 | 3.0 | 17.0 | 5 | 250 | 0 |
| creamy (*Bolthouse Farms* Yogurt) .... | 70 | 1.0 | 2.0 | 7.0 | 10 | 105 | 0 |
| creamy (*Ken's*) ...... | 120 | 0 | 3.0 | 13.0 | 0 | 300 | 0 |
| creamy (*Kraft*) ...... | 100 | 0 | 2.0 | 11.0 | 0 | 250 | 0 |
| creamy (*Marzetti*) .... | 120 | 0 | 2.0 | 13.0 | 5 | 370 | 0 |
| creamy (*Wish-Bone*) .. | 110 | <1.0 | 4.0 | 10.0 | 0 | 240 | 0 |
| garlic (*Pfeiffer* Zesty) ............. | 100 | 0 | 4.0 | 10.0 | 0 | 600 | 0 |
| garlic, creamy (*Marie's*) ......... | 180 | 1.0 | 1.0 | 19.0 | 15 | 135 | 0 |
| garlic, roasted, vinaigrette (*Marzetti*) | 90 | 0 | 2.0 | 9.0 | 0 | 530 | 0 |

| Food and Measure | cal. | prot. (gms) | carbo. (gms) | fat (gms) | chol. (mgs) | sod. (mgs) | fiber (gms) |
|---|---|---|---|---|---|---|---|
| garlic and asiago | | | | | | | |
| (*Ken's*) . . . . . . . . . | 110 | 0 | 7.0 | 12.0 | 0 | 420 | 0 |
| herb, sweet | | | | | | | |
| (*Bernstein's*) . . . . . . | 130 | 0 | 8.0 | 11.0 | 0 | 380 | 0 |
| red wine and garlic | | | | | | | |
| (*Bernstein's*) . . . . . . | 110 | 0 | 2.0 | 11.0 | 0 | 250 | 0 |
| roasted red pepper | | | | | | | |
| Parmesan (*Kraft*) . . | 40 | 0 | 5.0 | 2.0 | 0 | 440 | 0 |
| Romano (*Girard's*) . . . | 130 | 1.0 | 2.0 | 13.0 | 0 | 500 | 0 |
| Romano (*Ken's*) . . . . . | 120 | 0 | 2.0 | 12.0 | 0 | 300 | 0 |
| Romano and red | | | | | | | |
| pepper (*Ken's* | | | | | | | |
| *Healthy Options*) . . | 45 | 0 | 2.0 | 4.0 | 0 | 230 | 0 |
| Italian vinaigrette: | | | | | | | |
| (*Good Seasons*) . . . . . | 60 | 0 | 3.0 | 4.5 | 0 | 300 | 0 |
| (*Kraft* Classic) . . . . . . . | 60 | 0 | 5.0 | 4.0 | 0 | 430 | 0 |
| (*Litehouse* Zesty) . . . . | 60 | 0 | 3.0 | 5.0 | 0 | 340 | 0 |
| (*Marie's*) . . . . . . . . . . | 80 | 0 | 3.0 | 8.0 | 0 | 360 | 0 |
| herb (*Seeds of | | | | | | | |
| Change* Organic) . . | 60 | 0 | 5.0 | 4.5 | 0 | 260 | 0 |
| lemon: | | | | | | | |
| chive (*Annie's | | | | | | | |
| Naturals*) . . . . . . . . | 150 | 0 | 1.0 | 16.0 | 0 | 150 | 0 |
| tarragon (*Brianna's*) . . | 35 | 0 | 8.0 | 0 | 0 | 150 | 0 |
| lime vinaigrette | | | | | | | |
| (*Newman's Own | | | | | | | |
| Lighten Up!*) . . . . . . . . | 60 | 0 | 4.0 | 6.0 | 0 | 320 | 0 |
| mango vinaigrette: | | | | | | | |
| (*Annie's Naturals* | | | | | | | |
| Nonfat) . . . . . . . . . | 20 | 0 | 5.0 | 0 | 0 | 5 | 0 |
| (*Bolthouse Farms*) . . . | 30 | 0 | 5.0 | 1.5 | 0 | 95 | 0 |
| melon cucumber | | | | | | | |
| (*Teresa's*) . . . . . . . . . | 100 | 0 | 5.0 | 9.0 | 0 | 130 | 0 |
| oil and vinegar: | | | | | | | |
| (*Annie's Naturals* | | | | | | | |
| Organic) . . . . . . . . . | 120 | 0 | 1.0 | 13.0 | 0 | 220 | 0 |
| olive oil (*Ken's | | | | | | | |
| Healthy Options*) . . | 50 | 0 | 3.0 | 4.0 | 0 | 240 | 0 |
| olive oil (*Newman's | | | | | | | |
| Own*) . . . . . . . . . . . | 150 | 0 | 1.0 | 16.0 | 0 | 150 | 0 |
| olive oil vinaigrette: | | | | | | | |
| (*Ken's* Lite) . . . . . . . . | 60 | 0 | 3.0 | 6.0 | 0 | 240 | 0 |
| (*Wish-Bone*) . . . . . . . . | 60 | 0 | 4.0 | 5.0 | 0 | 250 | 0 |

| Food and Measure | cal. | prot. (gms) | carbo. (gms) | fat (gms) | chol. (mgs) | sod. (mgs) | fiber (gms) |
|---|---|---|---|---|---|---|---|
| **Salad dressing** *(cont.)* | | | | | | | |
| onion, Vidalia: | | | | | | | |
| (*Ken's* Golden) ...... | 120 | 0 | 10.0 | 9.0 | 0 | 95 | 0 |
| sweet (*Ken's* Lite) .... | 80 | 0 | 11.0 | 4.5 | 0 | 120 | 0 |
| sweet (*Marzetti*) ..... | 130 | 0 | 8.0 | 11.0 | 10 | 300 | 0 |
| sweet, vinaigrette (*Ken's Healthy Options*) ......... | 60 | 0 | 7.0 | 4.0 | 0 | 210 | 0 |
| vinaigrette (*Teresa's*) . | 130 | 0 | 8.0 | 11.0 | 0 | 200 | 0 |
| vinaigrette, roasted red pepper (*Kraft*) . | 80 | 0 | 8.0 | 5.0 | 0 | 320 | 0 |
| orange: | | | | | | | |
| citrus (*Litehouse* Tangy) .......... | 50 | 0 | 13.0 | 0 | 0 | 190 | 0 |
| ginger (*Newman's Own*) ............ | 80 | 0 | 9.0 | 4.5 | 0 | 340 | 0 |
| papaya poppy seed (*Annie's Naturals* Organic) .......... | 120 | 0 | 4.0 | 11.0 | 0 | 180 | 0 |
| Parmesan: | | | | | | | |
| creamy, cracked peppercorn (*Ken's* Lite) ....... | 110 | 1.0 | 3.0 | 9.0 | 10 | 290 | 0 |
| peppercorn (*Ken's Healthy Options*) .. | 60 | 1.0 | 3.0 | 4.0 | 10 | 250 | <1.0 |
| and roasted garlic (*Newman's Own*) .. | 110 | 1.0 | 2.0 | 11.0 | 0 | 340 | 0 |
| Parmesan Romano (*Kraft* Special Collection) ......... | 140 | 1.0 | 2.0 | 14.0 | 10 | 360 | 0 |
| peanut, Thai: | | | | | | | |
| (*Litehouse*) ......... | 60 | 1.0 | 6.0 | 3.0 | 0 | 280 | 1.0 |
| (*Marzetti*) .......... | 140 | 0 | 6.0 | 11.0 | 0 | 250 | 0 |
| pear vinaigrette (*Cardini's*) .......... | 100 | 0 | 6.0 | 9.0 | 0 | 150 | 0 |
| peppercorn: | | | | | | | |
| Parmesan (*Cains*) .... | 150 | 1.0 | 2.0 | 15.0 | 5 | 360 | 0 |
| vinaigrette (*Marzetti*) . | 140 | 0 | 5.0 | 13.0 | 0 | 300 | 0 |
| pomegranate: | | | | | | | |
| blueberry vinaigrette (*Litehouse* Organic) | 25 | 0 | 6.0 | 0 | 0 | 130 | 0 |
| vinaigrette (*Annie's Naturals* Organic) .. | 80 | 0 | 2.0 | 7.0 | 0 | 270 | 0 |

| Food and Measure | cal. | prot. (gms) | carbo. (gms) | fat (gms) | chol. (mgs) | sod. (mgs) | fiber (gms) |
|---|---|---|---|---|---|---|---|
| poppy seed: | | | | | | | |
| (*Brianna's*) ......... | 160 | 0 | 7.0 | 14.0 | 0 | 220 | 0 |
| (*Litehouse*) ......... | 60 | 0 | 6.0 | 4.0 | 10 | 220 | 0 |
| (*Marie's*) ........... | 150 | 0 | 8.0 | 13.0 | 10 | 170 | 0 |
| (*Marzetti* 15 oz.) ..... | 140 | 0 | 8.0 | 13.0 | 5 | 200 | 0 |
| (*Marzetti* 16 oz.) ..... | 160 | 0 | 11.0 | 13.0 | 10 | 310 | 0 |
| (*Newman's Own*) .... | 140 | 0 | 5.0 | 13.0 | 0 | 220 | 0 |
| (*Pfeiffer*) ........... | 160 | 0 | 11.0 | 13.0 | 10 | 310 | 0 |
| citrus (*Marzetti* Light) ............. | 80 | 0 | 6.0 | 6.0 | 0 | 190 | 0 |
| creamy (*Kraft*) ...... | 130 | 0 | 8.0 | 11.0 | 5 | 260 | 0 |
| sweet (*Bolthouse Farms* Yogurt) .... | 70 | 1.0 | 8.0 | 4.5 | 5 | 120 | 0 |
| potato salad: | | | | | | | |
| (*Marie's* Classic) ..... | 170 | 0 | 0 | 19.0 | 15 | 190 | 0 |
| (*Marie's* German) .... | 110 | 0 | 3.0 | 11.0 | 0 | 200 | 0 |
| (*Marzetti*) .......... | 160 | 0 | 6.0 | 15.0 | 20 | 340 | 0 |
| Dijon herb (*Marie's*) .. | 140 | 1.0 | 1.0 | 15.0 | 15 | 190 | 0 |
| ranch: | | | | | | | |
| (*Annie's Naturals* Cowgirl) ......... | 120 | 1.0 | 3.0 | 11.0 | 10 | 260 | 0 |
| (*Bolthouse Farms* Yogurt) .......... | 80 | 1.0 | 3.0 | 7.5 | 5 | 290 | 0 |
| (*Cains Light*) ........ | 80 | 0 | 6.0 | 6.0 | 5 | 310 | 0 |
| (*Ken's*) ............ | 140 | 0 | 2.0 | 15.0 | 10 | 310 | 0 |
| (*Ken's Healthy Options*) ......... | 60 | 0 | 6.0 | 4.0 | 10 | 190 | 0 |
| (*Ken's Lite*) ......... | 90 | 0 | 5.0 | 7.0 | 10 | 320 | 0 |
| (*Kraft*) ............. | 120 | 0 | 3.0 | 12.0 | 0 | 370 | 0 |
| (*Kraft Light*) ........ | 80 | 0 | 7.0 | 6.0 | 10 | 440 | 0 |
| (*Kraft Free*) ........ | 50 | 0 | 11.0 | 0 | 0 | 330 | 0 |
| (*Litehouse*) ......... | 120 | 1.0 | 2.0 | 12.0 | 10 | 200 | 0 |
| (*Litehouse* Homestyle) | 120 | 0 | 2.0 | 12.0 | 10 | 240 | 0 |
| (*Litehouse* Lite) ..... | 60 | 1.0 | 3.0 | 6.0 | 0 | 230 | 0 |
| (*Litehouse* Organic) .. | 130 | 1.0 | 2.0 | 13.0 | 10 | 190 | 0 |
| (*Litehouse* Yogurt Kefir) ........... | 60 | 1.0 | 3.0 | 5.0 | 5 | 220 | 0 |
| (*Marie's* Yogurt) ..... | 70 | 1.0 | 2.0 | 7.0 | 5 | 180 | 0 |
| (*Marzetti*) .......... | 120 | 0 | 2.0 | 13.0 | 10 | 240 | 0 |
| (*Marzetti* Classic) .... | 160 | 1.0 | 1.0 | 17.0 | 10 | 200 | 0 |
| (*Marzetti* Classic Light) ............ | 80 | 1.0 | 2.0 | 8.0 | 10 | 250 | 0 |
| (*Newman's Own*) .... | 150 | 0 | 2.0 | 16.0 | 10 | 310 | 0 |
| (*Pfeiffer*) ........... | 120 | 0 | 2.0 | 13.0 | 10 | 240 | 0 |

| Food and Measure | cal. | prot. (gms) | carbo. (gms) | fat (gms) | chol. (mgs) | sod. (mgs) | fiber (gms) |
|---|---|---|---|---|---|---|---|
| **Salad dressing, ranch** *(cont.)* | | | | | | | |
| (*Pfeiffer* Garden) . . . . . | 130 | 0 | 2.0 | 13.0 | 10 | 240 | 0 |
| (*Pfeiffer* Light) . . . . . . | 80 | 0 | 4.0 | 7.0 | 10 | 300 | 1.0 |
| (*Pfeiffer* Nonfat) . . . . . | 25 | 0 | 7.0 | 0 | 0 | 390 | 1.0 |
| (*Wish-Bone*) . . . . . . . . | 130 | 0 | 2.0 | 13.0 | 5 | 250 | 0 |
| (*Wish-Bone* Light) . . . | 40 | 0 | 5.0 | 2.0 | 0 | 290 | 0 |
| (*Wish-Bone* Nonfat) . . | 30 | 0 | 6.0 | 0 | 0 | 280 | <1.0 |
| ancho chipotle | | | | | | | |
| (*Marzetti* Light) . . . | 70 | 1.0 | 2.0 | 6.0 | 10 | 240 | 0 |
| w/bacon (*Kraft*) . . . . . | 150 | 1.0 | 2.0 | 16.0 | 10 | 300 | 0 |
| barbecue (*Litehouse*) . | 110 | 0 | 4.0 | 10.0 | 10 | 290 | 0 |
| buttermilk (*Brianna's*) . | 160 | 1.0 | 2.0 | 17.0 | 0 | 280 | 0 |
| buttermilk (*Ken's Farmhouse*) . . . . . . | 160 | 0 | 2.0 | 16.0 | 5 | 260 | 0 |
| buttermilk (*Kraft*) . . . . | 150 | 0 | 3.0 | 16.0 | 10 | 320 | 0 |
| buttermilk (*Litehouse*) | 120 | 0 | 2.0 | 12.0 | 10 | 210 | 0 |
| buttermilk (*Marie's*) . . | 150 | 0 | 1.0 | 16.0 | 5 | 260 | 0 |
| 3 cheese (*Kraft*) . . . . . | 120 | 1.0 | 3.0 | 12.0 | 0 | 360 | 0 |
| 3 cheese (*Kraft* Light) . . . . . . . . . . | 80 | 0 | 2.0 | 8.0 | 0 | 450 | 0 |
| chipotle (*Cains*) . . . . . | 170 | 0 | 3.0 | 17.0 | 5 | 230 | 0 |
| chipotle, creamy (*Marie's*) . . . . . . . . | 170 | 0 | 1.0 | 19.0 | 15 | 150 | 0 |
| creamy (*Litehouse* Lite) . . . . . . . . . . . | 70 | 0 | 2.0 | 6.0 | 5 | 240 | 0 |
| creamy (*Marie's*) . . . . . | 170 | 1.0 | 1.0 | 19.0 | 15 | 150 | 0 |
| creamy (*Marie's* Lite) . . . . . . . . . . . | 60 | 1.0 | 2.0 | 6.0 | 5 | 200 | 0 |
| garlic (*Kraft*) . . . . . . . . | 120 | 0 | 3.0 | 12.0 | 0 | 360 | 0 |
| garlic (*Wish-Bone*) . . . | 150 | 0 | 2.0 | 15.0 | 0 | 310 | 0 |
| jalapeño (*Litehouse*) . . | 120 | 0 | 2.0 | 12.0 | 10 | 220 | 0 |
| jalapeño (*Marie's*) . . . | 160 | 1.0 | 1.0 | 17.0 | 10 | 220 | 0 |
| Parmesan (*Marie's*) . . | 170 | 1.0 | 1.0 | 19.0 | 15 | 160 | 0 |
| Parmesan (*Marzetti* Organic) . | 140 | 1.0 | 2.0 | 14.0 | 5 | 310 | 0 |
| Parmesan, aged (*Cardini's*) . . . . . . . | 150 | 1.0 | 1.0 | 16.0 | 10 | 300 | 0 |
| Parmesan, aged (*Marzetti*) . . . . . . . . | 140 | 1.0 | 2.0 | 14.0 | 10 | 290 | 0 |
| Parmesan garlic *Bernstein's* Light Fantastic) . . . . . . . . | 50 | 1.0 | 6.0 | 2.5 | 5 | 330 | 0 |
| Parmesan peppercorn (*Wish-Bone* Light) . | 45 | 0 | 7.0 | 2.0 | <5 | 270 | <1.0 |

| Food and Measure | cal. | prot. (gms) | carbo. (gms) | fat (gms) | chol. (mgs) | sod. (mgs) | fiber (gms) |
|---|---|---|---|---|---|---|---|
| peppercorn (*Ken's*) ... | 180 | 0 | 1.0 | 19.0 | 5 | 280 | 0 |
| peppercorn (*Kraft*) ... | 120 | 0 | 2.0 | 12.0 | 0 | 320 | 0 |
| peppercorn (*Pfeiffer*) . | 170 | 0 | 2.0 | 18.0 | 10 | 220 | 0 |
| salsa (*Litehouse* Lite) . | 60 | 0 | 2.0 | 5.0 | 5 | 200 | 0 |
| raspberry: | | | | | | | |
| (*Girard's*) .......... | 120 | 0 | 9.0 | 10.0 | 0 | 65 | 0 |
| cranberry (*Marzetti* Organic) | 100 | 0 | 6.0 | 8.0 | 0 | 65 | 0 |
| pecan (*Ken's* Nonfat) . | 50 | 0 | 12.0 | 0 | 0 | 280 | 0 |
| walnut (*Ken's Healthy* Options) ........ | 60 | 0 | 6.0 | 3.5 | 0 | 180 | 0 |
| walnut (*Newman's Own Lighten Up!*) .. | 70 | 0 | 7.0 | 5.0 | 0 | 120 | 0 |
| raspberry vinaigrette: | | | | | | | |
| (*Cains*) ............. | 80 | 0 | 6.0 | 6.0 | 0 | 130 | 0 |
| (*Cains* Light ...... | 80 | 0 | 11.0 | 4.0 | 0 | 20 | 0 |
| (*Kraft* Light) ....... | 60 | 0 | 5.0 | 4.0 | 0 | 270 | 0 |
| (*Marie's*) .......... | 50 | 0 | 7.0 | 3.0 | 0 | 100 | 0 |
| balsamic (*Annie's Naturals* Nonfat) ... | 30 | 0 | 7.0 | 0 | 0 | 10 | 0 |
| Cabernet (*Marzetti* Light) | 60 | 0 | 7.0 | 3.5 | 0 | 200 | 0 |
| hazelnut (*Wish-Bone*) . | 80 | 0 | 8.0 | 5.0 | 0 | 260 | 0 |
| lime (*Litehouse* Organic) ........ | 45 | 0 | 5.0 | 2.5 | 0 | 60 | 0 |
| Merlot, olive oil (*Bolthouse Farms*) . | 30 | 0 | 6.0 | .5 | 0 | 50 | 0 |
| pomegranate (*Cardini's*) | 100 | 0 | 5.0 | 8.0 | 0 | 150 | 0 |
| red, w/poppy seeds (*Good Seasons*) ... | 60 | 0 | 5.0 | 4.0 | 0 | 270 | 0 |
| walnut (*Ken's* Lite) ... | 80 | 0 | 7.0 | 6.0 | 0 | 120 | 0 |
| walnut (*Litehouse*) ... | 100 | 0 | 5.0 | 9.0 | 0 | 75 | 0 |
| walnut (*Wish-Bone* Light) .......... | 80 | 0 | 7.0 | 5.0 | 0 | 260 | 0 |
| raspberry white balsamic (*Teresa's*) ... | 100 | 0 | 5.0 | 9.0 | 0 | 190 | 0 |
| red pepper, roasted, vinaigrette: | | | | | | | |
| (*Annie's Naturals*) .... | 70 | 0 | 3.0 | 6.0 | 0 | 240 | 0 |
| (*Seeds of Change* Organic) ......... | 50 | 0 | 5.0 | 3.5 | 0 | 240 | 0 |
| red wine vinaigrette: (*Kraft Light Done Right*) .......... | 45 | 0 | 3.0 | 4.0 | 0 | 310 | 0 |

| Food and Measure | cal. | prot. (gms) | carbo. (gms) | fat (gms) | chol. (mgs) | sod. (mgs) | fiber (gms) |
|---|---|---|---|---|---|---|---|
| **Salad dressing, red wine vinaigrette** *(cont.)* | | | | | | | |
| (*Marie's*) .......... | 60 | 0 | 6.0 | 4.0 | 0 | 200 | 0 |
| (*Pfeiffer*) .......... | 90 | 0 | 3.0 | 9.0 | 0 | 450 | 0 |
| (*Seven Seas*) ....... | 90 | 0 | 2.0 | 9.0 | 0 | 470 | 0 |
| (*Seven Seas* Less Fat) ............. | 45 | 0 | 3.0 | 4.0 | 0 | 320 | 0 |
| (*Wish-Bone*) ........ | 70 | 0 | 6.0 | 5.0 | 0 | 230 | 0 |
| (*Wish-Bone* Nonfat) .. | 35 | 0 | 7.0 | 0 | 0 | 230 | 0 |
| olive oil (*Annie's Naturals* Organic) .. | 140 | 0 | 0 | 15.0 | 0 | 190 | 0 |
| olive oil (*Litehouse*) .. | 90 | 0 | 2.0 | 9.0 | 0 | 140 | 0 |
| red wine vinegar/oil: | | | | | | | |
| (*Ken's*) ............. | 120 | 0 | 2.0 | 12.0 | 0 | 360 | 0 |
| (*Newman's Own Lighten Up!*) ...... | 50 | 0 | 2.0 | 4.5 | 0 | 390 | 0 |
| Romano basil vinaigrette (*Wish-Bone*) | 60 | 0 | 2.0 | 5.0 | 0 | 330 | 0 |
| Russian: | | | | | | | |
| (*Ken's*) ............. | 140 | 0 | 5.0 | 14.0 | 15 | 280 | 0 |
| (*Wish-Bone*) ........ | 110 | 0 | 14.0 | 6.0 | 0 | 340 | 0 |
| sesame, Asian: | | | | | | | |
| (*Annie's Naturals* Organic) .......... | 130 | 0 | 4.0 | 12.0 | 0 | 300 | 0 |
| (*Ken's* Lite) ......... | 70 | 0 | 8.0 | 4.0 | 0 | 440 | 0 |
| roasted (*Cardini's*) ... | 120 | 0 | 7.0 | 10.0 | 0 | 360 | 0 |
| toasted (*Kraft*) ...... | 90 | 1.0 | 8.0 | 6.0 | 0 | 360 | 0 |
| vinaigrette (*Wish-Bone* Light) . | 70 | 0 | 5.0 | 5.0 | 0 | 300 | 0 |
| sesame ginger: | | | | | | | |
| (*Good Seasons*) ..... | 110 | 0 | 7.0 | 9.0 | 0 | 300 | 0 |
| (*Litehouse*) ......... | 40 | 1.0 | 9.0 | 0 | 0 | 270 | 0 |
| (*Marie's*) ........... | 100 | 0 | 7.0 | 8.0 | 0 | 250 | 0 |
| (*Marzetti*) .......... | 110 | 1.0 | 6.0 | 9.0 | 0 | 330 | 0 |
| (*Newman's Own Lighten Up!*) ...... | 35 | 0 | 5.0 | 1.5 | 0 | 390 | 0 |
| vinaigrette, w/ chamomile (*Annie's Naturals* Organic) .. | 100 | 1.0 | 4.0 | 9.0 | 0 | 240 | 0 |
| shiitake and sesame: | | | | | | | |
| (*Annie's Naturals*) .... | 130 | 1.0 | 1.0 | 14.0 | 0 | 270 | 0 |
| vinaigrette (*Annie's Naturals* Organic) .. | 120 | 0 | 1.0 | 13.0 | 0 | 270 | 0 |
| spinach: | | | | | | | |
| (*Girard's*) .......... | 70 | 1.0 | 14.0 | 2.0 | 0 | 250 | 0 |

| Food and Measure | cal. | prot. (gms) | carbo. (gms) | fat (gms) | chol. (mgs) | sod. (mgs) | fiber (gms) |
|---|---|---|---|---|---|---|---|
| (*Marzetti*) . . . . . . . . . | 70 | 0 | 13.0 | 1.5 | 0 | 250 | 0 |
| salad (*Litehouse*) . . . . | 70 | 1.0 | 14.0 | .5 | 0 | 340 | 0 |
| salad (*Marie's*) . . . . . . | 70 | 1.0 | 13.0 | 1.5 | 0 | 230 | 0 |
| strawberry vinaigrette: | | | | | | | |
| (*Marzetti*) . . . . . . . . . | 110 | 0 | 6.0 | 10.0 | 0 | 150 | 0 |
| Chardonnay | | | | | | | |
| (*Marzetti*) . . . . . . . . | 100 | 0 | 6.0 | 8.0 | 0 | 140 | 0 |
| sweet and sour: | | | | | | | |
| (*Litehouse*) . . . . . . . . | 70 | 0 | 9.0 | 3.5 | 5 | 240 | 0 |
| (*Marzetti*) . . . . . . . . . | 150 | 0 | 11.0 | 11.0 | 0 | 220 | 0 |
| (*Marzetti* Nonfat) . . . . | 45 | 0 | 12.0 | 0 | 0 | 290 | 0 |
| (*Pfeiffer*) . . . . . . . . . | 160 | 0 | 10.0 | 13.0 | 0 | 220 | 0 |
| tamari: | | | | | | | |
| ginger (*San-J*) . . . . . . | 25 | <1.0 | 5.0 | 0 | 0 | 490 | 0 |
| peanut (*San-J*) . . . . . . | 70 | 3.0 | 9.0 | 2.0 | 0 | 230 | <1.0 |
| sesame (*San-J*) . . . . . | 40 | 2.0 | 5.0 | 2.0 | 0 | 570 | 0 |
| Thousand Island: | | | | | | | |
| (*Annie's Naturals* | | | | | | | |
| Organic) . . . . . . . . . | 80 | 0 | 4.0 | 7.0 | 5 | 250 | 0 |
| (*Bolthouse Farms* | | | | | | | |
| Yogurt) . . . . . . . . . | 70 | 1.0 | 4.0 | 5.5 | 5 | 180 | <1.0 |
| (*Ken's*) . . . . . . . . . . . | 140 | 0 | 4.0 | 13.0 | 15 | 300 | 0 |
| (*Kraft*) . . . . . . . . . . . | 110 | 0 | 5.0 | 10.0 | 0 | 330 | 0 |
| (*Kraft* Light) . . . . . . . | 60 | 0 | 11.0 | 3.0 | 0 | 340 | 0 |
| (*Litehouse*) . . . . . . . . | 130 | 0 | 3.0 | 13.0 | 10 | 250 | 0 |
| (*Litehouse* Family) . . . | 120 | 0 | 3.0 | 12.0 | 10 | 240 | 0 |
| (*Litehouse* Lite) . . . . . | 70 | 0 | 4.0 | 7.0 | 5 | 240 | 0 |
| (*Marie's*) . . . . . . . . . | 150 | 0 | 4.0 | 15.0 | 15 | 190 | 0 |
| (*Marzetti* 16 oz.) . . . . . | 110 | 0 | 4.0 | 11.0 | 5 | 230 | 0 |
| (*Pfeiffer*) . . . . . . . . . | 140 | 0 | 4.0 | 14.0 | 10 | 240 | 0 |
| (*Pfeiffer* Light) . . . . . . | 70 | 0 | 6.0 | 5.0 | 15 | 360 | 0 |
| (*Wish-Bone*) . . . . . . . | 130 | 0 | 6.0 | 12.0 | 10 | 300 | 0 |
| (*Wish-Bone* Light) . . . | 60 | 0 | 9.0 | 2.0 | 5 | 280 | 0 |
| w/bacon (*Kraft*) . . . . . | 100 | 0 | 7.0 | 8.0 | 0 | 220 | 0 |
| tomato, basil, mozzarella | | | | | | | |
| (*Marie's* Caprese) . . . . | 110 | 0 | 2.0 | 11.0 | 0 | 85 | 0 |
| tomato, sun-dried: | | | | | | | |
| (*Newman's Own* | | | | | | | |
| *Lighten Up!*) . . . . . . | 60 | 0 | 5.0 | 4.0 | 0 | 380 | 0 |
| vinaigrette (*Ken's* | | | | | | | |
| Nonfat) . . . . . . . . . | 70 | 0 | 17.0 | 0 | 0 | 260 | 0 |
| vinaigrette (*Kraft*) . . . . | 60 | 0 | 4.0 | 5.0 | 0 | 350 | 0 |
| vinaigrette (*Teresa's*) . | 130 | 0 | 7.0 | 11.0 | 0 | 320 | 0 |

| Food and Measure | cal. | prot. (gms) | carbo. (gms) | fat (gms) | chol. (mgs) | sod. (mgs) | fiber (gms) |
|---|---|---|---|---|---|---|---|
| **Salad dressing, tomato, sundried** *(cont.)* | | | | | | | |
| vinaigrette, roasted red pepper (*Good Seasons*) ........ | 60 | 0 | 4.0 | 5.0 | 0 | 340 | 0 |
| tomato bacon (*Kraft* Tangy) ........ | 100 | 0 | 10.0 | 6.0 | 0 | 350 | 0 |
| **Salad dressing mix** (*Good Seasons*), dry, ⅛ pkt.: | | | | | | | |
| Caesar, gourmet ....... | 15 | 0 | 2.0 | 0 | 0 | 300 | 0 |
| cheese garlic .......... | 5 | 0 | 1.0 | 0 | 0 | 330 | 0 |
| garlic and herb ........ | 5 | 0 | 1.0 | 0 | 0 | 340 | 0 |
| Italian ............... | 5 | 0 | 1.0 | 0 | 0 | 320 | 0 |
| Italian, fat free ......... | 10 | 0 | 3.0 | 0 | 0 | 290 | 0 |
| Italian, mild .......... | 10 | 0 | 2.0 | 0 | 0 | 370 | 0 |
| Italian, zesty .......... | 5 | 0 | 1.0 | 0 | 0 | 220 | 0 |
| sesame, Asian ......... | 15 | 0 | 3.0 | 0 | 0 | 350 | 0 |
| **Salad seasoning** (*McCormick Perfect Pinch* Salad Supreme), ¼ tsp. .... | 0 | 0 | 0 | 0 | 0 | 55 | 0 |
| **Salad toppers** (see also "Croutons" and specific listings), ¼ oz., except as noted: | | | | | | | |
| (*McCormick Salad Toppins*), 1⅓ tbsp. .... | 35 | 2.0 | 3.0 | 1.5 | 0 | 70 | 0 |
| almonds (*Fresh Gourmet*), sliced: | | | | | | | |
| garlic, roasted ....... | 40 | 1.0 | 1.0 | 3.5 | 0 | 30 | 1.0 |
| honey-roasted ...... | 40 | 1.0 | 3.0 | 3.0 | 0 | 20 | 1.0 |
| ranch ............ | 40 | 1.0 | 1.0 | 3.5 | 0 | 50 | 1.0 |
| toasted ............ | 40 | 2.0 | 1.0 | 3.5 | 0 | 0 | 1.0 |
| bacon almond crunch (*Marzetti* Salad Accents), 1 tbsp. .... | 35 | 2.0 | 3.0 | 2.0 | 0 | 60 | 1.0 |
| cranberries: | | | | | | | |
| (*Fresh Gourmet*) ..... | 20 | 1.0 | 5.0 | 0 | 0 | 0 | 0 |
| and glazed walnuts (*Fresh Gourmet*) .. | 30 | 0 | 4.0 | 1.5 | 0 | 5 | 1.0 |
| fruit and nut (*Marzetti* Salad Accents), 1 tbsp. ............ | 45 | 1.0 | 5.0 | 2.0 | 0 | 25 | 1.0 |

| Food and Measure | cal. | prot. (gms) | carbo. (gms) | fat (gms) | chol. (mgs) | sod. (mgs) | fiber (gms) |
|---|---|---|---|---|---|---|---|
| garden vegetable (*McCormick Salad Toppins*), 1⅓ tbsp. .... | 35 | 2.0 | 3.0 | 1.5 | 0 | 50 | 0 |
| jalapeños, crispy (*Fresh Gourmet*) .......... | 40 | 0 | 3.0 | 3.0 | 0 | 30 | 0 |
| onions, crispy: | | | | | | | |
| (*Fresh Gourmet* Lightly Salted) .... | 40 | 0 | 4.0 | 2.5 | 0 | 35 | 0 |
| garlic pepper (*Fresh Gourmet*) ......... | 35 | 0 | 4.0 | 2.0 | 0 | 50 | 0 |
| pecan pieces, honey-roasted (*Fresh Gourmet*) .......... | 45 | 1.0 | 2.0 | 4.5 | 0 | 15 | 1.0 |
| raisins, golden: | | | | | | | |
| (*Fresh Gourmet*) ..... | 20 | 0 | 5.0 | 0 | 0 | 0 | 0 |
| and glazed pecans (*Fresh Gourmet*) .. | 35 | 0 | 4.0 | 2.0 | 0 | 10 | 0 |
| red pepper, crispy (*Fresh Gourmet*) ....... | 45 | 0 | 3.0 | 4.0 | 0 | 15 | 0 |
| sesame, Asian (*Marzetti* Salad Accents), 1 tbsp. .... | 40 | 1.0 | 3.0 | 2.5 | 0 | 55 | 1.0 |
| tortilla strips: | | | | | | | |
| (*Fresh Gourmet* Lightly Salted) .... | 35 | .5 | 4.0 | 1.5 | 0 | 15 | 0 |
| (*Fresh Gourmet* Santa Fe) ........ | 30 | 0 | 4.0 | 1.5 | 0 | 25 | 0 |
| chili lime (*New York* Texas Toast) ...... | 35 | <1.0 | 4.0 | 2.0 | 0 | 50 | 0 |
| chipotle cheddar (*New York* Texas Toast) ........... | 35 | <1.0 | 4.0 | 2.0 | 0 | 45 | 0 |
| tri-color (*Fresh Gourmet*) ........ | 35 | 0 | 4.0 | 1.5 | 0 | 15 | 0 |
| walnut pieces, glazed (*Fresh Gourmet*) ..... | 45 | 1.0 | 2.0 | 4.0 | 0 | 15 | 0 |
| wonton strips (*Fresh Gourmet*): | | | | | | | |
| authentic ........... | 35 | 1.0 | 4.0 | 1.5 | 0 | 40 | 0 |
| garlic ginger ........ | 35 | 1.0 | 4.0 | 2.0 | 0 | 35 | 0 |
| wasabi ranch ....... | 35 | 1.0 | 4.0 | 2.0 | 0 | 85 | 0 |
| **Salami**: | | | | | | | |
| beef: | | | | | | | |
| (*Boar's Head*), 2 oz. .. | 120 | 10.0 | 0 | 9.0 | 35 | 470 | 0 |

| Food and Measure | cal. | prot. (gms) | carbo. (gms) | fat (gms) | chol. (mgs) | sod. (mgs) | fiber (gms) |
|---|---|---|---|---|---|---|---|
| **Salami, beef** *(cont.)* | | | | | | | |
| (*Hebrew National*), 2 oz. | 150 | 8.0 | 0 | 13.0 | 35 | 420 | 0 |
| (*Hebrew National* Lean), 2 oz. ...... | 90 | 9.0 | 1.0 | 5.0 | 25 | 480 | 0 |
| (*Oscar Mayer*), 1 oz. ... | 80 | 4.0 | 0 | 7.0 | 20 | 400 | 0 |
| (*Oscar Mayer* Thin Sliced), 1.75 oz. ... | 150 | 8.0 | 0 | 13.0 | 35 | 640 | 0 |
| cooked, 2 oz.: | | | | | | | |
| (*Boar's Head*) ....... | 130 | 8.0 | 0 | 11.0 | 40 | 590 | 0 |
| (*Thumann's*) ........ | 110 | 9.0 | 1.0 | 7.0 | 30 | 440 | 0 |
| cotto (*Oscar Mayer*), 1 oz. .............. | 70 | 4.0 | 1.0 | 6.0 | 25 | 280 | 0 |
| dry, Italian, 1 oz.: | | | | | | | |
| (*Applegate Farms* Salame di Caprino) . | 110 | 8.0 | 0 | 8.0 | 30 | 480 | 0 |
| (*Boar's Head Bianco D'Oro*) .......... | 110 | 7.0 | 1.0 | 8.0 | 25 | 470 | 0 |
| (*Di Lusso*) .......... | 110 | 6.0 | 1.0 | 9.0 | 30 | 480 | 0 |
| (*Hormel*) ........... | 110 | 6.0 | 1.0 | 9.0 | 30 | 480 | 0 |
| herb or peppered (*Applegate Farms*) . | 70 | 5.0 | 1.0 | 4.5 | 20 | 240 | 0 |
| Genoa: | | | | | | | |
| (*Applegate Farms* Deli/Natural), 1 oz. . | 110 | 7.0 | 0 | 9.0 | 20 | 520 | 0 |
| (*Applegate Farms* Organic), 1 oz. .... | 100 | 7.0 | 0 | 7.0 | 25 | 400 | 0 |
| (*Applegate Farms* Salametti), 1 oz. ... | 70 | 9.0 | 0 | 4.0 | 30 | 450 | 0 |
| (*Black Bear*), 1 oz. ... | 90 | 8.0 | 1.0 | 7.0 | 23 | 500 | 0 |
| (*Boar's Head*), 2 oz. .. | 190 | 12.0 | 1.0 | 15.0 | 50 | 920 | 0 |
| (*Di Lusso*), 2 oz. ...... | 210 | 12.0 | 0 | 18.0 | 50 | 940 | 0 |
| (*Di Lusso* Natural Casing), 1 oz. ...... | 170 | 12.0 | 0 | 14.0 | 50 | 910 | 0 |
| (*Hormel San Remo Brand*), 2 oz. ..... | 210 | 11.0 | 0 | 18.0 | 55 | 940 | 0 |
| (*Thumann's*), 1 oz. ... | 120 | 6.0 | 0 | 10.0 | 45 | 450 | 0 |
| hot (*Applegate Farms*), 1 oz. ............. | 100 | 7.0 | 0 | 8.0 | 20 | 540 | 0 |
| hard, 1 oz.: | | | | | | | |
| (*Black Bear*) ........ | 110 | 6.0 | 1.0 | 10.0 | 30 | 450 | 0 |
| (*Boar's Head*) ....... | 110 | 6.0 | <1.0 | 9.0 | 30 | 490 | 0 |
| (*Di Lusso*) .......... | 110 | 5.0 | 0 | 10.0 | 35 | 450 | 0 |
| (*Hormel Homeland*) .. | 110 | 6.0 | 0 | 10.0 | 30 | 450 | 0 |
| (*Oscar Mayer*) ....... | 100 | 7.0 | 1.0 | 8.0 | 25 | 510 | 0 |

| Food and Measure | cal. | prot. (gms) | carbo. (gms) | fat (gms) | chol. (mgs) | sod. (mgs) | fiber (gms) |
|---|---|---|---|---|---|---|---|
| (*Thumann's*) ........ | 110 | 6.0 | 1.0 | 9.0 | 25 | 490 | 0 |
| uncured (*Hormel* | | | | | | | |
|   *Natural Choice*) ... | 110 | 6.0 | 0 | 10.0 | 30 | 450 | 0 |
| **"Salami," vegetarian** | | | | | | | |
| (*Yves*), 4 slices, 2.2 oz. | 80 | 15.0 | 4.0 | 0 | 0 | 480 | 0 |
| **Salisbury steak**, see | | | | | | | |
|   "Beef entree" | | | | | | | |
| **Salmon**, meat only: | | | | | | | |
| raw, 4 oz.: | | | | | | | |
|   Atlantic, farmed ..... | 207 | 22.6 | 0 | 12.3 | 67 | 66 | 0 |
|   Atlantic, wild ........ | 161 | 22.5 | 0 | 7.2 | 62 | 50 | 0 |
|   Chinook .......... | 204 | 22.8 | 0 | 11.9 | 75 | 53 | 0 |
|   chum ............. | 136 | 22.8 | 0 | 4.3 | 84 | 112 | 0 |
|   coho, farmed ...... | 182 | 24.1 | 0 | 8.7 | 58 | 53 | 0 |
|   coho, wild ......... | 158 | 26.6 | 0 | 4.9 | 62 | 66 | 0 |
|   pink ............. | 132 | 22.6 | 0 | 3.9 | 59 | 76 | 0 |
|   sockeye .......... | 191 | 24.2 | 0 | 9.7 | 70 | 53 | 0 |
| baked or broiled, 4 oz.: | | | | | | | |
|   Atlantic, farmed ..... | 234 | 25.0 | 0 | 14.0 | 71 | 69 | 0 |
|   Atlantic, wild ........ | 206 | 28.8 | 0 | 9.2 | 81 | 64 | 0 |
|   Chinook .......... | 262 | 29.2 | 0 | 15.2 | 96 | 68 | 0 |
|   chum ............. | 175 | 29.3 | 0 | 5.5 | 108 | 73 | 0 |
|   coho, farmed ...... | 202 | 27.6 | 0 | 9.3 | 71 | 59 | 0 |
|   coho, wild ......... | 165 | 25.0 | 0 | 6.7 | 51 | 53 | 0 |
|   pink ............. | 169 | 29.0 | 0 | 5.0 | 76 | 98 | 0 |
|   sockeye .......... | 245 | 31.0 | 0 | 12.4 | 99 | 75 | 0 |
| boiled, poached, or | | | | | | | |
|   steamed, coho, 4 oz. . | 209 | 31.0 | 0 | 8.5 | 65 | 60 | 0 |
| **Salmon, can/pouch,** | | | | | | | |
|   in water, ¼ cup, | | | | | | | |
|   except as noted: | | | | | | | |
| Atlantic (*Bumble Bee* | | | | | | | |
|   *Prime Fillet* Can) ..... | 80 | 12.0 | 0 | 4.0 | 30 | 180 | 0 |
| chum, drained, 4 oz. .... | 160 | 24.3 | 0 | 6.2 | 44 | 552 | 0 |
| keta (*Bumble Bee*) ...... | 70 | 14.0 | 0 | 2.0 | 75 | 200 | 0 |
| pink: | | | | | | | |
|   (*Bumble Bee*) ....... | 80 | 12.0 | 0 | 3.0 | 50 | 270 | 0 |
|   (*Chicken of the Sea*) .. | 90 | 12.0 | 0 | 5.0 | 40 | 270 | 0 |
|   (*Roland*) ........... | 90 | 12.0 | 0 | 5.0 | 40 | 270 | 0 |
| pink, skin/boneless: | | | | | | | |
|   (*Bumble Bee*) ....... | 60 | 12.0 | 0 | 1.5 | 30 | 180 | 0 |
|   (*Bumble Bee Prime* | | | | | | | |
|     *Fillet* Pouch) ...... | 60 | 14.0 | 0 | 1.5 | 30 | 180 | 0 |
|   (*Chicken of the Sea*) .. | 60 | 10.0 | 0 | 2.0 | 20 | 280 | 0 |

| Food and Measure | cal. | prot. (gms) | carbo. (gms) | fat (gms) | chol. (mgs) | sod. (mgs) | fiber (gms) |
|---|---|---|---|---|---|---|---|
| **Salmon, can/pouch, pink** *(cont.)* | | | | | | | |
| (*Chicken of the Sea*), | | | | | | | |
|   3-oz. can . . . . . . . . | 80 | 14.0 | 0 | 2.0 | 30 | 390 | 0 |
| (*Chicken of the Sea*), | | | | | | | |
|   2.6-oz. pouch . . . . . | 90 | 15.0 | 0 | 3.0 | 30 | 420 | 0 |
| red: | | | | | | | |
|   (*Bumble Bee*) . . . . . . . | 100 | 13.0 | 0 | 5.0 | 40 | 220 | 0 |
|   (*Chicken of the Sea*) . . | 110 | 13.0 | 0 | 7.0 | 40 | 270 | 0 |
|   (*Roland* Sockeye) . . . . | 110 | 13.0 | 0 | 7.0 | 40 | 270 | 0 |
|   (*Rubinstein's* | | | | | | | |
|     Blueback) . . . . . . . . | 110 | 13.0 | 0 | 7.0 | 40 | 270 | 0 |
| red sockeye, drained, | | | | | | | |
|   w/bone, 4 oz. . . . . . . . | 174 | 23.2 | 0 | 8.3 | 50 | 611 | 0 |
| seasoned, mango chipotle | | | | | | | |
| (*SeaKist Salmon Creations*), | | | | | | | |
|   ½ of 4-oz. pouch . . . . | 60 | 10.0 | 2.0 | 1.0 | 20 | 300 | 0 |
| **Salmon, frozen/chilled** | | | | | | | |
| (see also "Salmon | | | | | | | |
| entree, frozen"): | | | | | | | |
| bites (*Blue Horizon*), | | | | | | | |
|   4 pcs., 2 oz. . . . . . . . . | 160 | 10.0 | 2.0 | 12.0 | 50 | 170 | 0 |
| burger, 1 pc.: | | | | | | | |
|   (*Blue Horizon* | | | | | | | |
|     Sockeye), 3.2 oz. . . | 157 | 18.2 | 2.0 | 8.5 | 54 | 312 | .1 |
|   (*SeaPak*), 3.2 oz. . . . . | 110 | 18.0 | 1.0 | 3.0 | 60 | 380 | 0 |
|   (*Vita*), 4 oz. . . . . . . . . | 120 | 18.0 | 5.0 | 3.5 | 50 | 540 | 0 |
| cake: | | | | | | | |
|   (*Phillips*), 3-oz. pc. . . . | 260 | 17.0 | 5.0 | 19.0 | 85 | 480 | 0 |
|   breaded (*Dr.* | | | | | | | |
|     *Praeger's*), 2.9-oz. pc. | 190 | 10.0 | 15.0 | 10.0 | 15 | 350 | 3.0 |
| fillet, 5 oz.: | | | | | | | |
|   barbecue (*SeaPak*) . . . | 230 | 24.0 | 9.0 | 11.0 | 85 | 530 | <1.0 |
|   herb butter (*SeaPak*) . | 350 | 23.0 | 3.0 | 26.0 | 105 | 280 | 0 |
| fillet, grilled, 3.1 oz.: | | | | | | | |
|   (*Gorton's* Classic) . . . . | 100 | 15.0 | 2.0 | 3.0 | 35 | 270 | 0 |
|   lemon (*Gorton's*) . . . . | 100 | 17.0 | 1.0 | 3.0 | 40 | 300 | 0 |
| fillet, wild, ready-to- | | | | | | | |
| cook (*Vita* Simply | | | | | | | |
| Salmon), 6 oz.: | | | | | | | |
|   cracked peppercorn . . | 170 | 33.0 | 3.0 | 2.0 | 75 | 770 | 0 |
|   lemon pepper . . . . . . . | 170 | 31.0 | 4.0 | 3.5 | 70 | 825 | 0 |
| sticks, wild Alaskan | | | | | | | |
| (*Blue Horizon*), | | | | | | | |
|   3 pcs., 3 oz. . . . . . . . . | 260 | 12.0 | 24.0 | 13.0 | 45 | 480 | 1.0 |

| Food and Measure | cal. | prot. (gms) | carbo. (gms) | fat (gms) | chol. (mgs) | sod. (mgs) | fiber (gms) |
|---|---|---|---|---|---|---|---|
| **Salmon, marinated**: | | | | | | | |
| (*Vita* Jar), ¼ cup ....... | 100 | 7.0 | 9.0 | 6.0 | 25 | 400 | 0 |
| gravlax (*Spence & Co.*), | | | | | | | |
| 2 oz. .............. | 120 | 13.0 | <1.0 | 7.0 | 30 | 910 | <1.0 |
| steak (*Bumble Bee Prime Fillet*), 4-oz. pouch: | | | | | | | |
| lemon dill .......... | 150 | 25.0 | 2.0 | 4.5 | 45 | 600 | 0 |
| teriyaki ........... | 160 | 24.0 | 8.0 | 3.0 | 45 | 690 | 0 |
| **Salmon, smoked**, 2 oz.: | | | | | | | |
| Chinook. ............. | 66 | 10.4 | 0 | 2.4 | 13 | 445 | 0 |
| coho, wild (*Vita* Gold) ... | 70 | 13.0 | 2.0 | 1.0 | 30 | 720 | 0 |
| king, Alaska, wild (*SeaBear*) .......... | 110 | 13.0 | 0 | 7.0 | 60 | 380 | 0 |
| lox (*Vita*) .............. | 80 | 17.0 | <1.0 | 1.0 | 30 | 1080 | 0 |
| Nova: | | | | | | | |
| (*SeaBear*) .......... | 90 | 14.0 | 1.0 | 3.0 | 20 | 560 | 0 |
| (*Vita* Classic) ....... | 100 | 12.0 | 0 | 6.0 | 25 | 650 | 0 |
| (*Vita* Wild) ......... | 80 | 17.0 | 1.0 | 1.0 | 30 | 990 | 0 |
| pastrami style (*A&B Famous*) ........... | 110 | 10.0 | 1.0 | 7.0 | 20 | 880 | 0 |
| peppered (*Vita*) ........ | 100 | 12.0 | 0 | 6.0 | 25 | 650 | 0 |
| sockeye, wild (*Vita* Gold) | 70 | 12.0 | <1.0 | 1.5 | 30 | 950 | 0 |
| **Salmon, smoked, can/ pouch**, 3 oz.: | | | | | | | |
| in oil, drained (*Bumble Bee* 3.75 oz. can) .... | 160 | 20.0 | 0 | 8.0 | 35 | 390 | 0 |
| Pacific (*Chicken of the Sea* Pouch) ......... | 120 | 21.0 | 1.0 | 3.5 | 45 | 490 | 0 |
| **Salmon, smoked, spread**: | | | | | | | |
| (*SeaBear*), 1 tbsp. ...... | 35 | 2.0 | 0 | 3.0 | 10 | 85 | 0 |
| (*Vita* Jar), ¼ cup ....... | 310 | 6.0 | 2.0 | 31.0 | 40 | 460 | 0 |
| cheese, w/dill (*Goldy's*), 2 tbsp. .... | 90 | 2.0 | 1.0 | 8.0 | 30 | 160 | 0 |
| cream cheese (*Vita*), 2 tbsp. | 100 | 2.0 | 1.0 | 9.0 | 30 | 150 | 0 |
| pâté (*Trois Petits Cochons*), 2 oz. ..... | 110 | 5.0 | 2.0 | 9.0 | 35 | 250 | 0 |
| **Salmon cake**, see "Salmon, frozen" and "Salmon entree, frozen" | | | | | | | |
| **Salmon cake mix**: | | | | | | | |
| (*Old Bay Salmon Classic*), 1⅔ tbsp. ..... | 35 | 0 | 4.0 | 1.0 | 45 | 90 | 0 |
| (*Zatarain's*), 4 tbsp. ...... | 110 | 4.0 | 23.0 | 1.0 | 0 | 440 | 2.0 |

| Food and Measure | cal. | prot. (gms) | carbo. (gms) | fat (gms) | chol. (mgs) | sod. (mgs) | fiber (gms) |
|---|---|---|---|---|---|---|---|
| **Salmon entree, frozen** (see also "Salmon, frozen/chilled"), 1 pkg., except as noted: | | | | | | | |
| Alaskan, wild (*Organic Bistro*), 11.3 oz. . . . . . | 390 | 28.0 | 43.0 | 13.0 | 70 | 65 | 6.0 |
| w/basil (*Lean Cuisine Spa Cuisine*), 9.5 oz. . . | 220 | 16.0 | 26.0 | 6.0 | 20 | 600 | 5.0 |
| cake, Alaskan (*Organic Bistro*), 10 oz. . . . . . . | 410 | 28.0 | 39.0 | 16.0 | 70 | 250 | 8.0 |
| grilled, 3.1-oz. fillet: | | | | | | | |
| (*Gorton's* Classic) . . . . | 100 | 15.0 | 2.0 | 3.0 | 35 | 270 | 0 |
| lemon butter (*Gorton's*) . . . . . . . . | 100 | 17.0 | 1.0 | 3.0 | 40 | 300 | 0 |
| lemon dill (*StarKist SeaSations*), 9 oz. . . . . | 290 | 14.0 | 45.0 | 5.0 | 25 | 570 | 3.0 |
| primavera (*StarKist SeaSations*), 9 oz. . . . . | 280 | 17.0 | 38.0 | 6.0 | 25 | 720 | 8.0 |
| stuffed, spinach/cheese: | | | | | | | |
| (*Oven Poppers*), 5-oz. pc. . . . . . . . . . | 290 | 18.0 | 10.0 | 18.0 | 60 | 440 | 0 |
| (*Oven Poppers Qwickies*), 3-oz. pc. | 140 | 10.0 | 7.0 | 8.0 | 25 | 250 | 0 |
| teriyaki (*StarKist SeaSations*), 9 oz. . . . . | 270 | 13.0 | 50.0 | 2.5 | 20 | 970 | 2.5 |
| **Salmon franks**, see "Frankfurter" | | | | | | | |
| **Salmon gefilte fish**, see "Gefilte fish, frozen" | | | | | | | |
| **Salmon oil**, see "Oil" | | | | | | | |
| **Salmon pâté**, see "Salmon, smoked, spread" | | | | | | | |
| **Salmon salami** (*A&B Famous*), 2 oz. . . . . . . | 120 | 7.0 | 2.0 | 9.0 | 20 | 470 | 0 |
| **Salsa** (see also "Picante sauce" and specific sauces), 2 tbsp., except as noted: | | | | | | | |
| (*Chi-Chi's* Garden) . . . . . . | 10 | 0 | 3.0 | 0 | 0 | 150 | 0 |
| (*Emeril's* Kicked Up Chunky) . . . . . . . . . . . | 15 | 0 | 3.0 | 0 | 0 | 160 | 0 |
| (*Emeril's* Original) . . . . . . | 10 | 0 | 3.0 | 0 | 0 | 190 | 0 |

| Food and Measure | cal. | prot. (gms) | carbo. (gms) | fat (gms) | chol. (mgs) | sod. (mgs) | fiber (gms) |
|---|---|---|---|---|---|---|---|
| (*Herdez* Casera) ....... | 10 | 0 | 1.0 | 0 | 0 | 240 | 0 |
| (*Herdez* Chile de Arbol) .. | 10 | 0 | 2.0 | 0 | 0 | 220 | 0 |
| (*Herdez* Ranchera) ..... | 15 | 0 | 1.0 | 0 | 0 | 220 | 0 |
| (*Herdez* Taquera) ....... | 10 | 0 | 2.0 | 0 | 0 | 250 | 0 |
| (*Herdez* Verde) ........ | 10 | 0 | 1.0 | 0 | 0 | 310 | 0 |
| (*Mission* Chunky) ...... | 10 | 0 | 2.0 | 0 | 0 | 170 | 0 |
| (*Mission* Verde) ....... | 10 | 0 | 2.0 | 0 | 0 | 160 | 0 |
| (*Newman's Own* Farmer's Garden) .... | 15 | 1.0 | 4.0 | 0 | 0 | 220 | 0 |
| (*Old El Paso* Thick 'n Chunky) ......... | 10 | 0 | 2.0 | 0 | 0 | 230 | 0 |
| (*Pace* Chunky) ........ | 10 | 0 | 3.0 | 0 | 0 | 230 | 1.0 |
| (*Pace* Salsa Verde) ..... | 15 | 0 | 2.0 | .5 | 0 | 230 | 0 |
| (*Rosarita* Mexicana) .... | 10 | 0 | 2.0 | 0 | 0 | 200 | 0 |
| (*Rosarita* Salsa Verde) .. | 10 | 0 | 2.0 | 0 | 0 | 200 | 1.0 |
| (*Rosarita* Taquera) ..... | 10 | 0 | 2.0 | 0 | 0 | 180 | 1.0 |
| (*Tostitos* Restaurant Style) ............. | 15 | <1.0 | 3.0 | 0 | 0 | 210 | <1.0 |
| all varieties: | | | | | | | |
| (*Tostitos* All Natural) .. | 10 | 0 | 2.0 | 0 | 0 | 25 | <.0 |
| (*Wise*) ............. | 10 | 0 | 2.0 | 0 | 0 | 250 | <1.0 |
| black bean (*Mrs. Renfro's*) ........... | 15 | 1.0 | 3.0 | 0 | 0 | 230 | 0 |
| black bean and corn: | | | | | | | |
| (*Amy's* Organic) ..... | 15 | 1.0 | 3.0 | 0 | 0 | 170 | <1.0 |
| (*Chi-Chi's*) ......... | 10 | 0 | 3.0 | 0 | 0 | 150 | 0 |
| (*Muir Glen* Organic) .. | 20 | <1.0 | 4.0 | 0 | 0 | 135 | <1.0 |
| (*Newman's Own*) .... | 20 | 1.0 | 5.0 | 0 | 0 | 140 | 2.0 |
| (*Pace*) | 25 | 1.0 | 5.0 | 0 | 0 | 150 | 1.0 |
| cheese (salsa con queso), see "Cheese dip" | | | | | | | |
| chilis, 5 (*Herdez*) ....... | 15 | 0 | 2.0 | .5 | 0 | 330 | .5 |
| chipotle: | | | | | | | |
| (*Herdez*) ........... | 15 | 0 | 2.0 | 0 | 0 | 350 | 0 |
| (*Muir Glen* Organic) .. | 10 | 0 | 2.0 | 0 | 0 | 140 | 0 |
| corn (*Mrs. Renfro's*) .. | 15 | 0 | 3.0 | 0 | 0 | 230 | 0 |
| garlic (*Margaritaville* Peppadew) ....... | 10 | 0 | 2.0 | 0 | 0 | 100 | 0 |
| spicy (*Amy's* Organic) | 10 | 0 | 2.0 | 0 | 0 | 160 | 0 |
| cilantro, mild or medium (*La Victoria*) ........ | 5 | 0 | 1.0 | 0 | 0 | 200 | 0 |
| fruit (*Neera's* Caribbean), 1 tbsp. .... | 25 | 0 | 7.0 | 0 | 0 | 60 | 0 |

| Food and Measure | cal. | prot. (gms) | carbo. (gms) | fat (gms) | chol. (mgs) | sod. (mgs) | fiber (gms) |
|---|---|---|---|---|---|---|---|
| **Salsa** *(cont.)* | | | | | | | |
| garlic: | | | | | | | |
| (*Emeril's* Gaaahlic | | | | | | | |
| Lovers) .......... | 15 | 0 | 3.0 | 0 | 0 | 200 | 0 |
| (*Mrs. Renfro's*) ...... | 10 | 0 | 2.0 | 0 | 0 | 220 | 0 |
| cilantro (*Muir Glen* | | | | | | | |
| Organic) ......... | 10 | 0 | 2.0 | 0 | 0 | 130 | 0 |
| garlic, roasted: | | | | | | | |
| chunky (*Newman's* | | | | | | | |
| *Own*) ........... | 10 | 1.0 | 2.0 | 0 | 0 | 150 | <1.0 |
| medium (*Ortega*) .... | 10 | 0 | 2.0 | 0 | 0 | 240 | <1.0 |
| ghost pepper (*Mrs.* | | | | | | | |
| *Renfro's*) .......... | 15 | 0 | 3.0 | 0 | 0 | 310 | 0 |
| green chili (*Ortega*) ..... | 10 | 0 | 2.0 | 0 | 0 | 200 | 0 |
| habanero: | | | | | | | |
| (*Mrs. Renfro's*) ...... | 15 | 0 | 3.0 | 0 | 0 | 310 | 0 |
| mango (*Mrs. Renfro's*) | 15 | 0 | 4.0 | 0 | 0 | 170 | 0 |
| hot: | | | | | | | |
| (*Chi-Chi's*) ......... | 10 | 0 | 2.0 | 0 | 0 | 220 | 0 |
| (*Herdez* Casera) ..... | 10 | 0 | 1.0 | 0 | 0 | 270 | 0 |
| (*La Victoria* | | | | | | | |
| Ranchera/Victoria) . | 10 | 0 | 2.0 | 0 | 0 | 200 | 0 |
| (*La Victoria* Thick 'N | | | | | | | |
| Chunky) ......... | 10 | 0 | 2.0 | 0 | 0 | 220 | 0 |
| (*Mrs. Renfro's*) ...... | 15 | 0 | 3.0 | 0 | 0 | 310 | 0 |
| (*Mrs. Renfro's* | | | | | | | |
| Mexican Sauce) ... | 15 | 0 | 2.0 | 0 | 0 | 210 | 0 |
| (*Newman's Own*) .... | 10 | 0 | 2.0 | 0 | 0 | 150 | <1.0 |
| jalapeño: | | | | | | | |
| green (*Mrs. Renfro's*) . | 10 | 0 | 2.0 | 0 | 0 | 390 | 0 |
| green, extra hot (*La* | | | | | | | |
| *Victoria*) ......... | 10 | 0 | 2.0 | 0 | 0 | 260 | 0 |
| red, extra hot (*La* | | | | | | | |
| *Victoria*) ......... | 10 | 0 | 2.0 | 0 | 0 | 170 | 0 |
| mango: | | | | | | | |
| (*Margaritaville*) ...... | 10 | 0 | 3.0 | 0 | 0 | 75 | 0 |
| (*Newman's Own*) .... | 20 | 0 | 5.0 | 0 | 0 | 180 | 0 |
| medium: | | | | | | | |
| (*Herdez*) ........... | 10 | 0 | 1.0 | 0 | 0 | 270 | 0 |
| (*La Victoria* Suprema) | 10 | 0 | 2.0 | 0 | 0 | 150 | 0 |
| (*La Victoria* Thick 'N | | | | | | | |
| Chunky) ......... | 10 | 0 | 2.0 | 0 | 0 | 210 | 0 |
| (*La Victoria* Thick 'N | | | | | | | |
| Chunky Verde) .... | 10 | 0 | 2.0 | 0 | 0 | 220 | 0 |

| Food and Measure | cal. | prot. (gms) | carbo. (gms) | fat (gms) | chol. (mgs) | sod. (mgs) | fiber (gms) |
|---|---|---|---|---|---|---|---|
| (*Margaritaville*) ...... | 10 | 0 | 2.0 | 0 | 0 | 0 | .4 |
| (*Mrs. Renfro's*) ...... | 15 | 0 | 3.0 | 0 | 0 | 280 | 0 |
| (*Newman's Own*) .... | 10 | 0 | 2.0 | 0 | 0 | 105 | <1.0 |
| (*Ortega* Restaurant) .. | 10 | 0 | 2.0 | 0 | 0 | 230 | 0 |
| (*Ortega* Thick & Chunky) ......... | 10 | 0 | 2.0 | 0 | 0 | 180 | <1.0 |
| medium or mild: | | | | | | | |
| (*Amy's* Organic) ..... | 10 | 0 | 2.0 | 0 | 0 | 190 | 0 |
| (*Chi-Chi's*) ......... | 10 | 0 | 2.0 | 0 | 0 | 150 | 0 |
| (*El Torito* Original) ... | 10 | 0 | 2.0 | 0 | 0 | 180 | 0 |
| (*Herdez* Casera) ..... | 10 | 0 | 1.0 | 0 | 0 | 270 | 0 |
| (*Margaritaville* Peppadew) ....... | 10 | 0 | 2.0 | 0 | 0 | 105 | 0 |
| (*Muir Glen* Organic) .. | 10 | 0 | 3.0 | 0 | 0 | 130 | 0 |
| (*Ortega* Garden/ Homestyle) ....... | 10 | <1.0 | 2.0 | 0 | 0 | 220 | <1.0 |
| (*Taco Bell* Thick 'N Chunky) ......... | 15 | 1.0 | 3.0 | 0 | 0 | 210 | 0 |
| mild: | | | | | | | |
| (*La Victoria* Suprema) | 5 | 0 | 2.0 | 0 | 0 | 108 | 0 |
| (*La Victoria* Thick 'N Chunky Verde) .... | 10 | 0 | 2.0 | 0 | 0 | 180 | 0 |
| (*Mrs. Renfro's*) ...... | 10 | 0 | 2.0 | 0 | 0 | 240 | 0 |
| (*Mrs. Renfro's* Mexican Sauce) ... | 10 | 0 | 3.0 | 0 | 0 | 240 | 0 |
| (*Newman's Own*) .... | 10 | 0 | 2.0 | 0 | 0 | 65 | <1.0 |
| (*Ortega* Mexican) .... | 15 | 1.0 | 3.0 | 0 | 0 | 180 | 1.0 |
| (*Ortega* Thick & Chunky) ......... | 10 | <1.0 | 2.0 | 0 | 0 | 210 | <1.0 |
| peach: | | | | | | | |
| (*Mrs. Renfro's*) ...... | 10 | 0 | 3.0 | 0 | 0 | 170 | 0 |
| (*Newman's Own*) .... | 25 | 0 | 6.0 | 0 | 0 | 90 | <1.0 |
| pico de gallo (*Pace*) .... | 10 | 0 | 3.0 | 0 | 0 | 150 | 0 |
| pineapple: | | | | | | | |
| (*Mrs. Renfro's*) ...... | 15 | 0 | 4.0 | 0 | 0 | 105 | 0 |
| (*Newman's Own*) .... | 15 | 0 | 3.0 | 0 | 0 | 90 | <1.0 |
| mango chipotle (*Pace*) | 20 | 0 | 4.0 | 0 | 0 | 130 | 0 |
| pomegranate (*Mrs. Renfro's*) ........... | 20 | 0 | 5.0 | 0 | 0 | 90 | 0 |
| raspberry chipotle (*Mrs. Renfro's*) ...... | 15 | 0 | 4.0 | 0 | 0 | 70 | 0 |
| roasted (*Mrs. Renfro's*) .. | 10 | 0 | 2.0 | 0 | 0 | 220 | 0 |
| Southwest (*Emeril's*) .... | 15 | 0 | 4.0 | 0 | 0 | 105 | 0 |

| Food and Measure | cal. | prot. (gms) | carbo. (gms) | fat (gms) | chol. (mgs) | sod. (mgs) | fiber (gms) |
|---|---|---|---|---|---|---|---|
| **Salsa** *(cont.)* | | | | | | | |
| tequila: | | | | | | | |
| (*Mrs. Renfro's*) . . . . . . | 15 | 0 | 3.0 | 0 | 0 | 140 | 0 |
| lime (*Newman's Own*) | 15 | 0 | 3.0 | 0 | 0 | 170 | 0 |
| **Salsa, chilled**, all styles | | | | | | | |
| (*Emerald Valley* | | | | | | | |
| *Organic*), 2 tbsp. . . . . . | 10 | 0 | 2.0 | 0 | 0 | 140 | 0 |
| **Salsa dip** (see also | | | | | | | |
| "Cheese dip"), | | | | | | | |
| 2 tbsp.: | | | | | | | |
| (*Cabot* Grande) . . . . . . . . | 50 | 1.0 | 1.0 | 5.0 | 15 | 130 | 0 |
| (*Heluva Good!* Fiesta) . . . | 60 | 1.0 | 3.0 | 5.0 | 20 | 230 | 0 |
| **Salsify**: | | | | | | | |
| raw: | | | | | | | |
| (*Frieda's*), 3 oz. . . . . . . | 70 | 3.0 | 16.0 | 0 | 0 | 15 | 3.0 |
| untrimmed, 1 lb. . . . . . | 325 | 13.0 | 73.4 | .8 | 0 | 79 | 13.0 |
| sliced, ½ cup . . . . . . . | 55 | 2.2 | 12.5 | .1 | 0 | 13 | 2.2 |
| boiled, drained, | | | | | | | |
| sliced, ½ cup . . . . . . | 46 | 1.9 | 10.5 | .1 | 0 | 11 | 2.1 |
| **Salsify, canned**, cut | | | | | | | |
| (*Roland*), ½ cup . . . . . | 35 | 1.0 | 7.0 | 0 | 0 | 280 | 3.0 |
| **Salt**, ¼ tsp.: | | | | | | | |
| (*Morton*) . . . . . . . . . . . . | 0 | 0 | 0 | 0 | 0 | 590 | 0 |
| kosher (*Diamond Crystal*) | 0 | 0 | 0 | 0 | 0 | 280 | 0 |
| sea salt: | | | | | | | |
| (*Eden* French) . . . . . . . | 0 | 0 | 0 | 0 | 0 | 392 | 0 |
| (*Eden* Portuguese) . . . | 0 | 0 | 0 | 0 | 0 | 408 | 0 |
| (*McCormick* Grinder) . | 0 | 0 | 0 | 0 | 0 | 400 | 0 |
| all varieties (*Roland*) . . | 0 | 0 | 0 | 0 | 0 | 400 | 0 |
| sesame, see "Sesame | | | | | | | |
| seed condiment" | | | | | | | |
| **Salt, seasoned** (see also | | | | | | | |
| specific listings), ¼ tsp.: | | | | | | | |
| (*Lawry's*) . . . . . . . . . . . . | 0 | 0 | 0 | 0 | 0 | 380 | 0 |
| black pepper (*Lawry's*) . . | 0 | 0 | 0 | 0 | 0 | 170 | 0 |
| **Salt, substitute**, ¼ tsp. . . | 0 | 0 | 0 | 0 | 0 | 0 | 0 |
| **Salt pork**: | | | | | | | |
| (*Farmer John*), 2 oz. . . . . | 250 | 7.0 | 1.0 | 24.0 | 35 | 1560 | 0 |
| raw, 1 oz. . . . . . . . . . . . . | 212 | 1.4 | 0 | 22.8 | 25 | 404 | 0 |
| **Sandwich sauce**, canned, | | | | | | | |
| ¼ cup: | | | | | | | |
| (*Hormel Not-So-Sloppy-Joe*) | 70 | 1.0 | 15.0 | .5 | 0 | 810 | 1.0 |
| sloppy Joe: | | | | | | | |
| (*Del Monte*) . . . . . . . . | 50 | 1.0 | 11.0 | 0 | 0 | 620 | 0 |

| Food and Measure | cal. | prot. (gms) | carbo. (gms) | fat (gms) | chol. (mgs) | sod. (mgs) | fiber (gms) |
|---|---|---|---|---|---|---|---|
| (*Manwich* Bold) ..... | 70 | 1.0 | 15.0 | 0 | 0 | 800 | 2.0 |
| (*Manwich* Original) ... | 40 | <1.0 | 9.0 | 0 | 0 | 410 | 2.0 |
| (*Manwich* Thick & Chunky) ......... | 45 | <1.0 | 10.0 | 0 | 0 | 430 | 2.0 |
| hickory (*Del Monte*) .. | 60 | 1.0 | 14.0 | 0 | 0 | 660 | 0 |
| **Sandwich sauce, chilled** (*Manwich* Heat & Serve), ¼ cup ....... | 70 | 5.0 | 6.0 | 3.0 | 5 | 310 | 2.0 |
| **Sandwich sauce mix** (*Fantastic* Sloppy Joe), 3 tbsp. ........ | 80 | 9.0 | 12.0 | 0 | 0 | 530 | 1.0 |
| **Sandwich sauce seasoning**, see "Sloppy Joe seasoning" | | | | | | | |
| **Sandwich spread** (see also "Meat spread," and specific listings), mayonnaise style: | | | | | | | |
| (*Cains*), 1 tbsp. ........ | 70 | 0 | 2.0 | 7.0 | 5 | 130 | 0 |
| (*Blue Plate*), 1 tbsp. .... | 75 | 0 | 3.0 | 7.0 | 5 | 105 | 0 |
| (*Hellmann's/Best Foods*), 1 tbsp. ....... | 60 | 0 | 2.0 | 5.0 | <5 | 200 | 0 |
| **Sandwiches**, see "Panini," "Wraps, filled," and specific listings | | | | | | | |
| **Sangria drink mixer**, red (*Stirrings*), 3 fl. oz. ............. | 60 | 0 | 15.0 | 0 | 0 | 0 | 0 |
| **Sapodilla:** | | | | | | | |
| (*Frieda's*), 3-oz. fruit .... | 70 | 0 | 17.0 | 1.0 | 0 | 10 | 5.0 |
| 1 medium, 3" x 2½" ..... | 140 | .7 | 33.9 | 1.9 | 0 | 20 | 9.0 |
| ½ cup ............... | 100 | .5 | 24.1 | 1.3 | 0 | 15 | 6.4 |
| **Sapote:** | | | | | | | |
| (*Frieda's* White), 5 oz. ... | 190 | 3.0 | 47.0 | 1.0 | 0 | 15 | 4.0 |
| 11.2-oz. fruit, 7.9 oz. trimmed ............. | 301 | 4.8 | 76.0 | 1.4 | 0 | 23 | 5.9 |
| trimmed, 1 oz. ......... | 38 | .6 | 9.6 | .2 | 0 | 3 | .7 |
| **Sardine**, fresh, see "Herring" | | | | | | | |
| **Sardine, canned** (see also "Herring, canned"), 3.75-oz. can drained, except as noted: | | | | | | | |

| Food and Measure | cal. | prot. (gms) | carbo. (gms) | fat (gms) | chol. (mgs) | sod. (mgs) | fiber (gms) |
|---|---|---|---|---|---|---|---|
| **Sardine, canned** (cont.) | | | | | | | |
| Atlantic, in oil: | | | | | | | |
| drained, 2 oz. ........ | 118 | 14.8 | 0 | 6.5 | 81 | 286 | 0 |
| 2 medium, 3" long ... | 50 | 5.9 | 0 | 2.8 | 34 | 121 | 0 |
| in balsamic vinaigrette | | | | | | | |
| (*King Oscar* Brisling) . | 150 | 14.0 | 0 | 11.0 | 120 | 340 | 0 |
| in chipotle sauce (*King* | | | | | | | |
| *Oscar* Brisling) ...... | 167 | 12.0 | 2.0 | 12.0 | 40 | 340 | 0 |
| in hot sauce: | | | | | | | |
| (*Bumble Bee*) ....... | 150 | 18.0 | 2.0 | 8.0 | 110 | 420 | 0 |
| (*Chicken of the Sea*) .. | 130 | 17.0 | 2.0 | 6.0 | 60 | 490 | 2.0 |
| (*Crown Prince* Louisiana), | | | | | | | |
| 4.25-oz. can ...... | 230 | 24.0 | 0 | 15.0 | 65 | 190 | <1.0 |
| in lemon and oil (*Vigo*), | | | | | | | |
| 2 pcs. ............. | 125 | 11.0 | 0 | 8.0 | 20 | 250 | 0 |
| Mediterranean style | | | | | | | |
| (*King Oscar* Brisling) . | 150 | 13.0 | 0 | 10.0 | 110 | 320 | 0 |
| in mustard sauce: | | | | | | | |
| (*Bumble Bee*) ....... | 140 | 17.0 | 2.0 | 10.0 | 100 | 460 | 0 |
| (*Chicken of the Sea*) .. | 150 | 17.0 | 2.0 | 8.0 | 60 | 490 | 2.0 |
| (*Crown Prince*), | | | | | | | |
| 4.25-oz, can ...... | 190 | 21.0 | 5.0 | 9.0 | 55 | 730 | 0 |
| (*Crown Prince* | | | | | | | |
| Brisling) ......... | 210 | 14.0 | <1.0 | 16.0 | 45 | 710 | <1.0 |
| Dijon (*King Oscar* | | | | | | | |
| Brisling) ......... | 160 | 14.0 | 0 | 11.0 | 125 | 710 | 0 |
| dill (*Brunswick*) ..... | 150 | 16.0 | 3.0 | 8.0 | 100 | 580 | 0 |
| in olive oil, drained: | | | | | | | |
| (*Brunswick*) ....... | 190 | 20.0 | 0 | 13.0 | 110 | 250 | 0 |
| (*Crown Prince* | | | | | | | |
| Brisling) ......... | 210 | 16.0 | 1.0 | 15.0 | 65 | 500 | <1.0 |
| (*King Oscar* Brisling) . | 150 | 14.0 | 0 | 11.0 | 120 | 340 | 0 |
| (*Roland*), 2 pcs., 2 oz. | 100 | 13.0 | 0 | 5.0 | 35 | 260 | 0 |
| skin/boneless (*Crown* | | | | | | | |
| *Prince*) .......... | 220 | 26.0 | 0 | 12.0 | 15 | 280 | 0 |
| skin/boneless | | | | | | | |
| (*Granadaisa*) ..... | 206 | 23.5 | 0 | 12.5 | 40 | 400 | 0 |
| in oil, drained: | | | | | | | |
| (*Bumble Bee*) ....... | 190 | 20.0 | 0 | 13.0 | 110 | 230 | 0 |
| (*Crown Prince*), | | | | | | | |
| 4.25-oz. can ...... | 210 | 23.0 | 0 | 13.0 | 35 | 210 | 0 |
| (*Crown Prince* | | | | | | | |
| Brisling) ......... | 210 | 15.0 | 0 | 17.0 | 50 | 320 | 0 |

| Food and Measure | cal. | prot. (gms) | carbo. (gms) | fat (gms) | chol. (mgs) | sod. (mgs) | fiber (gms) |
|---|---|---|---|---|---|---|---|
| (*Crown Prince* Brisling No Salt) ... | 230 | 17.0 | 0 | 18.0 | 45 | 125 | 0 |
| (*King Oscar* Brisling Low Sodium) ..... | 140 | 13.0 | 0 | 10.0 | 110 | 200 | 0 |
| (*King Oscar* Brisling Spirit of Norway) .. | 150 | 14.0 | 0 | 11.0 | 120 | 340 | 0 |
| (*Vigo*), 2 pcs. ....... | 130 | 11.0 | 0 | 9.0 | 20 | 250 | 0 |
| w/green chilies (*Crown Prince* 4.25 oz.), 3.3 oz. ... | 200 | 22.0 | 0 | 12.0 | 55 | 170 | <1.0 |
| w/chili peppers (*Roland*), 2 oz. .... | 110 | 13.0 | 0 | 6.0 | 40 | 370 | 0 |
| hot, spiced (*Vigo*), 2 pcs. ........... | 130 | 11.0 | 0 | 9.0 | 20 | 250 | 0 |
| w/hot tabasco pepper (*Brunswick*) ...... | 190 | 20.0 | 0 | 12.0 | 110 | 280 | 0 |
| lightly smoked (*Roland*), 3 pcs. ... | 110 | 13.0 | 0 | 6.0 | 41 | 370 | 0 |
| skin/boneless (*Crown Prince*) .......... | 220 | 24.0 | 0 | 14.0 | 35 | 360 | 0 |
| skin/boneless (*Roland*), 3 pcs. ... | 120 | 13.0 | 0 | 7.0 | 20 | 350 | 0 |
| skin/boneless (*Vigo*), 3 pcs. ........... | 130 | 14.0 | 1.0 | 8.0 | 20 | 250 | 0 |
| smoked (*Chicken of the Sea*) ........ | 190 | 12.0 | 2.0 | 14.0 | 45 | 430 | 0 |
| spiced (*Roland*) ..... | 120 | 14.0 | 0 | 8.0 | 10 | 110 | 0 |
| in tomato sauce: | | | | | | | |
| (*Chicken of the Sea*) .. | 130 | 17.0 | 2.0 | 6.0 | 60 | 490 | 2.0 |
| (*Chicken of the Sea* 15 oz.), 2 oz. ..... | 90 | 10.0 | 1.0 | 5.0 | 35 | 260 | 1.0 |
| (*Consul*), 2 oz. ....... | 80 | 10.0 | 1.0 | 4.0 | 36 | 170 | 1.0 |
| (*Crown Prince*), 4.25-oz. can ...... | 180 | 21.0 | 6.0 | 8.0 | 55 | 320 | 1.0 |
| (*Crown Prince* Brisling) .......... | 210 | 16.0 | 0 | 16.0 | 50 | 600 | <1.0 |
| (*Crown Prince* Oval Morocco), 2 oz. ... | 90 | 8.0 | 2.0 | 5.0 | 40 | 240 | 1.0 |
| (*Crown Prince* Oval Thailand), 2 oz. ... | 60 | 8.0 | 1.0 | 2.0 | 35 | 300 | <1.0 |
| (*King Oscar* Brisling) . | 170 | 14.0 | 0 | 12.0 | 110 | 420 | 0 |
| (*Roland*), ¼ cup ..... | 90 | 10.0 | 1.0 | 5.0 | 40 | 220 | 0 |
| (*Vigo*), ½ of 4⅜-oz. can ............. | 100 | 9.0 | 0 | 7.0 | 20 | 250 | 0 |

| Food and Measure | cal. | prot. (gms) | carbo. (gms) | fat (gms) | chol. (mgs) | sod. (mgs) | fiber (gms) |
|---|---|---|---|---|---|---|---|
| **Sardine, canned, in tomato sauce** *(cont.)* | | | | | | | |
| basil (*Brunswick*) . . . . | 150 | 16.0 | 3.0 | 8.0 | 100 | 530 | 0 |
| w/chili (*Roland*), | | | | | | | |
| ¼ cup . . . . . . . . . . | 50 | 9.0 | 1.0 | 1.0 | 45 | 280 | 0 |
| Pacific, 2 oz. . . . . . . . | 101 | 9.3 | n.a. | 6.8 | 35 | 235 | <1.0 |
| in water, drained: | | | | | | | |
| (*Bumble Bee*) . . . . . . . | 140 | 19.0 | 0 | 7.5 | 100 | 270 | 0 |
| (*Brunswick* No Salt) . . | 140 | 19.0 | 0 | 7.0 | 100 | 200 | 0 |
| (*Chicken of the Sea*) . . | 100 | 13.0 | 2.0 | 4.0 | 45 | 430 | 0 |
| (*King Oscar* Brisling | | | | | | | |
| Low Sodium) . . . . . | 140 | 13.0 | 0 | 10.0 | 110 | 200 | 0 |
| (*Roland* Low Sodium), | | | | | | | |
| ¼ cup, 2 oz. . . . . . . | 70 | 12.0 | 0 | 2.0 | 70 | 45 | 0 |
| skin/boneless | | | | | | | |
| (*Roland* Low | | | | | | | |
| Sodium), ¼ cup . . . | 90 | 12.0 | 0 | 5.0 | 25 | 35 | 0 |
| **Sardine oil**, see "Oil" | | | | | | | |
| **Satsuma**, see "Tangerine" | | | | | | | |
| **Sauce**, see "Finishing | | | | | | | |
| sauce" and specific | | | | | | | |
| sauce listings | | | | | | | |
| **Sauerkraut**, 2 tbsp., | | | | | | | |
| except as noted: | | | | | | | |
| (*Boar's Head*) . . . . . . . . . | 5 | 0 | 1.0 | 0 | 0 | 180 | <1.0 |
| (*Del Monte*) . . . . . . . . . . . | 0 | 0 | <1.0 | 0 | 0 | 180 | <1.0 |
| (*Del Monte* Bavarian) . . . | 15 | 0 | 4.0 | 0 | 0 | 180 | 0 |
| (*Eden* Organic), ½ cup . . | 25 | 2.0 | 4.0 | 0 | 0 | 580 | 3.0 |
| (*S&W*) . . . . . . . . . . . . . . . | 0 | 0 | 1.0 | 0 | 0 | 180 | <1.0 |
| **Sausage** (see also | | | | | | | |
| specific sausage | | | | | | | |
| listings), cooked, | | | | | | | |
| except as noted: | | | | | | | |
| beef, smoked: | | | | | | | |
| (*Hillshire Farm/ | | | | | | | |
| Hillshire Farm Hot | | | | | | | |
| Links*), 2.3-oz. link . | 200 | 8.0 | 3.0 | 16.0 | 40 | 760 | 1.0 |
| (*Hillshire Farm Lit'l | | | | | | | |
| Smokies*), 5 links . . | 160 | 7.0 | 2.0 | 14.0 | 40 | 550 | 0 |
| hot (*Johnsonville | | | | | | | |
| Bold*), 2.3-oz. link . . | 210 | 8.0 | 3.0 | 18.0 | 40 | 700 | 0 |
| beef patty (*Banquet | | | | | | | |
| Brown 'n Serve*), | | | | | | | |
| 2 pcs., 1.6 oz. . . . . . . | 160 | 6.0 | 1.0 | 14.0 | 15 | 350 | 0 |

| Food and Measure | cal. | prot. (gms) | carbo. (gms) | fat (gms) | chol. (mgs) | sod. (mgs) | fiber (gms) |
|---|---|---|---|---|---|---|---|
| chicken, 1 link, 3 oz., except as noted: | | | | | | | |
| apple (*Applegate Farms* Organic) ... | 140 | 14.0 | 6.0 | 6.0 | 65 | 500 | 1.0 |
| apple (*Aidells/Aidells* Organic) ........ | 180 | 14.0 | 3.0 | 13.0 | 80 | 690 | <1.0 |
| apple (*Al Fresco*) .... | 160 | 14.0 | 10.0 | 7.0 | 60 | 480 | 0 |
| apple, minis (*Aidells*), 5 links, 2 oz. ...... | 110 | 9.0 | 2.0 | 7.0 | 60 | 500 | 0 |
| Andouille (*Aidells* Organic) ........ | 160 | 13.0 | 2.0 | 10.0 | 90 | 700 | 0 |
| artichoke garlic (*Aidells*) ........ | 170 | 15.0 | 1.0 | 12.0 | 50 | 620 | <1.0 |
| Buffalo style (*Al Fresco*) .......... | 130 | 13.0 | 4.0 | 6.0 | 60 | 620 | 0 |
| chipotle chorizo (*Al Fresco*) .......... | 140 | 15.0 | 5.0 | 7.0 | 65 | 550 | 0 |
| garlic, roasted (*Al Fresco*) .......... | 140 | 15.0 | 3.0 | 7.0 | 70 | 480 | 0 |
| garlic, roasted, basil (*Aidells* Organic) .. | 160 | 13.0 | 3.0 | 11.0 | 65 | 700 | <1.0 |
| habanero green chile (*Aidells*) ........ | 180 | 14.0 | 3.0 | 13.0 | 80 | 690 | <1.0 |
| hardwood smoked (*Hillshire Farm*), 2 oz. ............. | 90 | 8.0 | 3.0 | 5.0 | 35 | 440 | <1.0 |
| Italian, w/mozzarella (*Aidells*) ........ | 170 | 14.0 | 2.0 | 12.0 | 70 | 670 | <1.0 |
| Italian, sweet (*Al Fresco*) .......... | 130 | 15.0 | 1.0 | 7.0 | 65 | 480 | 0 |
| jalapeño, spicy (*Al Fresco*) .......... | 130 | 15.0 | 2.0 | 7.0 | 65 | 480 | 0 |
| mango (*Aidells*) ..... | 170 | 13.0 | 4.0 | 11.0 | 95 | 670 | <1.0 |
| pineapple, mini (*Aidells* Hawaiian), 5 pcs., 2 oz. ...... | 120 | 7.0 | 6.0 | 8.0 | 50 | 420 | <1.0 |
| pineapple bacon (*Aidells*) ......... | 210 | 12.0 | 8.0 | 14.0 | 80 | 690 | <1.0 |
| roasted pepper asiago (*Al Fresco*) ......... | 140 | 15.0 | 1.0 | 8.0 | 70 | 550 | 0 |
| spinach feta (*Aidells* Organic) ......... | 140 | 13.0 | 2.0 | 9.0 | 90 | 600 | <1.0 |
| spinach feta (*Al Fresco*) .......... | 130 | 15.0 | 1.0 | 7.0 | 65 | 540 | 0 |

| Food and Measure | cal. | prot. (gms) | carbo. (gms) | fat (gms) | chol. (mgs) | sod. (mgs) | fiber (gms) |
|---|---|---|---|---|---|---|---|
| **Sausage, chicken** *(cont.)* | | | | | | | |
| sun-dried tomato | | | | | | | |
| (*Aidells* Organic) .. | 150 | 13.0 | 3.0 | 9.0 | 85 | 770 | <1.0 |
| sun-dried tomato | | | | | | | |
| basil (*Al Fresco*) ... | 140 | 15.0 | 2.0 | 7.0 | 70 | 480 | 0 |
| chicken, breakfast: | | | | | | | |
| apple (*Aidells*), 2 oz. .. | 140 | 8.0 | 2.0 | 8.0 | 50 | 440 | 0 |
| apple (*Aidells* | | | | | | | |
| Organic), 2 oz. .... | 120 | 9.0 | 2.0 | 8.0 | 50 | 440 | 0 |
| apple (*Applegate* | | | | | | | |
| Farms), 2 links, | | | | | | | |
| 1.6 oz. .......... | 100 | 7.0 | 2.0 | 7.0 | 35 | 260 | 0 |
| apple maple (*Al* | | | | | | | |
| *Fresco*), 1.2-oz. link | 60 | 6.0 | 4.0 | 2.5 | 25 | 160 | 0 |
| blueberry (*Al Fresco*), | | | | | | | |
| 1.2-oz. link ....... | 70 | 6.0 | 5.0 | 3.0 | 25 | 160 | 0 |
| country (*Al Fresco*), | | | | | | | |
| 1.2-oz. link ....... | 50 | 6.0 | 0 | 3.0 | 30 | 170 | 0 |
| maple (*Applegate* | | | | | | | |
| Farms), 2 links, | | | | | | | |
| 1.6 oz. .......... | 100 | 7.0 | 2.0 | 7.0 | 40 | 270 | 0 |
| sage (*Applegate Farms*), | | | | | | | |
| 2 links, 1.6 oz. .... | 100 | 7.0 | 2.0 | 7.0 | 35 | 270 | 0 |
| chicken, raw (*Al Fresco*), | | | | | | | |
| 1 link: | | | | | | | |
| apple, sweet, 3 oz. ... | 160 | 14.0 | 10.0 | 7.0 | 60 | 480 | 0 |
| Buffalo style, 3 oz. ... | 130 | 13.0 | 4.0 | 6.0 | 60 | 620 | 0 |
| Italian, sweet, 3 oz. ... | 130 | 15.0 | 1.0 | 7.0 | 65 | 480 | 0 |
| mango chipotle, 3.2 oz. | 170 | 21.0 | 8.0 | 6.0 | 50 | 670 | 0 |
| chicken/turkey, see | | | | | | | |
| "turkey/chicken," | | | | | | | |
| below | | | | | | | |
| crumbles (*Jimmy Dean* | | | | | | | |
| Cooked), ⅔ cup: | | | | | | | |
| original ............ | 210 | 14.0 | 2.0 | 19.0 | 35 | 620 | 0 |
| hot, hearty ........ | 200 | 8.0 | 1.0 | 18.0 | 45 | 610 | 0 |
| turkey, hearty ....... | 90 | 11.0 | 2.0 | 4.0 | 20 | 500 | 0 |
| pork: | | | | | | | |
| link, raw, 1 oz. ...... | 118 | 3.3 | .3 | 11.4 | 19 | 189 | 0 |
| link, cooked, .5 oz. ... | 105 | 6.6 | .6 | 22.8 | 39 | 378 | 0 |
| patty, raw, 2-oz. pc. ... | 286 | 6.6 | .6 | 22.8 | 39 | 378 | 0 |
| pork, chub/roll, 2 oz.: | | | | | | | |
| (*Bob Evans* Naturally) . | 190 | 12.0 | 0 | 16.0 | 30 | 420 | 0 |
| (*Bob Evans* Original) .. | 180 | 11.0 | 0 | 15.0 | 30 | 460 | 0 |

| Food and Measure | cal. | prot. (gms) | carbo. (gms) | fat (gms) | chol. (mgs) | sod. (mgs) | fiber (gms) |
|---|---|---|---|---|---|---|---|
| (*Jimmy Dean*) . . . . . . . | 180 | 8.0 | 1.0 | 16.0 | 40 | 450 | 0 |
| (*Jimmy Dean* All | | | | | | | |
|    Natural) . . . . . . . . . | 190 | 12.0 | 1.0 | 15.0 | 55 | 520 | 0 |
| (*Jimmy Dean* Light) . . | 140 | 9.0 | 1.0 | 11.0 | 35 | 350 | 0 |
| all varieties | | | | | | | |
|    (*Johnsonville*) . . . . | 180 | 11.0 | 0 | 15.0 | 35 | 420 | 0 |
| hot (*Bob Evans* Zesty) | 180 | 11.0 | 0 | 15.0 | 30 | 510 | 0 |
| hot (*Jimmy Dean*) . . . . | 180 | 8.0 | 1.0 | 16.0 | 40 | 490 | 0 |
| Italian (*Bob Evans*) . . | 180 | 11.0 | 0 | 15.0 | 30 | 600 | 0 |
| Italian (*Jimmy Dean*) . | 190 | 8.0 | 1.0 | 17.0 | 40 | 320 | 0 |
| maple (*Jimmy Dean*) . | 180 | 8.0 | 1.0 | 16.0 | 40 | 450 | 0 |
| mild (*Jimmy Dean* | | | | | | | |
|    Country) . . . . . . . . . | 200 | 9.0 | 1.0 | 21.0 | 35 | 380 | 0 |
| sage (*Bob Evans*) . . . . | 180 | 11.0 | 0 | 15.0 | 30 | 570 | 0 |
| sage (*Jimmy Dean*) . . | 180 | 8.0 | 1.0 | 16.0 | 40 | 420 | 0 |
| pork, breakfast links, | | | | | | | |
| 3 links, except as | | | | | | | |
| noted: | | | | | | | |
| (*Banquet Brown 'N* | | | | | | | |
|    *Serve* Country) . . . . | 200 | 7.0 | 3.0 | 18.0 | 30 | 510 | 1.0 |
| (*Banquet Brown 'N* | | | | | | | |
|    *Serve* Original) . . . . | 200 | 8.0 | 2.0 | 18.0 | 30 | 490 | 1.0 |
| (*Bob Evans* Fully | | | | | | | |
|    Cooked), 2 links . . . | 130 | 8.0 | 0 | 10.0 | 25 | 290 | 0 |
| (*Bob Evans* Original) . . | 140 | 9.0 | 0 | 11.0 | 25 | 330 | 0 |
| (*Jimmy Dean* Heat | | | | | | | |
|    'n Serve Bag) . . . . . | 210 | 9.0 | 1.0 | 19.0 | 65 | 580 | 0 |
| (*Jimmy Dean* Original) | 170 | 7.0 | 1.0 | 14.0 | 35 | 350 | 0 |
| (*Jimmy Dean* Original | | | | | | | |
|    Fully Cooked) . . . . . | 240 | 9.0 | 1.0 | 22.0 | 45 | 450 | 0 |
| (*Johnsonville*) . . . . . . . | 180 | 11.0 | 2.0 | 14.0 | 35 | 610 | 0 |
| (*Little Sizzlers*) . . . . . . | 200 | 8.0 | 0 | 19.0 | 40 | 580 | 0 |
| (*Little Sizzlers* Heat | | | | | | | |
|    & Serve) . . . . . . . . . | 200 | 8.0 | 0 | 19.0 | 40 | 620 | 0 |
| (*Organic Prairie* | | | | | | | |
|    Brown & Serve), | | | | | | | |
|    2 links . . . . . . . . . . | 150 | 9.0 | 0 | 13.0 | 40 | 500 | 0 |
| brown sugar honey | | | | | | | |
|    (*Johnsonville*) . . . . | 170 | 8.0 | 4.0 | 13.0 | 35 | 480 | 0 |
| cheddar (*Johnsonville*) | 170 | 8.0 | 2.0 | 14.0 | 35 | 510 | 0 |
| hot (*Jimmy Dean* | | | | | | | |
|    Heat 'n Serve) . . . . | 210 | 9.0 | 2.0 | 19.0 | 65 | 580 | 0 |
| maple (*Banquet Brown* | | | | | | | |
|    *'N Serve*) . . . . . . . . | 210 | 8.0 | 2.0 | 19.0 | 25 | 520 | 0 |

| Food and Measure | cal. | prot. (gms) | carbo. (gms) | fat (gms) | chol. (mgs) | sod. (mgs) | fiber (gms) |
|---|---|---|---|---|---|---|---|
| **Sausage, pork, breakfast links** *(cont.)* | | | | | | | |
| maple (*Bob Evans* Fully | | | | | | | |
| Cooked), 2 links ... | 130 | 7.0 | 2.0 | 11.0 | 25 | 270 | 0 |
| maple (*Jimmy Dean* | | | | | | | |
| Fully Cooked) ..... | 170 | 7.0 | 2.0 | 14.0 | 35 | 400 | 0 |
| maple (*Jimmy Dean* | | | | | | | |
| Heat 'n Serve) .... | 220 | 9.0 | 4.0 | 18.0 | 60 | 560 | 0 |
| maple (*Little Sizzlers*) . | 210 | 8.0 | 2.0 | 19.0 | 40 | 580 | 0 |
| pork, breakfast patties, | | | | | | | |
| 2 pcs., except as | | | | | | | |
| noted: | | | | | | | |
| (*Banquet Brown 'N* | | | | | | | |
| *Serve* Original) .... | 170 | 6.0 | 2.0 | 15.0 | 25 | 410 | <1.0 |
| (*Bob Evans* Fully | | | | | | | |
| Cooked) ......... | 160 | 9.0 | 0 | 12.0 | 30 | 360 | 0 |
| (*Bob Evans* Original) .. | 160 | 11.0 | 0 | 13.0 | 30 | 380 | 0 |
| (*Bob Evans* | | | | | | | |
| Sandwich Size), 1 pc. | 140 | 10.0 | 0 | 11.0 | 25 | 340 | 0 |
| (*Jimmy Dean* Fully | | | | | | | |
| Cooked/Original) .. | 240 | 9.0 | 1.0 | 23.0 | 50 | 610 | 0 |
| (*Jimmy Dean* Heat 'N | | | | | | | |
| Serve) .......... | 200 | 8.0 | 1.0 | 17.0 | 60 | 560 | 0 |
| (*Jimmy Dean* | | | | | | | |
| Sandwich Size Fully | | | | | | | |
| Cooked), 1 pc. .... | 160 | 6.0 | 0 | 15.0 | 30 | 400 | 0 |
| (*Johnsonville* 9 oz.) .. | 210 | 12.0 | 2.0 | 17.0 | 45 | 510 | 0 |
| (*Johnsonville* 12 oz.) . | 180 | 10.0 | 1.0 | 15.0 | 40 | 450 | 0 |
| (*Little Sizzlers*) ...... | 200 | 8.0 | 0 | 19.0 | 40 | 580 | 0 |
| hot (*Jimmy Dean* | | | | | | | |
| Fully Cooked) ..... | 250 | 9.0 | 1.0 | 23.0 | 50 | 540 | 0 |
| maple (*Bob Evans*) ... | 180 | 10.0 | 3.0 | 14.0 | 30 | 360 | 0 |
| maple (*Jimmy Dean*) . | 170 | 7.0 | 2.0 | 14.0 | 35 | 410 | 0 |
| maple (*Jimmy Dean* | | | | | | | |
| Fully Cooked) ..... | 250 | 8.0 | 3.0 | 22.0 | 45 | 510 | 0 |
| maple (*Johnsonville* | | | | | | | |
| Vermont 9 oz.) .... | 210 | 12.0 | 2.0 | 17.0 | 45 | 580 | 0 |
| maple (*Johnsonville* | | | | | | | |
| Vermont 12 oz.) ... | 190 | 10.0 | 3.0 | 15.0 | 40 | 510 | 0 |
| pork, Italian, 1 link: | | | | | | | |
| cheese, 4 | | | | | | | |
| (*Johnsonville*), 3 oz. | 270 | 13.0 | 3.0 | 23.0 | 55 | 630 | 0 |
| hot, mild, or sweet | | | | | | | |
| (*Johnsonville*), 3 oz. | 270 | 15.0 | 3.0 | 22.0 | 60 | 710 | 0 |

| Food and Measure | cal. | prot. (gms) | carbo. (gms) | fat (gms) | chol. (mgs) | sod. (mgs) | fiber (gms) |
|---|---|---|---|---|---|---|---|
| hot and spicy, smoked (*Hillshire Farm*), 2.7 oz. .......... | 250 | 8.0 | 4.0 | 22.0 | 50 | 670 | 1.0 |
| hot or sweet (*Thumann's*), 3.2 oz. | 290 | 19.0 | 0 | 25.0 | 65 | 750 | 0 |
| smoked (*Hillshire Farm*), 2 oz. ...... | 190 | 7.0 | 4.0 | 16.0 | 35 | 410 | <1.0 |
| pork, Italian, ground: hot (*Johnsonville*), 2 oz. ............ | 170 | 10.0 | 1.0 | 13.0 | 40 | 400 | 0 |
| mild or sweet (*Johnsonville*), 2 oz. | 170 | 10.0 | 1.0 | 13.0 | 40 | 480 | 0 |
| pork, smoked, 1 link, except as noted: (*Boar's Head* Natural Casing), 4 oz. ..... | 310 | 15.0 | 2.0 | 27.0 | 65 | 920 | 0 |
| Andouille (*Aidells* Cajun), 3 oz. ...... | 170 | 15.0 | 1.0 | 12.0 | 50 | 620 | <1.0 |
| Andouille (*Applegate Farms* Organic), 3 oz. ............ | 200 | 12.0 | 2.0 | 15.0 | 50 | 510 | 1.0 |
| Andouille (*Johnsonville* New Orleans), 2.7 oz. ... | 230 | 9.0 | 2.0 | 20.0 | 40 | 630 | 0 |
| hot (*Boar's Head*), 3.2 oz. .......... | 250 | 12.0 | 1.0 | 22.0 | 55 | 740 | 0 |
| pork, smoked, cheddar/ cheese, 1 link: (*Black Bear* Cheddar-wurst), 3.2 oz. .... | 270 | 12.0 | 4.0 | 23.0 | 40 | 750 | 0 |
| (*Hillshire Farm CheddarWurst*), 2.3 oz. .......... | 220 | 9.0 | 4.0 | 19.0 | 45 | 700 | <1.0 |
| (*Johnsonville* Bedder w/Cheddar), 2.3 oz. | 210 | 8.0 | 3.0 | 18.0 | 40 | 630 | 0 |
| pork/beef, raw, .5-oz. link .......... | 112 | 3.9 | .8 | 10.3 | 20 | 228 | 0 |
| smoked (see also specific sausage): (*Hillshire Farm*), 2 oz. . | 190 | 7.0 | 3.0 | 16.0 | 35 | 480 | <1.0 |
| (*Hillshire Farm* Lite), 2 oz. ....... | 110 | 9.0 | 0 | 8.0 | 30 | 490 | <1.0 |
| (*Hillshire Farm Lit'l Smokies*), 5 links .. | 160 | 7.0 | 2.0 | 14.0 | 40 | 550 | 0 |

| Food and Measure | cal. | prot. (gms) | carbo. (gms) | fat (gms) | chol. (mgs) | sod. (mgs) | fiber (gms) |
|---|---|---|---|---|---|---|---|
| **Sausage, smoked** *(cont.)* | | | | | | | |
| (*Hillshire Farm Hot* | | | | | | | |
| Links), 2.7-oz. link . | 250 | 8.0 | 4.0 | 22.0 | 50 | 670 | 1.0 |
| chili cheese | | | | | | | |
| (*Johnsonville* Bold), | | | | | | | |
| 2.3-oz. link . . . . . . . | 210 | 8.0 | 3.0 | 18.0 | 40 | 490 | 0 |
| hot (*Hillshire Farm*), | | | | | | | |
| 2 oz. . . . . . . . . . . . . | 190 | 6.0 | 3.0 | 17.0 | 35 | 450 | <1.0 |
| Italian (*Hillshire* | | | | | | | |
| Farm), 2 oz. . . . . . . | 190 | 7.0 | 4.0 | 16.0 | 35 | 410 | <1.0 |
| jalapeño cheese | | | | | | | |
| (*Johnsonville* Bold), | | | | | | | |
| 2.3 oz. . . . . . . . . . . | 210 | 8.0 | 1.0 | 18.0 | 40 | 490 | 0 |
| turkey, breakfast: | | | | | | | |
| (*Banquet Brown 'N* | | | | | | | |
| *Serve*), 3 links . . . . | 110 | 9.0 | 2.0 | 7.0 | 40 | 390 | 0 |
| (*Banquet Brown 'N* | | | | | | | |
| *Serve*), 2 patties . . . | 90 | 8.0 | 2.0 | 6.0 | 35 | 320 | 0 |
| (*Bob Evans*), 2 patties | 90 | 11.0 | 0 | 4.5 | 40 | 420 | 0 |
| (*Jennie-O* Links), 2 oz. | 140 | 9.0 | 0 | 11.0 | 45 | 360 | 0 |
| (*Jennie-O* Patties), | | | | | | | |
| 2.25 oz. . . . . . . . . . | 160 | 10.0 | 0 | 12.0 | 50 | 410 | 0 |
| (*Jennie-O* Roll), 4 oz. . | 270 | 16.0 | 0 | 21.0 | 80 | 720 | 0 |
| (*Jennie-O Breakfast* | | | | | | | |
| *Lover's* Links), 2 oz. | 130 | 8.0 | 0 | 10.0 | 45 | 310 | 0 |
| (*Jimmy Dean* Fully | | | | | | | |
| Cooked), 3 links | | | | | | | |
| or 2 patties . . . . . . . | 120 | 13.0 | 1.0 | 7.0 | 55 | 490 | 0 |
| (*Shady Brook Farms*), | | | | | | | |
| 2 links . . . . . . . . . . | 120 | 13.0 | 1.0 | 7.0 | 45 | 470 | 0 |
| roll (*Shady Brook* | | | | | | | |
| Farms), ⅙ pkg. . . . . | 100 | 12.0 | 1.0 | 5.0 | 40 | 320 | 0 |
| turkey, breakfast, raw: | | | | | | | |
| (*Jennie-O* Links), | | | | | | | |
| 2 oz. . . . . . . . . . . . . | 140 | 9.0 | 0 | 11.0 | 45 | 360 | 0 |
| (*Jennie-O* Patties), | | | | | | | |
| 2.25 oz. . . . . . . . . . | 160 | 10.0 | 0 | 12.0 | 50 | 410 | 0 |
| (*Jennie-O Breakfast* | | | | | | | |
| *Lover's* links), 2 oz. | 130 | 8.0 | 0 | 10.0 | 45 | 310 | 0 |
| (*Perdue* Tube), 2 oz. . . | 80 | 9.0 | 0 | 5.0 | 30 | 350 | 0 |
| (*Shady Brook Farms*). | | | | | | | |
| 2 links, 2.6 oz. . . . . | 130 | 13.0 | 2.0 | 7.0 | 45 | 480 | 0 |
| Italian, sweet | | | | | | | |
| (*Perdue* Tube), 2 oz. | 90 | 9.0 | 2.0 | 5.0 | 40 | 270 | 0 |

| Food and Measure | cal. | prot. (gms) | carbo. (gms) | fat (gms) | chol. (mgs) | sod. (mgs) | fiber (gms) |
|---|---|---|---|---|---|---|---|
| roll (*Jennie-O*), 4 oz. . . | 270 | 16.0 | 0 | 21.0 | 80 | 720 | 0 |
| roll (*Shady Brook Farms*), ⅙ pkg. . . . . | 100 | 13.0 | 1.0 | 4.5 | 40 | 350 | 0 |
| turkey, Italian, raw, 1 link: | | | | | | | |
| hot (*Shady Brook Farms*), 3.3 oz. . . . . | 160 | 16.0 | 2.0 | 9.0 | 55 | 620 | 0 |
| hot, lean (*Jennie-O*), 3.8 oz. . | 160 | 17.0 | 0 | 10.0 | 70 | 890 | 0 |
| sweet, lean (*Jennie-O*), 3.8 oz. . | 160 | 17.0 | 0 | 10.0 | 65 | 650 | 0 |
| turkey, Italian, roll (*Shady Brook Farms*), 2.5 oz., cooked . . . . . . | 100 | 12.0 | 1.0 | 5.0 | 40 | 420 | 0 |
| turkey, smoked: | | | | | | | |
| (*Hillshire Farm*), 2 oz. . | 90 | 9.0 | 3.0 | 5.0 | 30 | 460 | <1.0 |
| (*Hillshire Farm Lit'l Smokies*), 5 links . . | 80 | 8.0 | 4.0 | 4.0 | 25 | 480 | <1.0 |
| (*Jennie-O*), 2 oz. . . . . . | 100 | 9.0 | 3.0 | 3.0 | 40 | 550 | 0 |
| (*Johnsonville*), 2.25-oz. link . . . . . . | 110 | 10.0 | 4.0 | 6.0 | 45 | 710 | 0 |
| (*Oscar Mayer*), 2 oz. . . | 90 | 8.0 | 2.0 | 5.0 | 35 | 770 | 0 |
| cheddar (*Johnsonville*), 2.25-oz. link . . . . . . | 120 | 10.0 | 4.0 | 6.0 | 45 | 740 | 0 |
| turkey/chicken, 1 link, 3 oz., except as noted: | | | | | | | |
| Andouille (*Applegate Farms* Organic) . . . | 120 | 13.0 | 3.0 | 6.0 | 60 | 620 | 1.0 |
| Andouille, minis (*Aidells* Cajun), 5 links, 2 oz. . . . . . . | 100 | 11.0 | 1.0 | 6.0 | 45 | 490 | 1.0 |
| garlic, roasted, gruyere (*Aidells*) . . | 190 | 14.0 | 2.0 | 14.0 | 85 | 700 | 2.0 |
| garlic, roasted, gruyere (*Aidells* Fresh) | 180 | 14.0 | 3.0 | 13.0 | 80 | 690 | <1.0 |
| Italian, sweet (*Applegate Farms* Organic) . . . | 130 | 15.0 | 2.0 | 7.0 | 70 | 500 | 1.0 |
| mango jalapeño, spicy (*Aidells*) . . . . . . . . | 180 | 10.0 | 11.0 | 10.0 | 70 | 640 | <1.0 |
| mango jalapeño, spicy (*Aidells* Fresh) . . . . | 180 | 14.0 | 3.0 | 13.0 | 80 | 690 | <1.0 |
| maple, smoked bacon (*Aidells* Breakfast), 2 oz. . . . . . . . . . . . | 100 | 10.0 | 2.0 | 6.0 | 45 | 490 | <1.0 |

| Food and Measure | cal. | prot. (gms) | carbo. (gms) | fat (gms) | chol. (mgs) | sod. (mgs) | fiber (gms) |
|---|---|---|---|---|---|---|---|
| **Sausage, turkey/chicken** *(cont.)* | | | | | | | |
| portobello (*Aidells*) ... | 150 | 14.0 | 1.0 | 10.0 | 70 | 650 | 0 |
| roasted red pepper (*Applegate Farms* | | | | | | | |
| Organic) ......... | 120 | 14.0 | 2.0 | 6.0 | 65 | 500 | 1.0 |
| spinach feta (*Aidells*) . | 180 | 14.0 | 3.0 | 13.0 | 80 | 690 | <1.0 |
| spinach feta (*Applegate Farms* Organic) ... | 120 | 13.0 | 2.0 | 7.0 | 60 | 470 | 0 |
| sun-dried tomato, w/ mozzerella (*Aidells*) | 170 | 13.0 | 3.0 | 12.0 | 75 | 710 | 2.0 |
| **Sausage, canned** | | | | | | | |
| (*Libby's* Vienna), 3 links: | | | | | | | |
| barbecue, w/sauce ..... | 140 | 5.0 | 4.0 | 12.0 | 40 | 430 | 1.0 |
| chicken ............. | 100 | 5.0 | 1.0 | 8.0 | 50 | 410 | 0 |
| original ............. | 120 | 5.0 | 1.0 | 12.0 | 40 | 260 | 0 |
| **"Sausage," vegetarian, canned**: | | | | | | | |
| (*Loma Linda* Little Links), 2 pcs., 1.6 oz. | 90 | 8.0 | 3.0 | 5.0 | 0 | 250 | 2.0 |
| (*Worthington Saucettes*), 1.3-oz. pc. ......... | 90 | 6.0 | 1.0 | 6.0 | 0 | 200 | 1.0 |
| **"Sausage," vegetarian, frozen**: | | | | | | | |
| crumbles (*MorningStar Farms Meal Starters Grillers Recipe Crumbles*), ⅔ cup .... | 90 | 11.0 | 5.0 | 2.5 | 0 | 420 | 3.0 |
| links, 2-oz. pc., except as noted: | | | | | | | |
| apple, spiced (*Veggie Patch*) .......... | 110 | 7.0 | 7.0 | 6.0 | 0 | 300 | 0 |
| jalapeño cheddar (*Veggie Patch*) .... | 100 | 8.0 | 3.0 | 6.0 | 5 | 440 | <1.0 |
| smoked (*Boca*), 2.5 oz. | 130 | 14.0 | 6.0 | 6.0 | 0 | 680 | 1.0 |
| sun-dried tomato artichoke (*Veggie Patch*) .......... | 100 | 8.0 | 5.0 | 6.0 | 0 | 340 | 1.0 |
| links, breakfast 2 pcs., 1.6 oz., except as noted: | | | | | | | |
| (*Boca* Breakfast) ..... | 70 | 8.0 | 5.0 | 3.0 | 0 | 330 | 2.0 |
| (*Boca* Breakfast Organic) ......... | 90 | 10.0 | 5.0 | 3.0 | 0 | 370 | 2.0 |
| (*MorningStar Farms*) . | 80 | 9.0 | 3.0 | 3.0 | 0 | 300 | 2.0 |

| Food and Measure | cal. | prot. (gms) | carbo. (gms) | fat (gms) | chol. (mgs) | sod. (mgs) | fiber (gms) |
|---|---|---|---|---|---|---|---|
| (*Tofurky* Breakfast) . . . | 120 | 10.0 | 6.0 | 6.0 | 0 | 320 | 2.0 |
| (*Worthington Prosage*) | 80 | 9.0 | 3.0 | 3.0 | 0 | 320 | 2.0 |
| link, Italian, 1 link: | | | | | | | |
| (*Boca*), 2.5 oz. . . . . . . | 130 | 13.0 | 6.0 | 6.0 | 0 | 650 | 1.0 |
| (*MorningStar Farms Meal Starters*), | | | | | | | |
| 2.25 oz. . . . . . . . . | 120 | 10.0 | 7.0 | 6.0 | 0 | 350 | 1.0 |
| (*Tofurky*), 3.5 oz. . . . . | 270 | 29.0 | 12.0 | 13.0 | 0 | 620 | 8.0 |
| patties, 1.3-oz. pc., except as noted: | | | | | | | |
| (*Boca* Breakfast Organic) . . . . . . . . . | 70 | 8.0 | 5.0 | 2.5 | 0 | 310 | 2.0 |
| (*MorningStar Farms*) . | 80 | 10.0 | 3.0 | 3.0 | 0 | 260 | 1.0 |
| (*MorningStar Farms* w/Organic Soy) . . . | 80 | 8.0 | 4.0 | 3.0 | 0 | 240 | 1.0 |
| (*Yves*), 2 pcs., 2 oz. . . | 80 | 11.0 | 4.0 | 2.0 | 0 | 350 | 2.0 |
| hot and spicy (*MorningStar Farms*) | 70 | 8.0 | 3.0 | 3.0 | 0 | 230 | 1.0 |
| maple (*MorningStar Farms*) . . . . . . . . . . | 80 | 10.0 | 5.0 | 3.0 | 0 | 250 | <1.0 |
| roll (*Worthington Prosage*), 2 oz. . . . . . . | 140 | 11.0 | 3.0 | 10.0 | 0 | 380 | 2.0 |
| **Sausage entree, frozen**, 1 pkg., except as noted: | | | | | | | |
| and chicken gumbo (*Zatarain's*), 12 oz. . . . | 300 | 14.0 | 36.0 | 14.0 | 30 | 1330 | 2.0 |
| Italian: | | | | | | | |
| penne and (*Michelina's Budget Gourmet*), 8 oz. . . . | 280 | 10.0 | 41.0 | 7.0 | 10 | 410 | 3.0 |
| rigatoni (*Contessa* MicroSteam), 1 cup* | 300 | 12.0 | 41.0 | 11.0 | 20 | 540 | 3.0 |
| spicy (*Macaroni Grill* Pomodoro), ½ of 24-oz. pkg. . . . . . . . | 460 | 20.0 | 48.0 | 21.0 | 35 | 820 | 6.0 |
| **Sausage entree, microwave**, spicy Italian, pasta (*Hormel Compleats*), 10-oz. pkg. | 360 | 14.0 | 37.0 | 17.0 | 20 | 920 | 2.0 |
| **Sausage gravy**, see "Gravy, country" | | | | | | | |
| **Savory**, ground, 1 tsp. . . | 4 | .1 | 1.0 | .1 | 0 | <1 | <1.0 |

| Food and Measure | cal. | prot. (gms) | carbo. (gms) | fat (gms) | chol. (mgs) | sod. (mgs) | fiber (gms) |
|---|---|---|---|---|---|---|---|
| **Scallion**, see "Onion, green" | | | | | | | |
| **Scallop**, meat only: | | | | | | | |
| raw, 4 oz. . . . . . . . . . . . . | 100 | 19.0 | 2.7 | .9 | 38 | 183 | 0 |
| raw, 2 large or | | | | | | | |
|    5 small, 1.1 oz. . . . . . . | 26 | 5.0 | .7 | .2 | 10 | 48 | 0 |
| steamed, 4 oz. . . . . . . . . | 127 | 26.3 | 0 | 1.6 | 60 | 301 | 0 |
| **Scallop, frozen**: | | | | | | | |
| bacon wrapped | | | | | | | |
|   (*Original Rangoon*), | | | | | | | |
|   4 pcs., 3.5 oz. . . . . . . . | 190 | 16.0 | 1.0 | 14.0 | 45 | 440 | 0 |
| fried (*Mrs. Paul's*). | | | | | | | |
|   13 pcs., 3.7 oz. . . . . . . | 280 | 13.0 | 30.0 | 12.0 | 15 | 700 | <1.0 |
| **"Scallop," imitation**, | | | | | | | |
|   from surimi, 4 oz. . . . . | 112 | 14.5 | 12.1 | .5 | 25 | 902 | 0 |
| **"Scallop," vegetarian**, | | | | | | | |
|   canned (*Worthington* | | | | | | | |
|   *Skallops*), ½ cup . . . . | 90 | 17.0 | 4.0 | 1.0 | 0 | 390 | 3.0 |
| **Scallop squash** (see | | | | | | | |
|   also "Sunburst | | | | | | | |
|   Squash"), ½ cup: | | | | | | | |
| raw, sliced . . . . . . . . . . . | 12 | .8 | 2.5 | .1 | 0 | 1 | 1.2 |
| boiled, drained, sliced . . . | 14 | .9 | 3.0 | .2 | 0 | 1 | 1.1 |
| boiled, drained, mashed . | 19 | 1.2 | 4.0 | .2 | 0 | 1 | 1.4 |
| **Scampi sauce**, see | | | | | | | |
|   "Seafood sauce" | | | | | | | |
| **Scrapple**, 2 oz.: | | | | | | | |
| (*Hatfield*) . . . . . . . . . . . . . | 90 | 5.0 | 5.0 | 5.0 | 35 | 310 | 0 |
| beef (*Hatfield*) . . . . . . . . . | 90 | 4.0 | 7.0 | 5.0 | 15 | 320 | 0 |
| **Scrod**, fresh, see | | | | | | | |
|   "Cod, Atlantic" | | | | | | | |
| **Scup**, meat only: | | | | | | | |
| raw, 4 oz. . . . . . . . . . . . . | 119 | 21.4 | 0 | 3.1 | 59 | 48 | 0 |
| baked or broiled, 4 oz. . . | 153 | 27.5 | 0 | 4.0 | 76 | 61 | 0 |
| **Sea bass**, meat only: | | | | | | | |
| raw, 4 oz. . . . . . . . . . . . . | 110 | 20.9 | 0 | 2.3 | 47 | 77 | 0 |
| baked or broiled, 4 oz. . . | 141 | 26.8 | 0 | 2.9 | 60 | 99 | 0 |
| **Sea bass, Chilean**, | | | | | | | |
|   frozen (*Seamazz*), 4 oz. | 270 | 16.0 | 5.0 | 20.0 | 35 | 75 | 0 |
| **Sea trout**, meat only: | | | | | | | |
| raw, 4 oz. . . . . . . . . . . . . | 118 | 19.0 | 0 | 4.1 | 94 | 66 | 0 |
| baked or broiled, 4 oz. . . | 151 | 24.3 | 0 | 5.3 | 120 | 84 | 0 |
| **Sea vegetables**, see | | | | | | | |
|   "Seaweed" | | | | | | | |

| Food and Measure | cal. | prot. (gms) | carbo. (gms) | fat (gms) | chol. (mgs) | sod. (mgs) | fiber (gms) |
|---|---|---|---|---|---|---|---|
| **Seafood**, see specific listings | | | | | | | |
| **Seafood coating mix** (see also "Batter/ breading mix"): | | | | | | | |
| (*Golden Dipt* Fish Fry), 2 tbsp. ........ | 60 | 1.0 | 13.0 | 0 | 0 | 580 | 0 |
| (*Golden Dipt* Seafood Fry), 2 tbsp. . | 60 | 1.0 | 13.0 | 0 | 0 | 630 | 0 |
| (*Oven Fry* Fish), 1 tbsp. ... | 45 | 1.0 | 9.0 | .5 | 0 | 290 | 0 |
| (*Zatarain's* Bake & Crisp Seafood), 2 tbsp. | 60 | 1.0 | 9.0 | 2.0 | 0 | 430 | 0 |
| (*Zatarain's Fish-Fri*), 1½ tbsp. ........... | 45 | 1.0 | 10.0 | 0 | 0 | 0 | 0 |
| (*Zatarain's Shrimp-Fri*), 1½ tbsp. ........... | 40 | <1.0 | 9.0 | 0 | 0 | 460 | 0 |
| beer batter (*Golden Dipt*), ¼ cup ........ | 90 | 1.0 | 21.0 | 0 | 0 | 890 | 0 |
| Cajun: | | | | | | | |
| (*Golden Dipt* Fry Mix), 2 tbsp. ...... | 60 | 1.0 | 13.0 | 0 | 0 | 490 | 0 |
| (*Oven Easy*), ¼ cup .. | 80 | 2.0 | 14.0 | 1.5 | 0 | 500 | 1.0 |
| cracker meal (*Golden Dipt* Seafood Fry), ¼ cup .............. | 130 | 3.0 | 24.0 | 1.0 | 0 | 10 | 0 |
| fish and chips, ¼ cup: | | | | | | | |
| (*Don's Chuck Wagon*) . | 100 | 3.0 | 21.0 | 0 | 0 | 740 | 1.0 |
| (*Golden Dipt* Seafood Batter) ... | 100 | 1.0 | 21.0 | 0 | 0 | 1000 | 0 |
| fish mix, batter (*Don's Chuck Wagon*), ¼ cup | 95 | 4.0 | 21.0 | 0 | 0 | 710 | 1.0 |
| garlic (*Zatarian's Fish-Fri*), 1½ tbsp. ... | 40 | <1.0 | 9.0 | 0 | 0 | 580 | 0 |
| lemon pepper: | | | | | | | |
| (*Oven Easy*), ¼ cup .. | 80 | 2.0 | 14.0 | 1.0 | 0 | 500 | <1.0 |
| (*Zatarain's Fish-Fri*), 1½ tbsp. ......... | 40 | <1.0 | 9.0 | 0 | 0 | 830 | 0 |
| Southern (*Zatarain's Fish-Fri*), 2 tbsp. ..... | 50 | <1.0 | 11.0 | 0 | 0 | 520 | <1.0 |
| tempura (*Golden Dipt* Seafood), ¼ cup ..... | 100 | 2.0 | 21.0 | 0 | 0 | 150 | 0 |
| **Seafood entree**, see specific listings | | | | | | | |

| Food and Measure | cal. | prot. (gms) | carbo. (gms) | fat (gms) | chol. (mgs) | sod. (mgs) | fiber (gms) |
|---|---|---|---|---|---|---|---|
| **Seafood salad kit** | | | | | | | |
| (*Bumble Bee*): | | | | | | | |
| 2.75-oz. can salad . . . | 90 | 4.0 | 15.0 | 1.0 | 10 | 550 | 1.0 |
| 6 crackers, .6 oz. . . . . | 90 | 2.0 | 12.0 | 4.5 | 0 | 180 | 0 |
| **Seafood sauce** (see also | | | | | | | |
| "Marinade seasoning | | | | | | | |
| mix," "Tartar sauce" | | | | | | | |
| and specific listings): | | | | | | | |
| (*Marinade Bay* Baja), | | | | | | | |
| 1 tbsp. . . . . . . . . . . . . | 15 | 0 | 4.0 | 0 | 0 | 180 | 0 |
| (*McCormick* Santa | | | | | | | |
| Fe Style), 2 tbsp. . . . . . | 20 | 0 | 4.0 | 0 | 0 | 380 | 0 |
| Asian (*McCormick*), | | | | | | | |
| 2 tbsp. . . . . . . . . . . . | 50 | <1.0 | 7.0 | 1.5 | 0 | 470 | 0 |
| Cajun: | | | | | | | |
| (*Louisiana*), 1 tbsp. . . | 30 | 0 | 7.0 | 0 | 0 | 160 | 0 |
| (*McCormick*), 2 tbsp. . | 15 | 0 | 3.0 | 0 | 0 | 370 | 0 |
| cocktail, ¼ cup, except | | | | | | | |
| as noted: | | | | | | | |
| (*Crosse & Blackwell*) . | 100 | 1.0 | 25.0 | 0 | 0 | 750 | <1.0 |
| (*Del Monte*) . . . . . . . . | 100 | 1.0 | 24.0 | 0 | 0 | 910 | 0 |
| (*Golden Dipt*) . . . . . . . | 90 | 1.0 | 19.0 | .5 | 0 | 970 | 1.0 |
| (*Marinade Bay*), | | | | | | | |
| 2 tbsp. . . . . . . . . . . | 25 | 0 | 6.0 | 0 | 0 | 250 | 0 |
| (*McCormick* | | | | | | | |
| Original/Extra Hot) . | 90 | 1.0 | 19.0 | .5 | 0 | 970 | 1.0 |
| (*Old Bay*) . . . . . . . . . . | 110 | 0 | 18.0 | .5 | 0 | 960 | 0 |
| (*Zatarain's*) . . . . . . . . . | 70 | <1.0 | 17.0 | 0 | 0 | 950 | 0 |
| Creole (*Crosse &* | | | | | | | |
| *Blackwell*), ¼ cup . . . . | 45 | 1.0 | 9.0 | 0 | 0 | 410 | 1.0 |
| lemon butter dill: | | | | | | | |
| (*McCormick*), 2 tbsp. . | 100 | 0 | 4.0 | 9.0 | <5 | 190 | 0 |
| (*McCormick* Fat | | | | | | | |
| Free), 2 tbsp. . . . . . | 30 | 0 | 7.0 | 0 | 0 | 210 | 2.0 |
| lemon dill (*Crosse* | | | | | | | |
| *& Blackwell*), ¼ cup . . | 130 | 0 | 33.0 | 0 | 0 | 15 | 0 |
| lemon herb | | | | | | | |
| (*McCormick*), 2 tbsp. . | 140 | 0 | <1.0 | 15.0 | 0 | 220 | 0 |
| Mediterranean | | | | | | | |
| (*McCormick*), 2 tbsp. . | 20 | 0 | 4.0 | 0 | 0 | 380 | 0 |
| scampi: | | | | | | | |
| (*Crosse & Blackwell*), | | | | | | | |
| ¼ cup . . . . . . . . . . . | 260 | 1.0 | 7.0 | 25.0 | 0 | 450 | 0 |

| Food and Measure | cal. | prot. (gms) | carbo. (gms) | fat (gms) | chol. (mgs) | sod. (mgs) | fiber (gms) |
|---|---|---|---|---|---|---|---|
| (*Marinade Bay*), | | | | | | | |
| 1 tbsp. . . . . . . . . . | 15 | <1.0 | <1.0 | 1.0 | 0 | 130 | 0 |
| (*McCormick*), 2 tbsp. . | 160 | 0 | 2.0 | 17.0 | 0 | 220 | 0 |
| shrimp (*Crosse &* | | | | | | | |
| *Blackwell* Zesty), | | | | | | | |
| ¼ cup . . . . . . . . . . | 110 | 1.0 | 25.0 | 0 | 0 | 780 | 0 |
| **Seafood seasoning** (see | | | | | | | |
| also "Rubs," | | | | | | | |
| "Seafood coating mix," | | | | | | | |
| and specific listings): | | | | | | | |
| (*Old Bay*), ¼ tsp. . . . . . . . | 0 | 0 | 0 | 0 | 0 | 160 | 0 |
| (*Old Bay* 30% Less | | | | | | | |
| Sodium), ¼ tsp. . . . . . | 0 | 0 | 0 | 0 | 0 | 95 | 0 |
| (*Old Bay* Seafood | | | | | | | |
| Steamers), 2 tsp. . . . . | 15 | 0 | 2.0 | 0 | 0 | 640 | 0 |
| blackened (*Old Bay*), | | | | | | | |
| ½ tsp. . . . . . . . . . . . . | 0 | 0 | 0 | 0 | 0 | 95 | 0 |
| garlic butter | | | | | | | |
| (*McCormick* Seafood | | | | | | | |
| Steamers), 1 tbsp. . . . | 40 | <1.0 | 2.0 | 2.5 | 10 | 380 | 0 |
| w/garlic and herb | | | | | | | |
| (*Old Bay*), ¼ tsp. . . . . | 0 | 0 | 0 | 0 | 0 | 100 | 0 |
| lemon garlic | | | | | | | |
| (*McCormick* Seafood | | | | | | | |
| Steamers), 1 tbsp. . . . | 25 | 0 | 4.0 | .5 | 0 | 400 | 0 |
| w/lemon and herb | | | | | | | |
| (*Old Bay*), ¼ tsp. . . . . | 0 | 0 | 0 | 0 | 0 | 150 | 0 |
| **Seasoning** (see also | | | | | | | |
| specific listings) | | | | | | | |
| (*Maull's* Homestyle), | | | | | | | |
| ¼ tbsp. . . . . . . . . . . . | 5 | 0 | 1.0 | 0 | 0 | 420 | 0 |
| **Seaweed:** | | | | | | | |
| agar: | | | | | | | |
| (*Eden* Agar Agar), | | | | | | | |
| .25-oz. bar . . . . . . | 25 | 0 | 5.0 | 0 | 0 | 0 | 5.0 |
| (*Roland* Agar | | | | | | | |
| Agar), ½ cup . . . . . | 20 | 0 | 5.0 | 0 | 0 | 15 | 0 |
| dried, 1 oz. . . . . . . . . | 87 | 1.8 | 22.9 | .1 | 0 | 29 | 2.2 |
| flakes (*Eden* Agar | | | | | | | |
| Agar), 1 tbsp. . . . . . | 0 | 0 | 1.0 | 0 | 0 | 10 | 1.0 |
| raw, 2 tbsp. . . . . . . . . | 3 | .5 | .7 | 0 | 0 | 1 | <.1 |
| strips, white (*Roland*), | | | | | | | |
| ½ cup . . . . . . . . . . . | 20 | 0 | 5.0 | 0 | 0 | 15 | 0 |

| Food and Measure | cal. | prot. (gms) | carbo. (gms) | fat (gms) | chol. (mgs) | sod. (mgs) | fiber (gms) |
|---|---|---|---|---|---|---|---|
| **Seaweed** *(cont.)* | | | | | | | |
| arame, wild *(Eden)*, | | | | | | | |
| ½ cup ............. | 30 | 1.0 | 7.0 | 0 | 0 | 120 | 7.0 |
| dulse flakes *(Eden* | | | | | | | |
| Organic), 1 tsp. ...... | 3 | 0 | 0 | 0 | 0 | 15 | 0 |
| hiziki, wild *(Eden)*, | | | | | | | |
| ½ cup ............. | 5 | 1.0 | 0 | 0 | 0 | 160 | 6.0 |
| hodai, dried *(Roland)*, | | | | | | | |
| 2 pcs., .5 oz. ........ | 50 | 1.0 | 11.0 | 0 | 0 | 405 | 5.0 |
| Irish moss, raw, 1 oz. ... | 14 | .4 | 3.5 | <.1 | 0 | 19 | .4 |
| kelp, raw, 1 oz. ....... | 12 | .5 | 2.7 | .2 | 0 | 66 | .4 |
| kombu, wild *(Eden)*, | | | | | | | |
| ½ of 7" pc. ......... | 5 | 0 | 1.0 | 0 | 0 | 90 | 1.0 |
| laver, raw, 1 oz. ....... | 10 | 1.6 | 1.4 | .1 | 0 | 1 | 4.1 |
| nori, 1 sheet, except | | | | | | | |
| as noted: | | | | | | | |
| *(Eden)* ............. | 10 | 1.0 | 0 | 0 | 0 | 5 | 1.0 |
| *(Eden* Sushi) ........ | 5 | 1.0 | 0 | 0 | 0 | 5 | 1.0 |
| *(Eden* Sushi | | | | | | | |
| 50-sheet Pkg.) .... | 10 | 1.0 | 0 | 0 | 0 | 5 | 1.0 |
| *(Roland)* ........... | 10 | 1.0 | 1.0 | 0 | 0 | 0 | 1.0 |
| roasted, dried | | | | | | | |
| *(Roland)* ......... | 10 | 1.0 | 1.0 | 0 | 0 | 20 | 0 |
| toasted krinkles | | | | | | | |
| *(Eden)*, ½ cup .... | 10 | 1.0 | 1.0 | 0 | 0 | 5 | 1.0 |
| toasted strips, spicy | | | | | | | |
| *(Eden* 5-sheet | | | | | | | |
| Pkg.) ........... | 0 | <1.0 | <1.0 | 0 | 0 | 20 | <1.0 |
| spirulina, 1 oz.: | | | | | | | |
| raw ............... | 8 | 1.7 | .7 | .1 | 0 | 28 | n.a. |
| dried ............. | 82 | 16.3 | 6.8 | 2.2 | 0 | 297 | 1.0 |
| wakame: | | | | | | | |
| *(Eden)*, ½ cup ....... | 25 | 2.0 | 4.0 | 0 | 0 | 660 | 4.0 |
| *(Eden* Mekabu), 1 tsp. | 0 | 0 | 0 | 0 | 0 | 35 | 0 |
| flakes *(Eden)*, 1 tsp. ... | 0 | 0 | 0 | 0 | 0 | 90 | 0 |
| raw, 1 oz. ........... | 13 | .9 | 2.6 | .2 | 0 | 247 | .1 |
| **Seaweed chips** *(Eden* | | | | | | | |
| Organic Sea Vegetable), | | | | | | | |
| 25 pcs., 1.1 oz. ...... | 140 | <1.0 | 23.0 | 5.0 | 0 | 220 | 0 |
| **Seaweed snack** *(Annie* | | | | | | | |
| *Chun's)*, 10 sheets: | | | | | | | |
| sesame ............. | 25 | 1.0 | 1.0 | 1.5 | 0 | 150 | 1.0 |
| wasabi ............. | 30 | 1.0 | 1.0 | 2.0 | 0 | 65 | 0 |

| Food and Measure | cal. | prot. (gms) | carbo. (gms) | fat (gms) | chol. (mgs) | sod. (mgs) | fiber (gms) |
|---|---|---|---|---|---|---|---|
| **Seitan** (*White Wave*): | | | | | | | |
| traditional, 3 oz. . . . . . . . | 90 | 18.0 | 3.0 | 1.0 | 0 | 380 | 1.0 |
| chicken style, 3 oz. . . . . . | 130 | 24.0 | 9.0 | 0 | 0 | 270 | 3.0 |
| stir-fry strips, 3 oz. . . . . . | 110 | 22.0 | 2.0 | 1.5 | 0 | 420 | 1.0 |
| **Semolina**, whole | | | | | | | |
| grain, 1 cup . . . . . . . . | 601 | 21.2 | 121.6 | 1.8 | 0 | 2 | 6.5 |
| **Semolina flour** | | | | | | | |
| (*Hodgson Mill* | | | | | | | |
| Pasta), <¼ cup . . . . . . | 105 | 4.0 | 21.0 | 0 | 0 | 0 | 1.0 |
| **Sesame flour**, 1 oz.: | | | | | | | |
| high fat . . . . . . . . . . . . . | 149 | 8.7 | 7.6 | 10.5 | 0 | 12 | 1.8 |
| partially defatted . . . . . . . | 108 | 11.4 | 10.0 | 3.4 | 0 | 12 | 1.7 |
| low fat . . . . . . . . . . . . . . | 95 | 14.2 | 10.1 | .5 | 0 | 11 | 1.4 |
| **Sesame meal**, | | | | | | | |
| partially defatted, 1 oz. | 161 | 4.8 | 7.4 | 13.6 | 0 | 11 | 1.1 |
| **Sesame nut mix** | | | | | | | |
| (*Planters*), 1 oz. . . . . . | 160 | 5.0 | 9.0 | 13.0 | 0 | 240 | 2.0 |
| **Sesame paste** (see also | | | | | | | |
| "Tahini"), from | | | | | | | |
| whole seeds, 1 tbsp. . . . | 95 | 2.9 | 4.1 | 8.1 | 0 | 2 | .9 |
| **Sesame seed condiment**: | | | | | | | |
| (*Eden Shake* Organic | | | | | | | |
| Furikake), ½ tsp. . . . . . | 5 | 0 | 1.0 | 0 | 0 | 25 | 1.0 |
| salt (*Eden* Organic | | | | | | | |
| Gomasio), 1 tsp.: | | | | | | | |
| black/black and tan . . . | 20 | <1.0 | <1.0 | 1.5 | 0 | 80 | 0 |
| regular, garlic, or | | | | | | | |
| seaweed . . . . . . . . . | 15 | <1.0 | <1.0 | 1.5 | 0 | 80 | 0 |
| **Sesame seeds**: | | | | | | | |
| whole: | | | | | | | |
| (*Arrowhead Mills* | | | | | | | |
| Organic), ¼ cup . . . | 190 | 6.0 | 8.0 | 17.0 | 0 | 0 | 4.0 |
| black (*Roland*), 1 tsp. . | 20 | 0 | 0 | 2.0 | 0 | 1 | 0 |
| brown (*Bob's Red* | | | | | | | |
| Mill), 2 tbsp. . . . . . . . | 70 | 3.0 | 4.0 | 1.0 | 0 | 2 | 2.0 |
| dried, 1 tbsp. . . . . . . . | 52 | 1.6 | 2.1 | 4.5 | 0 | 1 | 1.1 |
| roasted, toasted, 1 oz . | 160 | 4.8 | 7.3 | 13.6 | 0 | 3 | 4.0 |
| kernels, hulled: | | | | | | | |
| (*Arrowhead Mills* | | | | | | | |
| Organic), ¼ cup . . . | 210 | 9.0 | 3.0 | 19.0 | 0 | 15 | 1.0 |
| dried, 1 tsp. . . . . . . . . | 16 | .7 | .3 | 1.5 | 0 | 1 | <1.0 |
| toasted, 1 oz. . . . . . . . | 161 | 4.8 | 7.4 | 13.6 | 0 | 11 | 4.8 |
| white (*Bob's Red Mill*), | | | | | | | |
| 2 tbsp. . . . . . . . . . . | 92 | 3.0 | 4.0 | 8.0 | 0 | 2 | 2.0 |

| Food and Measure | cal. | prot. (gms) | carbo. (gms) | fat (gms) | chol. (mgs) | sod. (mgs) | fiber (gms) |
|---|---|---|---|---|---|---|---|
| **Sesame seeds, flavored** (*Roland*), 1 tsp.: | | | | | | | |
| curry or wasabi | 30 | 1.0 | 2.0 | 2.0 | 0 | 45 | 0 |
| garlic | 30 | 1.0 | 2.0 | 2.0 | 0 | 50 | 0 |
| plum | 30 | 1.0 | 2.0 | 2.0 | 0 | 70 | 0 |
| soy sauce | 30 | 1.0 | 2.0 | 2.0 | 0 | 100 | 0 |
| **Sesame stick snack,** spelt (*VitaSpelt*): | | | | | | | |
| Cajun, 1 oz. | 150 | 3.0 | 15.0 | 9.0 | 0 | 240 | 1.0 |
| cheddar, 1 oz. | 150 | 3.0 | 16.0 | 9.0 | 0 | 230 | 1.0 |
| garlic, 1 oz. | 150 | 3.0 | 15.0 | 9.0 | 0 | 220 | 2.0 |
| salted, 1 oz. | 150 | 3.0 | 15.0 | 9.0 | 0 | 230 | 1.0 |
| sour cream/onion, 1 oz. | 150 | 3.0 | 15.0 | 9.0 | 0 | 270 | 1.0 |
| whole grain, 1 oz. | 150 | 3.0 | 14.0 | 9.0 | 0 | 220 | 2.0 |
| wild rice, 1 oz. | 140 | 3.0 | 17.0 | 7.0 | 0 | 230 | 1.0 |
| **Sesbania flower:** | | | | | | | |
| raw, 1 cup | 5 | .3 | 1.4 | <.1 | 0 | 3 | n.a. |
| steamed, ½ cup | 11 | .6 | 2.7 | <.1 | 0 | 6 | n.a. |
| **Shad**, meat only: | | | | | | | |
| raw, 4 oz. | 223 | 19.2 | 0 | 15.6 | 85 | 58 | 0 |
| baked or broiled, 4 oz. | 286 | 24.6 | 0 | 20.0 | 109 | 74 | 0 |
| **Shallot**, fresh: | | | | | | | |
| peeled, 1 oz. | 20 | .7 | 4.8 | <.1 | 0 | 3 | <1.0 |
| chopped (*Frieda's*), 1 tbsp., .4 oz. | 7 | 0 | 2.0 | 0 | 0 | 1 | 0 |
| chopped, 1 tbsp. | 7 | .3 | 1.7 | <.1 | 0 | 1 | <1.0 |
| **Shallot, freeze-dried**, 1 tbsp. | 3 | .1 | .7 | tr. | 0 | 1 | <1.0 |
| **Shark**, meat only, raw, 4 oz. | 148 | 23.8 | 0 | 5.1 | 58 | 90 | 0 |
| **Sheepshead**, meat only: | | | | | | | |
| raw, 4 oz. | 123 | 22.9 | 0 | 2.7 | 56 | 81 | 0 |
| baked or broiled, 4 oz. | 143 | 29.5 | 0 | 1.8 | 73 | 83 | 0 |
| **Shellie beans**, canned w/liquid, ½ cup | 37 | 2.1 | 7.6 | .2 | 0 | 408 | 4.1 |
| **Shells, pasta, entree, frozen**, 1 pkg., except as noted: | | | | | | | |
| and cheese, jalapeños (*Michelina's*), 8 oz. | 320 | 10.0 | 41.0 | 12.0 | 25 | 690 | 2.0 |
| cheese stuffed, 10 oz., except as noted: | | | | | | | |
| (*Amy's* Bowls) | 310 | 19.0 | 30.0 | 13.0 | 30 | 740 | 5.0 |

| Food and Measure | cal. | prot. (gms) | carbo. (gms) | fat (gms) | chol. (mgs) | sod. (mgs) | fiber (gms) |
|---|---|---|---|---|---|---|---|
| (*Celentano*) . . . . . . . . | 410 | 17.0 | 51.0 | 14.0 | 30 | 990 | 6.0 |
| (*Celentano*), ½ of 14-oz. pkg. . . . . . . . | 310 | 14.0 | 41.0 | 10.0 | 25 | 700 | 4.0 |
| (*Celentano* Light) . . . . | 340 | 17.0 | 53.0 | 6.0 | 20 | 800 | 7.0 |
| broccoli (*Celentano* Light) . . . . . . . . . . | 330 | 16.0 | 53.0 | 5.0 | 15 | 630 | 8.0 |
| cheese stuffed, w/out sauce (*Celentano*), ½ of 12.5-oz. pkg. . . . | 330 | 18.0 | 42.0 | 9.0 | 40 | 690 | 2.0 |
| pesto (*Blue Horizon*), ¼ of 32-oz. pkg. . . . . | 280 | 17.0 | 38.0 | 6.0 | 40 | 420 | 3.0 |
| soy ricotta (*Rising Moon Organics*), 10 oz. . . . | 370 | 16.0 | 54.0 | 10.0 | 0 | 470 | 6.0 |
| vegetables and, garlic butter sauce (*Birds Eye*), 9 oz. . . . . . . . . . | 270 | 6.0 | 32.0 | 13.0 | 15 | 430 | 3.0 |
| **Shells, pasta, mix**, cheddar, 1 cup\*, except as noted: | | | | | | | |
| (*Annie's* Deluxe Real Aged) . . . . . . . . . . . | 330 | 12.0 | 48.0 | 9.0 | 25 | 740 | 2.0 |
| (*Annie's* Real Aged/ White) . . . . . . . . . . . | 280 | 11.0 | 48.0 | 4.5 | 15 | 550 | 2.0 |
| (*Annie's* Real Aged/ White Organic) . . . . . . | 270 | 11.0 | 48.0 | 4.0 | 10 | 580 | 2.0 |
| (*Velveeta*), ⅓ pkg. . . . . . | 360 | 13.0 | 49.0 | 12.0 | 20 | 940 | 2.0 |
| (*Velveeta* 2%), ⅓ pkg. . . | 330 | 14.0 | 58.0 | 4.5 | 15 | 990 | 2.0 |
| (*Velveeta* Cup), 2 oz. . . . | 220 | 8.0 | 29.0 | 8.0 | 10 | 640 | 1.0 |
| (*Velveeta* Cup), 4 oz. . . . | 360 | 13.0 | 49.0 | 12.0 | 20 | 940 | 2.0 |
| whole wheat (*Annie's* Deluxe) . . . . . . . . . . | 260 | 11.0 | 47.0 | 4.0 | 10 | 680 | 7.0 |
| Alfredo (*Annie's* Organic) . . . . . . . . . . | 270 | 11.0 | 47.0 | 4.0 | 10 | 680 | 2.0 |
| white cheddar: | | | | | | | |
| (*Annie's* Organic Family) . . . . . . . . . | 280 | 11.0 | 48.0 | 4.0 | 10 | 580 | 2.0 |
| (*Pasta Roni*) . . . . . . . | 290 | 9.0 | 38.0 | 12.0 | 5 | 730 | 2.0 |
| whole wheat (*Annie's* Organic) . . . . . . . . | 260 | 10.0 | 44.0 | 4.5 | 10 | 580 | 5.0 |
| **Shepherd's pie**, see "Beef entree," "Lamb entree," and "Vegetable entree" | | | | | | | |

| Food and Measure | cal. | prot. (gms) | carbo. (gms) | fat (gms) | chol. (mgs) | sod. (mgs) | fiber (gms) |
|---|---|---|---|---|---|---|---|
| **Sherbet** (see also "Sorbet"), ½ cup: | | | | | | | |
| berry rainbow (*Dreyer's/Edy's*) . . . . . | 130 | 1.0 | 29.0 | 2.0 | 5 | 35 | 0 |
| orange: | | | | | | | |
| (*Land O Lakes*) . . . . . . | 130 | 2.0 | 28.0 | 1.5 | 5 | 35 | 0 |
| (*Turkey Hill* Grove) . . . | 120 | 1.0 | 26.0 | 1.0 | 5 | 20 | 0 |
| orange, w/vanilla ice cream: | | | | | | | |
| (*Dreyer's/Edy's*) . . . . . | 120 | 2.0 | 23.0 | 2.0 | 10 | 40 | 0 |
| swirl (*Turkey Hill*) . . . . | 130 | 2.0 | 19.0 | 6.0 | 20 | 35 | 0 |
| rainbow (*Turkey Hill*) . . . . | 120 | 1.0 | 26.0 | 1.0 | 5 | 15 | 0 |
| tropical rainbow (*Dreyer's/Edy's*) . . . . . | 130 | 1.0 | 29.0 | 1.0 | 0 | 35 | 0 |
| **Sherbet bar**, see "Iced confection bar" | | | | | | | |
| **Shiitaki soy ginger sauce** (*Annie Chun's*), 1 tbsp. . . . . . . . . . . . | 15 | 0 | 4.0 | 0 | 0 | 180 | 0 |
| **Shiso leaf powder** (*Eden*), 1 tsp. . . . . . . . | 0 | 0 | 0 | 0 | 0 | 200 | 0 |
| **Shortening**, all varieties (*Crisco*), 1 tbsp. . . . . . | 110 | 0 | 0 | 12.0 | 0 | 0 | 0 |
| **Shrimp**, meat only: | | | | | | | |
| raw, 4 oz. . . . . . . . . . . . . . | 120 | 23.0 | 1.0 | 2.0 | 173 | 168 | 0 |
| raw, 4 large, 1 oz. . . . . . . | 30 | 5.7 | .3 | .5 | 43 | 42 | 0 |
| boiled or steamed: | | | | | | | |
| 4 oz. . . . . . . . . . . . . . . | 112 | 23.7 | 0 | 1.2 | 221 | 254 | 0 |
| 4 large, .8 oz. . . . . . . . | 22 | 4.6 | 0 | .2 | 43 | 49 | 0 |
| **Shrimp, canned**: | | | | | | | |
| (*Roland* Picnic), ½ cup, 2 oz. . . . . . . . . | 45 | 10.0 | 1.0 | 0 | 35 | 250 | 0 |
| all varieties, 2 oz.: | | | | | | | |
| (*Bumble Bee*) . . . . . . . | 40 | 10.0 | 0 | 0 | 115 | 430 | 0 |
| (*Chicken of the Sea*) . . | 45 | 10.0 | 1.0 | .5 | 145 | 400 | 0 |
| canned, 1 cup . . . . . . . . . | 154 | 29.6 | 1.3 | 2.5 | 222 | 216 | 0 |
| **Shrimp, frozen** (see also "Shrimp entree"): | | | | | | | |
| balsamic glazed (*Contessa* MicroSteam), ½ of 9-oz. pkg. . . . . . . | 120 | 13.0 | 10.0 | 3.0 | 100 | 740 | .5 |
| barbecue (*Contessa*), | | | | | | | |
| 4 pcs., w/sauce . . . . . . | 150 | 17.0 | 6.0 | 7.0 | 135 | 960 | 0 |
| 4 pcs., w/out sauce . . . | 120 | 17.0 | 3.0 | 4.0 | 135 | 490 | 0 |

| Food and Measure | cal. | prot. (gms) | carbo. (gms) | fat (gms) | chol. (mgs) | sod. (mgs) | fiber (gms) |
|---|---|---|---|---|---|---|---|
| battered, beer (*Gorton's*), | | | | | | | |
| 5 pcs., 3.5 oz. ....... | 240 | 7.0 | 25.0 | 12.0 | 40 | 670 | 0 |
| breaded: | | | | | | | |
| (*Phillips*), 5 pcs., | | | | | | | |
| 3.1 oz. .......... | 230 | 12.0 | 20.0 | 13.0 | 50 | 620 | 2.0 |
| (*Seamazz*), 4 oz. ..... | 150 | 11.0 | 23.0 | 1.5 | 55 | 580 | 0 |
| (*SeaPak* Tossers), | | | | | | | |
| 9 pcs. and ¼ sauce | | | | | | | |
| pkt., 4 oz. ........ | 290 | 9.0 | 21.0 | 19.0 | 60 | 650 | 1.0 |
| garlic herb (*Blue* | | | | | | | |
| *Horizon*), 3.5 oz. .. | 160 | 15.0 | 22.0 | 2.0 | 80 | 360 | 1.0 |
| breaded, butterfly: | | | | | | | |
| (*Gorton's*), 5 pcs., | | | | | | | |
| 3.5 oz. .......... | 250 | 11.0 | 27.0 | 11.0 | 55 | 430 | 4.0 |
| (*SeaPak* Oven Crispy), | | | | | | | |
| 3 oz. ........... | 210 | 10.0 | 20.0 | 10.0 | 60 | 480 | <1.0 |
| (*SeaPak* Ready to | | | | | | | |
| Fry), 8 pcs., 4 oz. .. | 150 | 11.0 | 22.0 | 1.0 | 70 | 680 | 1.0 |
| (*Van de Kamp's*), | | | | | | | |
| 7 pcs., 4 oz. ...... | 330 | 16.0 | 31.0 | 16.0 | 85 | 620 | 1.0 |
| Buffalo: | | | | | | | |
| (*Contessa* Dragon Tail | | | | | | | |
| MicroSteam), ½ of | | | | | | | |
| 9-oz. pkg. ........ | 120 | 13.0 | 5.0 | 5.0 | 116 | 870 | .5 |
| (*Phillips*), 5 pcs., | | | | | | | |
| 3 oz., ¾ oz. sauce . | 260 | 12.0 | 26.0 | 13.0 | 50 | 920 | 2.0 |
| cheese and jalapeño | | | | | | | |
| stuffed (*Margaritaville* | | | | | | | |
| Volcano), 3 oz. ...... | 220 | 7.0 | 20.0 | 13.0 | 40 | 430 | <1.0 |
| chili (*Tiger Thai* Bistro), | | | | | | | |
| 5–6 pcs., 3 oz. ...... | 280 | 10.0 | 20.0 | 18.0 | 55 | 370 | 2.0 |
| chili sauce, 1.1 oz. ... | 100 | 0 | 32.0 | 0 | 0 | 410 | 2.0 |
| cocktail, w/cocktail | | | | | | | |
| sauce (*Chicken of the* | | | | | | | |
| *Sea* Ring), 3 oz. ..... | 100 | 16.0 | 6.0 | .5 | 130 | 580 | 0 |
| coconut: | | | | | | | |
| (*Contessa*), 5 pcs. | | | | | | | |
| w/sauce .......... | 270 | 9.0 | 29.0 | 14.0 | 75 | 440 | 3.0 |
| w/out sauce ...... | 230 | 8.0 | 18.0 | 14.0 | 75 | 390 | 1.0 |
| (*Margaritaville* | | | | | | | |
| Calypso), 4 pc., 3 oz. | 230 | 8.0 | 20.0 | 13.0 | 60 | 330 | 1.0 |
| sauce, 2 tbsp. ...... | 50 | 0 | 12.0 | 0 | 0 | 90 | 0 |
| (*Phillips*), 5 pcs., | | | | | | | |
| 3.4 oz. .......... | 330 | 11.0 | 27.0 | 20.0 | 100 | 420 | 1.0 |

| Food and Measure | cal. | prot. (gms) | carbo. (gms) | fat (gms) | chol. (mgs) | sod. (mgs) | fiber (gms) |
|---|---|---|---|---|---|---|---|
| **Shrimp, frozen, coconut** *(cont.)* | | | | | | | |
| (*SeaPak*), 4 pcs., | | | | | | | |
| w/sauce, 3.7 oz. ... | 310 | 12.0 | 36.0 | 14.0 | 65 | 140 | 1.0 |
| (*Tiger Thai*), 4 pcs., | | | | | | | |
| 3 oz. ........... | 260 | 10.0 | 15.0 | 17.0 | 70 | 200 | 1.0 |
| sauce, 1.4 oz. ..... | 135 | <1.0 | 26.0 | 1.0 | 0 | 210 | <1.0 |
| cooked, peeled, 3 oz.: | | | | | | | |
| (*Chicken of the Sea*) . | 80 | 18.0 | 0 | .5 | 130 | 190 | 0 |
| black tiger (*Seamazz*) . | 60 | 13.0 | 0 | .5 | 80 | 610 | 0 |
| white (*Seamazz*) ..... | 50 | 12.0 | 0 | .5 | 85 | 390 | 0 |
| cracker crumb (*SeaPak* | | | | | | | |
| Light & Crispy), 3 oz. . | 190 | 10.0 | 13.0 | 10.0 | 70 | 810 | 0 |
| crunchy (*Tiger Thai*), | | | | | | | |
| 3 pcs., 3 oz. ........ | 280 | 10.0 | 17.0 | 19.0 | 50 | 140 | 1.0 |
| curry, Thai (*Contessa*), | | | | | | | |
| 5 pcs., w/sauce ...... | 290 | 7.0 | 34.0 | 14.0 | 65 | 1070 | 1.0 |
| w/out sauce ........ | 210 | 7.0 | 15.0 | 14.0 | 60 | 790 | 1.0 |
| garlic herb (*Phillips* | | | | | | | |
| *Steamer Creations*), | | | | | | | |
| 8 pcs., 4 oz. ........ | 180 | 20.0 | 3.0 | 9.0 | 165 | 390 | 0 |
| grilled (*Gorton's* | | | | | | | |
| Classic), 8 pcs., 4 oz. . | 110 | 18.0 | 5.0 | 1.5 | 50 | 920 | 0 |
| honey chipotle | | | | | | | |
| (*Phillips Steamer* | | | | | | | |
| *Creations*), 8 pcs., 4 oz. | 180 | 20.0 | 5.0 | 8.0 | 160 | 420 | 0 |
| honey-roasted (*Contessa* | | | | | | | |
| MicroSteam), | | | | | | | |
| ½ of 9-oz. pkg. ...... | 120 | 12.0 | 9.0 | 3.0 | 95 | 650 | .5 |
| jerk (*Margaritaville* | | | | | | | |
| Jammin'), 7 pcs., 4 oz. | 210 | 12.0 | 4.0 | 10.0 | 120 | 1040 | 1.0 |
| lime (*Margaritaville* | | | | | | | |
| Island), 6 pcs., 4 oz. .. | 240 | 12.0 | 5.0 | 11.0 | 115 | 330 | 0 |
| Marsala (*Contessa*), | | | | | | | |
| 10 pcs., w/sauce ..... | 230 | 11.0 | 28.0 | 7.0 | 105 | 560 | 1.0 |
| w/out sauce ........ | 130 | 11.0 | 17.0 | 1.5 | 100 | 440 | 1.0 |
| orange: | | | | | | | |
| (*Contessa*), 10 pcs., | | | | | | | |
| w/sauce ......... | 180 | 11.0 | 29.0 | 2.0 | 100 | 750 | 2.0 |
| w/out sauce ...... | 130 | 11.0 | 17.0 | 1.5 | 100 | 440 | 1.0 |
| mandarin (*Tiger Thai*), | | | | | | | |
| 7 pcs., 3.5 oz. .... | 200 | 11.0 | 28.0 | 5.0 | 70 | 210 | 2.0 |
| sauce, 2 oz. ...... | 100 | <1.0 | 22.0 | 1.0 | 0 | 150 | <1.0 |
| panko (*Blue Horizon*), | | | | | | | |
| 3.5 oz. ........... | 160 | 15.0 | 22.0 | 1.5 | 80 | 360 | 1.0 |

| Food and Measure | cal. | prot. (gms) | carbo. (gms) | fat (gms) | chol. (mgs) | sod. (mgs) | fiber (gms) |
|---|---|---|---|---|---|---|---|
| plum (*Margaritaville* | | | | | | | |
| Crazy), 7 pcs., 3 oz. .. | 210 | 8.0 | 19.0 | 12.0 | 55 | 520 | 1.0 |
| sauce, 2 tbsp. ........ | 60 | 0 | 14.0 | 0 | 0 | 250 | 0 |
| popcorn, breaded: | | | | | | | |
| (*Blue Horizon*), | | | | | | | |
| 3.5 oz. .......... | 160 | 15.0 | 22.0 | 2.0 | 80 | 360 | 1.0 |
| (*Gorton's*), 22 pcs., | | | | | | | |
| 3.5 oz. .......... | 260 | 10.0 | 26.0 | 13.0 | 60 | 680 | 0 |
| (*SeaPak*), 3 oz. ...... | 210 | 10.0 | 20.0 | 10.0 | 60 | 480 | 1.0 |
| (*Tiger Thai*), 7–8 pcs., | | | | | | | |
| 3 oz. ............ | 260 | 10.0 | 20.0 | 18.0 | 55 | 370 | 2.0 |
| scampi: | | | | | | | |
| (*Contessa*), 8 pcs., | | | | | | | |
| 4 oz. ............ | 240 | 10.0 | 6.0 | 19.0 | 105 | 540 | 1.0 |
| (*Gorton's*), 4 oz. ..... | 120 | 10.0 | 8.0 | 6.0 | 65 | 630 | <1.0 |
| (*Margaritaville* Sun- | | | | | | | |
| set), 7 pcs., 4 oz. .. | 340 | 11.0 | 2.0 | 28.0 | 145 | 460 | 0 |
| (*SeaPak* Tail Off), | | | | | | | |
| 8 pcs., 4 oz. ...... | 350 | 15.0 | 2.0 | 29.0 | 155 | 460 | 0 |
| (*SeaPak* Tail On), | | | | | | | |
| 6 pcs., 4 oz. ...... | 310 | 13.0 | 4.0 | 26.0 | 145 | 830 | <1.0 |
| grilled (*Gorton's*), | | | | | | | |
| 8 pcs., 4 oz. ...... | 130 | 19.0 | 3.0 | 4.5 | 110 | 860 | 0 |
| lemon (*Gorton's*), | | | | | | | |
| 4 oz. ............ | 120 | 8.0 | 8.0 | 6.0 | 65 | 740 | <1.0 |
| spiced, steamed | | | | | | | |
| (*Phillips Steamer* | | | | | | | |
| *Creations*), 8 pcs., 4 oz. | 120 | 22.0 | 2.0 | 2.0 | 160 | 560 | 0 |
| tempura: | | | | | | | |
| (*Blue Horizon*), 3.5 oz. | 160 | 15.0 | 22.0 | 1.5 | 85 | 290 | 1.0 |
| (*Chicken of the Sea*), | | | | | | | |
| 3 pcs., w/sauce ... | 200 | 9.0 | 14.0 | 13.0 | 50 | 245 | 0 |
| (*SeaPak*), 4 pcs., | | | | | | | |
| w/sauce, 4.1 oz. ... | 240 | 9.0 | 35.0 | 8.0 | 35 | 570 | 7.0 |
| (*Tiger Thai*), 1 pc. ..... | 70 | 3.0 | 7.0 | 3.0 | 15 | 50 | <1.0 |
| sauce, 1 oz. ....... | 30 | <1.0 | 7.0 | 0 | 0 | 670 | 0 |
| tikka Masala (*Contessa* | | | | | | | |
| MicroSteam), ½ of | | | | | | | |
| 9-oz. pkg. .......... | 170 | 13.0 | 6.0 | 10.0 | 130 | 700 | .5 |
| vegetable nests (*Tiger* | | | | | | | |
| *Thai*), 4 pcs., 3.7 oz. .. | 210 | 10.0 | 27.0 | 11.0 | 35 | 160 | 5.0 |
| wontons (*Original* | | | | | | | |
| *Rangoon*), 3 pcs., 3 oz. | 220 | 12.0 | 29.0 | 5.0 | 25 | 580 | <1.0 |

| Food and Measure | cal. | prot. (gms) | carbo. (gms) | fat (gms) | chol. (mgs) | sod. (mgs) | fiber (gms) |
|---|---|---|---|---|---|---|---|
| **Shrimp coating**, see "Seafood coating mix" | | | | | | | |
| **Shrimp cocktail**, see "Shrimp, frozen" | | | | | | | |
| **Shrimp entree**, frozen (see also "Shrimp, frozen"), 1 pkg. except as noted: | | | | | | | |
| Alfredo: | | | | | | | |
| (*Lean Cuisine* Cafe), 9 oz. | 250 | 18.0 | 32.0 | 5.0 | 60 | 590 | 3.0 |
| (*Zatarain's*), 10.5 oz. | 470 | 23.0 | 44.0 | 21.0 | 120 | 840 | 2.0 |
| penne (*Blue Horizon Organic*), ½ of 10-oz. pkg. | 430 | 17.0 | 39.0 | 22.0 | 115 | 380 | 2.0 |
| angel-hair pasta (*Lean Cuisine* Cafe), 10 oz. | 230 | 14.0 | 34.0 | 4.0 | 50 | 610 | 2.0 |
| arrabiata (*SeaKist SeaSations*), 9 oz. | 210 | 12.0 | 33.0 | 3.5 | 45 | 590 | 6.0 |
| barbecue, Southwest (*SeaKist SeaSations*), 9 oz. | 310 | 10.0 | 60.0 | 3.5 | 45 | 1020 | 3.0 |
| fried rice, see "Rice entree, frozen" | | | | | | | |
| garlic: | | | | | | | |
| (*Birds Eye Voila!*), 1 cup* | 230 | 10.0 | 27.0 | 9.0 | 50 | 410 | 2.0 |
| (*Stouffer's Easy Express* Skillets), ½ of 22-oz. pkg. | 310 | 15.0 | 40.0 | 10.0 | 50 | 1110 | 5.0 |
| herb (*Healthy Choice Steam*), 8.5 oz. | 260 | 11.0 | 37.0 | 7.0 | 30 | 600 | 5.0 |
| garlic butter (*SeaKist SeaSations*), 9 oz. | 260 | 14.0 | 35.0 | 7.0 | 60 | 1100 | 6.0 |
| Jamaican (*Organic Bistro*), 10 oz. | 320 | 18.0 | 49.0 | 7.0 | 75 | 105 | 6.0 |
| lemon garlic (*Lean Cuisine Dinnertime Cuisine*), 12 oz. | 280 | 18.0 | 39.0 | 6.0 | 75 | 830 | 5.0 |
| lo mein: | | | | | | | |
| (*Smart Ones Dragon*), 9.25 oz. | 220 | 11.0 | 38.0 | 3.0 | 30 | 540 | 4.0 |
| (*Wanchai Ferry*), ½ of 24-oz. pkg.* | 600 | 20.0 | 92.0 | 18.0 | 85 | 1600 | 6.0 |

| Food and Measure | cal. | prot. (gms) | carbo. (gms) | fat (gms) | chol. (mgs) | sod. (mgs) | fiber (gms) |
|---|---|---|---|---|---|---|---|
| marinara, w/linguine (*Smart Ones*), 9 oz. | 190 | 10.0 | 34.0 | 2.0 | 20 | 650 | 4.0 |
| Mediterranean (*Contessa On the Stove*), ⅓ pkg.: | | | | | | | |
| w/sauce, 7.8 oz. | 180 | 11.0 | 26.0 | 3.0 | 45 | 900 | 3.0 |
| w/out sauce | 150 | 9.0 | 22.0 | 2.5 | 40 | 740 | 2.0 |
| w/pasta, vegetables (*Michelina's Lean Gourmet*), 8 oz. | 260 | 11.0 | 39.0 | 6.0 | 45 | 620 | 2.0 |
| penne alla vodka (*Blue Horizon* Organic), ½ of 10-oz. pkg. | 270 | 17.0 | 38.0 | 6.0 | 75 | 280 | 3.0 |
| pesto farfalle w/ (*Blue Horizon* Organic), ½ of 10-oz. pkg. | 280 | 17.0 | 38.0 | 6.0 | 70 | 430 | 3.0 |
| primavera (*Contessa On the Stove*), ⅓ pkg.: | | | | | | | |
| w/sauce, 7 oz. | 290 | 13.0 | 30.0 | 13.0 | 65 | 770 | 3.0 |
| w/out sauce | 180 | 13.0 | 29.0 | 1.0 | 60 | 260 | 3.0 |
| rotini w/ (*Blue Horizon* Organic), ½ of 10-oz. pkg. | 410 | 18.0 | 44.0 | 19.0 | .85 | 640 | 4.0 |
| and scallop bake (*Blue Horizon*), ¼ of 28-oz. pkg. | 270 | 14.0 | 33.0 | 9.0 | 50 | 560 | 1.0 |
| scampi: | | | | | | | |
| (*Birds Eye Voila!*), 1 cup* | 190 | 11.0 | 31.0 | 2.5 | 60 | 540 | 3.0 |
| (*Lean Cuisine Market Creations*), 10.5 oz. | 250 | 15.0 | 32.0 | 7.0 | 58 | 690 | 4.0 |
| (*Marie Callender's*), 13 oz. | 380 | 16.0 | 45.0 | 15.0 | 70 | 1200 | 4.0 |
| (*Michelina's Lean Gourmet*), 8 oz. | 280 | 11.0 | 44.0 | 6.0 | 40 | 610 | 2.0 |
| and linguine (*Contessa* MicroSteam), 1 cup* | 310 | 12.0 | 37.0 | 12.0 | 60 | 450 | 3.0 |
| w/pasta (*Zatarain's*), 10.5 oz. | 380 | 22.0 | 50.0 | 10.0 | 95 | 1260 | 2.0 |
| roasted garlic (*Macaroni Grill*), ½ of 24-oz. pkg.* | 410 | 16.0 | 51.0 | 16.0 | 105 | 1090 | 3.0 |
| sesame ginger (*StarKist SeaSations*), 9 oz. | 270 | 11.0 | 44.0 | 5.0 | 50 | 620 | 4.0 |

| Food and Measure | cal. | prot. (gms) | carbo. (gms) | fat (gms) | chol. (mgs) | sod. (mgs) | fiber (gms) |
|---|---|---|---|---|---|---|---|
| **Shrimp entree** *(cont.)* | | | | | | | |
| Shanghai (*Lean Cuisine* Market Creations), 10.5 oz. .. | 250 | 14.0 | 41.0 | 3.0 | 55 | 700 | 4.0 |
| spicy, diavolo (*Healthy Choice* Complete), 11.5 oz. ........... | 250 | 13.0 | 42.0 | 2.5 | 70 | 550 | 7.0 |
| stir-fry (*Contessa On the Stove*), ⅓ pkg.: | | | | | | | |
| w/sauce, 8 oz. ....... | 130 | 9.0 | 22.0 | 0 | 50 | 670 | 3.0 |
| w/out sauce ........ | 80 | 8.0 | 9.0 | 0 | 50 | 230 | 3.0 |
| sweet and sour (*Contessa On the Stove*): | | | | | | | |
| w/sauce, 10 oz. ...... | 250 | 14.0 | 46.0 | .5 | 65 | 490 | 4.0 |
| w/out sauce ........ | 200 | 13.0 | 34.0 | 0 | 65 | 310 | 3.0 |
| sweet and spicy (*Wanchai Ferry*), ½ of 24-oz. pkg.* .... | 420 | 14.0 | 76.0 | 7.0 | 85 | 1600 | 2.0 |
| Szechuan stir-fry, w/ (*Lean Cuisine Spa Cuisine*), 9 oz. .... | 230 | 12.0 | 41.0 | 2.0 | 50 | 570 | 5.0 |
| **Shrimp entree mix** citrus glazed, w/angel hair (*Good Earth Restaurant Favorites*), 1 cup* ............ | 290 | 14.0 | 38.0 | 9.0 | 90 | 360 | 4.0 |
| **Shrimp sauce**, see "Seafood sauce" | | | | | | | |
| **Shrimp seasoning mix**, Szechuan (*Kikkoman*), 1⅓ tbsp. ........... | 30 | <1.0 | 5.0 | 1.0 | <5 | 620 | <1. |
| **Sloppy Joe sauce**, see "Sandwich sauce" | | | | | | | |
| **Sloppy Joe seasoning:** | | | | | | | |
| (*Lawry's*), 2 tsp. ....... | 20 | 0 | 5.0 | 0 | 0 | 480 | 0 |
| (*McCormick*), 1 tsp. .... | 20 | 0 | 3.0 | 0 | 0 | 300 | 0 |
| **Smelt**, rainbow, meat only: | | | | | | | |
| raw, 4 oz. ............ | 110 | 20.0 | 0 | 2.8 | 80 | 68 | 0 |
| baked or broiled, 4 oz. .. | 141 | 25.6 | 0 | 3.5 | 102 | 87 | 0 |
| **Smoke, liquid** (*Colgin*), 1 tsp. ...... | 0 | 0 | 0 | 0 | 0 | 10 | 0 |
| **Snack bars**, see "Granola/cereal bars" | | | | | | | |

| Food and Measure | cal. | prot. (gms) | carbo. (gms) | fat (gms) | chol. (mgs) | sod. (mgs) | fiber (gms) |
|---|---|---|---|---|---|---|---|
| **Snack chips/crisps** (see also "Snack mix," "Corn chips/crisps" "Crackers," etc.), 1 oz., except as noted: | | | | | | | |
| (*Ritz* Toasted) ......... | 130 | 2.0 | 21.0 | 4.5 | 0 | 250 | 1.0 |
| cheddar: | | | | | | | |
| (*Herr's Friez*) ........ | 150 | 2.0 | 16.0 | 8.0 | 0 | 320 | 1.0 |
| (*Ritz* Toasted) ....... | 130 | 2.0 | 19.0 | 6.0 | 0 | 290 | 0 |
| garlic, roasted, rye (*Gardetto's* Special Request), 1.1 oz. .... | 160 | 2.0 | 16.0 | 10.0 | 0 | 340 | 1.0 |
| hot (*Herr's Friez* Hot Hot Hot!*) ....... | 150 | 2.0 | 16.0 | 8.0 | 0 | 330 | 1.0 |
| multigrain: | | | | | | | |
| (*Genisoy Crisps* Lightly Salted) .... | 110 | 3.0 | 22.0 | 2.0 | 0 | 180 | 2.0 |
| (*Genisoy Crisps* Naked) .......... | 110 | 3.0 | 22.0 | 2.0 | 0 | 40 | 2.0 |
| (*Pringles* Original) ... | 140 | 1.0 | 16.0 | 8.0 | 0 | 150 | 1.0 |
| (*Wheat Thins* Toasted Great Plains) ..... | 120 | 2.0 | 20.0 | 4.0 | 0 | 240 | 1.0 |
| cheddar (*Pringles*) ... | 140 | 1.0 | 16.0 | 8.0 | 0 | 190 | 1.0 |
| ranch (*Pringles*) ..... | 140 | 1.0 | 16.0 | 8.0 | 0 | 170 | 1.0 |
| rosemary and olive oil (*Genisoy Crisps*) .. | 120 | 3.0 | 21.0 | 3.0 | 0 | 180 | 2.0 |
| onion rings (*Treat*) ..... | 130 | 2.0 | 19.0 | 6.0 | 0 | 290 | 1.0 |
| sour cream/onion (*Ritz* Toasted) ....... | 130 | 2.0 | 19.0 | 6.0 | 0 | 270 | 0 |
| vegetable (*Wheat Thins* Toasted) ...... | 130 | 2.0 | 19.0 | 5.0 | 0 | 290 | 1.0 |
| **Snack mix** (see also "Trail mix"), ½ cup, except as noted: | | | | | | | |
| (*Annie's* Bunnies Organic), 1.1 oz. ..... | 140 | 3.0 | 20.0 | 5.0 | 0 | 290 | 0 |
| (*Beer Nuts* Bar Mix), 1 oz. ............. | 140 | 4.0 | 15.0 | 7.0 | 0 | 220 | 1.0 |
| (*Cheerios* Original), ⅔ cup ............. | 130 | 3.0 | 22.0 | 3.5 | 0 | 290 | 1.0 |
| (*Cheez-It* Original) ...... | 130 | 3.0 | 21.0 | 3.5 | 0 | 390 | 2.0 |
| (*Chex Mix* Bold Party Blend) ............. | 120 | 2.0 | 20.0 | 4.0 | 0 | 190 | 1.0 |

| Food and Measure | cal. | prot. (gms) | carbo. (gms) | fat (gms) | chol. (mgs) | sod. (mgs) | fiber (gms) |
|---|---|---|---|---|---|---|---|
| **Snack mix** *(cont.)* | | | | | | | |
| (*Chex Mix* Sweet 'n | | | | | | | |
| Salty Trail Mix) ...... | 150 | 3.0 | 24.0 | 5.0 | 0 | 95 | 1.0 |
| (*Chex Mix* Traditional) ... | 120 | 2.0 | 20.0 | 4.0 | 0 | 210 | 1.0 |
| (*Gardetto's* Original) .... | 150 | 3.0 | 18.0 | 7.0 | 0 | 260 | 1.0 |
| (*Gardetto's* Reduced | | | | | | | |
| Fat) .............. | 140 | 3.0 | 20.0 | 5.0 | 0 | 310 | 1.0 |
| (*Munchies Flamin'* | | | | | | | |
| *Hot*), 1 oz., ¾ cup .... | 140 | 2.0 | 18.0 | 7.0 | 0 | 200 | 1.0 |
| (*Nabisco Mixers* | | | | | | | |
| Traditional), 1 oz. .... | 130 | 2.0 | 21.0 | 5.0 | 0 | 360 | 1.0 |
| (*Treat* Party Mix), | | | | | | | |
| 1 oz. .............. | 140 | 2.0 | 18.0 | 6.0 | 0 | 270 | 1.0 |
| assortment (*Cheez-It*) ... | 130 | 3.0 | 20.0 | 4.5 | 0 | 330 | 1.0 |
| barbecue: | | | | | | | |
| (*Chex Mix*) ......... | 120 | 2.0 | 21.0 | 4.0 | 0 | 160 | 1.0 |
| cheddar (*Cheez-It*) ... | 130 | 3.0 | 20.0 | 4.5 | 0 | 430 | 1.0 |
| caramel crunch (*Chex* | | | | | | | |
| *Mix* Sweet 'n Salty) ... | 120 | 2.0 | 21.0 | 3.5 | 0 | 120 | 1.0 |
| cheddar: | | | | | | | |
| (*Annie's* Bunnies | | | | | | | |
| Organic), 1.1 oz. .. | 140 | 3.0 | 20.0 | 5.0 | 0 | 300 | 0 |
| (*Cheerios*), ⅔ cup .... | 130 | 3.0 | 21.0 | 4.0 | 0 | 280 | 1.0 |
| (*Chex Mix*), ⅔ cup ... | 130 | 2.0 | 21.0 | 4.0 | 0 | 220 | 1.0 |
| (*Munchies* Ultimate), | | | | | | | |
| ¾ cup, 1 oz. ...... | 130 | 2.0 | 19.0 | 4.5 | 0 | 230 | 1.0 |
| (*Nabisco Mixers*), | | | | | | | |
| 1 oz. ............ | 130 | 2.0 | 19.0 | 4.5 | 0 | 340 | 1.0 |
| cheese: | | | | | | | |
| (*Munchies* Cheese | | | | | | | |
| Fix), ¾ cup ....... | 140 | 2.0 | 18.0 | 7.0 | 0 | 250 | 1.0 |
| double (*Cheez-It*) .... | 130 | 2.0 | 19.0 | 5.0 | 0 | 470 | 1.0 |
| Italian blend | | | | | | | |
| (*Gardetto's*) ...... | 150 | 3.0 | 20.0 | 6.0 | 0 | 290 | <1.0 |
| chipotle cheddar (*Chex* | | | | | | | |
| *Mix*), ⅔ cup ........ | 130 | 2.0 | 24.0 | 4.5 | 0 | 260 | 2.0 |
| chocolate: | | | | | | | |
| dark (*Chex Mix*) ..... | 140 | 1.0 | 23.0 | 4.5 | 0 | 60 | <1.0 |
| peanut butter (*Chex* | | | | | | | |
| *Mix*) ............. | 160 | 3.0 | 24.0 | 6.0 | 0 | 85 | 1.0 |
| turtle (*Chex Mix*) ..... | 130 | 2.0 | 20.0 | 5.0 | <5 | 115 | <1.0 |
| green tea (*Ka•Me*), | | | | | | | |
| ¼ cup, 1.1 oz. ....... | 160 | 6.0 | 12.0 | 10.0 | 0 | 120 | 3.0 |

| Food and Measure | cal. | prot. (gms) | carbo. (gms) | fat (gms) | chol. (mgs) | sod. (mgs) | fiber (gms) |
|---|---|---|---|---|---|---|---|
| honey nut: | | | | | | | |
| (*Cheerios*), ⅔ cup .... | 130 | 2.0 | 23.0 | 3.5 | 0 | 220 | 1.0 |
| (*Chex Mix* Sweet | | | | | | | |
| 'n Salty) ......... | 130 | 2.0 | 22.0 | 4.0 | 0 | 140 | 1.0 |
| hot/spicy (*Chex Mix*) .... | 120 | 2.0 | 21.0 | 3.5 | 0 | 290 | 1.0 |
| jalapeño: | | | | | | | |
| (*Beer Nuts*), 1 oz. .... | 160 | 4.0 | 13.0 | 10.0 | 0 | 260 | 1.0 |
| cheddar (*Chex Mix*) .. | 120 | 2.0 | 21.0 | 4.0 | 0 | 280 | 1.0 |
| multigrain (*SunChips*), | | | | | | | |
| 1 oz.: | | | | | | | |
| chipotle, spicy ...... | 130 | 2.0 | 17.0 | 6.0 | 0 | 135 | 2.0 |
| *Harvest Cheddar* ..... | 140 | 2.0 | 19.0 | 6.0 | 0 | 200 | 3.0 |
| onion, French ....... | 140 | 2.0 | 18.0 | 6.0 | 0 | 170 | 3.0 |
| original ........... | 140 | 2.0 | 19.0 | 6.0 | 0 | 120 | 3.0 |
| peppercorn ranch .... | 140 | 2.0 | 17.0 | 6.0 | 0 | 160 | 3.0 |
| salsa, garden ....... | 140 | 2.0 | 19.0 | 6.0 | 0 | 170 | 3.0 |
| peanut lovers (*Chex* | | | | | | | |
| *Mix*) ............. | 140 | 3.0 | 19.0 | 6.0 | 0 | 200 | 1.0 |
| ranch (*Munchies* | | | | | | | |
| Totally Ranch), ¾ cup . | 140 | 2.0 | 19.0 | 6.0 | 0 | 260 | 1.0 |
| sour cream and onion | | | | | | | |
| (*Chex Mix*) ......... | 120 | 2.0 | 20.0 | 4.0 | 0 | 280 | 1.0 |
| wasabi peas mix | | | | | | | |
| (*Ka•Me*), ⅓ cup ..... | 150 | 5.0 | 17.0 | 7.0 | 0 | 200 | 2.0 |
| **Snail**, fresh, raw, | | | | | | | |
| 1 oz. ............. | 26 | 4.6 | <.1 | .4 | 14 | 20 | 0 |
| **Snail, canned** (*Roland* | | | | | | | |
| Extra Large/Giant/ | | | | | | | |
| Helix), ½ cup ....... | 50 | 10.0 | 1.0 | 1.0 | 135 | 150 | 1.0 |
| **Snail, sea**, see "Whelk" | | | | | | | |
| **Snapper**, meat only: | | | | | | | |
| raw, 4 oz. .......... | 113 | 23.3 | 0 | 1.5 | 42 | 73 | 0 |
| baked or broiled, 4 oz. .. | 145 | 30.0 | 0 | 2.0 | 53 | 65 | 0 |
| **Snow peas**, see "Peas, | | | | | | | |
| edible-podded" | | | | | | | |
| **Soft drinks**, 12 fl. oz., | | | | | | | |
| except as noted: | | | | | | | |
| apple: | | | | | | | |
| (*Fanta*), 8 fl. oz. ..... | 120 | 0 | 33.0 | 0 | 0 | 35 | 0 |
| (*Goya*) ............ | 150 | 0 | 37.0 | 0 | 0 | 10 | 0 |
| (*Izze*) ............ | 130 | 0 | 33.0 | 0 | 0 | 20 | 0 |
| (*R.W. Knudsen* | | | | | | | |
| Spritzer Organic) .. | 170 | <1.0 | 44.0 | 0 | 0 | 35 | 0 |
| cider, spiced (*Reed's*) . | 160 | 0 | 41.2 | 0 | 0 | 6 | 0 |

| Food and Measure | cal. | prot. (gms) | carbo. (gms) | fat (gms) | chol. (mgs) | sod. (mgs) | fiber (gms) |
|---|---|---|---|---|---|---|---|
| **Soft drinks** *(cont.)* | | | | | | | |
| berry: | | | | | | | |
| (*Fanta*), 8 fl. oz. ..... | 117 | 0 | 32.0 | 0 | 0 | 22 | 0 |
| (*Vault Red Blitz*) ..... | 180 | 0 | 47.0 | 0 | 0 | 45 | 0 |
| wild (*Blue Sky* | | | | | | | |
| Energy), 8 fl. oz. ... | 120 | 0 | 29.0 | 0 | 0 | 200 | 0 |
| blackberry (*Izze*) ....... | 130 | 0 | 31.0 | 0 | 0 | 25 | 0 |
| blueberry (*Izze*) ....... | 130 | 0 | 33.0 | 0 | 0 | 30 | 0 |
| boysenberry (*R.W.* | | | | | | | |
| *Knudsen* Spritzer) .... | 160 | <1.0 | 40.0 | 0 | 0 | 20 | <1.0 |
| cherry (*Santa Cruz* | | | | | | | |
| *Organic*) ........... | 140 | 0 | 34.0 | 0 | 0 | 20 | 0 |
| cherry, black: | | | | | | | |
| (*Blue Sky* Natural) ... | 140 | 0 | 37.0 | 0 | 0 | 10 | 0 |
| (*Blue Sky* Organic | | | | | | | |
| Cherish) .......... | 150 | 0 | 37.0 | 0 | 0 | 10 | 0 |
| (*Fanta*), 8 fl. oz. ..... | 110 | 0 | 29.0 | 0 | 0 | 35 | 0 |
| (*R.W. Knudsen* | | | | | | | |
| Spritzer) ......... | 180 | <1.0 | 46.0 | 0 | 0 | 30 | 0 |
| (*R.W. Knudsen* | | | | | | | |
| Spritzer Light) .... | 100 | <1.0 | 26.0 | 0 | 0 | 30 | 0 |
| cherry vanilla crème | | | | | | | |
| (*Blue Sky*) .......... | 170 | 0 | 46.0 | 0 | 0 | 10 | 0 |
| citrus: | | | | | | | |
| (*Fanta*), 8 fl. oz. ..... | 91 | 0 | 25.0 | 0 | 0 | 16 | 0 |
| (*Mello Yello*), | | | | | | | |
| 8 fl. oz. .......... | 118 | 0 | 32.0 | 0 | 0 | 33 | 0 |
| (*Mountain Dew/* | | | | | | | |
| *Mountain Dew* | | | | | | | |
| Livewire/Voltage) .. | 170 | 0 | 46.0 | 0 | 0 | 65 | 0 |
| (*Mountain Dew Code* | | | | | | | |
| Red) ............ | 170 | 0 | 46.0 | 0 | 0 | 105 | 0 |
| (*7Up/7Up* Cherry), | | | | | | | |
| 8 fl. oz. .......... | 100 | 0 | 26.0 | 0 | 0 | 25 | 0 |
| (*Sun Drop*) ......... | 180 | 0 | 46.0 | 0 | 0 | 55 | 0 |
| (*Sun Drop* Caffeine | | | | | | | |
| Free) ............ | 190 | 0 | 51.0 | 0 | 0 | 30 | 0 |
| (*Vault*) ............ | 180 | 0 | 47.0 | 0 | 0 | 45 | 0 |
| cherry lemon (*Sun* | | | | | | | |
| Drop) ............ | 180 | 0 | 46.0 | 0 | 0 | 55 | 0 |
| clementine (*Izze*) ....... | 120 | 0 | 30.0 | 0 | 0 | 25 | 0 |
| coconut (*Goya*) ........ | 200 | 0 | 45.0 | 0 | 0 | 65 | 0 |
| cola: | | | | | | | |
| (*Blue Sky* Natural) ... | 160 | 0 | 42.0 | 0 | 0 | 10 | 0 |

| Food and Measure | cal. | prot. (gms) | carbo. (gms) | fat (gms) | chol. (mgs) | sod. (mgs) | fiber (gms) |
|---|---|---|---|---|---|---|---|
| (*Blue Sky* Organic New Century) . . . . . | 160 | 0 | 40.0 | 0 | 0 | 10 | 0 |
| (*Coca-Cola* Classic) . . | 140 | 0 | 39.0 | 0 | 0 | 45 | 0 |
| (*Coca-Cola* Classic/ Free), 8 fl. oz. . . . . . | 100 | 0 | 27.0 | 0 | 0 | 30 | 0 |
| (*Dr Pepper/Dr Pepper* Free), 8 fl. oz. . . . . . | 100 | 0 | 27.0 | 0 | 0 | 35 | 0 |
| (*Goya* Champagne) . . . | 200 | 0 | 47.0 | 0 | 0 | 60 | 0 |
| (*Inca Kola*), 8 fl. oz. . . | 96 | 0 | 26.0 | 0 | 0 | 31 | 0 |
| (*Pepsi* Natural) . . . . . . | 150 | 0 | 39.0 | 0 | 0 | 35 | 0 |
| (*Pepsi* Throwback) . . . | 150 | 0 | 40.0 | 0 | 0 | 40 | 0 |
| (*Pepsi/Pepsi* Free) . . . | 150 | 0 | 41.0 | 0 | 0 | 30 | 0 |
| berry (*Blue Sky* Dr. Becker) . . . . . . . | 140 | 0 | 38.0 | 0 | 0 | 10 | 0 |
| cherry (*Coca-Cola*) . . . | 150 | 0 | 42.0 | 0 | 0 | 35 | 0 |
| cherry (*Dr Pepper*), 8 fl. oz. . . . . . . . . . | 110 | 0 | 29.0 | 0 | 0 | 40 | 0 |
| cherry (*R.W. Knudsen* Spritzer) . . . . . . . . . | 170 | <1.0 | 41.0 | 0 | 0 | 25 | 0 |
| cherry, wild (*Pepsi*) . . | 160 | 0 | 42.0 | 0 | 0 | 30 | 0 |
| cherry vanilla (*Dr Pepper*), 8 fl. oz. . . . | 100 | 0 | 26.0 | 0 | 0 | 40 | 0 |
| ginseng (*Blue Sky*) . . . | 170 | 0 | 42.0 | 0 | 0 | 10 | 0 |
| ginseng (*Natural Brew*) . . . . . . . . . . . | 170 | 0 | 42.0 | 0 | 0 | 20 | 0 |
| w/lime (*Coca-Cola*), 8 fl. oz. . . . . . . . . | 98 | 0 | 27.0 | 0 | 0 | 25 | 0 |
| vanilla (*Coca-Cola*) . . . | 150 | 0 | 42.0 | 0 | 0 | 35 | 0 |
| cranberry: | | | | | | | |
| (*R.W. Knudsen* Spritzer) . . . . . . . . | 190 | 1.0 | 46.0 | 0 | 0 | 65 | 0 |
| (*Sierra Mist* Splash) . . | 160 | 0 | 42.0 | 0 | 0 | 35 | 0 |
| cream: | | | | | | | |
| (*A&W*), 8 fl. oz. . . . . . . | 120 | 0 | 31.0 | 0 | 0 | 30 | 0 |
| (*Barq's* Red), 8 fl. oz. . | 115 | 0 | 31.0 | 0 | 0 | 43 | 0 |
| (*Blue Sky*) . . . . . . . . . | 170 | 0 | 48.0 | 0 | 0 | 10 | 0 |
| (*Mug*) . . . . . . . . . . . . | 180 | 0 | 47.0 | 0 | 0 | 60 | 0 |
| vanilla (*Barq's* French), 8 fl.oz. . . . . . . . . . | 112 | 0 | 30.0 | 0 | 0 | 44 | 0 |
| vanilla crème (*Natural Brew*) . . . . . . . . . . . | 170 | 0 | 42.0 | 0 | 0 | 20 | 0 |
| vanilla crème (*R.W. Knudsen* Spritzer) . | 160 | <1.0 | 38.0 | 0 | 0 | 25 | 0 |

| Food and Measure | cal. | prot. (gms) | carbo. (gms) | fat (gms) | chol. (mgs) | sod. (mgs) | fiber (gms) |
|---|---|---|---|---|---|---|---|
| **Soft drinks, cream** *(cont.)* | | | | | | | |
| vanilla crème (*Santa Cruz Organic*) ..... | 160 | 0 | 38.0 | 0 | 0 | 10 | 0 |
| fruit punch (*Goya*) ...... | 190 | 0 | 49.0 | 0 | 0 | 40 | 0 |
| ginger ale: | | | | | | | |
| (*Blue Sky* Jamaican) .. | 140 | 0 | 37.0 | 0 | 0 | 10 | 0 |
| (*Blue Sky* Organic) ... | 160 | 0 | 39.0 | 0 | 0 | 10 | 0 |
| (*Canada Dry*) ....... | 120 | 0 | 33.0 | 0 | 0 | 40 | 0 |
| (*Natural Brew*) ...... | 170 | 0 | 42.0 | 0 | 0 | 20 | 0 |
| (*R.W. Knudsen* Spritzer) ......... | 160 | <1.0 | 39.0 | 0 | 0 | 20 | 0 |
| (*Reed's* Jamaican) ... | 145 | 0 | 47.5 | 0 | 0 | 5 | 0 |
| (*Santa Cruz Organic*) . | 150 | 0 | 37.0 | 0 | 0 | 10 | 0 |
| (*Schweppes*), 8 fl. oz. .. | 80 | 0 | 23.0 | 0 | 0 | 40 | 0 |
| cherry (*Reed's*) ...... | 150 | 0 | 38.5 | 0 | 0 | 5 | 0 |
| green tea (*Canada Dry*) | 140 | 0 | 36.0 | 0 | 0 | 65 | 0 |
| raspberry (*Reed's*) ... | 145 | 0 | 37.4 | 0 | 0 | 5 | 0 |
| ginger beer: | | | | | | | |
| (*Goya*) ............ | 190 | 0 | 43.0 | 0 | 0 | 30 | 0 |
| (*Reed's* Jamaican Brew Premium/ Extra Ginger) ..... | 145 | 0 | 37.4 | 0 | 0 | 5 | 0 |
| golden (*Goya* El Dorado) ............ | 160 | 0 | 39.0 | 0 | 0 | 30 | 0 |
| grape: | | | | | | | |
| (*Blue Sky*) .......... | 130 | 0 | 36.0 | 0 | 0 | 10 | 0 |
| (*Crush*), 8 fl. oz. ..... | 130 | 0 | 35.0 | 0 | 0 | 45 | 0 |
| (*Fanta*), 8 fl. oz. ..... | 120 | 0 | 33.0 | 0 | 0 | 25 | 0 |
| (*Goya*) ............ | 230 | 0 | 57.0 | 0 | 0 | 5 | 0 |
| (*R.W. Knudsen* Spritzer) ......... | 180 | <1.0 | 45.0 | 0 | 0 | 20 | 0 |
| (*Santa Cruz Organic* Concord) ........ | 150 | 0 | 36.0 | 0 | 0 | 15 | 0 |
| (*Slice*) ............. | 190 | 0 | 50.0 | 0 | 0 | 65 | 0 |
| (*Tropicana Twister*) ... | 190 | 0 | 50.0 | 0 | 0 | 65 | 0 |
| grapefruit: | | | | | | | |
| (*Blue Sky*) .......... | 140 | 0 | 38.0 | 0 | 0 | 10 | 0 |
| (*Fanta*), 8 fl. oz. ..... | 100 | 0 | 28.0 | 0 | 0 | 45 | 0 |
| (*Goya*) ............ | 180 | 0 | 46.0 | 0 | 0 | 35 | 0 |
| (*Izze*) ............. | 120 | 0 | 31.0 | 0 | 0 | 20 | 0 |
| (*Sierra Mist* Ruby Splash) .......... | 150 | 0 | 39.0 | 0 | 0 | 35 | 0 |
| pink (*Fanta*), 8 fl. oz. .. | 113 | 0 | 30.0 | 0 | 0 | 30 | 0 |
| guava (*Goya*) ......... | 170 | 0 | 42.0 | 0 | 0 | 30 | 0 |

| Food and Measure | cal. | prot. (gms) | carbo. (gms) | fat (gms) | chol. (mgs) | sod. (mgs) | fiber (gms) |
|---|---|---|---|---|---|---|---|
| lemon (*Fanta*), 8 fl. oz. | 112 | 0 | 30.0 | 0 | 0 | 30 | 0 |
| lemon, bitter | | | | | | | |
| (*Stirrings*), 6.3 fl. oz. | 50 | 0 | 13.0 | 0 | 0 | 0 | 0 |
| lemon lime: | | | | | | | |
| (*Blue Sky* Natural) | 130 | 0 | 35.0 | 0 | 0 | 10 | 0 |
| (*Goya*) | 170 | 0 | 42.0 | 0 | 0 | 35 | 0 |
| (*R.W. Knudsen* | | | | | | | |
| Spritzer) | 170 | <1.0 | 41.0 | 0 | 0 | 25 | 0 |
| (*Santa Cruz Organic*) | 140 | 0 | 36.0 | 0 | 0 | 10 | 0 |
| (*Sierra Mist*) | 150 | 0 | 39.0 | 0 | 0 | 35 | 0 |
| (*Sprite*), 8 fl. oz. | 96 | 0 | 26.0 | 0 | 0 | 47 | 0 |
| lemonade (see also | | | | | | | |
| "Lemonade"): | | | | | | | |
| (*R.W. Knudsen* | | | | | | | |
| Spritzer Light) | 90 | <1.0 | 22.0 | 0 | 0 | 20 | 0 |
| (*Santa Cruz Organic*) | 150 | 0 | 38.0 | 0 | 0 | 0 | 0 |
| Jamaican (*R.W.* | | | | | | | |
| *Knudsen* Spritzer) | 160 | <1.0 | 40.0 | 0 | 0 | 20 | 0 |
| raspberry (*Santa Cruz* | | | | | | | |
| *Organic*) | 120 | 0 | 29.0 | 0 | 0 | 10 | 0 |
| lime (*Izze*) | 130 | 0 | 31.0 | 0 | 0 | 15 | 0 |
| mandarin lime (*R.W.* | | | | | | | |
| *Knudsen* Spritzer) | 170 | <1.0 | 40.0 | 0 | 0 | 30 | 0 |
| mango: | | | | | | | |
| (*Fiesta Mirinda*) | 140 | 0 | 38.0 | 0 | 0 | 45 | 0 |
| (*R.W. Knudsen* | | | | | | | |
| Spritzer) | 170 | <1.0 | 42.0 | 0 | 0 | 20 | 0 |
| (*R.W. Knudsen* | | | | | | | |
| Spritzer Light) | 110 | <1.0 | 27.0 | 0 | 0 | 20 | 0 |
| orange: | | | | | | | |
| (*Blue Sky* Organic | | | | | | | |
| Divine) | 180 | 0 | 44.0 | 0 | 0 | 10 | 0 |
| (*Crush*), 8 fl. oz. | 130 | 0 | 35.0 | 0 | 0 | 50 | 0 |
| (*Fanta*), 8 fl. oz. | 110 | 0 | 30.0 | 0 | 0 | 35 | 0 |
| (*Goya* Mandarin) | 170 | 0 | 44.0 | 0 | 0 | 35 | 0 |
| (*Mirinda*), 8 fl. oz. | 120 | 0 | 32.0 | 0 | 0 | 25 | 0 |
| (*Slice*) | 180 | 0 | 48.0 | 0 | 0 | 35 | 0 |
| (*Tropicana Twister*) | 190 | 0 | 52.0 | 0 | 0 | 35 | 0 |
| cream (*Blue Sky*) | 160 | 0 | 44.0 | 0 | 0 | 10 | 0 |
| orange mango (*Santa* | | | | | | | |
| *Cruz Organic*) | 130 | 0 | 33.0 | 0 | 0 | 10 | 0 |
| orange passion fruit | | | | | | | |
| (*R.W. Knudsen* | | | | | | | |
| Spritzer) | 160 | <1.0 | 38.0 | 0 | 0 | 20 | 0 |

| Food and Measure | cal. | prot. (gms) | carbo. (gms) | fat (gms) | chol. (mgs) | sod. (mgs) | fiber (gms) |
|---|---|---|---|---|---|---|---|
| **Soft drinks** *(cont.)* | | | | | | | |
| peach: | | | | | | | |
| (*Crush*), 8 fl. oz. ..... | 120 | 0 | 33.0 | 0 | 0 | 40 | 0 |
| (*Fanta*), 8 fl. oz. ..... | 110 | 0 | 29.0 | 0 | 0 | 30 | 0 |
| (*Izze*) ............ | 130 | 0 | 32.0 | 0 | 0 | 20 | 0 |
| (*R.W. Knudsen* Spritzer) ......... | 160 | <1.0 | 39.0 | 0 | 0 | 25 | 0 |
| (*Slice*) ............ | 180 | 0 | 51.0 | 0 | 0 | 65 | 0 |
| pineapple: | | | | | | | |
| (*Crush*), 8 fl. oz. ..... | 130 | 0 | 35.0 | 0 | 0 | 45 | 0 |
| (*Fiesta Mirinda*) ..... | 140 | 0 | 38.0 | 0 | 0 | 45 | 0 |
| (*Fanta*), 8 fl. oz. ..... | 120 | 0 | 33.0 | 0 | 0 | 35 | 0 |
| (*Goya*) ............ | 170 | 0 | 43.0 | 0 | 0 | 40 | 0 |
| pomegranate (*Izze*) ..... | 120 | 0 | 31.0 | 0 | 0 | 15 | 0 |
| raspberry: | | | | | | | |
| (*Blue Sky*) .......... | 170 | 0 | 45.0 | 0 | 0 | 10 | 0 |
| (*R.W. Knudsen* Spritzer) ......... | 200 | <1.0 | 46.0 | 0 | 0 | 25 | 0 |
| root beer: | | | | | | | |
| (*A&W*), 8 fl. oz. ...... | 120 | 0 | 31.0 | 0 | 0 | 30 | 0 |
| (*Barq's*), 8 fl. oz. ..... | 110 | 0 | 30.0 | 0 | 0 | 50 | 0 |
| (*Blue Sky* Natural) ... | 160 | 0 | 43.0 | 0 | 0 | 10 | 0 |
| (*Blue Sky* Organic Encore) ......... | 170 | 0 | 43.0 | 0 | 0 | 10 | 0 |
| (*Mug*) ............ | 160 | 0 | 43.0 | 0 | 0 | 65 | 0 |
| (*Natural Brew* Draft) .. | 180 | 0 | 44.0 | 0 | 0 | 0 | 0 |
| (*Santa Cruz Organic*) . | 150 | 0 | 36.0 | 0 | 0 | 10 | 0 |
| sangria (*Señorial*) ...... | 180 | 0 | 44.0 | 0 | 0 | 70 | 0 |
| strawberry: | | | | | | | |
| (*Crush*), 8 fl. oz. ..... | 120 | 0 | 31.0 | 0 | 0 | 45 | 0 |
| (*Fanta*), 8 fl. oz. ..... | 120 | 0 | 33.0 | 0 | 0 | 30 | 0 |
| (*R.W. Knudsen* Spritzer) | 160 | <1.0 | 39.0 | 0 | 0 | 20 | 0 |
| (*Slice*) ............ | 160 | 0 | 43.0 | 0 | 0 | 65 | 0 |
| (*Tropicana Twister*) ... | 160 | 0 | 43.0 | 0 | 0 | 50 | 0 |
| tangerine: | | | | | | | |
| (*Fanta*), 8 fl. oz. ..... | 123 | 0 | 33.0 | 0 | 0 | 40 | 0 |
| (*R.W. Knudsen* Spritzer) ......... | 200 | <1.0 | 48.0 | 0 | 0 | 25 | 0 |
| (*Santa Cruz Organic*) . | 160 | 0 | 39.0 | 0 | 0 | 15 | 0 |
| tea soda, all varieties (*Blue Sky*) .......... | 130 | 0 | 33.0 | 0 | 0 | 10 | 0 |
| tonic, 8 fl. oz.: | | | | | | | |
| (*Canada Dry*) ....... | 90 | 0 | 24.0 | 0 | 0 | 35 | 0 |
| (*Schweppes*) ....... | 90 | 0 | 23.0 | 0 | 0 | 35 | 0 |

| Food and Measure | cal. | prot. (gms) | carbo. (gms) | fat (gms) | chol. (mgs) | sod. (mgs) | fiber (gms) |
|---|---|---|---|---|---|---|---|
| vanilla crème, see "cream," above | | | | | | | |
| **Sofrito**, in jars (*Goya*), 1 tsp. . . . . . . . | 0 | 0 | 0 | 0 | 0 | 45 | 0 |
| **Sole**, see "Flatfish" | | | | | | | |
| **Sole entree**, frozen, stuffed (*Oven Poppers*), 5-oz. pc., except as noted: | | | | | | | |
| crab . . . . . . . . . . . . . . . . | 240 | 17.0 | 15.0 | 13.0 | 35 | 400 | 0 |
| crab, lump . . . . . . . . . | 200 | 18.0 | 9.0 | 10.0 | 80 | 430 | 0 |
| crab *Qwickies*, 3 oz. . . . . | 150 | 10.0 | 9.0 | 8.0 | 20 | 250 | 0 |
| garlic/shrimp/ almonds . . . . . . . . . . | 260 | 16.0 | 16.0 | 14.0 | 60 | 380 | 0 |
| shrimp/lobster, in Newburg sauce . . . . . . | 170 | 21.0 | 6.0 | 6.0 | 130 | 540 | 0 |
| spinach, cheese . . . . . . . | 210 | 15.0 | 13.0 | 10.0 | 55 | 270 | 0 |
| ***Sonic*** Drive-In: | | | | | | | |
| breakfast: | | | | | | | |
| *Breakfast Toaster*: | | | | | | | |
| w/bacon . . . . . . . . . | 530 | 21.0 | 39.0 | 33.0 | 325 | 1460 | 2.0 |
| w/ham . . . . . . . . . | 490 | 24.0 | 39.0 | 27.0 | 325 | 1720 | 2.0 |
| w/sausage . . . . . . . | 520 | 21.0 | 39.0 | 42.0 | 340 | 1400 | 2.0 |
| breakfast burrito: | | | | | | | |
| w/bacon . . . . . . . . . | 470 | 19.0 | 37.0 | 28.0 | 300 | 1470 | 1.0 |
| w/ham . . . . . . . . . | 460 | 25.0 | 37.0 | 23.0 | 310 | 1810 | 1.0 |
| w/sausage . . . . . . . | 500 | 18.0 | 37.0 | 31.0 | 300 | 1380 | 1.0 |
| Jr. . . . . . . . . . . . . . . . . | 340 | 12.0 | 24.0 | 21.0 | 220 | 930 | 0 |
| steak and egg . . . . . | 590 | 28.0 | 45.0 | 33.0 | 320 | 1450 | 3.0 |
| *SuperSonic* . . . . . . | 590 | 18.0 | 47.0 | 36.0 | 300 | 1830 | 3.0 |
| *CroisSonic*: | | | | | | | |
| w/bacon . . . . . . . . . | 510 | 19.0 | 28.0 | 36.0 | 320 | 1410 | 0 |
| w/ham . . . . . . . . . | 430 | 21.0 | 24.0 | 27.0 | 355 | 1520 | 1.0 |
| w/sausage . . . . . . . | 600 | 19.0 | 28.0 | 46.0 | 340 | 1350 | 0 |
| French toast sticks . . . | 500 | 7.0 | 49.0 | 31.0 | 15 | 490 | 2.0 |
| syrup . . . . . . . . . . . | 90 | 0 | 22.0 | 0 | 0 | 0 | 0 |
| *Sausage Biscuit Dippers*, w/gravy . . | 690 | 15.0 | 57.0 | 44.0 | 60 | 1770 | 0 |
| burgers: | | | | | | | |
| *Sonic* burger: | | | | | | | |
| w/mayo . . . . . . . . | 800 | 36.0 | 55.0 | 49.0 | 110 | 740 | 5.0 |
| w/mustard . . . . . . . | 700 | 36.0 | 54.0 | 38.0 | 100 | 770 | 5.0 |
| w/ketchup . . . . . . . | 710 | 36.0 | 57.0 | 38.0 | 100 | 840 | 5.0 |

| Food and Measure | cal. | prot. (gms) | carbo. (gms) | fat (gms) | chol. (mgs) | sod. (mgs) | fiber (gms) |
|---|---|---|---|---|---|---|---|
| **Sonic, burgers** *(cont.)* | | | | | | | |
| *Sonic* cheeseburger: | | | | | | | |
| w/mayo ......... | 860 | 39.0 | 55.0 | 54.0 | 130 | 1070 | 5.0 |
| w/mayo, bacon .... | 930 | 44.0 | 56.0 | 60.0 | 140 | 1330 | 5.0 |
| w/mustard ....... | 770 | 39.0 | 54.0 | 43.0 | 120 | 1100 | 5.0 |
| w/ketchup ....... | 770 | 40.0 | 58.0 | 43.0 | 120 | 1170 | 5.0 |
| *SuperSonic:* | | | | | | | |
| w/mayo ......... | 1270 | 68.0 | 56.0 | 87.0 | 245 | 1500 | 5.0 |
| w/mustard ....... | 1180 | 68.0 | 55.0 | 76.0 | 235 | 1530 | 5.0 |
| w/ketchup ....... | 1190 | 68.0 | 58.0 | 76.0 | 235 | 1600 | 5.0 |
| *SuperSonic*, jalapeño . | 1180 | 67.0 | 54.0 | 76.0 | 235 | 1660 | 5.0 |
| burger: | | | | | | | |
| jalapeño ......... | 700 | 36.0 | 53.0 | 38.0 | 100 | 900 | 5.0 |
| Jr. .............. | 310 | 15.0 | 30.0 | 15.0 | 35 | 610 | 3.0 |
| Jr. deluxe ........ | 350 | 15.0 | 28.0 | 20.0 | 40 | 440 | 3.0 |
| Thousand Island ... | 760 | 36.0 | 56.0 | 44.0 | 110 | 830 | 5.0 |
| cheeseburger: | | | | | | | |
| California ....... | 450 | 39.0 | 56.0 | 50.0 | 125 | 1100 | 5.0 |
| chili ........... | 800 | 42.0 | 55.0 | 47.0 | 125 | 1020 | 5.0 |
| green chili ....... | 770 | 39.0 | 55.0 | 43.0 | 120 | 1100 | 5.0 |
| hickory .......... | 780 | 39.0 | 60.0 | 43.0 | 120 | 1200 | 5.0 |
| jalapeño ......... | 760 | 39.0 | 52.0 | 43.0 | 120 | 960 | 5.0 |
| Jr. bacon ........ | 410 | 20.0 | 30.0 | 23.0 | 60 | 1070 | 3.0 |
| Jr. double ........ | 570 | 31.0 | 31.0 | 36.0 | 110 | 1330 | 3.0 |
| upgrades: | | | | | | | |
| bacon ........... | 70 | 4.0 | 0 | 5.0 | 15 | 260 | 0 |
| cheese ......... | 70 | 4.0 | 1.0 | 6.0 | 20 | 330 | 0 |
| chili ........... | 50 | 3.0 | 2.0 | 3.5 | 10 | 160 | 1.0 |
| green chilies ...... | 5 | 0 | 1.0 | 0 | 0 | 5 | 0 |
| jalapeños ........ | 5 | 0 | 1.0 | 0 | 0 | 280 | 1.0 |
| onions, grilled .... | 25 | 0 | 2.0 | 2.0 | 0 | 200 | 1.0 |
| slaw ........... | 45 | 0 | 4.0 | 3.0 | 0 | 45 | 1.0 |
| *Toaster* sandwiches: | | | | | | | |
| bacon cheeseburger .. | 820 | 39.0 | 51.0 | 51.0 | 130 | 1500 | 3.0 |
| BLT .............. | 490 | 14.0 | 39.0 | 31.0 | 40 | 960 | 2.0 |
| chicken club ........ | 740 | 30.0 | 54.0 | 46.0 | 80 | 1760 | 4.0 |
| steak, country fried ... | 670 | 14.0 | 71.0 | 37.0 | 50 | 1370 | 4.0 |
| wraps: | | | | | | | |
| chicken, crispy ...... | 490 | 21.0 | 49.0 | 23.0 | 40 | 1280 | 3.0 |
| chicken, grilled ...... | 390 | 28.0 | 39.0 | 14.0 | 80 | 1420 | 2.0 |
| *Fritos* chili cheese .... | 700 | 21.0 | 65.0 | 39.0 | 25 | 1600 | 4.0 |
| salads: | | | | | | | |
| crispy chicken ....... | 340 | 20.0 | 24.0 | 19.0 | 50 | 970 | 5.0 |
| grilled chicken ...... | 250 | 29.0 | 12.0 | 10.0 | 100 | 1070 | 3.0 |

| Food and Measure | cal. | prot. (gms) | carbo. (gms) | fat (gms) | chol. (mgs) | sod. (mgs) | fiber (gms) |
|---|---|---|---|---|---|---|---|
| *Marzetti* dressing: | | | | | | | |
| buttermilk ranch ... | 210 | 1.0 | 2.0 | 22.0 | 10 | 370 | 0 |
| Dijon honey ...... | 180 | 0 | 8.0 | 16.0 | 15 | 260 | 0 |
| Italian, fat free .... | 25 | 0 | 5.0 | 0 | 0 | 390 | 0 |
| ranch, light ....... | 70 | 1.0 | 8.0 | 4.0 | 0 | 310 | 0 |
| Thousand Island .. | 220 | 0 | 7.0 | 21.0 | 25 | 350 | 0 |
| chicken: | | | | | | | |
| bacon ranch, crispy .. | 610 | 30.0 | 47.0 | 35.0 | 75 | 1750 | 4.0 |
| bacon ranch, grilled .. | 470 | 36.0 | 34.0 | 22.0 | 105 | 1630 | 3.0 |
| sandwich, crispy ..... | 550 | 22.0 | 46.0 | 32.0 | 45 | 1070 | 4.0 |
| sandwich, grilled .... | 400 | 28.0 | 32.0 | 19.0 | 80 | 960 | 3.0 |
| strip dinner, 4 ....... | 970 | 37.0 | 106.0 | 45.0 | 65 | 1970 | 8.0 |
| *Jumbo Popcorn*, large | 560 | 27.0 | 41.0 | 32.0 | 65 | 1890 | 5.0 |
| *Jumbo Popcorn*, small | 380 | 18.0 | 27.0 | 22.0 | 45 | 1250 | 3.0 |
| BBQ sauce ....... | 45 | 0 | 11.0 | 0 | 0 | 390 | 0 |
| honey mustard .... | 90 | 0 | 7.0 | 7.0 | 10 | 190 | 0 |
| ranch sauce ...... | 150 | 0 | 1.0 | 16.0 | 10 | 230 | 0 |
| coney, regular ...... | 400 | 16.0 | 32.0 | 23.0 | 45 | 1210 | 2.0 |
| coney, footlong ....... | 830 | 32.0 | 55.0 | 53.0 | 90 | 1980 | 4.0 |
| corn dog ............ | 210 | 6.0 | 23.0 | 11.0 | 20 | 530 | 2.0 |
| snacks/sides: | | | | | | | |
| apple slices ......... | 35 | 0 | 9.0 | 0 | 0 | 0 | 2.0 |
| w/caramel sauce .. | 110 | 0 | 28.0 | 0 | 0 | 60 | 2.0 |
| *Ched 'R' Bites*, 12 .. | 280 | 13.0 | 22.0 | 15.0 | 30 | 740 | 1.0 |
| *Ched 'R' Peppers*, 4 .. | 330 | 6.0 | 36.0 | 17.0 | 25 | 1110 | 2.0 |
| chili pie, *Fritos:* | | | | | | | |
| large ............ | 970 | 25.0 | 71.0 | 64.0 | 35 | 1780 | 6.0 |
| medium ......... | 510 | 14.0 | 36.0 | 34.0 | 15 | 1000 | 3.0 |
| fish sandwich ....... | 650 | 22.0 | 71.0 | 31.0 | 40 | 1160 | 7.0 |
| fries: | | | | | | | |
| large ............ | 450 | 5.0 | 67.0 | 18.0 | 0 | 600 | 5.0 |
| medium ......... | 330 | 4.0 | 48.0 | 13.0 | 0 | 440 | 4.0 |
| small ........... | 200 | 2.0 | 30.0 | 8.0 | 0 | 270 | 2.0 |
| fries, w/cheese: | | | | | | | |
| large ............ | 740 | 14.0 | 92.0 | 36.0 | 35 | 1480 | 7.0 |
| medium ......... | 460 | 9.0 | 55.0 | 23.0 | 30 | 990 | 4.0 |
| small ........... | 330 | 6.0 | 40.0 | 16.0 | 20 | 680 | 3.0 |
| chili, large ....... | 850 | 19.0 | 96.0 | 43.0 | 25 | 1680 | 8.0 |
| chili, medium ..... | 540 | 13.0 | 59.0 | 28.0 | 15 | 1100 | 5.0 |
| chili, small ....... | 360 | 8.0 | 42.0 | 18.0 | 10 | 720 | 3.0 |
| mozzarella sticks .... | 440 | 19.0 | 40.0 | 22.0 | 45 | 1050 | 2.0 |
| onion rings, large .... | 640 | 9.0 | 80.0 | 31.0 | 0 | 630 | 4.0 |
| onion rings, medium . | 440 | 6.0 | 55.0 | 21.0 | 0 | 430 | 3.0 |
| *Pickle-O's* .......... | 310 | 5.0 | 36.0 | 16.0 | 0 | 1020 | 2.0 |

| Food and Measure | cal. | prot. (gms) | carbo. (gms) | fat (gms) | chol. (mgs) | sod. (mgs) | fiber (gms) |
|---|---|---|---|---|---|---|---|
| **Sonic**, snacks/sides *(cont.)* | | | | | | | |
| tots: | | | | | | | |
| large .............. | 640 | 9.0 | 80.0 | 31.0 | 0 | 630 | 4.0 |
| medium ......... | 200 | 2.0 | 20.0 | 13.0 | 0 | 440 | 2.0 |
| small .......... | 130 | 1.0 | 13.0 | 8.0 | 0 | 270 | 1.0 |
| tots, w/cheese: | | | | | | | |
| large ............. | 540 | 10.0 | 42.0 | 37.0 | 35 | 1550 | 4.0 |
| medium ......... | 300 | 7.0 | 21.0 | 21.0 | 25 | 940 | 2.0 |
| small .......... | 190 | 4.0 | 13.0 | 14.0 | 20 | 600 | 1.0 |
| chili, large ....... | 680 | 17.0 | 49.0 | 46.0 | 25 | 1820 | 6.0 |
| chili, medium ..... | 390 | 11.0 | 25.0 | 27.0 | 20 | 1100 | 3.0 |
| chili, small ...... | 230 | 6.0 | 15.0 | 16.0 | 10 | 660 | 2.0 |
| **Sopressata**, 1 oz.: | | | | | | | |
| (*Applegate Farms*) ...... | 110 | 7.0 | 0 | 9.0 | 20 | 520 | 0 |
| (*Di Lusso*) ............ | 110 | 7.0 | 0 | 9.0 | 30 | 400 | 0 |
| hot (*Applegate Farms*) .. | 100 | 7.0 | 0 | 9.0 | 20 | 500 | 0 |
| hot or sweet (*Boar's Head*) ............. | 100 | 8.0 | 0 | 7.0 | 25 | 500 | 0 |
| sweet (*Thumann's*) ..... | 90 | 8.0 | 1.0 | 6.0 | 20 | 510 | 0 |
| **Sorbet** (see also "Sherbet"), ½ cup: | | | | | | | |
| banana mango (*Ciao Bella*) ......... | 110 | 1.0 | 27.0 | 0 | 0 | 10 | 1.0 |
| berry, mixed (*Sharon's*) . | 100 | 0 | 24.0 | 0 | 0 | 0 | 0 |
| blackberry Cabernet (*Ciao Bella*) ......... | 130 | 1.0 | 29.0 | 0 | 0 | 0 | 2.0 |
| blueberry: | | | | | | | |
| (*Sharon's*) ........... | 80 | 0 | 21.0 | 0 | 0 | 0 | 1.0 |
| w/blackberry (*Ben & Jerry's Berried Treasure*) ........ | 110 | 0 | 29.0 | 0 | 0 | 5 | 1.0 |
| wild (*Ciao Bella*) ..... | 70 | 0 | 17.0 | 0 | 0 | 0 | 1.0 |
| chocolate: | | | | | | | |
| (*Häagen-Dazs*) ...... | 130 | 2.0 | 28.0 | .5 | 0 | 70 | 2.0 |
| (*Sharon's*) .......... | 110 | 0 | 20.0 | 3.5 | 0 | 15 | 0 |
| dark (*Ciao Bella*) ..... | 200 | 5.0 | 21.0 | 10.0 | 0 | 15 | 2.0 |
| coconut: | | | | | | | |
| (*Ciao Bella*) ......... | 190 | 1.0 | 28.0 | 9.0 | 0 | 15 | 0 |
| (*Palapa Azul*) ........ | 110 | 1.0 | 15.0 | 6.0 | 0 | 15 | 0 |
| (*Sharon's*) .......... | 140 | 0 | 25.0 | 4.0 | 0 | 15 | 0 |
| (*Whole Fruit*) ....... | 180 | 0 | 41.0 | 2.5 | 5 | 25 | <1.0 |
| cranberry blueberry (*Häagen-Dazs*) ...... | 100 | 0 | 25.0 | 0 | 0 | 0 | <1.0 |

| Food and Measure | cal. | prot. (gms) | carbo. (gms) | fat (gms) | chol. (mgs) | sod. (mgs) | fiber (gms) |
|---|---|---|---|---|---|---|---|
| hibiscus: | | | | | | | |
| (*Palapa Azul*) ....... | 110 | 1.0 | 28.0 | 0 | 0 | 0 | 0 |
| (*So Delicious*) ....... | 100 | 0 | 26.0 | 0 | 0 | 160 | 3.0 |
| lemon: | | | | | | | |
| (*Ciao Bella* Zest) ..... | 130 | 0 | 32.0 | 0 | 0 | 0 | 0 |
| (*Häagen-Dazs* Zesty) . | 110 | 0 | 28.0 | 0 | 0 | 25 | <1.0 |
| (*Sharon's*) .......... | 100 | 0 | 26.0 | 0 | 0 | 0 | 0 |
| (*Whole Fruit*) ....... | 140 | 0 | 35.0 | 0 | 0 | 20 | 0 |
| lemonade (*So Delicious*) . | 110 | 0 | 27.0 | 0 | 0 | 150 | 2.0 |
| mango: | | | | | | | |
| (*Ciao Bella*) ......... | 120 | 0 | 29.0 | 0 | 0 | 0 | 1.0 |
| (*Häagen-Dazs*) ...... | 120 | 0 | 37.0 | 0 | 0 | 10 | 0 |
| (*Palapa Azul*) ....... | 80 | 0 | 21.0 | 0 | 0 | 0 | 0 |
| (*Sharon's*) .......... | 100 | 0 | 25.0 | 0 | 0 | 0 | 1.0 |
| (*So Delicious*) ....... | 100 | 0 | 26.0 | 0 | 0 | 170 | 3.0 |
| (*Whole Fruit*) ....... | 150 | 0 | 38.0 | 0 | 0 | 10 | 0 |
| orange, blood (*Ciao Bella*) ............. | 60 | 0 | 16.0 | 0 | 0 | 0 | 0 |
| passion fruit: | | | | | | | |
| (*Ciao Bella*) ......... | 120 | 0 | 29.0 | 0 | 0 | 0 | 0 |
| (*Sharon's*) .......... | 80 | 1.0 | 25.0 | 0 | 0 | 0 | 0 |
| peach: | | | | | | | |
| (*Häagen-Dazs*) ...... | 130 | 0 | 33.0 | 0 | 0 | 0 | <1.0 |
| (*Whole Fruit*) ....... | 140 | 0 | 34.0 | 0 | 0 | 10 | 0 |
| peach ginger (*Ciao Bella*) ............. | 100 | 0 | 26.0 | 0 | 0 | 0 | 1.0 |
| pineapple, w/passion fruit (*Ben & Jerry's* Jamaican Me Crazy) .. | 130 | 0 | 33.0 | 0 | 0 | 10 | 1.0 |
| pomegranate blueberry acai (*Whole Fruit*) .... | 130 | 0 | 33.0 | 0 | 0 | 15 | <1.0 |
| prickly pear (*Ciao Bella*) ............. | 80 | 0 | 20.0 | 0 | 0 | 0 | 1.0 |
| raspberry: | | | | | | | |
| (*Ciao Bella*) ......... | 120 | 1.0 | 30.0 | 0 | 0 | 0 | 2.0 |
| (*Häagen-Dazs*) ...... | 120 | 0 | 30.0 | 0 | 0 | 0 | 2.0 |
| (*Sharon's*) .......... | 100 | 0 | 25.0 | 0 | 0 | 0 | 2.0 |
| (*So Delicious*) ....... | 110 | 0 | 27.0 | 0 | 0 | 150 | 2.0 |
| (*Whole Fruit*) ....... | 120 | 0 | 32.0 | 0 | 0 | 10 | <1.0 |
| strawberry: | | | | | | | |
| (*Ciao Bella*) ......... | 120 | 0 | 31.0 | 0 | 0 | 0 | 1.0 |
| (*Häagen-Dazs*) ...... | 120 | 0 | 31.0 | 0 | 0 | 0 | 1.0 |
| (*Sharon's*) .......... | 100 | 0 | 25.0 | 0 | 0 | 0 | 1.0 |
| (*Whole Fruit*) ....... | 120 | 0 | 31.0 | 0 | 0 | 10 | 1.0 |

| Food and Measure | cal. | prot. (gms) | carbo. (gms) | fat (gms) | chol. (mgs) | sod. (mgs) | fiber (gms) |
|---|---|---|---|---|---|---|---|
| **Sorbet bar** (see also "Fruit bar"), 1 bar: | | | | | | | |
| coffee, fudge (*Healthy Choice* Mocha Swirl) . | 90 | 3.0 | 17.0 | 1.0 | 5 | 40 | 1.0 |
| orange or raspberry, vanilla ice cream (*Healthy Choice*) ..... | 90 | 1.0 | 17.0 | 1.0 | 5 | 35 | 1.0 |
| **Sorghum**, whole-grain, 1 cup ............ | 650 | 21.7 | 143.3 | 6.3 | 0 | 12 | n.a. |
| **Sorghum flour** (*Bob's Red Mill* Gluten Free), ¼ cup ........ | 120 | 4.0 | 25.0 | 1.0 | 0 | 0 | 3.0 |
| **Sorghum syrup**: | | | | | | | |
| (*Eden* Organic), 1 tbsp. ............ | 60 | 0 | 14.0 | 0 | 0 | 0 | 0 |
| ½ cup ............... | 479 | 0 | 123.7 | 0 | 0 | 13 | 0 |
| 1 tbsp. ............. | 61 | 0 | 15.7 | 0 | 0 | 2 | 0 |
| **Sorrel**, see "Dock" | | | | | | | |
| **Soup**, ready-to-serve, 1 cup, except as noted: | | | | | | | |
| acorn squash and mango, creamy (*Imagine* Organic) .... | 70 | 1.0 | 14.0 | 1.5 | 0 | 430 | 2.0 |
| alphabet (*Amy's* Organic) ........... | 80 | 3.0 | 16.0 | 0 | 0 | 680 | 2.0 |
| bean: | | | | | | | |
| 5, vegetable (*Health Valley* Organic) .... | 100 | 5.0 | 23.0 | 0 | 0 | 480 | 6.0 |
| and ham (*Campbell's Chunky* Hearty) ... | 170 | 10.0 | 28.0 | 1.5 | 10 | 780 | 8.0 |
| and ham (*Healthy Choice*) .......... | 180 | 11.0 | 28.0 | 2.5 | 10 | 480 | 6.0 |
| and rice (*Amy's* Organic Tuscan) ... | 160 | 5.0 | 25.0 | 4.5 | 0 | 680 | 5.0 |
| bean, black: | | | | | | | |
| (*Health Valley* Organic No Salt) ... | 140 | 7.0 | 29.0 | 1.5 | 0 | 30 | 6.0 |
| (*Imagine Bistro* Organic Cuban) ... | 170 | 8.0 | 30.0 | 3.5 | 0 | 480 | 6.0 |
| (*Muir Glen* Organic Southwest) ....... | 130 | 7.0 | 25.0 | <1.0 | 0 | 680 | 8.0 |
| (*Progresso* Hearty) ... | 160 | 8.0 | 29.0 | 1.0 | <5 | 690 | 8.0 |

| Food and Measure | cal. | prot. (gms) | carbo. (gms) | fat (gms) | chol. (mgs) | sod. (mgs) | fiber (gms) |
|---|---|---|---|---|---|---|---|
| jalapeños (*Progresso* Fijoles Negros) .... | 130 | 7.0 | 30.0 | 1.0 | 0 | 690 | 7.0 |
| spicy (*Pacific* Organic) ......... | 80 | 4.0 | 14.0 | 1.0 | 0 | 590 | 4.0 |
| vegetable (*Amy's* Organic) ......... | 140 | 6.0 | 26.0 | 1.5 | 0 | 620 | 5.0 |
| vegetable (*Health Valley* Organic) .... | 110 | 5.0 | 25.0 | 0 | 0 | 480 | 5.0 |
| bean, white: | | | | | | | |
| (*Imagine* Organic Tuscan) ......... | 160 | 8.0 | 28.0 | 2.5 | 0 | 840 | n.a. |
| w/roasted ham (*Campbell's Select Harvest* Savory) ... | 170 | 9.0 | 30.0 | 1.5 | 5 | 480 | 7.0 |
| w/smoked bacon (*Pacific* Organic) .. | 220 | 13.0 | 27.0 | 7.0 | 10 | 780 | 7.0 |
| beef: | | | | | | | |
| and dumplings (*Campbell's Chunky*) | 130 | 8.0 | 20.0 | 1.5 | 25 | 800 | 3.0 |
| noodle (*Campbell's Chunky* Hearty) ... | 100 | 7.0 | 15.0 | 1.0 | 20 | 850 | 2.0 |
| rib roast, w/potato (*Campbell's Chunky*) | 110 | 7.0 | 17.0 | 1.0 | 10 | 890 | 2.0 |
| w/rice, white/wild (*Campbell's Chunky*) | 140 | 8.0 | 24.0 | 1.5 | 10 | 890 | 2.0 |
| slow-roasted, w/ mushrooms (*Campbell's Chunky*) | 120 | 8.0 | 18.0 | 1.5 | 15 | 830 | 3.0 |
| slow-roasted, and vegetables (*Campbell's Select Harvest*) .... | 100 | 7.0 | 17.0 | .5 | 10 | 480 | 2.0 |
| tips, roasted, w/ vegetables (*Campbell's Chunky*) | 130 | 8.0 | 20.0 | 1.5 | 15 | 800 | 2.0 |
| and vegetable (*Muir Glen* Organic) ..... | 90 | 5.0 | 12.0 | 3.0 | 10 | 890 | 2.0 |
| vegetable (*Progresso* Micro) .......... | 110 | 8.0 | 16.0 | 1.5 | 15 | 690 | 2.0 |
| vegetable (*Progresso* Reduced Sodium) . | 110 | 7.0 | 16.0 | 2.5 | 15 | 480 | 1.0 |
| vegetable (*Progresso*) | 120 | 8.0 | 18.0 | 2.0 | 15 | 690 | 2.0 |
| w/vegetables, country (*Campbell's Chunky*) | 130 | 8.0 | 18.0 | 3.0 | 15 | 920 | 3.0 |

| Food and Measure | cal. | prot. (gms) | carbo. (gms) | fat (gms) | chol. (mgs) | sod. (mgs) | fiber (gms) |
|---|---|---|---|---|---|---|---|
| **Soup, beef** *(cont.)* | | | | | | | |
| w/vegetables, country (*Campbell's Chunky* Micro) .... | 150 | 9.0 | 21.0 | 3.0 | 15 | 890 | 3.0 |
| beef, w/barley: | | | | | | | |
| (*Campbell's Chunky*) .. | 160 | 9.0 | 28.0 | 2.0 | 10 | 790 | 4.0 |
| (*Muir Glen* Organic) .. | 100 | 5.0 | 17.0 | 2.0 | 10 | 850 | 3.0 |
| (*Progresso*) ........ | 120 | 8.0 | 17.0 | 2.5 | 15 | 690 | 2.0 |
| (*Progresso* 99% Fat Free) ......... | 120 | 7.0 | 20.0 | 1.5 | 10 | 720 | 4.0 |
| roasted (*Campbell's Select Harvest*) .... | 130 | 9.0 | 22.0 | 1.0 | 10 | 480 | 3.0 |
| vegetable (*Progresso* Rich/Hearty) ...... | 140 | 9.0 | 17.0 | 2.5 | 15 | 690 | 2.0 |
| beef, pot roast: | | | | | | | |
| (*Campbell's Chunky* Savory) ......... | 120 | 7.0 | 20.0 | 1.0 | 10 | 790 | 2.0 |
| (*Healthy Choice*) ..... | 100 | 6.0 | 18.0 | 1.0 | 5 | 430 | 3.0 |
| (*Healthy Choice* Micro) .......... | 110 | 7.0 | 19.0 | .5 | 10 | 470 | 3.0 |
| (*Progresso* Light) .... | 80 | 7.0 | 12.0 | 1.0 | 10 | 660 | 2.0 |
| (*Progresso* Rich/ Hearty) .......... | 120 | 8.0 | 16.0 | 2.0 | 15 | 690 | 2.0 |
| beef broth: | | | | | | | |
| (*College Inn*) ........ | 25 | 4.0 | 0 | 1.0 | 0 | 900 | 0 |
| (*College Inn* Fat Free/Lower Sodium) ......... | 15 | 4.0 | 0 | 1.0 | 0 | 450 | 0 |
| (*College Inn* Organic) . | 15 | 2.0 | 2.0 | .5 | 0 | 490 | 0 |
| (*Health Valley* Organic No Salt) ... | 10 | 3.0 | 0 | 0 | 0 | 120 | 0 |
| (*Imagine* Organic) .... | 20 | 2.0 | 1.0 | 1.0 | 5 | 700 | 0 |
| (*Imagine* Organic Low Sodium) ..... | 15 | 1.0 | 1.0 | 1.0 | <5 | 140 | 0 |
| (*Pacific*) ............ | 20 | 4.0 | 1.0 | 0 | 0 | 570 | 0 |
| (*Pacific* Low Sodium) . | 15 | 3.0 | 1.0 | 0 | 0 | 140 | 0 |
| (*Pacific* Organic) ..... | 20 | 2.0 | 1.0 | 1.0 | 5 | 570 | 0 |
| (*Progresso*) ........ | 20 | 1.0 | 3.0 | 0 | 0 | 850 | 0 |
| (*Swanson*) ......... | 15 | 2.0 | 1.0 | 0 | 0 | 890 | 0 |
| (*Swanson* 50% Less Sodium) .......... | 15 | 3.0 | 1.0 | 0 | 0 | 440 | 0 |
| (*Swanson* Organic) ... | 15 | 2.0 | 1.0 | .5 | 0 | 550 | 0 |
| (*Tabatchnick*), ⅔ cup . | 5 | 0 | 0 | 0 | 0 | 560 | 0 |

| Food and Measure | cal. | prot. (gms) | carbo. (gms) | fat (gms) | chol. (mgs) | sod. (mgs) | fiber (gms) |
|---|---|---|---|---|---|---|---|
| beef stock: | | | | | | | |
| (*College Inn* Bold) .... | 45 | 7.0 | 4.0 | 0 | 0 | 730 | 0 |
| (*Imagine* Organic) .... | 15 | 3.0 | 1.0 | 0 | 0 | 630 | 0 |
| (*Imagine* Organic Low Sodium) ..... | 10 | 2.0 | <1.0 | 0 | 0 | 140 | 0 |
| (*Kitchen Basics*) ..... | 20 | 5.0 | 1.0 | 0 | 0 | 430 | 0 |
| (*Kitchen Basics* Unsalted) ........ | 20 | 5.0 | 1.0 | 0 | 0 | 190 | 0 |
| broccoli: | | | | | | | |
| cream of (*Campbell's Soup at Hand*), 1 cont. .......... | 160 | 3.0 | 15.0 | 10.0 | 5 | 970 | 3.0 |
| creamy (*Imagine* Organic) ......... | 60 | 3.0 | 10.0 | 1.5 | 0 | 470 | 2.0 |
| creamy, garden (*Imagine* Organic Light Sodium) .... | 70 | 2.0 | 12.0 | 1.5 | 0 | 200 | n.a. |
| garden (*Campbell's V8*) ............. | 90 | 3.0 | 15.0 | 2.0 | 5 | 480 | 3.0 |
| butternut squash: | | | | | | | |
| (*Amy's* Organic Light Sodium) ......... | 100 | 2.0 | 20.0 | 2.0 | 0 | 290 | 2.0 |
| creamy (*Imagine* Organic) ......... | 90 | 0 | 18.0 | 2.0 | 0 | 460 | 2.0 |
| creamy (*Pacific* Organic) ......... | 90 | 2.0 | 17.0 | 2.0 | 0 | 550 | 3.0 |
| creamy (*Pacific* Organic Low Sodium) ......... | 90 | 2.0 | 17.0 | 2.0 | 0 | 280 | 3.0 |
| golden (*Campbell's V8*) | 90 | 2.0 | 18.0 | 1.0 | 5 | 480 | 3.0 |
| carrot, cashew ginger creamy (*Pacific*) ..... | 120 | 1.0 | 19.0 | 5.0 | 0 | 650 | 3.0 |
| celery, cream of (*Health Valley* Organic) ...... | 90 | 2.0 | 11.0 | 5.0 | 0 | 680 | 1.0 |
| cheddar cheese (*Tabatchnick*), ⅔ cup . | 150 | 1.0 | 10.0 | 11.0 | 0 | 970 | 0 |
| chicken: | | | | | | | |
| (*Healthy Choice* Hearty) .......... | 130 | 8.0 | 18.0 | 2.0 | 15 | 480 | 3.0 |
| (*Progresso* Homestyle) | 100 | 7.0 | 14.0 | 2.0 | 10 | 690 | 1.0 |
| (*Progresso* Santa Fe Light) ............ | 80 | 5.0 | 12.0 | 1.0 | 10 | 670 | 2.0 |
| (*Progresso* Tuscany High Fiber) ....... | 130 | 9.0 | 20.0 | 3.0 | 15 | 690 | 7.0 |

| Food and Measure | cal. | prot. (gms) | carbo. (gms) | fat (gms) | chol. (mgs) | sod. (mgs) | fiber (gms) |
|---|---|---|---|---|---|---|---|
| **Soup, chicken** *(cont.)* | | | | | | | |
| Alfredo (*Campbell's Select Harvest*) .... | 220 | 10.0 | 15.0 | 13.0 | 20 | 480 | 1.0 |
| barley (*Progresso*) ... | 80 | 7.0 | 11.0 | 1.0 | 15 | 690 | 2.0 |
| w/beans, white, herbs (*Campbell's Select Harvest* Tuscany) .. | 90 | 7.0 | 12.0 | 1.5 | 10 | 480 | 4.0 |
| broccoli, cheese, and potato (*Campbell's Chunky*) | 210 | 7.0 | 20.0 | 11.0 | 20 | 880 | 3.0 |
| cheese enchilada (*Progresso*) ...... | 170 | 8.0 | 9.0 | 11.0 | 25 | 890 | 1.0 |
| cream of (*Health Valley* Organic) .... | 110 | 3.0 | 11.0 | 6.0 | 15 | 680 | 1.0 |
| creamy (*Campbell's Soup at Hand*), 1 cont. .......... | 150 | 3.0 | 13.0 | 9.0 | 5 | 880 | 2.0 |
| creamy (*Imagine* Organic) ......... | 70 | 3.0 | 12.0 | 1.5 | 5 | 680 | 1.0 |
| and dumplings (*Campbell's Chunky*) | 180 | 8.0 | 19.0 | 8.0 | 30 | 890 | 3.0 |
| and dumplings (*Campbell's Chunky* Micro) .......... | 190 | 8.0 | 18.0 | 9.0 | 30 | 890 | 3.0 |
| and dumplings (*Healthy Choice*) .. | 150 | 8.0 | 22.0 | 3.0 | 25 | 480 | 3.0 |
| and dumplings (*Progresso* Light) .. | 80 | 6.0 | 12.0 | 1.5 | 20 | 690 | 2.0 |
| and dumplings, herb (*Progresso*) ...... | 100 | 5.0 | 13.0 | 2.5 | 25 | 650 | 1.0 |
| fajita, w/rice, beans (*Campbell's Chunky*) | 130 | 7.0 | 23.0 | 1.5 | 15 | 850 | 2.0 |
| fajita, spicy (*Pacific* Organic) ......... | 160 | 8.0 | 26.0 | 2.5 | 5 | 710 | 5.0 |
| grilled, w/vegetables, pasta (*Campbell's Chunky*) ......... | 110 | 6.0 | 14.0 | 2.5 | 15 | 880 | 2.0 |
| gumbo (*Glen Muir* Organic Cajun) .... | 90 | 4.0 | 14.0 | <1.0 | 10 | 810 | 1.0 |
| gumbo (*Progresso* Reduced Sodium) . | 110 | 7.0 | 18.0 | 1.5 | 15 | 450 | 2.0 |
| w/meatballs (*Progresso* Chickarina) ....... | 130 | 8.0 | 14.0 | 5.0 | 20 | 690 | 1.0 |

| Food and Measure | cal. | prot. (gms) | carbo. (gms) | fat (gms) | chol. (mgs) | sod. (mgs) | fiber (gms) |
|---|---|---|---|---|---|---|---|
| w/penne (*Pacific* Organic) ......... | 80 | 5.0 | 14.0 | 1.0 | 15 | 790 | 1.0 |
| pot pie (*Progresso* Rich/Hearty) ...... | 140 | 7.0 | 19.0 | 4.0 | 10 | 770 | 2.0 |
| rotini (*Progresso*) .... | 100 | 7.0 | 13.0 | 2.0 | 15 | 690 | 1.0 |
| Southwest (*Progresso*) | 120 | 6.0 | 18.0 | 2.0 | 10 | 740 | 2.0 |
| and stars (*Campbell's Soup at Hand*), 1 cont. ......... | 70 | 3.0 | 10.0 | 2.0 | 5 | 960 | 1.0 |
| chicken, roasted: | | | | | | | |
| garlic (*Progresso*) .... | 100 | 7.0 | 13.0 | 2.0 | 20 | 690 | 1.0 |
| w/Italian herbs (*Campbell's Select Harvest* Light) .... | 80 | 6.0 | 9.0 | 2.5 | 10 | 480 | 3.0 |
| rotini (*Progresso*) .... | 80 | 5.0 | 10.0 | 2.0 | 10 | 670 | <1.0 |
| w/rotini and penne (*Campbell's Select Harvest*) ......... | 90 | 7.0 | 13.0 | 1.5 | 10 | 480 | 1.0 |
| chicken broth/stock: | | | | | | | |
| (*Campbell's* Low Sodium), 1 can ... | 30 | 3.0 | 1.0 | 1.0 | 5 | 140 | 0 |
| (*College Inn*) ........ | 15 | 1.0 | 0 | 1.0 | 0 | 930 | 0 |
| (*College Inn* Light & Fat Free) ....... | 5 | 1.0 | 0 | 0 | 0 | 450 | 0 |
| (*College Inn* Organic) . | 15 | 2.0 | <1.0 | 0 | 0 | 510 | 0 |
| (*Health Valley* Organic) ......... | 25 | 6.0 | 0 | 0 | 0 | 390 | 0 |
| (*Health Valley* Organic No Salt) ... | 35 | 5.0 | 0 | 1.5 | 0 | 130 | 0 |
| (*Imagine* Organic) .... | 10 | 1.0 | 1.0 | 0 | 0 | 570 | 0 |
| (*Imagine* Organic Low Sodium) ..... | 20 | 1.0 | 1.0 | 1.0 | 5 | 95 | 0 |
| (*Pacific/Pacific/ Organic*) ......... | 10 | 1.0 | 1.0 | 0 | 0 | 570 | 0 |
| (*Pacific* Organic Low Sodium) ..... | 15 | 2.0 | 1.0 | 0 | 0 | 70 | 0 |
| (*Progresso*) ........ | 20 | 3.0 | 1.0 | 0 | 0 | 850 | 0 |
| (*Progresso* Reduced Sodium) ........ | 20 | 3.0 | 2.0 | 0 | 0 | 560 | 0 |
| (*Swanson*) ........ | 10 | 1.0 | 1.0 | .5 | 5 | 860 | 0 |
| (*Swanson* Organic) ... | 15 | 1.0 | 1.0 | .5 | 0 | 550 | 0 |
| (*Swanson Natural Goodness*) ....... | 15 | 2.0 | 1.0 | 0 | 0 | 570 | 0 |
| (*Tabatchnick*), ⅔ cup . | 5 | 0 | 0 | 0 | 0 | 550 | 0 |

| Food and Measure | cal. | prot. (gms) | carbo. (gms) | fat (gms) | chol. (mgs) | sod. (mgs) | fiber (gms) |
|---|---|---|---|---|---|---|---|
| **Soup, chicken broth/stock** *(cont.)* | | | | | | | |
| (*Tabatchnick* Kosher/ Organic), ⅔ cup ... | 10 | 0 | 1.0 | 0 | 0 | 590 | 0 |
| w/roasted garlic (*College Inn*) ..... | 20 | 1.0 | 3.0 | 0 | 0 | 1000 | 0 |
| w/roasted vegetables, herbs (*College Inn*) | 20 | 1.0 | 3.0 | 0 | 0 | 1060 | 0 |
| stock (*Imagine* Organic) ......... | 15 | 3.0 | 1.0 | 0 | 0 | 610 | 0 |
| stock (*Imagine* Organic Low Sodium) | 15 | <1.0 | <1.0 | 1.0 | 0 | 140 | 0 |
| stock (*Kitchen Basics*) | 20 | 5.0 | 1.0 | 0 | 0 | 260 | 0 |
| stock (*Kitchen Basics* Unsalted) ........ | 20 | 5.0 | 1.0 | 0 | 0 | 150 | 0 |
| vegetarian (*Imagine* Organic No-Chicken) ...... | 10 | 1.0 | 2.0 | 0 | 0 | 450 | 0 |
| chicken noodle: | | | | | | | |
| (*Annie Chun's* Bowl), ½ cont. .......... | 130 | 4.0 | 26.0 | 1.0 | 0 | 500 | 1.0 |
| (*Campbell's* Low Sodium), 1 can ... | 160 | 12.0 | 17.0 | 4.5 | 30 | 140 | 2.0 |
| (*Campbell's* Micro) ... | 70 | 3.0 | 10.0 | 2.0 | 15 | 870 | 1.0 |
| (*Campbell's* Micro Homestyle) ....... | 70 | 3.0 | 10.0 | 2.0 | 10 | 890 | 0 |
| (*Campbell's Chunky* Classic) ......... | 120 | 8.0 | 14.0 | 3.0 | 25 | 790 | 2.0 |
| (*Campbell's Chunky* Micro) .......... | 110 | 6.0 | 14.0 | 3.0 | 25 | 790 | 2.0 |
| (*Campbell's Chunky Healthy Request* Classic) ......... | 120 | 8.0 | 17.0 | 2.5 | 20 | 410 | 2.0 |
| (*Campbell's Chunky Healthy Request* Classic Micro) .... | 120 | 7.0 | 17.0 | 3.0 | 20 | 410 | 1.0 |
| (*Health Valley* Organic) ......... | 80 | 4.0 | 11.0 | 2.5 | 15 | 480 | 3.0 |
| (*Healthy Choice* Old Fashioned) | 100 | 8.0 | 12.0 | 1.5 | 15 | 460 | 2.0 |
| (*Healthy Choice* Old Fashioned Micro) .. | 90 | 7.0 | 14.0 | 2.0 | 15 | 460 | 2.0 |
| (*Imagine* Organic) .... | 90 | n.a. | 12.0 | 2.0 | 15 | 730 | n.a. |
| (*Muir Glen* Organic) .. | 70 | 4.0 | 10.0 | 2.0 | 10 | 800 | 1.0 |
| (*Progresso*) ........ | 100 | 7.0 | 12.0 | 2.5 | 20 | 690 | 1.0 |

| Food and Measure | cal. | prot. (gms) | carbo. (gms) | fat (gms) | chol. (mgs) | sod. (mgs) | fiber (gms) |
|---|---|---|---|---|---|---|---|
| (*Progresso* 99% Fat Free) . . . . . . . . | 90 | 6.0 | 12.0 | 2.0 | 20 | 670 | 1.0 |
| (*Progresso* Homestyle) | 110 | 8.0 | 14.0 | 2.5 | 20 | 690 | 1.0 |
| (*Progresso* Light) . . . . | 70 | 5.0 | 10.0 | 1.5 | 20 | 680 | 2.0 |
| (*Progresso* Micro) . . . | 90 | 6.0 | 10.0 | 2.5 | 20 | 690 | 1.0 |
| (*Progresso* Reduced Sodium) . . . . . . . . | 90 | 6.0 | 13.0 | 2.0 | 20 | 470 | 1.0 |
| egg noodle (*Campbell's Select Harvest*) . . . . | 100 | 8.0 | 11.0 | 3.0 | 25 | 480 | 1.0 |
| egg noodle (*Campbell's Select Harvest* Micro) . . . . . . . . . . | 110 | 8.0 | 13.0 | 3.0 | 25 | 480 | 1.0 |
| mini (*Campbell's Soup at Hand*), 1 cont. . . | 80 | 4.0 | 11.0 | 2.0 | 10 | 980 | 2.0 |
| mini (*Campbell's Soup at Hand* 25% Less Sodium), 1 cont. . . | 80 | 4.0 | 11.0 | 2.0 | 10 | 730 | 2.0 |
| chicken pot pie (*Imagine* Organic) . . . . | 160 | 7.0 | 22.0 | 4.5 | 20 | 670 | n.a. |
| chicken rice: |  |  |  |  |  |  |  |
| (*Health Valley* Organic) . . . . . . . . | 90 | 4.0 | 14.0 | 2.0 | 10 | 480 | 3.0 |
| (*Healthy Choice*) . . . . . | 120 | 6.0 | 14.0 | 1.5 | 15 | 460 | 2.0 |
| (*Healthy Choice* Fiesta) . . . . . . . . | 100 | 6.0 | 15.0 | 1.5 | 5 | 420 | 3.0 |
| (*Healthy Choice* Micro) . . . . . . . . . | 100 | 5.0 | 14.0 | 2.0 | 10 | 450 | 2.0 |
| long grain (*Campbell's Select Harvest* Can/Micro) | 110 | 6.0 | 18.0 | 1.0 | 15 | 480 | 1.0 |
| white/wild (*Campbell's Chunky* Savory) . . . | 110 | 6.0 | 18.0 | 2.0 | 10 | 810 | 2.0 |
| chicken rice, wild: |  |  |  |  |  |  |  |
| (*Imagine* Organic) . . . . | 100 | 4.0 | 15.0 | 2.0 | 5 | 710 | n.a. |
| (*Muir Glen* Organic) . . | 70 | 4.0 | 10.0 | 2.0 | 10 | 710 | 1.0 |
| (*Pacific* Organic Savory) . . . . . . . . . | 80 | 4.0 | 15.0 | 0 | 5.0 | 670 | 1.0 |
| (*Progresso*) . . . . . . . . | 100 | 6.0 | 15.0 | 1.5 | 15 | 650 | 1.0 |
| (*Progresso* Micro) . . . | 120 | 6.0 | 22.0 | 1.5 | 10 | 680 | 2.0 |
| (*Progresso* Reduced Sodium) . . . . . . . . | 120 | 6.0 | 20.0 | 2.0 | 15 | 470 | 1.0 |
| creamy (*Progresso* Rich/Hearty) . . . . . . | 140 | 6.0 | 18.0 | 5.0 | 15 | 860 | 1.0 |

| Food and Measure | cal. | prot. (gms) | carbo. (gms) | fat (gms) | chol. (mgs) | sod. (mgs) | fiber (gms) |
|---|---|---|---|---|---|---|---|
| **Soup** *(cont.)* | | | | | | | |
| chicken sausage gumbo: | | | | | | | |
| (*Progresso*) ........ | 130 | 6.0 | 18.0 | 3.5 | 15 | 650 | 1.0 |
| grilled (*Campbell's Chunky*) ......... | 140 | 7.0 | 21.0 | 3.0 | 20 | 850 | 2.0 |
| grilled (*Campbell's Chunky* Micro) .... | 140 | 7.0 | 18.0 | 4.0 | 15 | 780 | 1.0 |
| grilled (*Campbell's Chunky Healthy Request*) ........ | 140 | 8.0 | 21.0 | 3.0 | 15 | 410 | 3.0 |
| grilled (*Campbell's Chunky Healthy Request* Micro) ... | 130 | 7.0 | 18.0 | 3.0 | 10 | 410 | 2.0 |
| chicken tortilla: | | | | | | | |
| (*Glen Muir* Organic) .. | 120 | 6.0 | 17.0 | 3.0 | 10 | 830 | 3.0 |
| (*Healthy Choice*) ..... | 140 | 9.0 | 23.0 | 1.5 | 15 | 390 | 6.0 |
| (*Healthy Choice* Micro) .......... | 140 | 9.0 | 23.0 | 1.5 | 15 | 420 | 5.0 |
| (*Progresso* Tortilla y Pollo) ......... | 110 | 6.0 | 17.0 | 2.5 | 10 | 690 | 3.0 |
| Mexican (*Campbell's Select Harvest*) .... | 110 | 7.0 | 17.0 | 2.0 | 10 | 480 | 2.0 |
| Mexican (*Campbell's Select Harvest Healthy Request*) .. | 130 | 7.0 | 20.0 | 2.0 | 15 | 410 | 3.0 |
| chicken vegetable: | | | | | | | |
| (*Campbell's Chunky Hearty*) .......... | 110 | 6.0 | 17.0 | 2.0 | 15 | 710 | 3.0 |
| (*Campbell's Select Harvest* Light) .... | 80 | 5.0 | 14.0 | 1.0 | 10 | 480 | 2.0 |
| (*Campbell's Select Harvest* Medley) ... | 120 | 7.0 | 20.0 | 1.5 | 10 | 480 | 1.0 |
| (*Progresso* Caldo de Pollo) ........... | 90 | 5.0 | 14.0 | 1.5 | 10 | 690 | 1.0 |
| roasted (*Progresso* Light) ........... | 70 | 5.0 | 10.0 | 1.0 | 15 | 460 | 3.0 |
| rotini (*Progresso* Light) ........... | 70 | 5.0 | 11.0 | 1.0 | 10 | 660 | 2.0 |
| chickpea bisque (*Imagine Bistro* Organic Moroccan) ... | 120 | 5.0 | 16.0 | 4.0 | 0 | 660 | n.a. |
| chili (see also "Chili"), 3 bean, w/beef (*Progresso* High Fiber) | 140 | 8.0 | 23.0 | 4.0 | 10 | 480 | 7.0 |

| Food and Measure | cal. | prot. (gms) | carbo. (gms) | fat (gms) | chol. (mgs) | sod. (mgs) | fiber (gms) |
|---|---|---|---|---|---|---|---|
| clam chowder, Manhattan: | | | | | | | |
| (*Campbell's Chunky*) .. | 130 | 5.0 | 19.0 | 3.5 | 5 | 830 | 3.0 |
| (*Progresso*) ........ | 100 | 3.0 | 17.0 | 2.0 | 5 | 690 | 2.0 |
| clam chowder, New England: | | | | | | | |
| (*Campbell's Chunky*) .. | 230 | 7.0 | 20.0 | 13.0 | 10 | 890 | 3.0 |
| (*Campbell's Chunky* Micro) ......... | 200 | 6.0 | 17.0 | 12.0 | 10 | 870 | 3.0 |
| (*Campbell's Chunky* Healthy Request) .. | 130 | 5.0 | 20.0 | 3.0 | 10 | 410 | 2.0 |
| (*Campbell's Select* Harvest) ......... | 180 | 5.0 | 17.0 | 10.0 | 10 | 480 | 3.0 |
| (*Campbell's Select* Harvest 98% Fat Free) | 110 | 6.0 | 17.0 | 2.5 | 10 | 480 | 1.0 |
| (*Campbell's Soup at* Hand), 1 cont. .... | 150 | 3.0 | 13.0 | 10.0 | 5 | 890 | 3.0 |
| (*Healthy Choice*) ..... | 110 | 4.0 | 20.0 | 1.5 | 10 | 480 | 3.0 |
| (*Progresso*) ........ | 180 | 6.0 | 20.0 | 9.0 | 15 | 890 | 1.0 |
| (*Progresso* 99% Fat Free) ............ | 110 | 4.0 | 21.0 | 1.5 | 5 | 810 | 2.0 |
| (*Progresso* Light) .... | 100 | 3.0 | 20.0 | 2.5 | <5 | 690 | 4.0 |
| (*Progresso* Rich/ Hearty) .......... | 180 | 5.0 | 22.0 | 8.0 | 15 | 8640 | 2.0 |
| clam stock (*Kitchen Basics*) ............. | 20 | 3.0 | 1.0 | 0 | 0 | 600 | 0 |
| coconut, Thai (*Amy's*), ½ can ............. | 140 | 4.0 | 9.0 | 10.0 | 0 | 580 | 2.0 |
| corn: | | | | | | | |
| chipotle bisque (*Imagine Bistro* Organic) ......... | 100 | 3.0 | 22.0 | 1.0 | 0 | 590 | 2.0 |
| creamy, harvest (*Imagine* Organic Light Sodium) .... | 110 | 3.0 | 20.0 | 3.0 | 0 | 220 | n.a. |
| creamy, lemongrass (*Imagine* Organic) . | 120 | 4.0 | 20.0 | 3.0 | 0 | 450 | 3.0 |
| Southwest (*Campbell's* V8) ............. | 140 | 3.0 | 24.0 | 3.0 | 0 | 480 | 3.0 |
| and vegetable (*Amy's* Organic Summer) . | 150 | 4.0 | 23.0 | 6.0 | 15 | 680 | 3.0 |
| and vegetable (*Health Valley* Organic) .... | 100 | 3.0 | 22.0 | 0 | 0 | 460 | 4.0 |

|  | cal. | prot. (gms) | carbo. (gms) | fat (gms) | chol. (mgs) | sod. (mgs) | fiber (gms) |
|---|---|---|---|---|---|---|---|
| **Soup** *(cont.)* | | | | | | | |
| corn chowder: | | | | | | | |
| chicken (*Campbell's* *Chunky* Can/Micro) | 200 | 7.0 | 20.0 | 10.0 | 15 | 860 | 2.0 |
| chicken (*Campbell's* *Chunky Healthy* *Request*) ........ | 140 | 7.0 | 22.0 | 3.0 | 10 | 410 | 3.0 |
| chicken (*Progresso*) .. | 200 | 7.0 | 23.0 | 9.0 | 15 | 890 | 2.0 |
| poblano pepper and (*Pacific*) ......... | 190 | 3.0 | 22.0 | 10.0 | 35 | 700 | 1.0 |
| crab: | | | | | | | |
| cream of (*Chincoteague*) .... | 200 | 11.0 | 23.0 | 6.0 | 35 | 830 | 0 |
| Maryland style (*Campbell's Select* *Harvest* Light) .... | 80 | 3.0 | 16.0 | .5 | 5 | 480 | 2.0 |
| curry, Thai: | | | | | | | |
| green (*Tiger Tiger*) ... | 358 | 7.0 | 24.0 | 26.0 | 0 | 320 | <1.0 |
| red, spicy (*Tiger* *Tiger*), ½ cup ..... | 90 | <1.0 | 23.0 | 0 | 0 | 20 | 2.0 |
| garlic, roasted, and mushroom (*Pacific*) .. | 210 | 7.0 | 37.0 | 3.5 | 10 | 740 | 7.0 |
| gumbo (*Healthy* *Choice* Zesty) ....... | 100 | 5.0 | 15.0 | 2.0 | 10 | 460 | 2.0 |
| ham stock (*Kitchen* *Basics*) ............. | 20 | 3.0 | 1.0 | 0 | 0 | 480 | 0 |
| hot and sour, noodle (*Annie Chun's* Bowl), ½ cont. ...... | 140 | 4.0 | 28.0 | 1.0 | 0 | 450 | 1.0 |
| Italian style wedding: | | | | | | | |
| (*Campbell's Chunky*) .. | 160 | 8.0 | 24.0 | 3.0 | 15 | 650 | 3.0 |
| (*Campbell's Select* *Harvest* Can) ..... | 140 | 7.0 | 16.0 | 5.0 | 15 | 480 | 2.0 |
| (*Campbell's Select* *Harvest* Micro) .... | 120 | 7.0 | 15.0 | 3.0 | 15 | 840 | 2.0 |
| (*Campbell's Select* *Harvest Healthy* *Request*) ........ | 110 | 6.0 | 15.0 | 2.5 | 10 | 410 | 2.0 |
| (*Healthy Choice*) ..... | 120 | 9.0 | 16.0 | 2.5 | 10 | 430 | 4.0 |
| (*Healthy Choice* Micro) .......... | 140 | 11.0 | 19.0 | 2.5 | 10 | 480 | 3.0 |
| (*Progresso*) ........ | 120 | 7.0 | 11.0 | 4.0 | 15 | 690 | 2.0 |
| (*Progresso* Micro) ... | 120 | 6.0 | 13.0 | 4.5 | 15 | 690 | 1.0 |

| Food and Measure | cal. | prot. (gms) | carbo. (gms) | fat (gms) | chol. (mgs) | sod. (mgs) | fiber (gms) |
|---|---|---|---|---|---|---|---|
| (*Progresso* Reduced Sodium) | 120 | 6.0 | 16.0 | 3.0 | 5 | 480 | 2.0 |
| kimchi noodle (*Annie Chun's* Bowl), ½ cont. | 140 | 6.0 | 28.0 | 1.5 | 0 | 720 | 1.0 |
| lentil: | | | | | | | |
| (*Amy's* Organic) | 180 | 8.0 | 25.0 | 5.0 | 0 | 590 | 6.0 |
| (*Amy's* Organic Light Sodium) | 180 | 8.0 | 25.0 | 5.0 | 0 | 290 | 6.0 |
| (*Health Valley* Organic No Salt) | 140 | 9.0 | 27.0 | 1.5 | 0 | 30 | 8.0 |
| (*Healthy Choice* Micro Traditional) | 150 | 7.0 | 27.0 | 2.0 | 5 | 440 | 5.0 |
| (*Muir Glen* Organic Savory) | 130 | 6.0 | 23.0 | 2.0 | 0 | 950 | 3.0 |
| (*Progresso*) | 160 | 9.0 | 30.0 | 2.0 | 0 | 810 | 5.0 |
| (*Progresso* 99% Fat Free) | 140 | 8.0 | 25.0 | 1.5 | 0 | 500 | 3.0 |
| apple (*Imagine* Organic) | 150 | 6.0 | 29.0 | 5.0 | 0 | 680 | n.a. |
| and carrot (*Health Valley* Organic) | 110 | 8.0 | 24.0 | 0 | 0 | 450 | 8.0 |
| curried (*Amy's*) | 230 | 9.0 | 30.0 | 8.0 | 0 | 680 | 11.0 |
| curried, red (*Pacific*) | 140 | 5.0 | 19.0 | 4.5 | 0 | 720 | 5.0 |
| golden (*Amy's* Indian) | 220 | 9.0 | 25.0 | 9.0 | 0 | 680 | 7.0 |
| vegetable (*Amy's* Organic) | 160 | 7.0 | 24.0 | 4.0 | 0 | 680 | 8.0 |
| vegetable (*Amy's* Organic Light Sodium) | 160 | 7.0 | 24.0 | 4.0 | 0 | 340 | 8.0 |
| vegetable, roasted red pepper (*Pacific*) | 150 | 8.0 | 27.0 | .5 | 0 | 760 | 7.0 |
| macaroni and bean (*Progresso*) | 160 | 8.0 | 25.0 | 3.5 | 0 | 690 | 6.0 |
| meatball: | | | | | | | |
| (*Progresso* Italian Light) | 80 | 3.0 | 13.0 | 2.0 | 5 | 460 | 2.0 |
| w/bow-tie pasta (*Campbell's Select Harvest* Mediterranean) | 120 | 7.0 | 15.0 | 4.0 | 20 | 740 | 2.0 |
| and orzo (*Imagine* Organic) | 150 | 9.0 | 20.0 | 3.5 | 10 | 730 | n.a. |
| and rice (*Campbell's Select Harvest* Azteca) | 130 | 5.0 | 18.0 | 5.0 | 15 | 730 | 1.0 |

| Food and Measure | cal. | prot. (gms) | carbo. (gms) | fat (gms) | chol. (mgs) | sod. (mgs) | fiber (gms) |
|---|---|---|---|---|---|---|---|
| **Soup, meatball** *(cont.)* | | | | | | | |
| and rice (*Progresso* | | | | | | | |
| Albondigas) ...... | 130 | 5.0 | 18.0 | 4.5 | 20 | 690 | 2.0 |
| minestrone: | | | | | | | |
| (*Amy's* Organic) ..... | 90 | 3.0 | 17.0 | 1.5 | 0 | 580 | 3.0 |
| (*Amy's* Organic Light | | | | | | | |
| Sodium) ......... | 90 | 3.0 | 17.0 | 1.5 | 0 | 290 | 3.0 |
| (*Campbell's Select* | | | | | | | |
| *Harvest*) ........ | 100 | 5.0 | 20.0 | .5 | 0 | 480 | 3.0 |
| (*Campbell's Select* | | | | | | | |
| *Harvest* Light) .... | 80 | 4.0 | 14.0 | .5 | 0 | 480 | 4.0 |
| (*Health Valley* | | | | | | | |
| Organic) ......... | 110 | 6.0 | 26.0 | 0 | 0 | 470 | 7.0 |
| (*Health Valley* | | | | | | | |
| Organic No Salt) ... | 90 | 4.0 | 16.0 | 2.0 | 0 | 50 | 3.0 |
| (*Healthy Choice* | | | | | | | |
| Micro) .......... | 140 | 6.0 | 27.0 | 1.0 | 5 | 360 | 6.0 |
| (*Imagine* Organic) .... | 120 | 4.0 | 20.0 | 3.5 | 0 | 800 | n.a. |
| (*Muir Glen* Organic | | | | | | | |
| Classic) ......... | 110 | 4.0 | 19.0 | 2.0 | 0 | 960 | 5.0 |
| (*Progresso*) ........ | 100 | 4.0 | 20.0 | 2.0 | 0 | 690 | 4.0 |
| (*Progresso* 99% | | | | | | | |
| Fat Free) ......... | 100 | 5.0 | 19.0 | 1.0 | 0 | 600 | 5.0 |
| (*Progresso* Homestyle | | | | | | | |
| High Fiber) ....... | 110 | 5.0 | 24.0 | 2.0 | 0 | 690 | 7.0 |
| (*Progresso* Micro) ... | 90 | 4.0 | 17.0 | 1.5 | 0 | 690 | 4.0 |
| (*Progresso* Reduced | | | | | | | |
| Sodium) ......... | 120 | 5.0 | 22.0 | 2.0 | 0 | 470 | 4.0 |
| miso noodle (*Annie* | | | | | | | |
| *Chun's*), ½ cont. ..... | 110 | 3.0 | 23.0 | 1.0 | 0 | 450 | 1.0 |
| mushroom, cream of: | | | | | | | |
| (*Amy's* Organic) ..... | 150 | 3.0 | 13.0 | 9.0 | 10 | 590 | 2.0 |
| (*Campbell's* Low | | | | | | | |
| Sodium), 1 can ... | 160 | 3.0 | 19.0 | 8.0 | 15 | 60 | 0 |
| (*Health Valley* | | | | | | | |
| Organic) ......... | 100 | 2.0 | 11.0 | .5 | 15 | 680 | 1.0 |
| (*Tabatchnick*), ⅔ cup . | 30 | <1.0 | 3.0 | 2.0 | 5 | 490 | 0 |
| creamy (*Progresso*) .. | 120 | 2.0 | 9.0 | 8.0 | 5 | 890 | 1.0 |
| portobello, creamy | | | | | | | |
| (*Imagine*) ........ | 80 | 3.0 | 10.0 | 3.0 | 0 | 390 | 3.0 |
| mushroom barley | | | | | | | |
| (*Health Valley* Organic | | | | | | | |
| No Salt) ........... | 90 | 2.0 | 15.0 | 2.5 | 0 | 60 | 3.0 |

| Food and Measure | cal. | prot. (gms) | carbo. (gms) | fat (gms) | chol. (mgs) | sod. (mgs) | fiber (gms) |
|---|---|---|---|---|---|---|---|
| mushroom broth | | | | | | | |
| (*Pacific* Organic) ..... | 5 | 0 | 1.0 | 0 | 0 | 530 | 0 |
| noodle (*Amy's* No | | | | | | | |
| Chicken) .......... | 100 | 5.0 | 13.0 | 3.0 | 0 | 540 | 2.0 |
| onion, French: | | | | | | | |
| (*Campbell's Select* | | | | | | | |
| *Harvest*) ......... | 80 | 3.0 | 12.0 | 2.0 | 5 | 480 | 1.0 |
| (*Pacific* Organic) ..... | 30 | 1.0 | 5.0 | 1.0 | 0 | 720 | 0 |
| (*Progresso*) ........ | 50 | 2.0 | 9.0 | 1.0 | 0 | 690 | 1.0 |
| pasta and 3-bean | | | | | | | |
| (*Amy's* Organic) ..... | 150 | 5.0 | 22.0 | 4.0 | 0 | 680 | 4.0 |
| pea, split: | | | | | | | |
| (*Amy's* Organic) ..... | 100 | 7.0 | 19.0 | 0 | 0 | 670 | 6.0 |
| (*Amy's* Organic | | | | | | | |
| Light Sodium) .... | 100 | 7.0 | 19.0 | 0 | 0 | 330 | 6.0 |
| (*Health Valley* | | | | | | | |
| Organic No Salt) ... | 140 | 8.0 | 26.0 | 2.5 | 0 | 85 | 8.0 |
| (*Imagine* Organic | | | | | | | |
| Country) ........ | 180 | 9.0 | 30.0 | 2.5 | 5 | 760 | n.a. |
| (*Muir Glen* Organic | | | | | | | |
| Homestyle) ....... | 170 | 10.0 | 35.0 | 1.0 | 0 | 900 | 5.0 |
| w/bacon, Swiss cheese | | | | | | | |
| (*Pacific* Organic) .. | 260 | 13.0 | 29.0 | 10.0 | 20 | 640 | 11.0 |
| and carrot (*Health* | | | | | | | |
| *Valley* Organic) .... | 120 | 7.0 | 26.0 | 0 | 0 | 480 | 7.0 |
| green (*Progresso*) ... | 160 | 9.0 | 28.0 | 2.0 | 0 | 690 | 4.0 |
| and ham (*Campbell's* | | | | | | | |
| *Chunky*) ......... | 190 | 12.0 | 30.0 | 2.5 | 10 | 780 | 5.0 |
| w/ham (*Healthy* | | | | | | | |
| *Choice*) .......... | 160 | 12.0 | 27.0 | 2.5 | 10 | 470 | 6.0 |
| w/ham (*Progresso*) ... | 140 | 9.0 | 24.0 | 1.0 | 5 | 690 | 4.0 |
| w/ham, roasted | | | | | | | |
| (*Campbell's Select* | | | | | | | |
| *Harvest*) ......... | 150 | 9.0 | 29.0 | 1.0 | 5 | 480 | 5.0 |
| pea, sweet, creamy | | | | | | | |
| (*Imagine* Organic) .... | 80 | 4.0 | 14.0 | 1.5 | 0 | 570 | 3.0 |
| penne, in chicken | | | | | | | |
| broth (*Progresso*) .... | 80 | 3.0 | 14.0 | 1.0 | 0 | 710 | 1.0 |
| pork stock (*Kitchen* | | | | | | | |
| *Basics*) ............. | 20 | 3.0 | 1.0 | 0 | 0 | 480 | 0 |
| potato: | | | | | | | |
| broccoli cheese | | | | | | | |
| (*Campbell's* | | | | | | | |
| *Select Harvest*) .... | 160 | 3.0 | 17.0 | 9.0 | 5 | 480 | 3.0 |

| Food and Measure | cal. | prot. (gms) | carbo. (gms) | fat (gms) | chol. (mgs) | sod. (mgs) | fiber (gms) |
|---|---|---|---|---|---|---|---|
| **Soup** *(cont.)* | | | | | | | |
| broccoli cheese | | | | | | | |
|   chowder (*Progresso*) | 210 | 5.0 | 20.0 | 12.0 | 15 | 860 | 2.0 |
|   w/garlic, roasted | | | | | | | |
|     (*Imagine* Organic) . | 120 | 2.0 | 22.0 | 3.0 | 15 | 700 | n.a. |
|   w/garlic, roasted, creamy | | | | | | | |
|     (*Campbell's Select* | | | | | | | |
|     *Harvest*) . . . . . . . . | 180 | 3.0 | 20.0 | 10.0 | 10 | 480 | 2.0 |
|   rosemary (*Pacific*) . . . | 230 | 1.0 | 36.0 | 8.0 | 30 | 730 | 2.0 |
|   red bliss (*Imagine* | | | | | | | |
|     Organic) . . . . . . . . . | 100 | 3.0 | 18.0 | 2.5 | 0 | 220 | n.a. |
| potato, baked: | | | | | | | |
|   w/cheddar, bacon | | | | | | | |
|     bits (*Campbell's* | | | | | | | |
|     *Chunky*) . . . . . . . . . | 190 | 5.0 | 23.0 | 9.0 | 10 | 790 | 2.0 |
|   w/steak, cheese | | | | | | | |
|     (*Campbell's Chunky*) | 200 | 8.0 | 21.0 | 9.0 | 15 | 840 | 3.0 |
| potato ham chowder | | | | | | | |
|   (*Campbell's Chunky* | | | | | | | |
|   Old Fashioned) . . . . . . | 190 | 6.0 | 17.0 | 11.0 | 20 | 800 | 3.0 |
| potato leek, organic: | | | | | | | |
|   (*Health Valley* No | | | | | | | |
|   Salt) . . . . . . . . . . . . | 100 | 2.0 | 20.0 | 2.0 | 0 | 30 | 3.0 |
|   creamy (*Imagine*) . . . . | 70 | 3.0 | 12.0 | 1.5 | 5 | 680 | 3.0 |
| red pepper, roasted, | | | | | | | |
|   tomato: | | | | | | | |
|   (*Pacific* Organic) . . . . . | 110 | 5.0 | 16.0 | 2.0 | 10 | 720 | 1.0 |
|   (*Pacific* Organic | | | | | | | |
|     Light Sodium) . . . . | 110 | 5.0 | 16.0 | 2.0 | 10 | 360 | 1.0 |
|   (*Tabatchnick*), ⅔ cup . | 70 | 1.0 | 13.0 | 2.5 | 0 | 620 | 1.0 |
| red pepper, sweet | | | | | | | |
|   (*Campbell's V8*) . . . . . | 120 | 3.0 | 22.0 | 1.5 | 5 | 480 | 3.0 |
| rice and red bean | | | | | | | |
|   (*Amy's* Spanish) . . . . . | 140 | 5.0 | 24.0 | 2.5 | 0 | 690 | 5.0 |
| Salisbury steak, | | | | | | | |
|   mushrooms, onion | | | | | | | |
|   (*Campbell's Chunky*) . . | 140 | 7.0 | 19.0 | 4.5 | 15 | 800 | 2.0 |
| sausage: | | | | | | | |
|   Italian, w/pasta, | | | | | | | |
|     pepperoni (*Campbell's* | | | | | | | |
|     *Select Harvest*) . . . . | 160 | 7.0 | 18.0 | 7.0 | 15 | 480 | 2.0 |
|   and vegetable | | | | | | | |
|     (*Campbell's Select* | | | | | | | |
|     *Harvest* Savory) . . . | 90 | 4.0 | 12.0 | 3.0 | 10 | 480 | 2.0 |

| Food and Measure | cal. | prot. (gms) | carbo. (gms) | fat (gms) | chol. (mgs) | sod. (mgs) | fiber (gms) |
|---|---|---|---|---|---|---|---|
| seafood stock (*Kitchen Basics*) ............ | 10 | 2.0 | 0 | 0 | 0 | 480 | 0 |
| sirloin burger, w/ vegetables: | | | | | | | |
| (*Campbell's Chunky*) .. | 130 | 8.0 | 18.0 | 2.5 | 15 | 800 | 3.0 |
| (*Campbell's Chunky Micro*) .......... | 140 | 8.0 | 18.0 | 3.5 | 15 | 800 | 3.0 |
| (*Campbell's Chunky Healthy Request*) .. | 130 | 9.0 | 19.0 | 2.0 | 15 | 410 | 3.0 |
| steak, sirloin, w/vegetables: | | | | | | | |
| (*Progresso*) ........ | 130 | 8.0 | 19.0 | 2.0 | 10 | 690 | 2.0 |
| grilled (*Campbell's Chunky* Hearty) ... | 130 | 8.0 | 19.0 | 2.0 | 10 | 890 | 3.0 |
| steak and: | | | | | | | |
| noodles (*Healthy Choice* Micro) .... | 100 | 6.0 | 15.0 | 1.5 | 10 | 340 | 2.0 |
| noodles (*Progresso* Homemade) ...... | 110 | 8.0 | 14.0 | 2.5 | 20 | 690 | 1.0 |
| potato (*Campbell's Chunky*) ......... | 120 | 8.0 | 18.0 | 2.0 | 15 | 920 | 3.0 |
| roasted russet potato (*Progresso*) ...... | 130 | 8.0 | 20.0 | 2.0 | 10 | 690 | 1.0 |
| sweet potato: | | | | | | | |
| chipotle (*Pacific*) ..... | 220 | 4.0 | 40.0 | 4.0 | 15 | 730 | 3.0 |
| Thai (*Pacific*) ....... | 160 | 3.0 | 25.0 | 6.0 | 0 | 660 | 3.0 |
| sweet potato, creamy: | | | | | | | |
| (*Imagine* Organic) .... | 110 | 2.0 | 23.0 | 1.5 | 0 | 400 | 1.0 |
| (*Imagine* Organic Light Sodium) .... | 110 | 2.0 | 23.0 | 1.0 | 0 | 140 | 1.0 |
| Thai: | | | | | | | |
| (*Tiger Tiger* Tom Kha) ........... | 229 | 2.0 | 17.0 | 17.0 | 0 | 580 | 1.0 |
| (*Tiger Tiger* Tom Yum) .......... | 93 | 2.0 | 10.0 | 0 | 0 | 550 | 1.0 |
| noodle (*Annie Chun's Chun's* Tom Yum Bowl), ½ cont. .... | 150 | 5.0 | 30.0 | 1.5 | 0 | 730 | 1.0 |
| tomato: | | | | | | | |
| (*Campbell's* Micro) ... | 100 | 3.0 | 23.0 | 0 | 0 | 480 | 2.0 |
| (*Campbell's Soup at Hand*), 1 cont. .... | 140 | 3.0 | 30.0 | .5 | 0 | 645 | 2.0 |
| (*Campbell's Soup at Hand* 25% Less Sodium), 1 cont. ... | 140 | 3.0 | 33.0 | 0 | 0 | 480 | 2.0 |

| Food and Measure | cal. | prot. (gms) | carbo. (gms) | fat (gms) | chol. (mgs) | sod. (mgs) | fiber (gms) |
|---|---|---|---|---|---|---|---|
| **Soup, tomato** *(cont.)* | | | | | | | |
| *(Health Valley* | | | | | | | |
| Organic No Salt) ... | 100 | 1.0 | 19.0 | 2.5 | 5 | 60 | 3.0 |
| *(Imagine* Organic) .... | 100 | 1.0 | 19.0 | 2.5 | 5 | 610 | n.a. |
| *(Muir Glen* Organic | | | | | | | |
| Hearty) .......... | 130 | 5.0 | 25.0 | 2.0 | 0 | 880 | 2.0 |
| *(Progresso* Hearty) ... | 110 | 3.0 | 24.0 | .5 | 0 | 690 | 3.0 |
| basil *(Campbell's* | | | | | | | |
| *Select Harvest)* .... | 100 | 3.0 | 22.0 | 0 | 0 | 480 | 2.0 |
| basil *(Healthy* | | | | | | | |
| *Choice)* .......... | 130 | 3.0 | 28.0 | .5 | 5 | 470 | 3.0 |
| basil *(Healthy Choice* | | | | | | | |
| Micro) .......... | 130 | 4.0 | 28.0 | .5 | 5 | 470 | 3.0 |
| basil *(Progresso)* .... | 150 | 3.0 | 29.0 | 3.0 | 0 | 680 | 2.0 |
| garden *(Campbell's* | | | | | | | |
| *Select Harvest)* .... | 100 | 3.0 | 21.0 | .5 | 5 | 700 | 2.0 |
| herb *(Campbell's V8)* . | 90 | 3.0 | 19.0 | 0 | 0 | 480 | 3.0 |
| Parmesan *(Progresso* | | | | | | | |
| Reduced Sodium) . | 100 | 5.0 | 17.0 | 1.5 | 5 | 480 | 3.0 |
| w/pasta *(Campbell's* | | | | | | | |
| *Chunky* Hearty) ... | 140 | 5.0 | 28.0 | 1.0 | 5 | 650 | 3.0 |
| rotini *(Progresso)* .... | 130 | 4.0 | 28.0 | .5 | 0 | 690 | 4.0 |
| vegetable *(Health* | | | | | | | |
| *Valley* Organic) .... | 70 | 3.0 | 17.0 | 0 | 0 | 470 | 5.0 |
| tomato, cream/creamy: | | | | | | | |
| *(Amy's* Organic) ..... | 110 | 3.0 | 19.0 | 2.5 | 10 | 690 | 3.0 |
| *(Amy's* Organic | | | | | | | |
| Light Sodium) .... | 100 | 2.0 | 17.0 | 2.5 | 10 | 340 | 3.0 |
| *(Campbell's* Micro) ... | 160 | 3.0 | 25.0 | 5.0 | 5 | 480 | 3.0 |
| *(Campbell's Soup at* | | | | | | | |
| *Hand),* 1 cont. .... | 190 | 3.0 | 32.0 | 5.0 | 5 | 650 | 2.0 |
| *(Imagine* Organic) .... | 90 | 2.0 | 18.0 | 2.0 | 0 | 460 | 2.0 |
| *(Muir Glen* Organic) .. | 170 | 4.0 | 26.0 | 6.0 | 15 | 840 | 2.0 |
| *(Pacific* Organic) ..... | 100 | 5.0 | 16.0 | 2.0 | 10 | 750 | 1.0 |
| *(Pacific* Organic | | | | | | | |
| Light Sodium) .... | 100 | 5.0 | 16.0 | 2.0 | 10 | 380 | 1.0 |
| *(Tabatchnick),* ⅔ cup . | 70 | 1.0 | 14.0 | 2.0 | 5 | 620 | 1.0 |
| basil *(Imagine* | | | | | | | |
| Organic) ......... | 90 | 3.0 | 17.0 | 1.5 | 0 | 430 | 2.0 |
| basil *(Progresso* | | | | | | | |
| High Fiber) ....... | 130 | 3.0 | 26.0 | 4.0 | 5 | 520 | 7.0 |
| garden *(Imagine* | | | | | | | |
| Organic Light | | | | | | | |
| Sodium) ......... | 80 | 2.0 | 16.0 | 1.0 | 0 | 300 | 2.0 |

| Food and Measure | cal. | prot. (gms) | carbo. (gms) | fat (gms) | chol. (mgs) | sod. (mgs) | fiber (gms) |
|---|---|---|---|---|---|---|---|
| tomato bisque: | | | | | | | |
| (*Amy's* Organic) ..... | 130 | 3.0 | 21.0 | 3.5 | 10 | 680 | 3.0 |
| (*Amy's* Organic Light Sodium) ......... | 120 | 2.0 | 21.0 | 3.5 | 10 | 340 | 2.0 |
| (*Campbell's Select Harvest* Zesty) .... | 120 | 3.0 | 21.0 | 2.5 | 5 | 480 | 3.0 |
| (*Healthy Choice*) ..... | 130 | 3.0 | 28.0 | .5 | 5 | 470 | 3.0 |
| fire-roasted (*Imagine Bistro* Organic) .... | 120 | 2.0 | 24.0 | 2.5 | 0 | 670 | n.a. |
| Parmesan, creamy (*Campbell's Soup at Hand*), 1 cont. .... | 220 | 4.0 | 35.0 | 7.0 | 10 | 780 | 3.0 |
| tortilla (*Imagine* Organic Southwest) .. | 160 | 5.0 | 25.0 | 4.0 | 0 | 750 | n.a. |
| turkey: | | | | | | | |
| broth (*College Inn*) ... | 20 | 2.0 | 0 | 1.0 | 0 | 950 | 0 |
| noodle (*Progresso*) ... | 80 | 5.0 | 12.0 | 1.0 | 15 | 690 | 1.0 |
| stock (*Kitchen Basics*) | 20 | 3.0 | 2.0 | 0 | 0 | 430 | 0 |
| udon noodle (*Annie Chun's* Bowl), ½ cont. | 110 | 3.0 | 22.0 | .5 | 0 | 460 | 1.0 |
| veal stock (*Kitchen Basics*) ............ | 20 | 3.0 | 3.0 | 0 | 0 | 480 | 0 |
| vegetable: | | | | | | | |
| (*Amy's* Organic Chunky) ......... | 60 | 3.0 | 13.0 | 0 | 0 | 680 | 3.0 |
| (*Amy's* Organic French Country) ... | 180 | 5.0 | 23.0 | 8.0 | 0 | 640 | 5.0 |
| (*Amy's* Organic Rustic Italian) ..... | 140 | 4.0 | 18.0 | 6.0 | 0 | 680 | 4.0 |
| (*Campbell's* Micro) ... | 100 | 3.0 | 22.0 | .5 | 0 | 800 | 3.0 |
| (*Campbell's Chunky* Savory) ......... | 110 | 3.0 | 22.0 | 1.0 | 0 | 770 | 4.0 |
| (*Campbell's Chunky Healthy Request*) .. | 120 | 3.0 | 24.0 | 1.0 | 0 | 410 | 4.0 |
| (*Campbell's Select Harvest* Medley) ... | 80 | 3.0 | 16.0 | .5 | 0 | 480 | 3.0 |
| (*Health Valley* Organic No Salt) ... | 100 | 3.0 | 18.0 | 2.5 | 0 | 50 | 4.0 |
| (*Healthy Choice* Country) ......... | 100 | 4.0 | 20.0 | .5 | 5 | 480 | 5.0 |
| (*Healthy Choice* Country Micro) .... | 90 | 4.0 | 18.0 | .5 | 0 | 480 | 4.0 |
| (*Progresso*) ........ | 80 | 5.0 | 15.0 | 0 | 0 | 660 | 3.0 |
| (*Progresso* Italiano) .. | 100 | 4.0 | 20.0 | 1.5 | 0 | 770 | 2.0 |

| Food and Measure | cal. | prot. (gms) | carbo. (gms) | fat (gms) | chol. (mgs) | sod. (mgs) | fiber (gms) |
|---|---|---|---|---|---|---|---|
| **Soup, vegetable** *(cont.)* | | | | | | | |
| (*Progresso* Light) .... | 60 | 2.0 | 14.0 | 0 | 0 | 470 | 4.0 |
| (*Progresso* Micro) ... | 80 | 3.0 | 15.0 | .5 | 0 | 690 | 2.0 |
| barley (*Amy's* Organic) | 70 | 2.0 | 13.0 | 1.0 | 0 | 580 | 3.0 |
| barley (*Health Valley* Organic) ......... | 90 | 3.0 | 20.0 | .5 | 0 | 480 | 4.0 |
| barley (*Progresso* Light Savory) ..... | 60 | 2.0 | 14.0 | 0 | 0 | 690 | 4.0 |
| barley, hearty (*Healthy Choice* Micro) .... | 140 | 4.0 | 30.0 | 1.0 | 5 | 430 | 4.0 |
| barley, vegetarian (*Progresso*) ...... | 80 | 3.0 | 18.0 | 0 | 0 | 670 | 3.0 |
| crab, red (*Chincoteague*) .... | 90 | 5.0 | 12.0 | 2.5 | 15 | 880 | 2.0 |
| fire-roasted, Southwestern (*Amy's* Organic) ... | 140 | 4.0 | 21.0 | 4.0 | 0 | 680 | 4.0 |
| 14 garden (*Health Valley* Organic) .... | 80 | 3.0 | 18.0 | 0 | 0 | 480 | 4.0 |
| garden (*Healthy Choice*) .......... | 130 | 5.0 | 25.0 | .5 | 5 | 450 | 5.0 |
| garden (*Muir Glen* Organic) ......... | 80 | 3.0 | 16.0 | 1.0 | 0 | 960 | 3.0 |
| garden (*Progresso*) .. | 90 | 3.0 | 20.0 | 0 | 0 | 690 | 3.0 |
| garden (*Progresso* Reduced Sodium) . | 100 | 3.0 | 22.0 | 0 | 0 | 450 | 3.0 |
| garden, blend (*Campbell's V8*) ... | 120 | 5.0 | 23.0 | 1.0 | 5 | 480 | 3.0 |
| Italian style (*Campbell's Select Harvest* Light) .... | 50 | 3.0 | 12.0 | 0 | 0 | 480 | 4.0 |
| Italian style (*Progresso* Light) .......... | 60 | 2.0 | 14.0 | 0 | 0 | 470 | 4.0 |
| noodle (*Progresso* High Fiber) ....... | 90 | 4.0 | 18.0 | 1.5 | 5 | 690 | 7.0 |
| noodle (*Progresso* Light) .......... | 60 | 2.0 | 13.0 | .5 | 5 | 690 | 4.0 |
| w/noodles, mini round (*Campbell's Soup at Hand*), 1 cont. .. | 100 | 2.0 | 21.0 | .5 | 5 | 650 | 1.0 |
| and pasta (*Campbell's Select Harvest* Light) | 60 | 3.0 | 13.0 | 0 | 0 | 480 | 4.0 |
| and rice (*Progresso* Light Homestyle) .. | 60 | 2.0 | 14.0 | 0 | 0 | 690 | 4.0 |

| Food and Measure | cal. | prot. (gms) | carbo. (gms) | fat (gms) | chol. (mgs) | sod. (mgs) | fiber (gms) |
|---|---|---|---|---|---|---|---|
| Southwest (*Campbell's Select Harvest* Light) .......... | 50 | 2.0 | 13.0 | 0 | 0 | 480 | 4.0 |
| Southwest (*Campbell's Select Harvest* Light Micro) ...... | 50 | 2.0 | 13.0 | 0 | 0 | 400 | 4.0 |
| Southwest (*Progresso* Light) .......... | 60 | 3.0 | 12.0 | .5 | 0 | 690 | 4.0 |
| vegetable beef: | | | | | | | |
| (*Campbell's* Micro) ... | 80 | 5.0 | 15.0 | .5 | 10 | 880 | 3.0 |
| (*Campbell's Chunky Old Fashioned*) .... | 120 | 8.0 | 17.0 | 2.5 | 15 | 890 | 3.0 |
| (*Campbell's Chunky Old Fashioned Micro*) .......... | 100 | 7.0 | 14.0 | 1.5 | 10 | 880 | 3.0 |
| (*Campbell's Chunky Healthy Request Old Fashioned*) .... | 120 | 7.0 | 19.0 | 2.0 | 10 | 410 | 3.0 |
| (*Campbell's Soup at Hand*), 1 cont. .. | 70 | 3.0 | 11.0 | 1.0 | 5 | 930 | 1.0 |
| (*Healthy Choice*) ..... | 130 | 9.0 | 21.0 | 1.5 | 10 | 420 | 4.0 |
| barley (*Campbell's Select Harvest*) .... | 80 | 6.0 | 12.0 | 1.0 | 10 | 480 | 2.0 |
| slow-cooked (*Progresso*) ...... | 140 | 9.0 | 20.0 | 2.0 | 15 | 690 | 2.0 |
| vegetable broth: | | | | | | | |
| (*College Inn* Garden) . | 25 | 1.0 | 6.0 | 1.0 | 0 | 590 | 0 |
| (*Imagine* Organic) .... | 20 | 2.0 | 2.0 | 0 | 0 | 550 | 0 |
| (*Imagine* Organic Low Sodium) ..... | 20 | 0 | 3.0 | 0 | 0 | 140 | <1.0 |
| (*Pacific* Organic) ...... | 15 | 0 | 3.0 | 0 | 0 | 530 | 1.0 |
| (*Pacific* Organic Low Sodium) ..... | 15 | 0 | 3.0 | 0 | 0 | 140 | 1.0 |
| (*Swanson*) ......... | 15 | 0 | 3.0 | 0 | 0 | 940 | 0 |
| (*Swanson* Organic) ... | 15 | 0 | 3.0 | 0 | 0 | 550 | 0 |
| (*Tabatchnick*), ⅔ cup . | 10 | 0 | 2.0 | 0 | 0 | 550 | 0 |
| vegetable stock: | | | | | | | |
| (*Imagine* Organic) .... | 30 | 1.0 | 6.0 | 0 | 0 | 580 | 0 |
| (*Kitchen Basics*) ...... | 20 | 0 | 4.0 | 0 | 0 | 240 | 0 |
| Vietnamese noodle (*Annie Chun's* Pho Bowl), ½ cont. ...... | 220 | 6.0 | 45.0 | 1.0 | 0 | 970 | 2.0 |
| white wine and herb broth (*College Inn*) ... | 5 | 0 | 1.0 | .5 | 0 | 920 | 0 |

| Food and Measure | cal. | prot. (gms) | carbo. (gms) | fat (gms) | chol. (mgs) | sod. (mgs) | fiber (gms) |
|---|---|---|---|---|---|---|---|
| **Soup, condensed,** | | | | | | | |
| undiluted, ½ cup: | | | | | | | |
| (*Campbell's*): | | | | | | | |
| asparagus, cream of .. | 110 | 2.0 | 9.0 | 7.0 | 5 | 830 | 3.0 |
| bean, w/bacon ...... | 160 | 8.0 | 25.0 | 3.0 | 5 | 860 | 8.0 |
| beef, w/vegetables, | | | | | | | |
| barley ........... | 90 | 5.0 | 15.0 | 1.5 | 10 | 890 | 3.0 |
| beef broth .......... | 15 | 3.0 | 1.0 | 0 | 0 | 860 | 0 |
| beef consommé ..... | 20 | 4.0 | 1.0 | 0 | 0 | 810 | 0 |
| beef noodle ........ | 70 | 4.0 | 8.0 | 2.0 | 10 | 820 | 1.0 |
| broccoli, cream of .... | 90 | 2.0 | 12.0 | 5.0 | 5 | 750 | 1.0 |
| broccoli cheese ...... | 100 | 2.0 | 12.0 | 4.5 | 5 | 820 | 0 |
| 98% fat free ...... | 70 | 2.0 | 12.0 | 1.5 | 5 | 480 | 1.0 |
| celery, cream of ..... | 90 | 1.0 | 9.0 | 6.0 | 5 | 640 | 3.0 |
| 98% fat free ...... | 70 | 1.0 | 9.0 | 3.0 | 5 | 480 | 2.0 |
| cheddar cheese ...... | 100 | 2.0 | 11.0 | 5.0 | 5 | 650 | 1.0 |
| cheese, nacho, fiesta . | 120 | 3.0 | 10.0 | 8.0 | 10 | 790 | 1.0 |
| chicken, cream of .... | 120 | 2.0 | 10.0 | 8.0 | 10 | 870 | 2.0 |
| 98% fat free ...... | 70 | 2.0 | 10.0 | 2.5 | 5 | 480 | 1.0 |
| w/herbs ......... | 80 | 2.0 | 9.0 | 4.0 | 10 | 800 | 0 |
| and mushrooms ... | 100 | 2.0 | 9.0 | 6.0 | 10 | 830 | 4.0 |
| chicken alphabet ..... | 70 | 3.0 | 12.0 | 1.5 | 5 | 480 | 1.0 |
| chicken broth ....... | 20 | 1.0 | 1.0 | 1.0 | 5 | 770 | 0 |
| chicken broth, low | | | | | | | |
| sodium .......... | 30 | 3.0 | 1.0 | 1.0 | 5 | 140 | 0 |
| chicken gumbo ...... | 70 | 2.0 | 12.0 | 1.0 | 5 | 480 | 1.0 |
| chicken mushroom | | | | | | | |
| barley ........... | 70 | 2.0 | 14.0 | 1.0 | 5 | 480 | 2.0 |
| chicken noodle ...... | 60 | 3.0 | 8.0 | 2.0 | 15 | 890 | <1.0 |
| 25% less sodium .. | 60 | 3.0 | 8.0 | 2.0 | 15 | 660 | 1.0 |
| *Double Noodle* .... | 110 | 3.0 | 20.0 | 2.0 | 10 | 480 | 1.0 |
| *Noodle O's* ........ | 90 | 3.0 | 15.0 | 2.5 | 20 | 480 | 1.0 |
| creamy .......... | 120 | 4.0 | 11.0 | 7.0 | 15 | 870 | 4.0 |
| homestyle ....... | 70 | 4.0 | 10.0 | 2.0 | 10 | 650 | 1.0 |
| Mega ........... | 90 | 3.0 | 15.0 | 2.0 | 15 | 480 | 1.0 |
| chicken w/rice ....... | 70 | 2.0 | 13.0 | 1.5 | 5 | 610 | 1.0 |
| chicken rice, white | | | | | | | |
| and wild ......... | 70 | 3.0 | 13.0 | 1.5 | 5 | 480 | 1.0 |
| chicken stars ....... | 70 | 3.0 | 11.0 | 2.0 | 5 | 480 | 1.0 |
| chicken vegetable .... | 80 | 3.0 | 15.0 | 1.0 | 5 | 890 | 2.0 |
| chicken wonton ..... | 50 | 3.0 | 8.0 | 1.0 | 5 | 870 | 0 |
| clam chowder: | | | | | | | |
| Manhattan ....... | 60 | 2.0 | 12.0 | .5 | 0 | 880 | 2.0 |
| New England ..... | 90 | 4.0 | 13.0 | 2.5 | 5 | 650 | 1.0 |

| Food and Measure | cal. | prot. (gms) | carbo. (gms) | fat (gms) | chol. (mgs) | sod. (mgs) | fiber (gms) |
|---|---|---|---|---|---|---|---|
| Italian style wedding .. | 80 | 3.0 | 12.0 | 2.0 | 5 | 480 | 2.0 |
| lentil ............. | 140 | 8.0 | 24.0 | 1.0 | 0 | 800 | 5.0 |
| minestrone ........ | 90 | 4.0 | 17.0 | 1.0 | 5 | 650 | 3.0 |
| mushroom, beefy .... | 50 | 3.0 | 6.0 | 2.0 | 5 | 890 | 0 |
| mushroom, cream of . | 100 | 1.0 | 9.0 | 6.0 | 5 | 870 | 2.0 |
| 25% less sodium .. | 110 | 2.0 | 8.0 | 8.0 | 5 | 650 | 2.0 |
| 98% fat free ...... | 60 | 1.0 | 9.0 | 2.5 | 5 | 480 | 1.0 |
| low sodium ...... | 160 | 3.0 | 19.0 | 8.0 | 15 | 60 | 0 |
| w/roasted garlic ... | 70 | 2.0 | 10.0 | 2.5 | 5 | 480 | 2.0 |
| mushroom, golden ... | 80 | 2.0 | 10.0 | 3.5 | 0 | 650 | 1.0 |
| onion, cream of ..... | 100 | 1.0 | 10.0 | 6.0 | 5 | 800 | 3.0 |
| onion, French ....... | 70 | 2.0 | 12.0 | 1.5 | 5 | 650 | 1.0 |
| oyster stew ........ | 80 | 3.0 | 3.0 | 6.0 | 20 | 910 | 0 |
| pea, green ......... | 180 | 9.0 | 28.0 | 3.0 | 0 | 870 | 4.0 |
| pea, split, w/ham, and bacon ....... | 180 | 10.0 | 30.0 | 2.0 | 5 | 850 | 4.0 |
| potato, cream of ..... | 90 | 2.0 | 15.0 | 2.0 | 5 | 600 | 2.0 |
| shrimp, cream of .... | 100 | 3.0 | 8.0 | 6.0 | 20 | 860 | 0 |
| tomato ............ | 90 | 2.0 | 20.0 | 0 | 0 | 480 | 1.0 |
| tomato bisque ...... | 130 | 2.0 | 23.0 | 3.5 | 5 | 880 | 1.0 |
| tomato rice ........ | 110 | 1.0 | 23.0 | 2.0 | <5 | 770 | 1.0 |
| vegetable ......... | 100 | 4.0 | 21.0 | .5 | 5 | 650 | 3.0 |
| vegetable, old fashioned | 80 | 3.0 | 14.0 | 1.5 | 5 | 920 | 2.0 |
| vegetable beef ....... | 90 | 5.0 | 15.0 | 1.0 | 5 | 890 | 3.0 |
| vegetable orzo ...... | 80 | 3.0 | 15.0 | 1.0 | 5 | 480 | 2.0 |
| vegetarian vegetable .. | 90 | 3.0 | 18.0 | .5 | 0 | 480 | 2.0 |
| (Campbell's Healthy Request): | | | | | | | |
| celery, cream of ..... | 70 | 1.0 | 12.0 | 2.0 | <5 | 410 | 1.0 |
| chicken, cream of .... | 80 | 2.0 | 12.0 | 2.5 | 5 | 410 | 1.0 |
| chicken noodle ...... | 60 | 3.0 | 8.0 | 2.0 | 10 | 410 | 1.0 |
| chicken noodle, homestyle ....... | 60 | 3.0 | 10.0 | 1.5 | 10 | 410 | 1.0 |
| chicken w/rice ....... | 70 | 2.0 | 13.0 | 1.5 | 5 | 410 | 1.0 |
| minestrone ........ | 80 | 3.0 | 15.0 | .5 | 0 | 410 | 3.0 |
| mushroom, cream of . | 70 | 2.0 | 10.0 | 2.0 | 5 | 410 | 1.0 |
| tomato ............ | 90 | 2.0 | 17.0 | 1.5 | 0 | 410 | 1.0 |
| vegetable ......... | 100 | 4.0 | 20.0 | 1.0 | 0 | 410 | 3.0 |
| vegetable beef ....... | 90 | 5.0 | 15.0 | 1.0 | 5 | 410 | 3.0 |
| (Chincoteague): | | | | | | | |
| clam bisque ........ | 100 | 8.0 | 13.0 | 2.0 | 15 | 990 | 1.0 |
| clam chowder, Manhattan ....... | 100 | 8.0 | 13.0 | 2.0 | 15 | 990 | 1.0 |

| Food and Measure | cal. | prot. (gms) | carbo. (gms) | fat (gms) | chol. (mgs) | sod. (mgs) | fiber (gms) |
|---|---|---|---|---|---|---|---|
| **Soup, condensed (Chincoteague)** *(cont.)* | | | | | | | |
| clam chowder, New | | | | | | | |
| England . . . . . . . . . | 80 | 5.0 | 10.0 | 2.5 | 10 | 590 | <1.0 |
| 99% fat free . . . . . . | 70 | 2.0 | 12.0 | 1.0 | 5 | 610 | <1.0 |
| corn chowder . . . . . . . | 100 | 2.0 | 16.0 | 3.5 | 0 | 890 | 1.0 |
| crab, she . . . . . . . . . . | 70 | 4.0 | 7.0 | 3.0 | 20 | 770 | 0 |
| crab and cheddar . . . . | 90 | 4.0 | 10.0 | 3.5 | 20 | 590 | 0 |
| lobster bisque . . . . . . . | 90 | 4.0 | 10.0 | 4.0 | 15 | 650 | 0 |
| and cheddar . . . . . . | 110 | 4.0 | 10.0 | 6.0 | 20 | 610 | 0 |
| oyster stew . . . . . . . . . | 80 | 4.0 | 11.0 | 3.5 | 25 | 680 | 0 |
| shrimp bisque . . . . . . . | 80 | 2.0 | 10.0 | 3.0 | 20 | 590 | 0 |
| (*Pacific*): | | | | | | | |
| celery, cream of . . . . . | 70 | 1.0 | 11.0 | 2.5 | 10 | 760 | 0 |
| chicken, cream of . . . . | 70 | 1.0 | 11.0 | 2.5 | 10 | 760 | 0 |
| mushroom, cream of . | 100 | 2.0 | 18.0 | 2.5 | 10 | 740 | 1.0 |
| **Soup, frozen**, 7.5 oz., | | | | | | | |
| except as noted: | | | | | | | |
| bean: | | | | | | | |
| black (*Tabatchnick*) . . . | 230 | 13.0 | 39.0 | 2.5 | 0 | 420 | 9.0 |
| black (*Tabatchnick* | | | | | | | |
| Organic) . . . . . . . . . | 220 | 13.0 | 38.0 | 2.5 | 0 | 400 | 9.0 |
| white, vegetables | | | | | | | |
| (*Moosewood* Organic | | | | | | | |
| Tuscan), 1 cup . . . . | 130 | 6.0 | 23.0 | 2.0 | 0 | 770 | 5.0 |
| Southwest (*Tabatchnick*) | 220 | 11.0 | 35.0 | 5.0 | 0 | 440 | 9.0 |
| Yankee | | | | | | | |
| (*Tabatchnick*) . . . . . | 180 | 11.0 | 33.0 | 1.5 | 0 | 340 | 10.0 |
| broccoli, cream of | | | | | | | |
| (*Tabatchnick*) . . . . . . . | 90 | 3.0 | 12.0 | 4.0 | 5 | 440 | 3.0 |
| broccoli and cheese, | | | | | | | |
| creamy (*Moosewood* | | | | | | | |
| Organic), 1 cup . . . . . . | 170 | 6.0 | 18.0 | 9.0 | 20 | 850 | 2.0 |
| cabbage (*Tabatchnick*) . . | 90 | 2.0 | 21.0 | 1.0 | 0 | 160 | 1.0 |
| carrot and coriander | | | | | | | |
| (*Kettle Cuisine* | | | | | | | |
| Organic), 10 oz. . . . . . | 100 | 1.0 | 15.0 | 3.0 | 0 | 410 | 5.0 |
| chicken, 10 oz.: | | | | | | | |
| chili w/white beans | | | | | | | |
| (*Kettle Cuisine*) . . . | 330 | 21.0 | 27.0 | 15.0 | 70 | 660 | 3.0 |
| w/rice noodles | | | | | | | |
| (*Kettle Cuisine*) . . . | 140 | 15.0 | 12.0 | 3.0 | 45 | 560 | 1.0 |
| chicken broth: | | | | | | | |
| w/noodles, dumplings | | | | | | | |
| (*Tabatachnick*) . . . . | 150 | 5.0 | 19.0 | 6.0 | 65 | 740 | <1.0 |

| Food and Measure | cal. | prot. (gms) | carbo. (gms) | fat (gms) | chol. (mgs) | sod. (mgs) | fiber (gms) |
|---|---|---|---|---|---|---|---|
| w/noodles, vegetables (*Tabatachnick*) .... | 70 | 3.0 | 13.0 | 1.0 | 15 | 460 | 0 |
| chicken corn chowder, grilled (*Kettle Cuisine*), 10 oz. ...... | 270 | 13.0 | 27.0 | 12.0 | 55 | 570 | 3.0 |
| clam chowder: | | | | | | | |
| (*Kettle Cuisine*), 10 oz. ........... | 330 | 15.0 | 26.0 | 18.0 | 80 | 800 | 1.0 |
| (*Phillips*), 1 cup ..... | 280 | 12.0 | 19.0 | 17.0 | 80 | 940 | 1.0 |
| corn chowder (*Tabatchnick*) ....... | 130 | 4.0 | 21.0 | 4.5 | 10 | 390 | 2.0 |
| crab, 1 cup: | | | | | | | |
| cream of (*Phillips*) ... | 340 | 6.0 | 15.0 | 29.0 | 115 | 660 | 1.0 |
| Maryland (*Phillips*) ... | 100 | 5.0 | 14.0 | 2.5 | 15 | 940 | 3.0 |
| crab chowder, 1 cup: | | | | | | | |
| and corn (*Phillips*) ... | 220 | 8.0 | 17.0 | 13.0 | 55 | 670 | 1.0 |
| and shrimp (*Phillips*) . | 180 | 6.0 | 16.0 | 11.0 | 55 | 880 | 3.0 |
| lentil, Tuscany: | | | | | | | |
| (*Tabatchnick*) ....... | 160 | 11.0 | 29.0 | 0 | 0 | 360 | 8.0 |
| (*Tabatchnick* Organic) ......... | 160 | 11.0 | 30.0 | 0 | 0 | 370 | 8.0 |
| lobster bisque (*Phillips*), 1 cup ............. | 310 | 10.0 | 20.0 | 21.0 | 100 | 960 | 1.0 |
| minestrone (*Tabatchnick*) ....... | 100 | 5.0 | 18.0 | 1.5 | 0 | 320 | 4.0 |
| mushroom, cream of (*Tabatchnick*) ....... | 100 | 3.0 | 11.0 | 5.0 | 15 | 260 | <1.0 |
| mushroom barley: | | | | | | | |
| (*Moosewood* Organic), 1 cup ............ | 100 | 3.0 | 16.0 | 2.5 | 0 | 860 | 3.0 |
| (*Tabatchnick*) ....... | 80 | 3.0 | 17.0 | 1.0 | 0 | 420 | 3.0 |
| (*Tabatchnick* Low Sodium) ......... | 80 | 3.0 | 17.0 | 1.0 | 0 | 40 | 4.0 |
| mushroom and potato (*Kettle Cuisine* Organic), 10 oz. ..... | 140 | 4.0 | 14.0 | 8.0 | 15 | 670 | 4.0 |
| pea, split: | | | | | | | |
| (*Tabatchnick*) ....... | 140 | 13.0 | 34.0 | 0 | 0 | 380 | 13.0 |
| (*Tabatchnick* Low Sodium) ......... | 140 | 13.0 | 34.0 | 0 | 0 | 50 | 14.0 |
| potato: | | | | | | | |
| (*Tabatchnick* Old Fashioned) ....... | 100 | 3.0 | 21.0 | 1.5 | 0 | 330 | 2.0 |

| Food and Measure | cal. | prot. (gms) | carbo. (gms) | fat (gms) | chol. (mgs) | sod. (mgs) | fiber (gms) |
|---|---|---|---|---|---|---|---|
| **Soup, frozen, potato** *(cont.)* | | | | | | | |
| New England (*Tabatchnick*) . . . . . | 140 | 5.0 | 24.0 | 4.0 | 15 | 370 | 1.0 |
| potato corn chowder, creamy (*Moosewood Organic*), 1 cup . . . . . . | 170 | 5.0 | 28.0 | 6.0 | 15 | 410 | 3.0 |
| rice, wild (*Tabatchnick* Wilderness) . . . . . | 80 | 3.0 | 16.0 | .5 | 0 | 220 | 1.0 |
| shrimp bisque (*Phillips*), 1 cup . . . . . | 270 | 10.0 | 18.0 | 17.0 | 90 | 1000 | 1.0 |
| spinach, cream of (*Tabatchnick*) . . . . . . . | 90 | 3.0 | 11.0 | 4.0 | 5 | 390 | 2.0 |
| tempura udon (*Tiger Thai* Kit): | | | | | | | |
| ½ of 24-oz. pkg. . . . . . | 460 | 14.0 | 67.0 | 6.0 | 25 | 1690 | 6.0 |
| broth, ½ pkg. . . . . . . . | 30 | <1.0 | 7.0 | 0 | 0 | 670 | 0 |
| tomato rice, balsamic (*Tabatchnick*) . . . . . . . | 110 | 2.0 | 18.0 | 3.5 | 0 | 260 | 3.0 |
| tomato vegetable, garden (*Kettle Cuisine*), 10 oz. . . . . . . . . . . . . . | 110 | 3.0 | 14.0 | 4.0 | 0 | 780 | 5.0 |
| vegetable: | | | | | | | |
| (*Tabatchnick*) . . . . . . . | 90 | 3.0 | 17.0 | 1.5 | 0 | 350 | 4.0 |
| (*Tabatchnick* Low Sodium) . . . . . . . . . | 90 | 4.0 | 17.0 | 1.5 | 0 | 45 | 4.0 |
| roasted (*Kettle Cuisine*), 10 oz. . . . | 140 | 3.0 | 19.0 | 6.0 | 0 | 560 | 5.0 |
| **Soup, mix**, dry, 1 pkg. or cont., except as noted: | | | | | | | |
| asparagus, creamy (*Maggi*), ¼ pkt. . . . . . . | 60 | 1.0 | 10.0 | 1.5 | 0 | 1090 | 0 |
| bean: | | | | | | | |
| (*Alessi* Neapolitan), ¼ of 6-oz. pkg. . . . . | 140 | 6.0 | 29.0 | .5 | 0 | 680 | 6.0 |
| (*Alessi* Tuscan), ¼ of 6-oz. pkg. . . . . . . . . | 150 | 7.0 | 28.0 | .5 | 0 | 660 | 7.0 |
| chili (*Fantastic* Cha Cha), 1 cup* . . . . . | 110 | 6.0 | 20.0 | 1.5 | 0 | 580 | 7.0 |
| and ham (*Hormel* Micro) . . . . . . . . . . | 190 | 9.0 | 29.0 | 4.0 | 10 | 720 | 7.0 |
| bean, black: | | | | | | | |
| (*Vigo*), ¼ of 6-oz. pkg. . . . . . . . . | 150 | 8.0 | 28.0 | 0 | 0 | 750 | 9.0 |

| Food and Measure | cal. | prot. (gms) | carbo. (gms) | fat (gms) | chol. (mgs) | sod. (mgs) | fiber (gms) |
|---|---|---|---|---|---|---|---|
| w/rice (*Health Valley* Zesty), ⅓ cup . . . . . | 100 | 5.0 | 22.0 | 0 | 0 | 320 | 4.0 |
| bean, garbanzo (*Vigo* Spanish), ¼ of 6-oz. pkg. . . . . . . . . | 150 | 6.0 | 30.0 | 1.0 | 0 | 660 | 8.0 |
| beef: | | | | | | | |
| pasta (*Maggi*), ¼ pkt. . | 50 | 0 | 8.0 | 1.5 | 0 | 1180 | 0 |
| vegetable (*Hormel* Micro) | 90 | 6.0 | 16.0 | 1.0 | 10 | 790 | 1.0 |
| broccoli cheddar (*Vigo* Bison Canyon), 1 cup* . . . . . . . . . . . | 130 | 3.0 | 31.0 | 4.5 | 5 | 900 | 1.0 |
| broccoli cheese rice (*Uncle Ben's*), 1 oz. . . . | 110 | 3.0 | 43.0 | 2.0 | 5 | 680 | 1.0 |
| cheddar chipotle (*Vigo* Bison Canyon), 1 cup* . . . . . . . . . . . | 160 | 3.0 | 26.0 | 4.5 | 5 | 910 | 1.0 |
| chicken, cream of (*Cup-a-Soup*) . . . . . . . | 70 | 1.0 | 14.0 | 1.5 | 0 | 730 | 0 |
| chicken, creamy (*Maggi*), ¼ pkt. . . . . . . | 60 | 1.0 | 9.0 | 1.0 | 0 | 810 | 0 |
| chicken noodle: | | | | | | | |
| (*Alessi* Brodo di Pollo), ¼ of 6-oz. pkg. . . . . | 70 | 3.0 | 14.0 | 0 | 10 | 750 | 2.0 |
| (*Cup-a-Soup*) . . . . . . . | 80 | 2.0 | 17.0 | .5 | <5 | 920 | 0 |
| (*Hormel* Micro) . . . . . . . | 100 | 7.0 | 12.0 | 2.5 | 25 | 790 | 0 |
| (*Vigo* Bison Canyon), 1 cup* . . . . . . . . . . | 70 | 2.0 | 14.0 | 5 | 0 | 680 | 1.0 |
| chicken pasta, ¼ pkt.: | | | | | | | |
| (*Maggi*) . . . . . . . . . . . . | 50 | 1.0 | 9.0 | .5 | 0 | 880 | 0 |
| seashell (*Maggi*) . . . . . | 50 | 1.0 | 10.0 | .5 | 0 | 880 | 0 |
| chicken rice: | | | | | | | |
| (*Hormel* Micro) . . . . . . . | 110 | 4.0 | 18.0 | 3.0 | 10 | 850 | 1.0 |
| (*Maggi*), ¼ pkt. . . . . . . | 50 | 1.0 | 10.0 | .5 | 0 | 880 | 0 |
| chili (*Vigo* Bison Canyon), 1 cup* . . . . . | 100 | 6.0 | 18.0 | 1.0 | 0 | 390 | 5.0 |
| clam chowder, New England (*Hormel* Micro) . . . . . . . . . . . . . | 140 | 5.0 | 18.0 | 5.0 | 20 | 800 | 1.0 |
| collard greens (*Vigo*), ¼ of 6-oz. pkg. . . . . . . | 160 | 8.0 | 26.0 | 2.5 | 0 | 680 | n.a. |
| corn: | | | | | | | |
| (*Kikkoman* Egg Flower), 1 tsp. . . . . | 50 | 1.0 | 11.0 | 0 | 0 | 750 | <1.0 |
| creamy (*Maggi*), ¼ pkt. | 60 | 2.0 | 10.0 | 1.0 | 0 | 780 | 0 |

| Food and Measure | cal. | prot. (gms) | carbo. (gms) | fat (gms) | chol. (mgs) | sod. (mgs) | fiber (gms) |
|---|---|---|---|---|---|---|---|
| **Soup, mix** *(cont.)* | | | | | | | |
| crab flavor (*Kikkoman* Seafood), 3 tsp. ...... | 25 | 1.0 | 5.0 | 0 | 0 | 860 | <1.0 |
| hot and sour (*Kikkoman* Egg Flower), 2 tsp. ... | 30 | <1.0 | 6.0 | 0 | 0 | 880 | 0 |
| Japanese broth (*Kikkoman* Osuimono) | 0 | 0 | <1.0 | 0 | 0 | 660 | 0 |
| lentil (*Alessi* Sicilian), ¼ of 6-oz. pkg. ...... | 150 | 8.0 | 27.0 | 0 | 0 | 690 | 5.0 |
| miso: | | | | | | | |
| dark (*San-J*) ........ | 40 | 4.0 | 3.0 | 1.5 | 0 | 1150 | 1.0 |
| mild (*San-J*) ........ | 45 | 3.0 | 5.0 | 1.5 | 0 | 1360 | <1.0 |
| red (*Kikkoman* Aka) .. | 35 | 2.0 | 4.0 | 1.0 | 0 | 790 | 0 |
| tofu (*Kikkoman*) ..... | 35 | 3.0 | 3.0 | 1.0 | 0 | 740 | 0 |
| tofu spinach (*Kikkoman*) ...... | 35 | 3.0 | 4.0 | 1.0 | 0 | 790 | 0 |
| white (*Kikkoman* Shiro) | 35 | 3.0 | 4.0 | 1.0 | 0 | 820 | 0 |
| white (*San-J*) ....... | 40 | 3.0 | 3.0 | 1.5 | 0 | 860 | 0 |
| mushroom, creamy (*Maggi*), ¼ pkt. ...... | 60 | 1.0 | 9.0 | 3.0 | 0 | 990 | 0 |
| noodle, chicken flavor, w/vegetables (*Health Valley*), ½ cont. ..... | 110 | 5.0 | 24.0 | 0 | 0 | 390 | 3.0 |
| noodle, ramen, all flavors (*Roland*), 1 oz. .............. | 130 | 2.0 | 17.0 | 6.0 | 0 | 480 | 1.0 |
| noodle cup (*Roland*): | | | | | | | |
| beef .............. | 310 | 7.0 | 41.0 | 13.0 | 0 | 1100 | 0 |
| chicken ............ | 300 | 7.0 | 37.0 | 14.0 | 0 | 1100 | 0 |
| vegetable .......... | 300 | 7.0 | 39.0 | 13.0 | 0 | 930 | 0 |
| pea, split: | | | | | | | |
| (*Alessi* Sicilian), ¼ of 6-oz. pkg. ........ | 120 | 7.0 | 24.0 | .5 | 0 | 740 | 5.0 |
| (*Fantastic* Dutch), 1 cup* .......... | 120 | 8.0 | 21.0 | 1.0 | 0 | 590 | 5.0 |
| potato, creamy (*Fantastic* Blarneystone), 1 oz. ... | 110 | 9.0 | 28.0 | 2.0 | 5 | 760 | 3.0 |
| potato white bean (*Vigo* Bison Canyon), 1 cup* | 150 | 4.0 | 27.0 | 3.5 | 0 | 870 | 3.0 |
| scallop flavor (*Kikkoman* Seafood), 3 tsp. ..... | 35 | 1.0 | 7.0 | 0 | 0 | 1040 | <1.0 |
| seafood, creamy (*Maggi*), ¼ pkt. ...... | 80 | 2.0 | 11.0 | 2.5 | 20 | 1130 | 0 |

| Food and Measure | cal. | prot. (gms) | carbo. (gms) | fat (gms) | chol. (mgs) | sod. (mgs) | fiber (gms) |
|---|---|---|---|---|---|---|---|
| shrimp flavor (*Kikkoman* Seafood), 3 tsp. ..... | 30 | 1.0 | 5.0 | .5 | 0 | 770 | .3 |
| tomato, w/croutons (*Cup-a-Soup*) ....... | 90 | 1.0 | 16.0 | 2.5 | 0 | 870 | <1.0 |
| tomato, w/pasta, all styles (*Maggi*), ¼ pkt. | 60 | 2.0 | 13.0 | .5 | 0 | 1090 | 0 |
| udon noodle, chicken flavor (*Frieda's*), 3.5 oz. ............ | 132 | 3.0 | 28.0 | 1.0 | 0 | 675 | 0 |
| vegetable (*Kikkoman* Egg Flower), 1⅓ tsp. . | 40 | 1.0 | 7.0 | 1.0 | 0 | 870 | <1.0 |
| wakame: | | | | | | | |
| (*Kikkoman*) ......... | 15 | <1.0 | 3.0 | 0 | 0 | 700 | 0 |
| (*San-J*) ............ | 50 | <1.0 | 11.0 | 0 | 0 | 960 | <1.0 |
| **Soup base** (see also "Boullion"): | | | | | | | |
| beef: | | | | | | | |
| (*Glory* Cooking Base), 1 tsp. ...... | 15 | 1.0 | 1.0 | .5 | 0 | 670 | 0 |
| (*Roland*), ¾ tsp. ..... | 10 | 0 | 0 | 0 | 0 | 580 | 0 |
| chicken: | | | | | | | |
| (*Glory* Cooking Base), 1 tsp. ...... | 10 | 1.0 | 2.0 | 0 | 0 | 630 | 0 |
| (*Roland*), ½ tsp. ..... | 15 | 0 | 1.0 | 0 | 0 | 600 | 0 |
| clam (*Roland*), ½ tsp. ... | 10 | 0 | 0 | 0 | 0 | 590 | 0 |
| coconut ginger (*A Taste of Thai*), 1 tsp. ... | 8 | 0 | 2.0 | 0 | 0 | 720 | 0 |
| lobster (*Roland*), ½ tsp. . | 10 | 0 | 0 | 0 | 5 | 640 | 0 |
| noodle (*Kikkoman* Memmi), 2 tbsp. ...... | 40 | 2.0 | 7.0 | 0 | 0 | 2020 | 0 |
| vegetable: | | | | | | | |
| (*Roland*), ¾ tsp. ..... | 10 | 0 | 2.0 | 0 | 0 | 510 | 0 |
| roasted (*Glory* Cooking Base), 1 tsp. | 10 | 0 | 2.0 | 0 | 0 | 660 | 0 |
| **Soup seasoning mix** (*McCormick* Slow Cookers): | | | | | | | |
| chicken noodle, 2 tsp. ... | 10 | 0 | 2.0 | 0 | 0 | 790 | 0 |
| vegetable beef, 1 tsp. ... | 10 | 0 | 2.0 | 0 | 0 | 540 | 0 |
| **Sour cream**, see "Cream, sour" | | | | | | | |
| **Soursop**, ½ cup ....... | 75 | 1.1 | 18.9 | .3 | 0 | 16 | 3.7 |
| **Soy, cultured**, see "Yogurt, soy" | | | | | | | |

| Food and Measure | cal. | prot. (gms) | carbo. (gms) | fat (gms) | chol. (mgs) | sod. (mgs) | fiber (gms) |
|---|---|---|---|---|---|---|---|
| **Soy bean**, see "Soybean" | | | | | | | |
| **Soy beverage** (see also "Rice-soy beverage" and "Soy-milk beverage"), 8 fl. oz.: | | | | | | | |
| (*Edensoy* Organic Extra Original) . . . . . . . | 130 | 11.0 | 13.0 | 4.0 | 0 | 100 | <1.0 |
| (*Edensoy* Organic Original) . . . . . . . . . . . | 140 | 11.0 | 14.0 | 5.0 | 0 | 105 | <1.0 |
| (*Edensoy* Organic Unsweetened) . . . . . . . | 120 | 12.0 | 5.0 | 6.0 | 0 | 5 | <1.0 |
| (*8th Continent* Complete) | 80 | 6.0 | 8.0 | 2.5 | 0 | 95 | 3.0 |
| (*8th Continent* Original) . . . . . . . . . . . | 80 | 8.0 | 7.0 | 2.5 | 0 | 95 | 0 |
| (*8th Continent* Original Nonfat) . . . . . | 60 | 6.0 | 8.0 | 0 | 0 | 100 | 0 |
| (*8th Continent* Original Light) . . . . . . . | 50 | 6.0 | 2.0 | 2.0 | 0 | 115 | 0 |
| (*Pacific* Organic Unsweetened) . . . . . . . | 90 | 9.0 | 4.0 | 4.5 | 0 | 15 | 2.0 |
| (*Pacific* Select Low Fat) . . . . . . . . . . | 70 | 5.0 | 9.0 | 2.5 | 0 | 115 | 1.0 |
| (*Pacific* Ultra) . . . . . . . . . | 120 | 10.0 | 11.0 | 4.0 | 0 | 150 | 1.0 |
| (*Pearl* Organic Original) . . . . . . . . . . . | 110 | 7.0 | 12.0 | 3.0 | 0 | 110 | 1.0 |
| (*Pearl* Organic Unsweetened) . . . . . . . | 90 | 8.0 | 6.0 | 4.5 | 0 | 130 | 0 |
| (*Silk* DHA Omega-3/Calcium) . . . | 110 | 7.0 | 8.0 | 5.0 | 0 | 120 | 1.0 |
| (*Silk* Heart Health) . . . . . . | 80 | 6.0 | 10.0 | 1.5 | 0 | 95 | 1.0 |
| (*Silk* Light) . . . . . . . . . . | 70 | 6.0 | 8.0 | 2.0 | 0 | 120 | 1.0 |
| (*Silk* Original/ Original Organic) . . . . | 100 | 7.0 | 8.0 | 4.0 | 0 | 120 | 1.0 |
| (*Silk* Unsweetened Organic) . . . . . . . . . . | 80 | 7.0 | 4.0 | 4.0 | 0 | 85 | 1.0 |
| (*Soy Dream* Organic Original Classic Chilled) . . . . . . . . . . . . | 130 | 7.0 | 16.0 | 4.0 | 0 | 150 | 2.0 |
| (*Soy Dream* Organic Original Enriched) . . . . | 100 | 7.0 | 8.0 | 4.0 | 0 | 135 | 2.0 |
| (*Soy Dream* Organic Original Enriched Refrigerated) . . . . . . . | 100 | 8.0 | 9.0 | 3.5 | 0 | 140 | 2.0 |

| Food and Measure | cal. | prot. (gms) | carbo. (gms) | fat (gms) | chol. (mgs) | sod. (mgs) | fiber (gms) |
|---|---|---|---|---|---|---|---|
| carob (*Edensoy* Organic) | 170 | 7.0 | 28.0 | 4.0 | 0 | 95 | <1.0 |
| chocolate: | | | | | | | |
| (*Edensoy* Organic) ... | 180 | 8.0 | 28.0 | 4.0 | 0 | 105 | <1.0 |
| (*8th Continent*) ...... | 140 | 7.0 | 22.0 | 3.0 | 0 | 125 | 1.0 |
| (*8th Continent* Light) .......... | 90 | 7.0 | 12.0 | 1.5 | 0 | 120 | <1.0 |
| (*Odwalla Super Protein*) ......... | 170 | 10.0 | 24.0 | 3.5 | 0 | 240 | 0 |
| (*Pearl* Organic) ...... | 150 | 8.0 | 21.0 | 4.5 | 0 | 180 | 0 |
| (*Silk*) .............. | 140 | 5.0 | 23.0 | 3.0 | 0 | 100 | 2.0 |
| (*Silk* Light) ......... | 90 | 3.0 | 15.0 | 1.5 | 0 | 80 | 2.0 |
| (*Soy Dream* Organic Enriched) | 150 | 7.0 | 21.0 | 4.0 | 0 | 125 | 3.0 |
| coffee (*Pearl* Organic) ... | 150 | 6.0 | 24.0 | 4.0 | 0 | 190 | 0 |
| green tea (*Pearl* Organic) .......... | 110 | 7.0 | 13.0 | 3.5 | 0 | 95 | 1.0 |
| vanilla: | | | | | | | |
| (*Edensoy* Organic) ... | 150 | 7.0 | 24.0 | 3.0 | 0 | 85 | <1.0 |
| (*Edensoy* Organic Extra) ........... | 150 | 7.0 | 23.0 | 3.0 | 0 | 90 | <1.0 |
| (*Edensoy* Organic Light) .......... | 110 | 4.0 | 22.0 | 1.0 | 0 | 110 | 0 |
| (*8th Continent*) ...... | 100 | 6.0 | 11.0 | 3.0 | 0 | 105 | 0 |
| (*8th Continent* Light) . | 60 | 6.0 | 5.0 | 2.0 | 0 | 110 | 0 |
| (*8th Continent* Nonfat) .......... | 70 | 6.0 | 11.0 | 0 | 0 | 100 | 0 |
| (*Pacific* Select Low Fat) ......... | 80 | 5.0 | 11.0 | 2.5 | 0 | 115 | 1.0 |
| (*Pacific* Ultra) ....... | 130 | 10.0 | 14.0 | 4.0 | 0 | 150 | 1.0 |
| (*Pearl* Organic) ...... | 100 | 6.0 | 10.0 | 3.5 | 0 | 95 | 1.0 |
| (*Silk* Light) ......... | 80 | 6.0 | 10.0 | 2.0 | 0 | 95 | 1.0 |
| (*Silk* Original/ Organic) ......... | 100 | 6.0 | 11.0 | 3.5 | 0 | 95 | 1.0 |
| (*Silk* Very Vanilla) .... | 130 | 6.0 | 19.0 | 4.0 | 0 | 140 | 1.0 |
| (*Soy Dream* Organic Classic) ......... | 140 | 7.0 | 18.0 | 4.0 | 0 | 135 | 2.0 |
| (*Soy Dream* Organic Enriched) ........ | 120 | 7.0 | 14.0 | 4.0 | 0 | 135 | 2.0 |
| (*Soy Dream* Organic Enriched Chilled) .. | 120 | 8.0 | 14.0 | 3.5 | 0 | 130 | 2.0 |
| vanilla chai tea (*Bolthouse Farms Perfectly Protein*) .... | 160 | 10.0 | 25.0 | 3.0 | 0 | 60 | 0 |

| Food and Measure | cal. | prot. (gms) | carbo. (gms) | fat (gms) | chol. (mgs) | sod. (mgs) | fiber (gms) |
|---|---|---|---|---|---|---|---|
| **Soy crisps** (see also "Potato soy crisps") (*Genisoy*), 1 oz.: | | | | | | | |
| apple cinnamon, bag .... | 120 | 7.0 | 17.0 | 3.0 | 0 | 270 | 2.0 |
| barbecue ............. | 110 | 6.0 | 14.0 | 4.0 | 0 | 150 | 2.0 |
| barbecue, zesty ........ | 120 | 7.0 | 17.0 | 3.0 | 0 | 270 | 2.0 |
| cheddar ............. | 120 | 7.0 | 13.0 | 4.5 | 0 | 190 | 2.0 |
| cheddar, bag .......... | 110 | 7.0 | 14.0 | 3.0 | 0 | 270 | 2.0 |
| nacho cheese ........ | 120 | 7.0 | 14.0 | 4.0 | 0 | 170 | 2.0 |
| ranch ............... | 120 | 7.0 | 14.0 | 4.0 | 0 | 270 | 2.0 |
| roasted garlic onion .... | 100 | 7.0 | 14.0 | 2.0 | 0 | 280 | 2.0 |
| salt and vinegar ........ | 110 | 6.0 | 14.0 | 3.5 | 0 | 250 | 2.0 |
| salt and vinegar, bag .... | 110 | 7.0 | 14.0 | 3.0 | 0 | 270 | 2.0 |
| salted, deep sea ....... | 100 | 8.0 | 15.0 | 1.5 | 0 | 270 | 2.0 |
| **Soy flour**, see "Soybean flour" | | | | | | | |
| **Soy meal**, defatted, raw, 1 cup .......... | 414 | 54.8 | 49.0 | 2.9 | 0 | 3 | 14.0 |
| **Soy milk**, see "Soy beverage" | | | | | | | |
| **Soy-milk beverage** (*Odwalla Protein Monster*), 8 fl. oz.: | | | | | | | |
| chocolate ............ | 220 | 18.0 | 27.0 | 4.0 | 5 | 310 | 0 |
| strawberry ........... | 160 | 13.0 | 19.0 | 3.5 | 2 | 90 | 0 |
| vanilla ............... | 200 | 18.0 | 24.0 | 3.5 | 5 | 130 | 0 |
| **Soy nuts**, roasted: | | | | | | | |
| (*Frieda's* Salted), ⅓ cup, 1.1 oz. ....... | 140 | 11.0 | 9.0 | 7.0 | 0 | 50 | 5.0 |
| (*Genisoy* Deep Sea Salted), ¼ cup, 1 oz. . | 120 | 10.0 | 11.0 | 4.0 | 0 | 230 | 7.0 |
| (*Genisoy* Unsalted), ¼ cup, 1 oz. ........ | 120 | 11.0 | 10.0 | 5.0 | 0 | 10 | 5.0 |
| barbecue (*Genisoy*), ¼ cup, 1 oz. ........ | 120 | 10.0 | 11.0 | 4.0 | 0 | 230 | 7.0 |
| barbecue, honey, or wasabi (*Frieda's*), ¼ cup .............. | 140 | 10.0 | 11.0 | 7.0 | 0 | 110 | 5.0 |
| hickory smoked (*Genisoy*), ¼ cup, 1 oz. | 120 | 10.0 | 11.0 | 5.0 | 0 | 290 | 6.0 |
| toasted: | | | | | | | |
| 1 oz. or 95 kernels ... | 129 | 10.5 | 8.7 | 6.8 | 0 | 1 | 1.0 |
| whole, 1 cup ........ | 490 | 40.0 | 33.0 | 25.9 | 0 | 4 | 3.9 |

| Food and Measure | cal. | prot. (gms) | carbo. (gms) | fat (gms) | chol. (mgs) | sod. (mgs) | fiber (gms) |
|---|---|---|---|---|---|---|---|
| **Soy protein**, concentrate, 1 oz.: | | | | | | | |
| w/alcohol ............ | 94 | 16.5 | 8.8 | .1 | 0 | 1 | <2.0 |
| acid/water wash ....... | 94 | 16.5 | 8.8 | .1 | 0 | 255 | <2.0 |
| **Soy sauce**, 1 tbsp., except as noted: | | | | | | | |
| (*Angostura*) ........... | 10 | 1.0 | 1.0 | 0 | 0 | 670 | 0 |
| (*Angostura* Lite) ....... | 10 | 1.0 | 2.0 | 0 | 0 | 390 | 0 |
| (*House of Tsang* Less Sodium) .......... | 0 | 0 | 0 | 0 | 0 | 320 | 0 |
| (*Ka•Me*) .............. | 10 | <1.0 | 2.0 | 0 | 0 | 650 | 0 |
| (*Kikkoman*) ........... | 10 | 2.0 | 0 | 0 | 0 | 920 | 0 |
| (*Kikkoman* Less Sodium) | 10 | 1.0 | 1.0 | 0 | 0 | 575 | 0 |
| (*Kikkoman* Organic) .... | 10 | 2.0 | 1.0 | 0 | 0 | 1000 | 0 |
| (*La Choy*) ............. | 10 | 1.0 | 1.0 | 0 | 0 | 1160 | 0 |
| (*La Choy* Lite) ........ | 15 | 1.0 | 2.0 | 0 | 0 | 550 | 0 |
| (*Mee Tu* Light) ........ | 12 | .4 | 3.0 | 0 | 0 | 320 | 0 |
| (*Roland*) .............. | 10 | 1.0 | 2.0 | 0 | 0 | 820 | 0 |
| ginger flavor: | | | | | | | |
| (*House of Tsang*) .... | 20 | 1.0 | 4.0 | 0 | 0 | 760 | 0 |
| (*House of Tsang* Less Sodium) ..... | 10 | 0 | 2.0 | 0 | 0 | 330 | 0 |
| shoyu: | | | | | | | |
| (*Eden* Imported) ...... | 15 | 2.0 | 2.0 | 0 | 0 | 1010 | 0 |
| (*Eden* Organic) ...... | 15 | 2.0 | 2.0 | 0 | 0 | 1040 | 0 |
| (*Eden* Organic Imported Reduced Sodium) ......... | 10 | 2.0 | 2.0 | 0 | 0 | 500 | 0 |
| (*San-J* Organic) ..... | 10 | 2.0 | 1.0 | 0 | 0 | 960 | 0 |
| sushi and sashimi (*Kikkoman*) ......... | 15 | 1.0 | 2.0 | 0 | 0 | 870 | 0 |
| tamari: | | | | | | | |
| (*Eden* Organic) ...... | 15 | 2.0 | 2.0 | 0 | 0 | 860 | 0 |
| (*Eden* Organic Imported) | 10 | 2.0 | 2.0 | 0 | 0 | 990 | 0 |
| (*Kikkoman*) .......... | 15 | 2.0 | 1.0 | 0 | 0 | 980 | 0 |
| (*San-J* Organic Gluten Free) ...... | 10 | 2.0 | <1.0 | 0 | 0 | 940 | 0 |
| (*San-J* Premium) .... | 15 | 2.0 | 1.0 | 0 | 0 | 960 | 0 |
| (*San-J* Reduced Sodium) ......... | 15 | 2.0 | 1.0 | 0 | 0 | 700 | 0 |
| **Soybean**, fresh (see also "Edamame"): | | | | | | | |
| raw, shelled, ½ cup ..... | 188 | 16.6 | 14.1 | 8.7 | 0 | 19 | 5.4 |
| boiled, drained, ½ cup .. | 127 | 11.1 | 10.0 | 5.8 | 0 | 13 | 3.8 |

| Food and Measure | cal. | prot. (gms) | carbo. (gms) | fat (gms) | chol. (mgs) | sod. (mgs) | fiber (gms) |
|---|---|---|---|---|---|---|---|
| **Soybean, canned**, black (*Eden* Organic), ½ cup .......... | 120 | 11.0 | 8.0 | 6.0 | 0 | 30 | 7.0 |
| **Soybean, dried**: dry, ¼ cup, except as noted: | | | | | | | |
| (*Arrowhead Mills* Organic) ......... | 160 | 14.0 | 11.0 | 8.0 | 0 | 0 | 4.0 |
| (*Bob's Red Mill*) ..... | 180 | 16.0 | 13.0 | 9.0 | 0 | 0 | 4.0 |
| (*Bob's Red Mill* Organic), ½ cup ... | 190 | 17.0 | 14.0 | 9.0 | 0 | 0 | 4.0 |
| dry-roasted ......... | 194 | 17.0 | 14.1 | 9.3 | 0 | 1 | 3.5 |
| roasted ............ | 202 | 15.2 | 14.5 | 10.9 | 0 | 70 | 3.5 |
| boiled, ½ cup ........ | 149 | 14.3 | 8.5 | 7.7 | 0 | 1 | 5.2 |
| **Soybean, frozen**, see "Edamame" | | | | | | | |
| **Soybean flour**: | | | | | | | |
| (*Arrowhead Mills* Organic), ¼ cup ..... | 100 | 7.0 | 9.0 | 4.5 | 0 | 0 | 4.0 |
| (*Bob's Red Mill* Low Fat), 3 tbsp. ........ | 80 | 10.0 | 5.0 | 1.5 | 0 | 0 | 3.0 |
| (*Bob's Red Mill* Stoneground Regular/ Organic), ¼ cup ..... | 120 | 10.0 | 8.0 | 6.0 | 0 | 0 | 3.0 |
| (*Hodgson Mill*), <¼ cup ............ | 80 | 14.0 | 10.0 | 0 | 0 | 0 | 6.0 |
| (*Hodgson Mill* Organic), <¼ cup .... | 120 | 10.0 | 10.0 | 6.0 | 0 | 0 | 6.0 |
| stirred, ¼ cup: | | | | | | | |
| full fat, raw ......... | 93 | 7.4 | 7.5 | 4.4 | 0 | 3 | 2.1 |
| defatted ........... | 82 | 11.8 | 9.6 | .3 | 0 | 5 | 4.4 |
| low fat ............ | 72 | 10.2 | 8.4 | .6 | 0 | 4 | 2.3 |
| **Soybean kernels, roasted**, see "Soy nuts" | | | | | | | |
| **Soybean sprouts**, steamed, ½ cup ..... | 38 | 4.0 | 3.1 | 2.1 | 0 | 5 | .4 |
| **Spaghetti**, see "Pasta" | | | | | | | |
| **Spaghetti entree, canned** (see also "Pasta entree, canned") 1 cup: | | | | | | | |
| and meatballs: | | | | | | | |
| (*Chef Boyardee*) ..... | 260 | 10.0 | 30.0 | 11.0 | 15 | 750 | 4.0 |

| Food and Measure | cal. | prot. (gms) | carbo. (gms) | fat (gms) | chol. (mgs) | sod. (mgs) | fiber (gms) |
|---|---|---|---|---|---|---|---|
| (*Chef Boyardee* Big) .. | 270 | 12.0 | 28.0 | 12.0 | 25 | 980 | 3.0 |
| mini (*Chef Boyardee*) . | 240 | 10.0 | 28.0 | 10.0 | 15 | 750 | 3.0 |
| rings, mini (*Chef Boyardee*) ........ | 240 | 9.0 | 28.0 | 10.0 | 20 | 700 | 3.0 |
| tomato cheese sauce (*Campbell's*) ........ | 200 | 7.0 | 40.0 | 1.5 | 5 | 950 | 3.0 |
| **Spaghetti entree, frozen,** 1 pkg., except as noted: | | | | | | | |
| Bolognese (*Contessa* MicroSteam), 1 cup* . | 300 | 14.0 | 34.0 | 13.0 | 25 | 640 | 3.0 |
| cheesy (*Stouffer's* Bake), 12 oz. ........ | 460 | 21.0 | 39.0 | 24.0 | 120 | 950 | 4.0 |
| marinara, 8 oz.: | | | | | | | |
| (*Michelina's Authentico*) ...... | 250 | 8.0 | 47.0 | 2.0 | 0 | 430 | 3.0 |
| (*Michelina's Budget Gourmet*) ........ | 270 | 9.0 | 49.0 | 3.5 | 0 | 620 | 3.0 |
| w/meat sauce: | | | | | | | |
| (*Lean Cuisine*), 11.5 oz. | 300 | 15.0 | 49.0 | 4.0 | 15 | 690 | 4.0 |
| (*Marie Callender's*), 15 oz. ........... | 490 | 23.0 | 67.0 | 14.0 | 20 | 1030 | 7.0 |
| (*Michelina's Authentico*), 8.5 oz. | 300 | 11.0 | 46.0 | 7.0 | 10 | 750 | 4.0 |
| (*Michelina's Lean Gourmet*), 9 oz. ... | 320 | 12.0 | 49.0 | 7.0 | 15 | 560 | 4.0 |
| (*Smart Ones*), 11.5 oz. | 290 | 16.0 | 44.0 | 5.0 | 15 | 720 | 5.0 |
| (*Stouffer's*), 12 oz. ... | 350 | 17.0 | 44.0 | 12.0 | 30 | 660 | 5.0 |
| w/meatballs: | | | | | | | |
| (*Banquet*), 9 oz. ..... | 330 | 15.0 | 35.0 | 14.0 | 20 | 650 | 5.0 |
| (*Lean Cuisine*), 9.5 oz. | 270 | 16.0 | 38.0 | 6.0 | 25 | 580 | 3.0 |
| (*Michelina's Authentico*), 8 oz. .. | 270 | 12.0 | 37.0 | 8.0 | 15 | 710 | 3.0 |
| (*Stouffer's*), 12.6 oz. ... | 360 | 19.0 | 45.0 | 12.0 | 35 | 850 | 6.0 |
| w/popcorn chicken (*Banquet*), 7 oz. ..... | 270 | 12.0 | 37.0 | 8.0 | 10 | 580 | 4.0 |
| **Spaghetti entree, microwave,** 1 cont.: | | | | | | | |
| (*Hormel Compleats*), 10 oz. ............. | 250 | 15.0 | 29.0 | 8.0 | 40 | 590 | 3.0 |
| and meatballs: (*Chef Boyardee*), 7.2 oz. .......... | 190 | 8.0 | 21.0 | 8.0 | 15 | 740 | 2.0 |

| Food and Measure | cal. | prot. (gms) | carbo. (gms) | fat (gms) | chol. (mgs) | sod. (mgs) | fiber (gms) |
|---|---|---|---|---|---|---|---|
| **Spaghetti entree, microwave, and meatballs** *(cont.)* | | | | | | | |
| rings, mini (*Chef Boyardee*), 7.5 oz. . | 220 | 8.0 | 27.0 | 9.0 | 15 | 750 | 3.0 |
| w/meat sauce: | | | | | | | |
| (*Hormel* Microcup), 7.5 oz. . . . . . . . . . | 210 | 10.0 | 31.0 | 5.0 | 15 | 750 | 3.0 |
| (*Hormel Compleats*), 10 oz. . . . . . . . . . . | 290 | 15.0 | 36.0 | 9.0 | 30 | 800 | 3.0 |
| **Spaghetti entree mix** (*Kraft Spaghetti Classics*), ¼ pkg.: | | | | | | | |
| Italian, tangy . . . . . . . . . | 200 | 8.0 | 38.0 | 1.5 | 0 | 600 | 1.0 |
| w/meat sauce . . . . . . . . . | 330 | 12.0 | 46.0 | 11.0 | 15 | 830 | 3.0 |
| **Spaghetti sauce**, see "Pasta sauce" | | | | | | | |
| **Spaghetti sauce mix**: | | | | | | | |
| (*Lawry's*), 1½ tbsp. . . . . . | 25 | 0 | 6.0 | 0 | 0 | 600 | 0 |
| (*Lawry's* Extra Rich & Thick), 1 tbsp. . | 30 | <1.0 | 7.0 | 0 | 0 | 620 | <1.0 |
| (*McCormick* Thick & Zesty), 1 tbsp. . . . . . . | 35 | 0 | 7.0 | 0 | 0 | 530 | 0 |
| Italian style (*McCormick*), 1⅓ tbsp. . . . . . . . . . | 40 | 0 | 8.0 | 0 | 0 | 500 | 0 |
| **Spaghetti squash**: | | | | | | | |
| raw (*Frieda's*), 3 oz. . . . . . | 30 | 1.0 | 6.0 | 0 | 0 | 15 | 1.0 |
| baked or boiled, drained, ½ cup . . . . . . | 23 | .5 | 5.0 | .2 | 0 | 14 | 1.1 |
| **Spanakopita**, see "Spinach entree" | | | | | | | |
| **Spareribs**, see "Pork" | | | | | | | |
| **Spelt**, grain, ¼ cup: | | | | | | | |
| (*Bob's Red Mill* Berries) . . . . . . . . . . . | 150 | 6.0 | 32.0 | 1.5 | 0 | 0 | 4.0 |
| (*Bob's Red Mill* Organic Berries) . . . . . | 130 | 5.0 | 33.0 | 1.0 | 0 | 0 | 6.0 |
| (*VitaSpelt* Kernels Regular/Organic) . . . . | 130 | 7.0 | 32.0 | 1.0 | 0 | 0 | 8.0 |
| **Spelt flakes**, see "Cereal" | | | | | | | |
| **Spelt flour**: | | | | | | | |
| (*Arrowhead Mills* Organic), ⅓ cup . . . . . | 130 | 4.0 | 25.0 | 1.0 | 0 | 0 | 4.0 |

| Food and Measure | cal. | prot. (gms) | carbo. (gms) | fat (gms) | chol. (mgs) | sod. (mgs) | fiber (gms) |
|---|---|---|---|---|---|---|---|
| (*Bob's Red Mill* Light), ¼ cup | 100 | 4.0 | 21.0 | .5 | 0 | 0 | 2.0 |
| (*Bob's Red Mill* Organic), ¼ cup | 120 | 4.0 | 22.0 | 1.0 | 0 | 1 | 4.0 |
| white (*VitaSpelt* Organic), ¼ cup | 100 | 4.0 | 21.0 | .5 | 0 | 0 | 1.0 |
| whole grain (*VitaSpelt* Organic), ¼ cup | 110 | 5.0 | 23.0 | 1.0 | 0 | 0 | 2.0 |
| **Spinach**, fresh: | | | | | | | |
| raw, 3 oz., 3–4 cups: | | | | | | | |
| (*Dole/Dole* Baby) | 20 | 2.0 | 3.0 | 0 | 0 | 67 | 2.0 |
| (*Fresh Express*) | 20 | 2.0 | 3.0 | 0 | 0 | 65 | 2.0 |
| baby (*Fresh Express*) | 25 | 3.0 | 2.0 | 0 | 0 | 65 | 1.0 |
| baby (*Ready Pac*) | 20 | 2.0 | 3.0 | 0 | 0 | 65 | 2.0 |
| cooked, boiled, drained, ½ cup | 21 | 2.7 | 3.4 | .2 | 0 | 63 | 2.2 |
| **Spinach, canned**: | | | | | | | |
| leaf, ½ cup: | | | | | | | |
| (*Popeye* No Salt) | 40 | 4.0 | 5.0 | .5 | 0 | 30 | 2.0 |
| (*S&W*) | 30 | 2.0 | 4.0 | 0 | 0 | 360 | 2.0 |
| cut (*Freshlike*) | 45 | 5.0 | 5.0 | 1.0 | 0 | 200 | 3.0 |
| leaf or chopped, ½ cup: | | | | | | | |
| (*Del Monte*) | 30 | 2.0 | 4.0 | 0 | 0 | 360 | 2.0 |
| (*Popeye*) | 30 | 3.0 | 4.0 | 0 | 0 | 190 | 2.0 |
| seasoned, Southern (*Glory*), ½ cup | 20 | 2.0 | 4.0 | 0 | 0 | 510 | 2.0 |
| drained, ½ cup | 25 | 3.0 | 3.6 | .5 | 0 | 29 | 2.6 |
| **Spinach, frozen** (see also "Spinach dish"): | | | | | | | |
| leaf or chopped (*Birds Eye*), ⅓ cup | 30 | 2.0 | 3.0 | 0 | 0 | 125 | 1.0 |
| cut leaf: | | | | | | | |
| (*Birds Eye*), 1 cup | 30 | 2.0 | 3.0 | 0 | 0 | 120 | 1.0 |
| (*Cascadian Farm* Organic), ⅓ cup | 25 | 2.0 | 3.0 | 0 | 0 | 160 | 1.0 |
| chopped: | | | | | | | |
| (*C&W/Freshlike*), ⅓ cup | 30 | 2.0 | 3.0 | 0 | 0 | 125 | 1.0 |
| (*Green Giant*), ½ cup | 25 | 2.0 | 3.0 | 0 | 0 | 200 | 1.0 |
| baby (*C&W*), 1 cup | 30 | 2.0 | 3.0 | 0 | 0 | 120 | 1.0 |
| chopped or leaf, drained, ½ cup | 27 | 3.0 | 5.1 | .2 | 0 | 82 | 2.6 |
| in butter sauce, cut (*Green Giant*), ½ cup | 30 | 2.0 | 4.0 | 1.0 | <5 | 330 | 2.0 |

| Food and Measure | cal. | prot. (gms) | carbo. (gms) | fat (gms) | chol. (mgs) | sod. (mgs) | fiber (gms) |
|---|---|---|---|---|---|---|---|
| **Spinach, malabar**, cooked, 1 cup . . . . . . . | 10 | 1.3 | 1.2 | .4 | 0 | 24 | .9 |
| **Spinach, New Zealand**, chopped: | | | | | | | |
| raw, ½ cup, 1 oz. . . . . . . | 4 | .4 | .7 | .1 | 0 | 37 | n.a. |
| boiled, drained, ½ cup . . | 11 | 1.2 | 2.0 | .2 | 0 | 97 | n.a. |
| **Spinach appetizer**, see "Spinach dish" | | | | | | | |
| **Spinach dip**, 2 tbsp.: | | | | | | | |
| (*Cedar's*) . . . . . . . . . . . . | 50 | 1.0 | 2.0 | 4.5 | 5 | 85 | 0 |
| (*Tostitos* Creamy) . . . . . . | 50 | 1.0 | 2.0 | 4.0 | <5 | 200 | <1.0 |
| (*Marzetti*) . . . . . . . . . . . . | 130 | 1.0 | 2.0 | 13.0 | 20 | 250 | 0 |
| artichoke (*Health is Wealth*) | 30 | 1.0 | 3.0 | 1.5 | 5 | 50 | 0 |
| Parmesan (*Marie's*) . . . . . | 90 | 2.0 | 2.0 | 9.0 | 15 | 200 | 0 |
| **Spinach dip mix**, dry (*McCormick*), 1 tsp. . . | 5 | 0 | <1.0 | 0 | 0 | 95 | 0 |
| **Spinach dish**, frozen/ chilled: | | | | | | | |
| bites, 3 pcs., 2.6 oz., except as noted: | | | | | | | |
| (*Dr. Praeger's*), 2 pcs., 2 oz. . . . . . . | 110 | 3.0 | 17.0 | 3.0 | 0 | 230 | 2.0 |
| (*Veggie Patch*) . . . . . | 150 | 6.0 | 16.0 | 8.0 | 10 | 350 | 3.0 |
| and artichoke (*Bistro au Naturel*) . . . . . . . | 170 | 4.0 | 16.0 | 11.0 | 10 | 380 | 1.0 |
| 3 cheese (*Bistro au Naturel*) . . . . . . . . | 150 | 6.0 | 16.0 | 8.0 | 10 | 350 | 3.0 |
| bites, w/cheese (*Health is Wealth Munchees*), 6 pcs., 3 oz. . . . . . . . . | 180 | 7.0 | 25.0 | 7.0 | 0 | 320 | 1.0 |
| creamed, ½ cup, except as noted: | | | | | | | |
| (*Birds Eye* Real) . . . . . | 90 | 3.0 | 9.0 | 4.0 | 10 | 500 | 4.0 |
| (*Green Giant*) . . . . . . . | 70 | 3.0 | 9.0 | 2.5 | 0 | 510 | 1.0 |
| (*Popeye SteamSupreme*) . . . | 100 | 3.0 | 5.0 | 6.0 | 20 | 330 | 1.0 |
| (*Seabrook Farms*) . . . . | 120 | 4.0 | 10.0 | 6.0 | 15 | 450 | 3.0 |
| (*Stouffer's*), ½ of 9-oz. pkg. . . . . . . . . | 200 | 5.0 | 8.0 | 16.0 | 25 | 490 | 2.0 |
| (*Tabatchnick*), ¼ of 15-oz. pkg. . . . . . . . | 40 | 1.0 | 7.0 | 1.0 | 5 | 240 | 1.0 |
| w/feta, spanakopita: | | | | | | | |
| (*Athens/Apollo*), 2 pcs., 2 oz. . . . . . . . . . . . . | 160 | 4.0 | 17.0 | 8.0 | 20 | 240 | 1.0 |

| Food and Measure | cal. | prot. (gms) | carbo. (gms) | fat (gms) | chol. (mgs) | sod. (mgs) | fiber (gms) |
|---|---|---|---|---|---|---|---|
| (*Kontos*), 1-oz. pc. . . . | 60 | 3.0 | 6.0 | 3.0 | 10 | 150 | 0 |
| (*The Fillo Factory* 10 oz.), 4 pcs., 3.3 oz. . . . . | 210 | 7.0 | 26.0 | 9.0 | 10 | 340 | 2.0 |
| (*The Fillo Factory* 12 oz.), 3 pcs., 3 oz. | 190 | 6.0 | 20.0 | 9.0 | 20 | 260 | 1.0 |
| (*Yiayia's*), 3-oz. pc. . . . | 190 | 7.0 | 20.0 | 9.0 | 30 | 290 | 1.0 |
| w/feta, pie (*The Fillo Factory* Organic), ½ of 10-oz. pkg. . . . . . | 280 | 10.0 | 30.0 | 14.0 | 15 | 470 | 3.0 |
| nuggets, breaded (*Veggie Patch*), 4 pcs., 3 oz. . . | 150 | 6.0 | 19.0 | 7.0 | 0 | 390 | 3.0 |
| pancake, 1 pc.: |  |  |  |  |  |  |  |
| (*Dr. Praeger's*), 2 oz. . . | 80 | 2.0 | 9.0 | 4.0 | 0 | 190 | 2.0 |
| (*Golden*), 1.3 oz. . . . . . | 70 | 2.0 | 10.0 | 3.0 | <5 | 210 | <1.0 |
| soufflé (*Stouffer's*), ⅓ of 12-oz. pkg. . . . . . | 150 | 6.0 | 9.0 | 10.0 | 110 | 390 | 1.0 |
| **Spinach entree, frozen**, 1 pkg., except as noted: |  |  |  |  |  |  |  |
| w/cheese, palak paneer: |  |  |  |  |  |  |  |
| (*Amy's*), 10 oz. . . . . . . | 300 | 12.0 | 38.0 | 11.0 | 15 | 680 | 6.0 |
| (*Ethnic Gourmet*), 11 oz. . . . . . . . . . . . | 240 | 13.0 | 23.0 | 11.0 | 35 | 810 | 4.0 |
| and feta pie (*Cedarlane* Organic Spanakopita), ½ of 10-oz. pkg. . . . . . | 260 | 12.0 | 38.0 | 8.0 | 20 | 650 | 2.0 |
| ricotta bake (*Michelina's Lean Gourmet*), 8 oz. . . . . . . . . . . . . . . . | 290 | 10.0 | 47.0 | 7.0 | 15 | 570 | 3.0 |
| **Spinach entree, micro-wave** (*Tasty Bite*), ½ of 10-oz. pkg.: |  |  |  |  |  |  |  |
| w/lentils, dal . . . . . . . . . | 110 | 5.0 | 13.0 | 5.0 | 0 | 530 | 4.0 |
| w/cheese, Kashmir . . . . . | 130 | 6.0 | 8.0 | 8.0 | 0 | 690 | 3.0 |
| **Spinach pocket sandwich**, frozen, 1 pc.: |  |  |  |  |  |  |  |
| and feta: |  |  |  |  |  |  |  |
| (*Amy's*), 4.5 oz. . . . . . | 260 | 11.0 | 34.0 | 9.0 | 20 | 590 | 3.0 |
| (*Aunt Trudy's*), 5 oz. . . | 270 | 11.0 | 31.0 | 12.0 | 15 | 470 | 3.0 |
| and potato (*Aunt Trudy's* Organic), 5 oz. | 250 | 6.0 | 40.0 | 9.0 | 0 | 380 | 4.0 |
| **Spinach snacks**, see "Spinach dish" |  |  |  |  |  |  |  |

| Food and Measure | cal. | prot. (gms) | carbo. (gms) | fat (gms) | chol. (mgs) | sod. (mgs) | fiber (gms) |
|---|---|---|---|---|---|---|---|
| **Spiny lobster**, meat only: | | | | | | | |
| raw, 4 oz. ............ | 127 | 23.4 | 2.8 | 1.7 | 80 | 201 | 0 |
| boiled or steamed: | | | | | | | |
|   2 lbs. in shell ....... | 233 | 43.1 | 5.1 | 3.2 | 146 | 370 | 0 |
|   4 oz. ............. | 138 | 29.9 | 3.5 | 2.2 | 102 | 257 | 0 |
| **Spleen**, braised: | | | | | | | |
| beef, 4 oz. ............ | 164 | 28.5 | 0 | 4.8 | 394 | 65 | 0 |
| lamb, 4 oz. ........... | 177 | 30.0 | 0 | 5.4 | 437 | 66 | 0 |
| pork, 4 oz. ............ | 169 | 32.0 | 0 | 3.6 | 572 | 121 | 0 |
| veal, 4 oz. ............ | 146 | 27.3 | 0 | 3.3 | 507 | 66 | 0 |
| **Split peas**: | | | | | | | |
| dry, green, ¼ cup: | | | | | | | |
|   (*Arrowhead Mills* | | | | | | | |
|     Organic) ......... | 160 | 12.0 | 24.0 | 1.0 | 0 | 10 | 4.0 |
|   or yellow (*Bob's Red* | | | | | | | |
|     *Mill*) ............. | 170 | 13.0 | 31.0 | .5 | 0 | 10 | 13.0 |
| boiled, ½ cup .......... | 116 | 8.2 | 20.7 | .4 | 0 | 2 | 8.1 |
| **Sports drink**, all flavors, 8 fl. oz.: | | | | | | | |
| (*AriZona Hypotonic*) .... | 35 | 0 | 10.0 | 0 | 0 | 110 | 0 |
| (*Gatorade*) ............ | 50 | 0 | 14.0 | 0 | 0 | 110 | 0 |
| (*R.W. Knudsen* | | | | | | | |
|   *Recharge*) .......... | 70 | 0 | 18.0 | 0 | 0 | 25 | 0 |
| **Spot**, meat only: | | | | | | | |
| raw, 4 oz. ............ | 140 | 21.0 | 0 | 5.6 | 68 | 33 | 0 |
| baked or broiled, 4 oz. .. | 179 | 26.9 | 0 | 7.1 | 87 | 42 | 0 |
| **Sprats**, smoked | | | | | | | |
|   (*Roland*), 3-oz. can ... | 250 | 18.0 | 0 | 19.0 | 85 | 360 | 0 |
| **Spring roll** (see also "Egg roll"), frozen: | | | | | | | |
| crab and shrimp | | | | | | | |
|   (*Phillips*), 3 pcs, 3 oz., | | | | | | | |
|   ¾ oz. sauce ........ | 270 | 7.0 | 46.0 | 7.0 | 35 | 540 | 2.0 |
| shrimp, Chinese or | | | | | | | |
|   Thai (*Blue Horizon*), | | | | | | | |
|   3 pcs., 2.1 oz. ...... | 110 | 3.0 | 16.0 | 4.0 | 0 | 210 | 1.0 |
| steak/cheese (*Original* | | | | | | | |
|   *Rangoon*), 2-oz. pc. .. | 225 | 11.0 | 40.0 | 12.0 | 40 | 470 | 0 |
| vegan (*Health is Wealth*), | | | | | | | |
|   2 pcs., 1.6 oz.: | | | | | | | |
|   Thai ............... | 90 | 3.0 | 13.0 | 3.0 | 0 | 300 | 1.0 |
|   vegetable .......... | 90 | 3.0 | 12.0 | 2.0 | 0 | 290 | 2.0 |

| Food and Measure | cal. | prot. (gms) | carbo. (gms) | fat (gms) | chol. (mgs) | sod. (mgs) | fiber (gms) |
|---|---|---|---|---|---|---|---|
| vegetable, 3 pcs.: | | | | | | | |
| Thai (*Blue* Horizon Organic), 2.1 oz. | 130 | 3.0 | 15.0 | 4.0 | 0 | 250 | 1.0 |
| Indian (*Blue Horizon* Organic), 2.1 oz. | 110 | 3.0 | 15.0 | 4.0 | 0 | 250 | 1.0 |
| **Sprite melon** (*Frieda's*), 10.6-oz. melon | 115 | 0 | 29.0 | 0 | 0 | 190 | 2.0 |
| **Squab**, fresh, raw: | | | | | | | |
| meat w/skin, 4 oz. | 333 | 20.9 | 0 | 27.0 | 108 | 61 | 0 |
| breast meat only, 4 oz. | 161 | 19.8 | 0 | 8.5 | 102 | 62 | 0 |
| **Squash**, see specific listings | | | | | | | |
| **Squid**, fresh, meat only, raw, 4 oz. | 104 | 17.7 | 3.5 | 1.6 | 265 | 50 | 0 |
| **Squid, canned**, see "Cuttlefish" | | | | | | | |
| **Squirrel**, meat only, roasted, 4 oz. | 196 | 34.9 | 0 | 5.3 | 137 | 135 | 0 |
| **Sriracha sauce** (see also "Hot sauce") (*Ka•Me*), 1 tbsp. | 20 | 0 | 5.0 | 0 | 0 | 580 | 0 |
| **Star fruit**, see "Carambola" | | | | | | | |
| **Star spangled squash** (*Frieda's*), 3 oz. | 20 | 2.0 | 3.0 | 0 | 0 | 0 | 1.0 |
| **Steak sauce** (see also "Marinade"), 1 tbsp.: | | | | | | | |
| (*A.1.*) | 15 | 0 | 3.0 | 0 | 0 | 280 | 0 |
| (*A.1.* Bold & Spicy) | 20 | 0 | 5.0 | 0 | 0 | 260 | 0 |
| (*A.1.* Chicago) | 20 | 0 | 3.0 | 1.0 | 0 | 270 | 0 |
| (*A.1.* New York) | 20 | 0 | 5.0 | 0 | 0 | 230 | 0 |
| (*A.1.* Thick & Hearty) | 25 | 0 | 6.0 | 0 | 0 | 290 | 0 |
| (*Heinz 57*) | 20 | 0 | 4.0 | 0 | 0 | 190 | 0 |
| (*HP* Original) | 20 | 0 | 5.0 | 0 | 0 | 160 | 0 |
| (*Justin Wilson's*) | 15 | 0 | 4.0 | 0 | 0 | 300 | 0 |
| (*Kikkoman*) | 20 | 0 | 5.0 | 0 | 0 | 290 | 0 |
| (*London Pub*) | 15 | 0 | 4.0 | 0 | 0 | 210 | 0 |
| (*Newman's Own*) | 20 | 0 | 4.0 | .5 | 0 | 85 | 0 |
| (*Rio Grande*) | 30 | 0 | 7.0 | 0 | 0 | 115 | 0 |
| (*TryMe* Bullfighter) | 15 | 0 | 4.0 | 0 | 0 | 220 | 0 |
| Cajun (*A.1.* New Orleans) | 25 | 0 | 5.0 | 0 | 0 | 180 | 0 |
| cracked pepper (*A.1.*) | 15 | 0 | 0 | 0 | 0 | 230 | 0 |
| garlic (*A.1.* Supreme) | 25 | 0 | 5.0 | 0 | 0 | 240 | 0 |

| Food and Measure | cal. | prot. (gms) | carbo. (gms) | fat (gms) | chol. (mgs) | sod. (mgs) | fiber (gms) |
|---|---|---|---|---|---|---|---|
| **Steak sauce** *(cont.)* | | | | | | | |
| hickory, sweet *(A.1.* | | | | | | | |
| w/*Bull's Eye*) . . . . . . . . | 20 | 0 | 5.0 | 0 | 0 | 170 | 0 |
| Jamaican jerk *(A.1)* . . . . . | 25 | 0 | 5.0 | .5 | 0 | 190 | 0 |
| mesquite: | | | | | | | |
| *(A.1.* Texas) . . . . . . . . | 15 | 0 | 4.0 | 0 | 0 | 400 | 0 |
| smoky *(A.1.)* . . . . . . . . | 30 | 0 | 8.0 | 0 | 0 | 240 | 0 |
| spicy *(London Pub)* . . . . | 25 | 0 | 6.0 | 0 | 0 | 270 | 0 |
| teriyaki *(A.1.)* . . . . . . . . . | 25 | 0 | 4.0 | 0 | 0 | 280 | 0 |
| **Steak seasoning:** | | | | | | | |
| *(Grill Mates* Montreal), | | | | | | | |
| ¾ tsp. . . . . . . . . . . . . | 5 | 0 | <1.0 | 0 | 0 | 560 | 0 |
| *(Grill Mates* Montreal | | | | | | | |
| Less Sodium), ¾ tsp. . | 5 | 0 | 1.0 | 0 | 0 | 390 | 0 |
| *(McCormick* Steak- | | | | | | | |
| house Grinder), ¼ tsp. | 0 | 0 | 0 | 0 | 0 | 70 | 0 |
| *(McCormick Perfect* | | | | | | | |
| *Pinch)*, ¼ tsp. . . . . . . . | 0 | 0 | 0 | 0 | 0 | 260 | 0 |
| spicy *(Grill Mates)*, | | | | | | | |
| ¼ tsp. . . . . . . . . . . . . | 5 | 0 | <1.0 | 0 | 0 | 300 | 0 |
| **Stir-fry sauce** (see | | | | | | | |
| also "Marinade," | | | | | | | |
| and specific sauces), | | | | | | | |
| 1 tbsp., except as | | | | | | | |
| noted: | | | | | | | |
| *(Annie Chun's)* . . . . . . . . | 45 | 1.0 | 4.0 | 3.0 | 0 | 350 | 0 |
| *(Kikkoman)* . . . . . . . . . . . | 20 | <1.0 | 4.0 | 0 | 0 | 520 | 0 |
| *(House of Tsang* | | | | | | | |
| Classic) . . . . . . . . . . . . | 25 | 0 | 4.0 | 1.0 | 0 | 570 | 0 |
| *(House of Tsang* | | | | | | | |
| Bangkok Padang) . . . . | 45 | 1.0 | 4.0 | 2.5 | 0 | 240 | 0 |
| *(House of Tsang* | | | | | | | |
| Imperial Citrus) . . . . . . | 25 | 0 | 5.0 | 0 | 0 | 180 | 0 |
| *(House of Tsang* | | | | | | | |
| Saigon Sizzle) . . . . . . . | 45 | 0 | 7.0 | 2.0 | 0 | 380 | 0 |
| *(House of Tsang* | | | | | | | |
| Szechuan Spicy) . . . . . | 25 | 0 | 4.0 | 1.0 | 0 | 500 | 0 |
| *(Litehouse* Classic), | | | | | | | |
| 2 tbsp. . . . . . . . . . . . . | 60 | 2.0 | 7.0 | 2.0 | 0 | 670 | 0 |
| garlic ginger *(La Choy)* . . | 30 | 0 | 6.0 | 0 | 0 | 320 | 0 |
| oyster flavor *(House* | | | | | | | |
| *of Tsang)* . . . . . . . . . . | 30 | 0 | 7.0 | 0 | 0 | 600 | 0 |
| sweet and sour *(House* | | | | | | | |
| *of Tsang)* . . . . . . . . . . | 35 | 0 | 9.0 | 0 | 0 | 75 | 0 |

| Food and Measure | cal. | prot. (gms) | carbo. (gms) | fat (gms) | chol. (mgs) | sod. (mgs) | fiber (gms) |
|---|---|---|---|---|---|---|---|
| teriyaki: | | | | | | | |
| (*House of Tsang Korean*) ......... | 35 | 0 | 5.0 | 1.5 | 0 | 460 | 0 |
| (*La Choy*) .......... | 30 | 0 | 7.0 | 0 | 0 | 320 | 0 |
| (*Litehouse*), 2 tbsp. .. | 60 | 1.0 | 12.0 | .5 | 0 | 590 | 0 |
| **Stir-fry seasoning**: | | | | | | | |
| (*Kikkoman*), 1 tbsp. .... | 25 | 1.0 | 6.0 | 0 | 0 | 640 | 0 |
| broccoli-beef | | | | | | | |
| (*Kikkoman*), 2 tsp. ... | 15 | <1.0 | 3.0 | 0 | 0 | 440 | 0 |
| **Stomach**, pork, raw, 1 oz. ................ | 44 | 4.7 | 0 | 2.7 | 55 | 15 | 0 |
| **Strawberry**, fresh: | | | | | | | |
| whole (*Dole*), 1 cup ..... | 45 | <1.0 | 11.0 | 0 | 0 | 0 | 3.0 |
| halves, ½ cup ......... | 23 | .5 | 5.3 | .3 | 0 | 1 | 1.8 |
| pureed, ½ cup ......... | 35 | .7 | 8.1 | .4 | 0 | 1 | 2.7 |
| **Strawberry, canned**, in heavy syrup, ½ cup .. | 117 | .7 | 29.9 | .3 | 0 | 5 | 2.2 |
| **Strawberry, dried**: | | | | | | | |
| (*Frieda's*), ½ cup ....... | 150 | 1.0 | 34.0 | 0 | 0 | 0 | 3.0 |
| (*Mariani*), ¼ cup ....... | 130 | 0 | 33.0 | 0 | 0 | 10 | 1.0 |
| **Strawberry, frozen**: | | | | | | | |
| whole: | | | | | | | |
| (*Cascadian Farm Organic*), 1 cup ... | 45 | <1.0 | 13.0 | 0 | 0 | 0 | 3.0 |
| (*Dole*), 1 cup ........ | 50 | 0 | 13.0 | 0 | 0 | 0 | 3.0 |
| or sliced (*Birds Eye/ C&W*), 1¼ cup .... | 50 | 0 | 12.0 | 0 | 0 | 5 | 1.0 |
| sliced (*Dole*), 1 cup ... | 50 | 0 | 13.0 | 0 | 0 | 0 | 3.0 |
| unsweetened, ½ cup .... | 39 | .5 | 10.1 | .1 | 0 | 2 | 2.3 |
| **Strawberry drink blend**, 8 fl. oz.: | | | | | | | |
| (*Odwalla C Monster Smoothie*) .......... | 160 | 2.0 | 38.0 | 0 | 0 | 20 | 0 |
| acai (*Snapple Antioxidant Water*) ... | 50 | 0 | 13.0 | 0 | 0 | 0 | 0 |
| banana: | | | | | | | |
| (*SoBe Lizard Fuel*) ... | 120 | 0 | 30.0 | 0 | 0 | 25 | 0 |
| (*V8 Splash* Smoothies) | 90 | 3.0 | 20.0 | 0 | 0 | 70 | 0 |
| (*V8 V-Fusion Light*) .. | 50 | 0 | 12.0 | 0 | 0 | 40 | 0 |
| frozen* (*Chiquita* Smoothies) ...... | 115 | 0 | 27.0 | 0 | 0 | 50 | 0 |
| daiquiri (*SoBe Lizard Lava*) ............. | 130 | 0 | 31.0 | 0 | 0 | 20 | 0 |

| Food and Measure | cal. | prot. (gms) | carbo. (gms) | fat (gms) | chol. (mgs) | sod. (mgs) | fiber (gms) |
|---|---|---|---|---|---|---|---|
| **Strawberry drink blend** *(cont.)* | | | | | | | |
| kiwi: | | | | | | | |
| (*Minute Maid*) . . . . . . . | 80 | 0 | 20.0 | 0 | 0 | 20 | 0 |
| (*SoBe Lifewater*) . . . . . | 40 | 0 | 16.0 | 0 | 0 | 20 | 0 |
| (*Tropicana Twister* | | | | | | | |
| Cyclone) . . . . . . . . . | 120 | 0 | 30.0 | 0 | 0 | 25 | 0 |
| (*V8 Splash*) . . . . . . . . | 70 | 0 | 18.0 | 0 | 0 | 50 | 0 |
| lemonade (*Odwalla*) . . . . | 110 | 0 | 28.0 | 0 | 0 | 10 | 0 |
| melon (*Lipton Brisk*) . . . . | 80 | 0 | 22.0 | 0 | 0 | 75 | 0 |
| **Strawberry drink** | | | | | | | |
| **mix** (*Nesquik*), | | | | | | | |
| 2 tbsp. . . . . . . . . . . . | 60 | 0 | 15.0 | 0 | 0 | 0 | 0 |
| **Strawberry glaze:** | | | | | | | |
| (*Litehouse*), 3 tbsp. . . . . . | 70 | 0 | 17.0 | 0 | 0 | 50 | 0 |
| (*Marie's*), 2 tbsp. . . . . . . | 40 | 0 | 10.0 | 0 | 0 | 40 | 0 |
| (*Marzetti*), 3 tbsp. . . . . . . | 60 | 0 | 16.0 | 0 | 0 | 65 | 0 |
| sugar free: | | | | | | | |
| (*Litehouse*), 3 tbsp. . . | 35 | 0 | 8.0 | 0 | 0 | 55 | 0 |
| (*Marie's*), 2 tbsp. . . . . | 20 | 0 | 6.0 | 0 | 0 | 35 | 0 |
| (*Marzetti*), 3 tbsp. . . . . | 10 | 0 | 3.0 | 0 | 0 | 60 | 0 |
| **Strawberry juice**, | | | | | | | |
| sparkling (*R.W.* | | | | | | | |
| *Knudsen*), 8 fl. oz. . . . | 120 | 0 | 29.0 | 0 | 0 | 15 | 0 |
| **Strawberry juice** | | | | | | | |
| **blend**, 8 fl. oz., | | | | | | | |
| except as noted: | | | | | | | |
| banana (*V8 V-Fusion*) . . . | 120 | 1.0 | 28.0 | 0 | 0 | 70 | 0 |
| banana smoothie: | | | | | | | |
| (*Bolthouse Farms*) . . . | 120 | 1.0 | 29.0 | 0 | 0 | 10 | <1.0 |
| (*Odwalla*) . . . . . . . . . | 130 | 1.0 | 31.0 | 0 | 0 | 0 | 1.0 |
| kiwi: | | | | | | | |
| (*Apple & Eve*), | | | | | | | |
| 6.75 fl. oz. . . . . . . | 100 | 0 | 24.0 | 0 | 0 | 20 | 0 |
| (*Dole*) . . . . . . . . . . . . | 120 | 0 | 31.0 | 0 | 0 | 25 | 0 |
| (*Santa Cruz Organic*) . | 120 | 1.0 | 30.0 | 0 | 0 | 15 | 0 |
| (*Tropicana*) . . . . . . . . . | 120 | 0 | 30.0 | 0 | 0 | 25 | 0 |
| lime (*Snapple*), | | | | | | | |
| 11.5 fl. oz. . . . . . . . . | 170 | 0 | 42.0 | 0 | 0 | 15 | 0 |
| mango: | | | | | | | |
| (*Apple & Eve* Passion) | 120 | 0 | 30.0 | 0 | 0 | 25 | 0 |
| (*Apple & Eve Organics* | | | | | | | |
| Passion) . . . . . . . . . | 160 | 0 | 40.0 | 0 | 0 | 20 | 0 |
| orange (*Tropicana*) . . . . . | 140 | <1.0 | 34.0 | 0 | 0 | 10 | 0 |

| Food and Measure | cal. | prot. (gms) | carbo. (gms) | fat (gms) | chol. (mgs) | sod. (mgs) | fiber (gms) |
|---|---|---|---|---|---|---|---|
| **Strawberry milk**, see "Milk, flavored" | | | | | | | |
| **Strawberry syrup**, 2 tbsp., except as noted: | | | | | | | |
| (*Hershey's*) . . . . . . . . . . | 100 | 0 | 26.0 | 0 | 0 | 10 | 0 |
| (*Hershey's* Sugar Free) .. | 10 | 0 | 4.0 | 0 | 0 | 55 | 0 |
| (*Maple Grove Farms*), ¼ cup . . . . . . . . . . . . | 210 | 0 | 53.0 | 0 | 0 | 0 | 0 |
| (*Nesquik*), 1 tbsp. . . . . . . | 50 | 0 | 13.0 | 0 | 0 | 30 | 0 |
| (*Smucker's Sundae Syrup*) . . . . . . . . . . | 110 | 0 | 26.0 | 0 | 0 | 0 | 0 |
| **Strawberry topping**: | | | | | | | |
| (*Smucker's*), 2 tbsp. . . . . | 100 | 0 | 26.0 | 0 | 0 | 0 | 0 |
| (*Smucker's* Sugar Free), 2 tbsp. . . . . . . . | 25 | 0 | 9.0 | 0 | 0 | 0 | 0 |
| **String bean**, see "Green bean" | | | | | | | |
| **Stromboli**, frozen (*Stouffer's Corner Bistro*), 6-oz. pc.: | | | | | | | |
| chicken broccoli cheddar . . . . . . . . . . | 360 | 20.0 | 45.0 | 11.0 | 35 | 750 | 4.0 |
| Italian style supreme . . . . | 430 | 19.0 | 45.0 | 19.0 | 40 | 970 | 5.0 |
| pepperoni/provolone . . . . | 430 | 24.0 | 45.0 | 17.0 | 50 | 1110 | 5.0 |
| **Stuffing**, dry, except as noted: | | | | | | | |
| (*Arnold* Unspiced), ¾ cup . . . . . . . . . . . . | 110 | 3.0 | 20.0 | 1.0 | 0 | 210 | <1.0 |
| chicken: | | | | | | | |
| (*Stove Top*), 1 oz. . . . . | 110 | 3.0 | 20.0 | 1.0 | 0 | 430 | 1.0 |
| (*Stove Top* One Step), 1 oz. . . . . . . . | 110 | 3.0 | 20.0 | 2.5 | 0 | 460 | 1.0 |
| (*Stove Top* Quick Cup), 1 oz. . . . . . . . | 110 | 3.0 | 20.0 | 2.5 | 0 | 540 | 1.0 |
| w/whole wheat (*Stove Top*), 1 oz. . . . . . . . | 140 | 3.0 | 20.0 | 1.5 | 0 | 440 | 3.0 |
| cornbread: | | | | | | | |
| (*Arnold*), ¾ cup . . . . . | 100 | 3.0 | 19.0 | 1.5 | 0 | 350 | <1.0 |
| (*Pepperidge Farm*), ¾ cup . . . . . . . . . . . | 170 | 4.0 | 33.0 | 2.0 | 0 | 480 | 2.0 |
| (*Stove Top*), 1 oz. . . . . | 160 | 3.0 | 22.0 | 1.0 | 0 | 500 | 1.0 |
| (*Stove Top* Quick Cup), 1 oz. . . . . . . . | 120 | 3.0 | 20.0 | 2.5 | 0 | 560 | 1.0 |

| Food and Measure | cal. | prot. (gms) | carbo. (gms) | fat (gms) | chol. (mgs) | sod. (mgs) | fiber (gms) |
|---|---|---|---|---|---|---|---|
| **Stuffing, cornbread** *(cont.)* | | | | | | | |
| herb (*Arrowhead Mills* Organic), ⅓ cup ... | 130 | 3.0 | 21.0 | 4.0 | 0 | 250 | >1.0 |
| cubed (*Pepperidge Farm* Country), ¾ cup ..... | 140 | 5.0 | 27.0 | 1.0 | 0 | 380 | 2.0 |
| garlic herb (*Arrowhead Mills* Organic Stuffing Express), ½ cup ..... | 110 | 3.0 | 20.0 | 2.0 | 0 | 400 | 1.0 |
| herb: | | | | | | | |
| (*Arnold*), ¾ cup ..... | 100 | 3.0 | 20.0 | 1.0 | 0 | 390 | 1.0 |
| (*Arrowhead Mills* Organic Savory), ½ cup ... | 120 | 3.0 | 20.0 | 3.0 | 0 | 240 | 1.0 |
| (*Stove Top* Savory), 1 oz. | 160 | 3.0 | 21.0 | 1.0 | 0 | 450 | 1.0 |
| seasoned (*Pepperidge Farm*), ¾ cup ..... | 170 | 5.0 | 33.0 | 2.0 | 0 | 600 | 3.0 |
| seasoned, cubed (*Pepperidge Farm*), ¾ cup ........... | 140 | 4.0 | 28.0 | 1.0 | 0 | 530 | 2.0 |
| sage (*Stove Top* Traditional), 1 oz. .... | 110 | 3.0 | 21.0 | 1.0 | 0 | 440 | 1.0 |
| sage and onion, ¾ cup: | | | | | | | |
| (*Arnold*) ........... | 100 | 3.0 | 20.0 | 1.0 | 0 | 440 | 1.0 |
| (*Pepperidge Farm*) ... | 140 | 5.0 | 26.0 | 1.0 | 0 | 540 | 3.0 |
| seasoned (*Arnold*), ¾ cup | 100 | 3.0 | 20.0 | 1.0 | 0 | 370 | <1.0 |
| turkey (*Stove Top*), 1 oz. . | 160 | 3.0 | 21.0 | 1.0 | 0 | 440 | 1.0 |
| **Stuffing, chilled** (*Bob Evans* Homestyle), ½ cup .............. | 150 | 3.0 | 21.0 | 6.0 | 0 | 540 | 1.0 |
| **Sturgeon**, meat only: | | | | | | | |
| raw, 4 oz. ........... | 120 | 18.3 | 0 | 4.6 | 68 | 61 | 0 |
| baked or broiled, 4 oz. .. | 153 | 23.5 | 0 | 5.9 | 87 | 78 | 0 |
| smoked, 4 oz. ......... | 196 | 35.4 | 0 | 5.0 | 91 | 838 | 0 |
| *Subway:* | | | | | | | |
| breakfast, egg muffin melts, regular: | | | | | | | |
| bacon/egg/cheese .... | 220 | 16.0 | 18.0 | 10.0 | 95 | 640 | 5.0 |
| BMT .............. | 230 | 17.0 | 19.0 | 11.0 | 105 | 890 | 6.0 |
| egg/cheese ......... | 170 | 13.0 | 18.0 | 6.0 | 85 | 450 | 5.0 |
| ham/egg/cheese ..... | 180 | 15.0 | 18.0 | 7.0 | 95 | 650 | 5.0 |
| Mega ............. | 310 | 18.0 | 18.0 | 20.0 | 110 | 810 | 5.0 |
| sausage/egg/cheese .. | 290 | 16.0 | 18.0 | 18.0 | 105 | 710 | 5.0 |
| steak/egg/cheese .... | 190 | 16.0 | 19.0 | 7.0 | 95 | 600 | 6.0 |
| *Sunshine Subway* .... | 230 | 20.0 | 20.0 | 9.0 | 105 | 910 | 6.0 |
| Western/egg/cheese .. | 180 | 15.0 | 19.0 | 7.0 | 95 | 650 | 6.0 |

| Food and Measure | cal. | prot. (gms) | carbo. (gms) | fat (gms) | chol. (mgs) | sod. (mgs) | fiber (gms) |
|---|---|---|---|---|---|---|---|
| breakfast, 6" omelet sandwich, regular: | | | | | | | |
| bacon/egg/cheese .... | 520 | 29.0 | 47.0 | 25.0 | 210 | 1430 | 5.0 |
| BMT .............. | 560 | 32.0 | 49.0 | 28.0 | 220 | 1940 | 6.0 |
| egg/cheese ......... | 420 | 22.0 | 46.0 | 18.0 | 190 | 1060 | 5.0 |
| ham/egg/cheese ..... | 450 | 27.0 | 47.0 | 19.0 | 200 | 1450 | 5.0 |
| Mega ............. | 710 | 33.0 | 47.0 | 45.0 | 235 | 1770 | 5.0 |
| sausage/egg/cheese .. | 670 | 30.0 | 46.0 | 41.0 | 225 | 1580 | 5.0 |
| steak/egg/cheese .... | 490 | 31.0 | 48.0 | 20.0 | 210 | 1430 | 5.0 |
| Sunrise Subway ..... | 540 | 37.0 | 50.0 | 23.0 | 225 | 1980 | 55.0 |
| Western/egg/cheese .. | 450 | 27.0 | 47.0 | 19.0 | 200 | 1450 | 5.0 |
| breakfast, omelet on flatbread, regular: | | | | | | | |
| bacon/egg/cheese .... | 530 | 29.0 | 43.0 | 27.0 | 210 | 1470 | 3.0 |
| BMT .............. | 570 | 32.0 | 45.0 | 30.0 | 220 | 1970 | 3.0 |
| egg/cheese ......... | 440 | 22.0 | 42.0 | 20.0 | 190 | 1100 | 3.0 |
| ham/egg/cheese ..... | 460 | 27.0 | 43.0 | 21.0 | 200 | 1490 | 3.0 |
| Mega ............. | 730 | 33.0 | 43.0 | 47.0 | 235 | 1800 | 3.0 |
| sausage/egg/cheese .. | 680 | 30.0 | 43.0 | 44.0 | 230 | 1620 | 3.0 |
| steak/egg/cheese .... | 500 | 31.0 | 44.0 | 23.0 | 210 | 1460 | 3.0 |
| Sunshine Subway .... | 550 | 37.0 | 46.0 | 26.0 | 225 | 2010 | 3.0 |
| Western/egg/cheese .. | 470 | 27.0 | 44.0 | 21.0 | 200 | 1490 | 3.0 |
| breakfast hash browns .. | 150 | 1.0 | 17.0 | 9.0 | 0 | 440 | 2.0 |
| 6" sub: | | | | | | | |
| BLT .............. | 360 | 17.0 | 45.0 | 13.0 | 30 | 990 | 5.0 |
| chicken/bacon ranch .. | 570 | 35.0 | 48.0 | 28.0 | 95 | 1190 | 5.0 |
| cold cut combo ...... | 410 | 21.0 | 48.0 | 16.0 | 60 | 1450 | 5.0 |
| Italian, spicy ........ | 520 | 22.0 | 47.0 | 28.0 | 65 | 1830 | 5.0 |
| Italian BMT ......... | 450 | 24.0 | 48.0 | 20.0 | 55 | 1730 | 5.0 |
| meatball marinara .... | 580 | 24.0 | 70.0 | 23.0 | 45 | 1530 | 9.0 |
| Philly cheesesteak .... | 520 | 39.0 | 53.0 | 18.0 | 90 | 1570 | 6.0 |
| steak and cheese .... | 380 | 26.0 | 50.0 | 10.0 | 50 | 1230 | 5.0 |
| Subway Melt ........ | 380 | 25.0 | 48.0 | 11.0 | 45 | 1530 | 5.0 |
| tuna .............. | 530 | 21.0 | 45.0 | 30.0 | 45 | 930 | 5.0 |
| 6" sub, low fat: | | | | | | | |
| chicken, roasted ..... | 320 | 23.0 | 49.0 | 4.5 | 25 | 750 | 5.0 |
| chicken teriyaki ...... | 380 | 26.0 | 60.0 | 4.5 | 50 | 1010 | 5.0 |
| ham, Black Forest .... | 290 | 18.0 | 47.0 | 4.5 | 25 | 1200 | 5.0 |
| roast beef .......... | 310 | 26.0 | 45.0 | 4.5 | 25 | 800 | 5.0 |
| Subway Club ....... | 320 | 26.0 | 47.0 | 5.0 | 35 | 1140 | 5.0 |
| turkey breast ........ | 280 | 18.0 | 47.0 | 3.5 | 20 | 920 | 5.0 |
| turkey/ham ......... | 300 | 19.0 | 47.0 | 4.0 | 25 | 1140 | 5.0 |
| Veggie Delite ........ | 230 | 8.0 | 45.0 | 2.5 | 0 | 410 | 5.0 |

| Food and Measure | cal. | prot. (gms) | carbo. (gms) | fat (gms) | chol. (mgs) | sod. (mgs) | fiber (gms) |
|---|---|---|---|---|---|---|---|
| **Subway** (cont.) | | | | | | | |
| 6" flatbread, low fat: | | | | | | | |
| chicken, roasted ..... | 330 | 23.0 | 45.0 | 7.0 | 25 | 780 | 3.0 |
| chicken teriyaki ...... | 390 | 26.0 | 56.0 | 7.0 | 30 | 1050 | 3.0 |
| ham, Black Forest .... | 300 | 18.0 | 43.0 | 7.0 | 25 | 1240 | 3.0 |
| roast beef ........... | 320 | 26.0 | 42.0 | 7.0 | 25 | 840 | 3.0 |
| *Subway Club* ....... | 330 | 26.0 | 44.0 | 7.0 | 35 | 1180 | 3.0 |
| turkey breast ........ | 300 | 18.0 | 43.0 | 6.0 | 20 | 950 | 3.0 |
| turkey/ham .......... | 310 | 19.0 | 44.0 | 7.0 | 25 | 1180 | 3.0 |
| *Veggie Delite* ........ | 240 | 8.0 | 41.0 | 5.0 | 0 | 450 | 3.0 |
| *Footlong*, low fat sub: | | | | | | | |
| chicken, roasted ..... | 640 | 46.0 | 97.0 | 9.0 | 45 | 1490 | 11.0 |
| chicken teriyaki ...... | 760 | 51.0 | 120.0 | 9.0 | 100 | 2020 | 10.0 |
| ham, Black Forest .... | 570 | 35.0 | 94.0 | 9.0 | 50 | 2400 | 10.0 |
| roast beef ........... | 630 | 52.0 | 91.0 | 9.0 | 55 | 1600 | 11.0 |
| *Subway Club* ....... | 640 | 52.0 | 94.0 | 10.0 | 65 | 2270 | 10.0 |
| turkey breast ........ | 570 | 35.0 | 94.0 | 7.0 | 40 | 1830 | 10.0 |
| turkey/ham .......... | 590 | 38.0 | 95.0 | 8.0 | 50 | 2280 | 10.0 |
| *Veggie Delite* ........ | 460 | 17.0 | 90.0 | 5.0 | 0 | 830 | 10.0 |
| 6" limited/regional: | | | | | | | |
| barbecue chicken .... | 310 | 15.0 | 53.0 | 5.0 | 35 | 1010 | 6.0 |
| barbecue rib patty .... | 430 | 19.0 | 48.0 | 18.0 | 50 | 730 | 5.0 |
| buffalo chicken ...... | 420 | 25.0 | 47.0 | 15.0 | 55 | 1290 | 5.0 |
| low fat .......... | 370 | 25.0 | 54.0 | 6.0 | 55 | 1300 | 5.0 |
| chicken pizziola ...... | 450 | 31.0 | 51.0 | 15.0 | 75 | 1360 | 5.0 |
| The Feast .......... | 540 | 39.0 | 50.0 | 22.0 | 85 | 2450 | 5.0 |
| pastrami, w/cheese ... | 580 | 31.0 | 50.0 | 28.0 | 65 | 1810 | 5.0 |
| *Subway Seafood* | | | | | | | |
| *Sensation* ........ | 460 | 15.0 | 52.0 | 22.0 | 25 | 1050 | 5.0 |
| turkey/bacon/avocado | 420 | 24.0 | 51.0 | 15.0 | 40 | 1310 | 7.0 |
| veggie patty ........ | 390 | 23.0 | 57.0 | 7.0 | 10 | 930 | 8.0 |
| salads, no dressing: | | | | | | | |
| chicken, roasted ..... | 130 | 19.0 | 9.0 | 2.5 | 50 | 270 | 4.0 |
| chicken teriyaki ...... | 200 | 20.0 | 24.0 | 3.0 | 50 | 660 | 4.0 |
| ham, Black Forest .... | 110 | 12.0 | 11.0 | 3.0 | 25 | 850 | 4.0 |
| roast beef ........... | 140 | 20.0 | 10.0 | 3.5 | 25 | 450 | 4.0 |
| *Subway Club* ....... | 140 | 20.0 | 11.0 | 3.5 | 35 | 790 | 4.0 |
| turkey breast ........ | 110 | 12.0 | 11.0 | 2.0 | 20 | 570 | 4.0 |
| turkey/ham .......... | 120 | 13.0 | 12.0 | 3.0 | 25 | 790 | 4.0 |
| *Veggie Delite* ........ | 50 | 3.0 | 9.0 | 1.0 | 0 | 65 | 4.0 |
| salad dressing: | | | | | | | |
| Italian, fat free ....... | 35 | 1.0 | 7.0 | 0 | 0 | 720 | 0 |
| ranch ............. | 290 | 1.0 | 3.0 | 30.0 | 15 | 540 | 0 |

| Food and Measure | cal. | prot. (gms) | carbo. (gms) | fat (gms) | chol. (mgs) | sod. (mgs) | fiber (gms) |
|---|---|---|---|---|---|---|---|
| 8" pizza, regional: | | | | | | | |
| cheese | 680 | 32.0 | 96.0 | 22.0 | 40 | 1070 | 4.0 |
| cheese/veggies | 740 | 36.0 | 100.0 | 25.0 | 50 | 1270 | 5.0 |
| pepperoni | 790 | 38.0 | 96.0 | 32.0 | 60 | 1350 | 4.0 |
| sausage | 820 | 39.0 | 97.0 | 34.0 | 70 | 1420 | 4.0 |
| soup, 10 oz., regional: | | | | | | | |
| broccoli/cheese | 180 | 5.0 | 16.0 | 11.0 | 25 | 990 | 4.0 |
| chicken/corn chowder | 140 | 6.0 | 22.0 | 3.0 | 15 | 900 | 2.0 |
| chicken/dumpling | 170 | 8.0 | 23.0 | 5.0 | 35 | 810 | 2.0 |
| chicken/dumpling, rosemary | 90 | 6.0 | 14.0 | 1.5 | 25 | 810 | 1.0 |
| chicken noodle | 80 | 6.0 | 12.0 | 2.0 | 15 | 950 | 1.0 |
| chicken rice w/pork | 110 | 6.0 | 16.0 | 2.5 | 5 | 980 | 1.0 |
| chicken tortilla | 110 | 25.0 | 11.0 | 1.5 | 10 | 440 | 3.0 |
| chili con carne | 340 | 20.0 | 35.0 | 11.0 | 60 | 950 | 10.0 |
| clam chowder | 150 | 6.0 | 20.0 | 5.0 | 10 | 990 | 4.0 |
| minestrone | 90 | 4.0 | 17.0 | 1.0 | <5 | 910 | 3.0 |
| potato w/bacon | 240 | 5.0 | 26.0 | 13.0 | 15 | 870 | 3.0 |
| tomato/orzo | 130 | 6.0 | 24.0 | 1.0 | 5 | 410 | 2.0 |
| tomato/vegetable | 90 | 3.0 | 20.0 | .5 | 0 | 820 | 3.0 |
| vegetable beef | 100 | 5.0 | 17.0 | 2.0 | 10 | 960 | 3.0 |
| wild rice w/chicken | 230 | 6.0 | 26.0 | 11.0 | 50 | 900 | 1.0 |
| condiments/extras: | | | | | | | |
| bacon, 2 slices | 45 | 3.0 | 0 | 3.5 | 10 | 190 | 0 |
| chipotle sauce | 100 | 0 | 1.0 | 10.0 | 10 | 220 | 0 |
| honey mustard sauce | 30 | 0 | 7.0 | 0 | 0 | 120 | 0 |
| mayo, 1 tbsp. | 110 | 0 | 0 | 12.0 | 10 | 80 | 0 |
| mayo, light, 1 tbsp. | 50 | 0 | <1.0 | 5.0 | 5 | 100 | 0 |
| mustard, 2 tsp. | 5 | 0 | <1.0 | 0 | 0 | 115 | 0 |
| olive oil blend, 1 tsp. | 45 | 0 | 0 | 5.0 | 0 | 0 | 0 |
| onion sauce | 40 | 0 | 9.0 | 0 | 0 | 85 | 0 |
| ranch dressing | 120 | 0 | 1.0 | 11.0 | 5 | 200 | 0 |
| red wine vinaigrette | 30 | 0 | 6.0 | 0 | 0 | 340 | 0 |
| **Succotash, canned**: | | | | | | | |
| (*Allens* Triple), ½ cup | 70 | 3.0 | 16.0 | 0 | 0 | 430 | 2.0 |
| cream-style, ½ cup | 103 | 3.5 | 23.4 | .7 | 0 | 325 | 4.0 |
| **Succotash, frozen**, boiled, drained, ½ cup | 79 | 3.7 | 17.0 | .8 | 0 | 38 | 4.6 |
| **Sucker**, white, meat only: | | | | | | | |
| raw, 4 oz. | 105 | 19.0 | 0 | 2.6 | 47 | 45 | 0 |
| baked or broiled, 4 oz. | 135 | 24.4 | 0 | 3.4 | 60 | 58 | 0 |

| Food and Measure | cal. | prot. (gms) | carbo. (gms) | fat (gms) | chol. (mgs) | sod. (mgs) | fiber (gms) |
|---|---|---|---|---|---|---|---|
| **Sugar, beet or cane**: | | | | | | | |
| brown: | | | | | | | |
|   1 oz. . . . . . . . . . . . . | 107 | 0 | 27.6 | 0 | 0 | 11 | 0 |
|   1 cup, not packed . . . . | 546 | 0 | 141.0 | 0 | 0 | 57 | 0 |
|   1 cup, packed . . . . . . . | 828 | 0 | 214.0 | 0 | 0 | 86 | 0 |
| cubes, rough cut, | | | | | | | |
|   white, or Demerara | | | | | | | |
|   (*Roland*), 1 cube . . . . . | 20 | 0 | 5.0 | 0 | 0 | 0 | 0 |
| granulated: | | | | | | | |
|   1 oz. . . . . . . . . . . . . | 110 | 0 | 28.3 | 0 | 0 | <1 | 0 |
|   1 cup . . . . . . . . . . . . | 773 | 0 | 199.8 | 0 | 0 | <1 | 0 |
|   1 tbsp. . . . . . . . . . . . | 46 | 0 | 12.0 | 0 | 0 | <1 | 0 |
|   1 tsp. . . . . . . . . . . . . | 15 | 0 | 4.0 | 0 | 0 | <1 | 0 |
| powder/confectioner's: | | | | | | | |
|   1 cup, sifted . . . . . . . . | 389 | 0 | 99.5 | 0 | 0 | 1 | 0 |
|   1 tbsp., unsifted . . . . . | 31 | 0 | 8.0 | 0 | 0 | <1 | 0 |
| **Sugar, maple**, 1 oz. . . . . | 99 | 0 | 25.5 | 0 | 0 | 4 | 0 |
| **Sugar, substitute** | | | | | | | |
|   (*Equal*), 1 pkt. . . . . . . . . | 4 | 0 | <1.0 | 0 | 0 | 0 | 0 |
|   (*NutraSweet*), 1 tsp. . . . . | 2 | 0 | <1.0 | 0 | 0 | 0 | 0 |
|   (*Splenda*), 1 pkt. . . . . . . . | 0 | 0 | <1.0 | 0 | 0 | 0 | 0 |
|   (*Sweet 'N Low*), 1 pkt. . . | 4 | 0 | 1.0 | 0 | 0 | 0 | 0 |
| **Sugar apple**: | | | | | | | |
| 1 medium, 9.9 oz. . . . . . . | 146 | 3.2 | 36.6 | .5 | 0 | 15 | 6.8 |
| ½ cup . . . . . . . . . . . . . . | 118 | 2.6 | 29.6 | .4 | 0 | 12 | 5.5 |
| **Sugar snap peas**, see | | | | | | | |
|   "Peas, edible-podded" | | | | | | | |
| **Sukiyaki sauce** | | | | | | | |
|   (*Kikkoman*), 1 tbsp. . . | 20 | <1.0 | 4.0 | 0 | 0 | 460 | 0 |
| **Summer sausage**, | | | | | | | |
|   2 oz., except as | | | | | | | |
|   noted: | | | | | | | |
| (*Hillshire Farm*) . . . . . . . . | 190 | 10.0 | <1.0 | 16.0 | 45 | 690 | <1.0 |
| (*Oscar Mayer*), 1.6 oz. . . | 140 | 7.0 | 0 | 12.0 | 40 | 660 | 0 |
| all varieties: | | | | | | | |
|   (*Johnsonville*) . . . . . . . | 170 | 9.0 | 1.0 | 15.0 | 45 | 680 | 0 |
|   (*Johnsonville* Deli | | | | | | | |
|     Bites), 6 pcs., 1 oz. | 90 | 5.0 | 0 | 8.0 | 20 | 370 | 0 |
| beef: | | | | | | | |
|   (*Di Lusso*) . . . . . . . . . . | 210 | 9.0 | 0 | 19.0 | 60 | 860 | 0 |
|   (*Hillshire Farm/* | | | | | | | |
|     *Hillshire Farm* | | | | | | | |
|     *Yard-O-Beef*) . . . . . | 190 | 10.0 | <1.0 | 16.0 | 50 | 700 | <1.0 |

| Food and Measure | cal. | prot. (gms) | carbo. (gms) | fat (gms) | chol. (mgs) | sod. (mgs) | fiber (gms) |
|---|---|---|---|---|---|---|---|
| hickory smoked (*Di Lusso*) ............ | 210 | 10.0 | 0 | 18.0 | 60 | 940 | 0 |
| **Summer squash** (see also specific listings), all varieties: | | | | | | | |
| raw: | | | | | | | |
| (*Green Giant*), 3.5 oz. . | 15 | 1.0 | 3.0 | 0 | 0 | 0 | 1.0 |
| sliced, 1 cup ........ | 23 | 1.3 | 4.9 | .2 | 0 | 2 | 2.2 |
| boiled, drained, sliced, 1 cup ............. | 36 | 1.6 | 7.8 | .6 | 0 | 2 | 2.5 |
| **Sun choke**, see "Jerusalem artichoke" | | | | | | | |
| **Sunburst squash**, baby (*Frieda's*), sliced, 1 cup, 4.5 oz. .. | 23 | 2.0 | 5.0 | 0 | 0 | 1 | 0 |
| **Sunfish**, pumpkinseed, meat only: | | | | | | | |
| raw, 4 oz. ............ | 101 | 22.0 | 0 | .8 | 76 | 91 | 0 |
| baked or broiled, 4 oz. .. | 129 | 28.2 | 0 | 1.0 | 98 | 117 | 0 |
| **Sunflower seed butter**: | | | | | | | |
| (*MaraNatha*), 2 tbsp. .... | 180 | 9.0 | 8.0 | 12.0 | 0 | 65 | 4.0 |
| 1 tbsp. ............... | 93 | 3.2 | 4.4 | 7.6 | 0 | 1 | .8 |
| **Sunflower seed flour**, partially defatted, 1 cup ...... | 261 | 38.5 | 28.7 | 1.3 | 0 | 2 | 4.2 |
| **Sunflower seeds**, 1 oz., except as noted: | | | | | | | |
| (*Arrowhead Mills* Organic), ¼ cup ..... | 170 | 7.0 | 6.0 | 15.0 | 0 | 0 | 3.0 |
| (*David* Original), ¼ cup .. | 190 | 9.0 | 4.0 | 15.0 | 0 | 220 | 3.0 |
| (*Frito-Lay*) ............ | 190 | 6.0 | 5.0 | 16.0 | 0 | 90 | 3.0 |
| (*Spitz* Salted) ......... | 180 | 7.0 | 5.0 | 15.0 | 0 | 530 | 3.0 |
| raw, kernels (*Bob's Red Mill*), ¼ cup ........ | 150 | 6.0 | 7.0 | 11.0 | 0 | 0 | 3.0 |
| unsalted: | | | | | | | |
| dry-roasted ......... | 165 | 5.5 | 6.8 | 14.1 | 0 | 1 | 3.2 |
| oil-roasted ......... | 174 | 6.1 | 4.2 | 16.3 | 0 | 1 | 4.2 |
| toasted ............ | 176 | 4.9 | 5.8 | 16.1 | 0 | 1 | 3.3 |
| dry-roasted (*Planters*), 1.1 oz. ............. | 180 | 7.0 | 6.0 | 15.0 | 0 | 260 | 3.0 |
| roasted, salted: | | | | | | | |
| (*Planters*) .......... | 160 | 7.0 | 5.0 | 14.0 | 0 | 150 | 3.0 |
| (*Planters* 5 oz.) ...... | 160 | 5.0 | 7.0 | 14.0 | 0 | 45 | 3.0 |

| Food and Measure | cal. | prot. (gms) | carbo. (gms) | fat (gms) | chol. (mgs) | sod. (mgs) | fiber (gms) |
|---|---|---|---|---|---|---|---|
| **Sunflower seeds, roasted, salted** *(cont.)* | | | | | | | |
| (*Planters*), 1.75-oz. pkg. | 290 | 11.0 | 9.0 | 25.0 | 0 | 260 | 5.0 |
| (*Planters*), 3-oz. pkg. | 280 | 10.0 | 8.0 | 23.0 | 0 | 180 | 4.0 |
| (*Planters* Kernels) | 160 | 7.0 | 5.0 | 14.0 | 0 | 150 | 4.0 |
| **Sunflower seeds, flavored**: | | | | | | | |
| (*Spitz* Seasoned), 1 oz. | 180 | 7.0 | 5.0 | 15.0 | 0 | 580 | 3.0 |
| barbecue: | | | | | | | |
| (*David*), ¼ cup | 190 | 8.0 | 6.0 | 15.0 | 0 | 115 | 2.0 |
| smoky (*Spitz*), 1 oz. | 180 | 7.0 | 5.0 | 15.0 | 0 | 350 | 3.0 |
| chili lime: | | | | | | | |
| (*David*), ¼ cup | 190 | 9.0 | 4.0 | 16.0 | 0 | 35 | 3.0 |
| (*Spitz*), 1 oz. | 180 | 7.0 | 5.0 | 15.0 | 0 | 460 | 3.0 |
| cracked pepper (*Spitz*), 1 oz. | 180 | 7.0 | 5.0 | 15.0 | 0 | 600 | 3.0 |
| dill pickle: | | | | | | | |
| (*David*), ¼ cup | 190 | 9.0 | 5.0 | 14.0 | 0 | 110 | 4.0 |
| (*Spitz*), 1 oz. | 180 | 7.0 | 5.0 | 15.0 | 0 | 550 | 3.0 |
| jalapeño (*David*), ¼ cup | 180 | 8.0 | 6.0 | 14.0 | 0 | 105 | 2.0 |
| nacho (*David*), .8 oz. | 60 | 3.0 | 2.0 | 5.0 | 0 | 40 | <1.0 |
| ranch (*David*), ¼ cup | 180 | 8.0 | 6.0 | 13.0 | 0 | 90 | 2.0 |
| spicy (*Spitz*), 1 oz. | 180 | 7.0 | 5.0 | 15.0 | 0 | 380 | 3.0 |
| **Surimi**, pollock, 4 oz. | 112 | 17.2 | 7.8 | 1.0 | 34 | 162 | 0 |
| **Sushi wrap**: | | | | | | | |
| nori, see "Seaweed" | | | | | | | |
| w/out rice, 1 pc.: | | | | | | | |
| colored (*Freida's*) | 15 | 2.0 | 0 | 0 | 0 | 25 | 0 |
| green, orange, or sesame (*Roland*) | 10 | 2.0 | 0 | 0 | 0 | 14 | 0 |
| pink or yellow (*Roland*) | 10 | 2.0 | 0 | 0 | 0 | 25 | 0 |
| w/cooked rice (*Annie Chun's* Sushi Wraps): | | | | | | | |
| brown rice, sprouted, ½ of 7-oz. pkg. | 150 | 5.0 | 30.0 | .5 | 0 | 330 | 2.0 |
| sticky white rice ½ of 8-oz. pkg. | 160 | 4.0 | 34.0 | .5 | 0 | 330 | 1.0 |
| **Swamp cabbage**: | | | | | | | |
| raw, .6-oz. shoot | 2 | .3 | .4 | <.1 | 0 | 15 | .3 |
| boiled, drained, chopped, ½ cup | 10 | 1.0 | 1.8 | .1 | 0 | 60 | .9 |
| **Sweet dumpling squash** (*Frieda's*), ¾ cup, 3 oz. | 30 | 1.0 | 7.0 | 0 | 0 | 0 | 1.0 |

| Food and Measure | cal. | prot. (gms) | carbo. (gms) | fat (gms) | chol. (mgs) | sod. (mgs) | fiber (gms) |
|---|---|---|---|---|---|---|---|
| **Sweet peas**, see "Peas, green" | | | | | | | |
| **Sweet potato**: | | | | | | | |
| raw: | | | | | | | |
| (*Green Giant*), 4.6 oz. | 100 | 2.0 | 23.0 | 0 | 0 | 70 | 4.0 |
| 5" x 2" potato | 136 | 2.1 | 31.6 | .4 | 0 | 17 | 3.9 |
| cubed (*Glory*), 4.9 oz. | 140 | 2.0 | 36.0 | 0 | 0 | 50 | 4.0 |
| baked in skin: | | | | | | | |
| 5" x 2" potato | 118 | 2.0 | 27.7 | .1 | 0 | 12 | 3.4 |
| mashed, ½ cup | 103 | 1.7 | 24.3 | .1 | 0 | 10 | 3.0 |
| boiled w/out skin: | | | | | | | |
| 4 oz. | 86 | 1.6 | 20.1 | .2 | 0 | 31 | 2.8 |
| mashed, ½ cup | 125 | 2.5 | 31.7 | .3 | 0 | 48 | 4.5 |
| **Sweet potato, canned**, ½ cup, except as noted: | | | | | | | |
| candied: | | | | | | | |
| (*Glory* Yams) | 210 | 1.0 | 52.0 | 0 | 0 | 240 | 1.0 |
| (*Royal Prince*) | 210 | 1.0 | 50.0 | 0 | 0 | 30 | 2.0 |
| (*S&W* Yams) | 170 | 2.0 | 46.0 | 0 | 0 | 360 | 4.0 |
| mashed: | | | | | | | |
| (*Glory* Casserole) | 180 | 2.0 | 43.0 | 0 | 0 | 250 | 2.0 |
| (*Sugary Sam*), ⅔ cup | 120 | 1.0 | 28.0 | 0 | 0 | 30 | 3.0 |
| in syrup, light: | | | | | | | |
| (*Glory*), ⅔ cup | 160 | 3.0 | 37.0 | 0 | 0 | 35 | 2.0 |
| cut (*Princella/Sugary Sam*), ⅔ cup | 160 | 0 | 39.0 | 0 | 0 | 35 | 3.0 |
| in syrup, heavy: | | | | | | | |
| whole (*Royal Prince*), 3 pcs. | 200 | 1.0 | 48.0 | 0 | 0 | 40 | 4.0 |
| whole (*Trappey's*), 4 pcs. | 200 | 1.0 | 48.0 | 0 | 0 | 40 | 4.0 |
| drained | 106 | 1.3 | 24.9 | .3 | 0 | 38 | 2.9 |
| orange pineapple (*Royal Prince*) | 210 | 1.0 | 50.0 | 0 | 0 | 30 | 3.0 |
| **Sweet potato, frozen/ chilled** (see also "Sweet potato dish"): | | | | | | | |
| baked, cubed, ½ cup | 88 | 1.5 | 20.6 | .1 | 0 | 7 | 2.6 |
| fries, 3 oz.: | | | | | | | |
| (*McCain*) | 120 | 0 | 22.0 | 3.0 | 0 | 180 | 2.0 |
| (*Ore-Ida*) | 160 | 1.0 | 23.0 | 8.0 | 0 | 160 | 2.0 |
| julienne (*Alexia*) | 140 | 1.0 | 24.0 | 5.0 | 0 | 140 | 3.0 |
| spicy (*Alexia*) | 130 | 1.0 | 23.0 | 4.0 | 0 | 250 | 3.0 |

| Food and Measure | cal. | prot. (gms) | carbo. (gms) | fat (gms) | chol. (mgs) | sod. (mgs) | fiber (gms) |
|---|---|---|---|---|---|---|---|
| **Sweet potato, frozen/chilled** *(cont.)* | | | | | | | |
| mashed:, ½ cup: | | | | | | | |
| (*Bob Evans*) . . . . . . . . | 170 | 2.0 | 34.0 | 3.0 | 5 | 250 | 2.0 |
| (*Simply Potatoes*) . . . . | 90 | 2.0 | 18.0 | 1.0 | 2 | 100 | 2.0 |
| (*Simply Potatoes* Diner's Choice/ Family Size) . . . . . . | 140 | 2.0 | 30.0 | 1.0 | <5 | 100 | 2.0 |
| w/brown sugar (*Larry's*) . . . . . . . . . | 140 | 2.0 | 27.0 | 3.5 | 10 | 530 | 2.0 |
| mashing (*Ore-Ida Steam n' Mash*), ⅙ pkg. . . . . . . . . . . . | 90 | 1.0 | 20.0 | 0 | 0 | 30 | 3.0 |
| patties (*McKenzie's* Yam), 2-oz. pc. . . . . . . | 70 | <1.0 | 16.0 | 0 | 0 | 90 | 1.0 |
| **Sweet potato chips**, 1 oz.: | | | | | | | |
| (*Terra*) . . . . . . . . . . . . . . | 160 | 1.0 | 15.0 | 11.0 | 0 | 10 | 3.0 |
| (*Terra* Crinkles) . . . . . . . . | 160 | 1.0 | 15.0 | 11.0 | 0 | 90 | 3.0 |
| blends: | | | | | | | |
| (*Terra* Sweets & Beets) . . . . . . . . . | 150 | 2.0 | 15.0 | 9.0 | 0 | 5 | 1.0 |
| (*Terra* Sweets & Carrots) . . . . . . . | 150 | 2.0 | 15.0 | 9.0 | 0 | 20 | 5.0 |
| candied (*Terra* Crinkles) . . . . . . . . . . . | 160 | 1.0 | 15.0 | 11.0 | 0 | 10 | 3.0 |
| honey chipotle barbecue (*Pringles*) . . | 140 | 1.0 | 16.0 | 8.0 | 0 | 210 | 1.0 |
| spiced (*Terra*) . . . . . . . . . | 160 | 1.0 | 14.0 | 11.0 | 0 | 150 | 2.0 |
| **Sweet potato dish**, frozen/chilled: | | | | | | | |
| casserole (*Boston Market*), 5.6 oz. . . . . . | 320 | 3.0 | 44.0 | 15.0 | 5 | 200 | 3.0 |
| nuggets (*Dr. Praeger's* Bites), 2 pcs., 2 oz. . . . | 110 | 3.0 | 20.0 | 2.5 | 0 | 180 | 1.0 |
| pancake, 1 pc.: | | | | | | | |
| (*Dr. Praeger's*), 2 oz. . . | 80 | 2.0 | 12.0 | 2.0 | 0 | 140 | 3.0 |
| (*Golden*), 1.3 oz. . . . . . . | 80 | 1.0 | 10.0 | 4.0 | 0 | 20 | 0 |
| **Sweet potato dish mix**, mashed (*Betty Crocker*), ½ cup* . . . . | 170 | 3.0 | 28.0 | 5.0 | 0 | 360 | 1.0 |
| **Sweet potato leaf:** | | | | | | | |
| raw, chopped, ½ cup . . . | 6 | .7 | 1.1 | .1 | 0 | 2 | <1.0 |
| steamed, ½ cup . . . . . . . | 11 | .7 | 2.3 | .1 | 0 | 4 | .6 |

| Food and Measure | cal. | prot. (gms) | carbo. (gms) | fat (gms) | chol. (mgs) | sod. (mgs) | fiber (gms) |
|---|---|---|---|---|---|---|---|
| **Sweet potato pocket,** frozen (*Aunt Trudy's Organic*), 5-oz. pkg. ... | 310 | 5.0 | 45.0 | 12.0 | 0 | 270 | 4.0 |
| **Sweet and sour drink mixer** (*Angostura*), 2 fl. oz. ... | 70 | 0 | 18.0 | 0 | 0 | 5 | 0 |
| **Sweet and sour sauce,** 2 tbsp., except as noted: | | | | | | | |
| (*Ah-So/China Pride* Sweet & Pungent) ... | 80 | 0 | 19.0 | 0 | 0 | 260 | 1.0 |
| (*Contadina*), 1 tbsp. .... | 40 | 0 | 8.0 | 1.0 | 0 | 115 | 0 |
| (*Crosse & Blackwell*) .... | 90 | 0 | 23.0 | 0 | 0 | 30 | 0 |
| (*Ka•Me*) ............. | 60 | 0 | 14.0 | 0 | 0 | 270 | 0 |
| (*Kikkoman*), 1 tbsp. .... | 35 | 0 | 9.0 | 0 | 0 | 190 | 0 |
| (*Kikkoman* Dipping) .... | 70 | 0 | 17.0 | 0 | 0 | 250 | 0 |
| (*La Choy*) ........... | 60 | 0 | 14.0 | 0 | 0 | 110 | 0 |
| (*San-J* Sweet & Tangy) .. | 50 | <1.0 | 13.0 | 0 | 0 | 320 | 0 |
| (*Simply Tsang* Marinade), 1 tbsp. ... | 50 | 0 | 13.0 | 0 | 0 | 420 | 0 |
| (*World Harbors* Maui) ... | 60 | 0 | 14.0 | 0 | 0 | 250 | 0 |
| cooking (*Tiger Tiger*), ½ cup ............. | 124 | 0 | 31.0 | 0 | 0 | 625 | 0 |
| duck sauce: | | | | | | | |
| (*Ah-So*) ............. | 50 | 0 | 13.0 | 0 | 0 | 15 | 0 |
| (*Ka•Me*), 1 tbsp. ..... | 40 | 0 | 10.0 | 0 | 0 | 90 | 0 |
| (*La Choy*) .......... | 60 | 0 | 15.0 | 0 | 0 | 120 | 0 |
| (*Mee Tu/Dai Day*) .... | 80 | 0 | 19.0 | 0 | 0 | 260 | 1.0 |
| (*Roland*) ............ | 80 | 0 | 19.0 | 0 | 0 | 260 | 1.0 |
| (*Saucy Susan*) ...... | 80 | 0 | 19.0 | 0 | 0 | 260 | 1.0 |
| **Sweet and sour sauce mix** (*Kikkoman*), 1½ tsp. .......... | 60 | 0 | 14.0 | 0 | 0 | 280 | 0 |
| **Sweetbreads,** see "Pancreas" and "Thymus" | | | | | | | |
| **Swiss chard,** fresh: | | | | | | | |
| raw: | | | | | | | |
| (*Frieda's*), 3 oz. ...... | 15 | 2.0 | 3.0 | 0 | 0 | 180 | 1.0 |
| chopped, ½ cup ..... | 3 | .3 | .7 | <.1 | 0 | 38 | .3 |
| boiled, drained, chopped, ½ cup ..... | 18 | 1.7 | 3.6 | .1 | 0 | 158 | 1.8 |
| **Swordfish,** fresh, meat only: | | | | | | | |
| raw, 4 oz. ............ | 137 | 22.5 | 0 | 4.6 | 45 | 102 | 0 |
| baked or broiled, 4 oz. .. | 176 | 28.8 | 0 | 5.8 | 57 | 130 | 0 |

| Food and Measure | cal. | prot. (gms) | carbo. (gms) | fat (gms) | chol. (mgs) | sod. (mgs) | fiber (gms) |
|---|---|---|---|---|---|---|---|
| **Syrup**, see specific listings | | | | | | | |
| **Szechuan paste** (*Roland*), 1 tsp. ..... | 5 | 0 | 1.0 | 0 | 0 | 180 | 0 |
| **Szechuan sauce** (see also "Stir-fry sauce"): | | | | | | | |
| (*Ka•Me*), 2 tbsp. ....... | 45 | <1.0 | 9.0 | 1.0 | 0 | 450 | 0 |
| (*San-J*), 1 tsp. ......... | 5 | 0 | <1.0 | 0 | 0 | 170 | 0 |

# T

| Food and Measure | cal. | prot. (gms) | carbo. (gms) | fat (gms) | chol. (mgs) | sod. (mgs) | fiber (gms) |
|---|---|---|---|---|---|---|---|
| **Tabouli salad**, 2 tbsp.: | | | | | | | |
| (*Cedar's*) . . . . . . . . . . . . . | 30 | 1.0 | 4.0 | 1.5 | 0 | 95 | <1.0 |
| (*Joseph's*) . . . . . . . . . . . | 30 | 1.0 | 5.0 | 1.0 | 0 | 40 | 1.0 |
| **Tabouli salad mix**: | | | | | | | |
| (*Fantastic*), ⅓ cup . . . . . . | 150 | 5.0 | 33.0 | 1.0 | 0 | 590 | 6.0 |
| (*Near East*), 1 oz. . . . . . . | 80 | 3.0 | 21.0 | 0 | 0 | 270 | 5.0 |
| **Taco**, frozen, beef and cheese, mini (*José Olé*), 4 pcs., 3 oz. . . . . | 230 | 8.0 | 23.0 | 12.0 | 20 | 440 | 5.0 |
| *Taco Bell:* | | | | | | | |
| burritos: | | | | | | | |
| ½ lb. cheesy potato . . | 550 | 19.0 | 59.0 | 26.0 | 50 | 1500 | 7.0 |
| ½ lb. combo . . . . . . . . | 460 | 22.0 | 52.0 | 18.0 | 50 | 1520 | 10.0 |
| 7-layer . . . . . . . . . . . . | 510 | 18.0 | 69.0 | 18.0 | 20 | 1300 | 13.0 |
| bean . . . . . . . . . . . . . | 370 | 14.0 | 56.0 | 10.0 | 5 | 1150 | 11.0 |
| beefy 5-layer . . . . . . . . | 560 | 20.0 | 70.0 | 22.0 | 35 | 1470 | 10.0 |
| beefy crunch . . . . . . . . | 510 | 15.0 | 61.0 | 22.0 | 30 | 1250 | 5.0 |
| cheesy bean/rice . . . . . | 490 | 13.0 | 60.0 | 21.0 | 10 | 1260 | 8.0 |
| cheesy double beef . . . | 470 | 18.0 | 54.0 | 20.0 | 40 | 1460 | 6.0 |
| chili cheese . . . . . . . . . | 380 | 16.0 | 41.0 | 17.0 | 35 | 930 | 5.0 |
| double steak . . . . . . . . | 610 | 29.0 | 71.0 | 23.0 | 65 | 1720 | 5.0 |
| Fresco bean . . . . . . . . | 350 | 13.0 | 56.0 | 8.0 | 0 | 1170 | 12.0 |
| grilled chicken . . . . . . | 430 | 18.0 | 49.0 | 18.0 | 40 | 1160 | 3.0 |
| Grilled Stuft: | | | | | | | |
| beef . . . . . . . . . . . . | 700 | 27.0 | 80.0 | 30.0 | 60 | 1930 | 13.0 |
| chicken . . . . . . . . . | 660 | 34.0 | 77.0 | 24.0 | 70 | 2010 | 9.0 |
| chicken enchilada . . | 690 | 36.0 | 79.0 | 26.0 | 85 | 1970 | 6.0 |
| steak . . . . . . . . . . . | 640 | 29.0 | 76.0 | 25.0 | 50 | 1860 | 9.0 |
| *Quad Steak* . . . . . . . . . | 690 | 41.0 | 72.0 | 26.0 | 100 | 2210 | 5.0 |
| *Supreme*, beef . . . . . . | 420 | 17.0 | 53.0 | 15.0 | 35 | 1260 | 9.0 |
| *Supreme*, chicken . . . . | 400 | 21.0 | 52.0 | 12.0 | 40 | 1300 | 8.0 |
| *Supreme*, steak . . . . . . | 390 | 18.0 | 51.0 | 13.0 | 30 | 1230 | 8.0 |
| volcano . . . . . . . . . . . . | 790 | 24.0 | 81.0 | 41.0 | 70 | 1770 | 9.0 |

| Food and Measure | cal. | prot. (gms) | carbo. (gms) | fat (gms) | chol. (mgs) | sod. (mgs) | fiber (gms) |
|---|---|---|---|---|---|---|---|
| **Taco Bell** *(cont.)* | | | | | | | |
| chalupas: | | | | | | | |
| Baja, beef ......... | 410 | 13.0 | 31.0 | 26.0 | 35 | 730 | 5.0 |
| Baja, chicken ....... | 390 | 16.0 | 29.0 | 23.0 | 35 | 760 | 3.0 |
| Baja, steak ........ | 380 | 13.0 | 29.0 | 23.0 | 30 | 690 | 3.0 |
| nacho, beef ......... | 370 | 12.0 | 31.0 | 22.0 | 20 | 730 | 4.0 |
| nacho, chicken ...... | 340 | 15.0 | 30.0 | 18.0 | 25 | 770 | 3.0 |
| nacho, steak ........ | 330 | 12.0 | 30.0 | 19.0 | 15 | 700 | 3.0 |
| supreme, beef ....... | 370 | 13.0 | 31.0 | 21.0 | 35 | 600 | 4.0 |
| supreme, chicken .... | 350 | 17.0 | 30.0 | 18.0 | 35 | 640 | 3.0 |
| supreme, steak ...... | 340 | 14.0 | 29.0 | 18.0 | 30 | 570 | 3.0 |
| Fresco menu: | | | | | | | |
| bean burrito ........ | 350 | 13.0 | 56.0 | 8.0 | 0 | 1170 | 12.0 |
| *Supreme*, chicken .... | 350 | 19.0 | 50.0 | 8.0 | 25 | 1290 | 8.0 |
| *Supreme*, steak ...... | 340 | 16.0 | 50.0 | 8.0 | 15 | 1220 | 8.0 |
| taco, crunchy ....... | 150 | 7.0 | 13.0 | 7.0 | 20 | 350 | 3.0 |
| taco, soft ......... | 190 | 8.0 | 22.0 | 7.0 | 20 | 580 | 4.0 |
| taco, soft, chicken ... | 170 | 12.0 | 22.0 | 4.0 | 25 | 680 | 3.0 |
| taco, soft, steak ..... | 160 | 9.0 | 21.0 | 4.5 | 15 | 550 | 2.0 |
| gorditas: | | | | | | | |
| *Baja*, beef ......... | 340 | 13.0 | 30.0 | 18.0 | 35 | 710 | 4.0 |
| *Baja*, chicken ....... | 320 | 16.0 | 29.0 | 15.0 | 35 | 750 | 3.0 |
| *Baja*, steak ........ | 310 | 14.0 | 28.0 | 15.0 | 30 | 680 | 3.0 |
| nacho, beef ......... | 290 | 12.0 | 31.0 | 14.0 | 20 | 720 | 4.0 |
| nacho, chicken ...... | 270 | 15.0 | 30.0 | 10.0 | 25 | 760 | 2.0 |
| nacho, steak ........ | 260 | 12.0 | 29.0 | 11.0 | 15 | 690 | 2.0 |
| *Supreme*, beef ...... | 300 | 13.0 | 31.0 | 13.0 | 35 | 590 | 4.0 |
| *Supreme*, chicken .... | 270 | 17.0 | 29.0 | 10.0 | 35 | 630 | 2.0 |
| *Supreme*, steak ...... | 270 | 14.0 | 29.0 | 11.0 | 30 | 550 | 2.0 |
| nachos: | | | | | | | |
| cheesy ........... | 280 | 4.0 | 28.0 | 17.0 | 0 | 300 | 2.0 |
| nachos ........... | 190 | 4.0 | 31.0 | 21.0 | 0 | 520 | 2.0 |
| *BellGrande* ........ | 770 | 20.0 | 78.0 | 42.0 | 30 | 1300 | 15.0 |
| supreme .......... | 440 | 13.0 | 42.0 | 24.0 | 30 | 800 | 8.0 |
| volcano ........... | 980 | 22.0 | 88.0 | 61.0 | 40 | 1870 | 16.0 |
| salad/specialties: | | | | | | | |
| *Crunchwrap Supreme* . | 540 | 17.0 | 71.0 | 21.0 | 30 | 1220 | 7.0 |
| *Enchirito*, beef ...... | 370 | 19.0 | 35.0 | 17.0 | 45 | 1380 | 9.0 |
| *Enchirito*, chicken .... | 350 | 22.0 | 34.0 | 14.0 | 50 | 1410 | 7.0 |
| *Enchirito*, steak ..... | 340 | 20.0 | 34.0 | 14.0 | 45 | 1340 | 7.0 |
| Mexican pizza ....... | 540 | 21.0 | 47.0 | 30.0 | 45 | 1030 | 8.0 |
| *MexiMelt* ........... | 280 | 15.0 | 23.0 | 14.0 | 45 | 820 | 4.0 |
| quesadilla, cheese ... | 480 | 19.0 | 40.0 | 27.0 | 50 | 1000 | 4.0 |
| quesadilla, chicken ... | 530 | 28.0 | 41.0 | 28.0 | 75 | 1320 | 4.0 |

| Food and Measure | cal. | prot. (gms) | carbo. (gms) | fat (gms) | chol. (mgs) | sod. (mgs) | fiber (gms) |
|---|---|---|---|---|---|---|---|
| quesadilla, steak | 520 | 25.0 | 41.0 | 28.0 | 65 | 1250 | 4.0 |
| double | 660 | 34.0 | 59.0 | 32.0 | 80 | 1720 | 5.0 |
| *Quad* | 750 | 46.0 | 60.0 | 36.0 | 115 | 2210 | 5.0 |
| taco salad: | | | | | | | |
| chicken ranch | 910 | 34.0 | 70 | 55.0 | 70 | 1560 | 9.0 |
| chipotle steak | 900 | 28.0 | 68.0 | 57.0 | 65 | 1600 | 8.0 |
| express, w/chips | 660 | 24.0 | 66.0 | 33.0 | 60 | 1490 | 11.0 |
| fiesta | 770 | 27.0 | 73.0 | 42.0 | 60 | 1550 | 12.0 |
| taquitos, chicken | 320 | 18.0 | 36.0 | 11.0 | 40 | 880 | 3.0 |
| taquitos, steak | 310 | 15.0 | 37.0 | 11.0 | 30 | 810 | 3.0 |
| tostada | 250 | 11.0 | 29.0 | 10.0 | 15 | 730 | 10.0 |
| tacos: | | | | | | | |
| beef, soft | 210 | 10.0 | 21.0 | 9.0 | 30 | 560 | 3.0 |
| *Supreme* | 240 | 11.0 | 24.0 | 11.0 | 35 | 590 | 4.0 |
| chicken, soft | 190 | 14.0 | 20.0 | 6.0 | 30 | 600 | 2.0 |
| crunchy | 170 | 8.0 | 12.0 | 10.0 | 30 | 330 | 3.0 |
| crunchy, fresco | 150 | 7.0 | 13.0 | 7.0 | 20 | 350 | 3.0 |
| *Double Decker* | 330 | 14.0 | 39.0 | 13.0 | 30 | 760 | 8.0 |
| *Supreme* | 360 | 15.0 | 41.0 | 16.0 | 35 | 780 | 9.0 |
| potato, soft, crispy | 280 | 6.0 | 33.0 | 14.0 | 10 | 560 | 3.0 |
| steak, grilled, soft | 260 | 11.0 | 21.0 | 14.0 | 30 | 650 | 2.0 |
| *Taco Supreme* | 200 | 9.0 | 15.0 | 12.0 | 35 | 350 | 3.0 |
| volcano | 230 | 8.0 | 14.0 | 16.0 | 35 | 440 | 3.0 |
| sides/dessert: | | | | | | | |
| avocado ranch dressing | 80 | 0 | 1.0 | 8.0 | 10 | 120 | 0 |
| border sauce, fire | 0 | 0 | 0 | 0 | 0 | 60 | 0 |
| border sauce, hot | 0 | 0 | 0 | 0 | 0 | 45 | 0 |
| border sauce, mild | 0 | 0 | 0 | 0 | 0 | 35 | 0 |
| caramel apple empanada | 310 | 3.0 | 39.0 | 15.0 | 0 | 310 | 2.0 |
| cheese roll-up | 200 | 9.0 | 19.0 | 10.0 | 20 | 480 | 2.0 |
| cinnamon twists | 170 | 1.0 | 26.0 | 7.0 | 0 | 200 | 1.0 |
| guacamole | 35 | 0 | 2.0 | 3.0 | 0 | 85 | 1.0 |
| jalapeño sauce | 70 | 0 | 1.0 | 7.0 | 5 | 50 | 0 |
| pepper jack sauce | 70 | 0 | 1.0 | 7.0 | 5 | 85 | 0 |
| red sauce | 10 | 0 | 2.0 | 0 | 0 | 240 | 0 |
| salsa | 5 | 0 | 1.0 | 0 | 0 | 80 | 0 |
| salsa, fiesta | 5 | 0 | 1.0 | 0 | 0 | 60 | 1.0 |
| salsa, fire-roasted | 0 | 0 | 1.0 | 0 | 0 | 45 | 0 |
| salsa verde | 0 | 0 | 1.0 | 0 | 0 | 55 | 0 |
| sour cream, low fat | 30 | 1.0 | 2.0 | 2.0 | 5 | 20 | 0 |
| tomatillo sauce | 10 | 0 | 2.0 | 0 | 0 | 170 | 0 |
| zesty dressing | 200 | 1.0 | 3.0 | 20.0 | 0 | 250 | 0 |

| Food and Measure | cal. | prot. (gms) | carbo. (gms) | fat (gms) | chol. (mgs) | sod. (mgs) | fiber (gms) |
|---|---|---|---|---|---|---|---|
| **Taco entree kit**: | | | | | | | |
| (*Las Palmas*), ¼ pkg. . . . | 170 | 3.0 | 25.0 | 7.0 | 0 | 910 | 3.0 |
| (*Old El Paso*): | | | | | | | |
| ⅙ pkg. mix . . . . . . . . . | 130 | 2.0 | 18.0 | 5.0 | 0 | 760 | 1.0 |
| 2 tacos, w/chicken* . . | 230 | 19.0 | 18.0 | 9.0 | 45 | 820 | 1.0 |
| 2 tacos, w/lean beef* . | 260 | 16.0 | 18.0 | 14.0 | 45 | 810 | 1.0 |
| (*Old El Paso* Gordita): | | | | | | | |
| ⅛ pkg. mix . . . . . . . . . | 240 | 4.0 | 33.0 | 10.0 | 0 | 830 | 1.0 |
| 1 taco* . . . . . . . . . . . . | 340 | 22.0 | 34.0 | 13.0 | 50 | 920 | 1.0 |
| (*Old El Paso* Hard/Soft): | | | | | | | |
| hard, ⅓ pkg. mix . . . . | 130 | 2.0 | 18.0 | 5.0 | 0 | 760 | 1.0 |
| hard, 2 tacos* . . . . . . . | 260 | 16.0 | 18.0 | 14.0 | 45 | 810 | 1.0 |
| soft, ⅓ pkg. mix . . . . . | 180 | 4.0 | 31.0 | 5.0 | 0 | 1040 | 1.0 |
| soft, 2 tacos* . . . . . . . | 180 | 18.0 | 31.0 | 13.0 | 45 | 1090 | 1.0 |
| (*Old El Paso* Soft): | | | | | | | |
| ⅕ pkg. mix . . . . . . . . . | 180 | 4.0 | 32.0 | 5.0 | 0 | 1170 | 1.0 |
| 2 tacos, w/chicken* . . | 310 | 25.0 | 32.0 | 9.0 | 25 | 1240 | 1.0 |
| 2 tacos, w/lean beef* . | 350 | 20.0 | 32.0 | 15.0 | 55 | 1220 | 1.0 |
| (*Old El Paso Soft Taco Bake*): | | | | | | | |
| ¼ pkg. mix . . . . . . . . . | 190 | 3.0 | 29.0 | 7.0 | 0 | 860 | 1.0 |
| 1 taco* . . . . . . . . . . . . | 390 | 24.0 | 29.0 | 20.0 | 70 | 930 | 1.0 |
| (*Old El Paso Stand 'n Stuff*): | | | | | | | |
| ⅕ pkg. mix . . . . . . . . . | 160 | 3.0 | 23.0 | 6.0 | 0 | 900 | 2.0 |
| 2 tacos, w/chicken* . . | 280 | 23.0 | 23.0 | 11.0 | 55 | 970 | 2.0 |
| 2 tacos, w/lean beef* . | 320 | 18.0 | 23.0 | 17.0 | 55 | 960 | 2.0 |
| (*Ortega*), ⅙ pkg. . . . . . . . | 160 | 2.0 | 22.0 | 7.0 | 0 | 640 | 3.0 |
| (*Ortega*), ⅑ of 16.7-oz. pkg. . . . . . . . | 150 | 2.0 | 21.0 | 6.0 | 0 | 770 | 2.0 |
| (*Ortega* Hard/Soft): | | | | | | | |
| mix, w/2 tacos . . . . . . | 120 | 2.0 | 16.0 | 6.0 | 0 | 170 | 2.0 |
| mix, w/2 tortillas . . . . . | 210 | 5.0 | 35.0 | 4.5 | 0 | 590 | <1.0 |
| (*Ortega* Hard/Soft Grande): | | | | | | | |
| mix, w/2 tacos . . . . . . | 160 | 3.0 | 22.0 | 7.0 | 0 | 840 | 2.0 |
| mix, w/2 tortillas . . . . . | 250 | 6.0 | 42.0 | 6.0 | 0 | 1270 | <1.0 |
| (*Ortega* Whole Grain), ⅕ pkg. . . . . . . . . . . . . | 130 | 2.0 | 23.0 | 6.0 | 0 | 790 | 6.0 |
| (*Taco Bell*), ⅙ pkg. . . . . . | 130 | 2.0 | 20.0 | 4.5 | 0 | 530 | 2.0 |
| (*Taco Bell* Cheesy Double Decker), ⅙ pkg. . . . . . . . . . . . . | 230 | 5.0 | 30.0 | 9.0 | 5 | 960 | 2.0 |
| (*Taco Bell* Soft), ⅕ pkg. . | 230 | 6.0 | 40.0 | 5.0 | 0 | 1000 | 2.0 |

| Food and Measure | cal. | prot. (gms) | carbo. (gms) | fat (gms) | chol. (mgs) | sod. (mgs) | fiber (gms) |
|---|---|---|---|---|---|---|---|
| chicken, soft (*Old El Paso*), ⅕ pkg.: | | | | | | | |
| mix only . . . . . . . . . . | 170 | 4.0 | 30.0 | 4.5 | 0 | 960 | 1.0 |
| 2 tacos* . . . . . . . . . . | 320 | 24.0 | 33.0 | 10.0 | 55 | 1040 | 1.0 |
| blue or yellow corn (*Garden of Eatin'*), ⅙ pkg. . . . . . . . . . . | 150 | 2.0 | 20.0 | 6.0 | 0 | 600 | 1.0 |
| **Taco filling**, meatless: | | | | | | | |
| (*Frieda's*), 1 oz. . . . . . . . . | 50 | 4.0 | 3.0 | 3.0 | 0 | 180 | 2.0 |
| mix (*Fantastic*), ¼ cup . . | 100 | 12.0 | 12.0 | 1.0 | 0 | 520 | 2.0 |
| **Taco sauce**, 1 tbsp., except as noted: | | | | | | | |
| (*Ortega*) . . . . . . . . . . . . . | 10 | 0 | 1.0 | 0 | 0 | 60 | 0 |
| (*Pace*) . . . . . . . . . . . . . . | 10 | 0 | 2.0 | 0 | 0 | 130 | 0 |
| (*Taco Bell*), 2 tbsp. . . . . . | 10 | 0 | 2.0 | 0 | 0 | 210 | 0 |
| all styles (*Old El Paso*) . . | 5 | 0 | 1.0 | 0 | 0 | 90 | 0 |
| chipotle (*La Victoria*) . . . . | 5 | 0 | 1.0 | 0 | 0 | 130 | 0 |
| jalapeño, hot, chunky (*La Victoria*) . . . . . . . . | 5 | 0 | 1.0 | 0 | 0 | 190 | 0 |
| medium: | | | | | | | |
| green (*La Victoria*) . . . | 5 | 0 | 1.0 | 0 | 0 | 110 | 0 |
| red (*La Victoria*) . . . . . | 5 | 0 | 1.0 | 0 | 0 | 105 | 0 |
| mild: | | | | | | | |
| green (*La Victoria*) . . . | 5 | 0 | 1.0 | 0 | 0 | 140 | 0 |
| red (*La Victoria*) . . . . . | 5 | 0 | 1.0 | 0 | 0 | 100 | 0 |
| **Taco seasoning mix**, 2 tsp., except as noted: | | | | | | | |
| (*Chi-Chi's* Fiesta), ⅛ pkg. . . . . . . . . . . . . | 15 | 0 | 3.0 | 0 | 0 | 240 | 0 |
| (*Lawry's*) . . . . . . . . . . . . . | 15 | 0 | 3.0 | 0 | 0 | 340 | <1.0 |
| (*McCormick*) . . . . . . . . . . | 20 | 0 | 3.0 | 0 | 0 | 430 | 0 |
| (*McCormick* 30% Less Sodium) . . . . . . . | 20 | 0 | 3.0 | 0 | 0 | 300 | 0 |
| (*Old El Paso*) . . . . . . . . . . | 15 | 0 | 3.0 | 0 | 0 | 580 | 0 |
| (*Old El Paso* 40% Less Sodium) . . . . . . . | 15 | 0 | 3.0 | 0 | 0 | 330 | 0 |
| (*Ortega*), 1 tbsp. . . . . . . . | 20 | 0 | 4.0 | 0 | 0 | 430 | 0 |
| (*Ortega* 40% Less Sodium) . . . . . . . . . . . | 15 | 0 | 3.0 | 0 | 0 | 330 | 0 |
| (*Taco Bell*) . . . . . . . . . . . . | 20 | 1.0 | 3.0 | 0 | 0 | 370 | 1.0 |
| cheesy: | | | | | | | |
| (*McCormick*) . . . . . . . | 15 | 0 | 3.0 | 0 | 0 | 390 | 0 |
| (*Old El Paso*) . . . . . . . | 15 | 0 | 3.0 | 0 | 0 | 340 | 0 |

| Food and Measure | cal. | prot. (gms) | carbo. (gms) | fat (gms) | chol. (mgs) | sod. (mgs) | fiber (gms) |
|---|---|---|---|---|---|---|---|
| **Taco seasoning mix** *(cont.)* | | | | | | | |
| chicken: | | | | | | | |
| (*Lawry's*) . . . . . . . . . | 25 | 0 | 5.0 | 0 | 0 | 430 | 0 |
| (*McCormick*) . . . . . . . | 25 | 0 | 4.0 | 0 | 0 | 450 | 0 |
| chipotle: | | | | | | | |
| (*Ortega*), 1 tbsp. . . . . . | 20 | 0 | 4.0 | 0 | 0 | 350 | 0 |
| (*Taco Bell*) . . . . . . . . . | 20 | 1.0 | 3.0 | 0 | 0 | 370 | 1.0 |
| hot: | | | | | | | |
| (*Lawry's*) . . . . . . . . . | 15 | 0 | 3.0 | 0 | 0 | 370 | <1.0 |
| (*McCormick*) . . . . . . . | 20 | 0 | 3.0 | 0 | 0 | 430 | 0 |
| (*Ortega*), 1 tbsp. . . . . . | 20 | 0 | 4.0 | 0 | 0 | 350 | 0 |
| hot and spicy (*Old El Paso*) . . . . . . . . . . . | 15 | 0 | 3.0 | 0 | 0 | 580 | 0 |
| jalapeño and onion (*Ortega*), 1 tbsp. . . . . . | 15 | 0 | 3.0 | 0 | 0 | 430 | <1.0 |
| mild: | | | | | | | |
| (*McCormick*) . . . . . . . | 20 | <1.0 | 4.0 | 0 | 0 | 460 | 0 |
| (*Old El Paso*) . . . . . . . | 15 | 0 | 3.0 | 0 | 0 | 390 | 0 |
| **Taco shell** (see also "Tostada shell"): | | | | | | | |
| (*Mission*), 3 pcs. . . . . . . | 150 | 2.0 | 20.0 | 6.0 | 0 | 0 | 2.0 |
| (*Mission* Jumbo), 1 pc. . . | 90 | 2.0 | 13.0 | 4.0 | 0 | 0 | 1.0 |
| (*Old El Paso*), 3 pcs. . . . . | 150 | 2.0 | 20.0 | 7.0 | 0 | 135 | 1.0 |
| (*Old El Paso* Super Stuffer), 2 pcs. . . . . . | 180 | 3.0 | 22.0 | 8.0 | 0 | 160 | 1.0 |
| (*Old El Paso Stand 'n Stuff*), 2 pcs. . . . . . | 130 | 2.0 | 16.0 | 6.0 | 0 | 115 | 1.0 |
| (*Taco Bell*), 3 pcs. . . . . . . | 150 | 2.0 | 22.0 | 6.0 | 0 | 5 | 2.0 |
| blue or yellow corn (*Garden of Eatin'*), 2 pcs., 1 oz. . . . . . . . . | 140 | 2.0 | 17.0 | 7.0 | 0 | 5 | 1.0 |
| soft, see "Tortilla" | | | | | | | |
| white corn (*Old El Paso*), 3 pcs. . . . . . . . | 150 | 2.0 | 20.0 | 7.0 | 0 | 140 | 1.0 |
| white or yellow corn (*Ortega*), 2 pcs. . . . . . | 120 | 2.0 | 16.0 | 6.0 | 0 | 170 | 2.0 |
| yellow corn (*Las Palmas*), 2 pcs. . . . . . . | 120 | 2.0 | 16.0 | 6.0 | 0 | 170 | 2.0 |
| **Taco snack**, frozen (*Michelina's* Rockin' Tacos), 5.5-oz. pkg. . . | 340 | 11.0 | 33.0 | 17.0 | 20 | 830 | 2.0 |
| **Tahini**, sesame, 2 tbsp.: | | | | | | | |
| (*Arrowhead Mills* Organic) . . . . . . . . . . . | 190 | 8.0 | 3.0 | 18.0 | 0 | 10 | <1.0 |

| Food and Measure | cal. | prot. (gms) | carbo. (gms) | fat (gms) | chol. (mgs) | sod. (mgs) | fiber (gms) |
|---|---|---|---|---|---|---|---|
| (*MaraNatha*) . . . . . . . . . . | 190 | 6.0 | 7.0 | 17.0 | 0 | 75 | 1.0 |
| (*Roland*) . . . . . . . . . . . . | 210 | 6.0 | 5.0 | 19.0 | 0 | 10 | 3.0 |
| **Tahini dip** (*Sabra* Classic), 2 tbsp. . . . . | 80 | 2.0 | 2.0 | 8.0 | 0 | 150 | <1.0 |
| **Tamale, canned**, 2 pcs.: | | | | | | | |
| beef (*Hormel* Jumbo) . . . | 190 | 6.0 | 21.0 | 10.0 | 25 | 980 | 3.0 |
| beef (*Hormel/Hormel* Hot'N Spicy) . . . . . . . . | 140 | 4.0 | 15.0 | 7.0 | 15 | 710 | 2.0 |
| w/chili sauce (*El Rio* Hot), 5 oz. . . . . . . | 280 | 6.0 | 19.0 | 20.0 | 25 | 820 | 3.0 |
| **Tamale, frozen** (*El Monterey*), 1 pc.: | | | | | | | |
| beef, 4 oz. . . . . . . . . . | 250 | 10.0 | 24.0 | 13.0 | 15 | 580 | 3.0 |
| chicken, 4 oz. . . . . . . . . | 210 | 7.0 | 23.0 | 11.0 | 25 | 690 | 2.0 |
| **Tamale entree**, frozen, 1 pkg.: | | | | | | | |
| black bean (*Amy's* Verde), 10.25 oz. . . . . | 330 | 7.0 | 55.0 | 10.0 | 0 | 780 | 8.0 |
| cheese (*Amy's* Verde), 10.25 oz. . . . . . . . . | 400 | 13.0 | 51.0 | 16.0 | 20 | 780 | 7.0 |
| Monterey Jack (*Cedarlane*), 9 oz.: | | | | | | | |
| green chili . . . . . . . . . | 290 | 9.0 | 39.0 | 11.0 | 20 | 700 | 4.0 |
| mushroom . . . . . . . . | 280 | 11.0 | 41.0 | 9.0 | 15 | 730 | 4.0 |
| spinach . . . . . . . . . . . | 330 | 13.0 | 42.0 | 13.0 | 30 | 860 | 6.0 |
| pie, meatless (*Amy's* Mexican), 8 oz. . . . . . . | 150 | 5.0 | 27.0 | 3.0 | 0 | 590 | 4.0 |
| vegetable, roasted (*Amy's*), 10.25 oz. . . . | 280 | 9.0 | 44.0 | 7.0 | 20 | 740 | 10.0 |
| **Tamari sauce**, see "Soy sauce" | | | | | | | |
| **Tamarillo**, red or gold (*Frieda's*), 2 pcs., 4.2 oz. . . . . . . . | 40 | 2.0 | 9.0 | 0 | 0 | 0 | 4.0 |
| **Tamarind**: | | | | | | | |
| 1 fruit, 3" x 1" . . . . . . . . | 5 | .1 | 1.3 | <.1 | 0 | 1 | .1 |
| pulp, ½ cup . . . . . . . . . . | 144 | 1.7 | 37.5 | .4 | 0 | 17 | 3.1 |
| **Tamarind sauce** (*Neera's*), 2 tbsp. . . . | 61 | 0 | 16.0 | 0 | 0 | 110 | 0 |
| **Tamarindo** (*Frieda's*), pulp, ½ cup . . . . . . . . | 140 | 2.0 | 38.0 | 0 | 0 | 17 | 3.0 |
| **Tangelo** (*Green Giant*), 3.8-oz. fruit . . . . . . . . | 50 | 1.0 | 15.0 | 0 | 0 | 0 | 3.0 |

| Food and Measure | cal. | prot. (gms) | carbo. (gms) | fat (gms) | chol. (mgs) | sod. (mgs) | fiber (gms) |
|---|---|---|---|---|---|---|---|
| **Tangerine**, fresh: | | | | | | | |
| (*Frieda's* Delite/Pixie | | | | | | | |
| Mandarin), 1 cup, 5 oz. | 60 | 0 | 16.0 | 0 | 0 | 0 | 3.0 |
| (*Frieda's* Page | | | | | | | |
| Mandarin), 1 cup, 5 oz. | 60 | 0 | 12.0 | 0 | 0 | 0 | 3.0 |
| (*Frieda's* Satsuma), | | | | | | | |
| 1 cup, 5 oz. . . . . . . . . | 60 | 1.0 | 16.0 | 0 | 0 | 0 | 3.0 |
| (*Green Giant* Fresh), | | | | | | | |
| 3.8-oz. pc. | 50 | 1.0 | 15.0 | 0 | 0 | 0 | 3.0 |
| clementine, 2.6-oz. pc. . . | 35 | .6 | 8.9 | .1 | 0 | 1 | 1.3 |
| 1 large 2½" diam., | | | | | | | |
| 3.5 oz. . . . . . . . . . . . | 43 | .6 | 11.0 | .2 | 0 | 1 | 2.3 |
| sections, 1 cup . . . . . . . | 86 | 1.2 | 21.8 | .4 | 0 | 2 | 4.5 |
| **Tangerine, can/jar** | | | | | | | |
| (mandarin orange), | | | | | | | |
| ½ cup, except as | | | | | | | |
| noted: | | | | | | | |
| in juice: | | | | | | | |
| (*Del Monte Fruit* | | | | | | | |
| *Naturals*) . . . . . . . . | 70 | 0 | 17.0 | 0 | 0 | 10 | <1.0 |
| (*Roland*) . . . . . . . . . . | 60 | 1.0 | 14.0 | 0 | 0 | 10 | 1.0 |
| w/liquid . . . . . . . . . . . | 46 | .8 | 11.9 | <.1 | 0 | 6 | .9 |
| in light syrup: | | | | | | | |
| (*Del Monte*) . . . . . . . | 80 | 0 | 19.0 | 0 | 0 | 10 | <1.0 |
| (*Del Monte*), 4 oz. . . | 70 | 0 | 17.0 | 0 | 0 | 10 | <1.0 |
| (*Dole* Bowl), 4 oz. . . . | 80 | 0 | 19.0 | 0 | 0 | 5 | 0 |
| (*Dole* Can) . . . . . . . . | 80 | 0 | 19.0 | 0 | 0 | 10 | 1.0 |
| (*Roland* 15 oz.) . . . . . | 90 | 1.0 | 20.0 | 0 | 0 | 20 | 1.0 |
| (*Roland* Segments) . . . | 70 | 1.0 | 17.0 | 0 | 0 | 10 | 1.0 |
| (*Del Monte SunFresh*) | 70 | <1.0 | 17.0 | 0 | 0 | 10 | 0 |
| w/liquid . . . . . . . . . . . | 77 | .6 | 20.4 | .1 | 0 | 8 | .9 |
| in orange gelatin: | | | | | | | |
| (*Del Monte* Lite), | | | | | | | |
| 4.5-oz. cup . . . . . . . | 60 | 0 | 14.0 | 0 | 0 | 40 | 0 |
| (*Dole*), 4.3-oz. cup . . . | 90 | 0 | 23.0 | 0 | 0 | 55 | 1.0 |
| in water (*Roland*) . . . . . | 45 | 1.0 | 10.0 | 0 | 0 | 15 | 1.0 |
| **Tangerine drink**, | | | | | | | |
| sparkling (*Santa Cruz* | | | | | | | |
| *Organic*), 8 fl. oz. . . . | 110 | 0 | 26.0 | 0 | 0 | 10 | 0 |
| **Tangerine juice**, 8 fl. oz.: | | | | | | | |
| (*Bolthouse Farms*) . . . . | 110 | 2.0 | 29.0 | 0 | 0 | 0 | 0 |
| fresh . . . . . . . . . . . . . . | 106 | 1.2 | 25.0 | 1.2 | 0 | 2 | .5 |
| canned, sweetened . . . . . | 125 | 1.3 | 29.9 | .5 | 0 | 2 | .5 |
| frozen* . . . . . . . . . . . . | 111 | 1.0 | 26.7 | .3 | 0 | 2 | .5 |

| Food and Measure | cal. | prot. (gms) | carbo. (gms) | fat (gms) | chol. (mgs) | sod. (mgs) | fiber (gms) |
|---|---|---|---|---|---|---|---|
| **Tapenade**, see "Olive spread" | | | | | | | |
| **Tapioca**, fine ground (*Bob's Red Mill*), ¼ cup . . . . . . . . . . . . | 100 | 0 | 26.0 | 0 | 0 | 0 | 0 |
| **Tapioca pudding**, see "Pudding" | | | | | | | |
| **Taquito**, frozen: | | | | | | | |
| breakfast, egg/bacon/ cheese (*El Monterey*), 2 pcs., 3 oz. . . . . . . . . | 220 | 6.0 | 23.0 | 11.0 | 20 | 340 | 0 |
| corn wrap, 3 oz.: | | | | | | | |
| chicken (*El Monterey*), 2 pcs. . . . . . . . . . . . | 180 | 6.0 | 22.0 | 8.0 | 15 | 360 | 4.0 |
| chicken (*José Olé*), 3 pcs. . . . . . . . . . . . | 200 | 7.0 | 26.0 | 8.0 | 10 | 390 | 3.0 |
| steak, shredded (*El Monterey*), 2 pcs. . . . | 160 | 10.0 | 21.0 | 4.0 | 10 | 250 | 4.0 |
| steak, shredded (*José Olé*), 3 pcs. . . . . . . . | 210 | 6.0 | 25.0 | 9.0 | 10 | 420 | 3.0 |
| flour wrap: | | | | | | | |
| chicken breast, char- broiled (*El Monterey Mexican Grill*), 3 pcs., 5.1 oz. . . . . | 380 | 15.0 | 36.0 | 19.0 | 35 | 670 | 1.0 |
| chicken/cheese (*El Monterey* 10 Pc.), 3 pcs., 4.5 oz. . . . . | 350 | 10.0 | 36.0 | 18.0 | 15 | 650 | 2.0 |
| chicken/cheese (*El Monterey* 16 Pc.), 2 pcs., 3 oz. . . . . . . | 240 | 8.0 | 24.0 | 12.0 | 10 | 390 | 0 |
| chicken/cheese (*El Monterey* 40 Pc.), 3 pcs., 4.5 oz. . . . . | 350 | 11.0 | 36.0 | 19.0 | 20 | 680 | 2.0 |
| chicken/cheese (*José Olé*), 2 pcs., 3 oz. . . | 230 | 9.0 | 26.0 | 10.0 | 15 | 510 | 3.0 |
| steak/cheese (*José Olé*), 2 pcs., 3 oz. . . | 250 | 8.0 | 26.0 | 12.0 | 15 | 470 | 3.0 |
| steak/cheese, shredded (*El Monterey* 10 Pc.), 3 pcs., 4.5 oz. . . . . | 350 | 11.0 | 36.0 | 17.0 | 20 | 650 | 1.0 |
| steak/cheese, shredded (*El Monterey* 16 Pc.), 2 pcs., 3 oz. . . . . . . | 240 | 9.0 | 24.0 | 11.0 | 10 | 360 | 0 |

| Food and Measure | cal. | prot. (gms) | carbo. (gms) | fat (gms) | chol. (mgs) | sod. (mgs) | fiber (gms) |
|---|---|---|---|---|---|---|---|
| **Taquito** *(cont.)* | | | | | | | |
| flour, in batter (*El Monterey*), 2 pcs., 2.8 oz.: | | | | | | | |
| beef, taco/cheese .... | 220 | 6.0 | 20.0 | 10.0 | 10 | 360 | 0 |
| chicken, Southwest .. | 170 | 6.0 | 20.0 | 8.0 | 10 | 330 | 1.0 |
| **Taramosalata** (*Krinos*), 1 tbsp. ............ | 60 | 1.0 | 0 | 6.0 | 15 | 115 | 0 |
| **Taro**, fresh, ½ cup: | | | | | | | |
| raw: | | | | | | | |
| chopped (*Frieda's Root*), 1 cup ...... | 115 | 2.0 | 28.0 | 0 | 0 | 11 | 4.0 |
| sliced, ½ cup ....... | 56 | .8 | 13.8 | .1 | 0 | 6 | 2.1 |
| cooked, sliced, ½ cup ... | 94 | .3 | 22.8 | .1 | 0 | 10 | 3.4 |
| Tahitian: | | | | | | | |
| raw, sliced ......... | 25 | 1.7 | 4.3 | .6 | 0 | 31 | n.a. |
| cooked, sliced ....... | 30 | 2.8 | 4.7 | .5 | 0 | 37 | n.a. |
| **Taro chips**, 1 oz.: | | | | | | | |
| (*Terra* Original) ........ | 140 | 1.0 | 19.0 | 6.0 | 0 | 110 | 4.0 |
| spiced (*Terra*) ......... | 130 | 1.0 | 20.0 | 5.0 | 0 | 170 | 2.0 |
| **Taro leaf**: | | | | | | | |
| raw, ½ cup ........... | 6 | .7 | .9 | .1 | 0 | 1 | .5 |
| steamed, ½ cup ....... | 17 | 2.0 | 2.9 | .3 | 0 | 1 | 1.5 |
| **Taro shoots**, ½ cup: | | | | | | | |
| raw, sliced ........... | 5 | .4 | 1.0 | <.1 | 0 | <1 | n.a. |
| cooked, sliced ....... | 10 | .5 | 2.2 | .1 | 0 | 1 | n.a. |
| **Tarragon**, ground, 1 tsp. .. | 5 | .4 | .8 | .1 | 0 | 1 | .1 |
| **Tart shell**, see "Fillo dough" and "Pastry shell" | | | | | | | |
| **Tartar sauce**, 2 tbsp.: | | | | | | | |
| (*Cains*) .............. | 160 | 0 | 2.0 | 16.0 | 15 | 160 | 0 |
| (*Crosse & Blackwell*) .... | 110 | 0 | 7.0 | 9.0 | 10 | 270 | 0 |
| (*Hellmann's/Best Foods*) ............. | 80 | 0 | 4.0 | 7.0 | 5 | 330 | 0 |
| (*Kraft*) .............. | 60 | 0 | 4.0 | 4.5 | 5 | 230 | 0 |
| (*Marinade Bay*) ........ | 150 | 0 | 0 | 17.0 | 10 | 210 | 0 |
| (*McCormick*) .......... | 140 | 0 | 3.0 | 14.0 | 20 | 190 | 0 |
| (*McCormick* Fat Free) ... | 30 | 0 | 7.0 | 0 | 0 | 250 | 0 |
| (*Old Bay*) ............. | 130 | 0 | 3.0 | 12.0 | 15 | 210 | 0 |
| **Tea**, plain, regular or instant, all varieties, 1 bag or tsp. ........ | 0 | 0 | 0 | 0 | 0 | 0 | 0 |

| Food and Measure | cal. | prot. (gms) | carbo. (gms) | fat (gms) | chol. (mgs) | sod. (mgs) | fiber (gms) |
|---|---|---|---|---|---|---|---|
| **Tea, iced**, 8 fl. oz., except as noted: | | | | | | | |
| (*AriZona* Sweet Southern Style) ..... | 90 | 0 | 23.0 | 0 | 0 | 20 | 0 |
| (*Lipton* Sweet) ........ | 90 | 0 | 23.0 | 0 | 0 | 60 | 0 |
| (*Lipton PureLeaf* Extra Sweet) ........ | 110 | 0 | 28.0 | 0 | 0 | 0 | 0 |
| (*Turkey Hill* Iced) ....... | 90 | 0 | 21.0 | 0 | 0 | 20 | 0 |
| (*Turkey Hill* Sweet) ..... | 90 | 0 | 21.0 | 0 | 0 | 10 | 0 |
| all varieties: | | | | | | | |
| (*Santa Cruz Organic*) . | 60 | 0 | 15 | 0 | 0 | 0 | 0 |
| berry, Black Forest (*Honest Tea* Organic) . | 30 | 0 | 8.0 | 0 | 0 | 5 | 0 |
| black tea: | | | | | | | |
| (*Honest Tea* Organic Assam) ........... | 17 | 0 | 5.0 | 0 | 0 | 5 | 0 |
| (*Honest Tea* Organic Just Black) ....... | 0 | 0 | 0 | 0 | 0 | 5 | 0 |
| (*Snapple* Earl Grey) .. | 35 | 0 | 8.0 | 0 | 0 | 5 | 0 |
| (*Snapple* English Breakfast) ........ | 40 | 0 | 10.0 | 0 | 0 | 10 | 0 |
| cherry pomegranate (*Turkey Hill*) ...... | 120 | 0 | 28.0 | 0 | 0 | 10 | 0 |
| ginseng (*AriZona*) .... | 60 | 0 | 15.0 | 0 | 0 | 20 | 0 |
| lemon (*Honest Tea* Organic) ......... | 40 | 0 | 10.0 | 0 | 0 | 5 | 0 |
| lemon (*Snapple*) ..... | 80 | 0 | 21.0 | 0 | 0 | 65 | 0 |
| pomegranate blackberry (*Pom*ₓ) . | 80 | 0 | 20.0 | 0 | 0 | 5 | 0 |
| black and white tea (*AriZona*) ........ | 50 | 0 | 14.0 | 0 | 0 | 10 | 0 |
| fermented tea, all varieties (*Honest Kombucha* Organic) .. | 35 | 0 | 10.0 | 0 | 0 | 0 | 0 |
| green tea: | | | | | | | |
| (*AriZona* Energy) .... | 100 | 0 | 16.0 | 0 | 0 | 10 | 0 |
| (*AriZona* Extra Sweet) . | 90 | 0 | 23.0 | 0 | 0 | 0 | 0 |
| (*Honest Tea* Organic Community) ....... | 17 | 0 | 5.0 | 0 | 0 | 5 | 0 |
| (*Honest Tea* Organic Just Green) ...... | 0 | 0 | 0 | 0 | 0 | 5 | 0 |
| (*Lipton Brisk*) ....... | 90 | 0 | 25.0 | 0 | 0 | 65 | 0 |
| (*Pacific* Organic Unsweetened) .... | 0 | 0 | 0 | 0 | 0 | 10 | 0 |

| Food and Measure | cal. | prot. (gms) | carbo. (gms) | fat (gms) | chol. (mgs) | sod. (mgs) | fiber (gms) |
|---|---|---|---|---|---|---|---|
| **Tea, iced, green tea** *(cont.)* | | | | | | | |
| (*Snapple* Original) . . . . | 60 | 0 | 15.0 | 0 | 0 | 5 | 0 |
| (*SoBe*) . . . . . . . . . . . . | 100 | 0 | 25.0 | 0 | 0 | 10 | 0 |
| (*Turkey Hill*) . . . . . . . . | 70 | 0 | 17.0 | 0 | 0 | 20 | 0 |
| all fruit varieties (*Pacific* Simply Tea Organic) . . . . . . | 35 | 0 | 8.0 | 0 | 0 | 20 | 0 |
| all fruit varieties (*V8 V-Fusion* + Tea) . . . | 50 | 0 | 13.0 | 0 | 0 | 60 | 0 |
| apple, red (*AriZona*) . . | 70 | 0 | 19.0 | 0 | 0 | 20 | 0 |
| citrus (*Lipton*) . . . . . . . | 80 | 0 | 21.0 | 0 | 0 | 80 | 0 |
| ginseng w/honey: (*AriZona*) . . . . . . . . | 70 | 0 | 18.0 | 0 | 0 | 20 | 0 |
| (*AriZona* Organic) . | 50 | 0 | 14.0 | 0 | 0 | 10 | 0 |
| honey (*Honest Tea* Organic) . . . . . . . . . | 35 | 0 | 9.0 | 0 | 0 | 5 | 0 |
| w/honey (*Lipton* PureLeaf) . . . . . . . . | 60 | 0 | 16.0 | 0 | 0 | 0 | 0 |
| w/honey (*Newman's Own*) . . . . . . . . . . . | 70 | 0 | 18.0 | 0 | 0 | 5 | 0 |
| jasmine (*Honest Tea* Organic Energy) . . . | 17 | 0 | 5.0 | 0 | 0 | 5 | 0 |
| lemonade (*AriZona* Half & Half) . . . . . . | 50 | 0 | 14.0 | 0 | 0 | 25 | 0 |
| mandarin orange (*AriZona*) . . . . . . . . | 70 | 0 | 19.0 | 0 | 0 | 20 | 0 |
| mango (*Honest Tea* Organic) . . . . . . . . . | 40 | 0 | 10.0 | 0 | 0 | 5 | 0 |
| mango (*Turkey Hill*) . . | 90 | 0 | 21.0 | 0 | 0 | 10 | 0 |
| mango or Asian pear (*Snapple*) . . . . . . . . | 60 | 0 | 15.0 | 0 | 0 | 5 | 0 |
| mint (*Honest Tea* Organic Moroccan) | 17 | 0 | 5.0 | 0 | 0 | 5 | 0 |
| w/passion fruit (*Honest Tea* Organic Green Dragon) . . . . . . . . . | 30 | 0 | 8.0 | 0 | 0 | 5 | 0 |
| peach (*AriZona* Georgia) . . . . . . . . | 70 | 0 | 18.0 | 0 | 0 | 10 | 0 |
| peach (*Lipton Brisk*) . . | 80 | 0 | 22.0 | 0 | 0 | 75 | 0 |
| peach (*Snapple*) . . . . . | 80 | 0 | 21.0 | 0 | 0 | 60 | 0 |
| peach mango (*Lipton* Chilled) . . . . . . . . . . | 60 | 0 | 16.0 | 0 | 0 | 20 | 0 |
| plum, Asia (*AriZona*) . . | 70 | 0 | 18.0 | 0 | 0 | 20 | 0 |

| Food and Measure | cal. | prot. (gms) | carbo. (gms) | fat (gms) | chol. (mgs) | sod. (mgs) | fiber (gms) |
|---|---|---|---|---|---|---|---|
| pomegranate | | | | | | | |
| (*AriZona*) . . . . . . . . | 70 | 0 | 19.0 | 0 | 0 | 10 | 0 |
| pomegranate | | | | | | | |
| (*AriZona* Energy) . . | 70 | 0 | 18.0 | 0 | 0 | 10 | 0 |
| pomegranate | | | | | | | |
| (*AriZona* Organic) . | 50 | 0 | 13.0 | 0 | 0 | 10 | 0 |
| pomegranate hibiscus | | | | | | | |
| (*Pom*x Light) . . . . . | 35 | 0 | 16.0 | 0 | 0 | 0 | 0 |
| pomegranate lychee | | | | | | | |
| (*Pom*x) . . . . . . . . . . | 70 | 0 | 18.0 | 0 | 0 | 5 | 0 |
| yumberry (*AriZona* | | | | | | | |
| Organic) . . . . . . . . | 50 | 0 | 13.0 | 0 | 0 | 10 | 0 |
| green tea, decaf | | | | | | | |
| (*AriZona*): | | | | | | | |
| apple . . . . . . . . . . . . | 80 | 0 | 20.0 | 0 | 0 | 20 | 0 |
| pomegranate . . . . . . . | 80 | 0 | 20.0 | 0 | 0 | 10 | 0 |
| white grape . . . . . . . . | 80 | 0 | 21.0 | 0 | 0 | 10 | 0 |
| herbal (*AriZona*): | | | | | | | |
| Rx Energy . . . . . . . . . | 120 | 0 | 31.0 | 0 | 0 | 25 | 0 |
| Rx Stress . . . . . . . . . | 70 | 0 | 19.0 | 0 | 0 | 20 | 0 |
| hibiscus/juice blend: | | | | | | | |
| (*R.W. Knudsen* | | | | | | | |
| *Hibiscus Cooler*) . . | 100 | 0 | 25.0 | 0 | 0 | 10 | 0 |
| (*Santa Cruz Organic* | | | | | | | |
| *Hibiscus Cooler*) . . | 100 | <1.0 | 24.0 | 0 | 0 | 40 | 0 |
| lemon: | | | | | | | |
| (*AriZona*) . . . . . . . . . | 90 | 0 | 25.0 | 0 | 0 | 20 | 0 |
| (*Honest Tea* | | | | | | | |
| Organic Lori's) . . . . | 30 | 0 | 8.0 | 0 | 0 | 5 | 0 |
| (*Lipton*) . . . . . . . . . . | 60 | 0 | 16.0 | 0 | 0 | 65 | 0 |
| (*Lipton* Chilled) . . . . . . | 60 | 0 | 15.0 | 0 | 0 | 20 | 0 |
| (*Lipton Brisk*) . . . . . . . | 80 | 0 | 22.0 | 0 | 0 | 65 | 0 |
| (*Lipton PureLeaf*) . . . . | 60 | 0 | 18.0 | 0 | 0 | 0 | 0 |
| (*Nantucket Nectars* | | | | | | | |
| Squeezed) . . . . . . . | 80 | 0 | 22.0 | 0 | 0 | 25 | 0 |
| (*Newman's Own* | | | | | | | |
| Virgin Lemon- | | | | | | | |
| Aided) . . . . . . . . . . | 110 | 0 | 27.0 | 0 | 0 | 40 | 0 |
| (*Snapple*) . . . . . . . . . | 80 | 0 | 21.0 | 0 | 0 | 5 | 0 |
| lemon-limeade | | | | | | | |
| (*AriZona* Half & Half) . | 50 | 0 | 14.0 | 0 | 0 | 10 | 0 |
| lemonade: | | | | | | | |
| (*AriZona* Arnold | | | | | | | |
| Palmer) . . . . . . . . . | 50 | 0 | 14.0 | 0 | 0 | 25 | 0 |

| Food and Measure | cal. | prot. (gms) | carbo. (gms) | fat (gms) | chol. (mgs) | sod. (mgs) | fiber (gms) |
|---|---|---|---|---|---|---|---|
| **Tea, iced, lemonade** *(cont.)* | | | | | | | |
| (*Lipton* Half & Half) .. | 50 | 0 | 13.0 | 0 | 0 | 80 | 0 |
| (*Lipton Brisk*) ....... | 60 | 0 | 16.0 | 0 | 0 | 70 | 0 |
| (*Minute Maid*) ....... | 110 | 0 | 29.0 | 0 | 0 | 15 | 0 |
| (*Nantucket Nectars* Squeezed Half and Half ......... | 90 | 0 | 22.0 | 0 | 0 | 25 | 0 |
| (*Snapple*) .......... | 100 | 0 | 26.0 | 0 | 0 | 5 | 0 |
| (*Turkey Hill*) ........ | 100 | 0 | 24.0 | 0 | 0 | 15 | 0 |
| mango (*AriZona* Half & Half) ......... | 50 | 0 | 14.0 | 0 | 0 | 10 | 0 |
| mint (*Snapple*) ........ | 70 | 0 | 17.0 | 0 | 0 | 5 | 0 |
| oolong: | | | | | | | |
| peach (*Honest Tea* Organic Oo-la-long) ........... | 30 | 0 | 8.0 | 0 | 0 | 5 | 0 |
| pineapple each mango (*Snapple*) ........ | 80 | 0 | 21.0 | 0 | 0 | 60 | 0 |
| orange (*Turkey Hill*) ..... | 100 | 0 | 25.0 | 0 | 0 | 15 | 0 |
| peach: | | | | | | | |
| (*AriZona*) .......... | 70 | 0 | 18.0 | 0 | 0 | 10 | 0 |
| (*Lipton PureLeaf*) .... | 80 | 0 | 20.0 | 0 | 0 | 0 | 0 |
| (*Snapple*) .......... | 90 | 0 | 23.0 | 0 | 0 | 5 | 0 |
| pomegranate (*Minute Maid* Enhanced) ..... | 40 | 0 | 9.0 | 0 | 0 | 20 | 0 |
| raspberry: | | | | | | | |
| (*AriZona*) .......... | 90 | 0 | 23.0 | 0 | 0 | 25 | 0 |
| (*Lipton Brisk*) ....... | 90 | 0 | 23.0 | 0 | 0 | 50 | 0 |
| (*Lipton PureLeaf*) .... | 80 | 0 | 20.0 | 0 | 0 | 0 | 0 |
| (*Snapple*) .......... | 80 | 0 | 21.0 | 0 | 0 | 5 | 0 |
| (*Turkey Hill*) ........ | 110 | 0 | 28.0 | 0 | 0 | 10 | 0 |
| red tea: | | | | | | | |
| acai mixed berry (*Snapple* Immunity) | 40 | 0 | 10.0 | 0 | 0 | 0 | 0 |
| pomegranate w/goji berry (*Honest Tea* Organic) ......... | 35 | 0 | 9.0 | 0 | 0 | 5 | 0 |
| pomegranate raspberry (*Snapple*) ......... | 80 | 0 | 21.0 | 0 | 0 | 60 | 0 |
| tropical (*AriZona* Half & Half) ...... | 50 | 0 | 14.0 | 0 | 0 | 5 | 0 |
| white tea: | | | | | | | |
| apple plum (*Snapple*) . | 80 | 0 | 21.0 | 0 | 0 | 60 | 0 |
| blueberry (*AriZona*) .. | 50 | 0 | 14.0 | 0 | 0 | 10 | 0 |

| Food and Measure | cal. | prot. (gms) | carbo. (gms) | fat (gms) | chol. (mgs) | sod. (mgs) | fiber (gms) |
|---|---|---|---|---|---|---|---|
| mango acai (*Honest Tea* Organic) | 35 | 0 | 9.0 | 0 | 0 | 5 | 0 |
| nectarine or raspberry (*Snapple*) | 60 | 0 | 15.0 | 0 | 0 | 5 | 0 |
| peach or pomegranate (*Honest Tea* Organic) | 40 | 0 | 10.0 | 0 | 0 | 5 | 0 |
| pear (*Honest Tea Organic Pearfect*) | 35 | 0 | 9.0 | 0 | 0 | 5 | 0 |
| pomegranate peach passion (*Pomx*) | 80 | 0 | 19.0 | 0 | 0 | 10 | 0 |
| pomegranate wildberry (*Pomx Light*) | 35 | 0 | 16.0 | 0 | 0 | 5 | 0 |
| raspberry (*Lipton*) | 50 | 0 | 14.0 | 0 | 0 | 80 | 0 |
| yerba maté: | | | | | | | |
| (*Honest Mate* Organic Sublime/Tropical) | 35 | 0 | 9.0 | 0 | 0 | 5 | 0 |
| (*Pacific* Organic Traditional) | 30 | 1.0 | 7.0 | 0 | 0 | 35 | 0 |
| agave (*Honest Mate* Organic) | 17 | 0 | 5.0 | 0 | 0 | 5 | 0 |
| citrus lychee (*Pacific* Organic) | 35 | 1.0 | 9.0 | 0 | 0 | 35 | 0 |
| lemon ginger or peach passion (*Pacific* Organic) | 40 | 1.0 | 8.0 | 0 | 0 | 35 | 0 |
| **Teff**, grain (*Bob's Red Mill*), ¼ cup | 180 | 7.0 | 37.0 | 1.0 | 0 | 5 | 4.0 |
| **Teff flour** (*Bob's Red Mill*), ¼ cup | 113 | 4.0 | 22.0 | 1.0 | 0 | 5 | 4.0 |
| **Tekka** (*Eden*), 1 tsp. | 5 | <1.0 | <1.0 | 0 | 0 | 70 | 0 |
| **Tempeh:** | | | | | | | |
| 5 grain: | | | | | | | |
| (*Turtle Island Foods* Organic), 3 oz. | 170 | 13.0 | 15.0 | 6.0 | 0 | 0 | 5.0 |
| (*White Wave*), 2.7 oz. | 160 | 12.0 | 15.0 | 6.0 | 0 | 10 | 7.0 |
| soy: | | | | | | | |
| (*Turtle Island Foods* Organic), 3 oz. | 160 | 13.0 | 20.0 | 3.5 | 0 | 10 | 7.0 |
| (*White Wave*), 2.7 oz. | 180 | 16.0 | 12.0 | 8.0 | 0 | 10 | 7.0 |
| rice (*White Wave*), 2.7 oz. | 160 | 12.0 | 12.0 | 7.0 | 0 | 10 | 7.0 |
| spicy veggie (*Turtle Island Foods*), 3 oz. | 140 | 13.0 | 12.0 | 5.0 | 0 | 25 | 5.0 |
| 1 oz. | 55 | 5.3 | 2.7 | 3.1 | 0 | 3 | n.a. |

| Food and Measure | cal. | prot. (gms) | carbo. (gms) | fat (gms) | chol. (mgs) | sod. (mgs) | fiber (gms) |
|---|---|---|---|---|---|---|---|
| **Tempeh** *(cont.)* | | | | | | | |
| ½ cup ............... | 160 | 15.4 | 7.8 | 9.0 | 0 | 7 | n.a. |
| ***Temptation* melon** | | | | | | | |
| (*Frieda's*), ⅒ melon, | | | | | | | |
| 4.7 oz. ........... | 55 | 1.0 | 14.0 | 0 | 0 | 45 | 1.0 |
| **Tempura batter mix,** | | | | | | | |
| see "Batter/breading | | | | | | | |
| mix" and "Seafood | | | | | | | |
| coating mix" | | | | | | | |
| **Tempura dipping sauce** | | | | | | | |
| (*Kikkoman*), 1 tsp. ... | 5.0 | 0 | 1.0 | 0 | 0 | 340 | 0 |
| **Tenderizer**, see "Meat | | | | | | | |
| tenderizer" | | | | | | | |
| **Teriyaki sauce** (see | | | | | | | |
| also "Stir-fry sauce"), | | | | | | | |
| 1 tbsp., except as | | | | | | | |
| noted: | | | | | | | |
| (*Ah-So*) .............. | 30 | 0 | 6.0 | 0 | 0 | 280 | 0 |
| (*Angostura*) ........... | 20 | 0 | 4.0 | 0 | 0 | 350 | 0 |
| (*Annie Chun's*) ........ | 25 | 2.0 | 6.0 | 0 | 0 | 300 | 0 |
| (*Ka•Me* Glaze) .......... | 15 | 0 | 4.0 | 0 | 0 | 290 | 0 |
| (*Ken's*) .............. | 20 | 0 | 4.0 | 0 | 0 | 260 | 0 |
| (*Kikkoman*) ............ | 15 | 1.0 | 2.0 | 0 | 0 | 610 | 0 |
| (*Kikkoman* Baste & | | | | | | | |
| Glaze), 2 tbsp. ....... | 50 | 1.0 | 11.0 | 0 | 0 | 810 | 0 |
| (*Kikkoman* Gourmet) .... | 30 | 1.0 | 7.0 | 0 | 0 | 450 | 0 |
| (*Kikkoman* Less | | | | | | | |
| Sodium) .......... | 15 | 1.0 | 3.0 | 0 | 0 | 320 | 0 |
| (*Kikkoman Takumi*) ..... | 30 | 1.0 | 6.0 | 0 | 0 | 450 | 0 |
| (*La Choy*) ............ | 40 | <1.0 | 10.0 | 0 | 0 | 570 | 0 |
| (*Mee Tu*) ............. | 12 | .4 | 3.0 | 0 | 0 | 320 | 0 |
| (*Newman's Own*) ....... | 25 | 0 | 6.0 | 0 | 0 | 330 | 0 |
| (*San-J*) .............. | 20 | <1.0 | 4.0 | 0 | 0 | 390 | 0 |
| (*Simply Tsang*) ........ | 45 | 0 | 11.0 | 0 | 0 | 690 | 0 |
| (*World Harbors*), | | | | | | | |
| 2 tbsp. ............ | 70 | 0 | 17.0 | 0 | 0 | 270 | 0 |
| (*World Harbors* | | | | | | | |
| Angostura) .........., | 20 | 0 | 4.0 | 0 | 0 | 350 | 0 |
| (*Yamasa*) ............. | 10 | 1.0 | 3.0 | 0 | 0 | 460 | 0 |
| garlic, roasted | | | | | | | |
| (*Kikkoman*) ......... | 25 | 1.0 | 4.0 | 0 | 0 | 730 | 0 |
| garlic green onion | | | | | | | |
| (*Kikkoman Takumi*) ... | 35 | 1.0 | 6.0 | .5 | 0 | 300 | 0 |

| Food and Measure | cal. | prot. (gms) | carbo. (gms) | fat (gms) | chol. (mgs) | sod. (mgs) | fiber (gms) |
|---|---|---|---|---|---|---|---|
| ginger: | | | | | | | |
| (*Marinade Bay*) ...... | 20 | 1.0 | 3.0 | .5 | 0 | 470 | 0 |
| triple (*Kikkoman* Takumi*) ......... | 15 | 0 | 4.0 | 0 | 0 | 370 | 0 |
| w/honey: | | | | | | | |
| (*Ken's*) ............ | 25 | 0 | 6.0 | 0 | 0 | 250 | 0 |
| and pineapple (*Kikkoman* Baste & Glaze), 2 tbsp. .... | 80 | 1.0 | 18.0 | 0 | 0 | 770 | 0 |
| hot (*World Harbors*), 2 tbsp. .......... | 70 | 0 | 17.0 | 0 | 0 | 300 | 0 |
| mango (*Marinade Bay*) .. | 30 | 0 | 2.0 | 2.5 | 0 | 180 | 0 |
| miso, spicy (*Kikkoman* Takumi*) ........... | 40 | 1.0 | 8.0 | 0 | 0 | 440 | 0 |
| w/pinapple juice (*Lawry's*) ........... | 20 | 0 | 5.0 | 0 | 0 | 560 | 0 |
| spicy (*Mrs. Dash*) ...... | 25 | 0 | 4.0 | .5 | 0 | 0 | 0 |
| **Teriyaki sauce mix** (*Kikkoman*), 2 tsp. .... | 20 | 0 | 4.0 | 0 | 0 | 620 | 0 |
| **Texas toast**, see "Bread, frozen/chilled" | | | | | | | |
| **Thai sauce** (see also "Chili sauce, Asian," "Peanut sauce," and specific listings): | | | | | | | |
| (*Neera's* Sauce & Marinade), 1 tsp. .... | 29 | 0 | 8.0 | 1.0 | 0 | 164 | 0 |
| (*World Harbors*), 2 tbsp. ........... | 40 | 0 | 8.0 | 0 | 0 | 350 | 0 |
| pad Thai: | | | | | | | |
| (*Annie Chun's*), 1 tbsp. | 30 | 0 | 7.0 | .5 | 0 | 400 | 0 |
| (*A Taste of Thai*), 2 tbsp. .......... | 70 | 0 | 15.0 | 1.5 | 0 | 300 | 0 |
| paste (*Tiger Tiger*), 1 tbsp. ........... | 45 | 0 | 6.0 | 2.0 | 0 | 210 | 0 |
| paste (*Tiger Tiger* Tom Yam), 1 tbsp. ........ | 45 | 1.0 | 3.0 | 3.0 | 0 | 600 | 0 |
| plum (*Tiger Tiger* Dipping), 2 tbsp. ..... | 50 | 0 | 12.0 | 0 | 0 | 200 | 1.0 |
| **Thai sauce, simmer** (see also "Curry sauce"): | | | | | | | |
| hot and sour (*Tiger Tiger* Tom Yum), ½ cup ............. | 50 | 1.0 | 3.5 | 3.5 | 0 | 510 | <1.0 |

| Food and Measure | cal. | prot. (gms) | carbo. (gms) | fat (gms) | chol. (mgs) | sod. (mgs) | fiber (gms) |
|---|---|---|---|---|---|---|---|
| **Thai sauce, simmer** *(cont.)* | | | | | | | |
| pad Thai (*Tasty Bite*), | | | | | | | |
| 3.5 oz. . . . . . . . . . . . . | 200 | 4.0 | 28.0 | 10.0 | 0 | 5 | 2.0 |
| satay (*Tasty Bite* | | | | | | | |
| Partay), 3.5 oz. . . . . . . | 150 | 3.0 | 16.0 | 9.0 | 0 | 0 | 2.0 |
| **Thyme**, ground, 1 tsp. . . | 4 | .1 | .9 | .1 | 0 | 1 | .3 |
| **Thymus**, 4 oz.: | | | | | | | |
| beef, braised . . . . . . . . . . | 362 | 24.8 | 0 | 28.3 | 333 | 132 | 0 |
| veal, braised . . . . . . . . . . | 197 | 35.8 | 0 | 4.9 | 532 | 75 | 0 |
| **Tilapia**, fresh: | | | | | | | |
| raw, 4 oz. . . . . . . . . . . . . | 109 | 22.8 | 0 | 1.9 | 57 | 59 | 0 |
| baked or broiled, 4 oz. . . | 145 | 29.6 | 0 | 3.0 | 64 | 63 | 0 |
| **Tilapia, frozen**: | | | | | | | |
| fillet, breaded, 4 oz.: | | | | | | | |
| (*Gorton's*) . . . . . . . . . . | 250 | 12.0 | 23.0 | 12.0 | 25 | 480 | 1.0 |
| lightly (*Mrs. Paul's*) . . | 230 | 16.0 | 17.0 | 11.0 | 35 | 220 | <1.0 |
| fillet, grilled, 3.1 oz.: | | | | | | | |
| (*Gorton's* Signature) . . | 80 | 14.0 | <1.0 | 2.5 | 50 | 250 | 0 |
| lemon peppercorn | | | | | | | |
| (*Gorton's*) . . . . . . . . | 80 | 14.0 | <1.0 | 3.0 | 40 | 260 | 0 |
| roasted garlic and | | | | | | | |
| butter (*Gorton's*) . . | 80 | 14.0 | <1.0 | 2.5 | 50 | 150 | 0 |
| tenders, breaded | | | | | | | |
| (*SeaPak*), 2 pcs., 4 oz. | 280 | 14.0 | 24.0 | 14.0 | 25 | 460 | 1.0 |
| **Tilapia entree, frozen**: | | | | | | | |
| herb, Mediterranean | | | | | | | |
| (*StarKist SeaSations*), | | | | | | | |
| 9 oz. . . . . . . . . . . . . . | 290 | 13.0 | 45.0 | 7.0 | 20 | 600 | 3.0 |
| orange miso (*StarKist* | | | | | | | |
| *SeaSations*), 9 oz. . . . . | 280 | 16.0 | 45.0 | 4.0 | 20 | 560 | 3.0 |
| stuffed fillet (*Oven* | | | | | | | |
| *Poppers*), 5 oz.: | | | | | | | |
| Caribbean . . . . . . . . . . | 160 | 20.0 | 10.0 | 5.0 | 50 | 140 | 0 |
| ginger teriyaki sauce . . | 250 | 18.0 | 11.0 | 15.0 | 60 | 270 | 0 |
| lemon garlic sauce . . . | 240 | 19.0 | 4.0 | 16.0 | 55 | 240 | 0 |
| sun-dried tomato, | | | | | | | |
| shrimp, lobster . . . . | 180 | 19.0 | 8.0 | 8.0 | 80 | 320 | 0 |
| **Tilefish**, meat only: | | | | | | | |
| raw, 4 oz. . . . . . . . . . . . . | 109 | 19.9 | 0 | 2.6 | 57 | 60 | 0 |
| baked or broiled, 4 oz. . . | 167 | 27.8 | 0 | 5.3 | 73 | 67 | 0 |
| **Toaster pastry** (see | | | | | | | |
| also "Breakfast | | | | | | | |
| sandwich"), 1 pc.: | | | | | | | |

| Food and Measure | cal. | prot. (gms) | carbo. (gms) | fat (gms) | chol. (mgs) | sod. (mgs) | fiber (gms) |
|---|---|---|---|---|---|---|---|
| apple: | | | | | | | |
| (*Amy's* Toaster Pops) | 160 | 4.0 | 29.0 | 3.5 | 0 | 110 | 2.0 |
| (*Toaster Strudel*) ..... | 190 | 3.0 | 26.0 | 8.0 | 5 | 180 | <1.0 |
| baked (*Health Valley* | | | | | | | |
| Organic Tarts) .... | 150 | 2.0 | 29.0 | 3.0 | 0 | 90 | 3.0 |
| cream Danish (*Toaster* | | | | | | | |
| *Strudel*) ......... | 180 | 3.0 | 26.0 | 7.0 | 5 | 190 | <1.0 |
| apple cinnamon: | | | | | | | |
| (*Nature's Path* | | | | | | | |
| Organic) ......... | 210 | 3.0 | 40.0 | 4.5 | 0 | 150 | 1.0 |
| (*Thomas' Toast-* | | | | | | | |
| *R-Cakes*) ........ | 110 | 2.0 | 17.0 | 3.5 | 5 | 210 | <1.0 |
| apple strudel | | | | | | | |
| (*Pop•Tarts*) ......... | 200 | 2.0 | 35.0 | 5.0 | 0 | 160 | <1.0 |
| berry, wild (*Pop•Tarts*) .. | 210 | 2.0 | 39.0 | 5.0 | 0 | 170 | <1.0 |
| blueberry: | | | | | | | |
| (*Fiber One*) ......... | 180 | 3.0 | 36.0 | 4.0 | 0 | 130 | 5.0 |
| (*Health Valley* | | | | | | | |
| Organic Tarts) .... | 150 | 2.0 | 30.0 | 3.0 | 0 | 95 | 3.0 |
| (*Nature's Path* | | | | | | | |
| Organic) ......... | 210 | 3.0 | 40.0 | 4.5 | 0 | 150 | 1.0 |
| (*Pop•Tarts*) ......... | 210 | 2.0 | 37.0 | 5.0 | 0 | 180 | <1.0 |
| (*Toaster Strudel*) ..... | 180 | 3.0 | 27.0 | 7.0 | 5 | 190 | <1.0 |
| frosted (*Nature's* | | | | | | | |
| *Path* Organic) ..... | 200 | 2.0 | 38.0 | 4.0 | 0 | 125 | 1.0 |
| frosted (*Pop•Tarts*) ... | 200 | 2.0 | 38.0 | 5.0 | 0 | 170 | <1.0 |
| frosted, muffin | | | | | | | |
| (*Pop•Tarts*) ....... | 200 | 2.0 | 35.0 | 5.0 | 0 | 200 | <1.0 |
| Boston cream pie | | | | | | | |
| (*Toaster Strudel*) ..... | 180 | 3.0 | 26.0 | 7.0 | 5 | 190 | <1.0 |
| brown sugar cinnamon: | | | | | | | |
| (*Fiber One*) ......... | 180 | 3.0 | 36.0 | 4.0 | 0 | 130 | 5.0 |
| (*Pop•Tarts*) ......... | 210 | 2.0 | 34.0 | 8.0 | 0 | 190 | <1.0 |
| frosted (*Pop•Tarts*) ... | 210 | 2.0 | 34.0 | 7.0 | 0 | 170 | <1.0 |
| frosted (*Pop•Tarts* | | | | | | | |
| Low Fat) ......... | 180 | 2.0 | 38.0 | 3.0 | 0 | 210 | <1.0 |
| frosted (*Pop•Tarts* | | | | | | | |
| Whole Grain) ..... | 200 | 3.0 | 34.0 | 6.0 | 0 | 160 | 5.0 |
| maple (*Nature's Path* | | | | | | | |
| Organic) ......... | 210 | 3.0 | 37.0 | 5.0 | 0 | 135 | 1.0 |
| maple, frosted (*Nature's* | | | | | | | |
| *Path* Organic) ..... | 210 | 3.0 | 39.0 | 4.5 | 0 | 125 | 1.0 |
| cherry: | | | | | | | |
| (*Pop•Tarts*) ......... | 200 | 2.0 | 38.0 | 5.0 | 0 | 160 | <1.0 |

| Food and Measure | cal. | prot. (gms) | carbo. (gms) | fat (gms) | chol. (mgs) | sod. (mgs) | fiber (gms) |
|---|---|---|---|---|---|---|---|
| **Toaster pastry, cherry** *(cont.)* | | | | | | | |
| (*Toaster Strudel*) ..... | 190 | 3.0 | 26.0 | 8.0 | 5 | 180 | <1.0 |
| red (*Health Valley* | | | | | | | |
| Organic Tarts) .... | 150 | 2.0 | 29.0 | 3.0 | 0 | 90 | 3.0 |
| cherry pomegranate | | | | | | | |
| (*Nature's Path* | | | | | | | |
| *Pomegran* Organic) | 200 | 3.0 | 37.0 | 4.5 | 0 | 150 | 1.0 |
| chocolate (*Health Valley* | | | | | | | |
| Organic Tarts) ....... | 140 | 2.0 | 28.0 | 3.0 | 0 | 90 | 3.0 |
| chocolate chip: | | | | | | | |
| (*Pop•Tarts*) .......... | 210 | 3.0 | 36.0 | 6.0 | 0 | 240 | <1.0 |
| cookie dough | | | | | | | |
| (*Pop•Tarts*) ....... | 200 | 2.0 | 35.0 | 5.0 | 0 | 190 | <1.0 |
| chocolate fudge: | | | | | | | |
| (*Fiber One*) ......... | 180 | 3.0 | 35.0 | 4.0 | 0 | 140 | 5.0 |
| (*Pop•Tarts*) ......(... | 200 | 3.0 | 37.0 | 5.0 | 0 | 230 | 1.0 |
| (*Pop•Tarts* Whole | | | | | | | |
| Grain) ............ | 190 | 3.0 | 34.0 | 5.0 | 0 | 250 | 5.0 |
| cinnamon roll: | | | | | | | |
| (*Pop•Tarts*) .......-.. | 210 | 2.0 | 34.0 | 7.0 | 0 | 160 | <1.0 |
| (*Toaster Strudel*) ..... | 190 | 3.0 | 29.0 | 7.0 | 5 | 210 | 1.0 |
| cookies and cream | | | | | | | |
| (*Pop•Tarts*) ......... | 190 | 2.0 | 35.0 | 5.0 | 0 | 300 | <1.0 |
| corn (*Thomas'* | | | | | | | |
| *Toast-R-Cakes*) ...... | 110 | 2.0 | 17.0 | 3.5 | 5 | 190 | 0 |
| cream cheese: | | | | | | | |
| (*Toaster Strudel* | | | | | | | |
| Danish Style) ..... | 190 | 3.0 | 24.0 | 9.0 | 10 | 220 | <1.0 |
| strawberry (*Amy's* | | | | | | | |
| Toaster Pops) ..... | 160 | 4.0 | 29.0 | 3.5 | 0 | 110 | 2.0 |
| and strawberry | | | | | | | |
| (*Toaster Strudel*) .. | 180 | 3.0 | 25.0 | 8.0 | 5 | 200 | <1.0 |
| grape, wild (*Pop•Tarts*) .. | 200 | 2.0 | 36.0 | 5.0 | 0 | 170 | <1.0 |
| hot fudge sundae | | | | | | | |
| (*Pop•Tarts Ice Cream* | | | | | | | |
| *Shoppe*) ........... | 190 | 2.0 | 33.0 | 5.0 | 0 | 190 | 2.0 |
| ice cream sandwich | | | | | | | |
| (*Pop•Tarts Ice Cream* | | | | | | | |
| *Shoppe*) ........... | 190 | 2.0 | 33.0 | 5.0 | 0 | 180 | 2.0 |
| milkshake (*Pop•Tarts* | | | | | | | |
| *Ice Cream Shoppe*): | | | | | | | |
| strawberry ......... | 190 | 2.0 | 33.0 | 6.0 | 0 | 190 | 1.0 |
| vanilla ............. | 190 | 2.0 | 34.0 | 6.0 | 0 | 190 | 1.0 |

| Food and Measure | cal. | prot. (gms) | carbo. (gms) | fat (gms) | chol. (mgs) | sod. (mgs) | fiber (gms) |
|---|---|---|---|---|---|---|---|
| raspberry: | | | | | | | |
| (*Health Valley* Organic Tarts) .... | 150 | 2.0 | 29.0 | 3.0 | 0 | 95 | 3.0 |
| (*Pop•Tarts*) ......... | 200 | 2.0 | 38.0 | 5.0 | 0 | 160 | <1.0 |
| (*Toaster Strudel*) ..... | 180 | 3.0 | 27.0 | 7.0 | 5 | 190 | <1.0 |
| frosted (*Nature's Path* Organic) ......... | 210 | 3.0 | 39.0 | 5.0 | 0 | 150 | 1.0 |
| s'mores (*Pop•Tarts*) .... | 200 | 3.0 | 36.0 | 5.0 | 0 | 210 | <1.0 |
| strawberry: | | | | | | | |
| (*Fiber One*) ......... | 180 | 3.0 | 36.0 | 4.0 | 0 | 120 | 5.0 |
| (*Health Valley* Organic Tarts) .... | 150 | 2.0 | 29.0 | 3.0 | 0 | 95 | 3.0 |
| (*Nature's Path* Organic) ......... | 210 | 3.0 | 40.0 | 4.5 | 0 | 150 | 1.0 |
| (*Pop•Tarts*) ......... | 210 | 2.0 | 37.0 | 5.0 | 0 | 180 | <1.0 |
| (*Toaster Strudel*) ..... | 180 | 3.0 | 27.0 | 7.0 | 5 | 190 | <1.0 |
| frosted (*Nature's Path* Organic) ..... | 210 | 3.0 | 40.0 | 4.0 | 0 | 140 | 1.0 |
| frosted (*Pop•Tarts*) ... | 200 | 2.0 | 38.0 | 5.0 | 0 | 170 | <1.0 |
| frosted (*Pop•Tarts* Low Fat) ......... | 190 | 2.0 | 39.0 | 2.5 | 0 | 210 | <1.0 |
| frosted (*Pop•Tarts* Whole Grain) ..... | 190 | 2.0 | 35.0 | 5.0 | 0 | 150 | 5.0 |
| wildberry: | | | | | | | |
| (*Toaster Strudel*) ..... | 180 | 3.0 | 27.0 | 7.0 | 5 | 190 | <1.0 |
| acai, frosted (*Nature's Path* Organic) ..... | 210 | 3.0 | 39.0 | 5.0 | 0 | 130 | 1.0 |
| **Toffee**, see "Candy" | | | | | | | |
| **Toffee baking chips,** 1 tbsp., .5 oz.: | | | | | | | |
| (*Heath Bits 'O Brickle*) ............ | 80 | 0 | 9.0 | 5.0 | 5 | 75 | 0 |
| chocolate (*Heath*) ...... | 80 | 0 | 9.0 | 5.0 | 5 | 50 | 0 |
| **Toffee topping** (*Heath* Shell), 2 tbsp. ....... | 210 | 1.0 | 17.0 | 17.0 | 0 | 40 | 1.0 |
| **Tofu,** fresh, 3 oz., except as noted: | | | | | | | |
| cubed, super firm (*Nasoya*), 2.8 oz. .... | 100 | 10.0 | 3.0 | 5.0 | 0 | 0 | <2.0 |
| dried (*Eden* Organic), .4-oz. pc. .......... | 50 | 5.0 | 0 | 2.5 | 0 | 0 | 2.0 |
| extra firm: | | | | | | | |
| (*Azumaya*) ......... | 70 | 8.0 | 2.0 | 4.0 | 0 | 20 | 1.0 |
| (*Azumaya* Lite), 2.8 oz. | 60 | 7.0 | 3.0 | 2.0 | 0 | 30 | 1.0 |

| Food and Measure | cal. | prot. (gms) | carbo. (gms) | fat (gms) | chol. (mgs) | sod. (mgs) | fiber (gms) |
|---|---|---|---|---|---|---|---|
| **Tofu, extra firm** *(cont.)* | | | | | | | |
| (*Frieda's*) .......... | 90 | 10.0 | 1.0 | 5.0 | 0 | 10 | 0 |
| (*Frieda's* Organic) .... | 70 | 7.0 | 2.0 | 4.0 | 0 | 10 | 0 |
| (*Nasoya*), 2.8 oz. .... | 80 | 8.0 | 2.0 | 4.0 | 0 | 0 | 1.0 |
| (*Nasoya* TofuPlus | | | | | | | |
| Organic) ......... | 80 | 8.0 | 5.0 | 4.0 | 0 | 5 | 1.0 |
| (*White Wave* Vacuum) | 110 | 11.0 | 3.0 | 6.0 | 0 | 5 | 1.0 |
| (*White Wave* Vacuum | | | | | | | |
| Organic), 3.2 oz. .. | 110 | 11.0 | 3.0 | 6.0 | 0 | 5 | 1.0 |
| firm: | | | | | | | |
| (*Azumaya*) ......... | 70 | 7.0 | 2.0 | 3.5 | 0 | 20 | <1.0 |
| (*Frieda's*) .......... | 60 | 6.0 | 2.0 | 3.0 | 0 | 10 | 0 |
| (*Nasoya*), 2.8 oz. .... | 70 | 7.0 | 2.0 | 3.0 | 0 | 0 | <1.0 |
| (*Nasoya* Lite), 2.8 oz. . | 40 | 7.0 | 1.0 | 1.5 | 0 | 25 | <1.0 |
| (*Nasoya* TofuPlus | | | | | | | |
| Organic) ......... | 40 | 7.0 | 1.0 | 1.5 | 0 | 25 | <1.0 |
| (*White Wave* Organic), | | | | | | | |
| 3.2 oz. .......... | 110 | 11.0 | 3.0 | 6.0 | 0 | 5 | 1.0 |
| salted and fermented | | | | | | | |
| (fuyu), 1 oz. ........ | 33 | 2.3 | 1.5 | 2.3 | 0 | 814 | <1.0 |
| silken, 3.2 oz.: | | | | | | | |
| (*Azumaya*) ......... | 40 | 4.0 | 1.0 | 2.0 | 0 | 0 | <1.0 |
| (*Nasoya*) .......... | 45 | 4.0 | 1.0 | 2.0 | 0 | 0 | 0 |
| (*Nasoya* Lite) ....... | 30 | 6.0 | 0 | 1.0 | 0 | 65 | 0 |
| silken, chocolate (*Nasoya* | | | | | | | |
| Creations), ½ cup .... | 120 | 3.0 | 23.0 | 1.5 | 0 | 45 | 1.0 |
| soft: | | | | | | | |
| (*Frieda's*) .......... | 45 | 5.0 | 1.0 | 2.5 | 0 | 15 | 0 |
| (*Frieda's* Organic) .... | 50 | 5.0 | 2.0 | 2.5 | 0 | 10 | 0 |
| (*Nasoya*), 2.8 oz. .... | 60 | 6.0 | 1.0 | 3.0 | 0 | 0 | <1.0 |
| (*White Wave* Organic), | | | | | | | |
| 3.2 oz. .......... | 110 | 10.0 | 3.0 | 6.0 | 0 | 5 | 1.0 |
| sprouted (*Nasoya* | | | | | | | |
| Organic) ........... | 100 | 10.0 | 3.0 | 5.0 | 0 | 25 | 1.0 |
| **Tofu, baked**: | | | | | | | |
| (*Frieda's*), 3 oz.: | | | | | | | |
| garlic herb, 3 oz. ..... | 120 | 10.0 | 8.0 | 6.0 | 0 | 240 | 1.0 |
| sesame garlic, 3 oz. .. | 130 | 10.0 | 10.0 | 6.0 | 0 | 210 | 1.0 |
| (*White Wave*), 2-oz. pc.: | | | | | | | |
| garlic herb Italian .... | 90 | 9.0 | 2.0 | 5.0 | 0 | 240 | 1.0 |
| lemon pepper, zesty .. | 90 | 9.0 | 3.0 | 5.0 | 0 | 200 | 1.0 |
| sesame peanut Thai .. | 90 | 9.0 | 2.0 | 5.0 | 0 | 280 | 1.0 |
| teriyaki Oriental ...... | 100 | 9.0 | 4.0 | 5.0 | 0 | 240 | 2.0 |
| tomato basil Roma ... | 90 | 9.0 | 3.0 | 5.0 | 0 | 240 | 1.0 |

| Food and Measure | cal. | prot. (gms) | carbo. (gms) | fat (gms) | chol. (mgs) | sod. (mgs) | fiber (gms) |
|---|---|---|---|---|---|---|---|
| **Tofu, canned**, in water | | | | | | | |
| (*Roland*), 4 pcs. . . . . . | 60 | 6.0 | 2.0 | 3.0 | 0 | 292 | 1.0 |
| **Tofu, dessert**, peach | | | | | | | |
| mango (*Frieda's*), 3 oz. | 60 | 2.0 | 9.0 | 1.5 | 0 | 0 | 0 |
| **Tofu breakfast**, frozen | | | | | | | |
| (*Amy's* Tofu Scramble), | | | | | | | |
| 9-oz. pkg.: | | | | | | | |
| Mexican . . . . . . . . . . . . | 400 | 20.0 | 40.0 | 18.0 | 15 | 680 | 8.0 |
| tofu scramble . . . . . . . . | 320 | 22.0 | 19.0 | 19.0 | 0 | 580 | 4.0 |
| **Tofu dip**, 4 oz.: | | | | | | | |
| hot (*White Mountain*) . . . | 135 | 11.0 | 0 | 8.0 | 0 | 640 | 0 |
| onion (*White Mountain*) . | 160 | 14.0 | 0 | 10.0 | 0 | 535 | 0 |
| **Tofu dish**, grilled (*Tofu-* | | | | | | | |
| *Town Tofu Tenders*), | | | | | | | |
| ½ of 10-oz. pkg.: | | | | | | | |
| black bean, Havana . . . . . | 210 | 15.0 | 18.0 | 8.0 | 0 | 690 | 2.0 |
| sesame ginger teriyaki . . | 240 | 15.0 | 24.0 | 9.0 | 0 | 680 | 3.0 |
| tahini, Mediterranean . . . | 240 | 15.0 | 16.0 | 13.0 | 0 | 640 | 3.0 |
| tamari, light . . . . . . . . . | 120 | 14.0 | 15.0 | 7.0 | 0 | 640 | 2.0 |
| **Tofu salad** (*White Mountain* | | | | | | | |
| No-Egg), 4 oz. . . . . . . | 120 | 14.0 | 0 | 7.0 | 0 | 430 | 0 |
| **Tofu scrambler mix** | | | | | | | |
| (*Fantastic*), 1 tbsp. . . . | 35 | 1.0 | 7.0 | 0 | 0 | 250 | 1.0 |
| **Tomatillo**, fresh: | | | | | | | |
| 1 medium, 1⅝" diam. . . . | 11 | .3 | 2.0 | .4 | 0 | tr. | .6 |
| chopped: | | | | | | | |
| (*Frieda's*), ½ cup . . . . | 20 | 1.0 | 4.0 | 1.0 | 0 | 0 | 1.0 |
| ½ cup . . . . . . . . . . . . | 21 | .6 | 3.8 | .7 | 0 | 1 | 1.3 |
| **Tomatillo, canned**, | | | | | | | |
| crushed (*Las Palmas*), | | | | | | | |
| ½ cup . . . . . . . . . . . . | 45 | 1.0 | 7.0 | 1.5 | 0 | 0 | 2.0 |
| **Tomato**, fresh, ripe: | | | | | | | |
| raw: | | | | | | | |
| (*Frieda's* Baby Roma/ | | | | | | | |
| Teardrop), ⅔ cup, | | | | | | | |
| 3 oz. . . . . . . . . . . . | 20 | 1.0 | 4.0 | 0 | 0 | 10 | 1.0 |
| (*Green Giant* Fresh), | | | | | | | |
| 1 medium, 5.2 oz. . . | 25 | 1.0 | 6.0 | 0 | 0 | 5 | 2.0 |
| 2⅗" tomato . . . . . . . . | 26 | 1.0 | 5.7 | .4 | 0 | 11 | 1.4 |
| chopped, 1 cup . . . . . . | 38 | 1.5 | 8.4 | .6 | 0 | 16 | 2.0 |
| boiled: | | | | | | | |
| 2 medium, 8.8 oz. . . . . | 66 | 2.6 | 14.3 | 1.0 | 0 | 27 | 2.5 |
| 1 cup . . . . . . . . . . . . | 65 | 2.6 | 14.0 | 1.0 | 0 | 27 | 2.4 |

| Food and Measure | cal. | prot. (gms) | carbo. (gms) | fat (gms) | chol. (mgs) | sod. (mgs) | fiber (gms) |
|---|---|---|---|---|---|---|---|
| **Tomato** *(cont.)* | | | | | | | |
| orange: | | | | | | | |
|   3.9-oz. tomato ...... | 18 | 1.3 | 3.5 | .2 | 0 | 47 | 1.0 |
|   chopped, 1 cup ...... | 25 | 1.8 | 5.0 | .3 | 0 | 66 | 1.4 |
| yellow: | | | | | | | |
|   7.8-oz. tomato ...... | 32 | 2.1 | 6.3 | .6 | 0 | 49 | 1.5 |
|   chopped, 1 cup ...... | 21 | 1.4 | 4.1 | .4 | 0 | 32 | 1.0 |
| **Tomato, can/jar** (see also "Tomato paste," "Tomato puree," and "Tomato sauce"), ½ cup, except as noted: | | | | | | | |
| whole, peeled: | | | | | | | |
|   (*Eden* Organic) ...... | 30 | 1.0 | 4.0 | 0 | 0 | 10 | 1.0 |
|   (*Hunt's*) .......... | 25 | 1.0 | 5.0 | 0 | 0 | 180 | 2.0 |
|   (*Hunt's* No Salt) ..... | 25 | 1.0 | 5.0 | 0 | 0 | 30 | 2.0 |
|   (*Muir Glen* Organic/ Organic Plum) .... | 25 | 1.0 | 5.0 | 0 | 0 | 260 | 1.0 |
|   (*S&W*) ............. | 25 | 1.0 | 6.0 | 0 | 0 | 250 | 2.0 |
|   w/basil (*Eden* Organic) | 30 | 1.0 | 4.0 | 0 | 0 | 10 | 1.0 |
|   w/basil (*Muir Glen* Organic) .......... | 25 | 1.0 | 5.0 | 0 | 0 | 260 | 1.0 |
|   fire-roasted (*Muir Glen* Organic) ..... | 25 | 1.0 | 5.0 | 0 | 0 | 290 | 1.0 |
| wedges (*Del Monte*) .... | 35 | 1.0 | 9.0 | 0 | 0 | 380 | 2.0 |
| diced: | | | | | | | |
|   (*Contadina*) ......... | 30 | <1.0 | 6.0 | 0 | 0 | 200 | <1.0 |
|   (*Contadina* Petite) .... | 25 | 1.0 | 6.0 | 0 | 0 | 250 | 2.0 |
|   (*Del Monte/Del Monte* Petite) ..... | 25 | 1.0 | 6.0 | 0 | 0 | 250 | 2.0 |
|   (*Del Monte* No Salt) .. | 25 | 1.0 | 6.0 | 0 | 0 | 50 | 2.0 |
|   (*Eden* Organic) ...... | 30 | 1.0 | 6.0 | 0 | 0 | 5 | 2.0 |
|   (*Hunt's*) ............ | 25 | 1.0 | 6.0 | 0 | 0 | 310 | 2.0 |
|   (*Hunt's* Petite) ...... | 25 | 1.0 | 6.0 | 0 | 0 | 280 | 1.0 |
|   (*Muir Glen* Organic) .. | 30 | 1.0 | 6.0 | 0 | 0 | 290 | 1.0 |
|   (*Muir Glen* Organic No Salt) .......... | 30 | 1.0 | 6.0 | 0 | 0 | 15 | 1.0 |
|   (*Progresso*) ......... | 20 | 1.0 | 5.0 | 0 | 0 | 250 | 1.0 |
|   (*Ro*Tel*) ............ | 20 | <1.0 | 4.0 | 0 | 0 | 520 | 1.0 |
|   (*S&W* Petite-Cut/ Ready-Cut) ....... | 25 | 1.0 | 6.0 | 0 | 0 | 250 | 2.0 |
|   (*S&W* Ready-Cut No Salt) ......... | 25 | 1.0 | 6.0 | 0 | 0 | 50 | 2.0 |

| Food and Measure | cal. | prot. (gms) | carbo. (gms) | fat (gms) | chol. (mgs) | sod. (mgs) | fiber (gms) |
|---|---|---|---|---|---|---|---|
| chili style (*Del Monte* Zesty) ..... | 30 | 1.0 | 8.0 | 0 | 0 | 600 | 2.0 |
| chili style (*Ro*Tel* Chili Fixins) ...... | 35 | 2.0 | 8.0 | 1.0 | 0 | 540 | 3.0 |
| chunky, pasta style (*Del Monte*) ...... | 45 | 1.0 | 11.0 | 0 | 0 | 560 | 2.0 |
| w/basil or onion (*Eden* Organic) .... | 30 | 1.0 | 6.0 | 0 | 0 | 5 | 2.0 |
| w/basil/garlic or garlic/ onion (*Muir Glen* Organic) .......... | 30 | 1.0 | 6.0 | 0 | 0 | 290 | 1.0 |
| w/basil/garlic/oregano (*Del Monte*) ...... | 50 | 2.0 | 11.0 | 0 | 0 | 650 | <1.0 |
| w/basil/garlic/oregano (*Hunt's*) ......... | 35 | 1.0 | 7.0 | 0 | 0 | 330 | 2.0 |
| fire-roasted (*Hunt's*) .. | 30 | <1.0 | 6.0 | 0 | 0 | 310 | 2.0 |
| fire-roasted (*Muir Glen* Organic) ..... | 30 | 1.0 | 6.0 | 0 | 0 | 290 | 1.0 |
| fire-roasted garlic (*Hunt's*) ......... | 25 | 1.0 | 5.0 | 0 | 0 | 270 | 2.0 |
| fire-roasted, w/green chili (*Muir Glen* Organic) ......... | 30 | 1.0 | 6.0 | 0 | 0 | 420 | 1.0 |
| w/garlic, roasted (*Contadina*) ...... | 45 | 1.0 | 10.0 | 0 | 0 | 560 | <1.0 |
| w/garlic, roasted (*Hunt's*) ......... | 35 | 1.0 | 8.0 | 0 | 0 | 290 | 2.0 |
| w/garlic, roasted (*S&W Ready-Cut*) . | 30 | 2.0 | 5.0 | .5 | 0 | 240 | <1.0 |
| w/garlic/olive oil (*Del Monte* Petite) . | 45 | 1.0 | 10.0 | .5 | 0 | 620 | 1.0 |
| w/garlic/onion (*Del Monte*) .......... | 40 | 2.0 | 8.0 | .5 | 0 | 610 | <1.0 |
| w/green chili (*Eden* Organic) .......... | 30 | 2.0 | 5.0 | 0 | 0 | 35 | 2.0 |
| w/green chili (*Hunt's*) . | 30 | 1.0 | 6.0 | 0 | 0 | 290 | 1.0 |
| w/green chili (*Ro*Tel*) | 20 | <1.0 | 4.0 | 0 | 0 | 520 | 1.0 |
| w/green chili (*S&W Ready-Cut*) ....... | 30 | 1.0 | 6.0 | 0 | 0 | 500 | 1.0 |
| w/green chili, mild (*Del Monte*) ...... | 30 | 1.0 | 6.0 | 0 | 0 | 500 | 1.0 |
| w/green pepper/celery/ onion (*Hunt's*) .... | 45 | 1.0 | 10.0 | 0 | 0 | 280 | 2.0 |

| Food and Measure | cal. | prot. (gms) | carbo. (gms) | fat (gms) | chol. (mgs) | sod. (mgs) | fiber (gms) |
|---|---|---|---|---|---|---|---|
| **Tomato, can/jar, diced** *(cont.)* | | | | | | | |
| w/green pepper/onion | | | | | | | |
| (*Del Monte*) . . . . . . | 40 | 1.0 | 9.0 | 0 | 0 | 480 | 2.0 |
| hot (*Ro\*Tel*) . . . . . . . . | 20 | <1.0 | 4.0 | 0 | 0 | 520 | 1.0 |
| Italian (*S&W* | | | | | | | |
| *Ready-Cut*) . . . . . . . | 25 | 1.0 | 4.0 | 0 . | 0 | 190 | <1.0 |
| w/Italian herbs | | | | | | | |
| (*Contadina*) . . . . . . | 45 | 1.0 | 11.0 | 0 | 0 | 390 | 1.0 |
| w/Italian herbs (*Muir* | | | | | | | |
| *Glen* Organic) . . . . . | 30 | 1.0 | 6.0 | 0 | 0 | 350 | 1.0 |
| w/jalapeño (*Del* | | | | | | | |
| *Monte* Petite) . . . . . | 30 | 1.0 | 6.0 | 0 | 0 | 500 | 1.0 |
| w/jalapeño (*S&W* | | | | | | | |
| *Petite-Cut*) . . . . . . . | 30 | 1.0 | 7.0 | 0 | 0 | 380 | 2.0 |
| marinara (*Contadina*) . | 70 | 1.0 | 13.0 | 1.5 | 0 | 600 | 2.0 |
| Mexican (*Ro\*Tel*) . . . . | 30 | <1.0 | 6.0 | 0 | 0 | 540 | 1.0 |
| w/mushrooms/garlic | | | | | | | |
| (*Del Monte*) . . . . . . | 45 | 1.0 | 10.0 | 0 | 0 | 590 | 1.0 |
| w/onion, sweet | | | | | | | |
| (*Hunt's*) . . . . . . . . . | 45 | 1.0 | 9.0 | 0 | 0 | 360 | <1.0 |
| w/onion, sweet | | | | | | | |
| (*S&W Petite-Cut*) . . | 45 | 1.0 | 10.0 | 0 | 0 | 550 | 1.0 |
| w/onion/green pepper | | | | | | | |
| (*S&W Ready-Cut*) . | 40 | 1.0 | 9.0 | 0 | 0 | 480 | 2.0 |
| primavera (*Contadina*) | 60 | 1.0 | 13.0 | 0 | 0 | 560 | 2.0 |
| w/red pepper, roasted | | | | | | | |
| (*Contadina*) . . . . . . | 60 | 1.0 | 13.0 | 0 | 0 | 550 | 2.0 |
| in sauce (*Hunt's*) . . . . | 30 | <1.0 | 7.0 | 0 | 0 | 350 | 2.0 |
| seasoned, for chili | | | | | | | |
| (*Hunt's*), ¼ cup . . . | 25 | <1.0 | 5.0 | 0 | 0 | 360 | 2.0 |
| crushed, ¼ cup, | | | | | | | |
| except as noted: | | | | | | | |
| (*Contadina*) . . . . . . . . | 20 | <1.0 | 4.0 | 0 | 0 | 150 | 1.0 |
| (*Hunt's*), ½ cup . . . . . | 40 | 2.0 | 8.0 | 0 | 0 | 290 | 2.0 |
| (*Progresso*) . . . . . . . . | 20 | 1.0 | 4.0 | 0 | 0 | 95 | 1.0 |
| (*Eden* Organic) . . . . . . | 20 | 1.0 | 3.0 | 0 | 0 | 0 | 1.0 |
| w/basil (*Hunt's*), | | | | | | | |
| ½ cup . . . . . . . . . . . | 40 | 2.0 | 8.0 | 0 | 0 | 290 | 3.0 |
| w/basil (*Muir Glen* | | | | | | | |
| Organic) . . . . . . . . . | 25 | 1.0 | 5.0 | 0 | 0 | 190 | 1.0 |
| w/basil or onion/garlic | | | | | | | |
| (*Eden* Organic) . . . . | 20 | 1.0 | 3.0 | 0 | 0 | 0 | 1.0 |
| fire-roasted (*Muir* | | | | | | | |
| *Glen* Organic) . . . . . | 20 | <1.0 | 4.0 | 0 | 0 | 160 | 1.0 |

| Food and Measure | cal. | prot. (gms) | carbo. (gms) | fat (gms) | chol. (mgs) | sod. (mgs) | fiber (gms) |
|---|---|---|---|---|---|---|---|
| Italian (*S&W*) ....... | 20 | 1.0 | 4.0 | 0 | 0 | 95 | 1.0 |
| w/Italian herbs or roasted garlic (*Contadina*) ...... | 20 | <1.0 | 3.0 | 0 | 0 | 150 | <1.0 |
| in puree (*S&W*) ..... | 20 | 1.0 | 4.0 | 0 | 0 | 125 | 1.0 |
| ground (*Muir Glen* Organic), ¼ cup ..... | 20 | <1.0 | 4.0 | 0 | 0 | 190 | 1.0 |
| stewed: | | | | | | | |
| (*Del Monte*) ........ | 35 | 1.0 | 9.0 | 0 | 0 | 360 | 2.0 |
| (*Del Monte* No Salt) .. | 35 | 1.0 | 9.0 | 0 | 0 | 50 | 2.0 |
| (*Hunt's*) ........... | 30 | 1.0 | 7.0 | 0 | 0 | 370 | 1.0 |
| (*Hunt's* No Salt) ..... | 40 | 1.0 | 8.0 | 0 | 0 | 30 | 2.0 |
| (*Muir Glen* Organic) .. | 30 | 1.0 | 6.0 | 0 | 0 | 290 | 1.0 |
| (*S&W*) ............. | 35 | 1.0 | 7.0 | 0 | 0 | 270 | 2.0 |
| (*S&W* No Salt) ...... | 35 | 1.0 | 9.0 | 0 | 0 | 50 | 2.0 |
| Cajun (*Del Monte*) ... | 35 | 1.0 | 9.0 | 0 | 0 | 460 | 2.0 |
| Italian (*Del Monte*) ... | 30 | 1.0 | 8.0 | 0 | 0 | 420 | 2.0 |
| Italian or Mexican (*S&W*) .......... | 35 | 1.0 | 7.0 | 0 | 0 | 270 | 2.0 |
| w/Italian herbs (*Contadina*) ...... | 35 | 1.0 | 8.0 | 0 | 0 | 260 | 1.0 |
| Mexican (*Del Monte*) . | 35 | 1.0 | 9.0 | 0 | 0 | 400 | 2.0 |
| w/onions, celery, peppers (*Contadina*) | 35 | 1.0 | 9.0 | 0 | 0 | 220 | 1.0 |
| strained (*Alessi* Prima Passata) ........... | 25 | 2.0 | 4.0 | 0 | 0 | 170 | 2.0 |
| **Tomato, dried:** | | | | | | | |
| 1 oz. ............... | 73 | 4.0 | 15.8 | .8 | 0 | 594 | 3.5 |
| 1 pc., 32 pcs. per cup ... | 5 | .3 | 1.1 | .1 | 0 | 42 | .3 |
| ½ cup .............. | 70 | 3.8 | 15.3 | .8 | 0 | 566 | 3.3 |
| halves: | | | | | | | |
| (*Alessi*), 2 pcs. ...... | 20 | 1.0 | 4.0 | 0 | 0 | 45 | 1.0 |
| (*Mariani*), .5 oz. ..... | 40 | 1.0 | 8.0 | 0 | 0 | 30 | 2.0 |
| or chopped (*Frieda's*), ⅓ cup, 1.1 oz. .... | 100 | 2.0 | 19.0 | 1.0 | 0 | 10 | 2.0 |
| diced (*Roland*), 2 tbsp. .. | 15 | 0 | 3.0 | 0 | 0 | 80 | 1.0 |
| julienne: | | | | | | | |
| (*Mariani*), .5 oz. ..... | 40 | 1.0 | 8.0 | 0 | 0 | 30 | 2.0 |
| (*Roland*), 1 tsp. ..... | 15 | 1.0 | 3.0 | 0 | 0 | 30 | 1.0 |
| marinated, in oil: | | | | | | | |
| (*Alessi*), 1 half or 3 pcs. julienne .... | 35 | 1.0 | 3.0 | 2.0 | 0 | 450 | 1.0 |
| (*Roland* 10 oz.), 2 halves ......... | 25 | 1.0 | 3.0 | 2.0 | 0 | 40 | 1.0 |

| Food and Measure | cal. | prot. (gms) | carbo. (gms) | fat (gms) | chol. (mgs) | sod. (mgs) | fiber (gms) |
|---|---|---|---|---|---|---|---|
| **Tomato, dried, marinated, in oil** *(cont.)* | | | | | | | |
| diced (*Roland*), 1 tsp. . | 20 | 0 | 1.0 | 2.0 | 0 | 0 | 0 |
| drained, ½ cup . . . . . . | 117 | 2.8 | 12.8 | 7.7 | 0 | 146 | 3.2 |
| halves or julienne | | | | | | | |
| (*Frieda's*), 1 tbsp. . . | 35 | 1.0 | 4.0 | 2.0 | 0 | 60 | 1.0 |
| minced (*Roland*), 1 tsp. | 30 | 0 | 2.0 | 2.0 | 0 | 60 | 1.0 |
| strips, w/herbs (*Roland*), | | | | | | | |
| 15 pcs., .5 oz. . . . . | 35 | 0 | 5.0 | 1.0 | 0 | 170 | 0 |
| oven-roasted, w/garlic, | | | | | | | |
| oregano (*Roland*), | | | | | | | |
| 2 tbsp. . . . . . . . . . . . | 50 | 1.0 | 6.0 | 2.0 | 0 | 115 | 2.0 |
| **Tomato, dried, blend**, | | | | | | | |
| seasoned (*Frieda's* | | | | | | | |
| Tomato Toss), ½ cup, | | | | | | | |
| .75 oz. . . . . . . . . . . | 70 | 4.0 | 13.0 | 0 | 0 | 75 | 3.0 |
| **Tomato, green**, raw, | | | | | | | |
| 1 large, 6.4 oz. . . . . . | 44 | 2.2 | 9.3 | .4 | 0 | 24 | 2.0 |
| **Tomato, sun-dried**, | | | | | | | |
| see "Tomato, dried" | | | | | | | |
| **Tomato chutney**, see | | | | | | | |
| "Chutney" | | | | | | | |
| **Tomato juice**, 8 fl. oz., | | | | | | | |
| except as noted: | | | | | | | |
| (*Campbell's*) . . . . . . . . . | 50 | 2.0 | 10.0 | 0 | 0 | 680 | 2.0 |
| (*Campbell's* Low | | | | | | | |
| Sodium) . . . . . . . . . . | 50 | 2.0 | 10.0 | 0 | 0 | 140 | 2.0 |
| (*Campbell's Healthy* | | | | | | | |
| *Request*) . . . . . . . . . . . | 50 | 2.0 | 10.0 | 0 | 0 | 480 | 2.0 |
| (*Del Monte*) . . . . . . . . | 50 | 2.0 | 10.0 | 0 | 0 | 760 | 1.0 |
| (*R.W. Knudsen* Organic) . | 60 | 2.0 | 14.0 | 0 | 0 | 390 | 0 |
| (*Sacramento*) . . . . . . . . | 45 | 1.0 | 10.0 | 0 | 0 | 680 | 2.0 |
| (*Sacramento*), 6 fl. oz. . . | 35 | 1.0 | 8.0 | 0 | 0 | 560 | 1.0 |
| **Tomato paste**, 2 tbsp., | | | | | | | |
| except as noted: | | | | | | | |
| (*Amore* Tube), 1½ tbsp. . | 35 | 1.0 | 4.0 | 2.0 | 0 | 130 | 3.0 |
| (*Contadina*) . . . . . . . . . . | 30 | 2.0 | 6.0 | 0 | 0 | 20 | 1.0 |
| (*Hunt's*) . . . . . . . . . . . . | 25 | 1.0 | 6.0 | 0 | 0 | 105 | 2.0 |
| (*Hunt's* No Salt) . . . . . . | 30 | 1.0 | 6.0 | 0 | 0 | 15 | 2.0 |
| (*Muir Glen* Organic) . . . . | 30 | 2.0 | 6.0 | 0 | 0 | 20 | 1.0 |
| (*S&W*) . . . . . . . . . . . . | 30 | 2.0 | 6.0 | 0 | 0 | 20 | 1.0 |
| w/basil, garlic, | | | | | | | |
| oregano (*Hunt's*) . . . . . | 30 | 1.0 | 6.0 | 0 | 0 | 270 | 2.0 |
| w/Italian herbs | | | | | | | |
| (*Contadina*) . . . . . . . . . | 35 | 1.0 | 7.0 | .5 | 0 | 290 | 1.0 |

| Food and Measure | cal. | prot. (gms) | carbo. (gms) | fat (gms) | chol. (mgs) | sod. (mgs) | fiber (gms) |
|---|---|---|---|---|---|---|---|
| w/pesto (*Contadina*) .... | 35 | 1.0 | 5.0 | .5 | 0 | 300 | <1.0 |
| w/roasted garlic (*Contadina*) ........ | 35 | 1.0 | 5.0 | .5 | 0 | 330 | <1.0 |
| **Tomato pickle**, sweet, w/onion, peppers (*Mrs. Renfro's*), 1 oz. . | 25 | 0 | 6.0 | 0 | 0 | 75 | 0 |
| **Tomato puree**, ¼ cup: | | | | | | | |
| (*Contadina*) ........... | 30 | <1.0 | 4.0 | 0 | 0 | 15 | <1.0 |
| (*Hunt's*) ............. | 40 | 2.0 | 8.0 | 0 | 0 | 125 | 3.0 |
| (*Muir Glen Organic*) .... | 20 | 1.0 | 5.0 | 0 | 0 | 20 | 1.0 |
| (*Progresso*) ........... | 25 | 1.0 | 5.0 | 0 | 0 | 15 | 1.0 |
| (*S&W*) ............... | 30 | 1.0 | 6.0 | 0 | 0 | 15 | 2.0 |
| **Tomato relish**, 1 tbsp., except as noted: | | | | | | | |
| (*B&G* Piccalilli) ........ | 20 | 0 | 5.0 | 0 | 0 | 120 | 0 |
| hot (*Mrs. Renfro's*) ..... | 10 | 0 | 3.0 | 0 | 0 | 40 | 0 |
| mild (*Mrs. Renfro's*) .... | 10 | 0 | 3.0 | 0 | 0 | 45 | 0 |
| **Tomato sauce** (see also "Pasta sauce," "Pizza sauce," and "Tomato, canned"), ¼ cup: | | | | | | | |
| (*Contadina*) ........... | 15 | <1.0 | 3.0 | 0 | 0 | 280 | <1.0 |
| (*Contadina* Extra Thick & Zesty) ...... | 20 | 1.0 | 3.0 | .5 | 0 | 340 | 1.0 |
| (*Del Monte*) ........... | 20 | 1.0 | 4.0 | 0 | 0 | 340 | <1.0 |
| (*Doña Maria*) .......... | 20 | 1.0 | 3.0 | 0 | 0 | 210 | 1.0 |
| (*Hunt's*) .............. | 20 | <1.0 | 4.0 | 0 | 0 | 410 | 1.0 |
| (*Hunt's No Salt*) ....... | 20 | <1.0 | 5.0 | 0 | 0 | 20 | 2.0 |
| (*Muir Glen Organic*) .... | 20 | <1.0 | 5.0 | 0 | 0 | 310 | 1.0 |
| (*Muir Glen Organic* Chunky) ........... | 20 | <1.0 | 4.0 | 0 | 0 | 160 | 1.0 |
| (*Muir Glen Organic* No Salt) ............. | 20 | <1.0 | 5.0 | 0 | 0 | 30 | 1.0 |
| (*S&W* Homestyle) ...... | 20 | 1.0 | 4.0 | 0 | 0 | 260 | 1.0 |
| w/basil, garlic, oregano (*Hunt's*) ........... | 15 | <1.0 | 3.0 | 0 | 0 | 360 | 1.0 |
| chili, seasoned for (*Hunt's*) ............ | 25 | <1.0 | 5.0 | 0 | 0 | 360 | 2.0 |
| w/garlic, roasted (*Hunt's*) ............ | 15 | <1.0 | 3.0 | 0 | 0 | 390 | 2.0 |
| w/garlic and onion (*Contadina*) ......... | 20 | 1.0 | 4.0 | .5 | 0 | 270 | 1.0 |
| w/Italian herbs (*Contadina*) ......... | 15 | <1.0 | 4.0 | 0 | 0 | 320 | 1.0 |

| Food and Measure | cal. | prot. (gms) | carbo. (gms) | fat (gms) | chol. (mgs) | sod. (mgs) | fiber (gms) |
|---|---|---|---|---|---|---|---|
| **Tomato sauce** *(cont.)* | | | | | | | |
| for meat loaf (*Hunt's*) ... | 30 | <1.0 | 7.0 | 0 | 0 | 470 | 2.0 |
| for pizza, see | | | | | | | |
| "Pizza sauce" | | | | | | | |
| **Tongue**, braised: | | | | | | | |
| beef, 4 oz. ............ | 321 | 25.1 | .4 | 23.5 | 121 | 68 | 0 |
| lamb, 4 oz. ........... | 312 | 24.5 | 0 | 23.0 | 214 | 76 | 0 |
| pork, 4 oz. ............ | 307 | 27.3 | 0 | 21.1 | 166 | 124 | 0 |
| veal (calves), 4 oz. ..... | 229 | 29.3 | 0 | 11.5 | 270 | 73 | 0 |
| **Tongue lunch meat**, | | | | | | | |
| beef, 2 oz. ........ | 120 | 10.0 | 0 | 9.0 | 50 | 330 | 0 |
| **Topping, dessert**, see | | | | | | | |
| specific flavors | | | | | | | |
| **Tortellini, frozen/chilled** | | | | | | | |
| (see also "Tortelloni"), | | | | | | | |
| 1 cup, except as noted: | | | | | | | |
| cheese: | | | | | | | |
| (*Celentano*) ......... | 240 | 9.0 | 45.0 | 2.5 | 25 | 490 | 2.0 |
| (*Italian Village*) ...... | 260 | 10.0 | 46.0 | 3.0 | 15 | 440 | 2.0 |
| mixed (*Buitoni*) ..... | 320 | 15.0 | 49.0 | 7.0 | 45 | 530 | 3.0 |
| 3 (*Barilla*), ⅔ cup .... | 230 | 8.0 | 32.0 | 8.0 | 35 | 500 | 3.0 |
| 3 (*Buitoni*) ......... | 320 | 15.0 | 50.0 | 7.0 | 40 | 480 | 3.0 |
| 3, whole wheat | | | | | | | |
| pasta (*Buitoni*) .... | 340 | 16.0 | 44.0 | 11.0 | 65 | 480 | 8.0 |
| cheese and spinach | | | | | | | |
| (*Barilla*), ¾ cup ...... | 230 | 8.0 | 32.0 | 8.0 | 55 | 310 | 5.0 |
| herb chicken (*Buitoni*) ... | 350 | 13.0 | 52.0 | 10.0 | 40 | 380 | 2.0 |
| meat (*Italian Village*) .... | 300 | 11.0 | 45.0 | 8.0 | 25 | 230 | 2.0 |
| spinach cheese (*Buitoni*) . | 320 | 15.0 | 49.0 | 7.0 | 55 | 510 | 3.0 |
| **Tortellini, pkg.**, cheese | | | | | | | |
| and garlic (*Ronzoni*), | | | | | | | |
| 2 oz. uncooked ...... | 220 | 8.0 | 34.0 | 6.0 | 30 | 640 | 1.0 |
| **Tortellini entree,** | | | | | | | |
| **frozen**, 1 pkg.: | | | | | | | |
| Alfredo (*Michelina's*), 8 oz. | 280 | 12.0 | 26.0 | 15.0 | 50 | 1460 | 1.0 |
| pesto (*Amy's* Bowls), | | | | | | | |
| 9.5 oz. ............. | 430 | 20.0 | 45.0 | 19.0 | 40 | 640 | 3.0 |
| primavera Parmesan | | | | | | | |
| (*Healthy Choice*), | | | | | | | |
| 9 oz. .............. | 220 | 9.0 | 35.0 | 4.5 | 15 | 500 | 6.0 |
| Romano (*Marie | | | | | | | |
| Callender's* Pasta | | | | | | | |
| al Dente), 10 oz. ..... | 430 | 17.0 | 59.0 | 14.0 | 40 | 840 | 7.0 |

| Food and Measure | cal. | prot. (gms) | carbo. (gms) | fat (gms) | chol. (mgs) | sod. (mgs) | fiber (gms) |
|---|---|---|---|---|---|---|---|
| **Tortelloni, frozen or chilled** (see also "Tortellini"): | | | | | | | |
| cheese/roasted garlic (*Buitoni*), 1 cup ..... | 270 | 12.0 | 37.0 | 8.0 | 35 | 360 | 2.0 |
| chicken/proscuitto (*Buitoni*), 1 cup ..... | 330 | 15.0 | 46.0 | 9.0 | 40 | 650 | 2.0 |
| ricotta and spinach (*Barilla*), ¾ cup ...... | 230 | 8.0 | 32.0 | 8.0 | 55 | 310 | 5.0 |
| sausage, sweet Italian (*Buitoni*), 1 cup ..... | 330 | 12.0 | 48.0 | 10.0 | 35 | 300 | 3.0 |
| **Tortelloni entree, frozen** (*Lean Cuisine Market Creations*), 10-oz. pkg.: | | | | | | | |
| asiago cheese ......... | 270 | 14.0 | 39.0 | 7.0 | 40 | 670 | 5.0 |
| mushroom ........... | 280 | 15.0 | 43.0 | 7.0 | 30 | 690 | 5.0 |
| **Tortilla** (see also "Wraps"), 1 pc., except as noted: | | | | | | | |
| corn: | | | | | | | |
| (*Chi-Chi's* 6"), .9 oz. .. | 50 | 2.0 | 11.0 | 0 | 0 | 100 | 1.0 |
| (*Mission* Extra Thin), 2 pcs., 1.3 oz. .... | 80 | 2.0 | 16.0 | 1.0 | 0 | 10 | 2.0 |
| (*Mission* Super Size), 1.2 oz. .......... | 70 | 2.0 | 14.0 | 1.0 | 0 | 5 | 2.0 |
| white (*Mission*), 2 pcs., 1.5 oz. .......... | 90 | 2.0 | 18.0 | 1.0 | 0 | 10 | 3.0 |
| white (*Mission* Estilo Casero), 2 pcs., 2.2 oz. .......... | 130 | 3.0 | 27.0 | 2.0 | 0 | 15 | 4.0 |
| yellow (*Mission*), 2 pcs., 1.3 oz. .......... | 80 | 2.0 | 16.0 | 1.0 | 0 | 10 | 2.0 |
| flour: | | | | | | | |
| (*Chi-Chi's* 6"), 1 oz. ... | 80 | 2.0 | 14.0 | 2.0 | 0 | 240 | 0 |
| (*Chi-Chi's* 8"), 2 oz. ... | 160 | 4.0 | 28.0 | 4.0 | 0 | 490 | 1.0 |
| (*Mission* Homestyle), 2.2 oz. .......... | 180 | 5.0 | 31.0 | 4.0 | 0 | 490 | 3.0 |
| whole wheat (*Garden of Eatin'*) .. | 110 | 4.0 | 22.0 | 1.0 | 0 | 130 | 3.0 |
| flour, burrito: | | | | | | | |
| (*Chi-Chi's* 9"), 2.1 oz. . | 170 | 4.0 | 31.0 | 3.5 | 0 | 540 | 0 |
| (*Mission*), 2.5 oz. .... | 210 | 6.0 | 36.0 | 5.0 | 0 | 630 | 1.0 |

| Food and Measure | cal. | prot. (gms) | carbo. (gms) | fat (gms) | chol. (mgs) | sod. (mgs) | fiber (gms) |
|---|---|---|---|---|---|---|---|
| **Tortilla** *(cont.)* | | | | | | | |
| flour, fajitas: | | | | | | | |
| (*Chi-Chi's* 6"), 1 oz. . . . | 80 | 2.0 | 14.0 | 1.5 | 0 | 260 | 0 |
| (*Mission*), 1.3 oz. . . . . | 110 | 3.0 | 18.0 | 2.5 | 0 | 320 | 1.0 |
| whole wheat (*Chi-Chi's* 6"), 2 oz. . . . . | 160 | 5.0 | 27.0 | 4.0 | 0 | 480 | 3.0 |
| flour, gordita (*Mission Estilo Casero*), 1.8 oz. . | 170 | 4.0 | 24.0 | 6.0 | 0 | 420 | 3.0 |
| flour, soft tacos: | | | | | | | |
| (*Chi-Chi's* 8"), 2 oz. . . . | 160 | 4.0 | 29.0 | 3.5 | 0 | 510 | 0 |
| (*Mission*), 1.7 oz. . . . . | 150 | 4.0 | 25.0 | 3.5 | 0 | 440 | 1.0 |
| (*Old El Paso*), 2 pcs., 1.7 oz. . . . . | 150 | 3.0 | 25.0 | 4.5 | 0 | 360 | 0 |
| whole wheat (*Mission*), 1.6 oz. . . . . . . . . . | 130 | 3.0 | 22.0 | 3.0 | 0 | 390 | 3.0 |
| **Tortilla casserole**, frozen, and black beans (*Amy's* Bowls), 9.5-oz. pkg. . . . . . . . | 390 | 17.0 | 41.0 | 18.0 | 25 | 780 | 7.0 |
| **Tortilla chips**, see "Corn chips/crisps" | | | | | | | |
| **Tortilla chips, multigrain**, 1 oz.: | | | | | | | |
| (*Bachman*) . . . . . . . . . . | 140 | 2.0 | 19.0 | 6.0 | 0 | 95 | 5.0 |
| (*Herr's*) . . . . . . . . . . . . . | 140 | 2.0 | 18.0 | 7.0 | 0 | 180 | 2.5 |
| (*Kettle*) . . . . . . . . . . . . | 140 | 3.0 | 18.0 | 7.0 | 0 | 100 | 2.0 |
| (*Snyder's*) . . . . . . . . . . . | 150 | 2.0 | 19.0 | 7.0 | 0 | 80 | 3.0 |
| (*Tostitos*) . . . . . . . . . . . | 150 | 2.0 | 18.0 | 8.0 | 0 | 135 | 2.0 |
| everything or sea salt (*Garden of Eatin'*) . . . . | 140 | 2.0 | 19.0 | 7.0 | 0 | 140 | 3.0 |
| **Tortilla snack**, cheese filled (*Combos*, 1 oz.: | | | | | | | |
| jalapeño . . . . . . . . . . . . . | 140 | 2.0 | 17.0 | 7.0 | 0 | 310 | 1.0 |
| salsa, zesty . . . . . . . . . . | 140 | 2.0 | 17.0 | 7.0 | 0 | 370 | 1.0 |
| **Tortilla strips**, see "Salad toppers" | | | | | | | |
| **Tostada shell** (see also "Taco shell"): | | | | | | | |
| (*Mission* Estilo Casero), 1 pc. . . . . . . . . . . . . . | 170 | 4.0 | 24.0 | 6.0 | 0 | 420 | 3.0 |
| (*Mission* Nortenas Amarillas/Rojas), 2 pcs. | 110 | 2.0 | 15.0 | 5.0 | 0 | 200 | 1.0 |
| (*Ortega*), 2 pcs. . . . . . . . | 120 | 2.0 | 16.0 | 6.0 | 0 | 170 | 2.0 |

| Food and Measure | cal. | prot. (gms) | carbo. (gms) | fat (gms) | chol. (mgs) | sod. (mgs) | fiber (gms) |
|---|---|---|---|---|---|---|---|
| **Trail mix:** | | | | | | | |
| (*Back to Nature* Bar Harbor), 1 oz. . . . . . . . | 130 | 2.0 | 17.0 | 7.0 | 0 | 0 | 2.0 |
| (*Back to Nature* Harvest), 1.1 oz. . . . . . | 150 | 5.0 | 12.0 | 10.0 | 0 | 5 | 3.0 |
| (*Back to Nature* Nantucket), 1.1 oz. . . . | 140 | 3.0 | 16.0 | 8.0 | 0 | 20 | 2.0 |
| (*Back to Nature* Pacific Heights), 1.1 oz. | 160 | 4.0 | 13.0 | 11.0 | 0 | 30 | 3.0 |
| (*Back to Nature* Red Rock), 1.1 oz. . . . . . . . | 140 | 4.0 | 19.0 | 6.0 | 0 | 5 | 3.0 |
| (*Back to Nature* Sonoma), 1.4 oz. . . . . | 130 | 1.0 | 33.0 | .5 | 0 | 5 | 2.0 |
| (*Eden* Organic All Mixed Up), 1.1 oz. . . . | 160 | 8.0 | 7.0 | 12.0 | 0 | 70 | 4.0 |
| (*Eden* Organic All Mixed Up Too), 3 tbsp., 1.1 oz. . . . . . . | 140 | 5.0 | 10.0 | 11.0 | 0 | 15 | 4.0 |
| (*Frito-Lay* Original), 3 tbsp. . . . . . . . . . . . . | 160 | 4.0 | 14.0 | 9.0 | 0 | 45 | 2.0 |
| (*Planters* Energy Mix), 1.5-oz. pkg. . . . . | 240 | 6.0 | 14.0 | 19.0 | 0 | 135 | 3.0 |
| (*Planters* Golden Nut Crunch), 1.1 oz. . . . . . | 160 | 5.0 | 12.0 | 11.0 | 0 | 95 | 2.0 |
| (*Planters* Sweet & Nutty), 1.1 oz. . . . . . . . | 160 | 5.0 | 15.0 | 10.0 | 0 | 35 | 2.0 |
| berry, wild, mix (*Eden* Organic), 3 tbsp., 1.1 oz. . . . . . . | 150 | 5.0 | 13.0 | 8.0 | 0 | 10 | 4.0 |
| berry almond: | | | | | | | |
| (*Planters*), 1.1 oz. . . . . | 130 | 3.0 | 19.0 | 5.0 | 0 | 35 | 2.0 |
| (*Planters* Daybreak), 1.5-oz. pouch . . . . . | 180 | 3.0 | 27.0 | 7.0 | 0 | 55 | 3.0 |
| berry/nut/chocolate (*Planters*), 1 oz. . . . . . | 120 | 2.0 | 18.0 | 5.0 | 0 | 20 | 1.0 |
| cranberry mix: | | | | | | | |
| and chocolate (*Craisins*), 3 tbsp. . . | 140 | 3.0 | 16.0 | 8.0 | 0 | 100 | n.a. |
| fruit and nut (*Craisins*), 3 tbsp. . . . . . . . . . . | 140 | 2.0 | 18.0 | 6.0 | 0 | 35 | n.a. |
| fruit and nut: | | | | | | | |
| (*Planters*), 1 oz. . . . . . | 140 | 4.0 | 14.0 | 9.0 | 0 | 15 | 2.0 |
| (*Planters*), 2-oz. pkg. . | 270 | 7.0 | 27.0 | 17.0 | 0 | 30 | 3.0 |

| Food and Measure | cal. | prot. (gms) | carbo. (gms) | fat (gms) | chol. (mgs) | sod. (mgs) | fiber (gms) |
|---|---|---|---|---|---|---|---|
| **Trail mix, fruit and nut** *(cont.)* | | | | | | | |
| (*Planters* 9 oz.), | | | | | | | |
| .95 oz. . . . . . . . . . | 120 | 3.0 | 14.0 | 7.0 | 0 | 10 | 2.0 |
| honey nut medley | | | | | | | |
| (*Planters*), 1.1 oz. . . . . | 150 | 4.0 | 14.0 | 10.0 | 0 | 135 | 1.0 |
| nuts and: | | | | | | | |
| Cajun sticks, spicy | | | | | | | |
| (*Planters*), 1 oz. . . . | 150 | 5.0 | 10.0 | 11.0 | 0 | 270 | 2.0 |
| chocolate (*Frito-Lay*), | | | | | | | |
| 1 oz. . . . . . . . . . . . | 160 | 4.0 | 13.0 | 10.0 | 0 | 65 | 2.0 |
| chocolate (*Planters* | | | | | | | |
| 6 oz.), 1.1 oz. . . . . . | 150 | 4.0 | 14.0 | 9.0 | 0 | 20 | 2.0 |
| chocolate (*Planters*), | | | | | | | |
| 1.25-oz. pkg. . . . . . | 180 | 5.0 | 16.0 | 12.0 | 0 | 20 | 2.0 |
| fruit (*Frito-Lay*), | | | | | | | |
| 1 oz. . . . . . . . . . . . | 150 | 4.0 | 12.0 | 9.0 | 0 | 80 | 2.0 |
| mixed, raisins | | | | | | | |
| (*Planters*), 1.1 oz. . | 160 | 6.0 | 11.0 | 12.0 | 0 | 20 | 2.0 |
| seeds and raisins | | | | | | | |
| (*Planters*), 1.1 oz. . | 160 | 6.0 | 11.0 | 11.0 | 0 | 15 | 2.0 |
| **Trail mix bar** (see | | | | | | | |
| also "Granola/cereal | | | | | | | |
| bar"), 1.4-oz. bar: | | | | | | | |
| (*Mariani* HoneyBar) . . . . . | 190 | 6.0 | 18.0 | 12.0 | 0 | 0 | 2.0 |
| cranberry (*Mariani* | | | | | | | |
| HoneyBar) . . . . . . . . | 180 | 5.0 | 20.0 | 10.0 | 0 | 0 | 2.0 |
| sesame (*Mariani* | | | | | | | |
| HoneyBar) . . . . . . . . | 200 | 6.0 | 16.0 | 14.0 | 0 | 0 | 3.0 |
| **Tree fern**, cooked, | | | | | | | |
| chopped, ½ cup . . . . . | 28 | .2 | 7.8 | .1 | 0 | 3 | 2.6 |
| **Triple sec** drink mix | | | | | | | |
| (*Angostura*), 1 tsp. . . . | 15 | 0 | 0 | 0 | 0 | 5 | 0 |
| **Triticale**, whole-grain: | | | | | | | |
| berries (*Bob's Red* | | | | | | | |
| *Mill*), ¼ cup . . . . . . . | 150 | 6.0 | 32.0 | 1.0 | 0 | 2 | 7.0 |
| 1 cup . . . . . . . . . . . . . . | 646 | 25.1 | 138.5 | 4.0 | 0 | 10 | 34.8 |
| **Triticale flour**: | | | | | | | |
| (*Bob's Red Mill*), ¼ cup . | 110 | 4.0 | 23.0 | .5 | 0 | 02 | 5.0 |
| whole-grain, 1 cup . . . . . | 440 | 17.1 | 95.1 | 2.4 | 0 | 3 | 19.0 |
| **Trout**, meat only: | | | | | | | |
| mixed species, 4 oz.: | | | | | | | |
| raw . . . . . . . . . . . . . . | 168 | 23.6 | 0 | 7.5 | 66 | 59 | 0 |
| baked or broiled . . . . . | 215 | 30.2 | 0 | 9.6 | 84 | 76 | 0 |

| Food and Measure | cal. | prot. (gms) | carbo. (gms) | fat (gms) | chol. (mgs) | sod. (mgs) | fiber (gms) |
|---|---|---|---|---|---|---|---|
| rainbow, farmed, 4 oz.: | | | | | | | |
| raw | 156 | 23.7 | 0 | 6.1 | 67 | 40 | 0 |
| baked or broiled | 192 | 27.5 | 0 | 8.2 | 77 | 48 | 0 |
| rainbow, wild, 4 oz.: | | | | | | | |
| raw | 135 | 23.2 | 0 | 3.9 | 67 | 35 | 0 |
| baked or broiled | 170 | 26.0 | 0 | 6.6 | 78 | 64 | 0 |
| sea, see "Sea trout" | | | | | | | |
| **Trout, smoked**, 2 oz.: | | | | | | | |
| canned, in olive oil | | | | | | | |
| (*Roland*) | 130 | 14.0 | 0 | 8.0 | 45 | 300 | 0 |
| chilled (*Ducktrap River*) | 90 | 14.0 | 0 | 4.0 | 10 | 680 | 0 |
| **Truffle**, black, all | | | | | | | |
| varieties (*Roland*), | | | | | | | |
| .4 oz. | 10 | 0 | 1.0 | 0 | 0 | 50 | 1.0 |
| **Truffle cream**, see | | | | | | | |
| "cream sauce" | | | | | | | |
| **Truffle juice**, canned | | | | | | | |
| (*Roland*), 1 tsp. | 0 | 0 | 0 | 0 | 0 | 70 | 0 |
| **Tuna**, meat only: | | | | | | | |
| bluefin, 4 oz.: | | | | | | | |
| raw | 163 | 26.5 | 0 | 5.6 | 43 | 44 | 0 |
| baked or broiled | 209 | 33.9 | 0 | 7.1 | 56 | 57 | 0 |
| skipjack, 4 oz.: | | | | | | | |
| raw | 117 | 25.0 | 0 | 1.2 | 53 | 42 | 0 |
| baked or broiled | 150 | 32.0 | 0 | 1.5 | 68 | 53 | 0 |
| yellowfin, 4 oz.: | | | | | | | |
| raw | 123 | 26.5 | 0 | 1.1 | 51 | 42 | 0 |
| baked or broiled | 158 | 34.0 | 0 | 1.4 | 66 | 53 | 0 |
| **Tuna, can/pouch**, | | | | | | | |
| drained, 2 oz. or | | | | | | | |
| ¼ cup, except as | | | | | | | |
| noted: | | | | | | | |
| chunk light, in oil: | | | | | | | |
| (*Bumble Bee*) | 70 | 13.0 | 0 | .5 | 25 | 180 | 0 |
| (*Bumble Bee* 3 oz.), | | | | | | | |
| 2.6 oz. | 100 | 15.0 | 0 | 4.0 | 35 | 240 | 0 |
| (*Chicken of the Sea*) | 100 | 10.0 | 0 | 6.0 | 25 | 180 | 0 |
| (*StarKist* 5 oz.) | 80 | 10.0 | 0 | 4.0 | 20 | 170 | 0 |
| safflower (*StarKist* | | | | | | | |
| 6.4-oz. Pouch) | 120 | 13.0 | 0 | 8.0 | 25 | 220 | 0 |
| chunk light, in water: | | | | | | | |
| (*Bumble Bee*) | 50 | 13.0 | 0 | .5 | 30 | 180 | 0 |
| (*Bumble Bee* 3 oz.), | | | | | | | |
| 2.6 oz. | 70 | 15.0 | 0 | .5 | 40 | 240 | 0 |

| Food and Measure | cal. | prot. (gms) | carbo. (gms) | fat (gms) | chol. (mgs) | sod. (mgs) | fiber (gms) |
|---|---|---|---|---|---|---|---|
| **Tuna, can/pouch, chunk light, in water** *(cont.)* | | | | | | | |
| (*Bumble Bee "Touch of Lemon"*) ....... | 50 | 13.0 | 0 | .5 | 30 | 180 | 0 |
| (*Chicken of the Sea 5 oz.*) ........... | 50 | 11.0 | 0 | .5 | 25 | 180 | 0 |
| (*Chicken of the Sea 9 or 12 oz.*) ...... | 60 | 13.0 | 0 | .5 | 30 | 180 | 0 |
| (*Chicken of the Sea*), 3-oz. can ........ | 80 | 18.0 | 0 | 1.0 | 40 | 350 | 0 |
| (*Chicken of the Sea Low Sodium*) ..... | 50 | 11.0 | 0 | .5 | 25 | 90 | 0 |
| (*StarKist* 5 oz. can) ... | 50 | 10.0 | <1.0 | 1.0 | 25 | 180 | 0 |
| (*StarKist*), 2.6-oz. pouch) .......... | 80 | 18.0 | 0 | .5 | 35 | 300 | 0 |
| (*StarKist* Low Sodium), 2.6-oz. pouch ..... | 80 | 19.0 | .5 | .5 | 30 | 130 | .5 |
| (*StarKist Gourmet Choice* Select) .... | 50 | 12.0 | 0 | .5 | 25 | 170 | 0 |
| (*StarKist Gourmet Choice* Low Sodium) ......... | 60 | 15.0 | 0 | .5 | 25 | 100 | 0 |
| chunk white albacore, in oil (*Bumble Bee*) ... | 60 | 12.0 | 0 | 1.0 | 25 | 140 | 0 |
| chunk white albacore, in water: | | | | | | | |
| (*Bumble Bee*) ....... | 60 | 12.0 | 0 | 1.0 | 25 | 140 | 0 |
| (*Bumble Bee* 3 oz.), 2.6 oz. | 70 | 16.0 | 0 | 1.0 | 35 | 140 | 0 |
| (*Chicken of the Sea*) .. | 50 | 11.0 | 0 | 1.0 | 25 | 180 | 0 |
| (*Chicken of the Sea* Very Low Sodium) . | 50 | 12.0 | 0 | .5 | 25 | 35 | 0 |
| (*StarKist* 5 oz.) ...... | 60 | 12.0 | 0 | 1.5 | 25 | 180 | 0 |
| (*StarKist*), 2.6-oz pouch .......... | 90 | 18.0 | 1.0 | 2.0 | 30 | 310 | 1.0 |
| (*StarKist* Low Sodium), 2.6-oz pouch ..... | 90 | 21.0 | 0 | 1.0 | 30 | 70 | 0 |
| (*StarKist Gourmet Choice* Very Low Sodium) ......... | 70 | 16.0 | 0 | 1.0 | 25 | 35 | 0 |
| light, in water, pouch: | | | | | | | |
| (*Bumble Bee*) ....... | 60 | 13.0 | 0 | .5 | 30 | 180 | 0 |
| (*Chicken of the Sea*), 2.5 oz. .......... | 90 | 20.0 | 0 | 1.0 | 45 | 230 | 0 |

| Food and Measure | cal. | prot. (gms) | carbo. (gms) | fat (gms) | chol. (mgs) | sod. (mgs) | fiber (gms) |
|---|---|---|---|---|---|---|---|
| solid light, in olive oil: | | | | | | | |
| (*Bumble Bee Prime* | | | | | | | |
| *Fillet* Tonno) ...... | 110 | 15.0 | 0 | 5.0 | 30 | 220 | 0 |
| (*Genova* Tonno) ..... | 120 | 13.0 | 0 | 8.0 | 25 | 250 | 0 |
| (*Genova* Tonno), | | | | | | | |
| 3-oz. can ....... | 190 | 19.0 | 0 | 12.0 | 40 | 350 | 0 |
| (*Progresso*) ........ | 120 | 15.0 | 0 | 6.0 | 35 | 330 | 0 |
| solid white albacore, | | | | | | | |
| in oil: | | | | | | | |
| (*Bumble Bee*) ....... | 80 | 14.0 | 0 | 3.0 | 25 | 140 | 0 |
| (*Bumble Bee* 3 oz.), | | | | | | | |
| 2.7 oz. .......... | 110 | 19.0 | 0 | 4.0 | 35 | 140 | 0 |
| (*Chicken of the Sea*) .. | 90 | 13.0 | 0 | 4.0 | 25 | 180 | 0 |
| (*StarKist* 5 oz.) ...... | 90 | 13.0 | 0 | 4.0 | 25 | 210 | 0 |
| solid white albacore, | | | | | | | |
| in olive oil: | | | | | | | |
| (*Genova* Tonno) ..... | 110 | 13.0 | 0 | 6.0 | 25 | 250 | 0 |
| (*Progresso* Albacore) . | 90 | 16.0 | 0 | 3.0 | 20 | 330 | 0 |
| (*StarKist Gourmet* | | | | | | | |
| *Choice* Fillet) ..... | 120 | 14.0 | 0 | 7.0 | 25 | 160 | 0 |
| solid white, in water: | | | | | | | |
| (*Roland* Tongol | | | | | | | |
| Low Sodium) ..... | 50 | 12.0 | 0 | 0 | 25 | 30 | 0 |
| (*StarKist Gourmet* | | | | | | | |
| *Choice*) .......... | 60 | 15.0 | 0 | .5 | 30 | 150 | 0 |
| solid white albacore, | | | | | | | |
| in water: | | | | | | | |
| (*Bumble Bee*) ....... | 60 | 13.0 | 0 | 1.0 | 25 | 140 | 0 |
| (*Bumble Bee* 3 oz.), | | | | | | | |
| 2.7 oz. | 80 | 18.0 | 0 | 1.0 | 35 | 140 | 0 |
| (*Bumble Bee* Premium), | | | | | | | |
| 2.5-oz. pouch ..... | 80 | 16.0 | 0 | 2.0 | 35 | 140 | 0 |
| (*Bumble Bee* Premium | | | | | | | |
| Pouch) .......... | 70 | 13.0 | 0 | 1.5 | 30 | 140 | 0 |
| (*Bumble Bee Prime* | | | | | | | |
| *Fillet*) ........... | 70 | 16.0 | 0 | 1.0 | 25 | 140 | 0 |
| (*Bumble Bee Prime* | | | | | | | |
| *Fillet* Very Low | | | | | | | |
| Sodium) ......... | 70 | 16.0 | 0 | 1.0 | 25 | 35 | 0 |
| (*Chicken of the Sea* | | | | | | | |
| 5 oz.) ........... | 80 | 11.0 | 0 | 4.0 | 25 | 180 | 0 |
| (*Chicken of the Sea*), | | | | | | | |
| 2.5-oz. pouch ..... | 100 | 20.0 | 0 | 1.5 | 40 | 230 | 0 |

| Food and Measure | cal. | prot. (gms) | carbo. (gms) | fat (gms) | chol. (mgs) | sod. (mgs) | fiber (gms) |
|---|---|---|---|---|---|---|---|
| **Tuna, can/pouch, solid white albacore** *(cont.)* | | | | | | | |
| (*StarKist Gourmet Choice* Fillet) ..... | 60 | 15.0 | 0 | .5 | 25 | 170 | 0 |
| yellowfin, in olive oil (*StarKist*), 2.6-oz. pouch ............ | 190 | 18.0 | .5 | 13.0 | 35 | 300 | .5 |
| yellowtail fillets, in olive oil (*Roland*) .... | 100 | 15.0 | 0 | 4.0 | 5 | 400 | 0 |
| **Tuna, can/pouch, seasoned**, 1 can or pkg.: | | | | | | | |
| (*Bumble Bee Prime Fillet* Albacore Steak), 4-oz. pouch: | | | | | | | |
| lemon cracked pepper | 170 | 28.0 | 0 | 5.0 | 40 | 370 | 0 |
| mesquite grilled ..... | 160 | 30.0 | 0 | 4.0 | 50 | 370 | 0 |
| (*Bumble Bee Sensations* Medley), 3-oz. pkg. w/ or w/out crackers: | | | | | | | |
| lemon pepper ....... | 110 | 18.0 | 2.0 | 3.0 | 25 | 350 | 0 |
| sun-dried tomato basil | 110 | 16.0 | 2.0 | 4.0 | 25 | 300 | 0 |
| spicy Thai chili ...... | 160 | 15.0 | 9.0 | 7.0 | 35 | 470 | 1.0 |
| crackers only, 6 pcs. .. | 90 | 1.0 | 11.0 | 4.5 | 0 | 110 | 0 |
| (*StarKist Tuna Creations* Pouch), 2 oz.: | | | | | | | |
| lemon pepper, zesty .. | 60 | 14.0 | 0 | .5 | 25 | 220 | 0 |
| hickory smoked ..... | 80 | 14.0 | <1.0 | 2.5 | 30 | 230 | 0 |
| sweet and spicy ..... | 70 | 11.0 | 4.0 | .5 | 25 | 270 | 0 |
| tomato pesto (*StarKist Albacore Creations* Pouch), 2 oz. ....... | 70 | 13.0 | <1.0 | 2.0 | 15 | 190 | 0 |
| yellowfin, marinated in olive oil (*StarKist Gourmet Choice*): | | | | | | | |
| roasted garlic ....... | 140 | 12.0 | 0 | 10.0 | 20 | 150 | 0 |
| lemon dill .......... | 120 | 12.0 | <1.0 | 8.0 | 25 | 230 | <1.0 |
| **Tuna, frozen** (see also "Tuna entree"): | | | | | | | |
| bites (*Blue Horizon*), 4 pcs., 2 oz. ........ | 110 | 6.0 | 6.0 | 7.0 | 15 | 300 | 0 |
| burger (*Blue Horizon* Albacore), 3.2-oz. pc. . | 102 | 18.5 | 1.4 | 2.4 | 39 | 230 | .3 |
| fillet (*StarKist SeaSations*), 5.7-oz. pc.: | | | | | | | |
| lemon herb, savory ... | 130 | 19.0 | 6.0 | 4.0 | 50 | 600 | 2.0 |

| Food and Measure | cal. | prot. (gms) | carbo. (gms) | fat (gms) | chol. (mgs) | sod. (mgs) | fiber (gms) |
|---|---|---|---|---|---|---|---|
| teriyaki orange ginger . | 130 | 20.0 | 8.0 | 2.0 | 60 | 710 | .5 |
| Thai w/basil ........ | 130 | 18.0 | 4.0 | 4.5 | 55 | 525 | 1.0 |
| tomato basil ........ | 110 | 18.0 | 3.0 | 2.5 | 50 | 390 | 1.0 |
| steaks (*SeaPak* Ahi), |  |  |  |  |  |  |  |
| 4.5-oz. pc. ......... | 240 | 24.0 | 2.0 | 14.0 | 45 | 840 | 0 |
| **Tuna, smoked** (*Acme/* |  |  |  |  |  |  |  |
| *Blue Hill Bay*), 2 oz. .. | 70 | 13.0 | 2.0 | 1.0 | 20 | 1 | 0 |
| **Tuna cake mix** |  |  |  |  |  |  |  |
| (*Old Bay Tuna* |  |  |  |  |  |  |  |
| *Classic*), 1⅓ tbsp. .:... | 30 | 1.0 | 3.0 | 1.0 | 35 | 90 | 0 |
| **Tuna entree, frozen,** |  |  |  |  |  |  |  |
| noodle, 1 pkg.: |  |  |  |  |  |  |  |
| casserole: |  |  |  |  |  |  |  |
| (*Stouffer's*), 12 oz. ... | 450 | 22.0 | 45.0 | 20.0 | 70 | 990 | 3.0 |
| creamy (*StarKist* |  |  |  |  |  |  |  |
| *SeaSations*), 9 oz. . | 300 | 20.0 | 35.0 | 9.0 | 30 | 870 | 5.0 |
| gratin (*Smart Ones*), |  |  |  |  |  |  |  |
| 9 oz. .............. | 250 | 14.0 | 37.0 | 5.0 | 30 | 730 | 3.0 |
| **Tuna entree mix**, 1 cup*: |  |  |  |  |  |  |  |
| (*Tuna Helper* Skillet): |  |  |  |  |  |  |  |
| broccoli, creamy ..... | 290 | 14.0 | 34.0 | 12.0 | 20 | 870 | 2.0 |
| fettuccine Alfredo .... | 280 | 13.0 | 31.0 | 12.0 | 20 | 970 | 1.0 |
| Parmesan, creamy ... | 290 | 15.0 | 37.0 | 9.0 | 15 | 850 | 1.0 |
| pasta, cheesy ....... | 300 | 13.0 | 35.0 | 12.0 | 15 | 820 | 1.0 |
| pasta, creamy ....... | 280 | 13.0 | 30.0 | 12.0 | 15 | 830 | 1.0 |
| tetrazzini ........... | 310 | 14.0 | 33.0 | 14.0 | 20 | 780 | 1.0 |
| tuna melt .......... | 300 | 14.0 | 39.0 | 10.0 | 15 | 1050 | <1.0 |
| spirals, creamy |  |  |  |  |  |  |  |
| (*Annie's* Organic |  |  |  |  |  |  |  |
| Skillet Meal) ........ | 320 | 22.0 | 39.0 | 8.5 | 35 | 830 | 2.0 |
| **Tuna salad**, chilled |  |  |  |  |  |  |  |
| (*Thumann's*), 3.5 oz. . | 270 | 14.0 | 4.0 | 22.0 | 40 | 480 | 0 |
| **Tuna salad kit,** |  |  |  |  |  |  |  |
| w/crackers, 1 pkg.: |  |  |  |  |  |  |  |
| (*Bumble Bee* Original): |  |  |  |  |  |  |  |
| 2.9-oz. can salad .... | 220 | 7.0 | 7.0 | 18.0 | 15 | 320 | 1.0 |
| 6 crackers, .6 oz. .... | 80 | 1.0 | 11.0 | 4.0 | 0 | 115 | 1.0 |
| (*Bumble Bee* Fat Free): |  |  |  |  |  |  |  |
| 2.9-oz. can salad .... | 70 | 7.0 | 10.0 | 0 | 20 | 450 | 0 |
| 6 crackers, .6 oz. .... | 80 | 2.0 | 14.0 | 1.5 | 0 | 310 | 1.0 |
| (*Bumble Bee*), w/mayo: |  |  |  |  |  |  |  |
| 2.9-oz can chunk |  |  |  |  |  |  |  |
| light tuna ........ | 70 | 15.0 | 0 | .5 | 40 | 240 | 0 |

| Food and Measure | cal. | prot. (gms) | carbo. (gms) | fat (gms) | chol. (mgs) | sod. (mgs) | fiber (gms) |
|---|---|---|---|---|---|---|---|
| **Tuna salad kit, (Bumble Bee)** *(cont.)* | | | | | | | |
| mayo (*Hellmann's*), | | | | | | | |
| 3.7-oz. pkt. ....... | 260 | 17.0 | 12.0 | 17.0 | 45 | 610 | 0 |
| 6 crackers (*Keebler*) .. | 90 | 2.0 | 12.0 | 4.5 | 0 | 180 | 0 |
| (*Bumble Bee Lunch on the Run* Kit): | | | | | | | |
| components: | | | | | | | |
| tuna salad ....... | 230 | 7.0 | 7.0 | 19.0 | 15 | 330 | 1.0 |
| crackers ......... | 90 | 1.0 | 11.0 | 4.0 | 0 | 115 | 0 |
| diced peaches .... | 80 | 0 | 19.0 | 0 | 0 | 15 | 1.0 |
| cookie .......... | 110 | 1.0 | 15.0 | 5.0 | 10 | 80 | 0 |
| kit total ........... | 510 | 9.0 | 52.0 | 28.0 | 25 | 540 | 2.0 |
| (*StarKist Charlie's Lunch Kit*), 4.3 oz.: | | | | | | | |
| albacore ........... | 290 | 22.0 | 17.0 | 9.0 | 40 | 600 | 1.0 |
| chunk light ........ | 210 | 20.0 | 19.0 | 8.0 | 40 | 580 | 2.0 |
| chunk light (*StarKist*), | | | | | | | |
| 3-oz. pouch ........ | 100 | 13.0 | 4.0 | 3.0 | 30 | 410 | 1.0 |
| **Turban squash** | | | | | | | |
| (*Frieda's*), 3 oz. ...... | 30 | 1.0 | 7.0 | 0 | 0 | 0 | 1.0 |
| **Turbot,** European, meat only: | | | | | | | |
| raw, 4 oz. ............ | 108 | 18.2 | 0 | 3.4 | 54 | 170 | 0 |
| baked or broiled, 4 oz. .. | 138 | 23.3 | 0 | 4.3 | 70 | 218 | 0 |
| **Turkey** (see also "Turkey, frozen/ chilled"), fresh, roasted: | | | | | | | |
| meat w/skin, 4 oz. ...... | 236 | 31.9 | 0 | 11.0 | 93 | 77 | 0 |
| meat only: | | | | | | | |
| 4 oz. ............. | 193 | 3.2 | 0 | 5.6 | 86 | 79 | 0 |
| diced, 1 cup ........ | 238 | 41.0 | 0 | 7.0 | 107 | 99 | 0 |
| skin only, 1 oz. ........ | 125 | 5.6 | 0 | 11.2 | 32 | 15 | 0 |
| dark meat: | | | | | | | |
| w/skin, 4 oz. ....... | 251 | 31.2 | 0 | 13.1 | 101 | 86 | 0 |
| meat only, 4 oz. ..... | 212 | 32.4 | 0 | 8.2 | 96 | 90 | 0 |
| meat only, diced, 1 cup ........... | 262 | 40.0 | 0 | 10.1 | 119 | 110 | 0 |
| light meat: | | | | | | | |
| w/skin, 4 oz. ........ | 223 | 32.4 | 0 | 9.4 | 86 | 71 | 0 |
| meat only, 4 oz. ..... | 178 | 33.9 | 0 | 3.7 | 78 | 73 | 0 |
| meat only, diced, 1 cup ........... | 219 | 41.9 | 0 | 4.5 | 97 | 89 | 0 |

| Food and Measure | cal. | prot. (gms) | carbo. (gms) | fat (gms) | chol. (mgs) | sod. (mgs) | fiber (gms) |
|---|---|---|---|---|---|---|---|
| **breast, meat w/skin:** | | | | | | | |
| ½ breast, 1.9 lb., (4.2 lbs. raw w/bone) | 1637 | 248.1 | 0 | 64.1 | 643 | 541 | 0 |
| 4 oz. | 214 | 32.6 | 0 | 8.4 | 84 | 71 | 0 |
| ground, see "Turkey ground" | | | | | | | |
| **leg, meat w/skin:** | | | | | | | |
| 1.2 lb. (1.5 lbs. raw w/bone) | 1133 | 152.2 | 0 | 53.6 | 466 | 420 | 0 |
| 4 oz. | 236 | 31.6 | 0 | 11.1 | 96 | 87 | 0 |
| **wing, meat w/skin:** | | | | | | | |
| 6.6 oz. (9.9 oz. raw w/bone) | 426 | 50.9 | 0 | 23.1 | 150 | 114 | 0 |
| 4 oz. | 260 | 31.0 | 0 | 14.1 | 92 | 69 | 0 |
| **Turkey, canned,** chunk, 2 oz.: | | | | | | | |
| (*Hormel*) | 70 | 11.0 | 0 | 2.5 | 45 | 270 | 0 |
| white (*Hormel*) | 60 | 11.0 | 0 | 1.5 | 35 | 230 | 0 |
| white (*Valley Fresh*) | 80 | 12.0 | 0 | 3.0 | 40 | 150 | 0 |
| **Turkey, frozen/chilled, raw**, 4 oz., except as noted: | | | | | | | |
| whole, seasoned: | | | | | | | |
| (*Jennie-O Oven Ready* Homestyle) | 140 | 20.0 | 1.0 | 6.0 | 60 | 460 | 0 |
| basted (*Shady Brook Farms*) | 170 | 21.0 | 0 | 8.0 | 70 | 230 | 0 |
| boneless, w/out gravy (*Shady Brook Farms* Roast) | 140 | 20.0 | 1.0 | 10.0 | 55 | 540 | 0 |
| breast, bone-in: | | | | | | | |
| w/gravy (*Jennie-O*) | 140 | 20.0 | 1.0 | 6.0 | 50 | 600 | 0 |
| w/gravy (*Jennie-O* Premium Basted Young), 5 oz. | 155 | 20.0 | 5.0 | 5.0 | 55 | 660 | 0 |
| seasoned (*Jennie-O Oven Ready*) | 130 | 22.0 | 0 | 4.0 | 55 | 420 | 0 |
| breast, bone/skinless: | | | | | | | |
| cutlets (*Shady Brook Farms*) | 110 | 25.0 | 0 | .5 | 60 | 240 | 0 |
| cutlets or tenderloins (*Jennie-O*) | 120 | 26.0 | 0 | 1.5 | 50 | 75 | 0 |

| Food and Measure | cal. | prot. (gms) | carbo. (gms) | fat (gms) | chol. (mgs) | sod. (mgs) | fiber (gms) |
|---|---|---|---|---|---|---|---|
| **Turkey, frozen/chilled, raw, breast, bone/skinless** *(cont.)* | | | | | | | |
| seasoned (*Jennie-O Oven Ready*) ..... | 100 | 23.0 | 1.0 | 1.0 | 40 | 460 | 0 |
| breast tenderloin, marinated/seasoned: | | | | | | | |
| (*Shady Brook Farms Homestyle*) ........ | 130 | 21.0 | 3.0 | 3.5 | 50 | 440 | 0 |
| applewood smoked (*Jennie-O*) ........ | 110 | 23.0 | 3.0 | 1.0 | 40 | 290 | 0 |
| bacon ranch (*Shady Brook Farms*) ..... | 140 | 21.0 | 3.0 | 4.5 | 55 | 270 | 0 |
| balsamic rosemary (*Shady Brook Farms*) | 130 | 21.0 | 5.0 | 3.0 | 50 | 470 | 0 |
| basil pesto (*Shady Brook Farms*) ...... | 150 | 21.0 | 3.0 | 6.0 | 50 | 450 | 0 |
| Dijon, creamy (*Shady Brook Farms*) ..... | 140 | 21.0 | 4.0 | 4.0 | 50 | 500 | 0 |
| Italian herb (*Shady Brook Farms*) ..... | 130 | 21.0 | 4.0 | 3.5 | 50 | 490 | 0 |
| lemon garlic (*Jennie-O*) ........ | 100 | 22.0 | 2.0 | 1.0 | 45 | 570 | 0 |
| lemon garlic (*Shady Brook Farms*) ..... | 130 | 21.0 | 2.0 | .5 | 55 | 500 | 0 |
| pepper, cracked (*Shady Brook Farms*) .......... | 130 | 21.0 | 4.0 | 3.5 | 50 | 470 | 0 |
| rotisserie (*Shady Brook Farms*) ..... | 130 | 21.0 | 2.0 | .5 | 50 | 630 | 0 |
| savory (*Jennie-O*) .... | 100 | 22.0 | 1.0 | 1.0 | 45 | 510 | 0 |
| teriyaki (*Shady Brook Farms*) .......... | 140 | 21.0 | 5.0 | 3.5 | 50 | 530 | 0 |
| teriyaki sesame ginger (*Jennie-O*) ........ | 130 | 22.0 | 4.0 | 3.0 | 40 | 550 | 0 |
| w/gravy (*Jennie-O Pan Roast*), 6.7 oz.: | | | | | | | |
| white meat ......... | 210 | 21.0 | 4.0 | 12.0 | 70 | 1070 | 0 |
| white and dark meat .. | 240 | 22.0 | 4.0 | 14.0 | 80 | 1040 | 0 |
| ground or burger, see "Turkey, ground" | | | | | | | |
| **Turkey, frozen/chilled, cooked**, 3 oz., except as noted: | | | | | | | |
| whole, barbecued (*Empire Kosher*), 5 oz. | 230 | 24.0 | 8.0 | 11.0 | 85 | 790 | 0 |

| Food and Measure | cal. | prot. (gms) | carbo. (gms) | fat (gms) | chol. (mgs) | sod. (mgs) | fiber (gms) |
|---|---|---|---|---|---|---|---|
| breast, roast (*Jennie-O So Easy*), 5 oz. ...... | 110 | 18.0 | 7.0 | 1.5 | 35 | 760 | 0 |
| breast, rotisserie, bone-in, split (*Jennie-O*) | 130 | 23.0 | 0 | 4.0 | 55 | 400 | 0 |
| breast, seasoned, 2 oz.: | | | | | | | |
| (*Jennie-O* Extra Lean) ........... | 50 | 11.0 | 0 | .5 | 25 | 480 | 0 |
| hickory smoked (*Jennie-O* Extra Lean) | 50 | 11.0 | 0 | 1.0 | 20 | 510 | 0 |
| honey cured (*Jennie-O* Extra Lean) ....... | 60 | 12.0 | 1.0 | .5 | 25 | 440 | 0 |
| sun-dried tomato (*Jennie-O* Premium) | 50 | 12.0 | 1.0 | .5 | 25 | 460 | 0 |
| burger (*Applegate Farms* Organic), 3.9 oz. ..... | 190 | 22.0 | 0 | 11.0 | 75 | 70 | 0 |
| drumsticks, smoked (*Jennie-O*) ......... | 140 | 19.0 | 0 | 7.0 | 85 | 600 | 0 |
| w/gravy (*Bob* Evans), 5 oz. ............. | 100 | 18.0 | 4.0 | 1.0 | 45 | 660 | 0 |
| pot roast, slow roast (*Jennie-O*), 3 oz. ..... | 130 | 14.0 | 2.0 | 6.0 | 60 | 530 | 0 |
| roast, seasoned broth (*Hormel*), 5 oz. ...... | 140 | 28.0 | 0 | 3.0 | 65 | 620 | 0 |
| Salisbury w/gravy (*Jennie-O So Easy*), 5 oz. ...... | 190 | 20.0 | 3.0 | 10.0 | 70 | 850 | 0 |
| sliced, and gravy (*Hormel*), 5.7-oz. pc. . | 130 | 21.0 | 4.0 | 3.0 | 50 | 1150 | 4.0 |
| strips, carved breast (*Perdue Short Cuts*), ½ cup, 2.5 oz. ...... | 90 | 20.0 | 2.0 | 1.0 | 45 | 370 | 0 |
| Stroganoff (*Hormel*), 5 oz. ............. | 180 | 22.0 | 2.0 | 9.0 | 85 | 450 | 0 |
| wings (*Shady Brook Farms*): | | | | | | | |
| barbecue glazed ..... | 180 | 16.0 | 6.0 | 13.0 | 100 | 410 | 0 |
| Buffalo ............. | 160 | 16.0 | 2.0 | 10.0 | 105 | 440 | 0 |
| oven roasted ........ | 180 | 15.0 | 5.0 | 10.0 | 45 | 700 | 0 |
| **Turkey, ground**: | | | | | | | |
| raw, 4 oz.: | | | | | | | |
| (*Empire Kosher* Fresh) ........... | 220 | 19.0 | 0 | 16.0 | 85 | 200 | 0 |
| (*Jennie-O* 15% Fat) .. | 220 | 19.0 | 0 | 17.0 | 95 | 95 | 0 |
| (*Jennie-O* 15% Fat Roll) ............ | 220 | 20.0 | 0 | 17.0 | 85 | 85 | 0 |

| Food and Measure | cal. | prot. (gms) | carbo. (gms) | fat (gms) | chol. (mgs) | sod. (mgs) | fiber (gms) |
|---|---|---|---|---|---|---|---|
| **Turkey, ground, raw** *(cont.)* | | | | | | | |
| (*Oscar Mayer* Pure) .. | 190 | 20.0 | 0 | 12.0 | 90 | 140 | 0 |
| (*Shady Brook Farms* 85% Lean) ....... | 240 | 20.0 | 0 | 17.0 | 85 | 75 | 0 |
| breast (*Perdue Fit & Easy*) ......... | 120 | 27.0 | 0 | 1.5 | 65 | 60 | 0 |
| breast (*Shady Brook Farms* 99%) ...... | 120 | 28.0 | 0 | 1.0 | 70 | 55 | 0 |
| lean (*Jennie-O*) ...... | 170 | 21.0 | 0 | 8.0 | 80 | 80 | 0 |
| lean (*Perdue*) ....... | 160 | 24.0 | 0 | 8.0 | 100 | 100 | 0 |
| lean (*Shady Brook Farms* 93%) ...... | 160 | 22.0 | 0 | 8.0 | 80 | 85 | 0 |
| lean, extra (*Jennie-O*) . | 120 | 26.0 | 0 | 1.5 | 55 | 70 | 0 |
| seasoned, Italian (*Jennie-O*) ....... | 160 | 20.0 | 0 | 8.0 | 80 | 680 | 0 |
| seasoned, Italian (*Shady Brook Farms*) .......... | 160 | 22.0 | 1.0 | 8.0 | 80 | 580 | 0 |
| seasoned, taco, lean (*Jennie-O*) ....... | 170 | 20.0 | 0 | 9.0 | 70 | 540 | 0 |
| raw, patties, 4 oz., except as noted: | | | | | | | |
| (*Jennie-O* All Natural White Burger), 5.25 oz. ......... | 180 | 30.0 | 0 | 7.0 | 85 | 340 | 0 |
| (*Jennie-O* All Natural White Patties) | 140 | 24.0 | 0 | 5.0 | 65 | 270 | 0 |
| (*Jennie-O* All Natural ¼ lb. Burger) ..... | 160 | 18.0 | 0 | 9.0 | 95 | 85 | 1.0 |
| (*Perdue*) ........... | 160 | 21.0 | 0 | 8.0 | 90 | 75 | 0 |
| (*Shady Brook Farms* Burgers) ......... | 240 | 20.0 | 0 | 17.0 | 85 | 75 | 0 |
| lean (*Jennie-O* Burger) | 170 | 21.0 | 0 | 8.0 | 80 | 100 | 0 |
| lean, seasoned (*Jennie-O* Burger) . | 170 | 20.0 | 0 | 8.0 | 75 | 600 | 0 |
| savory seasoned (*Jennie-O* Burger) . | 160 | 18.0 | 0 | 9.0 | 95 | 270 | 1.0 |
| cooked burgers, see "Turkey, frozen/ chilled, cooked" | | | | | | | |
| **"Turkey," vegetarian, frozen:** | | | | | | | |
| (*Yves*), 4 slices, 2.2 oz. .. | 100 | 16.0 | 5.0 | 1.5 | 0 | 340 | 0 |

| Food and Measure | cal. | prot. (gms) | carbo. (gms) | fat (gms) | chol. (mgs) | sod. (mgs) | fiber (gms) |
|---|---|---|---|---|---|---|---|
| deli, 5 slices, 1.8 oz.: | | | | | | | |
| all varieties, except | | | | | | | |
| cranberry and | | | | | | | |
| Italian (*Tofurky*) ... | 100 | 13.0 | 6.0 | 3.0 | 0 | 300 | 3.0 |
| cranberry (*Tofurky*) ... | 100 | 11.0 | 8.0 | 3.0 | 0 | 370 | 3.0 |
| Italian (*Tofurky*) ..... | 110 | 11.0 | 7.0 | 4.0 | 0 | 360 | 4.0 |
| ground (*Yves*), ⅓ cup ... | 60 | 14.0 | 4.0 | 1.0 | 0 | 330 | 2.0 |
| smoked, roll (*Worthington*), | | | | | | | |
| ⅜" slice, 2 oz. ....... | 130 | 10.0 | 4.0 | 8.0 | 0 | 440 | 0 |
| **Turkey bacon**, see | | | | | | | |
| "Bacon" | | | | | | | |
| **Turkey bologna**: | | | | | | | |
| (*Applegate Farms* | | | | | | | |
| Deli/Natural), 2 oz. ... | 90 | 9.0 | 0 | 5.5 | 30 | 400 | 0 |
| (*Empire Kosher*), 2 oz. .. | 100 | 6.0 | .5 | 8.0 | 45 | 530 | 0 |
| (*Jennie-O*), 2 oz. ....... | 110 | 8.0 | 2.0 | 9.0 | 45 | 670 | 0 |
| (*Oscar Mayer* Lower | | | | | | | |
| Fat), 1 oz. .......... | 50 | 3.0 | 1.0 | 4.0 | 20 | 270 | 0 |
| **Turkey burger**, see | | | | | | | |
| "Turkey, ground" | | | | | | | |
| **Turkey corned beef** | | | | | | | |
| (*Jennie-O* Serve | | | | | | | |
| Like), 2 oz. ......... | 80 | 9.0 | 2.0 | 3.5 | 40 | 550 | 0 |
| **Turkey dinner**, see | | | | | | | |
| "Turkey entree" | | | | | | | |
| **Turkey entree, canned**, | | | | | | | |
| stew (*Dinty Moore*), | | | | | | | |
| 1 cup ............. | 140 | 10.0 | 19.0 | 3.0 | 20 | 910 | 2.0 |
| **Turkey entree, frozen**, | | | | | | | |
| (see also "Turkey, | | | | | | | |
| frozen/chilled, | | | | | | | |
| cooked"), 1 pkg., | | | | | | | |
| except as noted: | | | | | | | |
| breast: | | | | | | | |
| (*Banquet*), 9.25 oz. ... | 250 | 13.0 | 32.0 | 7.0 | 25 | 1060 | 5.0 |
| golden roasted (*Healthy* | | | | | | | |
| *Choice* Complete), | | | | | | | |
| 10.5 oz. ......... | 290 | 17.0 | 44.0 | 4.5 | 30 | 460 | 8.0 |
| and gravy (*Banquet* | | | | | | | |
| Family), 2 slices | | | | | | | |
| w/gravy ........ | 90 | 5.0 | 6.0 | 5.0 | 20 | 710 | <1.0 |
| grilled (*Organic Bistro* | | | | | | | |
| Savory), 10.5 oz. .. | 370 | 31.0 | 40.0 | 10.0 | 60 | 240 | 7.0 |

| Food and Measure | cal. | prot. (gms) | carbo. (gms) | fat (gms) | chol. (mgs) | sod. (mgs) | fiber (gms) |
|---|---|---|---|---|---|---|---|
| **Turkey entree, frozen, breast** *(cont.)* | | | | | | | |
| stuffed (*Smart Ones*), | | | | | | | |
| 9 oz. . . . . . . . . . . . | 260 | 14.0 | 39.0 | 5.0 | 20 | 700 | 4.0 |
| w/stuffing, potatoes | | | | | | | |
| (*Stouffer's*), 16 oz. . | 450 | 22.0 | 51.0 | 17.0 | 50 | 1400 | 4.0 |
| breast medallions: | | | | | | | |
| (*Boston Market*), 11 oz. | 290 | 22.0 | 27.0 | 11.0 | 55 | 1240 | 2.0 |
| (*Boston Market* | | | | | | | |
| Dinner), 15 oz. . . . . | 360 | 24.0 | 35.0 | 14.0 | 55 | 1570 | 5.0 |
| cranberry relish (*Boston* | | | | | | | |
| *Market*), 10 oz. . . . . | 470 | 18.0 | 69.0 | 14.0 | 40 | 800 | 4.0 |
| w/stuffing (*Boston* | | | | | | | |
| *Market* Dinner), | | | | | | | |
| 13.5 oz. . . . . . . . . | 410 | 32.0 | 44.0 | 12.0 | 55 | 1870 | 4.0 |
| cream sauce, w/pasta | | | | | | | |
| (*Michelina's Budget* | | | | | | | |
| *Gourmet*), 7.5 oz. . . . | 240 | 9.0 | 36.0 | 6.0 | 20 | 510 | 2.0 |
| Marsala (*Healthy* | | | | | | | |
| *Choice* Complete), | | | | | | | |
| 10.8 oz. . . . . . . . . . . | 250 | 17.0 | 36.0 | 4.0 | 35 | 450 | 5.0 |
| medallions: | | | | | | | |
| cranberry (*Smart* | | | | | | | |
| *Ones Fruit* | | | | | | | |
| *Inspirations*), 9 oz. . | 250 | 16.0 | 43.0 | 2.0 | 30 | 460 | 4.0 |
| mushroom gravy | | | | | | | |
| (*Smart Ones*), 9 oz. . | 220 | 13.0 | 38.0 | 2.0 | 55 | 550 | 3.0 |
| slow roast (*Healthy* | | | | | | | |
| *Choice*), 8.5 oz. . . . | 220 | 14.0 | 28.0 | 5.0 | 35 | 460 | 5.0 |
| pie/pot pie, 8 oz., | | | | | | | |
| except as noted: | | | | | | | |
| (*Banquet*), 7 oz. . . . . . | 370 | 10.0 | 35.0 | 21.0 | 30 | 980 | 3.0 |
| (*Blake's*) . . . . . . . . . . . | 370 | 15.0 | 40.0 | 16.0 | 20 | 380 | 3.0 |
| (*Marie Callender's*), | | | | | | | |
| 10 oz. . . . . . . . . . . . | 630 | 19.0 | 58.0 | 36.0 | 20 | 1180 | 4.0 |
| (*Pacific* Organic), | | | | | | | |
| 1 cup . . . . . . . . . . . | 400 | 15.0 | 46.0 | 19.0 | 70 | 850 | 7.0 |
| (*Stouffer's*), 10 oz. . . . | 710 | 23.0 | 61.0 | 41.0 | 70 | 1200 | 2.0 |
| all meat (*Blake's*) . . . . | 360 | 17.0 | 34.0 | 15.0 | 20 | 380 | 1.0 |
| roasted: | | | | | | | |
| breast (*Lean Cuisine* | | | | | | | |
| Comfort), 9.75 oz. . | 300 | 14.0 | 51.0 | 4.0 | 20 | 650 | 2.0 |
| breast (*Lean Cuisine* | | | | | | | |
| *Dinnertime Cuisine*), | | | | | | | |
| 14 oz. . . . . . . . . . . . | 290 | 19.0 | 38.0 | 7.0 | 30 | 890 | 5.0 |

| Food and Measure | cal. | prot. (gms) | carbo. (gms) | fat (gms) | chol. (mgs) | sod. (mgs) | fiber (gms) |
|---|---|---|---|---|---|---|---|
| honey (*Marie Callender's*), 13 oz. . | 320 | 25.0 | 31.0 | 11.0 | 60 | 920 | 7.0 |
| slow, breast (*Smart Ones*), 9 oz. . . . . . . | 200 | 17.0 | 18.0 | 7.0 | 40 | 710 | 2.0 |
| w/stuffing (*Marie Callender's*), 14 oz. . | 350 | 23.0 | 43.0 | 10.0 | 35 | 1200 | 9.0 |
| and vegetables (*Lean Cuisine*), 8 oz. . . . . | 190 | 17.0 | 18.0 | 6.0 | 25 | 480 | 4.0 |
| tenderloins, glazed (*Lean Cuisine Comfort*), 9 oz. . . . . . . | 250 | 13.0 | 38.0 | 5.0 | 25 | 660 | 3.0 |
| tetrazzini (*Stouffer's*), 12 oz. . . . . . . . . . . . . | 450 | 23.0 | 38.0 | 23.0 | 70 | 980 | 2.0 |
| **Turkey entree, microwave** (*Hormel Compleats*), 10-oz. cont.: | | | | | | | |
| and dressing w/gravy . . . | 290 | 20.0 | 31.0 | 9.0 | 45 | 960 | 2.0 |
| roasted, and vegetables . | 220 | 15.0 | 28.0 | 5.0 | 35 | 600 | 3.0 |
| and vegetables, hearty . . | 180 | 14.0 | 24.0 | 3.5 | 25 | 1200 | 4.0 |
| **Turkey fat**, 1 tbsp. . . . . . . | 115 | 0 | 0 | 12.8 | 13 | 0 | 0 |
| **Turkey franks**, see "Frankfurter" | | | | | | | |
| **Turkey giblets**: | | | | | | | |
| simmered, 4 oz. . . . . . . . | 189 | 30.1 | 2.4 | 5.8 | 474 | 67 | 0 |
| simmered, diced, 1 cup . . . . . . . . . . . . | 243 | 38.5 | 3.0 | 7.4 | 606 | 85 | 0 |
| **Turkey gravy**, ¼ cup: | | | | | | | |
| (*Campbell's*) . . . . . . . . . | 25 | 1.0 | 3.0 | 1.0 | 0 | 270 | 0 |
| (*Franco-American* Slow Roast) . . . . . . . . | 25 | 1.0 | 4.0 | 0 | <5 | 320 | 0 |
| (*Heinz* Home Style Roasted) . . . . . . . . . . | 25 | 1.0 | 3.0 | 1.0 | <5 | 290 | 0 |
| (*Imagine* Organic) . . . . . . | 20 | 0 | 4.0 | .5 | 0 | 210 | 0 |
| **Turkey gravy mix**: | | | | | | | |
| (*Lawry's*), ¼ cup* . . . . . . | 25 | <1.0 | 4.0 | 1.0 | 0 | 320 | 0 |
| (*McCormick*), ¼ cup* . . . | 20 | 0 | 4.0 | .5 | 0 | 390 | 0 |
| **Turkey ham**, 2 oz., except as noted: | | | | | | | |
| (*Jennie-O* Original) . . . . . | 60 | 8.0 | 2.0 | 3.0 | 30 | 510 | 0 |
| (*Jennie-O* Extra Lean 10% Water) . . . . . . . . | 70 | 10.0 | 1.0 | 3.0 | 40 | 650 | 0 |
| (*Jennie-O* Extra Lean 20% Water) . . . . . . . . | 70 | 9.0 | 1.0 | 3.0 | 35 | 500 | 0 |
| (*Oscar Mayer*), 1 oz. . . . . | 40 | 5.0 | 1.0 | 2.5 | 20 | 360 | 0 |

| Food and Measure | cal. | prot. (gms) | carbo. (gms) | fat (gms) | chol. (mgs) | sod. (mgs) | fiber (gms) |
|---|---|---|---|---|---|---|---|
| **Turkey kielbasa**, see "Kielbasa" | | | | | | | |
| **Turkey lunch meat** (see also "Turkey ham," etc.), breast, 2 oz., except as noted: | | | | | | | |
| (*Applegate Farms* No Salt) | 60 | 15.0 | 0 | 0 | 35 | 30 | 0 |
| (*Black Bear* Original/ Golden Brown/ Homestyle) | 60 | 11.0 | 1.0 | 1.0 | 20 | 430 | 0 |
| (*Boar's Head* All Natural) | 60 | 13.0 | 1.0 | 1.0 | 30 | 330 | 0 |
| (*Boar's Head* All Natural French Country) | 60 | 12.0 | 0 | 1.0 | 30 | 400 | 0 |
| (*Boar's Head* All Natural Tuscan) | 60 | 15.0 | 0 | 1.0 | 30 | 380 | 0 |
| (*Boar's Head* Golden Catering) | 60 | 13.0 | 0 | 1.0 | 25 | 340 | 0 |
| (*Boar's Head* Premium Lower Sodium Skin Off) | 60 | 12.0 | 0 | .5 | 20 | 340 | 0 |
| (*Di Lusso* Golden Brown) | 50 | 11.0 | 0 | 1.0 | 25 | 470 | 0 |
| (*Di Lusso* Reduced Sodium) | 60 | 13.0 | 0 | 1.0 | 25 | 280 | 0 |
| (*Thumann's* Filet) | 40 | 13.0 | 0 | .5 | 25 | 350 | 0 |
| Black Forest, hickory smoke (*Boar's Head*) | 60 | 13.0 | 0 | .5 | 25 | 360 | 0 |
| bourbon maple (*Jennie-O*) | 50 | 12.0 | 1.0 | .5 | 25 | 460 | 0 |
| browned, tender: | | | | | | | |
| (*Jennie-O* Original) | 50 | 10.0 | 1.0 | 1.0 | 20 | 430 | 0 |
| (*Jennie-O* Deli Favorites) | 50 | 10.0 | 1.0 | .5 | 25 | 440 | 0 |
| (*Jennie-O* Grand Champion/Premium Fresh) | 50 | 11.0 | 0 | 1.0 | 25 | 390 | 0 |
| (*Jennie-O* Grand Champion w/Skin) | 50 | 11.0 | 0 | 1.0 | 25 | 460 | 0 |
| (*Jennie-O* Natural Choice) | 60 | 13.0 | 0 | .5 | 25 | 440 | 0 |

| Food and Measure | cal. | prot. (gms) | carbo. (gms) | fat (gms) | chol. (mgs) | sod. (mgs) | fiber (gms) |
|---|---|---|---|---|---|---|---|
| Buffalo (*Jennie-O*) ...... | 60 | 12.0 | 1.0 | .5 | 25 | 600 | 0 |
| Cajun style: | | | | | | | |
| (*Boar's Head*) ....... | 60 | 13.0 | 1.0 | .5 | 25 | 750 | 0 |
| (*Di Lusso*) .......... | 60 | 11.0 | 1.0 | 1.0 | 25 | 630 | 0 |
| (*Jennie-O*) ......... | 50 | 12.0 | 1.0 | .5 | 25 | 610 | 0 |
| (*Thumann's*) ........ | 40 | 13.0 | 0 | .5 | 25 | 350 | 0 |
| fried (*Jennie-O Grand Champion/ Premium Fresh*) ... | 50 | 12.0 | 0 | 1.0 | 25 | 450 | 0 |
| cranberry sage (*Jennie-O*) ......... | 60 | 11.0 | 3.0 | .5 | 20 | 600 | 0 |
| garlic, roasted, Italian style (*Jennie-O*) ..... | 50 | 120 | 1.0 | .5 | 25 | 530 | 0 |
| garlic herb (*Jennie-O Regional Favorites* Mediterranean) ...... | 60 | 12.0 | 1.0 | .5 | 25 | 570 | 0 |
| herb: | | | | | | | |
| (*Applegate Farms*) ... | 50 | 12.0 | 0 | 0 | 30 | 360 | 0 |
| (*Applegate Farms* Deli Counter) ..... | 50 | 12.0 | 0 | 0 | 30 | 400 | 0 |
| (*Applegate Farms* Organic) ......... | 50 | 10.0 | 0 | 0 | 25 | 360 | 0 |
| honey/honey cured: | | | | | | | |
| (*Black Bear*) ........ | 70 | 11.0 | 3.0 | 1.0 | 20 | 400 | 0 |
| (*Di Lusso*) .......... | 70 | 11.0 | 3.0 | 1.0 | 20 | 480 | 0 |
| (*Hormel Natural Choice*) .......... | 60 | 10.0 | 2.0 | 1.0 | 25 | 470 | 0 |
| (*Jennie-O Grand Champion/Premium Fresh*) ............ | 60 | 11.0 | 2.0 | .5 | 25 | 410 | 0 |
| honey maple: | | | | | | | |
| (*Applegate Farms*) ... | 60 | 11.0 | 2.0 | 1.0 | 25 | 450 | 0 |
| (*Applegate Farms* Deli Counter) ..... | 50 | 12.0 | 0 | 0 | 25 | 450 | 0 |
| honey and molasses (*Thumann's*) ........ | 60 | 13.0 | 1.0 | .5 | 20 | 320 | 0 |
| hot pepper (*Jennie-O Regional Favorites* Rio Grande) ........ | 50 | 12.0 | 0 | 1.0 | 25 | 450 | 0 |
| Italian style: | | | | | | | |
| (*Black Bear*) ........ | 60 | 11.0 | 1.0 | 1.0 | 20 | 430 | 0 |
| (*Thumann's*) ........ | 40 | 13.0 | 0 | .5 | 25 | 350 | 0 |
| lemon pepper (*Thumann's*) ........ | 40 | 13.0 | 0 | .5 | 25 | 350 | 0 |

| Food and Measure | cal. | prot. (gms) | carbo. (gms) | fat (gms) | chol. (mgs) | sod. (mgs) | fiber (gms) |
|---|---|---|---|---|---|---|---|
| **Turkey lunch meat** *(cont.)* | | | | | | | |
| London broil (*Black Bear*) | 60 | 11.0 | 0 | 1.0 | 20 | 460 | 0 |
| maple glazed: | | | | | | | |
| (*Boar's Head Honey Coat*) | 70 | 14.0 | 2.0 | .5 | 30 | 440 | 0 |
| (*Thumann's*) | 60 | 13.0 | 1.0 | .5 | 20 | 320 | 0 |
| oven browned (*Jennie-O Premium Fresh*) | 50 | 11.0 | 0 | .5 | 20 | 580 | 0 |
| pan-roasted, oil browned (*Jennie-O Grand Champion*) | 50 | 11.0 | 0 | 1.0 | 25 | 390 | 0 |
| pastrami style, see "Turkey pastrami" | | | | | | | |
| pepper and garlic (*Black Bear*) | 60 | 11.0 | 1.0 | .5 | 20 | 460 | 0 |
| pepper/peppered: | | | | | | | |
| (*Applegate Farms Deli Counter*) | 50 | 12.0 | 0 | 0 | 30 | 360 | 0 |
| (*Jennie-O Natural Choice*) | 50 | 12.0 | 0 | .5 | 25 | 450 | 0 |
| black (*Black Bear Homestyle*) | 60 | 11.0 | 1.0 | 1.0 | 20 | 430 | 0 |
| cracked (*Boar's Head Pepper Mill*) | 60 | 13.0 | 0 | .5 | 30 | 460 | 0 |
| cracked (*Di Lusso*) | 60 | 12.0 | 0 | 1.0 | 25 | 460 | 0 |
| cracked (*Jennie-O*) | 50 | 12.0 | 1.0 | .5 | 25 | 450 | 0 |
| cracked (*Jennie-O Regional Favorites Smoky Mountain*) | 60 | 11.0 | 1.0 | .5 | 20 | 430 | 0 |
| cracked (*Oscar Mayer Deli Fresh Shaved*), ¼ of 8-oz. pkg. | 50 | 8.0 | 2.0 | 1.0 | 20 | 500 | 0 |
| cracked, and paprika (*Thumann's*) | 40 | 13.0 | 0 | .5 | 25 | 350 | 0 |
| roast/roasted: | | | | | | | |
| (*Applegate Farms*) | 50 | 12.0 | 0 | 0 | 30 | 360 | 0 |
| (*Applegate Farms Organic*) | 50 | 10.0 | 1.0 | 0 | 25 | 360 | 0 |
| (*Boar's Head Ovengold*) | 60 | 12.0 | 1.0 | 1.5 | 35 | 360 | 0 |
| (*Boar's Head Ovengold Skinless*) | 60 | 13.0 | 0 | 1.0 | 20 | 350 | 0 |
| herb (*Jennie-O Premium Fresh*) | 50 | 12.0 | 1.0 | .5 | 25 | 360 | 0 |

| Food and Measure | cal. | prot. (gms) | carbo. (gms) | fat (gms) | chol. (mgs) | sod. (mgs) | fiber (gms) |
|---|---|---|---|---|---|---|---|
| roasted, oven: | | | | | | | |
| (*Applegate Farms* | | | | | | | |
| Deli Counter) . . . . . | 50 | 12.0 | 0 | 0 | 30 | 400 | 0 |
| (*Black Bear*) . . . . . . . . | 60 | 11.0 | 1.0 | 1.0 | 20 | 320 | 0 |
| (*Hormel Natural* | | | | | | | |
| *Choice*) . . . . . . . . . . | 50 | 10.0 | 1.0 | 1.0 | 25 | 490 | 0 |
| (*Jennie-O* Original) . . . | 50 | 10.0 | 1.0 | .5 | 20 | 420 | 0 |
| (*Jennie-O* Blue | | | | | | | |
| Ribbon) . . . . . . . . . | 50 | 9.0 | 2.0 | 1.0 | 20 | 470 | 0 |
| (*Jennie-O* Deli | | | | | | | |
| Favorites) . . . . . . . . | 50 | 10.0 | 1.0 | 0 | 15 | 450 | 0 |
| (*Jennie-O* Deli | | | | | | | |
| Favorites | | | | | | | |
| Reduced Sodium) . | 50 | 11.0 | 0 | 1.0 | 20 | 260 | 0 |
| (*Jennie-O* Grand | | | | | | | |
| Champion) . . . . . . . | 50 | 11.0 | 0 | .5 | 20 | 580 | 0 |
| (*Oscar Mayer* 98% | | | | | | | |
| Fat Free), 2.2 oz. . . | 50 | 9.0 | 0 | 1.0 | 25 | 470 | 0 |
| (*Oscar Mayer* Deli | | | | | | | |
| Fresh), 1.8 oz. . . . . | 45 | 8.0 | 1.0 | .5 | 20 | 460 | 0 |
| (*Oscar Mayer* Deli | | | | | | | |
| Fresh Thick Carve) . | 50 | 11.0 | 0 | 1.0 | 25 | 470 | 0 |
| (*Oscar Mayer* Deli | | | | | | | |
| Fresh Thin Sliced) . | 50 | 9.0 | 1.0 | 1.0 | 25 | 520 | 0 |
| (*Oscar Mayer* Deli | | | | | | | |
| Fresh 98% Fat | | | | | | | |
| Free), 1 oz. . . . . . . . | 30 | 5.0 | 1.0 | .5 | 10 | 220 | 0 |
| (*Oscar Mayer* Family | | | | | | | |
| Size 98% Fat | | | | | | | |
| Free), 1 oz. . . . . . . . | 25 | 4.0 | 1.0 | 0 | 10 | 320 | 0 |
| (*Shady Brook Farms*) . | 60 | 10.0 | 2.0 | 0 | 30 | 410 | 0 |
| shaved (*Tyson*) . . . . . . | 60 | 10.0 | 2.0 | 1.0 | 20 | 640 | 0 |
| rotisserie flavor | | | | | | | |
| (*Thumann's* Filet) . . . . | 40 | 13.0 | 0 | .5 | 25 | 350 | 0 |
| Southwestern (*Boar's* | | | | | | | |
| *Head Salsalito*) . . . . . . | 60 | 13.0 | 1.0 | .5 | 25 | 480 | 0 |
| smoked: | | | | | | | |
| (*Applegate Farms*) . . . | 50 | 12.0 | 0 | 0 | 30 | 360 | 0 |
| (*Applegate Farms* | | | | | | | |
| Deli Counter) . . . . . | 50 | 12.0 | 0 | 0 | 30 | 400 | 0 |
| (*Applegate Farms* | | | | | | | |
| Organic) . . . . . . . . . | 50 | 10.0 | 1.0 | 0 | 25 | 360 | 0 |
| (*Black Bear*) . . . . . . . . | 60 | 11.0 | 1.0 | 1.0 | 20 | 400 | 0 |

| Food and Measure | cal. | prot. (gms) | carbo. (gms) | fat (gms) | chol. (mgs) | sod. (mgs) | fiber (gms) |
|---|---|---|---|---|---|---|---|
| **Turkey lunch meat, smoked** *(cont.)* | | | | | | | |
| (*Boar's Head* All Natural) .......... | 60 | 14.0 | 0 | 1.0 | 30 | 390 | 0 |
| (*Di Lusso*) .......... | 60 | 11.0 | 1.0 | 1.0 | 25 | 620 | 0 |
| (*Empire Kosher*) ..... | 45 | 9.0 | 0 | 0 | 20 | 490 | 0 |
| (*Hormel Natural Choice*) .......... | 50 | 10.0 | 1.0 | 1.0 | 25 | 450 | 0 |
| (*Oscar Mayer* 95% Fat Free), 1 oz. .... | 30 | 3.0 | 1.0 | 1.5 | 10 | 250 | 0 |
| (*Oscar Mayer* 98% Fat Free), 2.2 oz. .. | 50 | 10.0 | 1.0 | 1.0 | 25 | 720 | 0 |
| (*Oscar Mayer* Deli Fresh Shaved), 1.8 oz. .......... | 45 | 8.0 | 1.0 | .5 | 20 | 460 | 0 |
| (*Oscar Mayer* Deli Fresh Thin Sliced) . | 60 | 9.0 | 2.0 | 1.0 | 20 | 630 | 0 |
| (*Oscar Mayer* White), 1 oz. .......... | 30 | 3.0 | 1.0 | 1.5 | 10 | 250 | 0 |
| applewood (*Jennie-O Natural Choice*) ... | 60 | 13.0 | 1.0 | .5 | 25 | 440 | 0 |
| cured, white (*Jennie-O Blue Ribbon*) ..... | 60 | 7.0 | 2.0 | 3.0 | 25 | 500 | 0 |
| honey (*Empire Kosher*) | 45 | 8.0 | 0 | .5 | 15 | 510 | 0 |
| honey (*Oscar Mayer*), 1 oz. .......... | 35 | 3.0 | 2.0 | 2.0 | 15 | 250 | 0 |
| honey (*Oscar Mayer* Shaved), ⅕ of 9-oz. pkg. ........ | 50 | 9.0 | 2.0 | 1.0 | 20 | 470 | 0 |
| honey (*Oscar Mayer* Thin Sliced) ...... | 60 | 10.0 | 3.0 | 1.0 | 25 | 530 | 0 |
| smoked, hickory: | | | | | | | |
| (*Jennie-O* Original) ... | 50 | 10.0 | 1.0 | .5 | 20 | 540 | 0 |
| (*Jennie-O Blue Ribbon*) .......... | 50 | 9.0 | 1.0 | 2.0 | 20 | 590 | 0 |
| (*Jennie-O Deli Favorites*) ........ | 50 | 10.0 | 1.0 | 0 | 15 | 450 | 0 |
| (*Jennie-O Grand Champion/Premium Fresh*) ........... | 50 | 11.0 | 1.0 | .5 | 25 | 570 | 0 |
| (*Jennie-O Grand Champion* w/Skin) . | 50 | 11.0 | 0 | 1.0 | 25 | 530 | 0 |
| (*Oscar Mayer* 98% Fat Free), 1 oz. .... | 25 | 5.0 | 1.0 | 0 | 10 | 220 | 0 |

| Food and Measure | cal. | prot. (gms) | carbo. (gms) | fat (gms) | chol. (mgs) | sod. (mgs) | fiber (gms) |
|---|---|---|---|---|---|---|---|
| *(Oscar Mayer 98% Fat Free 6 oz.)*, 1 oz. . . . . . . . . . . . | 30 | 5.0 | 1.0 | 0 | 10 | 260 | 0 |
| *(Shady Brook Farms)* . | 60 | 11.0 | 1.0 | .5 | 30 | 540 | 0 |
| *(Thumann's)* . . . . . . . . | 40 | 13.0 | 0 | .5 | 25 | 350 | 0 |
| honey *(Jennie-O Grand Champion)* . . | 50 | 11.0 | 2.0 | 0 | 20 | 550 | 0 |
| honey *(Jennie-O Premium Fresh)* . . . | 60 | 11.0 | 2.0 | .5 | 25 | 410 | 0 |
| honey *(Shady Brook Farms)* . . . . . . . . . | 60 | 11.0 | 3.0 | 0 | 30 | 430 | 0 |
| smoked, mesquite: | | | | | | | |
| *(Black Bear)* . . . . . . . | 50 | 11.0 | 0 | .5 | 20 | 390 | 0 |
| *(Boar's Head Wood Smoked)* | 60 | 13.0 | 1.0 | .5 | 25 | 440 | 0 |
| *(Hormel Natural Choice)* . . . . . . . . . | 50 | 10.0 | 1.0 | 1.0 | 25 | 450 | 0 |
| *(Jennie-O Grand Champion/Premium Fresh)* . . . . . . . . . | 50 | 11.0 | 0 | .5 | 25 | 500 | 0 |
| *(Oscar Mayer Deli Fresh Thin Sliced)* . | 60 | 10.0 | 2.0 | 1.0 | 25 | 690 | 0 |
| *(Oscar Mayer Deli Fresh Thin Sliced)*, ⅛ of 9-oz. pkg. . . . . | 50 | 8.0 | 2.0 | 1.0 | 20 | 440 | 0 |
| *(Thumann's)* . . . . . . . . | 40 | 13.0 | 0 | .5 | 25 | 350 | 0 |
| honey *(Di Lusso)* . . . . | 70 | 11.0 | 3.0 | 1.0 | 20 | 480 | 0 |
| honey *(Jennie-O Original)* . . . . . . . . . | 50 | 10.0 | 2.0 | .5 | 20 | 500 | 0 |
| honey *(Jennie-O Blue Ribbon)* . . . . . | 60 | 9.0 | 2.0 | 2.0 | 20 | 550 | 0 |
| honey *(Jennie-O Deli Favorites)* . . . . . . . . | 50 | 10.0 | 3.0 | 0 | 20 | 410 | 0 |
| Southwestern *(Applegate Farms Deli)* | 50 | 11.0 | 1.0 | 0 | 25 | 420 | 0 |
| sun-dried tomato *(Jennie-O)* . . . . . . . . | 50 | 12.0 | 1.0 | .5 | 20 | 460 | 0 |
| Tex-Mex *(Black Bear)* . . . | 60 | 12.0 | 1.0 | .5 | 20 | 460 | 0 |
| **Turkey pastrami**, 2 oz.: | | | | | | | |
| *(Applegate Farms)* . . . . . . | 50 | 12.0 | 0 | 0 | 30 | 360 | 0 |
| *(Boar's Head)* . . . . . . . . . | 60 | 13.0 | 1.0 | .5 | 25 | 440 | 0 |
| *(Empire Kosher)* . . . . . . . | 60 | 9.0 | 0 | 3.0 | 40 | 460 | 0 |
| *(Jennie-O)* . . . . . . . . . . . . | 70 | 9.0 | 3.0 | 2.5 | 40 | 700 | 0 |
| *(Shady Brook Farms)* . . . | 70 | 11.0 | 0 | 2.5 | 40 | 790 | 0 |

| Food and Measure | cal. | prot. (gms) | carbo. (gms) | fat (gms) | chol. (mgs) | sod. (mgs) | fiber (gms) |
|---|---|---|---|---|---|---|---|
| **Turkey pepperoni** (*Hormel Pillow Pack*), 1 oz. ......... | 70 | 9.0 | 0 | 4.0 | 40 | 640 | 0 |
| **Turkey pie**, see "Turkey entree" | | | | | | | |
| **Turkey salami**: (*Applegate Farms/ Deli/Natural*), 2 oz. ... | 70 | 11.0 | 0 | 2.0 | 30 | 360 | 0 |
| (*Empire Kosher*), 2 oz. .. | 100 | 11.0 | 0 | 4.0 | 30 | 450 | 0 |
| (*Jennie-O*), 2 oz. ....... | 90 | 8.0 | 2.0 | 5.0 | 40 | 650 | 0 |
| cooked, 1 oz. ........... | 56 | 4.6 | .2 | 3.9 | 23 | 285 | 0 |
| cotto (*Oscar Mayer*), 1 oz. .............. | 45 | 4.0 | 0 | 3.0 | 20 | 310 | 0 |
| **Turkey sandwich** (see also "Panini" and "Wraps, filled"): cheddar Dijon (*Oscar Mayer Deli Creations*), 6.8 oz. ... | 430 | 26.0 | 48.0 | 15.0 | 50 | 1410 | 5.0 |
| Monterey (*Oscar Mayer Deli Creations*), 7.1 oz. ... | 450 | 25.0 | 50.0 | 17.0 | 55 | 1090 | 4.0 |
| Parmesan basil/ focaccia (*Oscar Mayer Deli Creations*), 5.75 oz. ........... | 370 | 24.0 | 45.0 | 10.0 | 40 | 1180 | 2.0 |
| **Turkey sausage**, see "Sausage" | | | | | | | |
| **Turmeric**, ground, 1 tsp. . | 8 | .2 | 1.4 | .2 | 0 | 1 | .5 |
| **Turnip**, root: raw, 1 large 6.5 oz. ..... | 49 | 1.7 | 11.4 | .2 | 0 | 123 | 11.4 |
| raw, cubed: (*Glory*), ½ cup ...... | 20 | 1.0 | 4.0 | 0 | 0 | 45 | 1.0 |
| (*Green Giant* Fresh Yellow), 3 oz. ...... | 30 | 1.0 | 6.0 | 0 | 0 | 40 | 2.0 |
| ½ cup .............. | 18 | .6 | 4.1 | .1 | 0 | 44 | 1.2 |
| boiled, drained: cubed, ½ cup ....... | 16 | .6 | 3.8 | .6 | 0 | 39 | 1.6 |
| mashed, ½ cup ...... | 24 | .8 | 5.6 | .9 | 0 | 58 | 2.3 |
| **Turnip, frozen**, ½ cup: cooked, seasoned (*McKenzie's* Southland Yellow) ... | 70 | 1.0 | 11.0 | 3.0 | 0 | 250 | 2.0 |
| boiled, drained ........ | 18 | 1.2 | 3.4 | .2 | 0 | 28 | 1.6 |

| Food and Measure | cal. | prot. (gms) | carbo. (gms) | fat (gms) | chol. (mgs) | sod. (mgs) | fiber (gms) |
|---|---|---|---|---|---|---|---|
| **Turnip greens**, fresh: | | | | | | | |
| raw: | | | | | | | |
| (*Glory*), 2 cups ...... | 20 | 1.0 | 5.0 | 0 | 0 | 30 | 3.0 |
| untrimmed, 1 lb. ..... | 85 | 4.8 | 18.2 | 1.0 | 0 | 126 | 7.6 |
| raw, chopped: | | | | | | | |
| (*Del Monte*), 2 cups .. | 25 | 1.0 | 5.0 | 0 | 0 | 30 | 1.0 |
| chopped, ½ cup ..... | 7 | .4 | 1.6 | .1 | 0 | 11 | .7 |
| boiled, chopped, | | | | | | | |
| ½ cup ............. | 15 | .8 | 3.1 | .2 | 0 | 21 | 2.2 |
| **Turnip greens,** | | | | | | | |
| **canned**, ½ cup: | | | | | | | |
| chopped: | | | | | | | |
| (*Allens* No Salt) ..... | 25 | 2.0 | 3.0 | .5 | 0 | 15 | 2.0 |
| (*Bush's*) ........... | 25 | 2.0 | 3.0 | 0 | 0 | 300 | 2.0 |
| w/diced turnip: | | | | | | | |
| (*Allens* No Salt) ..... | 30 | 1.0 | 5.0 | .5 | 0 | 20 | 3.0 |
| (*Bush's*) ........... | 30 | 1.0 | 5.0 | 0 | 0 | 380 | 2.0 |
| seasoned (*Allens*) .... | 35 | 2.0 | 6.0 | 0 | 0 | 330 | 3.0 |
| seasoned (*Glory*) .... | 35 | 2.0 | 3.0 | 0 | 0 | 490 | 1.0 |
| seasoned (*Sunshine*) . | 35 | 4.0 | 5.0 | .5 | 0 | 860 | 2.0 |
| seasoned, Southern: | | | | | | | |
| (*Allens*) ............. | 35 | 2.0 | 5.0 | .5 | 0 | 400 | 2.0 |
| (*Glory*) ............. | 35 | 1.0 | 4.0 | 0 | 0 | 490 | 2.0 |
| (*Glory* Sensibly) ..... | 20 | 1.0 | 4.0 | 0 | 0 | 240 | 2.0 |
| (*Sunshine*) ......... | 35 | 4.0 | 5.0 | .5 | 0 | 860 | 2.0 |
| turkey flavor (*Glory*) .... | 25 | 1.0 | 5.0 | 0 | 0 | 590 | 2.0 |
| **Turnip greens, frozen**, 1 cup: | | | | | | | |
| (*Allens*) .............. | 25 | 2.0 | 4.0 | 0 | 0 | 15 | 2.0 |
| chopped (*McKenzie's*) ... | 30 | 2.0 | 3.0 | 0 | 0 | 30 | 2.0 |
| w/diced turnips | | | | | | | |
| (*McKenzie's*) ........ | 25 | 1.0 | 3.0 | 0 | 0 | 30 | 2.0 |
| boiled, drained ........ | 28 | 3.4 | 4.7 | .3 | 0 | 24 | 2.9 |
| **Turnover**, frozen/ | | | | | | | |
| chilled, 1 pc., except | | | | | | | |
| as noted: | | | | | | | |
| apple: | | | | | | | |
| (*Pepperidge Farm*) ... | 270 | 4.0 | 31.0 | 15.0 | 0 | 230 | 1.0 |
| (*Pillsbury* Real) ...... | 170 | 2.0 | 24.0 | 8.0 | 0 | 260 | <1.0 |
| cherry: | | | | | | | |
| (*Pepperidge Farm*) ... | 270 | 4.0 | 31.0 | 15.0 | 0 | 230 | 1.0 |
| (*Pillsbury* Real) ...... | 180 | 2.0 | 24.0 | 8.0 | 0 | 250 | <1.0 |
| peach (*Pepperidge Farm*) | 280 | 4.0 | 34.0 | 15.0 | 0 | 230 | 1.0 |
| raspberry (*Pepperidge* | | | | | | | |
| *Farm*) ............. | 280 | 4.0 | 34.0 | 15.0 | 0 | 230 | 2.0 |

| Food and Measure | cal. | prot. (gms) | carbo. (gms) | fat (gms) | chol. (mgs) | sod. (mgs) | fiber (gms) |
|---|---|---|---|---|---|---|---|
| **Turtle**, green, raw, meat only, 4 oz. ..... | 101 | 22.5 | 0 | .6 | 57 | 68 | 0 |
| **Twists, pasta, entree** (*Blue Horizon*), ¼ of 32-oz. pkg. ......... | 270 | 17.0 | 38.0 | 6.0 | 75 | 280 | 3.0 |
| **Tzaziki** (*Cedar's*), 2 tbsp. ............ | 35 | 1.0 | 2.0 | 2.5 | 5 | 55 | 0 |

# U–V

| Food and Measure | cal. | prot. (gms) | carbo. (gms) | fat (gms) | chol. (mgs) | sod. (mgs) | fiber (gms) |
|---|---|---|---|---|---|---|---|
| **Ugli fruit** (*Frieda's*), ½ fruit, 4.3 oz. ...... | 45 | 1.0 | 11.0 | 0 | 0 | 0 | 2.0 |
| **Umeboshi plum,** pickled (*Eden*), .3-oz. pc. .......... | 5 | 0 | 1.0 | 0 | 0 | 710 | 0 |
| **Umeboshi plum paste** (*Eden*), 1 tsp. .. | 5 | 0 | 0 | 0 | 0 | 340 | 0 |
| **Uzbek melon** (*Frieda's*), 1 cup, 1.4 oz. ....... | 35 | 1.0 | 9.0 | 0 | 0 | 15 | 1.0 |
| **Vanilla extract,** imitation, 1 tbsp.: | | | | | | | |
| w/alcohol ............. | 31 | 0 | .3 | 0 | 0 | <1 | 0 |
| w/out alcohol ......... | 7 | 0 | 1.8 | 0 | 0 | <1 | 0 |
| **Vanilla topping** (*Smucker's PlateScrapers*), 2 tbsp. | 110 | 1.0 | 24.0 | 1.0 | 0 | 125 | 0 |
| **Veal**, meat only, 4 oz.: | | | | | | | |
| cubed, lean only, braised or stewed .... | 213 | 39.6 | 0 | 4.9 | 164 | 105 | 0 |
| ground, broiled ........ | 195 | 27.6 | 0 | 8.6 | 117 | 94 | 0 |
| leg: | | | | | | | |
| braised, lean w/fat ... | 239 | 41.0 | 0 | 7.2 | 152 | 76 | 0 |
| braised, lean only .... | 230 | 41.6 | 0 | 5.8 | 159 | 76 | 0 |
| roasted, lean w/fat ... | 181 | 31.4 | 0 | 5.3 | 117 | 77 | 0 |
| roasted, lean only .... | 170 | 31.8 | 0 | 3.8 | 117 | 77 | 0 |
| loin: | | | | | | | |
| braised, lean w/fat ... | 322 | 34.2 | 0 | 19.5 | 134 | 91 | 0 |
| braised, lean only .... | 256 | 38.1 | 0 | 10.4 | 142 | 95 | 0 |
| roasted, lean w/fat ... | 246 | 28.1 | 0 | 14.0 | 117 | 105 | 0 |
| roasted, lean only .... | 198 | 29.8 | 0 | 7.9 | 120 | 109 | 0 |
| rib: | | | | | | | |
| braised, lean w/fat ... | 285 | 36.8 | 0 | 14.2 | 158 | 108 | 0 |
| braised, lean only .... | 247 | 39.1 | 0 | 8.9 | 163 | 112 | 0 |

| Food and Measure | cal. | prot. (gms) | carbo. (gms) | fat (gms) | chol. (mgs) | sod. (mgs) | fiber (gms) |
|---|---|---|---|---|---|---|---|
| **Veal, rib** *(cont.)* | | | | | | | |
| roasted, lean w/fat ... | 259 | 27.2 | 0 | 15.8 | 125 | 104 | 0 |
| roasted, lean only .... | 201 | 29.2 | 0 | 8.4 | 130 | 110 | 0 |
| shank, braised: | | | | | | | |
| lean w/fat .......... | 217 | 35.8 | 0 | 7.0 | 141 | 105 | 0 |
| lean only .......... | 201 | 35.4 | 0 | 4.9 | 143 | 107 | 0 |
| shoulder, whole: | | | | | | | |
| braised, lean w/fat ... | 259 | 36.4 | 0 | 11.5 | 143 | 108 | 0 |
| braised, lean only .... | 226 | 38.2 | 0 | 6.9 | 147 | 110 | 0 |
| roasted, lean w/fat ... | 209 | 28.7 | 0 | 9.5 | 128 | 109 | 0 |
| roasted, lean only .... | 193 | 29.3 | 0 | 7.5 | 129 | 110 | 0 |
| shoulder, arm: | | | | | | | |
| braised, lean w/fat ... | 268 | 38.1 | 0 | 11.6 | 168 | 99 | 0 |
| braised, lean only .... | 228 | 40.5 | 0 | 6.0 | 176 | 102 | 0 |
| roasted, lean w/fat ... | 208 | 28.9 | 0 | 9.4 | 122 | 102 | 0 |
| roasted, lean only .... | 186 | 29.6 | 0 | 6.6 | 124 | 103 | 0 |
| shoulder, blade: | | | | | | | |
| braised, lean w/fat ... | 255 | 35.4 | 0 | 11.4 | 174 | 111 | 0 |
| braised, lean only .... | 224 | 37.0 | 0 | 7.3 | 179 | 115 | 0 |
| roasted, lean w/fat ... | 211 | 28.5 | 0 | 9.8 | 133 | 113 | 0 |
| roasted, lean only .... | 194 | 29.1 | 0 | 7.8 | 135 | 116 | 0 |
| sirloin: | | | | | | | |
| braised, lean w/fat ... | 286 | 35.4 | 0 | 14.9 | 122 | 90 | 0 |
| braised, lean only .... | 231 | 38.5 | 0 | 7.4 | 128 | 92 | 0 |
| roasted, lean w/fat ... | 229 | 28.5 | 0 | 11.9 | 116 | 94 | 0 |
| roasted, lean only .... | 191 | 29.8 | 0 | 7.1 | 118 | 96 | 0 |
| **Veal entree**, frozen, parmigiana, w/ spaghetti (*Stouffer's*), 11.63-oz. pkg. ...... | 430 | 20.0 | 46.0 | 18.0 | 60 | 970 | 5.0 |
| **Vegetable blends**, see "Vegetables, mixed" | | | | | | | |
| **Vegetable burger**, see "Burger, vegetarian" and "Burger patty, vegetarian" | | | | | | | |
| **Vegetable cake**, see "Burger patty, vegetarian" | | | | | | | |
| **Vegetable chips/crisps** (see also specific listings), 1 oz., except as noted: | | | | | | | |
| (*Eden*), 1.1 oz. ......... | 140 | <1.0 | 23.0 | 5.0 | 0 | 260 | 0 |

| Food and Measure | cal. | prot. (gms) | carbo. (gms) | fat (gms) | chol. (mgs) | sod. (mgs) | fiber (gms) |
|---|---|---|---|---|---|---|---|
| (*Garden of Eatin'* Veggie Medley) ...... | 140 | 2.0 | 19.0 | 6.0 | 0 | 120 | 2.0 |
| (*Terra* Mediterranean) ... | 150 | 1.0 | 16.0 | 9.0 | 0 | 150 | 3.0 |
| (*Terra* Original) ........ | 150 | 1.0 | 16.0 | 9.0 | 0 | 50 | 3.0 |
| beet garlic (*Garden of Eatin'* Chips) ...... | 140 | 2.0 | 19.0 | 6.0 | 0 | 120 | 2.0 |
| onion flavor: sweet (*Terra Exotic Harvest*) .... | 140 | 2.0 | 18.0 | 6.0 | 0 | 40 | 3.0 |
| strips, jalapeño or savory seasoned (*Alexia* Crunchy) .. | 150 | 2.0 | 18.0 | 8.0 | 0 | 200 | 1.0 |
| sea salt (*Terra Exotic Harvest*) ............ | 130 | 2.0 | 16.0 | 6.0 | 0 | 160 | 3.0 |
| tomato, zesty (*Terra*) .... | 150 | 1.0 | 16.0 | 9.0 | 0 | 190 | 3.0 |
| wasabi (*Eden*), 1.1 oz. ... | 130 | <1.0 | 24.0 | 4.0 | 0 | 260 | 0 |
| **Vegetable dip** (see also specific listings), 2 tbsp.: | | | | | | | |
| garden (*Cabot*) ........ | 50 | 1.0 | 2.0 | 5.0 | 15 | 125 | 0 |
| "liver," vegetarian (*Sabra*) ............ | 70 | 1.0 | 2.0 | 6.0 | 30 | 70 | 0 |
| sautéed (*Sabra* Meditarranean) ...... | 80 | 1.0 | 5.0 | 7.0 | 0 | 410 | <1.0 |
| **Vegetable dip mix** (*McCormick*), ½ tsp. . | 5 | 0 | <1.0 | 0 | 0 | 130 | 0 |
| **Vegetable dish**, frozen/ chilled (see also "Vegetable entree, frozen" and specific listings): | | | | | | | |
| balls (*Dr.* Praeger's California), 2 pcs., 2 oz. | 80 | 4.0 | 10.0 | 2.5 | 0 | 190 | 3.0 |
| dumplings (*Health is Wealth* Potstickers), 2 pcs., 1.6 oz. ...... | 90 | 6.0 | 13.0 | 2.5 | 0 | 280 | 2.0 |
| fritter (*Lupita's* Baja), 1.3-oz. pc. ......... | 100 | 2.0 | 14.0 | 4.0 | 10 | 200 | 1.0 |
| pancake, 1 pc.: (*Golden*), 1.3 oz. ..... | 70 | 2.0 | 10.0 | 3.0 | <5 | 210 | <1.0 |
| (*Old Fashioned Kitchen* 4 Pack), 2.5 oz. ... | 130 | 3.0 | 18.0 | 6.0 | 10 | 390 | <1.0 |
| (*Old Fashioned Kitchen* 12 Pack), 3 oz. .... | 160 | 4.0 | 22.0 | 7.0 | 10 | 470 | <1.0 |

| Food and Measure | cal. | prot. (gms) | carbo. (gms) | fat (gms) | chol. (mgs) | sod. (mgs) | fiber (gms) |
|---|---|---|---|---|---|---|---|
| **Vegetable entree, frozen** (see also "Vegetable entree mix," "Vegetarian entree," and specific vegetable listings), 1 pkg., except as noted: | | | | | | | |
| korma curry, w/rice: | | | | | | | |
| (*Amy's* Indian), 9.5 oz. | 310 | 9.0 | 41.0 | 12.0 | 0 | 680 | 7.0 |
| (*Ethnic Gourmet*), 11 oz. . . . . . . . . . . . | 300 | 8.0 | 52.0 | 6.0 | 0 | 680 | 4.0 |
| matter paneer, 10 oz.: | | | | | | | |
| (*Amy's* Indian) . . . . . . | 370 | 13.0 | 54.0 | 11.0 | 20 | 780 | 6.0 |
| (*Amy's* Indian Light Sodium) . . . . . . . . . | 320 | 11.0 | 54.0 | 8.0 | 20 | 390 | 6.0 |
| matter tofu (*Amy's* Indian), 9.5 oz. . . . . . . | 280 | 12.0 | 40.0 | 8.0 | 20 | 680 | 5.0 |
| paneer tikka (*Amy's* Indian), 9.5 oz. . . . . . . | 320 | 8.0 | 36.0 | 19.0 | 20 | 550 | 5.0 |
| pie/pot pie, 7.5 oz.: | | | | | | | |
| (*Amy's*) . . . . . . . . . . . | 420 | 9.0 | 54.0 | 19.0 | 50 | 590 | 4.0 |
| nondairy (*Amy's*) . . . . | 360 | 10.0 | 50.0 | 13.0 | 0 | 640 | 4.0 |
| shepherd's pie, 8 oz.: | | | | | | | |
| (*Amy's*) . . . . . . . . . . . . | 160 | 6.0 | 27.0 | 4.0 | 0 | 590 | 5.0 |
| (*Amy's* Light Sodium) . | 160 | 5.0 | 27.0 | 4.0 | 0 | 290 | 5.0 |
| Southern (*Amy's* Whole Meal), 10 oz. . . | 310 | 11.0 | 51.0 | 7.0 | 15 | 720 | 8.0 |
| stir-fry, Shanghai (*Contessa On the Stove*), 1½ cup* w/sauce . . . . | 60 | 2.0 | 13.0 | 0 | 0 | 250 | 2.0 |
| **Vegetable entree, microwave** (*Tasty Bite*), ½ of 10-oz. pkg.: | | | | | | | |
| w/cheese, Jaipur . . . . . . . | 160 | 5.0 | 13.0 | 10.0 | 10 | 550 | 2.0 |
| korma | 130 | 3.0 | 15.0 | 6.0 | 0 | 430 | 5.0 |
| spicy coconut, kerala . . . | 140 | 2.0 | 15.0 | 4.0 | 0 | 430 | 2.0 |
| w/tofu, Malaysian Lodeh . . . . . . . . . . . . | 120 | 3.0 | 13.0 | 6.0 | 0 | 420 | 2.0 |
| **Vegetable entree mix, frozen** (*Green Giant Create a Meal! Stir Fry*), frozen, no meat: | | | | | | | |
| lo mein, 1⅔ cups . . . . . . | 130 | 4.0 | 27.0 | 1.0 | 0 | 710 | 2.0 |
| sesame, 1¼ cups . . . . . . | 90 | 3.0 | 9.0 | 5.0 | 0 | 540 | 3.0 |

| Food and Measure | cal. | prot. (gms) | carbo. (gms) | fat (gms) | chol. (mgs) | sod. (mgs) | fiber (gms) |
|---|---|---|---|---|---|---|---|
| sweet/sour, 1¼ cups .... | 140 | 2.0 | 34.0 | 0 | 0 | 410 | 2.0 |
| Szechuan, 1⅓ cups ..... | 70 | 3.0 | 14.0 | 1.0 | 0 | 840 | 2.0 |
| teriyaki, 1¼ cups ....... | 60 | 3.0 | 14.0 | 0 | 0 | 700 | 2.0 |
| **Vegetable fritter or pancake**, see "Vegetable dish" | | | | | | | |
| **Vegetable juice**, 8 fl. oz., except as noted: | | | | | | | |
| (*Bolthouse Farms Vedge*) ........... | 60 | 3.0 | 12.0 | 0 | 0 | 450 | 0 |
| (*R.W. Knudsen Very Veggie* Low Sodium) . | 50 | 2.0 | 11.0 | 0 | 0 | 35 | 2.0 |
| (*R.W. Knudsen Very Veggie* Organic Low Sodium) ...... | 70 | 2.0 | 14.0 | 0 | 0 | 35 | 2.0 |
| (*R.W. Knudsen Very Veggie* Organic) ..... | 70 | 2.0 | 14.0 | 0 | 0 | 630 | 2.0 |
| (*R.W. Knudsen Very Veggie* Original) ..... | 50 | 2.0 | 11.0 | 0 | 0 | 580 | 2.0 |
| (*R.W. Knudsen Very Veggie* Untomato) .... | 70 | 2.0 | 16.0 | 0 | 0 | 130 | 2.0 |
| (*Sacramento*) ......... | 50 | 1.0 | 11.0 | 0 | 0 | 620 | 2.0 |
| (*V8*) ................. | 50 | 2.0 | 10.0 | 0 | 0 | 420 | 2.0 |
| (*V8* Essential Antioxidants) ....... | 50 | 2.0 | 11.0 | 0 | 0 | 480 | 2.0 |
| (*V8* High Fiber) ........ | 60 | 2.0 | 13.0 | 0 | 0 | 480 | 5.0 |
| (*V8* Low Sodium) ...... | 50 | 2.0 | 10.0 | 0 | 0 | 140 | 2.0 |
| spicy/spicy hot: | | | | | | | |
| (*R.W. Knudsen Very Veggie*) ...... | 50 | 2.0 | 11.0 | 0 | 0 | 590 | 2.0 |
| (*V8*) ............. | 50 | 2.0 | 10.0 | 0 | 0 | 480 | 2.0 |
| (*V8* Low Sodium) .... | 50 | 2.0 | 11.0 | 0 | 0 | 140 | 2.0 |
| **Vegetable juice drink** (*V8 V-Lite*), 8 fl. oz. .. | 35 | 1.0 | 7.0 | 0 | 0 | 360 | 1.0 |
| **Vegetable juice fruit blend** (*V8 V-Fusion*), 8 fl. oz.: | | | | | | | |
| acai mixed berry ....... | 110 | 0 | 27.0 | 0 | 0 | 70 | 0 |
| acai mixed berry light .............. | 50 | 0 | 13.0 | 0 | 0 | 45 | 0 |
| cranberry blackberry .... | 110 | 0 | 27.0 | 0 | 0 | 70 | 0 |
| goji raspberry ......... | 110 | 0 | 27.0 | 0 | 0 | 70 | 0 |
| peach mango ......... | 120 | 1.0 | 28.0 | 0 | 0 | 70 | 0 |

| Food and Measure | cal. | prot. (gms) | carbo. (gms) | fat (gms) | chol. (mgs) | sod. (mgs) | fiber (gms) |
|---|---|---|---|---|---|---|---|
| **Vegetable juice fruit blend** *(cont.)* | | | | | | | |
| peach mango, light ..... | 50 | 0 | 13.0 | 0 | 0 | 40 | 0 |
| passion fruit tangerine .. | 110 | 0 | 27.0 | 0 | 0 | 70 | 0 |
| pomegranate blueberry .. | 100 | 0 | 25.0 | 0 | 0 | 60 | 0 |
| pomegranate blueberry | | | | | | | |
| light ............. | 50 | 0 | 13.0 | 0 | 0 | 60 | 0 |
| strawberry banana ..... | 120 | 1.0 | 28.0 | 0 | 0 | 70 | 0 |
| strawberry banana, | | | | | | | |
| light ............. | 50 | 0 | 12.0 | 0 | 0 | 40 | 0 |
| tropical orange ........ | 120 | 1.0 | 28.0 | 0 | 0 | 80 | 0 |
| **Vegetable oyster**, see "Salsify" | | | | | | | |
| **Vegetable pie**, see "Vegetable entree, frozen" | | | | | | | |
| **Vegetable pocket sandwich** (see also specific listings), 1 pc.: | | | | | | | |
| (*Amy's* Pie), 5 oz. ...... | 300 | 8.0 | 45.0 | 9.0 | 0 | 490 | 3.0 |
| Asian (*Aunt Trudy's* Organic), 5 oz. ...... | 240 | 5.0 | 34.0 | 10.0 | 0 | 390 | 3.0 |
| California (*Dr. Praeger's*), 2.75 oz. ... | 150 | 5.0 | 22.0 | 5.0 | 0 | 240 | 5.0 |
| Mexicali (*Aunt Trudy's* Organic), 5 oz. | 230 | 6.0 | 38.0 | 7.0 | 0 | 350 | 3.0 |
| roasted (*Aunt Trudy's* Organic), 5 oz. ...... | 240 | 5.0 | 33.0 | 11.0 | 0 | 280 | 3.0 |
| samosa (*Aunt Trudy's* Organic), 5 oz. ...... | 260 | 5.0 | 39.0 | 10.0 | 0 | 320 | 3.0 |
| Tex-Mex (*Dr. Praeger's*), 2.75 oz. ... | 150 | 5.0 | 24.0 | 4.5 | 0 | 320 | 5.0 |
| **Vegetable seasoning**: | | | | | | | |
| (*McCormick Perfect Pinch*), ¼ tsp. ........ | 0 | 0 | 0 | 0 | 0 | 130 | 0 |
| cheddar (*McCormick Steamers*), 1 tbsp. ... | 20 | <1.0 | 3.0 | .5 | <5 | 350 | 0 |
| garlic basil (*McCormick Steamers*), 2 tsp. .... | 15 | 0 | 2.0 | .5 | 0 | 270 | 0 |
| **Vegetable spread**, roasted (*Va Va Pindjur*), 1 oz. ....... | 55 | 2.3 | 3.2 | 4.5 | 0 | 300 | <1.0 |
| **Vegetables**, see specific listings | | | | | | | |

| Food and Measure | cal. | prot. (gms) | carbo. (gms) | fat (gms) | chol. (mgs) | sod. (mgs) | fiber (gms) |
|---|---|---|---|---|---|---|---|
| **Vegetables, mixed** | | | | | | | |
| fresh, 3 oz., except as noted: | | | | | | | |
| (*Green Giant* Harvest Blend) . . . . . . . . . . . . | 35 | 1.0 | 8.0 | 0 | 0 | 35 | 2.0 |
| (*Green Giant* Medley) . . . | 30 | 2.0 | 6.0 | 0 | 0 | 25 | 2.0 |
| (*Green Giant* Mirepoix Blend) . . . . . | 30 | 1.0 | 6.0 | 0 | 0 | 40 | 2.0 |
| Alfredo (*Green Giant* Primavera), 1 cup . . . . | 90 | 3.0 | 8.0 | 6.0 | 15 | 280 | 3.0 |
| Asian blend (*Green Giant* Fresh) . . . . . . . . | 25 | 1.0 | 5.0 | 0 | 0 | 20 | 2.0 |
| w/chive butter (*Green Giant* Harvest Trio), ⅔ cup . . . . . . . . | 110 | 1.0 | 6.0 | 9.0 | 20 | 220 | 2.0 |
| chop suey (*Ready Pac Ready Fixin's*) . . . . . . . | 15 | 1.0 | 2.0 | 0 | 0 | 45 | 1.0 |
| primavera (*Green Giant*) . | 20 | 1.0 | 4.0 | 0 | 0 | 20 | 2.0 |
| stir-fry, 2 cups, except as noted: | | | | | | | |
| (*Ready Pac Ready Fixin's*), 3 oz. . . . . . | 20 | 1.0 | 4.0 | 0 | 0 | 35 | 2.0 |
| garlic Szechuan (*Green Giant*) . . . . . | 110 | 5.0 | 20.0 | 2.5 | 0 | 1040 | 3.0 |
| ginger, spicy (*Green Giant*) . . . . . . . . . . | 100 | 4.0 | 21.0 | 0 | 0 | 880 | 3.0 |
| sweet and sour (*Green Giant*) . . . . . . . . . . | 130 | 3.0 | 28.0 | 1.5 | 0 | 510 | 4.0 |
| teriyaki (*Green Giant*) . | 140 | 4.0 | 28.0 | 1.5 | 0 | 990 | 4.0 |
| **Vegetables, mixed**, can/jar, ½ cup, except as noted: | | | | | | | |
| (*Allens*) . . . . . . . . . . . . . | 40 | 1.0 | 8.0 | 0 | 0 | 290 | 2.0 |
| (*Del Monte*) . . . . . . . . . . | 40 | 2.0 | 8.0 | 0 | 0 | 360 | 2.0 |
| (*Del Monte Savory Sides* Homestyle Medley) . . . . . . . . . . | 70 | 1.0 | 11.0 | 2.5 | 0 | 380 | 2.0 |
| (*Freshlike*) . . . . . . . . . . . | 45 | 1.0 | 8.0 | .5 | 0 | 410 | 2.0 |
| (*S&W*) . . . . . . . . . . . . . . | 45 | 2.0 | 10.0 | 0 | 0 | 360 | 2.0 |
| (*Veg-All* Homestyle) . . . . | 40 | 1.0 | 8.0 | 0 | 0 | 350 | 2.0 |
| (*Veg-All* Original) . . . . . . | 40 | 1.0 | 8.0 | 0 | 0 | 290 | 2.0 |
| Cajun (*Veg-All*) . . . . . . . . | 50 | 2.0 | 10.0 | 0 | 0 | 410 | 3.0 |
| Chinese stir-fry (*Tiger Tiger*), 1 cup . . . . . . . . | 50 | 3.0 | 9.0 | 0 | 0 | 20 | 2.0 |

| Food and Measure | cal. | prot. (gms) | carbo. (gms) | fat (gms) | chol. (mgs) | sod. (mgs) | fiber (gms) |
|---|---|---|---|---|---|---|---|
| **Vegetables, mixed, can/jar** *(cont.)* | | | | | | | |
| chop suey (*La Choy*) .... | 15 | <1.0 | 3.0 | 0 | 0 | 640 | <1.0 |
| w/potato (*Del Monte*) ... | 45 | 2.0 | 10.0 | 0 | 0 | 360 | 2.0 |
| spiced (*Veg-All* Hot 'n Spicy) | 40 | 1.0 | 8.0 | 0 | 0 | 370 | 2.0 |
| stir-fry: | | | | | | | |
| (*Ka•Me*), 1 can | | | | | | | |
| drained, 8 oz. ..... | 20 | 1.0 | 4.0 | 0 | 0 | 10 | 2.0 |
| (*La Choy*) .......... | 15 | <1.0 | 3.0 | 0 | 0 | 180 | 2.0 |
| **Vegetables, mixed, frozen** | | | | | | | |
| (see also "Vegetable | | | | | | | |
| dish, frozen" and spe- | | | | | | | |
| cific vegetable listings): | | | | | | | |
| (*Birds Eye* Classic | | | | | | | |
| 1 lb.), ⅔ cup ........ | 60 | 2.0 | 12.0 | 0 | 0 | 60 | 2.0 |
| (*Birds Eye* Classic | | | | | | | |
| 16/32 oz.), ⅔ cup .... | 60 | 2.0 | 12.0 | 0 | 0 | 20 | 2.0 |
| (*Birds Eye Steamfresh*), | | | | | | | |
| ⅔ cup ............. | 60 | 2.0 | 12.0 | 0 | 0 | 20 | 2.0 |
| (*Cascadian Farm* | | | | | | | |
| Organic), ⅔ cup ..... | 60 | 2.0 | 12.0 | 0 | 0 | 20 | 2.0 |
| (*Cascadian Farm* | | | | | | | |
| Organic Gardener's | | | | | | | |
| Blend), ¾ cup ....... | 60 | 2.0 | 12.0 | 0 | 0 | 35 | 2.0 |
| (*Cascadian Farm Purely* | | | | | | | |
| *Steam* Organic Garden | | | | | | | |
| Medley), 1 cup ...... | 60 | 2.0 | 12.0 | .5 | 0 | 270 | 1.0 |
| (*C&W The Ultimate* | | | | | | | |
| *Early Harvest* | | | | | | | |
| *Blend*), ½ cup ....... | 60 | 3.0 | 9.0 | 2.0 | 0 | 190 | 2.0 |
| (*C&W The Ultimate* | | | | | | | |
| *Petite Mixed* | | | | | | | |
| *Vegetables*), ¾ cup ... | 50 | 2.0 | 10.0 | 0 | 0 | 70 | 2.0 |
| (*C&W The Ultimate* | | | | | | | |
| *Southwest Blend*), | | | | | | | |
| ⅔ cup ............. | 90 | 5.0 | 16.0 | 1.0 | 0 | 80 | 6.0 |
| (*C&W The Ultimate* | | | | | | | |
| *Stir Fry*), ¾ cup ..... | 30 | 1.0 | 5.0 | 0 | 0 | 15 | 1.0 |
| (*Freshlike*), ⅔ cup ...... | 60 | 2.0 | 11.0 | 0 | 0 | 75 | 2.0 |
| (*Green Giant* Garden | | | | | | | |
| Medley), ½ cup* .... | 70 | 2.0 | 14.0 | .5 | 0 | 220 | 2.0 |
| (*Green Giant Valley* | | | | | | | |
| *Fresh Steamers*), | | | | | | | |
| ½ cup* ............. | 50 | 2.0 | 12.0 | 0 | 0 | 20 | 2.0 |

| Food and Measure | cal. | prot. (gms) | carbo. (gms) | fat (gms) | chol. (mgs) | sod. (mgs) | fiber (gms) |
|---|---|---|---|---|---|---|---|
| (*Green Giant Valley Fresh Steamers Healthy Colors Market Blend*), ½ cup* | 40 | 1.0 | 7.0 | 1.0 | 0 | 210 | 2.0 |
| (*Green Giant Valley Fresh Steamers Healthy Colors Nature's Blend*), ½ cup* | 40 | 1.0 | 8.0 | 1.0 | 0 | 220 | 2.0 |
| (*Green Giant Valley Fresh Steamers Healthy Colors Valley Blend*), ½ cup* . | 40 | 1.0 | 8.0 | 1.0 | 0 | 270 | 2.0 |
| (*Green Giant Simply Steam* Garden Medley), ½ cup* .... | 50 | 2.0 | 11.0 | .5 | 0 | 280 | 1.0 |
| (*McKenzie's* Seasoning Blend), ½ cup ....... | 10 | 0 | 2.0 | 0 | 0 | 10 | 0 |
| (*Veg-All SteamSupreme* Original), ⅔ cup ..... | 45 | 1.0 | 10.0 | 0 | 0 | 15 | 2.0 |
| (*Veg-All SteamSupreme* Summer Blend), ⅔ cup | 25 | 1.0 | 5.0 | 0 | 0 | 15 | 2.0 |
| (*Veg-All SteamSupreme* Winter Blend), 1 cup .. | 25 | 2.0 | 4.0 | 0 | 0 | 5 | 2.0 |
| Alfredo (*Green Giant* Bag), ½ cup* ....... | 60 | 3.0 | 9.0 | 1.5 | 0 | 360 | 2.0 |
| Asian: (*C&W*), ¾ cup ...... | 60 | 3.0 | 9.0 | 1.0 | 0 | 180 | 2.0 |
| (*Green Giant Valley Fresh Steamers*), ½ cup* .......... | 50 | 2.0 | 8.0 | 1.5 | 0 | 135 | 2.0 |
| (*Veg-All SteamSupreme* Far East), 1 cup ........... | 90 | 4.0 | 15.0 | 1.0 | 0 | 320 | 3.0 |
| sesame ginger sauce (*Birds Eye*), 1 cup . | 60 | 2.0 | 12.0 | 1.0 | 0 | 630 | 2.0 |
| baby (*Green Giant Simply Steam* Garden Medley), ½ cup* .... | 50 | 2.0 | 11.0 | .5 | 0 | 280 | 1.0 |
| butter sauce (*Green Giant* Immunity Blend), 1 cup ....... | 70 | 1.0 | 11.0 | 2.5 | 5 | 190 | 2.0 |
| California blend: (*Birds Eye*), 1 cup .... | 25 | <1.0 | 4.0 | 0 | 0 | 30 | 1.0 |

| Food and Measure | cal. | prot. (gms) | carbo. (gms) | fat (gms) | chol. (mgs) | sod. (mgs) | fiber (gms) |
|---|---|---|---|---|---|---|---|
| **Vegetables, mixed, frozen, California blend** *(cont.)* | | | | | | | |
| (*Cascadian Farm Organic*), ⅔ cup ... | 25 | 1.0 | 5.0 | 0 | 0 | 25 | 2.0 |
| (*Freshlike*), 1 cup .... | 30 | 1.0 | 5.0 | 0 | 0 | 35 | 2.0 |
| cheddar sauce (*Birds Eye*), ½ cup ...... | 80 | 2.0 | 8.0 | 4.0 | 5 | 390 | 1.0 |
| Chinese stir-fry (*Cascadian Farm Organic*), 1 cup ...... | 25 | 1.0 | 5.0 | 0 | 0 | 15 | 2.0 |
| garlic herb sauce (*Green Giant* Digestive Health), ½ cup* ..... | 80 | 4.0 | 14.0 | 2.5 | 0 | 390 | 5.0 |
| gumbo mix (*McKenzie's*), ¾ cup .. | 45 | 1.0 | 9.0 | 0 | 0 | 20 | 2.0 |
| Italian blend (*Birds Eye Steamfresh*), ¾ cup ............. | 30 | 1.0 | 5.0 | 0 | 0 | 35 | 2.0 |
| Normandy blend (*Birds Eye*), 1 cup ......... | 25 | 1.0 | 5.0 | 0 | 0 | 35 | 2.0 |
| Oriental stir-fry (*Birds Eye*), 1 cup ......... | 50 | 2.0 | 9.0 | 0 | 0 | 300 | 2.0 |
| soup mix, ⅔ cup: | | | | | | | |
| (*Freshlike*) ......... | 50 | 1.0 | 9.0 | 0 | 0 | 40 | 2.0 |
| (*McKenzie's*) ........ | 45 | 1.0 | 9.0 | 0 | 0 | 40 | 2.0 |
| stew mix: | | | | | | | |
| (*Freshlike*), ⅔ cup ... | 45 | 1.0 | 9.0 | 0 | 0 | 45 | 1.0 |
| (*McKenzie's*), ¾ cup .. | 45 | <1.0 | 9.0 | 0 | 0 | 40 | 1.0 |
| Szechuan, sesame sauce (*Birds Eye*), 1 cup .... | 60 | 1.0 | 9.0 | 1.5 | 0 | 460 | 2.0 |
| teriyaki: | | | | | | | |
| (*Green Giant*), 1¼ cups | 40 | 2.0 | 9.0 | 0 | 0 | 400 | 2.0 |
| stir-fry (*Birds Eye*), 2 cups .......... | 170 | 6.0 | 33.0 | 1.0 | 0 | 540 | 3.0 |
| Thai stir-fry: | | | | | | | |
| (*Birds Eye*), 1 cup .... | 50 | 3.0 | 10.0 | .5 | 0 | 350 | 3.0 |
| (*Cascadian Farm Organic*), ¾ cup ... | 25 | 1.0 | 5.0 | 0 | 0 | 15 | 2.0 |
| Tuscan, herb sauce, tomato (*Birds Eye*), 1 cup ............. | 50 | 1.0 | 7.0 | 2.0 | 0 | 180 | 2.0 |
| **Vegetables, mixed, pickled**, giardiniera: | | | | | | | |
| (*B&G*), 2 pcs., 1 oz. .... | 7 | 0 | 1.0 | 0 | 0 | 420 | 0 |
| (*Roland*), 1 oz. ........ | 10 | 0 | 2.0 | 0 | 0 | 580 | 1.0 |

| Food and Measure | cal. | prot. (gms) | carbo. (gms) | fat (gms) | chol. (mgs) | sod. (mgs) | fiber (gms) |
|---|---|---|---|---|---|---|---|
| **Vegetarian dish** (see also "Vegetarian entree" and specific listings): | | | | | | | |
| canned: | | | | | | | |
| (*Loma Linda* Tender Bits), 6 pcs., 3 oz. | 120 | 13.0 | 7.0 | 4.0 | 0 | 440 | 3.0 |
| (*Loma Linda Tender Rounds*), 6 pcs. | 120 | 13.0 | 6.0 | 4.5 | 0 | 340 | 1.0 |
| (*Worthington Choplets*), 2 slices, 3.3 oz. | 90 | 18.0 | 4.0 | 1.0 | 0 | 500 | 2.0 |
| (*Worthington MultiGrain Cutlets*), 2 slices, 3.2 oz. | 100 | 17.0 | 5.0 | 1.0 | 0 | 290 | 3.0 |
| frozen (*Worthington Dinner Roast*), ¾" slice | 180 | 14.0 | 6.0 | 11.0 | 0 | 580 | 3.0 |
| **Vegetarian entree, frozen** (see also specific listings), 1 pkg.: | | | | | | | |
| basil pesto (*Healthy Choice*), 8 oz. | 250 | 10.0 | 36.0 | 7.0 | 10 | 450 | 5.0 |
| beans, red, vegetable casserole (*Moosewood Organic Chilaquile*), 10 oz. | 410 | 15.0 | 49.0 | 17.0 | 25 | 760 | 8.0 |
| Thai stir-fry (*Amy's*), 10 oz. | 310 | 8.0 | 45.0 | 11.0 | 0 | 420 | 5.0 |
| Tuscan bake (*Kashi*), 10 oz. | 260 | 7.0 | 42.0 | 9.0 | 0 | 700 | 8.0 |
| **Venison**, meat only, 4 oz.: | | | | | | | |
| roasted | 179 | 34.3 | 0 | 3.6 | 127 | 61 | 0 |
| ground, pan-broiled | 212 | 30.0 | 0 | 9.3 | 111 | 88 | 0 |
| **Vermicelli dish mix,** garlic/olive oil: | | | | | | | |
| (*Near East*), 2.5 oz. | 240 | 9.0 | 48.0 | 2.5 | 5 | 460 | 2.0 |
| (*Pasta Roni*), 1 cup* | 350 | 9.0 | 47.0 | 14.0 | 0 | 930 | 2.0 |
| **Vine spinach**, raw, untrimmed, 1 lb. | 86 | 8.2 | 15.4 | 1.4 | 0 | 109 | 4.0 |
| **Vinegar**, 1 tbsp., except as noted: | | | | | | | |
| apple cider: | | | | | | | |
| (*Eden* Organic) | 0 | 0 | 0 | 0 | 0 | 0 | 0 |
| (*Musselman's*) | 6 | 0 | 0 | 0 | 0 | 4 | 0 |

| Food and Measure | cal. | prot. (gms) | carbo. (gms) | fat (gms) | chol. (mgs) | sod. (mgs) | fiber (gms) |
|---|---|---|---|---|---|---|---|
| **Vinegar** *(cont.)* | | | | | | | |
| balsamic: | | | | | | | |
| (*Alessi*) . . . . . . . . . . . | 20 | 0 | 5.0 | 0 | 0 | 0 | 0 |
| (*Consul*) . . . . . . . . . . | 10 | 0 | 3.0 | 0 | 0 | 0 | 0 |
| (*Holland House*) . . . . . | 15 | 0 | 4.0 | 0 | 0 | 0 | 0 |
| (*Progresso*) . . . . . . . . | 10 | 0 | 2.0 | 0 | 0 | 0 | 0 |
| (*Regina*) . . . . . . . . . . | 20 | 0 | 3.5 | 0 | 0 | 2 | 0 |
| (*Roland* Gold Label/ | | | | | | | |
| Organic) . . . . . . . . . | 10 | 0 | 3.0 | 0 | 0 | 0 | 0 |
| (*Vigo*) . . . . . . . . . . . | 15 | 0 | 3.0 | 0 | 0 | 0 | 0 |
| fig, pear, or | | | | | | | |
| raspberry (*Alessi*) . | 20 | 0 | 5.0 | 0 | 0 | 0 | 0 |
| white (*Roland*) . . . . . . | 30 | 0 | 7.0 | 0 | 0 | 0 | 0 |
| white (*Vigo*) . . . . . . . . | 10 | 0 | 3.0 | 0 | 0 | 0 | 0 |
| balsamic glaze: | | | | | | | |
| (*Roland*) . . . . . . . . . . | 20 | 0 | 4.0 | 0 | 0 | 0 | 0 |
| ginger (*Roland*) . . . . . | 45 | 0 | 11.0 | 0 | 0 | 0 | 0 |
| fig, orange, or | | | | | | | |
| tamarind (*Roland*) . | 40 | 0 | 10.0 | 0 | 0 | 0 | 0 |
| pomegranate (*Roland*) | 20 | 0 | 4.0 | 0 | 0 | 0 | 0 |
| Chianti (*Roland*) . . . . . . . | 0 | 0 | 0 | 0 | 0 | 0 | 0 |
| fish and chips (*Crosse* | | | | | | | |
| *& Blackwell*) . . . . . . . . | 0 | 0 | 0 | 0 | 0 | 0 | 0 |
| malt (*Holland House*) . . . | 0 | 0 | 0 | 0 | 0 | 0 | 0 |
| muscatel (*Don Bruno*) . . . | 25 | 0 | 6.0 | 0 | 0 | 4 | 0 |
| red wine (*Regina* | | | | | | | |
| Velvet) . . . . . . . . . . . | 5 | 0 | 1.0 | 0 | 0 | 0 | 0 |
| red or white wine: | | | | | | | |
| (*Alessi/Vigo*) . . . . . . . . | 0 | 0 | 0 | 0 | 0 | 0 | 0 |
| (*Holland House*) . . . . . | 0 | 0 | 0 | 0 | 0 | 0 | 0 |
| (*Regina*) . . . . . . . . . . | 0 | 0 | <1.0 | 0 | 0 | 0 | 0 |
| plain or flavored | | | | | | | |
| (*Roland*) . . . . . . . . . | 0 | 0 | 0 | 0 | 0 | 0 | 0 |
| rice: | | | | | | | |
| (*Nakano*) . . . . . . . . . . | 0 | 0 | 0 | 0 | 0 | 0 | 0 |
| (*Roland*) . . . . . . . . . . | 5 | 0 | 1.0 | 0 | 0 | 30 | 0 |
| brown (*Eden* Organic) | 2 | 0 | 0 | 0 | 0 | 0 | 0 |
| w/basil and oregano, | | | | | | | |
| garlic, or red pepper | | | | | | | |
| (*Roland*) . . . . . . . . . | 10 | 0 | 3.0 | 0 | 0 | 0 | 0 |
| seasoned (*Roland*) . . . | 5 | 0 | 2.0 | 0 | 0 | 150 | 0 |
| seasoned (*Kikkoman*) . | 20 | 0 | 5.0 | 0 | 0 | 510 | 0 |
| seasoned (*Nakano*) . . . | 20 | 0 | 5.0 | 0 | 0 | 240 | 0 |

| Food and Measure | cal. | prot. (gms) | carbo. (gms) | fat (gms) | chol. (mgs) | sod. (mgs) | fiber (gms) |
|---|---|---|---|---|---|---|---|
| ume plum (*Eden*), 1 tsp. . | 2 | 0 | 0 | 0 | 0 | 1050 | 0 |
| wine (*Don Bruno* Pedro Ximenez) ..... | 15 | 0 | 3.0 | 0 | 0 | 0 | 0 |
| **Vinegar reduction**, wine, all varieties (*Roland*), 1 tbsp. .... | 45 | 0 | 11.0 | 0 | 0 | 0 | 0 |

# W

| Food and Measure | cal. | prot. (gms) | carbo. (gms) | fat (gms) | chol. (mgs) | sod. (mgs) | fiber (gms) |
|---|---|---|---|---|---|---|---|
| **Waffle**, frozen, 2 pcs., except as noted: | | | | | | | |
| (*Aunt Jemima* Homestyle) ......... | 170 | 4.0 | 27.0 | 5.0 | <5 | 480 | <1.0 |
| (*Aunt Jemima* Low-Fat) . | 160 | 4.0 | 27.0 | 3.0 | <5 | 470 | <1.0 |
| (*Eggo* Homestyle) ...... | 190 | 4.0 | 27.0 | 7.0 | 15 | 370 | <1.0 |
| (*Eggo* Homestyle Minis), 3 sets of 4 .... | 260 | 6.0 | 38.0 | 10.0 | 25 | 610 | 1.0 |
| (*GoLean* Original) ...... | 170 | 8.0 | 33.0 | 3.0 | 0 | 330 | 6.0 |
| (*Nature's Path* Homestyle Organic Gluten Free) ........ | 270 | 2.0 | 44.0 | 10.0 | 0 | 420 | 2.0 |
| (*Nature's Path Mesa Sunrise* Organic Gluten Free) .............. | 200 | 2.0 | 34.0 | 7.0 | 0 | 450 | 1.0 |
| (*Van's* Belgian) ........ | 210 | 3.0 | 29.0 | 9.0 | 0 | 430 | 1.0 |
| (*Van's* Gluten Free) ..... | 230 | 2.0 | 39.0 | 7.0 | 0 | 400 | 1.0 |
| (*Van's* Totally Natural Lite) .............. | 140 | 3.0 | 33.0 | 2.0 | 0 | 340 | 6.0 |
| (*Van's* Totally Natural Minis), 2 sets of 4 .... | 140 | 3.0 | 25.0 | 3.5 | 0 | 360 | <1.0 |
| (*Van's* Totally Natural Organics) .......... | 200 | 5.0 | 29.0 | 7.0 | 0 | 350 | 6.0 |
| (*Van's* Wheat Free Minis), 2 sets of 4 .... | 150 | 2.0 | 25.0 | 5.0 | 0 | 250 | 1.0 |
| apple cinnamon (*Van's* Gluten Free) ... | 230 | 2.0 | 39.0 | 7.0 | 0 | 390 | 1.0 |
| blueberry: | | | | | | | |
| (*Aunt Jemima*) ...... | 180 | 4.0 | 29.0 | 5.0 | <5 | 470 | <1.0 |
| (*Eggo*) ............ | 190 | 4.0 | 29.0 | 6.0 | 15 | 370 | <1.0 |
| (*Eggo Nutri-Grain*) ... | 180 | 4.0 | 31.0 | 5.0 | 0 | 370 | 3.0 |
| (*GoLean*) .......... | 170 | 8.0 | 33.0 | 3.0 | 0 | 300 | 6.0 |

| Food and Measure | cal. | prot. (gms) | carbo. (gms) | fat (gms) | chol. (mgs) | sod. (mgs) | fiber (gms) |
|---|---|---|---|---|---|---|---|
| (*Smucker's Snack'n Waffles*), 2-oz. pc. | 220 | 4.0 | 33.0 | 8.0 | 20 | 220 | 2.0 |
| (*Van's* Gluten Free) | 230 | 2.0 | 39.0 | 7.0 | 0 | 380 | 1.0 |
| (*Van's* Organics) | 210 | 5.0 | 31.0 | 7.0 | 0 | 340 | 6.0 |
| buckwheat: | | | | | | | |
| (*Van's* Gluten Free) | 240 | 2.0 | 42.0 | 7.0 | 0 | 370 | 3.0 |
| wildberry (*Nature's Path* Organic) | 190 | 2.0 | 33.0 | 7.0 | 0 | 330 | 1.0 |
| buttermilk: | | | | | | | |
| (*Aunt Jemima*) | 190 | 4.0 | 29.0 | 5.0 | <5 | 510 | <1.0 |
| (*Eggo*) | 200 | 5.0 | 27.0 | 8.0 | 20 | 370 | <1.0 |
| chocolate chip: | | | | | | | |
| (*Eggo*) | 210 | 4.0 | 32.0 | 7.0 | 15 | 380 | 1.0 |
| (*Smucker's Snack'n Waffles*), 2-oz. pc. | 220 | 5.0 | 32.0 | 8.0 | 25 | 230 | 2.0 |
| (*Van's* Mini), 2 sets of 4 | 150 | 3.0 | 27.0 | 4.0 | 0 | 350 | <1.0 |
| cinnamon: | | | | | | | |
| (*Smucker's Snack'n Waffles*), 2-oz. pc. | 210 | 5.0 | 31.0 | 8.0 | 25 | 240 | 2.0 |
| toast (*Eggo*), 3 sets of 4 | 300 | 5.0 | 45.0 | 11.0 | 20 | 490 | 1.0 |
| flax: | | | | | | | |
| (*Nature's Path Flax Plus* Organic) | 200 | 4.0 | 30.0 | 8.0 | 0 | 330 | 5.0 |
| (*Van's* Gluten Free) | 230 | 3.0 | 37.0 | 7.0 | 0 | 370 | 2.0 |
| (*Van's* Organics) | 200 | 5.0 | 27.0 | 8.0 | 0 | 320 | 6.0 |
| w/figs (*Nature's Path Flax Plus* Organic) | 190 | 4.0 | 25.0 | 9.0 | 0 | 340 | 4.0 |
| red berry (*Nature's Path Flax Plus* Organic) | 180 | 4.0 | 26.0 | 8.0 | 0 | 350 | 4.0 |
| French toast (*Eggo*), 1 pc. | 140 | 3.0 | 19.0 | 6.0 | 10 | 240 | <1.0 |
| hemp (*Nature's Path Hemp Plus* Organic) | 200 | 4.0 | 30.0 | 8.0 | 0 | 290 | 5.0 |
| honey oat (*Heart to Heart*) | 160 | 6.0 | 31.0 | 3.0 | 0 | 370 | 3.0 |
| maple (*Smucker's Snack'n Waffles*), 2-oz. pc. | 220 | 4.0 | 32.0 | 8.0 | 25 | 230 | 2.0 |
| maple cinnamon (*Nature's Path Maple Cinn* Organic) | 180 | 4.0 | 28.0 | 6.0 | 0 | 380 | 4.0 |

| Food and Measure | cal. | prot. (gms) | carbo. (gms) | fat (gms) | chol. (mgs) | sod. (mgs) | fiber (gms) |
|---|---|---|---|---|---|---|---|
| **Waffle** *(cont.)* | | | | | | | |
| multigrain: | | | | | | | |
| (*Van's* Belgian) ...... | 190 | 3.0 | 32.0 | 7.0 | 0 | 330 | 6.0 |
| 8 (*Van's*) .......... | 180 | 3.0 | 31.0 | 7.0 | 0 | 320 | 6.0 |
| 8, berry (*Van's*) ...... | 190 | 3.0 | 33.0 | 7.0 | 0 | 320 | 6.0 |
| 8, maple (*Van's*) ..... | 200 | 3.0 | 35.0 | 7.0 | 0 | 330 | 6.0 |
| pomegranate (*Nature's Path* | | | | | | | |
| *Pomagran Plus* Organic) | 160 | 4.0 | 27.0 | 4.5 | 0 | 360 | 4.0 |
| strawberry: | | | | | | | |
| (*Eggo*) ........... | 190 | 4.0 | 29.0 | 6.0 | 15 | 370 | <1.0 |
| flax (*GoLean*) ....... | 160 | 8.0 | 31.0 | 3.0 | 0 | 300 | 6.0 |
| whole wheat: | | | | | | | |
| (*Eggo Nutri-Grain*) ... | 170 | 5.0 | 26.0 | 6.0 | 0 | 400 | 3.0 |
| (*Eggo Nutri-Grain* | | | | | | | |
| Low Fat) ......... | 140 | 5.0 | 27.0 | 2.5 | 0 | 390 | 3.0 |
| **Waffle mix**, see | | | | | | | |
| "Pancake mix" | | | | | | | |
| **Walnut**, dried: | | | | | | | |
| (*Planters*), 1.1 oz. ...... | 210 | 5.0 | 4.0 | 20.0 | 0 | 0 | 2.0 |
| black: | | | | | | | |
| (*Planters*), 2-oz. pkg. . | 370 | 14.0 | 7.0 | 33.0 | 0 | 0 | 4.0 |
| shelled (*Diamond*), | | | | | | | |
| ¼ cup, 1.1 oz. ...... | 190 | 7.0 | 3.0 | 18.0 | 0 | 0 | 2.0 |
| shelled, 1 oz. ........ | 172 | 6.9 | 3.4 | 16.1 | 0 | <1 | 1.4 |
| chopped, 1 cup ...... | 759 | 30.4 | 15.1 | 70.7 | 0 | 2 | 6.3 |
| English or Persian: | | | | | | | |
| all varieties | | | | | | | |
| (*Diamond*), 1.1 oz. . | 200 | 5.0 | 4.0 | 20.0 | 0 | 0 | 2.0 |
| shelled, 1 oz. ....... | 182 | 4.1 | 5.2 | 17.6 | 0 | 3 | 1.4 |
| pieces., 1 cup ....... | 770 | 17.2 | 22.0 | 74.2 | 0 | 12 | 5.8 |
| halves, 1 cup ....... | 642 | 14.3 | 18.3 | 61.9 | 0 | 10 | 4.8 |
| pieces (*Planters*), 1 oz. .. | 210 | 5.0 | 4.0 | 19.0 | 0 | 0 | 2.0 |
| **Walnut topping**, in | | | | | | | |
| syrup (*Smucker's*), | | | | | | | |
| 2 tbsp. ............. | 150 | 2.0 | 20.0 | 7.0 | 0 | 0 | <1.0 |
| **Wasabi**, root, fresh, | | | | | | | |
| sliced, ½ cup ...... | 71 | 3.1 | 15.3 | .4 | 0 | 11 | 5.0 |
| **Wasabi paste** (*Roland*), | | | | | | | |
| 1 tsp. ............. | 15 | 0 | 2.0 | .5 | 0 | 95 | 0 |
| **Wasabi powder**: | | | | | | | |
| (*Eden*), 1 tsp. ......... | 10 | 0 | 1.0 | 0 | 0 | 0 | .5 |
| (*Roland*), ¼ tsp. ....... | 0 | 0 | 0 | 0 | 0 | 0 | 0 |
| **Wasabi sauce**, w/ginger | | | | | | | |
| (*Gold's*), 1 tsp. ...... | 15 | 0 | 1.0 | 1.5 | 5 | 15 | 0 |

| Food and Measure | cal. | prot. (gms) | carbo. (gms) | fat (gms) | chol. (mgs) | sod. (mgs) | fiber (gms) |
|---|---|---|---|---|---|---|---|
| **Water chestnut**, fresh: | | | | | | | |
| (*Frieda's*), sliced, | | | | | | | |
| 1 cup ............. | 120 | 2.0 | 30.0 | 0 | 0 | 17 | 4.0 |
| 4 medium, 1.3 oz. ...... | 35 | .5 | 8.6 | <.1 | 0 | 5 | 1.1 |
| sliced, ½ cup .......... | 60 | .9 | 14.8 | .1 | 0 | 9 | 1.9 |
| **Water chestnut,** | | | | | | | |
| **can/jar**: | | | | | | | |
| whole, 4 pcs., 1 oz. ..... | 14 | .3 | 3.5 | <.1 | 0 | 2 | .7 |
| whole or sliced: | | | | | | | |
| (*Ka•Me*), 1 can | | | | | | | |
| drained, | | | | | | | |
| 4.9 oz. .......... | 45 | 1.0 | 11.0 | 0 | 0 | 10 | 4.0 |
| (*Roland*), ½ cup ..... | 40 | 1.0 | 9.0 | 0 | 0 | 20 | 1.0 |
| sliced, ½ cup: | | | | | | | |
| (*Geisha*) .......... | 50 | 1.0 | 9.0 | 0 | 0 | 25 | 1.0 |
| (*La Choy*) .......... | 25 | 1.0 | 5.0 | 0 | 0 | 10 | 1.0 |
| w/liquid ............. | 35 | .5 | 8.7 | <.1 | 0 | 6 | 1.8 |
| **Watercress**: | | | | | | | |
| (*Frieda's*), 1 cup, | | | | | | | |
| 3 oz. ............. | 10 | 2.0 | 1.0 | 0 | 0 | 35 | 2.0 |
| 10 sprigs, 11¼" ........ | 3 | .6 | .3 | <.1 | 0 | 10 | .6 |
| chopped, ½ cup ....... | 2 | .4 | .2 | <.1 | 0 | 7 | .4 |
| **Watermelon**, fresh: | | | | | | | |
| (*Earthbound Farm* | | | | | | | |
| Organic), 10 oz. ..... | 80 | 1.0 | 21.0 | 0 | 0 | 0 | 1.0 |
| 1" slice, 10" diam. ...... | 152 | 3.0 | 34.6 | 2.0 | 0 | 10 | 2.4 |
| diced, ½ cup .......... | 25 | .5 | 5.7 | .3 | 0 | 2 | .4 |
| yellow, seedless | | | | | | | |
| (*Frieda's*), 3 oz. ...... | 25 | 1.0 | 6.0 | 0 | 0 | 0 | 0 |
| **Watermelon drink** | | | | | | | |
| **blend**, 8 fl. oz.: | | | | | | | |
| (*AriZona*) ............. | 100 | 0 | 25.0 | 0 | 0 | 10 | 0 |
| strawberry (*Nantucket* | | | | | | | |
| *Nectars*) ......... | 110 | 0 | 28.0 | 0 | 0 | 25 | 0 |
| **Watermelon seeds,** | | | | | | | |
| dried, 1 oz. ......... | 158 | 8.1 | 4.4 | 13.5 | 0 | 28 | n.a. |
| **Wax beans, canned**: | | | | | | | |
| (*Del Monte*), ½ cup ..... | 20 | 1.0 | 4.0 | 0 | 0 | 360 | 2.0 |
| cut (*S&W*), ½ cup ...... | 20 | 1.0 | 4.0 | 0 | 0 | 360 | 2.0 |
| **Wax gourd**, cubed: | | | | | | | |
| raw (*Frieda's*), 1 cup .... | 20 | 0 | 4.0 | 0 | 0 | 147 | 4.0 |
| raw, 1 cup ............ | 17 | .5 | 4.0 | .3 | 0 | 147 | 3.8 |
| boiled, drained, 1 cup ... | 23 | .7 | 5.3 | .4 | 0 | 187 | 1.8 |

| Food and Measure | cal. | prot. (gms) | carbo. (gms) | fat (gms) | chol. (mgs) | sod. (mgs) | fiber (gms) |
|---|---|---|---|---|---|---|---|
| **Welsh rarebit**, frozen (*Stouffer's*), ¼ of 10-oz. pkg. .......... | 140 | 6.0 | 6.0 | 10.0 | 20 | 270 | 0 |
| ***Wendy's:*** | | | | | | | |
| burgers: | | | | | | | |
|   bacon deluxe ....... | 670 | 35.0 | 47.0 | 38.0 | 115 | 1460 | 2.0 |
|     double .......... | 890 | 54.0 | 47.0 | 54.0 | 185 | 1630 | 2.0 |
|   *Baconator* .......... | 630 | 33.0 | 43.0 | 36.0 | 110 | 1250 | 1.0 |
|     double .......... | 940 | 55.0 | 45.0 | 59.0 | 195 | 1590 | 2.0 |
|   cheeseburger, Jr. ..... | 270 | 15.0 | 27.0 | 11.0 | 40 | 690 | 1.0 |
|     w/bacon .......... | 350 | 17.0 | 28.0 | 19.0 | 55 | 660 | 2.0 |
|     w/bacon, double ... | 440 | 25.0 | 28.0 | 25.0 | 80 | 730 | 2.0 |
|     deluxe .......... | 300 | 15.0 | 29.0 | 14.0 | 45 | 720 | 2.0 |
|   *Double Stack* ....... | 360 | 23.0 | 27.0 | 18.0 | 70 | 760 | 1.0 |
|   hamburger, Jr. ....... | 230 | 12.0 | 26.0 | 8.0 | 30 | 480 | 1.0 |
|   w/everything, cheese . | 550 | 31.0 | 44.0 | 28.0 | 95 | 1280 | 2.0 |
|     double w/cheese .. | 770 | 50.0 | 44.0 | 44.0 | 160 | 1450 | 2.0 |
|     triple w/cheese .... | 1030 | 71.0 | 44.0 | 62.0 | 240 | 1820 | 2.0 |
| chicken sandwich: | | | | | | | |
|   asiago ranch club: | | | | | | | |
|     grilled ........... | 560 | 41.0 | 43.0 | 24.0 | 125 | 1470 | 2.0 |
|     homestyle ....... | 660 | 33.0 | 55.0 | 34.0 | 85 | 1490 | 3.0 |
|     spicy .......... | 660 | 33.0 | 57.0 | 33.0 | 95 | 1660 | 3.0 |
|   crispy ............. | 330 | 16.0 | 34.0 | 14.0 | 35 | 680 | 1.0 |
|   homestyle fillet ...... | 470 | 26.0 | 52.0 | 18.0 | 50 | 1160 | 3.0 |
|   spicy fillet .......... | 460 | 26.0 | 54.0 | 16.0 | 60 | 1330 | 3.0 |
|   grill, ultimate ....... | 370 | 34.0 | 42.0 | 7.0 | 90 | 1150 | 2.0 |
|   go wrap, grilled ...... | 260 | 20.0 | 25.0 | 10.0 | 55 | 750 | 1.0 |
|     homestyle ....... | 320 | 15.0 | 29.0 | 16.0 | 35 | 760 | 1.0 |
|     spicy .......... | 320 | 15.0 | 30.0 | 16.0 | 40 | 840 | 1.0 |
| chicken nuggets: | | | | | | | |
|   5 pcs. ............. | 230 | 12.0 | 13.0 | 14.0 | 35 | 430 | 0 |
|   10 pcs. ............ | 450 | 23.0 | 25.0 | 29.0 | 70 | 850 | 0 |
|   barbecue sauce ...... | 45 | 0 | 11.0 | 0 | 0 | 120 | 0 |
|   honey mustard ....... | 80 | 0 | 7.0 | 6.0 | 10 | 220 | 0 |
|   sweet & sour ....... | 50 | 0 | 12.0 | 0 | 0 | 120 | 0 |
| wings, boneless: | | | | | | | |
|   honey BBQ ......... | 570 | 33.0 | 69.0 | 18.0 | 80 | 1950 | 3.0 |
|   spicy chipotle ....... | 500 | 33.0 | 48.0 | 20.0 | 80 | 1640 | 3.0 |
|   sweet & spicy ....... | 540 | 33.0 | 62.0 | 18.0 | 80 | 2490 | 3.0 |
|   ranch dipping sauce .. | 120 | 0 | 3.0 | 12.0 | 10 | 240 | 0 |
| *Garden Sensations* salad: | | | | | | | |
|   apple pecan chicken .. | 350 | 37.0 | 29.0 | 12.0 | 110 | 1210 | 5.0 |
|     roasted pecans .... | 110 | 1.0 | 5.0 | 9.0 | 0 | 60 | 1.0 |

| Food and Measure | cal. | prot. (gms) | carbo. (gms) | fat (gms) | chol. (mgs) | sod. (mgs) | fiber (gms) |
|---|---|---|---|---|---|---|---|
| vinaigrette ....... | 60 | 0 | 8.0 | 3.0 | 0 | 160 | 0 |
| Baja salad .......... | 550 | 33.0 | 36.0 | 33.0 | 85 | 1610 | 12.0 |
| tortilla strips ...... | 80 | 1.0 | 11.0 | 4.5 | 0 | 105 | 1.0 |
| jalapeño dressing .. | 100 | 1.0 | 2.0 | ·10.0 | 10 | 270 | 0 |
| BLT cobb ........ | 460 | 46.0 | 12.0 | 26.0 | 285 | 1490 | 3.0 |
| avocado dressing .. | 100 | 1.0 | 1.0 | 10.0 | 10 | 220 | 0 |
| chicken Caesar, spicy | 230 | 17.0 | 14.0 | 13.0 | 50 | 650 | 40 |
| croutons ......... | 80 | 2.0 | 13.0 | 3.0 | 0 | 190 | 0 |
| Caesar dressing ... | 110 | 2.0 | 2.0 | 11.0 | 10 | 180 | 0 |
| added salad dressings: | | | | | | | |
| French, fat free ...... | 40 | 0 | 9.0 | 0 | 0 | 95 | 0 |
| Italian vinaigrette .... | 70 | 0 | 4.0 | 6.0 | 0 | 180 | 0 |
| ranch, classic ....... | 110 | 1.0 | 1.0 | 11.0 | 10 | 190 | 0 |
| ranch, light ......... | 50 | 1.0 | 2.0 | 4.5 | 10 | 200 | 0 |
| Thousand Island ..... | 160 | 0 | 5.0 | 15.0 | 15 | 290 | 0 |
| sides: | | | | | | | |
| chili, large .......... | 330 | 28.0 | 32.0 | 10.0 | 50 | 1310 | 8.0 |
| chili, small ....... | 220 | 18.0 | 22.0 | 7.0 | 35 | 870 | 6.0 |
| cheddar ......... | 70 | 4.0 | 1.0 | 6.0 | 15 | 105 | 0 |
| hot seasoning .... | 5 | 0 | 1.0 | 0 | 0 | 270 | 0 |
| saltines, 2 ........ | 25 | 1.0 | 5.0 | 0 | 0 | 80 | 0 |
| fries, large ......... | 520 | 6.0 | 67.0 | 25.0 | 0 | 630 | 7.0 |
| medium ......... | 420 | 5.0 | 54.0 | 20.0 | 0 | 500 | 6.0 |
| small ........... | 320 | 4.0 | 41.0 | 15.0 | 0 | 380 | 5.0 |
| value ........... | 220 | 3.0 | 29.0 | 11.0 | 0 | 270 | 3.0 |
| ketchup pkt. ...... | 10 | 0 | 3.0 | 0 | 0 | 115 | 0 |
| mandarin orange cup . | 90 | 1.0 | 21.0 | 0 | 0 | 10 | 1.0 |
| potato, baked ....... | 270 | 7.0 | 61.0 | 0 | 0 | 25 | 7.0 |
| sour cream/chive .. | 320 | 8.0 | 63.0 | 3.5 | 10 | 50 | 7.0 |
| side salad, Caesar .... | 60 | 4.0 | 5.0 | 3.5 | 10 | 95 | 2.0 |
| side salad, garden .... | 25 | 1.0 | 5.0 | 0 | 0 | 30 | 2.0 |
| croutons ......... | 80 | 2.0 | 13.0 | 3.0 | 0 | 190 | 0 |
| *Frosty*, small: | | | | | | | |
| chocolate .......... | 310 | 8.0 | 52.0 | 8.0 | 25 | 140 | 0 |
| chocolate fudge shake | 410 | 11.0 | 94.0 | 11.0 | 35 | 190 | 1.0 |
| *Frosty*-cino ......... | 380 | 7.0 | 63.0 | 11.0 | 35 | 140 | 0 |
| strawberry shake .... | 390 | 7.0 | 66.0 | 11.0 | 35 | 140 | 0 |
| vanilla ............. | 310 | 8.0 | 52.0 | 8.0 | 30 | 150 | 0 |
| vanilla bean shake ... | 380 | 7.0 | 64.0 | 11.0 | 35 | 140 | 0 |
| **Wheat**, whole grain: | | | | | | | |
| (*Arrowhead Mills* | | | | | | | |
| Organic), ¼ cup ..... | 150 | 7.0 | 31.0 | .1.0 | 0 | 0 | 5.0 |
| durum, 1 cup ......... | 651 | 26.3 | 136.6 | 4.7 | 0 | 3 | n.a. |

| Food and Measure | cal. | prot. (gms) | carbo. (gms) | fat (gms) | chol. (mgs) | sod. (mgs) | fiber (gms) |
|---|---|---|---|---|---|---|---|
| **Wheat** *(cont.)* | | | | | | | |
| hard red: | | | | | | | |
| spring, 1 cup ....... | 632 | 29.6 | 130.6 | 3.7 | 0 | 4 | 24.2 |
| winter, 1 cup ........ | 628 | 24.2 | 136.7 | 3.0 | 0 | 4 | 24.2 |
| hard white, 1 cup ...... | 657 | 21.7 | 145.7 | 3.3 | 0 | 4 | n.a. |
| soft red winter, 1 cup ... | 556 | 17.4 | 124.7 | 2.6 | 0 | 4 | 21.0 |
| soft white, 1 cup ....... | 571 | 18.0 | 126.6 | 3.3 | 0 | 3 | 21.3 |
| **Wheat, parboiled,** see "Bulgur" | | | | | | | |
| **Wheat, sprouted**, 1 cup . | 214 | 8.1 | 45.9 | 1.4 | 0 | 18 | 1.2 |
| **Wheat berries**, see "Wheat kernels" | | | | | | | |
| **Wheat bran** (see also "Cereal"): | | | | | | | |
| (*Arrowhead Mills* Organic), ⅓ cup ..... | 60 | 3.0 | 10.0 | 1.0 | 0 | 0 | 6.0 |
| crude, unprocessed: | | | | | | | |
| (*Bob's Red Mill*), ¼ cup ........... | 30 | 2.0 | 10.0 | .5 | 0 | 0 | 6.0 |
| (*Hodgson Mill*), ¼ cup | 30 | 2.0 | 10.0 | 0 | 0 | 0 | 7.0 |
| 2 tbsp. ............ | 15 | 1.1 | 4.5 | .3 | 0 | <1 | 3.0 |
| **Wheat flour** (see also specific flour listings), ¼ cup, except as noted: | | | | | | | |
| all purpose, see "white," below | | | | | | | |
| baking blend (*Arrowhead Mills* Organic) ....... | 120 | 4.0 | 25.0 | 0 | 0 | 0 | 3.0 |
| bread: | | | | | | | |
| (*Gold Medal* Better for Bread) ........ | 110 | 4.0 | 22.0 | 0 | 0 | 0 | <1.0 |
| (*Hodgson Mill* Best for Bread) ....... | 100 | 4.0 | 22.0 | 0 | 0 | 0 | 1.0 |
| (*Pillsbury Best*) ...... | 110 | 4.0 | 22.0 | 0 | 0 | 0 | <1.0 |
| cake: | | | | | | | |
| (*Pillsbury Softasilk*) .. | 110 | 3.0 | 25.0 | 0 | 0 | 0 | <1.0 |
| (*Swans Down*) ...... | 100 | 2.0 | 22.0 | 0 | 0 | 0 | 0 |
| self-rising (*Presto*) ... | 90 | 3.0 | 20.0 | 0 | 0 | 0 | 1.0 |
| gluten, see "Wheat gluten" | | | | | | | |
| pasta, see "Semolina flour" | | | | | | | |

| Food and Measure | cal. | prot. (gms) | carbo. (gms) | fat (gms) | chol. (mgs) | sod. (mgs) | fiber (gms) |
|---|---|---|---|---|---|---|---|
| pastry: | | | | | | | |
| (*Arrowhead Mills* Organic), ⅓ cup ... | 110 | 4.0 | 23.0 | .5 | 0 | 0 | 3.0 |
| whole wheat (*Bob's Red Mill* Stoneground Regular/Organic) .. | 110 | 3.0 | 23.0 | .5 | 0 | 0 | 4.0 |
| whole wheat (*Hodgson Mill* Regular/ Organic), <¼ cup .. | 100 | 3.0 | 22.0 | .5 | 0 | 0 | 4.0 |
| seasoned (*Kentucky Kernel*), 4 tsp. ....... | 36 | 1.0 | 8.0 | 0 | 0 | 544 | 0 |
| self-rising: | | | | | | | |
| (*Gold Medal*) ........ | 100 | 3.0 | 23.0 | 0 | 0 | 400 | <1.0 |
| (*Martha White*) ...... | 110 | 3.0 | 23.0 | 0 | 0 | 390 | <1.0 |
| (*Pillsbury Best*) ...... | 100 | 3.0 | 22.0 | 0 | 0 | 370 | <1.0 |
| tortilla mix: | | | | | | | |
| (*Quaker* Harina Preparada), ¼ cup . | 160 | 4.0 | 26.0 | 5.0 | 0 | 370 | 1.0 |
| 1 cup ............. | 449 | 10.7 | 74.5 | 11.8 | 0 | 751 | n.a. |
| white, all-purpose: | | | | | | | |
| (*Gold Medal/Gold Medal* Organic/ Unbleached) ...... | 100 | 3.0 | 22.0 | 0 | 0 | 0 | <1.0 |
| (*Martha White*) ...... | 110 | 3.0 | 24.0 | 0 | 0 | 0 | <1.0 |
| (*Pillsbury Best*) ...... | 110 | 3.0 | 23.0 | 0 | 0 | 0 | <1.0 |
| quick mixing (*Wondra*) ........ | 100 | 3.0 | 23.0 | 0 | 0 | 0 | <1.0 |
| white, hard, stoneground (*Bob's Red Mill* Organic) .... | 120 | 4.0 | 24.0 | .5 | 0 | 0 | 4.0 |
| white, unbleached: | | | | | | | |
| (*Arrowhead Mills* Organic) ......... | 120 | 4.0 | 26.0 | .5 | 0 | 0 | <1.0 |
| (*Bob's Red Mill* Regular/Organic) .. | 124 | 4.0 | 25.0 | 1.0 | 0 | 1 | 1.0 |
| (*Hodgson Mill* All Purpose/Organic), <¼ cup .......... | 100 | 3.0 | 23.0 | 0 | 0 | 0 | 1.0 |
| (*Pillsbury Best*) ...... | 110 | 3.0 | 23.0 | 0 | 0 | 0 | <1.0 |
| whole-grain, 1 cup ..... | 407 | 16.4 | 87.1 | 2.2 | 0 | 1 | 15.1 |
| whole wheat: | | | | | | | |
| (*Arrowhead Mills* Organic Stoneground) | 130 | 5.0 | 26.0 | 1.0 | 0 | 0 | 4.0 |

| Food and Measure | cal. | prot. (gms) | carbo. (gms) | fat (gms) | chol. (mgs) | sod. (mgs) | fiber (gms) |
|---|---|---|---|---|---|---|---|
| **Wheat flour, whole wheat** *(cont.)* | | | | | | | |
| (*Bob's Red Mill* | | | | | | | |
| Stoneground Organic) | 110 | 4.0 | 23.0 | .5 | 0 | 0 | 4.0 |
| (*Gold Medal*) ........ | 100 | 4.0 | 21.0 | .5 | 0 | 0 | 3.0 |
| (*Hodgson Mill*), <¼ cup | 100 | 3.0 | 22.0 | 1.0 | 0 | 0 | 3.0 |
| (*Hodgson Mill* Organic), | | | | | | | |
| <¼ cup ........... | 100 | 4.0 | 22.0 | 1.0 | 0 | 0 | 4.0 |
| (*Pillsbury Best*) ...... | 100 | 4.0 | 22.0 | .5 | 0 | 0 | 3.0 |
| graham (*Bob's Red* | | | | | | | |
| *Mill* Regular/ | | | | | | | |
| Organic) ......... | 110 | 4.0 | 23.0 | .5 | 0 | 0 | 4.0 |
| white (*Hodgson Mill*) . | 100 | 4.0 | 21.0 | .5 | 0 | 0 | 3.0 |
| whole wheat and white | | | | | | | |
| (*Hodgson Mill* | | | | | | | |
| 50/50), <¼ cup ...... | 100 | 4.0 | 21.0 | .5 | 0 | 0 | 3.0 |
| **Wheat germ**, 2 tbsp., | | | | | | | |
| except as noted | | | | | | | |
| (*Hodgson Mill* | | | | | | | |
| Untoasted) ......... | 55 | 4.0 | 8.0 | 1.0 | 0 | 0 | 2.0 |
| (*Mother's*) ............ | 50 | 4.0 | 6.0 | 1.0 | 0 | 0 | 2.0 |
| w/cinnamon, flax | | | | | | | |
| (*Hodgson Mill*) ...... | 65 | 4.0 | 7.0 | 2.0 | 0 | 0 | 3.0 |
| crude, 1 oz. ........... | 102 | 6.6 | 14.7 | 2.8 | 0 | 3 | 3.7 |
| raw (*Arrowhead Mills*), | | | | | | | |
| 3 tbsp. ............ | 60 | 4.0 | 7.0 | 1.5 | 0 | 0 | 2.0 |
| raw (*Bob's Red Mill*) .... | 60 | 4.0 | 9.0 | 1.5 | 0 | 0 | 2.0 |
| toasted, 1 oz. ......... | 108 | 8.3 | 14.1 | 3.0 | 0 | 1 | 3.7 |
| **Wheat gluten**, vital: | | | | | | | |
| (*Arrowhead Mills*), | | | | | | | |
| 1 tbsp. ............ | 35 | 5 | 3.0 | 0 | 0 | 0 | 0 |
| (*Hodgson Mill*), 4 tsp. ... | 40 | 8.0 | 3.0 | 0 | 0 | 0 | 1.0 |
| **Wheat kernels**, ¼ cup: | | | | | | | |
| (*VitaSpelt* Organic) ..... | 160 | 6.0 | 34.0 | 1.0 | 0 | 0 | 7.0 |
| hard red: | | | | | | | |
| (*Bob's Red Mill* | | | | | | | |
| Berries) ......... | 150 | 6.0 | 32.0 | .5 | 0 | 0 | 6.0 |
| (*Bob's Red Mill* | | | | | | | |
| Organic Berries) ... | 170 | 7.0 | 33.0 | 1.0 | 0 | 1 | 6.0 |
| white: | | | | | | | |
| hard (*Bob's Red Mill* | | | | | | | |
| Organic Berries) ... | 160 | 6.0 | 34.0 | .5 | 0 | 0 | 6.0 |
| soft (*Bob's Red Mill* | | | | | | | |
| Berries) ......... | 160 | 70 | 330 | 1.0 | 0 | 0 | 6.0 |

| Food and Measure | cal. | prot. (gms) | carbo. (gms) | fat (gms) | chol. (mgs) | sod. (mgs) | fiber (gms) |
|---|---|---|---|---|---|---|---|
| **Wheat malt syrup**, see "Malt syrup" | | | | | | | |
| **Wheat pilaf mix** (*Near East* Whole Grain), 2 oz. . . . . . . . . | 170 | 7.0 | 40.0 | 1.0 | 0 | 640 | 8.0 |
| **Wheat snacks**, puffed, chili lime (*Sabritones*), 1 oz. . . . | 150 | 2.0 | 13.0 | 10.0 | 0 | 690 | 1.0 |
| **Wheels, pasta, entree,** frozen, cheese, 1 pkg.: | | | | | | | |
| (*Michelina's*), 8 oz. . . . . . | 350 | 13.0 | 48.0 | 11.0 | 20 | 780 | 2.0 |
| (*Michelina's Budget Gourmet*), 7.5 oz. . . . . | 320 | 10.0 | 43.0 | 10.0 | 20 | 620 | 2.0 |
| **Whelk**, meat only: | | | | | | | |
| raw, 4 oz. . . . . . . . . . . . | 156 | 27.0 | 8.8 | .5 | 74 | 234 | 0 |
| boiled, steamed, or poached, 4 oz. . . . . . . | 312 | 54.1 | 17.6 | .9 | 147 | 467 | 0 |
| **Whey**, fluid: | | | | | | | |
| acid, 1 cup . . . . . . . . . | 59 | 1.9 | 12.6 | .2 | 0 | 118 | 0 |
| sweet, 1 cup . . . . . . . . . | 66 | 2.1 | 12.6 | .9 | 5 | 132 | 0 |
| **Whey, protein**, dry (*Designer Whey*), 1 level scoop: | | | | | | | |
| chocolate, double . . . . . . | 100 | 18.0 | 3.0 | 2.0 | 60 | 80 | .5 |
| natural . . . . . . . . . . . . . . | 100 | 19.0 | 2.0 | 2.0 | 60 | 60 | 0 |
| vanilla, French . . . . . . . . | 100 | 18.0 | 3.0 | 2.0 | 55 | 60 | 0 |
| vanilla almond . . . . . . . . | 100 | 18.0 | 3.0 | 2.0 | 60 | 65 | 0 |
| **Whipped topping**, see "Cream topping" | | | | | | | |
| **White bean**, mature: | | | | | | | |
| boiled, ½ cup . . . . . . . | 125 | 8.6 | 22.6 | .3 | 0 | 6 | 5.7 |
| small, boiled, ½ cup . . . . | 124 | 8.7 | 22.5 | .3 | 0 | 5 | 5.6 |
| **White bean, canned**: | | | | | | | |
| (*S&W*), ½ cup . . . . . . . . | 110 | 7.0 | 19.0 | .5 | 0 | 480 | 6.0 |
| w/liquid, ½ cup . . . . . . . | 153 | 9.5 | 28.7 | .4 | 0 | 595 | 6.3 |
| **White bean flour** (*Bob's Red Mill*), ¼ cup . . . . . . . . . . . | 110 | 7.0 | 20.0 | 0 | 0 | 0 | 8.0 |
| **White bean seasoning** (*Zatarain's*), 1 tsp. . . . | 15 | 0 | 3.0 | 0 | 0 | 420 | 0 |
| **Whitefish**, meat only: | | | | | | | |
| raw, 4 oz. . . . . . . . . . . . | 153 | 21.7 | 0 | 6.7 | 68 | 58 | 0 |
| baked or broiled, 4 oz. . . | 195 | 27.7 | 0 | 8.5 | 87 | 74 | 0 |
| smoked, 4 oz. . . . . . . . . | 122 | 26.5 | 0 | 1.1 | 37 | 1156 | 0 |

| Food and Measure | cal. | prot. (gms) | carbo. (gms) | fat (gms) | chol. (mgs) | sod. (mgs) | fiber (gms) |
|---|---|---|---|---|---|---|---|
| **Whiting**, meat only: | | | | | | | |
| raw, 4 oz. . . . . . . . . . . | 102 | 20.8 | 0 | 1.5 | 76 | 82 | 0 |
| baked or broiled, 4 oz. . . | 130 | 26.6 | 0 | 1.9 | 95 | 150 | 0 |
| **Wiener**, see "Frankfurter" | | | | | | | |
| **Wild rice:** | | | | | | | |
| raw, ¼ cup: | | | | | | | |
| (*Eden*) . . . . . . . . . . . | 160 | 6.0 | 35.0 | .5 | 0 | 15 | 3.0 |
| (*Lundberg* Organic) . . | 150 | 6.0 | 33.0 | 1.0 | 0 | 0 | 2.0 |
| (*Lundberg* Organic Quick) . . . . . . . . . | 150 | 6.0 | 33.0 | .5 | 0 | 0 | 2.0 |
| (*Roland*) . . . . . . . . . . | 170 | 6.0 | 35.0 | 0 | 0 | 0 | 2.0 |
| cooked, 1 cup . . . . . . . . | 166 | 6.5 | 35.0 | .6 | 0 | 6 | 1.5 |
| **Wild rice blends**, see "Rice" | | | | | | | |
| **Wild rice dish**, see "Rice" | | | | | | | |
| **Wine**, 3.5 fl. oz., except as noted: | | | | | | | |
| dessert or apertif[1] . . . . . . | 158 | .2 | 12.2 | 0 | 0 | 9 | 0 |
| dry or table[2]: | | | | | | | |
| red . . . . . . . . . . . . . | 74 | .2 | 1.8 | 0 | 0 | 5 | 0 |
| rose . . . . . . . . . . . . . | 73 | .2 | 1.4 | 0 | 0 | 5 | 0 |
| white . . . . . . . . . . . . | 70 | .1 | .8 | 0 | 0 | 5 | 0 |
| sake, 1 fl. oz. . . . . . . . . . | 39 | .1 | .1 | 0 | 0 | <1 | 0 |
| **Wine, cooking**, 2 tbsp., except as noted: | | | | | | | |
| Burgundy (*Roland*) . . . . . | 20 | 0 | 1.0 | 0 | 0 | 230 | 0 |
| Marsala: | | | | | | | |
| (*Holland House*) . . . . . | 45 | 0 | 4.0 | 0 | 0 | 190 | 0 |
| (*Roland*) . . . . . . . . . . | 30 | 0 | 4.0 | 0 | 0 | 190 | 0 |
| red: | | | | | | | |
| (*Holland House*) . . . . . | 20 | 0 | 1.0 | 0 | 0 | 190 | 0 |
| (*Regina*) . . . . . . . . . . | 25 | 0 | 3.0 | 0 | 0 | 190 | 0 |
| rice, sweet, 1 tbsp.: | | | | | | | |
| (*Eden* Mirin) . . . . . . . . | 25 | 0 | 7.0 | 0 | 0 | 130 | 0 |
| (*Kikkoman* Mirin) . . . . | 40 | 0 | 10.0 | 0 | 0 | 15 | 0 |

[1] Includes fortified wines containing more than 15% alcohol, such as port, sherry, vermouth, etc.

[2] Includes wines containing less than 15% alcohol, such as burgundy, Chablis, champagne, etc.

| Food and Measure | cal. | prot. (gms) | carbo. (gms) | fat (gms) | chol. (mgs) | sod. (mgs) | fiber (gms) |
|---|---|---|---|---|---|---|---|
| seasoned (*Sun Luck*) . | 25 | 0 | 6.0 | 0 | 0 | 180 | 0 |
| Sauterne, sherry or Chablis (*Roland*) ..... | 17 | 0 | 4.0 | 0 | 0 | 190 | 0 |
| sherry: | | | | | | | |
| (*Holland House*) ..... | 45 | 0 | 2.0 | 0 | 0 | 190 | 0 |
| (*Regina*) ........... | 35 | 0 | 5.0 | 0 | 0 | 190 | 0 |
| vermouth (*Holland House*) ........... | 35 | 0 | 2.0 | 0 | 0 | 190 | 0 |
| white: | | | | | | | |
| (*Regina*) ........... | 20 | 0 | 3.0 | 0 | 0 | 190 | 0 |
| regular or lemon (*Holland House*) ... | 20 | 0 | 0 | 0 | 0 | 190 | 0 |
| **Wing sauce** (see also "Hot sauce"), 1 tbsp., except as noted: | | | | | | | |
| (*Di Lusso* Buffalo), 1 tsp. ........... | 0 | 0 | 0 | 0 | 0 | 170 | 0 |
| (*Frank's Red Hot* Buffalo) ........... | 0 | 0 | 0 | 0 | 0 | 460 | 0 |
| (*Ken's* Buffalo) ....... | 15 | 0 | 1.0 | 1.5 | 0 | 490 | 0 |
| barbecue (*Frank's Red Hot* Sweet Heat) ..... | 20 | 0 | 4.0 | 0 | 0 | 290 | 0 |
| hot (*Frank's Red Hot* Buffalo) ........... | 5 | 0 | 0 | 0 | 0 | 460 | 0 |
| **Winged bean**, fresh: | | | | | | | |
| raw, sliced, ½ cup ...... | 11 | 1.5 | 1.0 | .2 | 0 | 1 | n.a. |
| boiled, drained, ½ cup .. | 12 | 1.6 | 1.0 | .2 | 0 | 1 | n.a. |
| **Winged bean, mature:** | | | | | | | |
| dry, ½ cup ........... | 372 | 27.0 | 38.0 | 14.9 | 0 | 35 | 14.1 |
| boiled, ½ cup ......... | 126 | 9.1 | 12.8 | 5.0 | 0 | 11 | n.a. |
| **Winged bean leaves,** trimmed, 1 oz. ...... | 21 | 1.7 | 4.0 | .3 | 0 | 3. | n.a. |
| **Winged bean tuber,** trimmed, 1 oz. ...... | 45 | 3.3 | 8.0 | .3 | 0 | 10 | n.a. |
| **Winter melon,** see "Wax gourd" | | | | | | | |
| **Winter squash** (see also specific listings): | | | | | | | |
| (*Green Giant*), 4 oz. ..... | 40 | 1.0 | 10.0 | 0 | 0 | 0 | 2.0 |
| all varieties, cubed: | | | | | | | |
| raw, 1 cup .......... | 43 | 1.7 | 10.2 | .3 | 0 | 5 | 1.7 |
| boiled, drained, 1 cup . | 80 | 1.8 | 17.9 | 1.3 | 0 | 2 | 5.7 |

| Food and Measure | cal. | prot. (gms) | carbo. (gms) | fat (gms) | chol. (mgs) | sod. (mgs) | fiber (gms) |
|---|---|---|---|---|---|---|---|
| **Winter squash, frozen:** | | | | | | | |
| (*Birds Eye*), ½ cup* .... | 45 | 0 | 11.0 | 0 | 0 | 0 | 2.0 |
| (*Cascadian Farm* | | | | | | | |
| Organic), ½ cup ..... | 50 | 1.0 | 11.0 | 0 | 0 | 0 | 2.0 |
| **Witloof**, see "Chicory, | | | | | | | |
| witloof" | | | | | | | |
| **Wolf fish**, Atlantic, meat only: | | | | | | | |
| raw, 4 oz. ........... | 109 | 19.9 | 0 | 2.7 | 52 | 97 | 0 |
| baked or broiled, 4 oz. .. | 139 | 25.4 | 0 | 3.5 | 67 | 124 | 0 |
| **Wonton**, filled, frozen, | | | | | | | |
| mini (*Annie Chun's*), | | | | | | | |
| 4 pcs., 1.27 oz.: | | | | | | | |
| chicken and cilantro .... | 50 | 3.0 | 9.0 | .5 | 5 | 160 | 1.0 |
| chicken and garlic ...... | 60 | 3.0 | 9.0 | .5 | 5 | 150 | 1.0 |
| pork and ginger ........ | 100 | 4.0 | 14.0 | 3.5 | 10 | 230 | 1.0 |
| **Wonton wrapper** | | | | | | | |
| (*Frieda's*), 4 pcs., 1 oz. | 70 | 2.0 | 17.0 | 0 | 0 | 150 | 1.0 |
| **Worcestershire sauce**: | | | | | | | |
| (*Angostura*), 1 tsp. ..... | 5 | 0 | 1.0 | 0 | 0 | 20 | 0 |
| (*Annie's Naturals* | | | | | | | |
| Organic), 1 tsp. ...... | 5 | 0 | 1.0 | 0 | 0 | 75 | 0 |
| (*Crystal*), 1 tsp. ....... | 5 | 0 | 1.0 | 0 | 0 | 70 | 0 |
| (*French's* Reduced | | | | | | | |
| Sodium), 1 tsp. ...... | 0 | 0 | 1.0 | 0 | 0 | 45 | 0 |
| (*French's* Extra | | | | | | | |
| Tenderizing), 1 tsp. ... | 5 | 0 | 1.0 | 0 | 0 | 65 | 0 |
| (*Lea & Perrins*), 1 tsp. .. | 5 | 0 | 1.0 | 0 | 0 | 65 | 0 |
| (*Lea & Perrins* | | | | | | | |
| Reduced Sodium), 1 tsp. | 5 | 0 | 1.0 | 0 | 0 | 45 | 0 |
| (*Lea & Perrins* Thick | | | | | | | |
| Classic), 2 tbsp. ..... | 30 | 0 | 8.0 | 0 | 0 | 200 | 0 |
| **Wraps** (see also "Tortilla") | | | | | | | |
| (*Mission*), 2.5-oz. pc.: | | | | | | | |
| garlic herb, zesty ....... | 210 | 6.0 | 35.0 | 4.5 | 0 | 570 | 1.0 |
| jalapeño cheddar ....... | 210 | 5.0 | 35.0 | 4.5 | 0 | 850 | 1.0 |
| multigrain ............ | 210 | 6.0 | 32.0 | 6.0 | 0 | 660 | 7.0 |
| original ............. | 210 | 6.0 | 35.0 | 5.0 | 0 | 580 | 4.0 |
| spinach herb, garden ... | 210 | 6.0 | 35.0 | 4.5 | 0 | 510 | 1.0 |
| sun-dried tomato basil .. | 210 | 6.0 | 35.0 | 4.5 | 0 | 570 | 2.0 |
| **Wraps, filled** (see also | | | | | | | |
| "Melts"), 1 pc.: | | | | | | | |
| black bean chipotle | | | | | | | |
| (*Guiltless Gourmet*), | | | | | | | |
| 5.75 oz. ........... | 230 | 8.0 | 47.0 | 6.0 | 0 | 45 0 | 7.0 |

| Food and Measure | cal. | prot. (gms) | carbo. (gms) | fat (gms) | chol. (mgs) | sod. (mgs) | fiber (gms) |
|---|---|---|---|---|---|---|---|
| breakfast: | | | | | | | |
| egg/sausage/cheese (*El Monterey*), 4 oz. | 280 | 12.0 | 21.0 | 16.0 | 150 | 450 | 0 |
| tofu scramble (*Amy's*), 5.5 oz. | 380 | 21.0 | 30.0 | 19.0 | 10 | 490 | 4.0 |
| chicken, grilled, Caesar (*Oscar Mayer*), 7.5 oz. | 370 | 23.0 | 46.0 | 11.0 | 55 | 1050 | 2.0 |
| chicken mushroom Florentine, mini (*Smart Ones*), ½ pkg. | 220 | 12.0 | 30.0 | 5.0 | 15 | 510 | 7.0 |
| chicken ranchero, mini (*Smart Ones*), ½ pkg. | 220 | 12.0 | 30.0 | 5.0 | 20 | 590 | 7.0 |
| couscous/vegetable (*Cedarlane* Low-Fat Veggie), 6 oz. | 220 | 14.0 | 36.0 | 3.0 | 0 | 580 | 3.0 |
| Indian: | | | | | | | |
| samosa (*Amy's*), 5 oz. | 250 | 8.0 | 35.0 | 9.0 | 0 | 680 | 4.0 |
| spinach tofu (*Amy's*), 5.5 oz. | 270 | 10.0 | 28.0 | 13.0 | 0 | 690 | 6.0 |
| pizza (*Cedarlane* Lowfat Veggie), 6 oz. | 220 | 17.0 | 32.0 | 3.0 | 0 | 520 | 2.0 |
| spinach (*Guiltless Gourmet* Mediterranean), 5.75 oz. | 220 | 9.0 | 39.0 | 6.0 | 5 | 410 | 6.0 |
| teriyaki (*Amy's*), 5.5 oz. | 310 | 11.0 | 51.0 | 7.0 | 0 | 540 | 5.0 |
| turkey (*Oscar Mayer* Deli), 6.6 oz. | 480 | 22.0 | 55.0 | 19.0 | 35 | 1050 | 2.0 |
| vegetable (*Guiltless Gourmet* California), 5.75 oz. | 230 | 8.0 | 40.0 | 7.0 | 0 | 470 | 6.0 |

# X–Y

| Food and Measure | cal. | prot. (gms) | carbo. (gms) | fat (gms) | chol. (mgs) | sod. (mgs) | fiber (gms) |
|---|---|---|---|---|---|---|---|
| **Xanthan gum** (*Hodgson Mill* Gluten Free), 1 tbsp. . . . . . . . . . . . . | 30 | 3.0 | 7.0 | 0 | 0 | 200 | 7.0 |
| **Yachtwurst**, w/pista-chios, cooked, 2 oz. . . | 150 | 8.3 | .8 | 12.7 | 36 | 524 | 0 |
| **Yam** (see also "Name yam"), cubed: | | | | | | | |
| raw, ½ cup . . . . . . . . . . | 89 | 1.2 | 20.9 | .1 | 0 | 7 | 3.1 |
| baked or boiled, ½ cup . . | 79 | 1.0 | 18.8 | .1 | 0 | 6 | 2.7 |
| **Yam, canned/frozen**, see "Sweet potato" | | | | | | | |
| **Yam, mountain**, Hawaiian, cubed, steamed, ½ cup . . . . . | 59 | 1.2 | 14.4 | .1 | 0 | 9 | n.a. |
| **Yam bean**, tuber: | | | | | | | |
| raw (*Frieda's Jicama*), 1 cup, 4.2 oz. . . . . . . . | 50 | 1.0 | 11.0 | 0 | 0 | 5 | 6.0 |
| raw, sliced, ½ cup . . . . . . | 23 | .4 | 5.3 | .1 | 0 | 3 | 2.9 |
| boiled, drained, 4 oz. . . . . | 43 | .8 | 10.0 | .1 | 0 | 5 | n.a. |
| **Yard-long bean**, fresh: | | | | | | | |
| raw (*Frieda's Dow Gok*), 1 cup, 3.2 oz. . . | 40 | 3.0 | 8.0 | 0 | 0 | 0 | 0 |
| boiled, drained, sliced, ½ cup . . . . . . . . . . . . . | 25 | 1.3 | 4.8 | .1 | 0 | 2 | n.a. |
| **Yard-long bean, mature**, boiled, ½ cup | 102 | 7.1 | 18.1 | .4 | 0 | 4 | 1.4 |
| **Yeast**, baker's: | | | | | | | |
| active, dry: | | | | | | | |
| (*Hodgson Mill*), 1 pkt. . | 30 | 4.0 | 3.0 | 0 | 0 | 0 | 1.0 |
| 1 tbsp. . . . . . . . . . . . . | 35 | 3.4 | 4.6 | .6 | 0 | 6 | .3 |
| compressed, .6-oz. . . . . . | 6 | <.1 | 1.1 | 0 | 0 | 2 | <.1 |
| fast rise (*Hodgson Mill*), 1 pkt. . . . . . . . . . . . . | 25 | 3.0 | 4.0 | 0 | 0 | 0 | 1.0 |

| Food and Measure | cal. | prot. (gms) | carbo. (gms) | fat (gms) | chol. (mgs) | sod. (mgs) | fiber (gms) |
|---|---|---|---|---|---|---|---|
| **Yellow beans**, dried, boiled, ½ cup ....... | 127 | 8.1 | 22.2 | 1.0 | 0 | 4 | 9.2 |
| **Yellow squash**, fresh (see also "Crookneck squash"), sliced, ¾ cup: | | | | | | | |
| (*Glory*) .............. | 20 | 1.0 | 3.0 | 0 | 0 | 20 | 1.0 |
| and zucchini (*Glory*) .... | 25 | 2.0 | 6.0 | 0 | 0 | 0 | 3.0 |
| **Yellow squash, canned**, ½ cup: | | | | | | | |
| baby, cut (*Sunshine*) .... | 25 | 0 | 5.0 | 0 | 0 | 160 | 2.0 |
| w/Vidalia onion (*Allens*) . | 25 | 1.0 | 6.0 | 0 | 0 | 260 | 1.0 |
| **Yellowtail**, meat only: | | | | | | | |
| raw, 4 oz. ............. | 166 | 26.3 | 0 | 6.0 | 62 | 44 | 0 |
| baked or broiled, 4 oz. .. | 212 | 33.6 | 0 | 7.6 | 81 | 57 | 0 |
| **Yerba maté drink**, see "Tea, iced" | | | | | | | |
| **Yogurt**: | | | | | | | |
| plain, 8 oz., except as noted: | | | | | | | |
| (*Activia*) ........... | 170 | 11.0 | 20.0 | 4.5 | 15 | 170 | 0 |
| (*Chobani* Greek Lowfat), 6 oz. ..... | 130 | 17.0 | 7.0 | 3.5 | 10 | 70 | 0 |
| (*Chobani* Greek Nonfat), 6 oz. ..... | 100 | 18.0 | 7.0 | 0 | 0 | 80 | 0 |
| (*Dannon*) .......... | 160 | 9.0 | 12.0 | 8.0 | 20 | 120 | 0 |
| (*Dannon* Greek) ..... | 120 | 22.0 | 9.0 | 0 | 15 | 80 | 0 |
| (*Dannon* Low Fat), 6 oz. ............. | 100 | 8.0 | 12.0 | 2.5 | 10 | 115 | 0 |
| (*Dannon* Nonfat), 6 oz. ............. | 80 | 9.0 | 12.0 | 0 | 5 | 120 | 0 |
| (*Fage* Total Greek) ... | 300 | 15.0 | 7.0 | 23.0 | 40 | 65 | 0 |
| (*Fage* Total Greek 2%) ............. | 150 | 19.0 | 9.0 | 4.5 | 15 | 75 | 0 |
| (*Fage* Total Greek Nonfat) ........... | 120 | 20.0 | 9.0 | 0 | 0 | 85 | 0 |
| (*Friendship*) ........ | 150 | 12.0 | 18.0 | 3.0 | 15 | 190 | 0 |
| (*Oikos* Organic Greek) | 130 | 23.0 | 9.0 | 0 | 0 | 95 | 0 |
| (*Stonyfield* Organic Cream Top) ...... | 170 | 8.0 | 13.0 | 9.0 | 35 | 130 | 3.0 |
| (*Stonyfield* Organic Low Fat) ......... | 120 | 10.0 | 15.0 | 2.0 | 10 | 150 | 0 |
| (*Stonyfield* Organic Low Fat), 6 oz. .... | 90 | 7.0 | 11.0 | 1.5 | 5 | 110 | 0 |

| Food and Measure | cal. | prot. (gms) | carbo. (gms) | fat (gms) | chol. (mgs) | sod. (mgs) | fiber (gms) |
|---|---|---|---|---|---|---|---|
| **Yogurt, plain** *(cont.)* | | | | | | | |
| (*Stonyfield* Organic Nonfat) . . . . . . . . . . | 110 | 11.0 | 15.0 | 0 | 0 | 160 | 0 |
| (*Stonyfield* Organic Nonfat), 6 oz. . . . . . | 80 | 8.0 | 11.0 | 0 | 0 | 120 | 0 |
| (*Yoplait* Nonfat) . . . . . | 130 | 15.0 | 19.0 | 0 | 5 | 220 | 0 |
| (*Yoplait* Greek Nonfat), 6 oz. . . . . . | 100 | 14.0 | 10.0 | 0 | 10 | 90 | 0 |
| all flavors: | | | | | | | |
| (*Cabot* Nonfat), 6 oz. . | 120 | 7.0 | 23.0 | 0 | 10 | 95 | 0 |
| (*Dannon Light & Fit Carb & Sugar Control*), 4 oz. . . . . | 50 | 5.0 | 3.0 | 1.5 | 10 | 25 | 0 |
| (*Fiber One*), 4 oz. . . . . | 50 | 3.0 | 13.0 | 0 | <5 | 55 | 5.0 |
| (*Yoplait* Creamy Low Fat), 8 oz. . . . . | 200 | 7.0 | 39.0 | 1.5 | 5 | 115 | 9 |
| (*Yoplait* Fridge Pack Original), 6 oz. . . . . | 170 | 5.0 | 33.0 | 1.5 | 10 | 80 | 0 |
| (*Yoplait* Fridge Pack Light), 6 oz. . . . . . . | 100 | 5.0 | 19.0 | 0 | <5 | 85 | 0 |
| (*Yoplait* Fridge Pack Thick & Creamy), 6 oz. . . . . . . . . . . . | 190 | 7.0 | 32.0 | 3.5 | 15 | 100 | 0 |
| (*Yoplait* Thick & Creamy), 6 oz. . . . . | 180 | 7.0 | 31.0 | 2.5 | 15 | 110 | 0 |
| (*Yoplait* Thick & Creamy Light), 6 oz. | 100 | 5.0 | 20.0 | 0 | <5 | 90 | 0 |
| (*Yoplait Splitz*), 3.3 oz. | 90 | 3.0 | 17.0 | 1.0 | <5 | 60 | 0 |
| except honey vanilla (*Yoplait* Greek Nonfat), 6 oz. . . . . . | 160 | 14.0 | 25.0 | 0 | 10 | 100 | 0 |
| except lemon and piña colada (*Yoplait* Original), 6 oz. . . . . | 170 | 5.0 | 33.0 | 1.5 | 10 | 80 | 0 |
| except banana/Boston/ lemon pie, cake flavors, and vanilla (*Yoplait* Light), 6 oz. | 100 | 5.0 | 19.0 | 0 | <5 | 85 | 0 |
| except blueberry and honey (*Fage* Total Greek), 5.3 oz. . . . . | 210 | 8.0 | 18.0 | 12.0 | 20 | 35 | 0 |
| except blueberry and honey (*Fage* Total Greek 2%), 5.3 oz. . | 140 | 10.0 | 19.0 | 2.5 | 5 | 40 | 0 |

| Food and Measure | cal. | prot. (gms) | carbo. (gms) | fat (gms) | chol. (mgs) | sod. (mgs) | fiber (gms) |
|---|---|---|---|---|---|---|---|
| all fruit flavors, 4 oz.: | | | | | | | |
| (*Yoplait Whips!*) ..... | 140 | 5.0 | 25.0 | 2.5 | 10 | 75 | 0 |
| (*Yoplait Yo-Plus*) .... | 110 | 4.0 | 21.0 | 1.5 | 10 | 70 | 3.0 |
| apple cinnamon (*Dannon* Fruit on Bottom), 6 oz. ....... | 150 | 6.0 | 28.0 | 1.5 | 5 | 130 | <1.0 |
| banana, 6 oz.: | | | | | | | |
| (*Dannon Light & Fit*) .. | 80 | 5.0 | 16.0 | 0 | <5 | 75 | 0 |
| pie (*Yoplait Light*) .... | 110 | 6.0 | 20.0 | 0 | <5 | 90 | 0 |
| banana vanilla (*Stonyfield* Organic Low Fat BaNilla), 8 oz. .... | 200 | 9.0 | 35.0 | 2.5 | 10 | 135 | 0 |
| berry (*Stonyfield* Organic Low Fat B-Well Harvest), 4 oz. ...... | 80 | 4.0 | 15.0 | 1.0 | 5 | 75 | <1.0 |
| berry, mixed: | | | | | | | |
| (*Activia*), 4 oz. ...... | 120 | 3.0 | 23.0 | 2.0 | 5 | 60 | 0 |
| (*Breyers* Fruit on Bottom), 6 oz. .... | 160 | 5.0 | 31.0 | 1.0 | 10 | 75 | <1.0 |
| (*Breyers* Light), 6 oz. . | 80 | 6.0 | 12.0 | 0 | <5 | 85 | <1.0 |
| (*Dannon* Fruit on Bottom), 6 oz. .... | 150 | 6.0 | 27.0 | 1.5 | 5 | 120 | <1.0 |
| (*Dannon Light & Fit*), 6 oz. ........ | 80 | 5.0 | 15.0 | 0 | <5 | 85 | 0 |
| crème, triple (*Yoplait Delights*), 4 oz. .... | 100 | 5.0 | 16.0 | 1.5 | 5 | 80 | 0 |
| Black Forest cake or Boston cream pie (*Yoplait Light*), 6 oz. .. | 110 | 6.0 | 20.0 | 0 | <5 | 90 | 0 |
| blackberry (*Dannon Light & Fit*), 6 oz. ..... | 80 | 5.0 | 16.0 | 0 | <5 | 75 | 0 |
| blueberries/cream, 6 oz.: | | | | | | | |
| (*Breyers* Light) ...... | 80 | 6.0 | 12.0 | 0 | <5 | 105 | <1.0 |
| (*Breyers Crème Savers*) .......... | 160 | 6.0 | 31.0 | 1.5 | 10 | 170 | 0 |
| blueberry: | | | | | | | |
| (*Activia*), 4 oz. ...... | 120 | 3.0 | 23.0 | 2.0 | 5 | 55 | <1.0 |
| (*Activia* Light), 4 oz. .. | 70 | 4.0 | 13.0 | 0 | <5 | 65 | 2.0 |
| (*Breyers* Fruit on Bottom), 6 oz. .... | 160 | 5.0 | 32.0 | 1.0 | 10 | 75 | <1.0 |
| (*Chobani* Greek Nonfat), 6 oz. ..... | 140 | 14.0 | 20.0 | 0 | 0 | 65 | <1.0 |
| (*Dannon* Fruit on Bottom), 6 oz. .... | 140 | 6.0 | 26.0 | 1.5 | 5 | 130 | <1.0 |

| Food and Measure | cal. | prot. (gms) | carbo. (gms) | fat (gms) | chol. (mgs) | sod. (mgs) | fiber (gms) |
|---|---|---|---|---|---|---|---|
| **Yogurt, blueberry** *(cont.)* | | | | | | | |
| (*Dannon* Greek), | | | | | | | |
| 5.3 oz. . . . . . . . . . . | 120 | 12.0 | 17.0 | 0 | 10 | 50 | 0 |
| (*Dannon Light &* | | | | | | | |
| *Fit*), 6 oz. . . . . . . . | 80 | 5.0 | 16.0 | 0 | <5 | 75 | 0 |
| (*Fage* Total Greek), | | | | | | | |
| 5.3 oz. . . . . . . . . . | 200 | 8.0 | 16.0 | 12.0 | 20 | 35 | 0 |
| (*Fage* Total Greek | | | | | | | |
| 2%), 5.3 oz. . . . . . | 130 | 10.0 | 17.0 | 2.5 | 5 | 40 | 0 |
| (*Oikos* Organic Greek), | | | | | | | |
| 5.3 oz. . . . . . . . . . | 120 | 13.0 | 15.0 | 0 | 0 | 70 | 0 |
| (*Oikos* Organic Greek), | | | | | | | |
| 4 oz. . . . . . . . . . . | 90 | 10.0 | 12.0 | 0 | 0 | 40 | 0 |
| (*Stonyfield* Organic | | | | | | | |
| Low Fat), 8 oz. . . . . | 180 | 9.0 | 30.0 | 2.0 | 10 | 170 | 0 |
| (*Stonyfield* Organic | | | | | | | |
| Low Fat Fruit on | | | | | | | |
| Bottom), 6 oz. . . . . | 120 | 6.0 | 21.0 | 1.5 | 5 | 90 | <1.0 |
| (*Stonyfield* Organic | | | | | | | |
| Nonfat), 6 oz. . . . . . | 120 | 6.0 | 22.0 | 0 | 0 | 100 | <1.0 |
| acai (*Dannon Light* | | | | | | | |
| *& Fit*), 6 oz. . . . . . . | 80 | 5.0 | 16.0 | 0 | <5 | 75 | 0 |
| pomegranate (*Cabot* | | | | | | | |
| Greek), 6 oz. . . . . . . | 160 | 13.0 | 26.0 | 3.0 | 20 | 80 | 0 |
| blueberry cheesecake | | | | | | | |
| (*Activia*), 4 oz. . . . . . | 150 | 5.0 | 23.0 | 4.0 | 15 | 100 | <1.0 |
| boysenberry (*Dannon* | | | | | | | |
| Fruit on Bottom), | | | | | | | |
| 6 oz. . . . . . . . . . . . | 150 | 6.0 | 27.0 | 1.5 | 5 | 110 | <1.0 |
| caramel, 4 oz.: | | | | | | | |
| (*Oikos* Organic Greek) | 110 | 10.0 | 17.0 | 0 | 0 | 60 | 0 |
| crème (*Yoplait* | | | | | | | |
| *Delights* Parfait) . . . | 100 | 5.0 | 18.0 | 1.5 | 5 | 90 | 0 |
| cherry: | | | | | | | |
| (*Activia*), 4 oz. . . . . . | 120 | 3.0 | 23.0 | 2.0 | 5 | 55 | 0 |
| (*Dannon* Fruit on | | | | | | | |
| Bottom), 6 oz. . . . . | 140 | 6.0 | 26.0 | 1.5 | 5 | 120 | 0 |
| (*Dannon Light &* | | | | | | | |
| *Fit*), 6 oz. . . . . . . . | 80 | 5.0 | 16.0 | 0 | <5 | 75 | 0 |
| cherry, black, 6 oz.: | | | | | | | |
| (*Breyers* Fruit on | | | | | | | |
| Bottom) . . . . . . . . . | 160 | 5.0 | 32.0 | 1.0 | 10 | 80 | <1.0 |
| (*Breyers* Light | | | | | | | |
| Jubilee) . . . . . . . . . | 80 | 6.0 | 12.0 | 0 | <5 | 90 | 0 |

| Food and Measure | cal. | prot. (gms) | carbo. (gms) | fat (gms) | chol. (mgs) | sod. (mgs) | fiber (gms) |
|---|---|---|---|---|---|---|---|
| (*Stonyfield* Organic Nonfat) ......... | 120 | 6.0 | 22.0 | 0 | 0 | 100 | <1.0 |
| cherry chocolate chip (*Breyers* Inspirations), 4 oz. ............. | 140 | 4.0 | 23.0 | 3.0 | 5 | 65 | 0 |
| cherry vanilla, 6 oz.: | | | | | | | |
| (*Dannon Light & Fit*) .. | 80 | 5.0 | 16.0 | 0 | <5 | 80 | 0 |
| (*Stonyfield* Organic Low Fat) ......... | 130 | 7.0 | 23.0 | 1.5 | 56 | 110 | 0 |
| chocolate: | | | | | | | |
| (*Oikos* Organic Greek), 4 oz. ...... | 110 | 10.0 | 17.0 | 0 | 0 | 55 | <1.0 |
| (*Stonyfield* Organic Cream Top), 6 oz. .. | 220 | 6.0 | 38.0 | 5.0 | 20 | 90 | <1.0 |
| (*Stonyfield* Organic Nonfat), 6 oz. ..... | 180 | 7.0 | 37.0 | 0 | 0 | 105 | <1.0 |
| mousse (*Yoplait Whips!*), 4 oz. .... | 160 | 5.0 | 26.0 | 4.0 | 10 | 105 | 0 |
| chocolate chip, 4 oz.: | | | | | | | |
| (*Breyers* Inspirations) . | 140 | 4.0 | 22.0 | 3.5 | 5 | 65 | 0 |
| cookie dough (*Breyers* Inspirations) ...... | 140 | 4.0 | 23.0 | 3.5 | 5 | 55 | 0 |
| mint (*Breyers* Inspirations) ...... | 140 | 4.0 | 23.0 | 3.5 | 5 | 65 | 0 |
| chocolate raspberry: | | | | | | | |
| (*Breyers* Fruit on Bottom), 6 oz. .... | 170 | 5.0 | 34.0 | 1.0 | 10 | 75 | <1.0 |
| (*Cabot* Greek), 6 oz. .. | 170 | 14.0 | 25.0 | 3.5 | 20 | 75 | 0 |
| (*Yoplait Delights* Parfait), 4 oz. ..... | 100 | 5.0 | 18.0 | 1.5 | 5 | 90 | 0 |
| white (*Dannon Light & Fit*), 6 oz. ...... | 80 | 5.0 | 16.0 | 0 | <5 | 75 | 0 |
| white (*Stonyfield* Organic Cream Top), 6 oz. .. | 170 | 6.0 | 23.0 | 6.0 | 25 | 105 | 0 |
| coffee (*Dannon*), 6 oz. ... | 150 | 7.0 | 25.0 | 2.5 | 10 | 100 | 0 |
| honey, Greek: | | | | | | | |
| (*Cabot*), 6 oz. ........ | 160 | 13.0 | 25.0 | 3.0 | 20 | 75 | 0 |
| (*Chobani* Nonfat), 6 oz. ............. | 150 | 16.0 | 20.0 | 0 | 0 | 75 | 0 |
| (*Dannon*), 5.3 oz. .... | 140 | 12.0 | 23.0 | 0 | 10 | 50 | 0 |
| (*Fage* Total), 5.3 oz. .. | 250 | 8.0 | 28.0 | 12.0 | 20 | 35 | 0 |
| (*Fage* Total 2%), 5.3 oz. ......... | 180 | 10.0 | 29.0 | 2.5 | 5 | 40 | 0 |
| (*Oikos* Organic), 5.3 oz. | 110 | 13.0 | 16.0 | 0 | 0 | 80 | 0 |

| Food and Measure | cal. | prot. (gms) | carbo. (gms) | fat (gms) | chol. (mgs) | sod. (mgs) | fiber (gms) |
|---|---|---|---|---|---|---|---|
| **Yogurt, honey, Greek** *(cont.)* | | | | | | | |
| (*Oikos* Organic), 4 oz. . . | 90 | 10.0 | 13.0 | 0 | 0 | 40 | 0 |
| vanilla (*Yoplait* Nonfat), 6 oz. . . . . . | 150 | 14.0 | 22.0 | 0 | 10 | 120 | 0 |
| lemon, 6 oz.: | | | | | | | |
| (*Dannon*) . . . . . . . . . . | 150 | 7.0 | 25.0 | 2.5 | 10 | 100 | 0 |
| (*Stonyfield* Organic Nonfat) . . . . . . . . . . | 130 | 7.0 | 26.0 | 0 | 0 | 115 | 0 |
| (*Yoplait* Original) . . . . . | 180 | 5.0 | 36.0 | 1.5 | 10 | 85 | 0 |
| chiffon (*Breyers* Light) . . . . . . . . . . | 80 | 6.0 | 11.0 | 0 | <5 | 120 | 0 |
| chiffon (*Dannon Light & Fit*) . . . . . . . . . . | 80 | 5.0 | 15.0 | 0 | <5 | 80 | 0 |
| cream pie (*Yoplait* Light) . . . . . . . . . . | 110 | 6.0 | 20.0 | 0 | <5 | 90 | 0 |
| lemon torte (*Yoplait Delights* Parfait), 4 oz. | 100 | 5.0 | 16.0 | 1.5 | 5 | 80 | 0 |
| lime, Key, 6 oz.: | | | | | | | |
| (*Dannon Light & Fit*), 6 oz. . . . . . . . . | 80 | 5.0 | 16.0 | 0 | <5 | 95 | 0 |
| (*Stonyfield* Organic Nonfat) . . . . . . . . . . | 130 | 7.0 | 25.0 | 0 | 0 | 120 | 0 |
| pie (*Breyers* Light) . . . | 80 | 6.0 | 11.0 | 0 | <5 | 170 | 0 |
| mango honey (*Stonyfield* Organic), 6 oz. . . . . . . | 130 | 7.0 | 23.0 | 1.5 | 5 | 110 | 0 |
| orange, 6 oz.: | | | | | | | |
| (*Dannon Light & Fit* Bliss) . . . . . . . . . | 80 | 5.0 | 15.0 | 0 | <5 | 75 | 0 |
| and crème (*Breyers Crème* Savers) . . . . | 170 | 6.0 | 31.0 | 1.5 | 10 | 170 | 0 |
| peach: | | | | | | | |
| (*Activia*), 4 oz. . . . . . . | 120 | 3.0 | 22.0 | 2.0 | 5 | 60 | 0 |
| (*Activia* Fiber), 4 oz. . . | 110 | 3.0 | 20.0 | 2.0 | 5 | 60 | 3.0 |
| (*Activia* Light), 4 oz. . . | 70 | 4.0 | 12.0 | 0 | <5 | 65 | 2.0 |
| (*Breyers* Fruit on Bottom), 6 oz. . . . . | 160 | 5.0 | 31.0 | 1.0 | 10 | 75 | <1.0 |
| (*Cabot* Greek), 6 oz. . . | 160 | 13.0 | 25.0 | 3.0 | 20 | 80 | 0 |
| (*Chobani* Greek Nonfat), 6 oz. . . . . . | 140 | 14.0 | 20.0 | 0 | 0 | 65 | <1.0 |
| (*Dannon* Fruit on Bottom), 6 oz. . . . . | 150 | 6.0 | 28.0 | 1.5 | 5 | 95 | 0 |
| (*Dannon Light & Fit*), 6 oz. . . . . . . . . | 80 | 5.0 | 16.0 | 0 | <5 | 75 | 0 |

| Food and Measure | cal. | prot. (gms) | carbo. (gms) | fat (gms) | chol. (mgs) | sod. (mgs) | fiber (gms) |
|---|---|---|---|---|---|---|---|
| (*Stonyfield* Organic Low Fat), 6 oz. . . . . | 130 | 6.0 | 22.0 | 1.5 | 5 | 110 | 0 |
| (*Stonyfield* Organic Nonfat), 6 oz. . . . . . . | 130 | 7.0 | 25.0 | 0 | 0 | 110 | 0 |
| cobbler (*Activia*), 4 oz. . . . . . . . . . . . | 140 | 6.0 | 21.0 | 4.0 | 15 | 100 | 0 |
| peach orange mango (*Breyers* Fruit on Bottom), 6 oz. . . . . . . . | 160 | 5.0 | 31.0 | 1.0 | 10 | 75 | <1.0 |
| peaches/cream, 6 oz.: | | | | | | | |
| (*Breyers* Light) . . . . . . | 80 | 6.0 | 12.0 | 0 | <5 | 110 | <1.0 |
| (*Breyers* Crème Savers) . . . . . . . . . | 170 | 6.0 | 31.0 | 1.5 | 10 | 170 | 0 |
| piña colada (*Yoplait* Original), 6 oz. . . . . . . | 170 | 5.0 | 33.0 | 2.0 | 10 | 80 | 0 |
| pineapple, 6 oz.: | | | | | | | |
| (*Breyers* Fruit on Bottom) . . . . . . . . . | 150 | 5.0 | 31.0 | 1.0 | 10 | 75 | <1.0 |
| (*Chobani* Greek Low Fat) . . . . . . . . . | 160 | 13.0 | 21.0 | 2.5 | 5 | 65 | 0 |
| (*Dannon* Fruit on Bottom) . . . . . . . . . | 150 | 6.0 | 28.0 | 1.5 | 5 | 125 | 0 |
| coconut (*Dannon* Light & Fit) . . . . . . . | 80 | 5.0 | 16.0 | 0 | <5 | 75 | 0 |
| upside-down cake (*Yoplait* Light) . . . . | 110 | 6.0 | 20.0 | 0 | <5 | 90 | 0 |
| pomegranate (*Chobani* Greek Nonfat), 6 oz. . . | 140 | 14.0 | 21.0 | 0 | 0 | 75 | 0 |
| pomegranate berry: | | | | | | | |
| (*Dannon Light & Fit*), 6 oz. . . . . . . . . | 80 | 5.0 | 16.0 | 0 | <5 | 75 | 0 |
| (*Stonyfield* Organic Nonfat), 6 oz. . . . . . . | 130 | 7.0 | 25.0 | 0 | 0 | 115 | 0 |
| pomegranate raspberry acai (*Stonyfield* Organic Nonfat Super Fruits), 6 oz. . . . . . . . . | 120 | 6.0 | 22.0 | 0 | 0 | 130 | <1.0 |
| prune (*Activia*), 4 oz. . . . . | 120 | 3.0 | 22.0 | 2.0 | 5 | 55 | 0 |
| raspberries/cream, 6 oz.: | | | | | | | |
| (*Breyers* Light) . . . . . . | 80 | 6.0 | 12.0 | 0 | <5 | 100 | <1.0 |
| (*Breyers* Crème Savers) . . . . . . . . . | 170 | 6.0 | 31.0 | 1.5 | 10 | 170 | 0 |
| raspberry: | | | | | | | |
| (*Activia* Light), 4 oz. . . | 70 | 4.0 | 13.0 | 0 | <5 | 75 | 2.0 |

| Food and Measure | cal. | prot. (gms) | carbo. (gms) | fat (gms) | chol. (mgs) | sod. (mgs) | fiber (gms) |
|---|---|---|---|---|---|---|---|
| **Yogurt, raspberry** *(cont.)* | | | | | | | |
| (*Chobani* Greek Nonfat), 6 oz. ..... | 140 | 14.0 | 22.0 | 0 | 0 | 65 | 1.0 |
| (*Dannon* Fruit on Bottom), 6 oz. .... | 150 | 6.0 | 28.0 | 1.5 | 5 | 115 | <1.0 |
| (*Dannon Light & Fit*), 6 oz. ........ | 80 | 5.0 | 16.0 | 0 | <5 | 75 | 0 |
| (*Stonyfield* Organic Low Fat), 6 oz. .... | 130 | 7.0 | 23.0 | 1.5 | 5 | 110 | 0 |
| raspberry cheesecake (*Yoplait* Light), 6 oz. .. | 110 | 6.0 | 20.0 | 0 | <5 | 90 | 0 |
| raspberry goji (*Dannon Light & Fit*), 6 oz. .... | 80 | 5.0 | 16.0 | 0 | <5 | 75 | 0 |
| strawberries/cream: | | | | | | | |
| (*Breyers Crème Savers*), 6 oz. ...... | 170 | 6.0 | 31.0 | 1.5 | 10 | 170 | 0 |
| (*Stonyfield* Organic Cream Top), 6 oz. .. | 150 | 5.0 | 20.0 | 6.0 | 20 | 110 | <1.0 |
| strawberry: | | | | | | | |
| (*Activia*), 4 oz. ...... | 120 | 3.0 | 22.0 | 2.0 | 5 | 65 | 0 |
| (*Activia* Fiber), 4 oz. .. | 110 | 3.0 | 20.0 | 2.0 | 5 | 60 | 3.0 |
| (*Activia* Light), 4 oz. .. | 70 | 4.0 | 13.0 | 0 | <5 | 70 | 2.0 |
| (*Breyers* Fruit on Bottom), 6 oz. .... | 150 | 5.0 | 31.0 | 1.0 | 10 | 75 | <1.0 |
| (*Breyers* Inspirations), 4 oz. ............ | 110 | 4.0 | 22.0 | 1.0 | 5 | 65 | <1.0 |
| (*Breyers* Light), 6 oz. . | 80 | 6.0 | 12.0 | 0 | <5 | 105 | <1.0 |
| (*Breyers* Smooth & Creamy), 4 oz. .. | 110 | 3.0 | 23.0 | 1.0 | 10 | 50 | 0 |
| (*Cabot* Greek), 6 oz. .. | 160 | 13.0 | 25.0 | 3.0 | 20 | 80 | 0 |
| (*Chobani* Greek Nonfat), 6 oz. ..... | 140 | 14.0 | 20.0 | 0 | 0 | 65 | <1.0 |
| (*Dannon* Fruit on Bottom), 6 oz. .... | 150 | 6.0 | 28.0 | 1.5 | 5 | 110 | <1.0 |
| (*Dannon* Greek), 5.3 oz. .......... | 120 | 12.0 | 17.0 | 0 | 10 | 55 | 0 |
| (*Dannon Light & Fit*), 6 oz. ........ | 80 | 5.0 | 16.0 | 0 | <5 | 80 | 0 |
| (*Oikos* Organic Greek), 5.3 oz. .......... | 110 | 13.0 | 16.0 | 0 | 0 | 80 | 0 |
| (*Oikos* Organic Greek), 4 oz. ............ | 90 | 10.0 | 12.0 | 0 | 0 | 60 | 0 |
| (*Stonyfield* Organic Low Fat), 8 oz. .... | 200 | 9.0 | 35.0 | 2.5 | 10 | 135 | 0 |

| Food and Measure | cal. | prot. (gms) | carbo. (gms) | fat (gms) | chol. (mgs) | sod. (mgs) | fiber (gms) |
|---|---|---|---|---|---|---|---|
| - (*Stonyfield* Organic Low Fat), 6 oz. .... | 120 | 6.0 | 21.0 | 1.5 | 5 | 120 | <1.0 |
| (*Stonyfield* Organic Nonfat), 6 oz. ...... | 130 | 7.0 | 26.0 | 1.5 | 0 | 115 | 0 |
| (*Stonyfield* Organic Nonfat Fruit on Bottom), 6 oz. .... | 110 | 6.0 | 22.0 | 0 | 0 | 125 | <1.0 |
| (*Yoplait* Light Creamy), 8 oz. ............ | 140 | 7.0 | 27.0 | 0 | 5 | 115 | 0 |
| strawberry acai (*Stonyfield* Organic Low Fat B-Healthy), 4 oz. .. | 90 | 4.0 | 15.0 | 1.0 | 5 | 70 | <1.0 |
| strawberry banana, 6 oz., except as noted: | | | | | | | |
| (*Breyers* Fruit on Bottom) | 150 | 5.0 | 31.0 | 1.0 | 10 | 75 | <1.0 |
| (*Breyers* Smooth & Creamy), 4 oz. .. | 120 | 3.0 | 24.0 | 1.0 | 10 | 50 | 0 |
| (*Chobani* Greek Low-Fat) ......... | 160 | 14.0 | 19.0 | 3.0 | 5 | 65 | 1.0 |
| (*Dannon* Fruit on Bottom) ......... | 150 | 6.0 | 26.0 | 1.5 | 5 | 95 | <1.0 |
| (*Dannon Light & Fit*) .. | 80 | 5.0 | 15.0 | 0 | <5 | 75 | 0 |
| split (*Breyers* Light) .. | 80 | 6.0 | 12.0 | 0 | 5 | 105 | 0 |
| strawberry cheesecake: | | | | | | | |
| (*Activia*), 4 oz. ...... | 140 | 6.0 | 20.0 | 4.0 | 15 | 100 | 0 |
| (*Breyers* Light), 6 oz. . | 80 | 6.0 | 12.0 | 0 | <5 | 85 | <1.0 |
| (*Dannon Light & Fit*), 6 oz. ........ | 80 | 5.0 | 16.0 | 0 | <5 | 75 | 0 |
| strawberry kiwi (*Dannon Light & Fit*), 6 oz. .... | 80 | 5.0 | 16.0 | 0 | <5 | 75 | 0 |
| strawberry pomegranate (*Stonyfield* Organic Low Fat), 6 oz. ...... | 130 | 7.0 | 23.0 | 1.5 | 5 | 110 | 0 |
| strawberry shortcake (*Yoplait* Light), 6 oz. .. | 110 | 6.0 | 20.0 | 0 | <5 | 90 | 0 |
| vanilla: | | | | | | | |
| (*Activia*), 4 oz. ...... | 120 | 3.0 | 22.0 | 2.0 | 5 | 60 | 0 |
| (*Activia*), 8 oz. ...... | 230 | 7.0 | 43.0 | 4.0 | 15 | 115 | 0 |
| (*Activia* Fiber), 4 oz. .. | 110 | 3.0 | 19.0 | 2.0 | 5 | 60 | 3.0 |
| (*Activia* Light), 4 oz. .. | 70 | 5.0 | 14.0 | 0 | <5 | 70 | 3.0 |
| (*Chobani* Greek Nonfat), 6 oz. ...... | 120 | 16.0 | 13.0 | 0 | 0 | 75 | 0 |
| (*Dannon*), 6 oz. ....... | 150 | 7.0 | 25.0 | 2.5 | 10 | 100 | 0 |

| Food and Measure | cal. | prot. (gms) | carbo. (gms) | fat (gms) | chol. (mgs) | sod. (mgs) | fiber (gms) |
|---|---|---|---|---|---|---|---|
| **Yogurt, vanilla** *(cont.)* | | | | | | | |
| (*Dannon* Greek), | | | | | | | |
| 5.3 oz. . . . . . . . . . . | 110 | 12.0 | 17.0 | 0 | 10 | 50 | 0 |
| (*Dannon Light &* | | | | | | | |
| *Fit*), 6 oz. . . . . . . . | 80 | 5.0 | 16.0 | 0 | <5 | 75 | 0 |
| (*Oikos* Organic Greek), | | | | | | | |
| 5.3 oz. . . . . . . . . . . | 110 | 15.0 | 12.0 | 0 | 0 | 60 | 0 |
| (*Oikos* Organic Greek), | | | | | | | |
| 4 oz. . . . . . . . . . . . | 80 | 11.0 | 9.0 | 0 | 0 | 45 | 0 |
| (*Yoplait* Light Very), | | | | | | | |
| 6 oz. . . . . . . . . . . . | 110 | 6.0 | 20.0 | 0 | <5 | 90 | 0 |
| bean (*Activia*), 4 oz. . . | 140 | 6.0 | 21.0 | 4.0 | 15 | 100 | 0 |
| bean (*Breyers* | | | | | | | |
| Inspirations), 4 oz. . . | 110 | 4.0 | 21.0 | 1.0 | 5 | 60 | 0 |
| bean (*Breyers* Light) . . | 80 | 6.0 | 11.0 | 0 | <5 | 80 | 0 |
| bean (*Cabot* Greek), | | | | | | | |
| 6 oz. . . . . . . . . . . . | 160 | 13.0 | 25.0 | 3.0 | 20 | 75 | 0 |
| creamy (*Yoplait* | | | | | | | |
| Nonfat), 8 oz. . . . . . | 140 | 7.0 | 27.0 | 0 | 5 | 115 | 0 |
| crème (*Yoplait Whips!*), | | | | | | | |
| 4 oz. . . . . . . . . . . . | 160 | 5.0 | 25.0 | 4.0 | 15 | 105 | 0 |
| vanilla, French | | | | | | | |
| (*Stoneyfield* Organic): | | | | | | | |
| cream top, 8 oz. . . . . | 230 | 8.0 | 31.0 | 8.0 | 30 | 130 | 0 |
| cream top, 6 oz. . . . . | 170 | 6.0 | 23.0 | 6.0 | 25 | 95 | 0 |
| low fat, 8 oz. . . . . . . | 170 | 9.0 | 29.0 | 2.0 | 10 | 140 | 0 |
| low fat, 6 oz. . . . . . . | 130 | 7.0 | 22.0 | 1.5 | 5 | 105 | 0 |
| **Yogurt, frozen,** ½ cup: | | | | | | | |
| (*Ben & Jerry's* | | | | | | | |
| *Half Baked*) . . . . . . . . | 180 | 4.0 | 35.0 | 3.0 | 20 | 95 | 1.0 |
| (*Häagen-Dazs* Tart | | | | | | | |
| Natural) . . . . . . . . . . | 180 | 9.0 | 30.0 | 2.5 | 45 | 45 | 0 |
| banana split (*Turkey* | | | | | | | |
| *Hill*) . . . . . . . . . . . . . . | 110 | 3.0 | 21.0 | 1.5 | 0 | 55 | 1.0 |
| cappuccino chip | | | | | | | |
| (*Dreyer's/Edy's* | | | | | | | |
| *Slow Churned*) . . . . . . | 110 | 2.0 | 18.0 | 3.5 | 10 | 40 | 0 |
| caramel praline crunch | | | | | | | |
| (*Dreyer's/Edy's* | | | | | | | |
| *Slow Churned*) . . . . . . | 120 | 3.0 | 20.0 | 3.5 | 10 | 45 | 0 |
| cherry, black, vanilla | | | | | | | |
| swirl (*Dreyer's/Edy's* | | | | | | | |
| *Slow Churned*) . . . . . . | 100 | 2.0 | 17.0 | 3.0 | 10 | 35 | 0 |

| Food and Measure | cal. | prot. (gms) | carbo. (gms) | fat (gms) | chol. (mgs) | sod. (mgs) | fiber (gms) |
|---|---|---|---|---|---|---|---|
| cherry chocolate chip (*Ben & Jerry's Cherry Garcia*) ...... | 200 | 8.0 | 37.0 | 3.0 | 20 | 90 | <1.0 |
| chocolate (*Stonyfield* Organic Nonfat) ..... | 100 | 4.0 | 21.0 | 0 | <5 | 55 | 1.0 |
| chocolate chip, minty (*Stonyfield* Organic Low Fat) .......... | 140 | 4.0 | 25.0 | 2.5 | <5 | 50 | 1.0 |
| chocolate chip cookie dough (*Turkey Hill*) ... | 120 | 3.0 | 23.0 | 2.0 | 5 | 95 | 1.0 |
| chocolate marshmallow (*Turkey Hill* Nonfat) .. | 110 | 3.0 | 24.0 | 0 | 0 | 110 | 1.0 |
| chocolate vanilla swirl (*Dreyer's/Edy's Slow Churned*) ...... | 100 | 3.0 | 16.0 | 3.0 | 10 | 35 | 0 |
| coffee: (*Häagen-Dazs*) ...... | 200 | 8.0 | 31.0 | 4.5 | 65 | 50 | 0 |
| (*Stonyfield* Organic Nonfat Java) ...... | 100 | 4.0 | 21.0 | 0 | <5 | 65 | 0 |
| cookies and cream: (*Dreyer's/Edy's Slow Churned*) ........ | 120 | 3.0 | 20.0 | 4.0 | 10 | 55 | 0 |
| (*Stonyfield* Organic Low Fat) .......... | 130 | 4.0 | 25.0 | 2.0 | 0 | 110 | 0 |
| crème caramel (*Stonyfield* Organic Low Fat) .... | 130 | 4.0 | 26.0 | 1.5 | 5 | 95 | 0 |
| dulce de leche (*Häagen-Dazs*) ...... | 190 | 6.0 | 35.0 | 2.5 | 75 | 35 | 0 |
| fudge brownie: (*Ben & Jerry's Lighten Up!*) ...... | 170 | 5.0 | 34.0 | 2.5 | 15 | 95 | 1.0 |
| (*Dreyer's/Edy's Slow Churned*) ........ | 120 | 3.0 | 19.0 | 3.5 | 10 | 40 | 1.0 |
| fudge ripple (*Turkey Hill* Nonfat) ......... | 100 | 3.0 | 21.0 | 0 | 0 | 65 | 0 |
| honey vanilla granola (*Turkey Hill*) ........ | 150 | 3.0 | 23.0 | 6.0 | 5 | 80 | 1.0 |
| lemon pie (*Turkey Hill* Southern Nonfat) .... | 120 | 3.0 | 25.0 | 0 | 0 | 115 | 0 |
| mango, tart (*Dreyer's/ Edy's Slow Churned*) . | 100 | 2.0 | 19.0 | 2.0 | 5 | 40 | 0 |
| mint cookies and cream (*Turkey Hill*) ........ | 110 | 3.0 | 22.0 | 1.5 | 0 | 75 | 0 |

| Food and Measure | cal. | prot. (gms) | carbo. (gms) | fat (gms) | chol. (mgs) | sod. (mgs) | fiber (gms) |
|---|---|---|---|---|---|---|---|
| **Yogurt, frozen** *(cont.)* | | | | | | | |
| Neapolitan (*Turkey Hill* | | | | | | | |
| Nonfat) ............ | 90 | 3.0 | 19.0 | 0 | 0 | 55 | 1.0 |
| peach: | | | | | | | |
| (*Dreyer's/Edy's Slow* | | | | | | | |
| *Churned*) ........ | 100 | 2.0 | 17.0 | 2.0 | 10 | 30 | 0 |
| (*Häagen-Dazs*) ...... | 170 | 8.0 | 31.0 | 2.0 | 40 | 40 | 0 |
| peanut butter pie | | | | | | | |
| (*Turkey Hill*) ........ | 160 | 4.0 | 22.0 | 7.0 | 0 | 95 | 1.0 |
| strawberry: | | | | | | | |
| (*Dreyer's/Edy's Slow* | | | | | | | |
| *Churned*) ........ | 100 | 2.0 | 17.0 | 2.5 | 10 | 30 | 0 |
| (*Stonyfield* Organic | | | | | | | |
| Nonfat) .......... | 100 | 4.0 | 21.0 | 0 | <5 | 55 | 0 |
| strawberry banana | | | | | | | |
| (*Ben & Jerry's*) ...... | 150 | 3.0 | 32.0 | 1.5 | 15 | 50 | 0 |
| vanilla: | | | | | | | |
| (*Dreyer's/Edy's Slow* | | | | | | | |
| *Churned*) ........ | 100 | 2.0 | 17.0 | 3.0 | 10 | 35 | 0 |
| (*Dreyer's/Edy's Slow* | | | | | | | |
| *Churned* Nonfat) .. | 90 | 3.0 | 20.0 | 0 | 0 | 45 | 0 |
| (*Häagen-Dazs*) ...... | 200 | 9.0 | 31.0 | 4.5 | 65 | 55 | 0 |
| (*Stonyfield* Organic | | | | | | | |
| Nonfat) .......... | 100 | 4.0 | 20.0 | 0 | <5 | 65 | 0 |
| bean (*Turkey Hill* | | | | | | | |
| Nonfat) .......... | 100 | 3.0 | 19.0 | 0 | 0 | 60 | 0 |
| vanilla fudge swirl | | | | | | | |
| (*Stonyfield* Organic | | | | | | | |
| Nonfat) ............ | 120 | 4.0 | 25.0 | 0 | <5 | 65 | 0 |
| vanilla raspberry swirl | | | | | | | |
| (*Häagen-Dazs*) ...... | 170 | 4.0 | 32.0 | 2.5 | 25 | 35 | 0 |
| wildberry (*Häagen-Dazs*) | 180 | 7.0 | 34.0 | 2.0 | 35 | 40 | 0 |
| **Yogurt, nondairy,** | | | | | | | |
| **coconut milk** (*So* | | | | | | | |
| *Delicious*), 6 oz.: | | | | | | | |
| plain ............... | 130 | 1.0 | 16.0 | 7.0 | 0 | 10 | 3.0 |
| blueberry ........... | 140 | 1.0 | 24.0 | 6.0 | 0 | 30 | 2.0 |
| chocolate ........... | 170 | 2.0 | 28.0 | 6.0 | 0 | 5 | 3.0 |
| passionate mango ...... | 130 | 1.0 | 19.0 | 7.0 | 0 | 10 | 2.0 |
| piña colada ........... | 140 | 1.0 | 22.0 | 6.0 | 0 | 10 | 2.0 |
| raspberry ............ | 140 | 1.0 | 24.0 | 6.0 | 0 | 30 | 2.0 |
| strawberry ........... | 130 | 1.0 | 21.0 | 6.0 | 0 | 5 | 2.0 |
| strawberry banana ..... | 150 | 1.0 | 26.0 | 6.0 | 0 | 40 | 2.0 |
| vanilla .............. | 150 | 1.0 | 22.0 | 6.0 | 0 | 5 | 2.0 |

| Food and Measure | cal. | prot. (gms) | carbo. (gms) | fat (gms) | chol. (mgs) | sod. (mgs) | fiber (gms) |
|---|---|---|---|---|---|---|---|
| **Yogurt, nondairy, soy,** 6 oz., except as noted: | | | | | | | |
| plain: | | | | | | | |
|   (*Silk Live!*), 8 oz. . . . . | 150 | 6.0 | 22.0 | 4.0 | 0 | 30 | 1.0 |
|   (*So Delicious*) . . . . . . . | 110 | 3.0 | 20.0 | 2.5 | 0 | 160 | 6.0 |
| blueberry: | | | | | | | |
|   (*Silk Live*) . . . . . . . . . | 150 | 4.0 | 29.0 | 2.0 | 0 | 25 | 1.0 |
|   (*So Delicious*) . . . . . . . | 140 | 3.0 | 28.0 | 2.5 | 0 | 140 | 5.0 |
|   (*Stonyfield* O'Soy Organic) . . . . . . . . | 170 | 7.0 | 29.0 | 2.5 | 0 | 30 | 2.0 |
| cherry, black (*Silk Live!*) . . . . . . . . . . . . | 150 | 4.0 | 29.0 | 2.0 | 0 | 20 | 1.0 |
| chocolate (*Stonyfield* O'Soy Organic) . . . . . | 160 | 8.0 | 25.0 | 3.0 | 0 | 35 | 2.0 |
| lime, key (*Silk Live!*) . . . . | 150 | 4.0 | 30.0 | 2.0 | 0 | 25 | 1.0 |
| peach: | | | | | | | |
|   (*Silk Live!*) . . . . . . . . | 160 | 4.0 | 32.0 | 2.0 | 0 | 25 | 1.0 |
|   (*Stonyfield* O'Soy Organic) . . . . . . . . | 170 | 7.0 | 30.0 | 2.5 | 0 | 45 | 2.0 |
| peach and strawberry (*Stonyfield* O'Soy Organic), 4 oz. . . . . . . | 100 | 5.0 | 15.0 | 2.0 | 0 | 25 | 1.0 |
| raspberry: | | | | | | | |
|   (*Silk Live!*) . . . . . . . . | 210 | 7.0 | 36.0 | 4.0 | 0 | 120 | 3.0 |
|   (*Stonyfield* O'Soy Organic) . . . . . . . . | 170 | 7.0 | 29.0 | 2.5 | 0 | 75 | 2.0 |
| strawberry: | | | | | | | |
|   (*Silk Live!*) . . . . . . . . | 160 | 4.0 | 31.0 | 2.0 | 0 | 25 | 1.0 |
|   (*Stonyfield* O'Soy Organic) . . . . . . . . | 170 | 7.0 | 29.0 | 2.5 | 0 | 55 | 2.0 |
| strawberry banana (*Silk Live!*) . . . . . . . . | 150 | 4.0 | 29.0 | 2.0 | 0 | 25 | 1.0 |
| vanilla: | | | | | | | |
|   (*Silk Live!*) . . . . . . . . | 150 | 5.0 | 25.0 | 3.0 | 0 | 20 | 1.0 |
|   (*So Delicious*) . . . . . . . | 130 | 3.0 | 25.0 | 2.5 | 0 | 140 | 5.0 |
|   (*Stonyfield* O'Soy Organic) . . . . . . . . | 150 | 7.0 | 24.0 | 3.0 | 0 | 40 | 1.0 |
| **Yogurt dip,** see "Fruit dip" | | | | | | | |
| **Yogurt drink** (see also "Kefir"): | | | | | | | |
| berry, wild: | | | | | | | |
|   (*Stonyfield* Organic), 10 fl. oz. . . . . . . . . | 230 | 10.0 | 39.0 | 3.0 | 10 | 150 | <1.0 |

| Food and Measure | cal. | prot. (gms) | carbo. (gms) | fat (gms) | chol. (mgs) | sod. (mgs) | fiber (gms) |
|---|---|---|---|---|---|---|---|
| **Yogurt drink, berry, wild** *(cont.)* | | | | | | | |
| (*Stonyfield* Organic), | | | | | | | |
| 6 fl. oz. . . . . . . . . . . | 140 | 6.0 | 23.0 | 2.0 | 5 | 90 | 0 |
| blueberry (*DanActive*), | | | | | | | |
| 3.1 fl. oz. . . . . . . . . . | 80 | 3.0 | 14.0 | 1.0 | 5 | 45 | 0 |
| mango (*Activia*), | | | | | | | |
| 7 fl. oz. . . . . . . . . . . . | 170 | 6.0 | 28.0 | 3.0 | 10 | 75 | 0 |
| peach: | | | | | | | |
| (*Activia*), 7 fl. oz. . . . . | 170 | 6.0 | 28.0 | 3.0 | 10 | 75 — | 0 |
| (*Stonyfield* Organic), | | | | | | | |
| 10 fl. oz. . . . . . . . . | 230 | 10.0 | 41.0 | 3.0 | 10 | 140 | <1.0 |
| (*Stonyfield* Organic), | | | | | | | |
| 6 fl. oz. . . . . . . . . . | 140 | 6.0 | 24.0 | 2.0 | 5 | 85 | 0 |
| prune (*Activia*), 7 fl. oz. . . | 160 | 6.0 | 28.0 | 3.0 | 10 | 75 | 0 |
| raspberry (*Stonyfield* | | | | | | | |
| Organic), 10 fl. oz. . . . | 230 | 10.0 | 39.0 | 3.0 | 10 | 150 | <1.0 |
| strawberry: | | | | | | | |
| (*Activia*), 7 fl. oz. . . . . | 160 | 6.0 | 27.0 | 3.0 | 10 | 70 | 0 |
| (*DanActive*), 3.1 fl. oz. | 80 | 3.0 | 14.0 | 1.0 | 5 | 45 | 0 |
| (*Stonyfield* Organic), | | | | | | | |
| 10 fl. oz. . . . . . . . . | 230 | 10.0 | 39.0 | 3.0 | 10 | 150 | <1.0 |
| (*Stonyfield* Organic), | | | | | | | |
| 6 fl. oz. . . . . . . . . . | 140 | 6.0 | 23.0 | 2.0 | 5 | 90 | 0 |
| strawberry banana: | | | | | | | |
| (*Activia*), 7 fl. oz. . . . . | 160 | 6.0 | 27.0 | 3.0 | 10 | 70 | 0 |
| (*DanActive*), 3.1 fl. oz. | 80 | 3.0 | 14.0 | 1.0 | 5 | 40 | 0 |
| (*Stonyfield* Organic), | | | | | | | |
| 10 fl. oz. . . . . . . . . | 230 | 10.0 | 40.0 | 3.0 | 10 | 150 | <1.0 |
| vanilla: | | | | | | | |
| (*DanActive*), 3.1 fl. oz. | 70 | 3.0 | 11.0 | 1.5 | 5 | 40 | 0 |
| (*Stonyfield* Organic), | | | | | | | |
| 10 fl. oz. . . . . . . . . | 240 | 10.0 | 40.0 | 3.0 | 10 | 140 | <1.0 |
| **Yogurt drink mix, frozen** | | | | | | | |
| (*Yoplait* Smoothie), | | | | | | | |
| 1 pouch: | | | | | | | |
| berry, triple . . . . . . . . . . | 70 | 1.0 | 14.0 | 1.5 | <5 | 20 | 2.0 |
| blueberry pomegranate . . | 80 | 1.0 | 16.0 | 2.0 | <5 | 170 | 2.0 |
| strawberry banana or | | | | | | | |
| mango pineapple . . . . | 70 | 1.0 | 14.0 | 1.0 | <5 | 15 | 1.0 |
| **Yogurt seasoning** | | | | | | | |
| (*Neera's* Raita Mix | | | | | | | |
| No Salt), 1 tsp. . . . . . . | 6 | 0 | 2.0 | 0 | 0 | 2 | 0 |
| **Youngberry juice**, | | | | | | | |
| (*Ceres*), 8 fl. oz. . . . . . | 120 | 0 | 30.0 | 0 | 0 | 10 | 0 |

| Food and Measure | cal. | prot. (gms) | carbo. (gms) | fat (gms) | chol. (mgs) | sod. (mgs) | fiber (gms) |
|---|---|---|---|---|---|---|---|
| **Yu choy sum** (*Frieda's*), sliced, 1 cup ........ | 9 | 1.0 | 2.0 | 0 | 0 | 46 | 1.0 |
| **Yuca root** (*Frieda's*), sliced, ½ cup ........ | 165 | 1.0 | 39.0 | 0 | 0 | 14 | 2.0 |
| **Yumberry juice** (*R.W. Knudsen* Organic), 8 fl. oz. ............ | 120 | 1.0 | 32.0 | 0 | 0 | 20 | 1.0 |
| **Yumberry pomegranate drink** (*SoBe*), 8 fl. oz. ............ | 100 | 0 | 26.0 | 0 | 0 | 20 | 0 |

# Z

| Food and Measure | cal. | prot. (gms) | carbo. (gms) | fat (gms) | chol. (mgs) | sod. (mgs) | fiber (gms) |
|---|---|---|---|---|---|---|---|
| **Ziti entree, frozen**, 1 pkg., except as noted: | | | | | | | |
| baked: | | | | | | | |
| (*Amy's* Bowl), 9.5 oz. . | 390 | 9.0 | 62.0 | 12.0 | 0 | 590 | 5.0 |
| (*Celentano* 4.5 lb.), 8 oz. . . . . . . . . . . . | 330 | 13.0 | 39.0 | 13.0 | 25 | 600 | 4.0 |
| marinara, 3 cheese: | | | | | | | |
| (*Michelina's Lean Gourmet*), 9.5 oz. . . | 300 | 11.0 | 46.0 | 8.0 | 10 | 680 | 3.0 |
| (*Smart Ones*), 9 oz. . . | 320 | 14.0 | 47.0 | 8.0 | 10 | 590 | 4.0 |
| Parmesano (*Michelina's Budget Gourmet*), 8 oz. . . . . . . . . . . . | 250 | 10.0 | 37.0 | 7.0 | 10 | 500 | 3.0 |
| **Ziti entree, microwave**, meat sauce (*Healthy Choice Fresh Mixers*), 6.9-oz. cont. . . . . . . . | 340 | 15.0 | 56.0 | 6.0 | 20 | 600 | 8.0 |
| **Zucchini**, fresh, w/skin: | | | | | | | |
| raw: | | | | | | | |
| chopped, ½ cup . . . . . | 9 | .7 | 1.8 | .1 | 0 | 2 | .7 |
| sliced, ½ cup . . . . . . . | 8 | .7 | 1.6 | .1 | 0 | 2 | .7 |
| and yellow (*Green Giant* Squash Medley), 3 oz. . . . . | 15 | 1.0 | 4.0 | 0 | 0 | 0 | 2.0 |
| raw, baby: | | | | | | | |
| (*Frieda's*), 1 cup, 4.5 oz. . . . . . . . . . | 25 | 4.0 | 4.0 | .5 | 0 | 0 | 1.0 |
| 1 large, 3⅛" . . . . . . . . | 3 | .4 | .5 | <.1 | 0 | tr. | <.1 |
| boiled, drained: | | | | | | | |
| sliced, ½ cup . . . . . . . | 14 | .6 | 3.5 | <.1 | 0 | 2 | 1.3 |
| mashed, ½ cup . . . . . . | 19 | .8 | 4.7 | .1 | 0 | 3 | 1.7 |